Contributors

Jennifer L. Agnew-Coughlin, BScPT, BHK
Physiotherapist Division of Respiratory Medicine
Hospital for Sick Children
Toronto, Ontario
Canada

Jo A. Ashwell, BScPT
Physiotherapist, Paediatric and School Care Program
Comcare
Niagara Falls, Ontario
Canada

Donna Bernhardt-Bainbridge, PT, ATC, EdD
Clinical Faculty Affiliate, Department of Physical Therapy
Department of Drama Dance, The University of Montana
Missoula, Montana;
President
High Peaks Orthopedic & Sports Rehabilitation
Stevensville, Montana

Debra Ann Bleakney, PT
President, OPT Therapy Services, Inc.
Wilmington, Delaware

Nina S. Bradley, PT, PhD
Associate Professor
Department of Biokinesiology and Physical Therapy
University of Southern California
Los Angeles, California

Suzann K. Campbell, PT, PhD, FAPTA
Professor, Department of Physical Therapy
College of Health and Human Development Sciences
University of Illinois at Chicago
Chicago, Illinois

Shirley J. Carlson, PT, PCS, MS
Physical Therapist
Spokane Guilds' School and Neuromuscular Center
Spokane, Washington

Linda Ezelle Daniels, PT, MS
Dayton, Ohio

Kathryn Steyer David, PT, PCS, MS
Physical Therapist, Heartland Area Education Agency
Johnston, Iowa;
Consultant for Physical Therapy Services
Bureau of Children, Family and Community Services
Iowa Department of Education
Des Moines, Iowa

Maureen Donohoe, PT, PCS
Clinical Specialist, Alfred I. DuPont Hospital for Children
Wilmington, Delaware

Helene Dumas, MS, PT, PCS
Director, Rehabilitation Services
Franciscan Children's Hospital and Rehabilitation Center
Boston, Massachusetts

Susan K. Effgen, PT, PhD
Professor, Department of Rehabilitation Sciences
MCP Hahnemann University
Philadelphia, Pennsylvania

Carrie G. Gajdosik, PT, MS
Associate Professor, Physical Therapy Department
School of Pharmacy and Allied Health Sciences
The University of Montana
Missoula, Montana

Richard L. Gajdosik, PT, PhD
Professor, Physical Therapy Department
School of Pharmacy and Allied Health Sciences
The University of Montana
Missoula, Montana

Susan R. Harris, PT, PhD, FAPTA
Professor, Division of Physical Therapy
School of Rehabilitation Sciences
University of British Columbia;
Faculty Clinical Associate
Sunny Hill Health Centre for Children
Vancouver, British Columbia
Canada

Kathleen A. Hinderer, PT, MS, MPT
Doctoral Candidate, Department of Movement Science
Division of Kinesiology, University of Michigan
Ann Arbor, Michigan;
Senior Physical Therapist
Rehabilitation Institute of Michigan
Detroit, Michigan

Steven R. Hinderer, PT, MD, MS
Assistant Professor
Department of Physical Medicine and Rehabilitation
Wayne State University of Medicine;
Medical Director of Research and the Clinical
  Rehabilitation Research Unit
Rehabilitation Institute of Michigan
Detroit, Michigan

Betsy A. Howell, PT, MS
Clinical Specialist
Pediatric Cardiopulmonary Physical Therapist
University of Michigan Medical Center
Ann Arbor, Michigan

Linda Kahn-D'Angelo, PT, ScD
Professor of Physical Therapy
University of Massachusetts
Lowell, Massachusetts

M. Kathleen Kelly, MS, PT
Assistant Professor, Department of Physical Therapy
University of Pittsburgh;
Senior Physical Therapist
Children's Hospital of Pittsburgh
Pittsburgh, Pennsylvania

Ginette A. Kerkering, PT
Pediatric Physical Therapist
St. Luke's Rehabilitation Institute
Spokane, Washington

Thubi H.A. Kolobe, PT, PhD
Assistant Professor, Department of Physical Therapy
College of Associated Health Professions
University of Illinois at Chicago
Chicago, Illinois

Hélène M. Larin, PT, PhD
Assistant Professor, Faculty of Health Sciences
School of Rehabilitation Science, McMaster University
Hamilton, Ontario
Canada

Judy Leach, PT
San Diego, California

Benjamin R. Lovelace-Chandler, PT, PCS, PhD
President, Kids' SPOT
Little Rock, Arkansas

Venita S. Lovelace-Chandler, PT, PCS, PhD
Professor and Chairperson
Department of Physical Therapy
University of Central Arkansas
Little Rock, Arkansas

Cynthia L. Magee, PT, MS
Medford, New Jersey

Teresa L. Massagli, MD
Associate Professor
Departments of Rehabilitation Medicine and Pediatrics
University of Washington;
Attending Physician
Children's Hospital and Regional Medical Center;
Consulting Physician
University of Washington Medical Center
Harborview Medical Center
Seattle, Washington

Irene R. McEwen, PT, PhD
Presbyterian Health Foundation Presidential Professor
Department of Physical Therapy
University of Oklahoma Health Sciences Center
Oklahoma City, Oklahoma

Sandra M. McGee, PT
Pediatric Rehabilitation Coordinator
Children's Seashore House of the Children's Hospital of
  Philadelphia
Child Development Center at Marlton;
Consultant, Comprehensive Hemophilia Clinic
Children's Hospital of Philadelphia
Philadelphia, Pennsylvania

PHYSICAL THERAPY
FOR CHILDREN

PHYSICAL THERAPY FOR CHILDREN

Editor

SUZANN K. CAMPBELL, PT, PhD, FAPTA

Professor, Department of Physical Therapy
College of Health and Human Development Sciences
University of Illinois at Chicago
Chicago, Illinois

Associate Editors

DARL W. VANDER LINDEN, PT, PhD

Associate Professor, Department of Physical Therapy
Eastern Washington University
Spokane, Washington

ROBERT J. PALISANO, PT, ScD

Professor, MCP Hahnemann University
Department of Rehabilitation Sciences
Philadelphia, Pennsylvania

SECOND EDITION

SAUNDERS COMPANY
An Imprint of Elsevier Science

SAUNDERS
An Imprint of Elsevier

The Curtis Center
Independence Square West
Philadelphia, PA 19106

Editor-in-Chief: Andrew Allen
Senior Developmental Editor: Kellie White
Developmental Editor: Rae Robertson
Project Manager: Linda McKinley
Production Editor: Rich Barber
Production: Graphic World Publishing Services

Physical Therapy for Children ISBN 0-7216-8316-9

Printed in the United States of America.

Last digit is the print number: 9   8   7   6   5

Merilyn L. Moore, PT
Guest Lecturer, University of Puget Sound
Tacoma, Washington, and University of Washington;
OT/PT/TR Supervisor, Harborview Medical Center
Seattle, Washington

Ellen Stamos Norton, PT, PCS
President, Pediatric Private Practice
San Diego, California

Sandra J. Olney, BSc(P&OT), MEd, PhD
Professor and Director, Associate Dean (Health Sciences)
School of Rehabilitation Therapy, Queen's University
Kingston, Ontario
Canada

Robert J. Palisano, PT, ScD
Professor, MCP Hahnemann University
Department of Rehabilitation Sciences
Philadelphia, Pennsylvania

Cheryl Patrick, PT
Senior Physical Therapist
Children's Memorial Hospital
Chicago, Illinois

Wendy E. Phillips, PT, PCS, MA, MS
Physical Therapist
Hughes Spalding Children's Hospital/
    Grady Memorial Hospital;
Instructor in Physical Therapy, Georgia State University
Atlanta, Georgia

Carole Ramsey, OTR/L, ATP
Supervisor of Occupational Therapy
University Hospital School, University of Iowa
Iowa City, Iowa

Shirley Albinson Scull, PT, MS
Director of Physical Therapy & Ambulatory
    Rehabilitation
Children's Seashore House of the Children's Hospital of
    Philadelphia
Philadelphia, Pennsylvania

Kristine A. Shakhazizian, PT
Chief Clinical Therapist
Department of Rehabilitation Medicine
Children's Hospital and Regional Medical Center
Seattle, Washington

David B. Shurtleff, MD
Professor, Department of Pediatrics, and
    Chief, Birth Defects Clinic
University of Washington;
Staff, University Hospital
Seattle, Washington;
President, International Society for Research into
    Hydrocephalus and Spina Bifida 1998–2000

Teresa L. Southard, PT
Physical Therapist, Mapleton Rehabilitation Center
Boulder Community Hospital
Boulder, Colorado

Joyce Sparling, PT/OT, PhD
Associate Professor Emerita
Division of Physical Therapy
University of North Carolina at Chapel Hill
Chapel Hill, North Carolina

Michael L. Spotts, JD
Office of the General Counsel
Grady Health System
Atlanta, Georgia

Meg Stanger, PT, PCS, MS
Director of Occupational Therapy and Physical Therapy
Children's Hospital/The Children's Institute
Pittsburgh, Pennsylvania

Jean L. Stout, PT, MS
Research Physical Therapist, Motion Analysis Laboratory
Gillette Children's Hospital
St. Paul, Minnesota

Wayne A. Stuberg, PT, PhD, PCS
Associate Professor and Director of Physical Therapy &
    the Brace Place
Munroe-Meyer Institute for Genetics and Rehabilitation;
Associate Professor of Physical Therapy
Assistant Professor of Anatomy
University of Nebraska Medical Center
Omaha, Nebraska

Rachel A. Unanue, MSPT, PCS
Doctoral Candidate
Department of Rehabilitation Sciences
MCP Hahnemann University
Philadelphia, Pennsylvania

Darl W. Vander Linden, PT, PhD
Associate Professor, Department of Physical Therapy
Eastern Washington University
Spokane, Washington

Marilyn J. Wright, BScPT, MEd
Clinical Lecturer
McMaster University, Children's Hospital
Hamilton Health Sciences Corporation
Hamilton, Ontario
Canada

Preface to the Second Edition

Since publication of the first edition of *Physical Therapy for Children,* the editors are pleased to find that the disability model of the National Center for Medical Rehabilitation Research, which we used as a conceptual framework for the first edition, has now been incorporated in the Guide to Physical Therapist Practice of the American Physical Therapy Association.[1] The Guide goes further, however, in establishing standard terminology for the elements of patient management (examination, evaluation, diagnosis, prognosis, and intervention) and in documenting practice patterns for the field. The revised edition of Chapter 7 on decision making provides an introduction to the elements of the Guide and a description of the disability model, which continues to frame the presentation of our book. The development of practice guidelines necessitated the publication of a second edition of *Physical Therapy for Chil-*

dren, which would conform to the Guide but also challenge it when it failed to adequately address the practice of pediatric physical therapy.

I believe that the authors and editors have admirably met the challenge of incorporating Guide terminology and practice patterns while reflecting on how both practice and the Guide can be improved. The authors have also updated each chapter with the latest research on evidence-based practice and with new patient cases that reflect the evolution of the health care and public education systems. Finally, developments in the field have led to the inclusion of a new chapter on brachial plexus injury and torticollis. We are gratified by the response of students, clinicians, and researchers to the first edition and hope that this new version will continue to be a useful and comprehensive reference for the practice of pediatric physical therapy.

Suzann K. Campbell, PT, PhD, FAPTA

Editor, Chicago, Illinois
June 23, 1999

---

[1]Guide to Physical Therapist Practice. Physical Therapy, *77*:1163–1650, 1997.

Preface to the First Edition

As Cherry[1] said in a description of philosophy and science in pediatric physical therapy, specialty practice in pediatrics derives from the general philosophy of physical therapy but must address additional concerns that are different from those of physical therapy for adults. For example, clinical decision making must be guided by the knowledge that the natural development of children interacts with disability. As a result, physical therapists must anticipate and provide for children's changing needs. In addition, treatment must be adapted to children's attention to the here and now and to their dependence on adult caregivers. These significant adults must be intimately involved in both the planning of needed care and its implementation in natural settings for children—the home, school, and playground.

Another conceptual basis for the clinical practice of pediatric physical therapy is the model of the disabling process developed at the National Center for Medical Rehabilitation Research (NCMRR)[2] of the U.S. National Institutes of Health. This model defines a variety of dimensions of disablement, including (1) *impairments* of organ systems, such as deformities and limited strength, (2) *functional limitations* in whole body or body segment activity, such as locomotion or manipulation, and (3) *disabilities* in performing age-appropriate roles or activities, such as community mobility and play with peers, or independence in activities of daily living. The editors believe that all interventions that physical therapists provide should have as their ultimate goal the reduction of disability as defined in the NCMRR model. Use of this model is helpful in directing attention toward the real purpose of providing therapy for children; therefore, a focus is maintained in this book on prevention of disability throughout childhood and during the transition to living successfully as an adult.

The NCMRR model and the special needs of pediatric clients form the basis for this first comprehensive reference book for the practice of pediatric physical therapy. In the design of *Physical Therapy for Children*, the Associate Editors and I attempted to meet these needs through inclusion of (1) comprehensive coverage of the most common conditions seen in pediatric practice, (2) current information on the characteristics of best practice both from the research literature and from the experiences of the scientific practitioners who wrote each chapter, (3) delineation of critical issues during successive stages of living well with a disability from infancy to adulthood, and (4) a focus on the process of disablement from the organ systems level to functional capacities of the whole child and to disability in participating in role functions typical of children's daily interactions in natural settings.

To meet our goal of providing a comprehensive reference for pediatric practice, we believed that it was necessary to begin the book by addressing essential foundational knowledge in development, motor control, motor learning, and clinical decision making. Section One therefore begins the book with seven chapters on *understanding motor performance in children*. These chapters provide information on the development of *functional motor skills, gait, and the musculoskeletal structures; motor control; health-related physical fitness; and motor learning*. The final chapter on *clinical decision making* presents the model of the disabling process that was used as the conceptual basis for subsequent chapters on specific pediatric condi-

---

[1]Cherry, DB. Pediatric physical therapy: Philosophy, science, and techniques. Pediatric Physical Therapy, 3:70–75, 1991.

[2]National Institutes of Health. Research Plan for the National Center for Medical Rehabilitation Research. NIH Pub. No. 93-3509. Bethesda, MD: National Institutes of Health, 1993.

tions. Although the reader will find each chapter to be self-contained, an early reading of this chapter will facilitate understanding of the structure of the material that follows.

Sections Two through Four of the book describe the pathophysiology and physical therapy management of common pediatric *musculoskeletal, neurologic,* and *cardiopulmonary* conditions, respectively. Application of the content is illustrated with case histories from the authors' practice. Physical therapy concerns are presented in each chapter in a way that makes explicit the relationships and the differences among treatment goals aimed at impairments, functional limitations, and disabilities. The Editors of this book believe that a clear delineation of each of the dimensions of the disabling process will lead to improved patient care, development of measurement tools with a strong underlying conceptual basis, and clinical research that clarifies the linkages among the various dimensions to improve the effectiveness and efficiency of clinical practice.

Finally, Section Five of *Physical Therapy for Children* addresses *special settings and special considerations,* including *the burn unit, the special care nursery, family-centered early intervention, the educational environment, private practice,* and *medicolegal issues,* such as child abuse and neglect and public laws addressing disabilities in childhood.

Just as children's health and development depend on the presence of a supportive environment, the

completion of a project like this would not be possible without a variety of supports. I would like to thank my outstanding Associate Editors, Darl Vander Linden and Robert Palisano; the Senior Editor for Health-Related Professions at W.B. Saunders, Margaret Biblis, who pursued the initiation of this project until I could no longer say no and continued her support for making the book the best it could be; my husband, Richard Campbell, who has always encouraged me to do more than I thought I could do (and been right); and my Department Head at the University of Illinois at Chicago, Jules Rothstein, for allowing the time commitment this work involved. Partial support was also provided by the Maternal and Child Health Bureau of the U.S. Department of Health and Human Services, which has funded my work and that of my former graduate students (including the Associate Editors) over two decades of partnership in building the science and practice of pediatric physical therapy. Finally, I would like to thank my colleagues and mentors in pediatric physical therapy who have given me the knowledge and support to empower children with disabilities and their families to be all that they can be: Leila Green, Georgia Shambes, Margaret Moore, Mary Clyde Singleton, Marc Hansen, Ernest Kraybill, Earl Siegel, Irma Wilhelm, Carolyn Heriza, Janet Wilson, Gay Girolami, Hélène Larin, and Thubi Kolobe.

SKC

Contents

UNDERSTANDING MOTOR PERFORMANCE IN CHILDREN

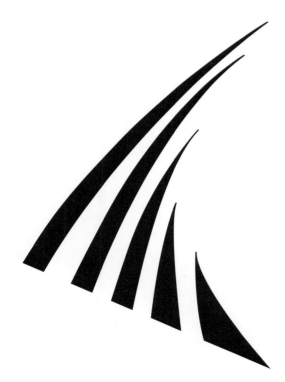

SUZANN K. CAMPBELL, PT, PhD, FAPTA

Section Editor

The Child's Development of Functional Movement

SUZANN K. CAMPBELL, PT, PhD, FAPTA

Working knowledge of motor development is the very basis of the practice of pediatric physical therapy. It provides the norms for functioning of children at various ages that guide diagnosis and treatment planning through emphasis on selection of age-appropriate skills as functional outcomes. Development of effective plans of care for children also requires knowledge of the cognitive milestones that must be recognized in order to provide intervention in a stimulating and motivating environment and to take advantage of interactions among cognitive, perceptual, and motor development. Developing such an environment for the provision of intervention typically involves use of adapted play activities at a cognitive level appropriate for an individual child, regardless of the child's level of motor development. The challenge is perhaps greatest when motor and cognitive levels in a particular child are exceedingly different.

Movement, on the other hand, also promotes cognitive and perceptual development (Bertenthal & Campos, 1987). The two go hand in hand to foster functional performance. Therapists must consider in their intervention planning how to structure therapy to facilitate best all aspects of their clients' development and to take advantage of the interactive nature of developmental subsystems, especially when functional limitations are present and likely to be lifelong. The "Guide to Physical Therapist Practice" (American Physical Therapy Association, 1997) suggests that *goals* of therapy should focus on treatment of impairments (e.g., strength, endurance, or range of motion), but anticipated *outcomes* of intervention should include minimization of functional limitations, optimization of health status, prevention of disability in daily life, and consumer satisfaction (see Chapter 7). Nevertheless, when to emphasize treatment of physical impairments and functional limitations through exercise and other therapeutic modalities, when to concentrate on finding compensatory means to prevent or limit disability in a variety of developmental areas, and when to combine the two are important considerations in an ongoing debate among practitioners.

In order to contribute to this debate, the specific purpose of this chapter is to describe the important milestones in the development of functional movement in children and to introduce a discussion of the processes by which development occurs, which will be elaborated on by Bradley in Chapter 2 on motor control. It seems appropriate first to define what is meant by functional movement. Fisher (1992) has reviewed the various meanings of the term *function* that rehabilitation professionals have used in the design and evaluation of tests and measures. Function is variously described as having a definite end or purpose and as being goal directed and meaningful. A functional limitation represents a failure of the individual's performance to meet a standard expectation. When permanent, functional limitations result in a reduction in behavioral skills, task accomplishment, or fulfillment of appropriate social roles. This chronic effect of functional limitations on behavior or social roles is defined for the purposes of this volume as constituting a disability (see Chapter 7 on clinical decision making for further elaboration of definitions). In rehabilitation, impaired functional performance resulting in disabilities is frequently evaluated by examining the degree of assistance the client needs to perform activities of daily living (ADL). The use of technology to compensate for functional limitations, however, means that disability in performing age-appropriate social roles can be avoided through alternative means for achieving independence in daily life functions (Butler, 1991).

Certainly all therapists would agree that ADL should be considered under the rubric of "functional." But children engage in many meaningful movement activities that appear to lack a well-defined goal. Spinning, bouncing, and endless repetition of newly learned movements, such as going up and down steps and putting things into containers and taking them out, are just a few examples (Shirley, 1931). We would probably call this "play" or "practice," but regardless of terminology, therapists surely see these activities as important aspects of motor development, motor learning, and environmental mastery. In other words, they are functional behaviors for the child's stage of development de-spite their lacking apparent goals. Repetition of motor behaviors might serve a variety of useful functions, such as muscle strengthening, trial of a variety of approaches to assembling effective task-related movements, testing the limits of balance, and learning to deal with the reactive forces produced elsewhere in the body by muscle contraction of prime movers for a particular activity. Certainly, children demonstrate a remarkable intensity of purpose when practicing emerging skills. Vander Linden (personal communication, 1993) provides several examples of his daughter Abby's development. Abby played almost compulsively with nesting cups for about 2 weeks, and when she could nest all 10, she was no longer interested in them. Similarly, she repeatedly went up and down a 4-inch step onto a screened porch in their home, insisting that her parents open the porch door for her to access the porch for stepping practice and resisting enticements to play with toys instead.

Based on many observations such as these, the definition provided by Fisher (1992) that I prefer is that function, or occupation, in the framework of occupational therapy theory and practice, is "what people do" (p. 184). These words imply that functional movements are self-chosen, self-directed, and, therefore, meaningful in the life of the individual at his or her particular place in the life cycle (Fisher, 1992; Oppenheim, 1981). Given this definition, our descriptive presentation will review information regarding what children do and the general order in which they do it, beginning with infants' spontaneously generated, that is, self-directed, movements and gradually incorporating information on tasks that are easier for adults to identify as purposeful and goal directed.

In keeping with the importance to pediatric physical therapists of knowledge of functional motor development, the main objectives of this chapter are to 1) briefly review the history of theories of motor development, 2) describe current information and hypotheses regarding general processes and principles of motor development, and 3) provide an overview of the developmental course of acquisition of upright posture and mobility and of object manipulation—the two most basic functions that underlie meaningful activity. Brief attention will be paid to issues in cognitive development, play, and the interaction of motor skill acquisition and perceptual-cognitive development, including memory for activities. The chapter concludes with an abbreviated review of tests of motor development and functional motor behavior of use to physical therapists from the point of view of the theoretic perspectives provided in earlier parts of the chapter.

MOTOR DEVELOPMENT THEORIES

Throughout the history of physical therapy, theories of child development have changed dramatically, eliciting successive revisions of intervention approaches to maximizing motor development and functional performance in children. Underlying the changes in developmental theory are differing conceptualizations of the respective roles of changing structure and function within the individual and of the influence of the environment on the developmental course. Thelen and colleagues (1987) summarized the major theoretic approaches as encompassing three theories: (1) neural-maturationist, (2) cognitive, and (3) dynamic systems. Each has an interesting history that in itself makes fascinating reading because of the strong role that changing biases and accumulation of new knowledge play in how research efforts are designed and how their results are interpreted and judged (Bergenn et al., 1992; Thelen & Adolph, 1992). These theories are reviewed briefly in this chapter, and their major distinguishing features are summarized in Table 1–1. Further elaboration can be found in Chapter 2 on motor control.

Neural-Maturationist Theories

The neural-maturationist point of view was pioneered by Gesell (1928a, 1928b, 1945; Gesell et al., 1934, 1940, 1975), Shirley (1931), and others. This view proposed that the ontogeny of behavior is "an intrinsic property of the organism, with maturation leading to an unfolding of predetermined patterns, supported, but not fundamentally altered by the environment" (Thelen et al., 1987, p. 40). According to this approach, functional behaviors appear as the nervous system matures, with more complex behaviors being based on the activity of progressively higher levels of the nervous system. This theory, therefore, depends on the assumption of hierarchic maturation of neural control structures.

Gesell's point of view and research findings resulted in the development of important tests of motor milestones and other adaptive behaviors that have had, and continue to have, a monumental influence on practice in the area of diagnosis of developmental delay or deviance (Thelen & Adolph, 1992). Virtually all subsequent tests of development contained items derived from Gesell's work. Gesell emphatically believed in stages of development as bio-

TABLE 1–1. Comparison of Developmental Theories

	Neural-Maturationist	Cognitive: Behavioral	Cognitive: Piagetian	Dynamical Systems
View on "stages"	Stages of motor development occur as a result of CNS maturation.	Stages are merely empirical descriptions of behavior.	Stages represent alternating periods of equilibrium and disequilibrium.	Apparent stages of development are actually states of relative stability arising from the self-organizing, emergent properties of a multitude of systems, each developing at its own continuous rate.
Driving forces for development	Development spirals with alternating periods of flexor vs. extensor dominance and symmetry vs. asymmetry based on maturation of the CNS.	Development occurs through interaction of the individual with the environment.	Development occurs through interaction between cognitive-neural structures and environmental opportunities for action.	The individual develops as the organism recognizes the affordances of the environment and selects (self-organizes) the most appropriate available responses to tasks.
Building blocks of development	Reflexes.	Pavlovian and operant responses to environmental stimuli.	First actions using reflexes and later from voluntary actions.	Multiple cooperating systems with individual rates of development and self-motivated exploration of the environment.

logic imperatives. Although he recognized that there are individual differences among children and was a strong believer in freedom of human action, he never resolved the paradox between these beliefs and his insistence on maturation as the predominant force driving development.

Thelen and Adolph (1992) pointed out, however, that among Gesell's less remembered contributions is the idea that the nature of development forms a spiraling function, with alternations between extremes in a variety of behavioral realms, including alternating dominance between flexor and extensor muscle activity. He believed in a principle of functional asymmetry in which the child must break free of symmetric movement patterns to achieve functional goals such as manipulation.

Pediatric physical therapy developed according to this theoretic model. As a result, emphasis was placed on examination of stages of reflex development and motor milestones as reflections of increasingly higher levels of neural maturation (Horak, 1991). Treatment of the child with central nervous system (CNS) dysfunction was organized around inhibition of primary reflexes that were believed to persist and produce functional limitations, along with facilitation of righting and equilibrium reactions that were supposedly the underlying coordinative structures for development of skilled voluntary motor behavior. It was generally assumed that functional outcomes would naturally follow.

Cognitive Theories

Behavioral Theory

Cognitive theories of motor skill development are of two types. Skinner (1972) developed a behavioral approach to development that emphasizes the importance of contingent learning and posits reinforcement from the environment as the motivator and shaper of both motor and cognitive development (see also Bijou, 1989; Catania & Harnad, 1988). In this theoretic approach, the environment is the site of developmental control.

In more contemporary developmental psychology, behavioral analysis theory was based on Skinner's later radical behaviorism and on the interbehaviorism of Kantor, in which the developing individual is conceived of as a pattern of psychologic responses in interaction with the functional environment (Bijou, 1989). Progressions in development depend on opportunities and circumstances inherent in the individual's makeup and in his or her past and present physical and social environments. Developmental progress occurs through Pavlovian responses to previous stimulation and by operant processes in

which responses are controlled by consequences. Operant responses are acquired and maintained by contingent stimuli with acquired or primary reinforcing functions, and the strength of these interactions is affected by conditions such as timing and frequency of reinforcements. Although sometimes misused, behavior modification approaches have greatly aided the training of specific skills for children with mental retardation (Bijou, 1989), and the knowledge base of the behavioral approach helped therapists to break down skills into component parts for easier learning by children with impaired neural control mechanisms. Clinical problems are approached based on the beliefs that each problem has its unique history and that the intervention program should be individually tailored to the specific problem behavior.

A frequently misunderstood aspect of behavioral analysis theory is the role of individuals in their own development. The individual is not perceived of as passive and responding only when stimulated. Rather, the individual is considered to be adjusting in continual interaction with the environment. The critical feature of this theory is that it is a psychology of the individual in interaction with the environment. Unlike Gesell's concept of development (Gesell, 1945), stages of development are considered to be merely empirical descriptions and not in any sense causal explanations of behavior. The research methodology of behavioral analysis is, therefore, one of single-subject designs or within-subject comparisons designed to demonstrate functional relationships rather than to test theories. The elaboration of such designs has been a significant contribution to clinical research science in physical therapy.

Piagetian Theory

A second cognitive theory based primarily on the work of Piaget (1952) emphasizes an interaction between maturation of cognitive-neural structures and environmental opportunities to promote action (Beilin, 1989; Flavell, 1963). Control functions are found in the development of higher-level plans based on biologic structures, termed *schemata* in Piagetian theory or *motor programs* or *subroutines* in motor control theory (Bruner, 1970; Connolly, 1970). Cognitive mechanisms of all types are believed to derive from knowledge gained through action based at first on innate hereditary reflexes and instinctual capacities and later on experience forming concrete intelligent operations. Cognitive development culminates in abstract intelligence based on coordination of fundamental cognitive operations.

Piagetian theory had little effect on pediatric physical therapy from the perspective of planning the motor aspects of therapeutic programming because it was primarily a cognitive theory and because it continued to emphasize the evolution of functional behaviors from reflexive movements. These movements were believed to be practiced and coordinated with developing mental structures. Adaptive responses were thought to develop through psychologic processes interacting with maturation of neural structures. In this view, the most important processes are successive equilibration, disequilibrium, and re-equilibration, resulting from the interaction of maturation and experience. An important aspect of Piagetian theory is the view of the individual as possessing a self-regulating system of psychologic processes that provides balance between assimilation of environmental experiences and accommodation of existing cognitive structures to that experience. The individual is a homeorrhetic system that, by virtue of its self-regulating characteristics, constantly adjusts itself to maintain equilibrium despite disturbances from the environment, thus driving developmental progress. Viewing the operation of these psychologic processes in children who were observed while solving interesting problems led to theories of the mental structures constructed by children as a result of their activity. Neo-Piagetian work has emphasized research on the functioning of these psychologic processes (Beilin, 1989).

The concept of stages played a major role in early Piagetian theory, although in his later conceptions of development, when faced with evidence contradicting some of his hypotheses, he realized that stage theory tended to lead one to think in terms of periods of rest or equilibrium, whereas development was, in fact, never static (Beilin, 1989). In later years, Piaget, like Gesell, tended to see development as a spiraling process, an important principle that we will return to later. Description of stages nonetheless forms the framework for discussions of development of cognitive systems in Piagetian theory.

Four main stages were posited, each with multiple substages. The first is the stage of sensorimotor intelligence from birth to about 18 to 24 months (Beilin, 1989). Repetition in action is a major factor in this stage, culminating in the major achievement of symbolic functioning. The second period of representational thought, from 1.5 to 2 through 6 years of age, involves the development of language and of one-way mappings of logical thought that allow classifications to be developed. (Current work on classifications suggests that they can be performed perceptually much earlier than Piaget projected, probably as early as 3 months of age in a primitive form [Hayne et al., 1987].) Experiments detailing the errors of logical thought in this period were influential in revealing the lack of sophistication in children's

mental constructions that was not previously obvious. In the third period of concrete operations, thought processes become reversible, allowing conservation of number, weight, and volume under transformation conditions. In the final period of cognitive development, formal operations beginning at about age 11 permit logical thinking in a hypothetico-deductive mode.

The impact of Piagetian theory on pediatric physical therapy was primarily on the inclusion of interesting spectacles and problem-solving activities in therapeutic programs to assist in the cognitive-motivational aspects of facilitating motor development. Therapists used problems such as the search for hidden objects (object permanence) and problems involving means-ends relationships and container-contained ideas as therapeutic media to motivate children to move and to examine and promote the perceptual-cognitive aspects of development and motor learning (Campbell & Wilson, 1976; Fetters, 1981).

Dynamical Systems Theory

Thelen and colleagues (Thelen, 1995; Thelen & Corbetta, 1994; Thelen & Ulrich, 1991; Thelen et al., 1987, 1989, 1993; Ulrich, 1989) have proposed a dynamical functional perspective on motor development that currently drives most research on motor development. Dynamical systems theory emphasizes process rather than product or hierarchically structured plans and places neural maturation on an equal plane with other structures and processes that interact to promote motor development. These "structures become progressively integrated with the self-organized properties of the system" (Thelen et al., 1987, p. 41) to gradually optimize skilled function. Cooperating systems include musculoskeletal components, sensory systems, central sensorimotor integrative mechanisms, and arousal and motivation (see Chapter 2) (Heriza, 1991; Horak, 1991; Shumway-Cook & Woollacott, 1985, 1993; Thelen et al., 1987). In this theoretic approach, both these internal components of the organism and the external context of the task are equivalent in determining the outcome of behavior because behavior is task specific. In this model of infant motor development, therefore, the environment is as important as the organism. Because, however, the infant's cooperating systems, such as those involving strength and postural control, do not develop at the same rate, certain components are seen as rate limiting or constraining to the performance of any specific behavior.

In a seminal paper in the physical therapy literature, Heriza (1991) described the basic concepts of dynamical systems theory and suggested various approaches to testing its utility in planning and assessing the outcomes of therapeutic interventions. For example, eight subsystems are postulated to be involved in the development of infant locomotion:

1. Pattern generation of the coordinative structure leading to reciprocal lower extremity activity, consisting primarily of alternating flexor muscle activation

2. Development of reciprocal muscle activity of flexor and extensor muscles

3. Strength of extensor muscles needed for opposing the force of gravity

4. Changes in body size and composition

5. Antigravity control of upright posture of the head and trunk

6. Appropriate decoupling of the tight synchronization characteristic of early reciprocal lower extremity movements, such that the knee moves out of phase with the hip and ankle

7. Visual flow sensitivity required to maintain posture while moving through the environment

8. Ability to recognize the requirements of the task and be motivated to move toward a goal

This listing makes it clear that the development of a particular motor pattern, in this case upright locomotion, depends on a combination of mechanical, neurologic, cognitive, and perceptual factors in addition to environmental contributions specific to both the task and the context of the infant's action. Each of the subsystems develops at its own rate but is constrained or supported by physical and environmental factors, such as opportunities to practice antigravity trunk extension while prone, standing upright, and stepping. For example, since the implementation of advice to encourage parents to have infants sleep on their back (American Academy of Pediatrics Task Force on Infant Positioning and SIDS, 1992), investigators have shown that back-sleeping infants are less likely to roll over at 4 months of age than infants who sleep in the prone position (Jantz et al., 1997) and have lower developmental scores at 6 months of age (Dewey et al., 1998), a difference that was no longer apparent at 18 months. Changing the environment available to the infant for practicing movements appears to have altered the timing of motor development.

In the dynamical systems view of development, the movements of locomotion are conceived not as derived from a set of instructions from the nervous system nor as built from chains of reflexes but as self-organizing and emergent as a result of the interaction of the subsystems described. The locus of control for function shifts over time, depending on the dominance or constraints of various subsystems.

Spontaneous exploration of movement possibilities and flexible selection of the most appropriate movement synergy for accomplishing goal-directed actions are key processes in development in the view of the proponents of dynamical systems theory (Thelen & Corbetta, 1994). Transitional periods, when movement patterns appear more variable, are thought to be sensitive periods in development when intervention might be particularly effective. Research is likely to identify these sensitive periods in the development of specific functional behaviors, thereby providing new knowledge to guide intervention by therapists.

Based on dynamical systems theory, developmental change is seen not as a series of discrete stages but as a series of states of stability, instability, and phase shifts in which new states become stable aspects of behavior (Thelen, 1995). Research involves the search for collective variables or patterns of behavior that reflect the action of the component parts involved in a particular environment or task context. An example of research designed to identify the collective variables that might show qualitative change as new movement patterns appear, as well as the control variables that limit or facilitate the transition between patterns, is work on the developmental transition between walking and running of Whitall and Getchell (1995).

Although running has generally been described as differing from walking in having a flight phase, Whitall and Getchell (1995) did not find this to be the case in the early development of running. Nor could they find another variable that differed significantly between the two patterns of movement, suggesting that the transition was really one between two similar movements and not two qualitatively different patterns at all. These researchers recommended that the search for a collective variable for describing the qualitative difference between walking and running should be continued by assessing the possible role of arm movements. Young runners had difficulty generating both horizontal forces (reflected in a small increase in stride length over that used in walking) and vertical forces (reflected in little flight and little hip extension in running). Whitall and Getchell (1995) surmised that the ability to produce or regulate force by the ankle extensors was a key control parameter for emergence of running. They suggested that another control parameter might be ability to organize posture during high-velocity movement.

A dynamical systems approach to studying the transition from reaching without grasping to reaching with grasping was more successful in showing a sharp transition from predominant use of one pattern to predominant use of the other over a period of approximately 1 to 2 weeks (Wimmers et al., 1998a, 1998b). In keeping with the prediction of dynamical systems theory, in the weeks just before the shift from predominance of one mode of reaching to the other, infants showed instability of mode choice; that is, they frequently switched between types of reaching during a single session of reaching opportunities (Wimmers et al., 1998a). Individual infants demonstrated the phase shift at different ages (usually between 13 and 20 weeks of age), and a search for control parameters driving the change showed that arm weight and arm circumference (which increased with age in a continuous, linear fashion) were significantly related to the change in preferred mode of reaching (Wimmers et al., 1998b).

Although use of dynamical systems theory to drive therapeutic theory and practice in physical therapy is still in its infancy, it is already clear that this model focuses the attention of the therapist on a number of important aspects of the therapeutic process of facilitating functional motor development. These aspects include (1) search for the constraints in subsystems that limit motor behavior, such as contractures or weakness, leading to treatment goals related to reduction of impairments; (2) creation of an environment that supports or compensates for weaker or less mature (rate-limiting) components of the systems that contribute to development of motor control; (3) attention to setting up a therapeutic environment that affords opportunities to practice tasks in a meaningful and functional context; (4) use of activities that promote exploration of a variety of movement patterns that might be appropriate for a task; and (5) search for control parameters, such as speed of movement or force production, that can be manipulated by intervention to facilitate the attainment of therapeutic goals, especially during sensitive periods of development during which behavior is less stable (Fetters, 1991a, 1991b; Heriza, 1991). Chapter 2 on motor control and Chapter 6 on motor learning explore these concepts as therapeutic guides in more detail.

Myrtle McGraw, although generally considered a member of the maturationist school, developed a theory of motor development in the 1930s that contained the rudiments of many of the components of the modern dynamical systems approach to understanding the development of motor skills (Bergenn et al., 1992; McGraw, 1935). McGraw was a psychologist who studied the effects of intensive intervention, beginning at 20 days of age, with Johnny, the weaker of twin boys named Johnny and Jimmy. Her research was conducted at the height of the nature-nurture controversy between maturationists and behaviorists. In summary, her work showed that providing up to 7 hours a day of exercise of newly emerging developmental skills in the first year of life did not increase the *rate* of motor development. Her anecdotal comments, however, indicated that the exercised twin had more relaxed muscle tone and better coordination of movement than the twin whose movements and exploration had been restricted to a crib for much of the day, with no interaction with people other than for needed care.

McGraw's work was interpreted at the time as supporting the maturationist theory that the environment had little effect on child development. In the second year of his life, however, McGraw provided Johnny with a stimulating environment and extensive practice opportunities (3 hours per day) for developing motor skills that were not otherwise likely to develop in a child younger than 2 years, such as roller skating, climbing inclines of 70°, and jumping off high pedestals. Under these conditions, Johnny excelled in physical growth, problem solving of difficult motor control situations, and attainment of skills that Jimmy refused even to try during the periodic testing sessions that occurred. McGraw also noted the remarkable persistence in tasks demonstrated by Johnny, as well as his extensive visual review of the situation before embarking on a task. Films of the twins at age 40 years, moreover, demonstrated that the twin who exercised intensively during the first 2 years had an impressive physique and elegantly coordinated movement compared with those of his twin.

Although the results of an analysis of two individual cases cannot be accepted as providing fundamental laws of motor development, McGraw's study makes it clear that we have little idea of the possibilities inherent in the very young child who is seldom stimulated to achieve the full potential of early motor skill development. By analogy, we can assume that we have barely scratched the surface in our understanding of how therapeutic intervention might be used to mitigate the effects of motor dysfunction. In recounting her life's work and its interpretation by herself and others, McGraw also illustrated how the biases of the times are reflected in how research results are interpreted and received.

DEVELOPMENTAL PROCESSES AND PRINCIPLES

Based on her study of Johnny and Jimmy, as well as 68 other babies studied longitudinally without special intervention, McGraw constructed a set of developmental principles, many of which remain current (or are once again current) today. She conceived of movements as behaviors within an action system in which objects in the environment are as important a part of the action system as the movements themselves. "Any activity is composed of many ingredients, some of which may for convenience be considered as external and others as internal with respect to the organism, but none of these factors can be considered as external to the behavior" (McGraw, 1935, p. 303). McGraw also recognized that multiple components are interwoven in the development of behavior patterns (McGraw, 1935, pp. 302–303):

> The growing of a behavior-pattern is likened to a design in the process of being woven, composed as it is of various colored threads. All of the threads do not move forward at the same time nor at the same rate. The weaver picks up the gold thread and weaves it back and forth, though at the same time steadily forward. Then he drops it in order to bring the blue thread forward a distance, until finally the two become united to make the pattern complete. The design is contingent upon the interrelation of the various threads. It is not the summation of the blue and gold threads but their position with respect to each other and to the piece as a whole which determines the design.

McGraw also described the uneven nature of development, in which a given behavior pattern has a period of "inception, incubation, consummation, and decline" (1935, p. 305). The results of her longitudinal studies on the intratask course of development of important motor patterns were published in 1945 (McGraw, 1963) and remain highly informative today (although her description of brain development itself has long been out of date). Because of her daily observations, she often saw a movement pattern appear only once or twice (examples of beginner's luck) and then disappear before becoming a stable part of the infant's repertoire. When first becoming stable, the activity seems overworked and exaggerated. Furthermore, she noted that "as the child begins to get control over a pattern or an aspect of a pattern, the activity itself becomes the incentive for repetition" (McGraw, 1935, p. 307). Thus, early in life, movement for the sake of movement is a functional activity.

Therapists who perceive these evanescent periods of self-driven motivation to practice emerging movements and who follow the lead of children in the flow of therapy are likely to be among those whose clients are both happy and productive in intervention sessions. Because children with disabilities may have fewer options for exploration of movement opportunities, it is important to note that research supports the importance of caregiver guidance in assisting children with self-discovery efforts. For example, young children with developmental disabilities do have mastery motivation (i.e., persistent task-directed behavior in moderately challenging problem-solving situations) that is similar to that of other children, but their level of motivation is related to their mental, rather than chronologic, age and is improved in those who experience high levels of adaptive interaction with their mothers (Blasco et al., 1990; Hauser-Cram, 1996).

McGraw suggested that a stable movement pattern may seem to disappear as a part of the child's repertoire, becoming superseded by some rapidly developing new behavior, but ultimately the movement is restricted to its most specific and economic form. She was among the first to note the presence of normal regressions in motor behavior and has been credited as one of the first developmental psychologists to recognize the bidirectionality of neural and behavioral development (Bergenn et al., 1992; Bevor, 1982; Oppenheim, 1981; Provost, 1981). A behavior may also become integrated with other behaviors to form a complex activity; thus, McGraw noted that the developmental course of a behavior may look quite different during different stages of its maturation. A "second wind" for a behavioral pattern in decline as a part of the movement repertoire was also noted.

Because McGraw noted these various characteristics across many developing movement patterns, she believed that fits and starts, spurts and regressions, and overlapping of patterns undergoing emergence, development, and decline were firm developmental principles and that snapshots of development, such as motor milestone tests, could not adequately reflect the underlying processes of development (Bergenn et al., 1992). McGraw firmly believed that there were sensitive periods (she actually used the term "critical period" but later regretted it because of its "use it or lose it permanently" interpretation in biology) in which interventions could produce the most influence on developing behavioral patterns. The period of greatest susceptibility to exercise was believed to be one in which the pattern was entering its most rapid phase of development. Delay did not mean that intervention could no longer affect the behavior pattern (the concept of critical period), but rather that the interference of other ongoing developmental programs, including changes in anthropometric configuration of the body with growth, can decrease effectiveness. Unfortunately, we still have little idea of how these developmental principles might be systematically applied in a therapeutic milieu, but dynamical systems theory has brought them back to the forefront of scientific thinking about the processes of motor development. When research provides prescriptions for most effectively structuring therapy based on a child's current repertoire and presence of instability in selection of behavioral response modes, readiness level for learning new skills, constraints that limit the possibility of change, and task or environmental characteristics that will be influential in evoking developmental progress, we are likely to make great strides in the efficient packaging of therapeutic programs (Bower & McLellan, 1992). Even more important will be knowledge that helps therapists to coach parents in effectively assisting children in their own self-initiated attempts to drive developmental progress.

McGraw ended her monumental study of human development by foreseeing the development and potential of dynamical systems–based motion analysis. "Perhaps the time will come when the movements of growth can be expressed in mathematical formulas as precisely as the movements of celestial bodies, but until that time arrives we shall have to be content with cumbersome descriptive analyses" (McGraw, 1935, p. 312). The work by Wimmers, Savelsbergh, van der Kamp, and Hartelman (1998b) on the transition between two modes of reaching is just one example of the elegant quantitative description of the process of change during motor development that McGraw predicted.

Although both McGraw and Gesell believed that neural maturation was the primary force driving development, the observations and theories of each pointed out the dynamic nature of motor development. The approach of dynamical systems analysis has added knowledge gained from many kinds of physical systems, including nonbiologic systems. In decades to come, we shall continue to see how this new approach contributes both to explaining the observations of the theorists who pioneered the study of motor development and to the development of new knowledge to guide therapeutic intervention.

Contemporary Issues in Understanding Principles of Motor Development

Despite a new theoretic perspective that models development as encompassing multiple organismic components in the creation of coordinative structures for posture and movement and emphasizes the crucial role of the environment and task characteristics in organizing emergent movements, certain principles of motor development have consistently appeared in the conceptual framework of various students of motor development. These include the notions that development of motor skills generally proceeds in a cephalocaudal and proximodistal direction, that neural maturation is an important component of unfolding skill development, and that motor development appears, at least on the surface, to be more stagelike than continuous, having a spiraling nature in which regressions, consolidations, and

reappearances of underlying fundamental processes occur (Bevor, 1982).

What is becoming clear is that these long-standing theoretic concepts must be expanded to incorporate a new understanding of the underlying developmental processes. For example, new research on developmental processes discussed in Chapter 2 on motor control has revealed that certain factors are rate limiting to motor development, with strength, postural control, and perceptual analysis capabilities being among the most important. When compensations are provided experimentally to eliminate the effects of these rate-limiting factors, the developing motor system may display previously unrecognized potential. Patterns of movement appear that seem precocious because they were previously denied expression owing to immaturity of certain of the cooperating systems.

Dynamical systems theory has also demonstrated that stagelike external behavior, such as the switch from reaching without grasping to reaching with grasping (Wimmers et al., 1998a, 1998b) can emerge from continuously changing underlying processes. Here a new stage seems to appear de novo only because the continuous developments of a number of cooperating systems finally merge in a way that allows the new behavior to appear. The behavior appears to reflect an entirely novel stage of development when in fact the underlying processes in multiple systems were developing continuously in a gradually accretive fashion. We will use more information about the development of eye-hand coordination to illustrate these points.

Cephalocaudal and Proximodistal Developmental Direction

The processes involved in functional reaching include (1) visual fixation to localize the object and choose a hand transport program, (2) foveal analysis for perceptual identification of the object needed for anticipatory adaptation of the action to fit the characteristics of the object, (3) manual capture, and (4) object manipulation (Hay, 1990). By the time of birth, a primitive body scheme has already developed that provides the infant with a hand transport program. Infants have been observed in utero during real-time ultrasound imaging to perform hand-to-mouth activities, touch other parts of their own bodies, and explore the uterine walls—all, of course, without visual guidance (Sparling, 1993). Shortly after birth, they are able to launch the hand toward a visualized object, preferring one that is moving (von Hofsten, 1982). (This competence fits well with the known characteristics of early development of the retina, which is more mature in the movement-sensitive periphery than in the foveal area [Abramov et al., 1982].) The hand, although open, does not engage in actual grasping in most cases, and the coordination of the movement does not include corrections of direction or hand-shaping for the object's properties during the course of the reach (Vinter, 1990). In fact, the entire arm is launched as a single unit in a pattern that can best be described as a swipe, a coordinative strategy that is quite unlike the lift-project strategy typical of more mature reaching.

Because we know that further development will include gradual refinement of hand use as part of reaching and grasping, this sequence of development would appear to follow the proximodistal developmental rule. The course of development, however, is much more complicated. First, reaching at 1 to 2 months is typically done with a fisted hand, rather than the open hand of the newborn, and reaching under visual control with an open hand begins anew at 4 to 5 months (Vinter, 1990). Furthermore, successful reach-and-grasp under visual control can often occur in the period from 1 to 2 months if the head is supported to eliminate a major problem in developing a successful coordinative strategy. Thus, when external controls are provided for the posturally incompetent head, the infant may be able to coordinate a reach-and-grasp successfully, even though, as we have seen, consistent use of reaching with grasping is not present until 13 to 20 weeks of age (Wimmers et al., 1998a).

These and other observations have led to the suggestions that postural control is a rate-limiting factor in early motor development (Shumway-Cook & Woollacott, 1993) and that distal competence may be masked by deficiencies in postural control of the head and neck. Although it seems readily apparent that the ability to control the head to maintain stability of visual perception is an important early competence in a general sequence of cephalocaudal progression of development, many aspects of proximal and distal control of the extremities are undergoing contemporaneous development that may not be overtly observable under normal conditions (see Fetters et al., 1989; Heriza, 1991; and Loria, 1980, for further examples). Many exceptions to a proximodistal progression of development have been found (Heriza, 1991).

An important consequence of understanding these new findings from research is that therapists should not conceive of individual body parts as developing independently, sequentially, or purely as a result of nervous system maturation when planning therapeutic intervention. Although various segments of the body may develop their patterns of control for any given task at different rates, any movement pattern is a composite, involving coordi-

nation of all of the body subsystems. Furthermore, the apparent directionality of development does not appear to be inherent only in the genetic direction of nervous system development, but rather is a result of the interactive functioning of the multiple systems children bring to exploration of the problems and possibilities inherent in a particular task at a particular point in their development (Thelen, 1990). The characteristics and demands of the task are critical in organizing the response of the subsystems, but each child's response is unique in its kinematics and time of appearance (Thelen et al., 1993; Wimmers et al., 1998a). In early infancy, for example, the enormous mass of the child's head relative to the size of the rest of the body places constraints on the functions that are possible. Lifting the head and sustaining its upright position while the body is prone therefore entails coordinating the trunk and extremities to create a stable base for head movement. The role of the neck extensor muscles may be comparatively minor, yet until the head can be adequately stabilized in space, other movement functions of the body in the prone position cannot be fully expressed. In attempts to lift the head while prone to look at an interesting object, each child produces a unique and specific pattern of movement that depends on individual anthropometric characteristics, muscle strength and limb compliance, visual acuity and perception, previous experience, and interest in the object.

What seems to play a major role, then, in the general observation of cephalocaudal progression of development are the infant's strength of key muscle groups and anthropometric characteristics, that is, the ability to control the large mass of the head relative to the rest of the body and cope with the high center of mass. Although cephalocaudal progression is a notion that seems to hold as an overall generalization regarding the postural control of the whole body, most movements used by infants entail the coordination of multiple body parts if they are to be effective. The coordination of a prone-on-elbows-with-head-turn strategy for responding to an interesting sound with visual fixation is a good example.

In developing items for the Test of Infant Motor Performance (Campbell et al., 1995), an interesting sequence of development was discovered in the organization of a response to a sound made behind an infant's head as the infant lay in the prone position (Campbell, 1998, unpublished data). An immature response involved dragging the face across the surface to turn the head toward the sound and visualize it. By four months of age, typically developing infants were able to support themselves on their elbows with head lifted and turn toward the sound. Over the course of weekly examinations, however, we noticed that infants tended to alternate for several weeks between the mature response described and one in which they lifted the head and extended the upper trunk, but seemed unable to turn their head toward the sound source despite obvious interest in the stimulus. After several weeks in which the two modes of response alternated, the individual infant's response stabilized in its most mature form. What intrigued us was why an infant who could lift his head, but apparently could not organize his posture so as to turn it toward an interesting sound, would not choose to go back to an earlier, successful response, that is, putting his head down on the surface to turn it. It appeared that once the infant had the ability to extend the neck and trunk in prone position, he would forego successful task accomplishment (i.e., seeing the interesting sound source) in favor of an unsuccessful head lifting strategy that was used repeatedly over a period of weeks until he could consistently put together all the components of the most mature response strategy using prone-on-elbows as a base of support. We also wondered why an infant who, for weeks, had used the drag-face-over-surface strategy to successfully find the interesting sound would suddenly move into a preference for using two head-and-trunk-extension strategies, one with support on elbows (successful) and one without (unsuccessful). By searching for correlates of the appearance of these two new strategies, we discovered that their appearance was preceded about a week earlier by the ability to perform full neck and trunk extension down to the lumbar area when the infant was held in prone suspension. Thus it appeared that strength or control of lumbar trunk extensors might be necessary for the elaboration of a controlled performance of head turning with thoracic spine extension, just as Tscharnuter (1993) has theorized, but we do not know yet what the control parameters might be that finally create consistent use of the prone-on-elbows strategy.

The examples given earlier illustrate the power of the dynamical systems perspective by pointing out that multiple systems and processes are developing at any given time, each at its own rate and instantaneous level of competence. What then appears to be a newly appearing "stage" may merely be the time at which one or more rate-limiting factors finally achieve a level of development in a continuous trajectory that supports the appearance of a new, stable form of behavior. The new behavior appears discontinuous with what went before only because the underlying continuous processes were not visible. In the example from research on the Test of Infant Motor Performance, it was only because both trunk extension in prone suspension and head turning in response to a sound were measured together on a weekly basis that the relationship between lumbar

trunk extension at one weekly examination and higher levels of performance in responding to sound the next week was identified. As a result, it can be recommended that a treatment plan for helping a child with motor dysfunction to achieve the ability to freely use head and later hands in a prone position might profitably include strengthening of *lower* trunk extensors and learning to organize the load-bearing parts of the lower body (Tscharnuter, 1993). Further research to identify the critical processes and subsystems that contribute to qualitative changes in infant behavior should be productive in refining intervention strategies to promote motor development in children with disabilities.

Nervous System Maturation as One Driving Force for Development

Although McGraw (1963), Gesell (1928a, 1928b), and Shirley (1931) emphasized brain maturation as being the major force driving development (despite their own contrary evidence for the important role of external factors), dynamical systems theory has sometimes seemed to view neural maturation with less credence than I believe it deserves. The nervous system in dynamical systems theory is described as merely another system in its developmental contribution, no more important than any other system. In children with mental retardation or cerebral motor dysfunction, however, therapists are well aware of the serious limitations in adapting movement to functional purposes imposed by a compromised CNS. In this chapter development and functions of the nervous system in movement are described; Chapter 4 provides information on another important cooperating component, the musculoskeletal system.

Research suggests that about 30% of the entire genome is expressed only in the brain (Nowakowski, 1987). Although it is true that we now know that experience drives brain development in just as important a way as do genetic programs (Greenough et al., 1987), the notion that no hierarchy of important functions or no unique function of structures exists is simply not true, especially in the human brain, with its highly encephalized processes. What is true is that lower levels of the nervous system, such as the midbrain and the spinal cord, have been recognized to be capable of controlling many finely coordinated movements, not only simple reflexes, and that vast amounts of the CNS are involved in the production and control of even the most basic movements. For example, animal research described by Bradley in Chapter 2 has revealed that well-coordinated stepping movements can be evoked from activation of spinal cord circuits. Involvement of higher levels of the nervous system, however, is necessary to control the body's overall equilibrium during gait and to express the intentionality of functional movements. The locus of control for a given movement varies, however, depending on task requirements and previous experience with similar tasks. Thus, environmental demands become a part of the neural ensemble for producing movement, and the infant's practice of movements creates inputs that drive brain development.

To return to the example of development of eye-hand coordination, humans display a major shift from subcortically organized movement in the first 3 to 4 months to increasing involvement of cortical circuits at 4 to 5 months (Paillard, 1990). Infants with later evidence of cortical blindness, for example, may be able to track an object visually in the newborn period, using brainstem processing mechanisms. Although the organism's own activity is influential in directing the early course of neural plasticity (Greenough et al., 1987), this example of deviant development reinforces the concept that the higher levels of the CNS are necessary (but not sufficient) for normal human development to occur. Visual functions involving binocularity seem particularly dependent on development of cortical visual circuits. For example, most infants can align their eyes appropriately in the first month of life, but only when visual cortex dominance columns have been refined do they gain control of both the sensory (optical fusion) and the motor (eye convergence) aspects of binocularity (Thorn et al., 1994).

Reaching, too, differs fundamentally in the newborn and the 6-month-old (Paillard, 1990). Reaching is a unitary action in the young infant; a differentiation among reach, grasp, manipulation, and release will later result from maturation of cortical systems in conjunction with anthropometric changes (Wimmers et al., 1998a, 1998b) and learning gained from experiences in the world of objects (Fentress, 1990). As seen in patients with a stroke that affects fine hand function, cortical activity is necessary for the more delicate aspects of motor control of the hand, and it cannot develop adequately unless the encephalic structures are intact. No examples have been reported in the literature of a capability of higher primates to develop or regain fine finger control in the absence of the primary motor cortex. In humans, individual finger movements cannot be evoked by electrical stimulation of the motor cortex before 3 months of age (Fentress, 1990).

Establishment of monosynaptic connections between the motor cortex and spinal cord motoneurons is associated with the appearance of selective control of digital movements in primates (Schoen, 1969); these connections are not present in neonatal monkeys and develop gradually during the first 8 months after birth. Improvement in monkeys' abilities to retrieve small pieces of food from indentations is seen when a wide range of rapid, small movements involving the forearm or shoulder joint appear to assist more efficient distal performance of the digits. This description is remarkably similar to descriptions of the development of fidgety movements in human infants at 2 to 3 months of age (Hadders-Algra & Prechtl, 1992). These movements herald the development of goal-directed movements, including the emergence of consistently effective reaching and grasping. These small synergistic movements in monkeys do not survive pyramidotomy, nor do selective digital movements.

At about the same time that fidgety movements develop, the appearance of ballistic movements (swipes and swats) heralds the switch from coactivation of muscle groups to the reciprocal coordination of muscle activity that characterizes more mature motor patterns (Hadders-Algra et al., 1992). Wimmers, Savelsbergh, van der Kamp, and Hartelman (1998b) suggest that use of coactivation patterns may also be correlated with reaching with a fisted hand and that the ability to reciprocally activate muscles may be related to both changes in arm circumference and the switch to reaching with an open hand. Although we do not know what leads to the appearance of reciprocal patterns of muscle activity, it is notable that this development does not seem to appear in children with cerebral palsy (CP) (Leonard et al., 1990).

According to Paillard (1990), four features characterize the evolution of the primate nervous system, culminating in the human brain, and promote use of the hand as an elaborate tool for manipulating the environment. These features are (1) extension of the precentral cortex developed principally for fine sensory-guided steering and control of the hand and digits; (2) enlargement of the lateral cerebellum, again relating to control of forelimb segments and to timing and smoothing of movements; (3) specialization of the parietal association cortex for precise visual guidance of goal-directed arm and hand movements; and (4) prominent development of the frontal association areas that funnel information to motor control regions, mainly through basal ganglia loops. Here we see an example of multiple subsystems in the brain cooperating with the musculoskeletal structures characteristic of the human organism to produce functional movement.

The frontal areas process information related to goal-directed behavior and anticipated consequences of intended acts involving the basic capacity to guide response choice by stored information (Goldman-Rakic, 1987; Paillard, 1990). Major developments in this area in the human infant begin at about

8 months and reach a maximum at 2 years of age. Activity in frontal areas cooperates in motor functions through basal ganglia circuits (Hoover & Strick, 1993). The basal ganglia are involved in the internal generation of automatic movements, the predictive monitoring of head and arm activities (Fentress, 1990), and the acquisition and learning of motor skills through their five parallel pallidal-thalamocortical loops, including projections to primary motor cortex, where the dynamics of movement patterns are selected (Georgopoulos et al., 1992).

Eye-head-body orientation activities and target-reaching activities have been shown in lower vertebrates to be coordinated primarily by brainstem centers, prominently involving the superior colliculus (Paillard, 1990). In keeping with identification of these behaviors in very young infants, arm projection at that age is possible without cerebral cortical control. Functional manipulation, such as the fine digital control involved in food taking in experimental primates, however, depends on the additional coordinated action of cortical pathways from higher centers (Fentress, 1990). Elegant hand-grasping and manipulation movements of the primate are dependent on inputs from cerebral cortical levels that are coordinated with lower-level eye-hand-head activity. Overall, however, the primary role of higher-level CNS structures is to tune, guide, learn, and select, adapt, or inhibit execution of basic movements by lower levels of the nervous system. The therapist views this as increasing ability to control movements selectively and adapt them to functional purposes.

Motor control functions are not assumed at successively higher hierarchic levels, leaving behind previously used primitive behaviors and control centers; rather, many levels of the nervous system cooperate in the production of movement behaviors. Typically, no single active site for any particular behavior can be identified; behavior is, rather, an emergent property of the cooperation of various subsystems, with task characteristics organizing the response (Thelen et al., 1993). That is, the characteristics of the task lead the nervous system with its distributed functions to select from a variety of currently available options for assembling a task-related action. The next section of this chapter elaborates on a theory of nervous system development and function that provides an appropriate explanatory model for how the developing organism actively constructs its own operating system for functional behavior.

The Theory of Neuronal Group Selection

According to a popular summary by Edelman (1992) of current theories of nervous system func-

tioning, previous psychologic theories have failed spectacularly in shedding light on how the human mind originates in the functioning of the physical brain because they have neglected the biology of the system. Popular models describing the brain as analogous to a computer with hardware (neurons) and software (motor programs) bear only superficial resemblance to the actual operation of the brain. Edelman's theory is based instead on facts that are garnered from biologic research but are also consistent with behavioral observations. Called the neuronal group selection theory, it has three basic tenets. These tenets describe how the anatomy of the brain is produced during development, how experience selects for strengthening certain patterns of responses from the anatomic structures, and how the resulting maps of the brain give rise to uniquely individual behavioral functions through a process called reentry. Sporns and Edelman (1993) further describe how such a system solves the problem of managing movement in an organism with multiple degrees of freedom.

The first tenet of Edelman's theory (1992) is concerned with developmental selection by which the characteristic neuroanatomy of a species is formed. The genetic code of the species does not specify the wiring diagram but instead inscribes the constraints of the process of formation of neural networks, resulting in a primary repertoire of species-specific behavior. In humans, for example, these behaviors appear to include rhythmic movements of the lower extremities, expressed in kicking and neonatal stepping (Thelen, 1990), mouth-to-hand behaviors, and visual following and projection of the arm toward moving objects (von Hofsten, 1982). An overproduction of early synaptic connections formed by activity and cell death or retraction of unexercised connections may explain why individual wiring diagrams vary somewhat yet still maintain the same general form across members of the species.

The second tenet of Edelman's (1992) neuronal group selection theory involves the development of a secondary repertoire of functional circuits from the basic neuroanatomic network through a process of selective activation that strengthens or weakens synaptic connections based on individual experience. The secondary repertoire includes mechanisms underlying skilled motor behavior, memory, and other important functions and is unique to the individual. In a movement system with multiple degrees of freedom, a variety of ways to accomplish the movements involved in functional tasks can arise (Sporns & Edelman, 1993), but to become incorporated into the secondary repertoire, the functional synergy selected must (1) accomplish the task, and (2) allow for postural stability of the body during the task.

Adolph (1997) showed that the first movement strategy selected for a risky task such as descending a steep slope is goal directed and may be highly inefficient, even foolhardy. During development, however, infants try out a variety of movement strategies that happen to occur to them, often accidentally, before readily selecting the most safe and economical one for the task at hand.

Edelman's third tenet describes how the first two selectional processes interact to connect biology with psychology. The primary and secondary repertoires of species-typical and uniquely individual functional neural circuits must form maps connected by massively parallel and reciprocal connections. Edelman gives the example that the visual system of the monkey consists of more than 30 different maps, each with a unique degree of functional segregation for orientation, color, movement, and other functions and each linked to the others by parallel and reciprocal connections that can be accessed by the reentry process. By this process, a nervous system with distributed functions is formed.

Selection occurs over neuronal groups from various maps throughout the region and the nervous system as a whole to produce a particular behavior. The behavior is unique to the individual in whom it occurs because of variations in maps caused by the effects of individual experience on their development. The combination of neuronal groups from selected multiple maps of an area's function (for example, the hand motor area of primary cerebral motor cortex combined with selections from maps that are concerned with receipt of visual and tactile information and ones concerned with postural function of the neck and shoulder) allows the production of a movement that is precisely tuned to the environmental demands for functional performance yet unique to the individual's capacity for processing sensory inputs and for combining selections of neuronal groups from his or her individual regional maps. A selectionist system with distributed functions requires a repertoire of variable actions in order to provide adaptability; that is, a variety of means for responding to environmental demands and internal changes such as growth must be available.

A selectionist model of the nervous system is consistent with the research of Keshner and colleagues (1989), demonstrating that when overtly similar movements are studied in a group of individuals, each person performs the movement with his or her own unique combination of synergistic muscle activation patterns. Thelen and colleagues (1993) have demonstrated similar findings in infants learning to reach. Although a group of infants tended to use a similar strategy of coactivating muscular antagonists when first learning to reach, each infant came at the task in a unique way based on preferred posture, movement, and energy level. Two quiet infants, for example, organized their reaches by lifting their arms and extending them slowly forward. Two other infants, who were highly active and frequently engaged in bilateral arm flapping, needed to damp down their oscillations to reach successfully. These infants used high-velocity swipes to orient their arms toward the toy. In testing infants on the Test of Infant Motor Performance, we also observed variations in how infants approached the orientation-to-sound task in the prone position, although typically developing infants used the two head-and-trunk-extension strategies described earlier. For example, one infant extended his neck and trunk when he heard the sound, but being unable to support himself on his elbows in order to turn his head, he instead flapped his arms and legs, causing his trunk to rock forward and backward, and eventually negotiated a partial turn of his trunk toward the sound source by pivoting on his abdomen (Campbell, 1998, unpublished data).

In keeping with each individual's march to a personal internal drum, each phenotypic neuronal group has a combination of excitatory and inhibitory connections, allowing the final motor output to be assembled selectively based on current demands and past experience with the task that has strengthened or weakened the tendencies to select particular groups from particular maps (Edelman, 1992; Thelen, 1990). Essential to this development is exposure of the nervous system to a sufficient sample of coactivated sensory signals to permit the neuronal groups to respond differentially to various objects and events in the environment (Sporns, 1994). Obtaining such a sampling of experience occurs during development when an infant spontaneously explores the environment through movement. To have adaptive value, the responding neuronal groups must also contribute to functional behavior in the organism. Resulting from these selections, higher-order dynamic structures called global maps are formed that link sensory and motor maps. Such correlated activity is essential to operation of a system based on variability in response units, which become strengthened through use and adaptive value. These global maps are able to interact with memory processes and other unmapped functions such as those of the basal ganglia and cerebellum. Global maps allow the connection between local maps and motor behavior, new sensory inputs, and further neural processing as important aspects of development and learning.

Neuronal group selection theory does not hold that *programs* are executed by the nervous system; rather, dynamic loops are created that continually match movements and postures to task-related sensory signals of multiple kinds. Functioning is based on statistical probabilities of signals, not coded signals or preformed programs. Georgopoulos and colleagues (1993), for example, have demonstrated that the precise directionality of a reaching movement can be specified by vectors calculated from the neural activity of large populations of cells in the motor cortex, each of which individually has a preferred directionality but also fires in relation to movements in multiple directions. Edelman (1992) further theorized that the system has biologic "values" that are species specific and drive the selective strengthening of synaptic activities based on experience. These values influence adaptive processes by linkage between the global mappings and activity in hedonic centers and the limbic system of the brain in a way that fulfills homeostatic needs of the organism that have been set through evolution.

In a computer model of a visual system with a set "value" that prefers light to no-light conditions in the center of a "visual" field (similar to that produced in humans by evolution), initially nondirected movements of an "arm" have been shaped to target an object (Edelman, 1992; Thelen, 1995). If one appreciates that newborn infants possess a primary repertoire that includes moving the mouth to the hand, seeking light, and producing head turns or arm projections in response to moving objects in the visual field, it is not difficult to perceive of the theory of neuronal group selection as an explanation for the gradual process of learning to reach successfully to grasp an object and put it into the mouth.

With repeated experience in reaching and grasping as an "individual problem-solver working each day" (Thelen et al., 1993), infants modulate their intrinsic dynamics, discovering the most stable trajectory, joint coordination, and patterns of muscle activation (Thelen et al., 1993), thereby creating their own personal maps. For example, Strick and Preston (1982a, 1982b) have suggested that separate representations of hand motor patterns at cerebral cortical levels may reflect the modular organization of sensorimotor units underlying the distinctive uses of the hand for power gripping or as a palpatory sensory surface. Dynamical systems theory, however, emphasizes that the nervous system is only one subsystem infants use to self-organize exploration of the environment.

Map creation through an individual's use of movement to drive brain plasticity can go awry. Byl and colleagues (1997), for example, reported that when a monkey was trained and reinforced for performing a stereotyped movement thousands of times, the simultaneous activation of muscles and tactile-kinesthetic receptors resulted in degradation of the primary sensory cortex maps. Neurons in the cortical area related to hand function become responsive to stimulation almost anywhere on the hand (even the back of the hand), a condition Byl and colleagues describe as a dedifferentiation of the normally exquisitely organized response patterns of the sensory cortex. They believe that this animal model may reflect the process of repetitive strain injury with focal dystonia in humans and that the findings support use of a sensorimotor retraining approach to treating this disorder in order to redifferentiate sensory maps in the cerebral cortex. If we think of the constrained and repetitive movements used by infants with CNS dysfunction, it is not hard to conceive of the possibility that they also have a poorly differentiated sensory cortex. The key to understanding and treating this type of problem is recognition that maps are formed connecting various areas of the brain based on the *simultaneous* activity of sensory and motor systems. We learn (and train the brain to select) what we do. Stereotyped simultaneous activity leads to poorly differentiated brain maps, whereas learning to use a variety of flexible patterns to accomplish common tasks leads to rich, complex brain organization compatible with adaptability to environmental demands and the internal changes accompanying growth.

Experience-Expectant and Experience-Dependent Neural Maturation

Greenough and colleagues (1987) have also discussed the importance of environmental experience in driving development of the brain, and their work provides further elaboration on Edelman's theory of neuronal group selection in a maturational context. Although no scientific evidence exists to suggest that training or an enriched environment leads to development of new neurons, extensive evidence documents the effect of training and environment on numbers and properties of synaptic connections among neural cells. Greenough and colleagues (1987) suggested that genetically specified directions lead to initial synaptic connectivities through a process of overproduction of populations of cells that are pruned by exposure to experiences common to all members of a species, such as the array of visual inputs to which infants are typically exposed. The result is species-typical behaviors akin to the primary repertoire described by Edelman (1992).

Greenough and colleagues (1987) called this process experience-expectant development and suggested that it occurs through the death of cells that do not establish productive connections. It has been discovered, however, that the genetic code may actually program cell death (Barinaga, 1993). If neurons have access to particular nerve growth factors, they may be able to escape their programmed fate. By such genetic-environmental interactions, development occurs by a size-matching process whereby the appropriate number of neurons survives to serve peripheral needs. By one's own developmental processes, therefore, each individual obtains a personal, unique structure and functional movement.

A second process, akin to Edelman's secondary repertoire and called experience-dependent neural maturation, is proposed to be the process by which each individual achieves further uniqueness in structure and function through exposure to an individualized set of experiences that establishes strong connectivities among cells based on strengthening of neural synapses that are "exercised" through both sensory and motor experiences (Greenough et al., 1987). The specific structure and function of a person therefore depend on both species-typical connectivities and the amount and strength of other connections resulting from personal experiences specific to each individual and his or her life history. Of most importance, in both aspects of neural plasticity, synaptic connectivity is linked to the individual's own activity in conjunction with genetic programs and environmental opportunities. Thus, the individual in a very real sense is the creator of his or her own unique brain and, by extension, functional motor behavior (Thelen, 1990).

Sensitive Periods in Development

Bertenthal and Campos (1987), in a commentary on Greenough and colleagues' theory, summarized research that may support the theory that experience-expectant and experience-dependent maturation of neural systems could be the basis of sensitive periods in development. They stressed that experience-dependent plasticity of the nervous system can initiate the generation of new synaptic connections and is available throughout the life span. The effects of experiences during a sensitive period, however, are expected to be qualitatively different from those at other points in the life span. The theory also predicts that sensitive periods in experience-expectant development can be extended by various means, including deprivation of sensory inputs that allow synaptic competition for connections to persist longer than is usual.

Most of the animal research on the influence of environmental stimuli on neural plasticity has been on cerebral cortical areas, especially those devoted to visual function. Research has documented the existence of sensitive and in some cases critical periods for development of visual perceptual skills (Thorn et al., 1994), once again suggesting the superior benefits of intervention earlier, rather than later, in life. Some evidence also exists to suggest effects of inter-

ventions on the sensory cortex, the motor cortex, and the cerebellum (Greenough et al., 1987; Nudo et al., 1996). For example, extensive practice of specific finger activities by monkeys led to enlarged areas of the motor cortex devoted to activation of the exercised fingers (Nudo et al., 1996).

Several sensitive periods in cognitive development have been demonstrated to occur during infancy (Fischer, 1987). At 2 to 4 months, infants demonstrate the ability to vary activity within a single action sequence to reach a simple goal, such as grasping a toy within reach. At 7 to 8 months, several actions can be related in a single functional unit, such as a delayed-response task, using vision to guide a manual manipulation or compare multiple objects, and using a string to activate a toy. By 12 to 13 months, a number of actions can be coordinated to perform a function such as putting a ball into a small hole in a toy box. At 18 to 21 months, symbolic representation is achieved in which a memory of an object can activate an action without the object's being present. Various types of evidence, such as changes in rates of synaptogenesis and electroencephalographic changes, show discontinuities at related time periods.

Unfortunately, only few data are available on the subject of sensitive periods as they affect motor skill development, particularly in children with acquired or congenital disabilities. Zelazo and colleagues (1972, 1983), however, demonstrated the effect of early stepping experience in human infants on maintenance of stepping behavior and earlier age of walking. Heriza (1991) has proposed that sensitive periods exist in the development of locomotor behavior that can be identified through kinematic analysis of rhythmic alternating movements of the legs based on dynamical systems theory and hypothesized that these transitional periods are important points for intervention in children at risk for developmental disabilities. Dynamical systems theory suggests that when children vary in their selection of a movement strategy in response to a particular task, this period of instability represents a special opportunity for directing development. Kanda and colleagues (1984) have also shown the superior benefits on quality of movement and walking in children with CP of early, as opposed to later, exposure to Vojta therapy, and Scherzer and colleagues (1976) suggested that children with CP who were treated at an earlier age than others also demonstrated greater benefits. These preliminary suggestions that intervention to promote motor development may vary in effectiveness based on timing of therapy are tantalizing, and further research on this topic is direly needed for improving the scheduling of intervention for maximizing outcomes. To be successful, however, research designs must be tailored specifically to the search for answers to the sensitive period question.

Periodic Equilibration in a Spiraling Pattern of Development

Piaget (1952) suggested that the experience of acting on the world (assimilation) with whatever sensorimotor schema is currently dominant was frequently met with resistance because the objects of interest were not easily adapted to the current schema (e.g., handling a soft cookie when the motor activity of crumpling or shaking was currently popular). This misfit between the child's current sensorimotor functioning and the response of handled objects leads to disequilibrium, which drives developmental progress through the child's persistence in gradually accommodating to the properties of objects eliciting interest. In so doing, the child eventually develops a different approach to handling the cookie and thereby alters the cognitive structure as well. I would suggest that our infants' alternation over several weeks between symmetric head and trunk extension versus supporting themselves on their elbows in response to a sound stimulus is an example of children learning to accommodate to new physical capabilities (head and trunk extension) while attempting to accomplish a task, in other words flexible problem solving.

Ames and colleagues (1979), following from Gesell's earlier observations, posited a similar process of alternating equilibrium and disequilibrium in behavioral characteristics that they believed cycled periodically. For example, toddlers at 18 months are likely to be trying to their parents because they have definite wants but few words with which to express them; they may communicate with crying and tantrums instead. (The reader should note that in this and other sections of the chapter, ages given are normative or average times of appearance of described behaviors; individual developmental rates may, of course, differ to some extent.) At 2 years, the child has developed more language and coordination and is emotionally on an even keel. Disequilibrium returns again at about 2.5 years, when this little person becomes more difficult to live with—bossy, rigid, and oppositional. Cooperation and sharing in play have not yet appeared, and the 2.5-year-old wants to hold onto any toy "he is playing with, has played with, or might in the future want to play with" (Ames et al., 1979, p. 28). The age of 3 years is again an easy time emotionally, whereas at 3.5 years children are insecure and anxious, yet determined and self-willed. At 3, children need their security blankets and thumbs a great deal. The 4-year-old is described as wild and wonderful. This child loves

humor and is secure and self-confident, although going overboard in either enthusiasm or anger, even threatening to run away when upset. Five-year-olds are more inwardly directed, prefer to stay within known boundaries, and have less interest in novel experiences. These children are careful to attempt only what can most definitely be achieved but are, nonetheless, expansive intellectually, loving to talk and learn about things. "Why?" is the word of choice. By 5.5 years, however, another period of disequilibrium seems to occur, but it is one characterized by extremes—shy at one moment, extremely bold the next. The child may seem to be in a constant state of tension, chewing on pencils and fidgeting. By 6.5 years, however, a calmer, more even-tempered child again emerges, moving toward the inner-directed 7-year-old.

Gesell (Heriza, 1991), Rood (Stengel et al., 1984), Bly (1983), and others have suggested that motor development also consists of an alternation and recombination of patterns of flexion, extension, and symmetry versus asymmetry, leading ever onward toward improved mobility and stability in posture and movement in opposition to the force of gravity. At different times, various patterns predominate, but an alternation between stability and instability of functioning characterized also by switches between symmetry and asymmetry is thought to be characteristic of normal developmental progression. Heriza has summarized these principles based on Gesell's early work as viewing growth "not as a linear process but a spiral one where structure and function jointly mature leading to regression, asymmetries, and reorganization. Although Gesell is best known for his principles of direction of development and individuating maturation, his principle of reciprocal interweaving . . . foreshadows [a] contemporary systems view of motor development" (Heriza, 1991, p. 102). As we have seen, McGraw (1935) held a similar view, but she and other early developmental researchers lacked the contemporary ability to reveal the underlying systems changes that produce these overtly observed patterns of development and tended to stress nervous system maturation as the driving force.

To summarize, studies have suggested that development proceeds in a continuous spiral characterized by "paired-but-opposed types of responses that occur in repeated alternation" (Ames et al., 1979, p. 4) and with relative periods of stability and instability (Heriza, 1991) that may reflect underlying developmental continuity within multiple subsystems involved in maturation. Regressions are also normal aspects of developmental processes (Bevor, 1982; Oppenheim, 1981; Provost, 1981). Ages 2, 5, 10, and 16 years are considered to be periods of emotional equilibrium; ages 3.5, 7, and 13 as periods of relative inwardness and withdrawal; and ages 4, 8, and 14 as periods of expansive behavior (Ames et al., 1979). More recent research has suggested that periods of rapid behavioral changes of many kinds occur at approximately 4, 6 to 7, 10 to 12, and 14 to 16 years (Fischer, 1987). Similarly, Shumway-Cook and Woollacott (1985) have suggested that motor patterns in the development of postural stability undergo a period of disequilibrium between 4 and 6 years, when a physical growth spurt occurs. Changes in perceptual functions during this period offer an alternative, or possibly an additional, explanation.

Whether these findings can be correlated with specific periods of brain growth is an interesting question. Epstein (1979) has found that there are major periods of accelerated brain growth (relative to body growth) in the periods from 3 to 10 months and from 2 to 4, 6 to 8, 10 to 12+, and 14 to 16+ years. Between 3 and 12 months, a major area of myelinization in the human is the inferior parietal cortex, a cross-modal association area. The cerebellum also shows its major, and virtually final, growth during this period, demonstrating an approximately threefold increase in DNA compared with the cerebrum. Except for the first period in infancy, however, brain growth is not accompanied by a net increase in brain DNA, so growth after about 1.5 years is assumed to be composed primarily of elaboration of networks of axons and dendrites and of axon myelinization. The latter is primarily associated with enhanced speed of neural processing.

Overall brain growth stages have been correlated with mind growth, a process called "phrenoblysis" (Epstein, 1979). Although Greenough and colleagues (1987) cautioned that spurts in growth of the whole brain or in head circumference may not be reflective of relative differences in timing of growth rates in the various regions of the brain, Goldman-Rakic (1987) has shown that concurrent spurts of synaptogenesis take place in many regions of the cerebral cortex of rhesus monkeys during the period of rapid behavioral growth in ability to perform delayed-response tasks. In humans, this stage occurs beginning at about 8 months, with rapid developments in understanding of object permanence, and can be correlated with rapid synaptogenesis in the visual cortex (Fischer, 1987; Goldman-Rakic, 1987). In humans, however, the prefrontal cortex, the area of the brain that has been related to delayed-response tasks, has an extensive period of synaptogenic development, peaking at 1 to 2 years and remaining high until about 7 years.

During the second postnatal brain growth stage (2 to 4 years), there are striking developments in sensory function, including binocularity, hearing, and language. Evidence suggests that earlier-occurring defects in these functions can be remedied only during the growth stage. For example, the fact that children with strabismus leading to amblyopia will never have normal binocularity if the strabismus is not corrected during the first 3 years of life is important evidence of a critical period in development (Banks et al., 1975; Hohmann & Creutzfeldt, 1975).

For cognitive function also, Epstein (1979) contended that mental age shows developmental stages that generally agree with those of brain growth. He suggested that the reason for successful enhancement of the cognitive development of children who begin attending the federally funded Head Start programs by age 2 versus those who do not begin until 4 to 6 years was that minimal brain growth occurs during the later period. Physical therapists, of course, have long suggested that treatment of developmental motor dysfunction, such as that found in CP, is more successful when begun during the first year of life, a period in which the cerebellum shows massive growth. As previously noted, however, only a small amount of suggestive evidence to support this conjecture is currently available (Kanda et al., 1984; Scherzer et al., 1976).

In summary, significant principles of motor development include (1) the concept that an apparent cephalocaudal progression results not from genetically directed brain development but rather from a process of coordination of a variety of subsystems in response to the affordances of the environment for action, (2) spiraling development characterized by periods of relative stability and instability and sensitive periods in which development is especially responsive to environmental influences and therapeutic intervention, and (3) self-regulating active construction of developmental progress on the part of the child. Developmental milestones that appear to reflect discontinuous stages may actually reflect underlying continuity of development in subsystems maturing at different rates. The finding of punctuated periods of rapid synaptogenesis in the brain may contradict this view at the cellular level, but these processes probably provide the means by which genetic programs provide a general framework for development of the individual. Each human brain is uniquely inscribed through active creation of functional networks of neuronal groups reinforced by species-typical values shaping selective processes driving development and learning. Most developmentalists would now agree that the individual is formed through interaction among genetically determined processes, individual history, and environmental opportunities at least partially created by the organism itself. Seen in this light, the infant's actions structure the organization and complexity of her or his brain, not the other way around.

"STAGES" OF MOTOR DEVELOPMENT

The next section will elaborate on the observable "stages" of gross and fine motor development that represent milestones of developmental progress toward achieving the goals of upright posture, mobility, and manipulation—essential elements of environmental mastery and control. As infants attain and perfect these major developmental motor skills, they are incorporated into functional ADL such as self-care, feeding, and play. Important milestones of motor development in later years of childhood will also be briefly addressed.

The major gross motor milestones of the first 12 to 18 months include achieving an indefinitely maintained upright head posture, attaining prone-on-elbows position, rolling from supine to prone, independent sitting, attaining hands-and-knees position, moving from sitting to four-point position and prone, creeping on hands and knees, pulling to a stand, standing independently, and walking independently (van Blankenstein et al., 1962). As each position or skill is attained, further development will entail the perfecting of postural control in these positions and the ability to make rapid, effortless transitions from one position to another. These developments are discussed by Bradley in Chapter 2.

Despite the greater complexity of our more recent view of the development of motor behavior, including the idea of underlying continuity of development in multiple systems, it is possible to summarize the perfection of use of various parts of the body in an overall schema of cephalocaudal direction. During the first quarter of the first year of life, infants develop the ability to control their heads in virtually all positions in space, although control will continue to be fine-tuned during successive months. As head control develops, load-bearing surfaces gradually shift caudally (Green et al., 1995). The second quarter reveals major advances in control of the arms and upper trunk, although once again continued refinements occur later. Arm movements are aided by increasing ability to control the destabilizing effects of arm movements on other parts of the body. During the third quarter, initial stages involving mastery of control of the lower trunk and pelvis in the upright position occur, and the final quarter of the first year reveals the development of milestones in mobility and control of the lower parts of the legs in conjunction with upright stance and overall postural control.

Infancy

Functional Head Control

At birth, infants already have the capacity to right the head from either full flexion or full extension when they are supported in an upright position. A stable vertical head position, however, cannot usually be sustained for more than a second or two, if at all. Supine, or with the head supported in a reclining position, head-turning to either side of midline can usually be elicited by attracting the infant's visual orientation to a moving object. At about 2 months, the infant can sustain the head in midline in the frontal plane during supported sitting but often appears to be looking down at his or her feet, so that the eyes are oriented about 30° below the horizontal plane as in Figure 1-1 (Campbell SK, Kolobe TH, Osten E, Girolami G, & Lenke M, unpublished research, 1992). Turning of the unsupported head in the upright position is not usually possible. If the child can be enticed to lift the head to the vertical

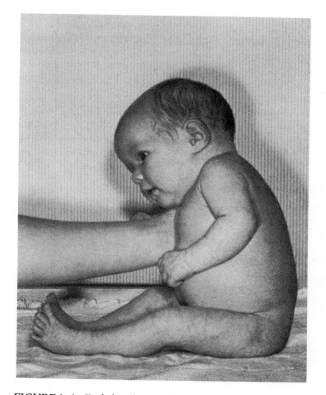

FIGURE 1-1. Early head control in space is characterized by ability to stabilize the head in midline but with eyes angled downward from the vertical. (From van Blankenstein, M, Welbergen, UR, & de Haas, JH. Le développement du nourrisson: Sa première année en 130 photographies. Paris: Presses Universitaires de France, 1962, p. 26.)

position, oscillations are typically seen with inability to maintain a stable upright posture. Finer synergistic control of neck flexor and extensor muscles typically appears in the third month, when the head is indefinitely stable in a vertical position and can be freely turned to follow visual stimulation, although sometimes with brief oscillations and loss of control.

When stabilizing control of the head in the upright position has been attained, the infant can typically organize head and trunk activity so that when placed prone with the arms extended along the sides of the body, the prone-on-elbows position is rapidly assumed by lifting the head and extending the thoracic spine while simultaneously bringing both arms up to rest on the elbows (Fig. 1–2). Given the large weight of the head relative to the rest of the body at this age, a stabilizing postural function of the legs and pelvis must provide a stable base of support for simultaneous neck and trunk extension with arm movement. Green and colleagues (1995) demonstrated that the developmental progression in both supine and prone positions involves a gradual shifting of the load-bearing surfaces in a caudal direction.

Turning the head to either side while prone on the elbows may still be difficult to coordinate at this stage, and lateral head-righting also remains imperfect. Nevertheless, by the end of the third or fourth postnatal month, the head, in conjunction with organized trunk and lower extremity extension, has largely perfected the maintenance of stable positioning in space appropriate for the further development of eye-head-hand control and of independent sitting to come (Fig. 1–3). Bushnell and Boudreau (1993)

believe that a stable head is a prerequisite for initial ability to perceive depth cues from kinetic information (movement of an object relative to its surround or to self), which is present by 3 months of age. Once established by 4 or 5 months of age, binocular vision is used to identify depth cues.

Commensurate with acquisition of functional control of head positioning are important developments in control of the arms. During the second and third months, generalized movements of the arms and body have altered their earlier writhing quality (Cioni & Prechtl, 1990). Small fidgety movements appear throughout the body, the arms and legs may show oscillations during movement, and ballistic swipes and swats with legs or arms appear for the first time (Hadders-Algra & Prechtl, 1992). For example, if the legs are flexed up to the chest and then released while the infant is supine, the legs may extend so that the heels pound the supporting surface, or when excited, the infant may make large arm-swiping movements in the air. As noted earlier, the first evidence of reciprocal activity of muscular antagonists about the shoulder underlies the ability to perform these ballistic movements (Hadders-Algra et al., 1992). Ferrari and colleagues (1990) suggested the importance of these developing qualitative changes in spontaneous movement by demonstrating that they herald the appearance of goal-directed reaching and by indicating that they do not appear in children destined to be diagnosed as having CP. Children with CNS dysfunction tend to move in tight ranges characterized by simultaneity of activity in multiple limbs, referred to as cramped synchrony.

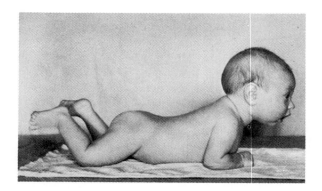

FIGURE 1–2. Early stage of prone-on-elbows posture with stable neck extension, elbows close to trunk, and flexed hips and knees. (From van Blankenstein, M, Welbergen, UR, & de Haas, JH. Le développement du nourrisson: Sa première année en 30 photographies. Paris: Presses Universitaires de France, 1962, p. 25.)

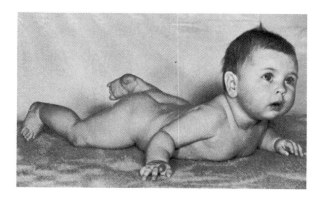

FIGURE 1–3. Advanced stage of prone-on-elbows posture, with free movement of head and arms and extended lower extremities. (From van Blankenstein, M, Welbergen, UR, & de Haas, JH. Le développement du nourrisson: Sa première année en 130 photographies. Paris: Presses Universitaires de France, 1962, p. 34.)

Upright Trunk Control

The initial ability to maintain sitting independently on propped arms when placed is achieved after the infant is able to (1) extend the head and trunk in prone position so as to use the legs and pelvis as the load-bearing surfaces and (2) control the pelvis and lower extremities while using the arms or moving the head in supine position, that is, has developed anticipatory stabilizing responses to counteract internally generated forces caused by movement (Green et al., 1995). Midway through the first year, the average child has achieved the ability to sit alone (Fig. 1–4) and can successfully manipulate an object with one hand while the other hand holds it, although sitting and manipulating at once may still be a challenge. Poking fingers explore crevices and crumbs and herald the fine selective digital control that characterizes the human organism. Strong extension throughout the body in the prone position allows significant freedom of action for the arms and head (Fig. 1–5). Bushnell and Boudreau (1993) be-

lieve that ability to perceive the characteristics of objects through their manipulation now allows the child to use configural cues from objects in depth perception. Despite these developments in arm control, the child in sitting lacks the fine pelvic and lower extremity control needed for moving into and out of the position or for turning the trunk freely on a stable base. Pelvic control functions begin to be developed at this time, however, in rolling from supine to prone position (Fig. 1–6), pivoting while prone, and playing with the legs and feet while supine.

Lower Trunk Control in the Upright Position

During the third quarter of the first year, functional movements free the child from a spot on which she or he is placed by others. Control of lower trunk and pelvis, combined with previously achieved upper body skills, provides new mobility when prone (Fig. 1–7), crawling and creeping (Fig. 1–8), pulling to a stand, moving from supine to four-point and

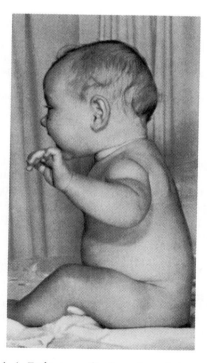

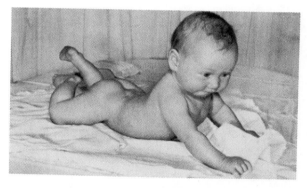

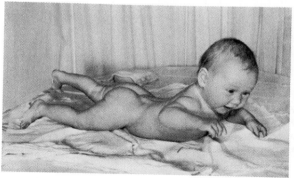

FIGURE 1–4. Early stage of independent sitting, with arms used for balance. (From van Blankenstein, M, Welbergen, UR, & de Haas, JH. Le développement du nourrisson: Sa première année en 130 photographies. Paris: Presses Universitaires de France, 1962, p. 39.)

FIGURE 1–5. In the most advanced stage of the prone posture, arms and legs move freely from a stable trunk. (From van Blankenstein, M, Welbergen, UR, & de Haas, JH. Le développement du nourrisson: Sa première année en 130 photographies. Paris: Presses Universitaires de France, 1962, p. 37.)

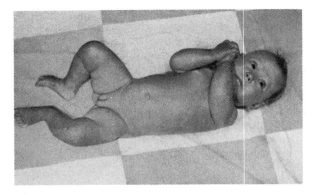

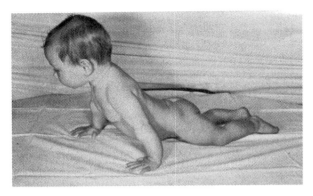

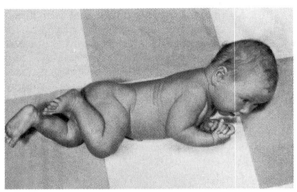

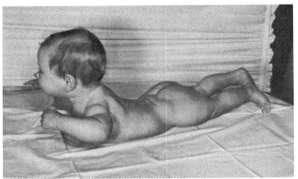

FIGURE 1–7. Dynamic play in prone position includes push-ups on extended arms and "flying" with strong trunk extension and scapular retraction. (From van Blankenstein, M, Welbergen, UR, & de Haas, JH. Le développement du nourrisson: Sa première année en 130 photographies. Paris: Presses Universitaires de France, 1962, p. 47.)

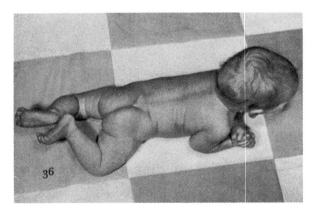

FIGURE 1–6. Rolling from supine to prone with head-righting. (From van Blankenstein, M, Welbergen, UR, & de Haas, JH. Le développement du nourrisson: Sa première année en 130 photographies. Paris: Presses Universitaires de France, 1962, p. 36.)

The presence of oscillations also continues to herald new developments. Rocking on four limbs before launching into creeping and bouncing while standing before beginning to cruise along furniture are examples of self-induced actions that appear to be important precursors of functional skills.

Fine Lower Extremity Control in the Upright Position

Once the child has attained competence at standing and cruising along furniture, the legs and feet move toward perfection of selective control because the trunk and pelvis are increasingly reliable supports that permit freedom of lower extremity activities. In creeping, pelvic swiveling motions give way to reciprocal hip flexion and extension activity, and creeping velocity increases because an arm and a leg on the same side of the body can be placed in simultaneous flight. The child can lower himself or herself

sitting positions, and moving down to hands and knees or prone position from sitting (Fig. 1–9). Inherent in each activity are freedom from a strong midline symmetry that previously characterized postural control and the continued refinement of rotational abilities within the axis of the trunk.

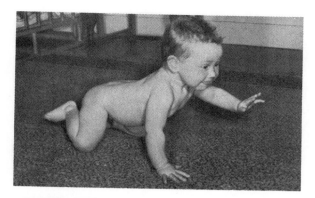

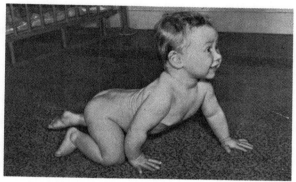

FIGURE 1–8. Creeping on hands and knees. (From van Blankenstein, M, Welbergen, UR, & de Haas, JH. Le développement du nourrisson: Sa première année en 130 photographies. Paris: Presses Universitaires de France, 1962, p. 53.)

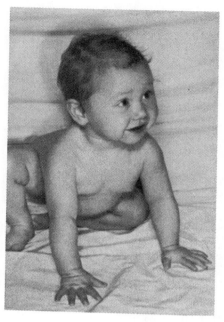

FIGURE 1–9. The infant moves from sitting to the four-point position over one leg. (From van Blankenstein, M, Welbergen, UR, & de Haas, JH. Le développement du nourrisson: Sa première année en 130 photographies. Paris: Presses Universitaires de France, 1962, p. 57.)

from standing (Fig. 1–10); bear-walk with dorsiflexed ankles, flexed hips, and partially extended knees (Fig. 1–11); and finally stand and walk independently at 9 to 15 months of age (Fig. 1–12).

The gradual refinement of gait is described by Stout in Chapter 3. During the first several months of walking experience, creeping is gradually abandoned and heel-strike in gait develops, allowing faster walking with longer strides. Roberton and Halverson (1984) hypothesized the following temporal sequence of development of foot locomotion patterns: walking; running; single leap, jumping down or bounce-jumping, and galloping (in uncertain order, but generally at about 2 to 2.5 years); hopping on dominant foot (seldom before age 3) and then nondominant foot; and skipping and sideways galloping or sliding. Although some children may manage a skip by age 4, many reach an early level of proficiency only by age 7. A rhythmic step-and-hop movement is even more difficult and does not appear until well into the primary school years, when it may be used in many dance forms. Before describing the

further development of gross motor skills in preschoolers, however, the sequence of development of functional hand use in infancy will be described.

Object Manipulation

Development of fine motor function entails two major features: control of the hand as a terminal device for reaching and grasping and object manipulation and release. Postural control for reaching and grasping will be detailed in Chapter 2; an excellent volume devoted to development of all aspects of the capacity to reach, grasp, and release, as well as the functional use of the hands, has been edited by Bard and colleagues (1990). This chapter emphasizes development of the manipulative functions of the hand.

Karniol (1989) has documented the stages of object manipulation in the first year of life. These stages of spontaneous behaviors observed in daily life occur in a hierarchic form that progresses from rotation (angular displacement) to translation (movement parallel to the object itself) to vibration (rapid per-

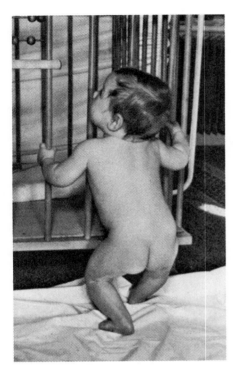

FIGURE 1–10. Lowering from standing to the floor with control. (From van Blankenstein, M, Welbergen, UR, & de Haas, JH. Le développement du nourrisson: Sa première année en 130 photographies. Paris: Presses Universitaires de France, 1962, p. 57.)

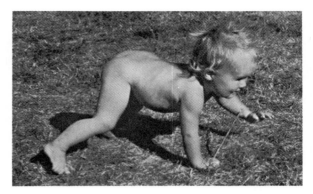

FIGURE 1–11. "Bear-walking" on hands and feet. (From van Blankenstein, M, Welbergen, UR, & de Haas, JH. Le développement du nourrisson: Sa première année en 130 photographies. Paris: Presses Universitaires de France, 1962, p. 54.)

iodic movements of either translation or rotation). Later stages involve combinations of these actions and bimanual activities. The invariant sequence of spontaneous behaviors documented by Karniol (1989) is as follows:

> *Stage 1, rotation of held objects—by 2 months.* With vision, holding objects becomes an intentional act. Objects are first held when they come directly into the infant's reach and are later (by 3 to 4 months) twisted while being held. Karniol (1989) indicated that through this action infants learn that objects can be held and their appearance transformed by rotation.
>
> *Stage 2, translation of grasped objects—by 3 months.* Typical of this stage is reaching for an object while in the prone position and bringing it to the mouth. The object may also be rotated. What the infant learns through these types of action is that he or she can translate objects in order to look at, or mouth, them and that it is not possible to reach objects further distant than the length of the arm.

> *Stage 3, vibration (shaking) of held objects—by 4 months.* In this stage infants learn that they can make interesting noises by rapidly flexing and extending their arms and can make the noise stop by holding still. If the object does not produce a noise, it may be translated or rotated and examined before being dropped, but visual attention is not a dominant part of this activity.
>
> *Stage 4, bilateral hold of two objects—by 4.5 months.* The infant may hold an object in one hand and shake an object held in the other, thereby learning that it is possible to do more than one thing at a time (Fig. 1–13).
>
> *Stage 5, two-handed hold of a single object—by 4.5 months.* First use of bimanual holding is to hold an object, such as a bottle, steady, but it rapidly advances to holding (and often rotating) large objects that require the use of two hands. These actions allow the child to learn that two hands can steady and rotate objects better than can one hand, as well as permit the holding of large objects.
>
> *Stage 6, hand-to-hand transfer of an object—at 4.5 to 6 months.* Transfer is usually followed by repeated actions on the object with the second hand, thereby learning that whatever can be done with the right hand can also be done with the left.
>
> *Stage 7, coordinated action with a single object in which one hand holds the object while the other manipulates or bangs it—at 5 to 6.5 months.* A quintessential example of this type of activity is holding a toy in one hand while picking at it with the other (Fig. 1–14). Displacements of the object caused by handling are followed by rotational read-

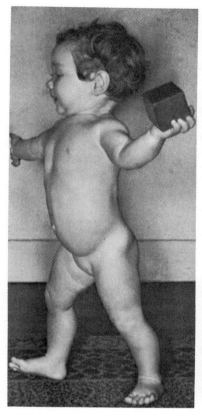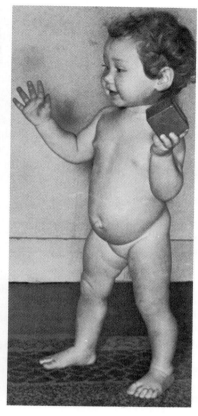

FIGURE 1–12. The infant walks and carries a toy, with wide-based gait and hands in "guard" position. (From van Blankenstein, M, Welbergen, UR, & de Haas, JH. Le développement du nourrisson: Sa première année en 130 photographies. Paris: Presses Universitaires de France, 1962, pp. 64–65.)

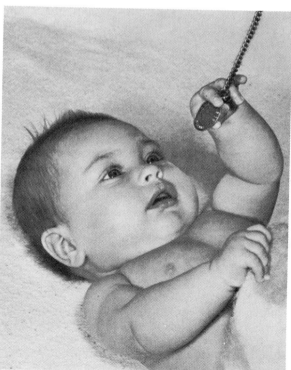

FIGURE 1–13. Bilateral hold of two objects: One hand holds the blanket, the other reaches for a keychain (stage 4 of Karniol, 1989). (From van Blankenstein, M, Welbergen, UR, & de Haas, JH. Le développement du nourrisson: Sa première année en 130 photographies. Paris: Presses Universitaires de France, 1962, p. 91.)

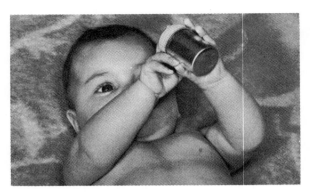

FIGURE 1-14. Coordinated action with a single object: holding a toy with one hand while poking at it with another (stage 7 of Karniol, 1989). (From van Blankenstein, M, Welbergen, UR, & de Haas, JH. Le développement du nourrisson: Sa première année en 130 photographies. Paris: Presses Universitaires de France, 1962, p. 93.)

justments of the hand that holds it. These activities teach the infant that two hands can do more than can one hand alone and that noise can be produced from striking objects that do not respond to vibrating.

Stage 8, coordinated action with two objects, such as striking two blocks together—at 6 to 8.5 months. Through these actions, the infant learns to produce interesting effects by moving one object toward another.

Stage 9, deformation of objects—at 7 to 8.5 months. At this stage, the infant learns that it is possible to alter the way things look or sound by ripping, bending, squeezing, or pulling them apart.

Stage 10, instrumental sequential actions—at 7.5 to 9.5 months. These activities involve the sequential use of two hands for goal-oriented functions, so that the infant learns that coordinated use of the hands leads to desired outcomes. The infant may, for example, open a box with one hand and take out its contents with the other.

The achievement of these stages completes the development of the essentials of manual manipulation. More complex actions follow that are related to the functional characteristics of objects or to imaginary play in which an object can be whatever one pretends it to be (Karniol, 1989). Manual manipulations become automatized, leaving attention to be directed more toward the functional use of objects.

Based on the previously discussed research of Edelman (1992), Thelen (1990), Thelen and colleagues (1993), and Keshner and colleagues (1989), we can hypothesize that, although functional hand use develops in a regular, invariant sequence, it is likely that each infant uses unique coordinative pat-

terns and kinetics to achieve manipulative goals that are circumscribed by individual variations in body structure, experiences, and rate of neural and physical maturation. Because the task characteristics structure the infant's unique response, parents play an important role in providing opportunities that support development.

Karniol (1989) suggested that parents and others who choose toys for infants have two important functions: (1) helping infants to master the abilities of each stage by providing objects that are appropriate for emerging skills and (2) facilitating infants' developing sense of capability to control their world by providing objects that are responsive to current manipulative abilities. Thus, Karniol and others believed that mastery of controlling objects in the environment is influential in development of the infant's general sense of competence and in providing initial sensorimotor knowledge of the permanence of objects and of cause-effect relationships. Karniol reviewed research demonstrating the influence on persistence at tasks and IQ at age 3 of play with objects that provide contingent feedback and are appropriate for the infant's manual manipulative competencies. Similarly, in a search for the correlates of performance of infants in descending slopes that varied in riskiness, Adolph (1997) found that experience in dealing with steps and backing off furniture at home was related to superior ability to negotiate risky slopes.

As each stage is attained, the presentation of any object results in action appropriate to the motor stage, whether or not the object lends itself well to that action. Thus, in stage 3, all objects are considered shakeable whether or not they make noise when shaken. Infants who could crawl plunged recklessly down slopes too steep to negotiate safely in order to get to their mothers at the landing (Adolph, 1997). With more experience crawling and walking, failures on risky slopes frequently led to accidental use of a different pattern (one that an infant already knew from previous activities) that was successful, such as sliding down the slope backwards or in sitting. The alternative mode then became one that children purposely selected for descending slopes they perceived to be risky. These facts are not well explained by developmental theories that suggest that children perceive the affordances of the environment and act on them (Fetters, 1991a, 1991b; Pick, 1992; Thelen, 1990), but this type of function was recognized by Piaget (Flavell, 1963) and included in his principle of assimilation. This principle states that when cognitive structures develop a particular schema, it is applied indiscriminately to objects in the environment, assimilating them to the existing cognitive structure. Piaget also posited that repeated experiences with attempted assimilations of inappropriate objects results in gradual accommodation to their properties and the appearance of both new behaviors and new cognitive structures.

On the other hand, a selectionist theory of motor development suggests that children must use on-line decision making to choose the appropriate motor synergy for use in a given situation (Adolph, 1997). Case-Smith and colleagues (1998) have shown that the characteristics of objects, such as differences in size and presence of moveable parts, lead to immediate use of distinct actions when grasping that are appropriate to the object's characteristics. For example, a given infant might display more mature patterns of grasp when handling a toy with moveable parts than when handling a pellet, so even infants do seem to have some capability to recognize the affordances for manipulation offered by different objects despite having preferred modes of operating on items in the environment. A surprising finding of Adolph's research on slope descent was that infants who had, week after week, practiced crawling down slopes that ranged from easy to hard, nevertheless did not transfer their experience with deciding which slopes were too risky to attempt to making the decision whether or not to traverse a risky slope once they learned to walk. Experienced crawlers, when faced as new walkers with slopes they had done over and over again for weeks on hands and knees, heedlessly plunged down slopes that were too risky for their immature walking skills. These infants did no better than control group subjects with no previous experience with slope descent. Only with more experience walking did infants become more cautious and choose to use an alternative mode of locomotion for difficult slopes. Because infants did make judgments indicating that they found some slopes too risky to attempt, Adolph surmised that children (1) used vision first to decide whether a slope was negotiable with just a quick glance, (2) then decided either to go or to take a longer look, and (3) then decided either to go or to use haptic exploration of the surface with actions such as a hand or foot pat, followed by (4) going using preferred current mode of locomotion (crawling or walking). With more experience, they became able to select an alternative, safer mode, such as sliding down backwards.

Because Adolph (1997) did not find that previous extensive experience with slopes of varying riskiness was useful when the means of preferred locomotion changed from crawling to walking, she believes that a selectionist view of what infants learn from experience with everyday problem-solving challenges is appropriate to describe what children have learned from the slope experiments. Each new presentation of a slope presented a choice: to go with the currently preferred mode of locomotion, to choose an alternative (presumably safer) mode of locomotion, or to avoid the situation, using a detour attempt or simply sitting down and waiting for the caretaker to come to the rescue. Notably, the latter was seldom selected with slopes that were moderately risky; it seemed that infants were goal oriented rather than safety oriented. Their choice was made based on first, visual information, and then if still uncertain, tactile and proprioceptive information. The choice was usually their preferred mode of locomotion until they had many weeks of experience and had, usually accidentally, discovered an already familiar motor strategy that appeared to be safer or more successful. As they gained experience crawling or walking, their choice was made more and more quickly; after many weeks of practice, a short glance was enough for making a decision. Near their ability boundary (slopes that generated less than predictable success in descending without falling), they appeared to have less than adequate knowledge of their own motor capabilities and instead made the decision based on desire to achieve the goal of returning to their caregiver and a quick judgment of whether or not to go based on visual or haptic information. Failure (i.e., falling) did not predict whether infants would choose to go on a subsequent trial, so they appeared to learn little between trials based on successful or unsuccessful outcomes. Adolph concludes that infants have extensive capability to use sensory inputs to make decisions about choice of motor actions although they are not always right about their motor capabilities for solving the problem at hand. They choose to act rather than avoid a challenging situation, do not engage in trial-and-error learning, but rather continue to rely on their visual-haptic analysis of whether or not to engage in risky behavior. When useful motor synergies happened serendipitously, however, they seemed to recognize the adaptability of such patterns and used them on subsequent trials as alternatives to generally preferred modes of locomotion that were riskier to use in a given situation. Goldfield (1997) summarizes Adolph's (1997) findings by indicating that "inexperienced infants tend to be drawn inexorably toward the goal, rather than stopping at a choice point, and apparently do not notice the available affordances.... Conversely, the experienced infant who has explored the available affordances may be overly conservative because the affordance information about slopes is inherently inhibitory; that is, it specifies ways for slowing, stopping, and changing direction" (p. 157). Thus it seems that infants generate information visually, use their preferred mode of locomotion if the choice is to go, and then over time learn, accidentally or through a general wealth of experience with variable-level surfaces, to select from a variety of possible choices the most efficacious method of traversing risky terrain. One must conclude that adaptive locomotion (i.e., selecting the most appropriate method for the task at hand) requires exploratory movements to obtain information and a repertoire of available movement synergies from which to select (Adolph, 1997). This research once again emphasizes that advances in motor behavior depend on having a variety of movement patterns from which to choose when faced with challenging new opportunities for action. As a result, children with disabilities, who generally have a limited vocabulary of movement synergies, are constrained in their motor development by a lack of experience with a variety of movement patterns and may also have limited perceptual capabilities for making on-line judgments about the likelihood of successfully accomplishing a motor task even when they have an intense interest in the goal.

The Preschool and Early School Years

Functional Motor Skills in Preschoolers

We return now to a description of the functional skills of preschool children, combining information on both gross and fine motor function in practical use. Toddlers operate with different anthropometric characteristics than infants. Toddlers gain about 5 pounds in weight and 2.5 inches in height each year, the latter resulting mostly from growth of the lower extremities (Colson & Dworkin, 1997). Fifty percent of adult height is reached between the ages of 2 to 2.5 years. In the second year, children walk well (although steps are still short and constrained) and enjoy the sheer pleasure of movement through running, climbing up and down stairs independently, and jumping off the bottom step (Ames et al., 1979). The 2-year-old child can kick a ball and steer a push-toy, and by 2.5 years the child can walk on tiptoes, jump with both feet, stand on one foot, and throw and catch a ball using arms and body together. Galloping may appear, but only leading with the preferred foot (Roberton & Halverson, 1984). The more practical pleasures of dressing independently (pulling on a simple garment at 2 years and pulling off pants and socks by 2.5 years) and eating with a spoon with little spilling also develop (Ames et al., 1979). Food preferences can become a touchy subject by around 2.5 years; nevertheless, the toddler is gradually developing impulse control (Colson & Dworkin, 1997).

The 3-year-old child can alternate feet easily when ascending stairs, can control speed of movement well, and takes pleasure in riding a tricycle (Ames et al., 1979). Hopping may emerge, although it is often a momentary, single hop on the preferred foot (Roberton & Halverson, 1984). Surprisingly, however, by 3.5 years, the child may seem less secure and physically coordinated, stumbling frequently and showing a fear of falling (Ames et al., 1979). Hands may show excessive dysmetria during block stacking. Nevertheless, typical 3-year-olds feed themselves well and can hold a glass with only one hand. At 3.5 years, mealtime may again become trying because the food must be put on the plate in a certain way and the sandwich has to be cut just so. The same may be true of the dressing process, with special objection being expressed against clothing that goes over the head. The typical 3-year-old can put on pants, socks, and shoes, but buttoning may be difficult. Nearly all 3-year-olds are consistently dry during the daytime, and bowel training is well established as the physical skills and the emotional willingness to participate in toilet training come together (Colson & Dworkin, 1997). The ability to delay gratification is developing, and toddlers strive for autonomy while continuing to intermittently seek reassurance from caregivers to whom they are securely attached.

Despite these generalizations, preschoolers exhibit a variety of individual behavioral styles (Colson & Dworkin, 1997). About 10% of children are considered "difficult" because of increased levels of activity, emotional negativity, and low adaptability. Another 15% of children are described as "slow to warm up" because they take a long time to adapt to new situations.

Typical 4-year-olds have been described by Ames and colleagues (1979) as characteristically out-of-bounds in their exuberance. Behavior in all spheres is frequently wild, and self-confidence and bragging seem endless. The 4-year-old can walk downstairs with one foot per step, catch with hands only, and learn to use roller skates or a small bicycle. (But remember McGraw's experiments demonstrating that learning these skills is possible much earlier.) Athletic activities are particularly enjoyed, especially running, jumping, and climbing. Four-year-olds can button large buttons and lace shoelaces, feed themselves independently except for cutting, and talk and eat at the same time. Most can take responsibility for washing hands and face and brushing teeth as well as dressing and undressing without help except for tying their shoes or differentiating front from back of some garments.

Five-year-olds tend to be more conforming than the exuberant 4-year-old (Ames et al., 1979). During the fifth year the child can skip, long jump about 2 feet, climb with sureness, jump rope, and do acrobatic tricks. Children begin to learn to dodge well at 5 years (Roberton & Halverson, 1984). Handedness is well established, and overhand throwing is accomplished (Ames et al., 1979). (Current research suggests that hand preference is already stable by 12 to 13 months in most children [Fagard, 1990].) The 5-year-old likes to help with household tasks, play with blocks, and build houses. Eating is independent, including using a knife except for cutting meat, although dawdling and wriggling in the chair may be trying to parents. The challenge of dressing oneself is past, so children age 5 may ask for more help than they need (usually only for tying shoes or buttoning difficult buttons), and overall, undressing is generally easier than dressing.

At age 6, children are constantly on the go, "lugging, tugging, digging, dancing, climbing, pushing, pulling" (Ames et al., 1979, p. 49). Six-year-olds seem to be consciously practicing body balance in climbing, crawling over and under things, and dancing about the room. They swing too high, build too tall, and try activities exceeding their ability. Indoors, awkwardness may cause accidents, and the child seems less coordinated than during the fifth year. Despite excellent eating skills, falling out of the chair or knocking over full glasses is not uncommon.

Steps in Motor Skill Development

In the various motor skills developed in the preschool and elementary school years, each body segment has its own developmental trajectory within the overall coordinative structure; one part can be at a different level of skill than another, although all parts tend to be at a primitive level early or at an advanced level when skills are well learned (Roberton & Halverson, 1984). Furthermore, when demands of the task change (increased height, distance, or accuracy requirements), or when fatigue sets in, one body component may regress in its action while another continues to perform at an advanced level of skill. Thus, task requirements are once again seen to be influential in determining the characteristics of motor responses. For hopping and other skills, such as catching, throwing, and jumping, Roberton and Halverson (1984) provided detailed analyses and photographs of the intratask developmental steps for each critical body component, instruction in how to make detailed observations to categorize the level of skill of body segments, and advice for guiding the learning of these childhood skills.

Physical therapists would find this information useful in planning intervention for children with mild physical disabilities or clumsiness. For example, as children learn to throw, the trunk goes through similar stages of development as those found in early developmental motor activities. The trunk is initially passive, then increasingly a stabilizer for the function of the extremities, and finally a participant in

actively imparting force to the flight of the ball. Jumping changes from a functional activity characterized best as falling and catching to one of projection, flight, and landing, each with components that add force and speed or shock absorption to lend elegance and style to the activity.

Although many tests of motor development include assessment of hopping skills, most therapists probably would not view this as a particularly functional activity because children seldom hop spontaneously (Roberton & Halverson, 1984). Physical educators, however, believe that hopping is an important developmental skill because a hop is often required in situations such as controlling momentum during sudden stops and in handling unexpected perturbations to balance, as well as for pleasurable play activities such as skipping. Hopping is also an excellent activity for describing the development of various strategies leading, finally, to skillful action.

Skillful hopping requires projected flight off the supporting leg and a pumping action of the swinging leg that assists in force production. Initial prehop attempts involve extension of the supporting leg as the child tries to lift off with the nonsupporting leg raised high. The first successful strategy, however, is usually a quick hip-and-knee flexion that pulls the supporting leg off the floor and into momentary flight (actually falling off balance and flexing the leg) while the swing leg remains inactive. At the next level of skill, the supporting leg again extends but with limited range and early timing relative to the point of takeoff. In skillful hopping, the swinging leg leads the takeoff, and extension of the supporting leg occurs late; thus the action becomes one of "land, ride, and extend" (Roberton & Halverson, 1984, p. 62). Just as with infants learning to descend risky slopes (Adolph, 1997), children learn through practice how to control their intrinsic dynamics to produce efficient movements that accomplish intended goals.

Sports and playground games become increasingly important parts of children's motor activities when they enter school and when complex feats of coordination become possible. Children have, however, individual rates of development of the components of motor skill, some undoubtedly innate, some based on cultural characteristics and family interest in development of physical skills. McGraw's (1935) work demonstrates, for example, that toddlers can develop motor skills that are usually considered inappropriate, primarily because of safety issues. Furthermore, research has generally supported the belief that African-American children have superior motor skills, especially those involving speed and agility, relative to white children (Cintas, 1988; Lee, 1980; Plimpton & Regimbal, 1992). Although most authors have explained these differences on the basis of socioeconomic status and differences in permissiveness of child rearing (Williams & Scott, 1953), we found differences among ethnic groups that approached statistical significance on test scores of the Test of Infant Motor Performance (TIMP) in infants younger than 3.5 months (Campbell et al., 1995). Both African-American and Latino infants scored slightly better on the TIMP than did white infants.

Interactions between Perceptual-Cognitive Development and Motor Development

The work of Bertenthal and Campos (1987) is significant in demonstrating that experience, not maturation alone, drives perceptual-cognitive development and that self-induced movement is critical in evoking advancements in a number of important cognitive processes. Through ingenious studies that varied locomotor experience levels by studying natural differences, such as length of time infants had been creeping, and unusual childhood events, such as being confined to a cast for a long period or being given a walker to induce locomotion before it occurred independently, Bertenthal and Campos have shown that self-induced locomotion is a critical ingredient in the development of depth perception that mediates avoidance of heights when a child is placed on a visual cliff. This behavior normally develops between 7 and 9 months of age but is related more to degree of locomotor experience than to age at locomotion. Bertenthal and Campos also reviewed other evidence that self-produced locomotion promotes developmental progress in functions such as memory for locations and ability to localize objects objectively with reference to external landmarks rather than egocentrically. Children who did not creep have also been demonstrated to be cognitively delayed when compared with children with creeping experience (McEwan et al., 1991). Adolph (1997) found that only 2 of 24 infants in her study of slope descent were able to transfer what they had learned from crawling on slopes to the choice of whether to traverse risky slopes as new walkers. Those infants were younger and smaller at crawling onset but older and more maturely proportioned at walking onset than infants who did not show transfer of learning from crawling on slopes to the decision regarding traversal by walking. These infants therefore had more experience with crawling than other infants. Infants who spent a long time as belly-crawlers also were able to descend steeper slopes than other infants. Two infants in the study who were consistently reckless (i.e., traversed hopelessly risky slopes despite repeated experiences of falling) were infants who spent little time as crawlers and walked very early.

These findings call into question the previous assumption that varying patterns of development of locomotion are merely that, variations without developmental significance for learning and future motor performance.

In general, therapists must take into account in treatment planning not only the precocity of an infant's abilities to perceive the basic affordances of the environment in terms of action possibilities but also the long period of development of motor skills and spatial-cognitive and other perceptual functions for fine-tuning choices regarding how to act on objects. For example, infants can adapt their reaching to the actual distance of an object at 3.5 to 5.5 months (Vinter, 1990). Depth perception is based on kinetic information at 3 months, binocular information at 5 months, and pictorial information at 7 to 9 months. Children preform the hand for the anticipated shape of an object at about 9 to 10 months and can adapt for anticipated weight by 14 to 16 months (Corbetta & Mounoud, 1990). Children under the approximate age of 6 are not able to conserve the amount of a substance when the shape of its container is altered (Beilin, 1989). By 7 or 8 years of age, however, they recognize that pouring water from a wide container to one that is narrower has not increased the amount of water (Roberton & Halverson, 1984). Weight, however, is not conserved until 9 or 10 years, and volume not until 11 or 12. As mentioned earlier, Bushnell and Boudreau (1993) propose that motor development is a rate-limiting factor in many of these perceptual-cognitive skills because movements make available information needed for the acquisition of related perceptual abilities. Although they believe that self-generated movements are the typical means for acquiring these abilities, they think that assistance with the necessary movements may also help infants to learn, an obvious area for research on intervention with children with disabilities.

Gibson used the term *differentiation* to describe the improvements that occur in perception over the course of development (Pick, 1992). According to Pick, Gibson stated that "progressive differentiation occurs with respect to information specifying the meaningful properties of the world" (Pick, 1992, p. 789). Gibson believed that perception involves an active effort to make sense of the world, but the action is exploratory, not executive in the sense of using physical manipulation. Perception improves because we detect more of the aspects, features, and nuances that convey the meaning of objects and events, such as how risky it might be to descend a steep slope. It seems likely that the alternations in apparent self-confidence, coordination, and other characteristics of children reported by Ames and colleagues (1979) and Adolph (1997) are related to their best attempts to make sense of the world as physical characteristics and control over intrinsic dynamics of the body, neural maturation, perceptual abilities, and other developmental subsystems change with growth and experience.

Although the importance of motor experience in the longitudinal development of many of the perceptual functions described earlier has not, to my knowledge, been explored by researchers aside from Adolph's inquiry regarding decisions about traversible slopes (1997), the finding that self-directed activity is influential in some spatial-cognitive functions suggests the need to pay attention to providing compensations for functional limitations that may hinder children's development when physical disabilities are present. Bertenthal and Campos (1987), for example, have shown that use of a walker before endogenously produced locomotion was present positively affected performance on the visual cliff problem. Thus, maneuvering under self-control appears to be more important than does locomotor movement per se. Perhaps therapists should reconsider prohibitions regarding the use of walkers for children with developmental disabilities if safety during usage can be assured.

Bushnell and Boudreau (1993) propose that if infants are unable to engage in motor activities necessary to the acquisition or practice of specific perceptual or cognitive skills, the motor problem may block mental development. An example is that lack of self-generated mobility may lead to failure to begin to code spatial location based on environmental landmarks rather than in relation to self. In their review of the development of haptic perception (ability to acquire information about objects with the hands and to discriminate and recognize objects from handling them as opposed to looking at them), Bushnell and Boudreau (1993) noticed a developmental timetable suggesting that infants under 7 months of age can already distinguish objects by characteristics such as temperature and hardness, that from 6 months on they can distinguish textures, and that ability to perceive weight emerges at about 9 months of age. Finally, distinguishing objects by configurational shape emerges sometime after 12 to 15 months. These authors believe that this timetable is explained by constraints placed on infants by their motor development, specifically the exploratory procedures or hand movements they are capable of making at various ages. Rubbing with the fingers, for example, is typically used to assess the texture of an object, and repeatedly lifting and lowering an object is used to gauge weight. Until an infant can use the property most appropriate for gaining knowledge about an object's multiple characteristics, such perceptual knowledge cannot be gained or used. Tem-

perature and hardness can be appraised by static contact or pressure, thus these properties of objects would logically be among the first to be recognized by an infant. In Adolph's (1997) study of slope behavior, it may be that infants used their vision and patting abilities only to decide that a risky slope provided a stable continuous path toward a landing below but were unable to consider whether their physical capabilities included sufficient balance to control gravitational and inertial forces that would result from their attempts to descend until they had sufficient experience with a variety of other movement patterns to help them learn about controlling intrinsic dynamics.

Gross Motor Activity in a Functional Context: Play

Research on childrens' activity memory, or ability to explicitly recall activities they observe or create, is helpful in considering how to structure therapeutic exercise to promote memory regarding what has been experienced. Ratner and Foley (1994) reviewed the literature on activity memory and suggest that children remember activities better if (1) there was a clear outcome of the activity, (2) actions within the activity were logically sequenced such that cause and effect were obvious throughout the activity, and (3) the child engaged in planning of the actions involved in the activity in advance of carrying it out (not just mental imaging of it) or were asked to plan to remember what happened. Young children do not always profit from external memory cues, at least not until 3 years of age or older, depending on the type of cue. Nevertheless, childrens' behaviors show that they both consciously and verbally anticipate the unfolding and outcomes of activities by at least 2 years of age, even telling themselves "no, no" when about to perform some forbidden action (Ratner & Foley, 1994). At this point, imaginary play with objects that are not present appears, and children express surprise when outcomes of actions are not what they expected. Play then provides the opportunity for children to voluntarily act out intentions and to learn the difference between plans and outcomes. By 20 months of age, children are able to work toward a concrete goal, such as building a house from blocks, exhibit checking behaviors, correct mistakes, and acknowledge successful achievement of the goal. Repetition of an activity typically enhances memory of it when recall support is provided, and even infants 4 to 6 months of age can be shown to have some retrospective processing of events in that experiments demonstrate that they actively notice properties of an activity that were previously not noticed. Preschoolers allowed to demonstrate what happened will recall far more of an activity than if only verbal recall is elicited. Therapists should consider the mental ages of the children they treat with a mind toward creating therapeutic activities that provide children with disabilities the opportunity to develop cognitive skills such as planning and activity memory as they engage in exercise to reduce impairments.

When seen in its functional context as a learning device, motor activity can also be seen to have a stagelike character. Physical activity play (i.e., play with a vigorous physical component) has three developmental stages (Pellegrini & Smith, 1998). In infancy, babies engage in what Thelen (1995) has called rhythmic stereotypies or repetitive gross motor activities without any obvious purpose, including body rocking, foot kicking, and leg waving. Whole-body, self-motion play is also called peragration, and Adolph (1997) suggests that such activities are the most direct route to knowledge—infants plunge in and obtain important information as a result. These behaviors peak around the midpoint of the first year of life with as much as 40% of a 1-hour observation at 6 months being composed of such play (Pellegrini & Smith, 1998).

A second stage called *exercise play* begins at the end of the first year (Pellegrini & Smith, 1998). Such play can be solitary or with others, increases from the toddler to the preschool periods, and then declines during the primary school years. It accounts for about 7% of behavior observed in child care settings. Activities included in exercise play include running, chasing, and climbing. Children with physical disabilities may need alternatives for participating in such play, particularly with other children.

The third phase of physical activity play is rough-and-tumble play such as wrestling, kicking, and tumbling in a social context. Often this type of play appears first in interaction with a parent, typically a father. Rough-and-tumble play increases through the preschool and primary school years and peaks just before early adolescence. No gender differences are noted in peragration activities, but males engage in more exercise play and rough-and-tumble play than females.

The functional benefits of physical activity play may be deferred or immediate. Pellegrini and Smith (1998) suggest that the benefits of rhythmic play in infants is immediate in improving control of specific motor patterns, that is, the primary repertoire in Edelman's terms. Through active self-generated body movement, infants create perturbations to balance for which they gradually learn to accommodate or plan; such play also provides interesting visual and perhaps auditory spectacles for development of perceptual systems. Strength and endurance are also developed through such activities. Pellegrini and Smith (1998) posit that the function of exercise play is specifically to promote muscle differentiation, strength, and endurance. Chapter 5 provides further information on health-related physical fitness, which may have its roots in early play behavior. Pellegrini and Smith (1998) describe animal research on the juvenile period suggesting that it is a sensitive period for such development (recall McGraw's experiment with Johnny and Jimmy and their respective adult physiques). Play may also have cognitive benefits in terms of providing a break from attention-demanding activities, thus leading to distributed practice and creating an enhanced arousal level of benefit to subsequent engagement in mental activities. Seen in this light, recess becomes something more than a meaningless break in the routine.

Pellegrini & Smith (1998) hypothesize that rough-and-tumble play serves a social function, especially for boys, related to establishing and maintaining dominance in social groups (girls are believed to use verbal skills more than boys in establishing dominance hierarchies). As a by-product, children also may use rough-and-tumble play as a way to code and decode social signals. For example, in early rough-and-tumble play with parents, children learn that this is "play" and not aggression. Rosenbaum (1998) suggests that this view of motor activity raises the question of what goals we should pursue in therapeutic interventions. Is it more important to provide opportunities to "travel" than to concentrate on improving gait? Do children with disabilities benefit from adapted recreational activities such as horseback riding in terms of social skills and cognitive function, as well as in motor skills per se? What is lost in terms of self-esteem or ability to decode social signals in children with disabilities if they are "protected" from rough-and-tumble play?

Using Developmental Sequences as a Therapeutic Framework

Most of our contemporary clinical approaches to developing intervention plans for children with disabilities were originally based on use of the developmental sequence as the primary framework for planning intervention. New theoretic models for understanding the achievement of functional motor skills suggest that this framework, as a rigid structure for approaching intervention, is inadequate. Atwater (1991), for example, suggested that a number of issues must be considered when deciding whether to follow a normal developmental sequence in planning treatment. These issues include the knowledge that (1) multiple underlying processes involving both distal and proximal function develop contemporaneously; (2) motor milestones and their components develop in overlapping sequences, with spurts and regressions being common; (3) many variations in the development of motor milestones occur in perfectly normal children, and thus motor milestones cannot be considered to be an invariant sequence leading to skill; (4) development in multiple domains must be considered; (5) the age of the child and the extent and type of disability are important considerations in determining which skills will be most functional for a child at any given time; and (6) child and family involvement in decisions regarding the goals of therapy must be considered. The discussion earlier in the chapter regarding contemporary theories of development and neural plasticity provides additional information in support of Atwater's suggestion (1991). She aptly quotes Bobath and Bobath (1984) in stating that

> treatment should not attempt to follow the sequence of development . . . regardless of the age and physical condition of the individual child. Rather, it should be decided what each child needs most urgently at any one stage or age, and what is absolutely necessary for him to participate for future functional skills, or for improving the skills he has but performs abnormally (Atwater, 1991, p. 91).

I would add the suggestion that an emphasis on processes underlying developmental progress, such as the role of self-induced exploratory movement in both motor learning and cognitive development, and the motivation on the part of children to engage in repetitive, apparently goal-less, practice of activities during sensitive periods of development, should be considered in treatment planning. Further information on sensitive periods of development for basic motor functions will be needed to target times appropriately for most effective intervention, especially for children with disabilities.

Also of great importance is identification of the most effective strategies for promoting the attainment of functional goals involving motor activity. Based on research on facilitation of cognitive development in disadvantaged children, early learning environments, and basic learning strategies, Ramey and Ramey (1992) have identified the following essential daily ingredients to promote intellectual development in children: (1) encouragement of exploration; (2) mentoring in basic skills such as labeling, sequencing, and noting means-ends relations; (3) celebration of developmental advances; (4) guided rehearsal and extension of new skills; (5) protection from inappropriate disapproval, teasing, or punishment; and (6) provision of a rich and responsive language environment. Many of these ingredients are likely to be equally important in promoting motor development in children with physically challenging conditions; research on the design of specific teaching and learning strategies for such children is direly needed. Chapter 6 reviews what is known.

Atwater (1991) recommended that treatment planning should focus on encouragement of functional independence to prevent cognitive retardation and learned helplessness that will be highly disabling in adolescence and adulthood, even when this means giving up goals for improving movement quality. Fetters (1991c) and Harris (1990) agree, suggesting that ecologically valid treatment programs have as their goals the movements that are necessary and useful to humans as they move about in their environment. Fetters (1991c), however, emphasized that there may be trade-offs inherent in working for function of which therapists should be cognizant. Independence in ambulation may be accomplished only with high physiologic cost; the achievement of faster reaching may result in poorer trunk control.

Although I agree wholeheartedly with the recommendations and observations of these three thoughtful scientific practitioners, I have also argued that therapists must choose wisely when making decisions regarding use of compensatory patterns or assistive devices to facilitate functioning of children with CNS dysfunction. Wise decision making involves giving due consideration to whether use of compensatory patterns may lead to later secondary impairments of a musculoskeletal nature that could also be severely disabling in the future (Campbell, 1991). It is not acceptable to include in a treatment plan a goal for functional movement that does not also meet a requirement that working toward such an objective will not be likely to contribute to potential future deformity, skin breakdown, osteoporosis, or other preventable secondary impairment (Campbell, 1997). A focus on health promotion and disease prevention, in addition to a focus on functional improvement for current and future needs, is required. Research presented here on the processes of motor development also suggests that children (1) should have the opportunity to make decisions about choosing how to act (rather than being assisted or guided) when a task is presented so that they can exercise their perceptual capabilities, (2) need to engage in exploration through movement in order to develop their appreciation for the affordances of objects and the environment and for whether they possess the motor skill for successful action, and (3) benefit from having a variety of movement synergies available from which to select the most appropriate adaptive strategy in an on-line process of making decisions about how to achieve immediate task goals.

To accomplish these objectives and provide children with a variety of movement strategies with which they can approach the world of infinite possibilities for meaningful activity, we need both our extensive knowledge of biomechanics and more information on the natural history of conditions we treat. Indeed, I believe that the combination of attention to assisting persons with disabilities to improve their functional capabilities through promoting achievement of useful, meaningful activities performed as efficiently as possible, along with prevention of musculoskeletal and other complications, constitutes the unique features of physical therapy. In Chapter 7 and throughout this book, we therefore recommend that therapists use a framework for describing the disabling process developed by the National Center for Medical Rehabilitation Research that approaches disability from the perspective of the multiple, interacting dimensions of the human organism, from the cellular to the societal (National Advisory Board on Medical Rehabilitation Research, 1993).

Such a comprehensive approach to clinical decision making requires the use of appropriate assessments on which to base treatment planning and outcome evaluation. Tests of motor development and functional skills that meet appropriate psychometric standards and are useful in clinical settings are discussed in the next section.

TESTS OF MOTOR DEVELOPMENT AND FUNCTIONAL PERFORMANCE

Physical therapists use motor milestone and functional performance tests to document children's developmental level in relation to age norms and to observe the functional limitations that may be present. Tests of specific functional skills, such as dressing and feeding, are also used to assess current levels of functioning and to document developmental progress and achievement of expected treatment outcomes. Constraints causing functional limitations can be assessed with various tests of impairment. Those related to postural control and musculoskeletal impairment are described in Chapters 2 and 4. In conjunction with family interviews and sometimes home observations, therapists can examine competencies in fulfilling age-appropriate roles and identify areas of disability that should be addressed with a therapeutic program in consultation with other professionals and the family.

Although all tests to be described in this chapter are standardized scales with acceptable psychometric properties according to the American Physical Therapy Association's Standards for Tests and Measurements in Physical Therapy (Task Force on Standards

for Measurement in Physical Therapy, 1991), some tests remain under development, so complete information is not available. Those selected for brief discussion include the TIMP, Alberta Infant Motor Scale, Harris Infant Neuromotor Test, Miller First Step, Bayley Infant Neurodevelopmental Screener, Bayley II, Peabody Developmental Motor Scales, Toddler and Infant Motor Evaluation, Bruininks-Oseretsky Test of Motor Proficiency, Gross Motor Function Measure, Pediatric Evaluation of Disability Inventory, and Functional Independence Measure for Children. Tests selected for discussion were limited by space, and commonly used tests such as the Denver II (Frankenburg et al., 1990, 1992) and the Gesell Revised Developmental Schedules (Knobloch et al., 1980) are not included because of poor specificity (43%) with high overreferral rates (Glascoe et al., 1992) and out-of-date norms, respectively. The reader may consult Palisano (1993) or Stengel (1991) for more information on these and other tests. Finally, the Pediatric Clinical Test of Sensory Interaction for Balance is briefly described as an example of a test of children's capability to use perception to control movement responses.

Although the tests described are at various stages of development, none is a test of disability in daily life in which observations take place in an ecologically valid setting. Those that purport to assess disability do so through report of a knowledgeable informant, such as the parent, guardian, or teacher. Some tests assess spontaneously generated or self-chosen movements; others specify the tasks a child is to perform in a particular way. Some are more useful for individual treatment planning, others for comparing global performance to age norms for diagnostic and classification purposes or for programmatic assessment of overall rehabilitation outcomes. Use of a combination of the tests would provide comprehensive assessment of functional skills in children with physical disabilities, although improved tests and well-thought-out, comprehensive protocols are still needed (Campbell, 1989, 1996; Fetters, 1991c; Haley et al., 1993; Long & Tieman, 1998).

Screening Tests

The Alberta Infant Motor Scale (AIMS) is an observational scale for assessing gross motor milestones in infants from birth through the stage of independent walking (Piper & Darrah, 1994; Piper et al., 1992). Function in this test is defined as spontaneously engendered motor behaviors performed with a specified level of postural control. The test's 58 items are scored dichotomously based on descriptors that specify demonstration of weight bearing, posture, and antigravity movement in prone, supine, sitting, and standing positions. The test was normed on 2202 infants in the Canadian province of Alberta, and the discriminative validity for identifying abnormal infants as abnormal was 89%. Predictive validity of assessments at 4 and 8 months for identifying delayed motor development at 18 months revealed sensitivity and specificity of 77% and 82%, respectively, using scores below the 10th percentile at 4 months, and 86% and 93%, respectively, at 8 months for scores below the 5th percentile (Darrah et al., 1998). In an assessment of the effect of anthropometric characteristics on motor development, Bartlett (1998) found that typically developing infants with larger heads had lower AIMS scores at 6 weeks than those with smaller head circumference, but there were no effects on later motor development. The test takes 10 to 20 minutes to administer and is noninvasive because only observation is involved.

The Harris Infant Neuromotor Test (HINT) (Harris & Daniels, 1996) is a 22-item screening test to identify developmental delay in infants from 3 to 12 months of age. The test includes items to assess neuromotor milestones, active and passive muscle tone, head circumference, stereotypic movement patterns, behavioral interactions, and the caregiver's assessment of the infant's development. Rather than reflecting a specific developmental theme, items were selected specifically because of research evidence suggesting sensitivity to delayed development. In a study of 54 high-risk infants (Harris & Daniels, 1999, under review), concurrent validity with the Bayley II motor scale in the first year of life was −0.89 (high scores on the HINT indicate poorer performance, accounting for the negative correlation). The predictive validity of the HINT in the first year to Bayley II motor scale scores at 17 to 22 months was −0.49, accounting for 24% of the variance in Bayley II scores. The test has not been normed, and a classification analysis for diagnostic purposes (sensitivity and specificity) has not been reported. The test takes less than 30 minutes to administer and score.

The Miller First Step Screening Test for Evaluating Preschoolers (Miller, 1992) is a screening test to identify children at risk for developmental delays. The test is appropriate for assessing cognitive, communicative, physical, social-emotional, and adaptive function in children from 2 years 9 months to 6 years 2 months of age. Function is defined as performance on games using toys that are entertaining and exciting for children in this age group. The test was normed on a U.S. sample of 100 boys and 100 girls in each 6-month age grouping. It takes 17 minutes to administer and score performance on the 18 games.

The Bayley Infant Neurodevelopmental Screener (BINS) (Aylward, 1992) was originally published as the Early Neuropsychologic Optimality Rating Scales (ENORS) and actually has no direct relationship to the Bayley Scales of Infant Development (Bayley, 1969, 1993). The purpose of the test is to assess brain-behavior relationships in the context of developmental change and maturation, expressed in tests for use at 3, 6, 9, 12, 18, and 24 months (±1 month). Functions are assessed in five neuropsychologic areas: basic neurologic function or intactness (tone, reflexes, signs); receptive functions (visual, auditory, verbal); expressive functions (fine motor and oral motor, gross motor); processing of higher-order functions (memory, problem solving, object permanence); and mental activity (goal-directed behavior, attention). Scoring of 16 to 22 items at each age is based on the optimality concept, and percentage scores (the number optimal divided by the sum of the number optimal and the number nonoptimal) are used as cutoff values for delay-nondelay. Sensitivity is highest at 24 months (92%, with 76% specificity) when compared with concurrently obtained Bayley scores, and specificity values peak at 12 months (94%, with sensitivity only 68%). The time required to complete a test at any age is about 15 minutes.

Comprehensive Developmental Assessment

The Bayley II (Bayley, 1993) is a revised and renormed version of the Bayley Scales of Infant Development (BSID) (Bayley, 1969), necessitated by changes in infants' developmental rate since 1969 (Campbell et al., 1986). The scales contain norm-referenced (based on a sample of 1700 U.S. children) motor and mental scales for children from birth to 42 months of age and a criterion-referenced behavioral scale for examining such areas as affect, attention, exploration, and fearfulness. Functions on the mental scale include object permanence, memory, problem solving, and complex language. The motor scale assesses both fine and gross motor function, including fine manipulative skills, coordination of large muscle groups, dynamic movement, postural imitation, and stereognosis.

Scores of infants tested longitudinally in the first year with the 1969 motor scale have not been demonstrated to be stable (Coryell et al., 1989), and Bayley herself recommended that three consecutive tests should be used to estimate performance during the first 15 months of life (Rosenblith, 1992). Because of the recent publication of the Bayley II, little research is available on predictive validity. Recently, however, Harris and Daniels (1999, under review) reported the correlation between Bayley II motor scale scores in the first year of life with scores at 17 to 22 months of age to be only 0.34. Therapists are advised to be conservative in assuming predictive capabilities of the new test until further research is available. The Bayley II takes about 45 to 60 minutes to administer.

Motor Assessments

The TIMP (Campbell et al., 1993, 1995) is a test for infants younger than age 4 months, including prematurely born infants as young as 32 weeks of postconceptional age. Function on this scale is defined as the postural and selective control needed for functional movements in early infancy, including head and trunk control in prone, supine, and upright positions. The test has 28 items scored pass-fail on the basis of observations of spontaneous activity and 31 scaled items administered by the examiner according to a standardized format. Elicited items present the infant with problems to solve that require organization of head and trunk posture in space to orient to interesting spectacles, interact with the tester, or regain a preferred postural configuration. Scores are correlated with age (0.83) and are sensitive to degree of medical complications experienced in the newborn period ($R^2 = 0.72, p < 0.00001$, when age and risk are used to predict test performance). Test-retest reliability over a 3-day period for infants across the age range of the test was 0.89 (Campbell, 1999), and at 3 months of age scores above and below 0.50 standard deviation below the mean on the TIMP identified 80% of the same children identified as above or below the 10th percentile on the AIMS at the same age (Campbell & Kolobe, 1999, under review). Ecologic validity of the TIMP has been demonstrated by research indicating that 98% of TIMP item-handling procedures are similar to demands for movement placed on infants by their caregivers in dressing, bathing, and play interactions (Murney & Campbell, 1998). The test has not yet been normed and predictive validity has not been reported. The test takes 25 to 45 minutes to administer.

The Peabody Developmental Motor Scales (PDMS) (Folio & Fewell, 1983; Hinderer et al., 1989) contain separate scales for gross and fine motor assessment for children from birth to 83 months of age. Functions examined by the gross motor scale include reflexes, balance, nonlocomotor and locomotor activities, and receipt and propulsion of objects. The fine motor scale examines grasp, hand functions, eye-hand coordination, and manual dexterity. The PDMS was normed on 617 U.S. children, and relatively small numbers of children were assessed at any given age level. Fine motor ratings were reported to be more reliable for children with delays (0.96) than for those without delays (0.76), but these results were related more to the statistical effect created by the greater variability of the delayed group than to actual disagreements between raters (Stokes et al., 1990). Kolobe and colleagues (1998) examined the sensitivity to change in children with motor delay or CP of the gross motor scale and found it to be as sensitive to change over a 6-month period as the Gross Motor Function Measure (Russell et al., 1989) described in the next section. The test takes 45 to 60 minutes to administer.

The Toddler and Infant Motor Evaluation (TIME) (Miller & Roid, 1994) is a comprehensive qualitative motor assessment for children from birth to 42 months with suspected motor delay or dysfunction. In addition to subtests of mobility, stability, motor organization, functional performance, and social/emotional abilities, optional clinical subtests examine atypical positions, quality, and movement components. Testing is based on parent-elicited play and naturalistic observations of movement. The test was normed on 731 U.S. children. The TIME takes 10 to 40 minutes depending on age, with an additional 15 minutes needed for the functional performance subtest administered by parent interview.

The Bruininks-Oseretsky Test of Motor Proficiency is a test of gross and fine motor function for children from 4.5 to 14.5 years of age (Bruininks, 1978). The test has subscales for running speed and agility, balance, bilateral coordination, strength, upper limb coordination, response speed, visual-motor control, and upper limb speed and dexterity. Although the test is largely one of coordination and balance (Krus et al., 1981), several subtests have items that are clearly related to functional demands for school-age children, such as cutting within lines and ball activities and physical education skills such as sit-ups, shuttle-runs, and long jumping. The test was normed on 765 U.S. subjects. The test takes 45 to 60 minutes to administer (a 15- to 20-minute short form is available).

Assessments Designed for Children with Disabilities

The Gross Motor Function Measure (GMFM) (Rosenbaum et al., 1990; Russell et al., 1989) is a test specifically designed and validated for measuring change over time in gross motor function in children with CP. Function in this test is defined as the child's degree of achievement of a motor behavior (regardless of quality) when instructed to perform or when placed in a particular position. Spontaneously chosen movements are not assessed. The test's items are distributed over five dimensions to measure how much children can do, not the quality with which they do it. These dimensions include lying and rolling; sitting; crawling and kneeling; standing; and walking, running, and jumping. The test was validated for sensitivity to change over a 6-month period in children with CP from 5 months to 16 years of age. Change judged from blind evaluation of videotapes was correlated with GMFM test scores at 0.82. Kolobe and colleagues (1998) found that, as would be expected, children with motor delay changed more on the GMFM over a 6-month period than did children with CP. The test has not been normed on a sample of able-bodied children, but generally all items are achievable by 5-year-olds with normal motor function. The test requires 45 to 60 minutes to administer.

The GMFM has been extensively used in research on interventions such as intensive physical therapy and selective dorsal rhizotomy, documenting its value for use in clinical practice and decision making (for a summary, see Bjornson et al., 1998a). Because children with CP are generally considered to be highly variable in performance from day to day, Bjornson and colleagues (1998b) studied test-retest reliability over a 1-week period and found intraclass correlations for all subsections to be at least 0.80. Russell and colleagues (1998) assessed the responsivity of the GMFM to change in children with Down syndrome below age 6. They found that, although children showed significant changes in scores over a 6-month period that were also greater for the youngest children than those demonstrated by the Bayley II, the correlation between GMFM scores and parents' or therapists' judgments of change was poor and lower than that obtained in studies of change responsivity in children with CP. Correlations were improved if raters accepted parents' reports of item achievement when the child did not demonstrate the behavior during testing. Finally, scores on the total GMFM and on the subsections using predominantly the legs are correlated with independently obtained assessments of leg strength, accounting for 55 to 65% of the common variance, but are not correlated with aerobic power or with arm strength (Parker et al., 1993). The Gross Motor Performance Measure, a companion test of postural control in items from the GMFM (Boyce et al., 1991), is described in the next chapter. A gross motor disability classification system for grouping children by level of disability, similar in nature to a disease staging system, which was recently developed by the same research group (Palisano et al., 1997), is described in Chapter 7 on clinical decision making.

The Pediatric Evaluation of Disability Inventory (PEDI) is a discriminative device for detecting functional limitations and disability in age-appropriate independence and a tool for program evaluation in tracking progress in individual children with disabil-

ities (Feldman et al., 1990; Haley et al., 1991, 1992). Function in this scale is defined as ability to perform ADL with or without modifications or assistance as reported by a knowledgeable informant. On the PEDI, 197 items measure functional skills in self-care, mobility, and social function, and 20 items assess the extent of caregiver assistance and modifications needed to reduce or eliminate disabilities in each domain. The test was normed on 412 nondisabled U.S. children, and initial validity for discriminating function and assistance needed was derived from a clinical sample of 102 children with various disabilities (Feldman et al., 1990). Both normative standard scores and scaled scores are provided for each of its three domains. The test takes 20 to 30 minutes to complete by therapists or teachers and 45 to 60 minutes by structured parent interview. Hey and colleagues at Boston Children's Hospital have developed a parent self-administered version of the PEDI that took an average of 35 minutes to complete in a sample of 110 parents (Hey LA, Kasser J, Rosenthal R, Ramsing N, & Katz J, unpublished data, 1992). Scoring software to obtain Rasch logit measures is available. Direct testing of children's performance in an ecologically valid setting is not specified but could be done.

The Functional Independence Measure for Children (WeeFIM) is a discipline-free test of disability for assessing functions in self-care, sphincter control, mobility, locomotion, and communication and social cognition (Granger et al., 1989; Msall et al., 1992a). Function in this scale is defined as caregiver assistance needed to accomplish daily tasks. The WeeFIM is descriptive of caretaker and special resources required because of functional limitations and is useful in tracking outcomes over time across health, developmental, and community settings. Although insufficient detail is provided to be useful in making treatment decisions, it is an excellent tool for description of overall rehabilitation outcomes, for use in program evaluation, and for cross-disciplinary communication. The test has 18 items measured on a seven-point ordinal scale for use with children with developmental disabilities from 6 months to 12 years of age. Pilot normative work on a sample of 222 children demonstrated significant correlations between total WeeFIM scores and age ($r = .80$) (Msall et al., 1992b). The test has been used with children with extreme prematurity, CP, Down syndrome, congenital limb disorders, myelodysplasia, and traumatic brain injury (Msall ME, personal communication, 1992). The test requires 20 to 30 minutes to complete.

Finally, given the evidence from studies such as Adolph's (1997), which illustrates how children use their perception of the affordances of the environment, one test that assesses childrens' ability to use their multiple senses to solve problems involving conflicting information for control of upright posture will be briefly mentioned. Deitz and colleagues (1996) developed the Pediatric Clinical Test of Sensory Interaction for Balance in order to assess children's standing stability under varying sensory conditions, including standing on stable versus foam surfaces, with and without vision, and with information from body sway relative to the surround occluded. Children must "select" the right sensory inputs to interpret their stability situation correctly, and these researchers have shown that children with learning disabilities and motor delays perform more poorly on the test than typically developing children. Tests of impairment such as this should be useful clinically to differentiate movement problems caused by sensory processing difficulties from problems with coordination of the motor ensemble.

In summary, a number of well-designed tests are available for screening and examining functional motor performance in children, and several new tests assess specific motor constructs or functional limitations of children with disabilities. Many of these new tests remain to be validated in clinical practice, but early results are promising. No standardized tests have yet emerged from the new interest in contemporary theories of motor development and motor control, perhaps because dynamical systems theory emphasizes the process rather than products of development. Measures derived from dynamical systems theory should (1) include examination of a variety of subsystems related to the motor ensemble, such as the musculoskeletal system, perception, and movement patterns; and (2) use age-appropriate tasks and variation in the environment (Heriza, 1991). Measurement of periods of instability in patterns of movement selected by the child in response to tasks in varying contexts is deemed to be important.

Long and Tieman (1998) recently reviewed two tests, the AIMS and the TIME, for conformity to the challenges of a dynamical systems perspective as outlined by Heriza (1991). They found that the tests examine age-appropriate tasks and some subsystems but do not specifically address contextual variations. Infant comfort in both tests is ensured by emphasis on spontaneous activity or activity in interaction with a caregiver. Neither test, however, is designed to search for the instability of selection of movement patterns just before systematic appearance of a qualitatively new motor behavior, a key issue in assessment of motor development from a dynamical systems perspective because such periods of instability are believed to be sensitive periods for effective intervention. We believe the TIMP *does* meet this criterion.

Evaluation of the results of tests of function and disability gives the therapist knowledge of what the child can do, with or without assistance from technology or caregivers. These results are important in diagnosis of developmental delay or deviance and for providing basic information regarding the child's motor competencies for accomplishing the important tasks of childhood play and for experiencing the joy of movement used for pleasure and for purposeful exploration of the world. More information, however, is needed for planning intervention when functional limitations are identified. Roberton and Halverson (1984) have described, in a beautifully succinct way, the process of developing a plan for helping a child to learn movement. Once having observed in what way and how the child responds to a movement task believed to be developmentally appropriate, the prospective coach must consider what the environment demands for the child to succeed at the task and also must interpret the child's response. "What is the meaning of a child's solution to a particular movement problem? Does it indicate a more advanced form of movement? Does it suggest improved perceptual functioning? Is the solution a cognitive attempt to avoid a balance-threatening position? Does the child's response suggest that the task is too stressful, too complex at that particular moment—that the child is not 'ready' for it?" (Roberton & Halverson, 1984, p. 3). According to dynamical systems theory, we would also ask what constraints in a variety of cooperating subsystems might be limiting performance and whether the child's selected movement strategy is stable or in transition. Based on task analysis and an interpretation of the child's solution, the teacher must decide whether to intervene or to leave the child and the environment alone. If the decision is to intervene, the teacher must decide whether to redesign the physical environment, verbally or physically coach the child, or show the child a possible solution. After implementing the decision, reexamination is used to evaluate the effectiveness of the intervention. The chapters that follow in this section provide further information to aid the physical therapist with these basic processes of clinical instruction and decision making. These chapters include information on the development of gait, motor control and motor learning processes and principles, physical growth and fitness, and suggestions for structuring clinical decision making using a scientific approach. The information provided in these chapters will enable pediatric physical therapists to apply current concepts and research for the benefit of our clients—children with disabilities and their families.

ACKNOWLEDGMENTS

Partial support for work described in this paper was provided by the Foundation for Physical Therapy and the National Center for Medical Rehabilitation Research of the U.S. National Institutes of Health.

References

Abramov, I, Gordon, J, Hendrickson, A, Hainline, L, Dobson, V, & LaBossiere, E. The retina of the human infant. Science, *217*:265–267, 1982.

Adolph, KE. Learning in the development of infant locomotion. Monographs of the Society for Research in Child Development, *62*(3):1–140, 1997.

American Academy of Pediatrics Task Force on Infant Positioning and SIDS. Positioning and SIDS. Pediatrics, *89*:1120–1126, 1992.

American Physical Therapy Association. Guide to physical therapist practice. Physical Therapy, *77*(11): 1997.

Ames, LB, Gillespie, C, Haines, J, & Ilg, FL. The Gesell Institute's Child from One to Six: Evaluating the Behavior of the Preschool Child. New York: Harper & Row, 1979.

Atwater, SW. Should the normal motor developmental sequence be used as a theoretical model in pediatric physical therapy? In Lister, MJ (Ed.), Contemporary Management of Motor Control Problems: Proceedings of the II STEP Conference. Alexandria, VA: Foundation for Physical Therapy, 1991, pp. 89–93.

Aylward, GP. Bayley Infant Neurodevelopmental Screener Manual. San Antonio, TX: Psychological Corporation, 1992.

Banks, M, Aslin, R, & Letson, R. Sensitive period for the development of human binocular vision. Science, *190*:675–677, 1975.

Bard, C, Fleury, M, & Hay, L (Eds.). Development of Eye-Hand Coordination across the Life Span. Columbia, SC: University of South Carolina Press, 1990.

Barinaga, M. Death gives birth to the nervous system. But how? Science, *259*:762–763, 1993.

Bartlett, DJ. Relationship between selected anthropometric characteristics and gross motor development among infants developing typically. Pediatric Physical Therapy, *10*:114–119, 1998.

Bayley, N. Manual for the Bayley Scales of Infant Development. New York: Psychological Corporation, 1969.

Bayley, N. Bayley II. San Antonio: Psychological Corporation, 1993.

Beilin, H. Piagetian theory. In Vasta, R (Ed.), Annals of Child Development, Vol. 6. Greenwich, CT: JAI Press, 1989, pp. 85–131.

Bergenn, VW, Dalton, TC, & Lipsitt, LP. Myrtle B. McGraw: A growth scientist. Developmental Psychology, *28*:381–395, 1992.

Bertenthal, BI, & Campos, JJ. New directions in the study of early experience. Child Development, *58*:560–567, 1987.

Bevor, TG. Regressions in Mental Development: Basic Phenomena and Theories. Hillsdale, NJ: Lawrence Erlbaum Associates, 1982.

Bijou, SW. Behavior analysis. In Vasta, R (Ed.), Annals of Child Development, Vol. 6. Greenwich, CT: JAI Press, 1989, pp. 61–83.

Bjornson, KF, Graubert, CS, Buford, VL, & McLaughlin, J. Validity of the Gross Motor Function Measure. Pediatric Physical Therapy, *10*:43–47, 1998a.

Bjornson, KF, Graubert, CS, McLaughlin, JF, Kerfeld, CI, & Clark, EM. Test-retest reliability of the Gross Motor Function Measure in children with cerebral palsy. Physical and Occupational Therapy in Pediatrics, *18*(2):51–61, 1998b.

Blasco, PM, Hrncir, EJ, & Blasco, PA. The contribution of maternal involvement to mastery performance in infants with cerebral palsy. Journal of Early Intervention, *14*:161–174, 1990.

Bly, L. The Components of Normal Movement during the First Year of Life and Abnormal Motor Development. Oak Park, IL: Neuro-Developmental Treatment Association, 1983.

Bobath, B, & Bobath, K. The neuro-developmental treatment. In Scrutton, D (Ed.), Management of the Motor Disorders of Children with Cerebral Palsy. London: Spastics International Medical Publications, 1984, pp. 6–18.

Bower, E, & McLellan, DL. Effect of increased exposure to physiotherapy on skill acquisition of children with cerebral palsy. Developmental Medicine and Child Neurology, *34*:25–39, 1992.

Boyce, W, Gowland, C, Hardy, S, Rosenbaum, P, Lane, M, Plews, N, Goldsmith, C, & Russell, D. Development of a quality of movement measure for children with cerebral palsy. Physical Therapy, *71*:820–832, 1991.

Bruininks, RH. Bruininks-Oseretsky Test of Motor Proficiency: Examiner's Manual. Circle Pines, MN: American Guidance Service, 1978.

Bruner, JS. The growth and structure of skill. In Connolly, K (Ed.), Mechanisms of Motor Skill Development. New York: Academic Press, 1970, pp. 63–94.

Bushnell, EW, & Boudreau, JP. Motor development and the mind: The potential role of motor abilities as a determinant of aspects of perceptual development. Child Development, *64*:1005–1021, 1993.

Butler, C. Augmentative mobility: Why do it? Physical Medicine and Rehabilitation Clinics of North America, *2*(4):801–815, 1991.

Byl, NN, Merzenich, MM, Cheung, S, Bedenbaugh, P, Nagarajan, SS, & Jenkins, WM. A primate model for studying focal dystonia and repetitive strain injury: Effects on the primary somatosensory cortex. Physical Therapy, *77*:269–284, 1997.

Campbell, SK. Measurement in developmental therapy: Past, present, and future. In Miller, LJ (Ed.), Developing Norm Referenced Standardized Tests. Binghamton, NY: Haworth Press, 1989, pp. 1–13.

Campbell, SK. Framework for the measurement of neurologic impairment and disability. In Lister, MJ (Ed.), Contemporary Management of Motor Control Problems: Proceedings of the II STEP Conference. Alexandria, VA: Foundation for Physical Therapy, 1991, pp. 143–153.

Campbell, SK. Quantifying the effects of interventions for movement disorders resulting from cerebral palsy. Journal of Child Neurology, *11*(suppl 1):S61–S70, 1996.

Campbell, SK. Therapy programs for children that last a lifetime. Physical and Occupational Therapy in Pediatrics *17*(1):1–15, 1997.

Campbell, SK. Test-retest reliability of the Test of Infant Motor Performance. Pediatric Physical Therapy, *11*:60–66, 1999.

Campbell, SK, & Kolobe, THA. Concurrent validity of the Test of Infant Motor Performance with the Alberta Infant Motor Scale. Pediatric Physical Therapy, 1999, under review.

Campbell, SK, Kolobe, THA, Osten, E, Lenke, M, & Girolami, GL. Construct validity of the Test of Infant Motor Performance. Physical Therapy, *75*:585–596, 1995.

Campbell, SK, Osten, ET, Kolobe, THA, & Fisher, AG. Development of the Test of Infant Motor Performance. In Granger, CV, & Gresham, GE (Eds.), New Developments in Functional Assessment. Philadelphia: WB Saunders, 1993, pp. 541–550.

Campbell, SK, Siegel, E, Parr, CA, & Ramey, CT. Evidence for the need to renorm the Bayley Scales of Infant Development based on the performance of a population-based sample of twelve-month-old infants. Topics in Early Childhood Special Education, *6*(2):83–96, 1986.

Campbell, SK, & Wilson, JM. Planning infant learning programs. Physical Therapy, *56*:1347–1357, 1976.

Case-Smith, J, Bigsby, R, & Clutter, J. Perceptual-motor coupling in the development of grasp. American Journal of Occupational Therapy, *52*:102–110, 1998.

Catania, A, & Harnad, S (Eds.). The Selection of Behavior—The Operant Behaviorism of B.F. Skinner: Comments and Consequences. New York: Cambridge University Press, 1988.

Cintas, HM. Cross-cultural variation in infant motor development. Physical and Occupational Therapy in Pediatrics, *8*(4):1–20, 1988.

Cioni, G, & Prechtl, HFR. Preterm and early postterm behaviour in low-risk premature infants. Early Human Development, 23:159–191, 1990.

Colson, ER, & Dworkin, PH. Toddler development. Pediatrics in Review, 18:255–259, 1997.

Connolly, K. Skill development: Problems and plans. In Connolly, K (Ed.), Mechanisms of Motor Skill Development. New York: Academic Press, 1970, pp. 3–21.

Corbetta, D, & Mounoud, P. Early development of grasping and manipulation. In Bard, C, Fleury, M, & Hay, L (Eds.), Development of Eye-Hand Coordination across the Life Span. Columbia, SC: University of South Carolina Press, 1990, pp. 188–213.

Coryell, J, Provost, BM, Wilhelm, IJ, & Campbell, SK. Stability of Bayley Motor Scale scores in the first two years. Physical Therapy, 69:834–841, 1989.

Darrah, J, Piper, M, & Watt, MJ. Assessment of gross motor skills of at-risk infants: Predictive validity of the Alberta Infant Motor Scale. Developmental Medicine and Child Neurology, 40:485–491, 1998.

Deitz, JC, Richardson, P, Crowe, TK, & Westcott, SL. Performance of children with learning disabilities and motor delays on the Pediatric Clinical Test of Sensory Interaction for Balance (P-CTSIB). Physical and Occupational Therapy in Pediatrics, 16(3):1–21, 1996.

Dewey, C, Fleming, P, & Golding, J. Does the supine sleeping position have any adverse effects on the child? II. Development in the first 18 months. Pediatrics (CZE), 101:E5, 1998.

Edelman, GM. Bright Air, Brilliant Fire: On the Matter of the Mind. New York: Basic Books, 1992.

Epstein, HT. Correlated brain and intelligence development in humans. In Hahn, ME, Jensen, C, & Dudek, BC (Eds.), Development and Evolution of Brain Size: Behavioral Implications. New York: Academic Press, 1979, pp. 111–131.

Fagard, J. The development of bimanual coordination. In Bard, C, Fleury, M, & Hay, L (Eds.), Development of Eye-Hand Coordination across the Life Span. Columbia, SC: University of South Carolina Press, 1990, pp. 262–282.

Feldman, AB, Haley, SM, & Coryell, J. Concurrent and construct validity of the Pediatric Evaluation of Disability Inventory. Physical Therapy, 70:602–610, 1990.

Fentress, JC. Animal and human models of coordination development. In Bard, C, Fleury, M, & Hay, L (Eds.), Development of Eye-Hand Coordination across the Life Span. Columbia, SC: University of South Carolina Press, 1990, pp. 3–25.

Ferrari, F, Cioni, G, & Prechtl, HRF. Qualitative changes of general movements in preterm infants with brain lesions. Early Human Development, 23:193–231, 1990.

Fetters, L. Object permanence development in infants with motor handicaps. Physical Therapy, 61:327–333, 1981.

Fetters, L. Foundations for therapeutic intervention. In Campbell, SK (Ed.), Pediatric Neurologic Physical Therapy. New York: Churchill Livingstone, 1991a, pp. 19–32.

Fetters, L. Cerebral palsy: Contemporary treatment concepts. In Lister, MJ (Ed.), Contemporary Management of Motor Control Problems: Proceedings of the II STEP Conference. Alexandria, VA: Foundation for Physical Therapy, 1991b, pp. 219–224.

Fetters, L. Measurement and treatment in cerebral palsy: An argument for a new approach. Physical Therapy, 71:244–247, 1991c.

Fetters, L, Fernandez, B, & Cermak, S. The relationship of proximal and distal components in the development of reaching. Journal of Human Movement Studies, 17:283–297, 1989.

Fischer, KW. Relations between brain and cognitive development. Child Development, 58:623–632, 1987.

Fisher, AG. Functional measures, Part 1: What is function, what should we measure, and how should we measure it? American Journal of Occupational Therapy, 46:183–185, 1992.

Flavell, JH. The Developmental Psychology of Jean Piaget. Princeton, NJ: Van Nostrand, 1963.

Folio, M, & Fewell, R. Peabody Developmental Motor Scales and Activity Cards. Allen, TX: DLM Teaching Resources, 1983.

Frankenburg, WK, Dodds, J, Archer, P, Bresnick, B, Maschka, P, Edelman, N, & Shapiro, H. Denver II. Denver: Denver Developmental Materials, 1990.

Frankenburg, WK, Dodds, J, Archer, P, Shapiro, H, & Bresnick, B. The Denver II. A major revision and restandardization of the DDST. Pediatrics, 89:91–97, 1992.

Georgopoulos, AP, Ashe, J, Smyrnis, M, & Taira, M. The motor cortex and the coding of force. Science, 256:1692–1695, 1992.

Georgopoulos, AP, Taira, M, & Lukashin, A. Cognitive neurophysiology of the motor cortex. Science, 260:47–52, 1993.

Gesell, A. Infancy and Human Growth. New York: Macmillan, 1928a.

Gesell, A. The Mental Growth of the Pre-school Child: A Psychological Outline of Normal Development from Birth to the Sixth Year, Including a System of Developmental Diagnosis. New York: Macmillan, 1928b.

Gesell, A. The Embryology of Behavior. New York: Harper & Row, 1945.

Gesell, A, Amatruda, CS, Castner, BM, & Thompson, H. Biographies of Child Development: The Mental Growth Careers of Eighty-four Infants and Children. New York: Arno Press, 1975.

Gesell, A, Halverson, HM, Thompson, H, Ilg, FL, Castner, BM, Ames, LB, & Amatruda, CS. The First Five Years of Life. New York: Harper & Row, 1940.

Gesell, A, Thompson, H, & Amatruda, CS. Infant Behavior: Its Genesis and Growth. New York: McGraw-Hill, 1934.

Glascoe, FP, Byrne, KE, Ashford, LG, Johnson, KL, Chang, B, & Strickland, B. Accuracy of the Denver-II in developmental screening. Pediatrics, 89:1221–1225, 1992.

Goldfield, EC. Toward a developmental ecological psychology. Monographs of the Society for Research in Child Development, 62(3):152–158, 1997.

Goldman-Rakic, PS. Development of cortical circuitry and cognitive function. Child Development, 58:601–622, 1987.

Granger, CV, Hamilton, BB, & Kayton, R. Guide for the Use of the Functional Independence Measure (WeeFIM) of the Uniform Data Set for Medical Rehabilitation. Buffalo, NY: Research Foundation, State University of New York, 1989.

Green, EM, Mulcahy, CM, & Pountney, TE. An investigation into the development of early postural control. Developmental Medicine and Child Neurology, 37:437–448, 1995.

Greenough, WT, Black, JE, & Wallace, CS. Experience and brain development. Child Development, 58:539–559, 1987.

Hadders-Algra, M, & Prechtl, HFR. Developmental course of general movements in early infancy. I. Descriptive analysis of change in form. Early Human Development, 28:201–213, 1992.

Hadders-Algra, M, Van Eykern, LA, Klip-van den Nieuwendijk, AWJ, & Prechtl, HFR. Developmental course of general movements in early infancy. II. EMG correlates. Early Human Development, 28:231–253, 1992.

Haley, SM, Baryza, MJ, & Blanchard, Y. Functional and naturalistic frameworks in assessing physical and motor disablement. In Wilhelm, IJ (Ed.), Physical Therapy Assessment in Early Infancy. New York: Churchill Livingstone, 1993, pp. 225–256.

Haley, SM, Coster, WJ, & Faas, RM. A content validity study of the Pediatric Evaluation of Disability Inventory. Pediatric Physical Therapy, 3:177–184, 1991.

Haley, SM, Coster, WJ, Ludlow, LH, Haltiwanger, JT, & Andrellos, PJ. The Pediatric Evaluation of Disability Inventory: Development Standardization and Administration Manual. Boston: New England Medical Center Publications, 1992.

Harris, SR. Efficacy of physical therapy in promoting family functioning and functional independence for children with cerebral palsy. Pediatric Physical Therapy, 2:160–164, 1990.

Harris, SR, & Daniels, LE. Content validity of the Harris Infant Neuromotor Test. Physical Therapy, 76:727–737, 1996.

Harris, SR, & Daniels, LE. Reliability and validity of the Harris Infant Neuromotor Test. Journal of Developmental and Behavioral Pediatrics, unpublished data, 1999.

Hauser-Cram, P. Mastery motivation in toddlers with developmental disabilities. Child Development, 67:236–248, 1996.

Hay, L. Developmental changes in eye-hand coordination behaviors: Preprogramming versus feedback control. In Bard, C, Fleury, M, & Hay, L (Eds.), Development of Eye-Hand Coordination across the Life Span. Columbia, SC: University of South Carolina Press, 1990, pp. 217–244.

Hayne, H, Rovee-Collier, C, & Perris, EE. Categorization and memory retrieval by three-month-olds. Child Development, 58:750–767, 1987.

Heriza, C. Motor development: Traditional and contemporary theories. In Lister, MJ (Ed.), Contemporary Management of Motor Control Problems: Proceedings of the II STEP Conference. Alexandria, VA: Foundation for Physical Therapy, 1991, pp. 99–126.

Hinderer, KA, Richardson, PK, & Atwater, SW. Clinical implications of the Peabody Developmental Motor Scales: A constructive review. Physical and Occupational Therapy in Pediatrics, 9(2):81–106, 1989.

Hohmann, A, & Creutzfeldt, OD. Squint and the development of binocularity in humans. Nature, 254:613–614, 1975.

Hoover, JE, & Strick, PL. Multiple output channels in the basal ganglia. Science, 259:819–821, 1993.

Horak, FB. Assumptions underlying motor control for neurologic rehabilitation. In Lister, MJ (Ed.), Contemporary Management of Motor Control Problems: Proceedings of the II STEP Conference. Alexandria, VA: Foundation for Physical Therapy, 1991, pp. 11–27.

Jantz, JW, Blosser, CD, & Fruechting, LA. A motor milestone change noted with a change in sleep position. Archives of Pediatrics and Adolescent Medicine, 151:565–568, 1997.

Kanda, T, Yuge, M, Yamori, Y, Suzuki, J, & Fukase, H. Early physiotherapy in the treatment of spastic diplegia. Developmental Medicine and Child Neurology, 26:438–444, 1984.

Karniol, R. The role of manual manipulative stages in the infant's acquisition of perceived control over objects. Developmental Review, 9:205–233, 1989.

Keshner, EA, Campbell, D, Katz, R, & Peterson, BW. Neck muscle activation patterns in humans during isometric head stabilization. Experimental Brain Research, 75:335–364, 1989.

Knobloch, H, Stevens, F, & Malone, AF. Manual of Developmental Diagnosis, rev. ed. New York: Harper & Row, 1980.

Kolobe, THA, Palisano, RJ, & Stratford, PW. Comparison of two outcome measures for infants with cerebral palsy and infants with motor delays. Physical Therapy, 78:1062–1072, 1998.

Krus, PH, Bruininks, RH, & Robertson, G. Structure of motor abilities in children. Perceptual and Motor Skills, 52:119–129, 1981.

Lee, AM. Child-rearing practices and motor performance of black and white children. Research Quarterly for Exercise and Sport, 51:494–500, 1980.

Leonard, CT, Moritani, T, Hirschfeld, H, & Forssberg, H. Deficits in reciprocal inhibition of children with cerebral palsy as revealed by H reflex testing. Developmental Medicine and Child Neurology, 32:974–984, 1990.

Long, TM, & Tieman, B. Review of two recently published measurement tools: The AIMS and the TIME. Pediatric Physical Therapy, 10:62–66, 1998.

Loria, C. Relationship of proximal and distal function in motor development. Physical Therapy, 60:167–172, 1980.

McEwan, MH, Dihoff, RE, & Brosvic, GM. Early infant crawling experience is reflected in later motor skill development. Perceptual and Motor Skills, 72:75–79, 1991.

McGraw, MB. Growth: A Study of Johnny and Jimmy. New York: Appleton-Century, 1935.

McGraw, MB. The Neuromuscular Maturation of the Human Infant. New York: Hafner, 1963. (Original work published by Columbia University Press, 1945.)

Miller, LJ. The Miller First Step (Screening Test for Evaluating Preschoolers). New York: Psychological Corporation, 1992.

Miller, LJ, & Roid, GH. The TIME. Toddler and Infant Motor Evaluation: A Standardized Assessment. Tucson, AZ: Therapy Skill Builders, 1994.

Msall, ME, Braun, S, Duffy, L, DiGaudio, K, LaForest, S, & Granger, C. Normative sample of the Pediatric Functional Independence Measure: A uniform data set for tracking disability (Abstract). Developmental Medicine and Child Neurology, 34(suppl 66):19, 1992a.

Msall, ME, Braun, S, Granger, C, DiGaudio, K, & Duffy, L. The Functional Independence Measure for Children (WeeFIM), Developmental Edition (Version 1.5). Buffalo, NY: Uniform Data Set for Medical Rehabilitation, 1992b.

Murney, ME, & Campbell, SK. The ecological relevance of the Test of Infant Motor Performance Elicited Scale items. Physical Therapy, 78:479–489, 1998.

National Advisory Board on Medical Rehabilitation Research. Research Plan for the National Center for Medical Rehabilitation Research. NIH Publication No. 93-3509. Bethesda, MD: National Institutes of Health, 1993.

Nowakowski, RS. Basic concepts of CNS development. Child Development, 58:568–595, 1987.

Nudo, RJ, Milliken, GW, Jenkins, WM, & Merzenich, MM. Use-dependent alterations of movement representations in primary motor cortex of adult squirrel monkeys. Journal of Neuroscience, 16:785–807, 1996.

Oppenheim, RW. Ontogenetic adaptations and retrogressive processes in the development of the nervous system and behavior: A neuroembryological perspective. In Connolly, K, & Prechtl, HFR (Eds.), Maturation and Development: Biological and Psychological Perspectives. Philadelphia: JB Lippincott, 1981, pp. 73–109.

Paillard, J. Basic neurophysiological structures of eye-hand coordination. In Bard, C, Fleury, M, & Hay, L (Eds.), Development of Eye-Hand Coordination across the Life Span. Columbia, SC: University of South Carolina Press, 1990, pp. 26–74.

Palisano, RJ. Neuromotor and developmental assessment. In Wilhelm, IJ (Ed.), Physical Therapy Assessment in Early Infancy. New York: Churchill Livingstone, 1993, pp. 173–224.

Palisano, R, Rosenbaum, P, Walter, S, Russell, D, Wood, E, & Galuppi, B. Development and reliability of a system to classify gross motor function in children with cerebral palsy. Developmental Medicine and Child Neurology, 39:214–223, 1997.

Parker, DF, Carriere, L, Hebestreit, H, Salsberg, A, & Bar-Or, O. Muscle performance and gross motor function of children with spastic cerebral palsy. Developmental Medicine and Child Neurology, 35:17–23, 1993.

Pellegrini, AD, & Smith, PK. Physical activity play: The nature and function of a neglected aspect of play. Child Development, 69:577–598, 1998.

Piaget, J. The Origins of Intelligence in Children. New York: International Universities Press, 1952.

Pick, HL, Jr. Eleanor J. Gibson. Learning to perceive and perceiving to learn. Developmental Psychology, 28:787–794, 1992.

Piper, MC, Darrah, J. Motor Assessment of the Developing Infant. Philadelphia: WB Saunders, 1994.

Piper, MC, Pinnell, LE, Darrah, J, Maguire, T, & Byrne, PJ. Construction and validation of the Alberta Infant Motor Scale (AIMS). Canadian Journal of Public Health, 83(suppl 2):S46–S50, 1992.

Plimpton, CE, & Regimbal, C. Differences in motor proficiency according to gender and race. Perceptual and Motor Skills, 74:399–402, 1992.

Provost, B. Normal development from birth to 4 months: Extended use of the NBAS-K. Part II. Physical and Occupational Therapy in Pediatrics, 1(3):19–34, 1981.

Ramey, CT, & Ramey, SL. Effective early intervention. Mental Retardation, 30(6):337–345, 1992.

Ratner, HH, & Foley, MA. A unifying framework for the development of children's activity memory. Advances in Child Development and Behavior, 25:33–105, 1994.

Roberton, MA, & Halverson, LE. Developing Children--Their Changing Movement. A Guide for Teachers. Philadelphia: Lea & Febiger, 1984.

Rosenbaum, P. Physical activity play in children with disabilities: A neglected opportunity for research? Child Development, 69:607-608, 1998.

Rosenbaum, P, Russell, D, Cadman, D, Gowland, C, Jarvis, S, & Hardy, S. Issues in measuring change in motor function in children with cerebral palsy: A special communication. Physical Therapy, 70:125-131, 1990.

Rosenblith, JF. A singular career: Nancy Bayley. Developmental Psychology, 28:747-758, 1992.

Russell, D, Palisano, R, Walter, S, Rosenbaum, P, Gemus, M, Gowland, C, Galuppi, B, & Lane, M. Evaluating motor function in children with Down syndrome: Validity of the GMFM. Developmental Medicine and Child Neurology, 40:693-701, 1998.

Russell, D, Rosenbaum, P, Cadman, D, Gowland, C, Hardy, S, & Jarvis, S. The Gross Motor Function Measure: A means to evaluate the effects of physical therapy. Developmental Medicine and Child Neurology, 31:341-352, 1989.

Scherzer, AL, Mike, V, & Ilson, J. Physical therapy as a determinant of change in the cerebral palsied infant. Pediatrics, 58:47-52, 1976.

Schoen, JHR. The corticofugal projection to the brain stem and spinal cord in man. Psychiatry, Neurology and Neurosurgery, 72:121-128, 1969.

Shirley, MM. The First Two Years: A Study of Twenty-five Babies. Vol. I. Postural and Locomotor Development. Minneapolis, MN: University of Minnesota Press, 1931.

Shumway-Cook, A, & Woollacott, M. The growth of stability: Postural control from a developmental perspective. Journal of Motor Behavior, 17:131-147, 1985.

Shumway-Cook, A, & Woollacott, M. Theoretical issues in assessing postural control. In Wilhelm, IJ (Ed.), Physical Therapy Assessment in Early Infancy. New York: Churchill Livingstone, 1993, pp. 161-171.

Skinner, BF. Cumulative Record: A Selection of Papers, 3rd ed. New York: Meredith, 1972.

Sparling, JW (Ed.). Concepts in Fetal Movement Research. New York: Haworth Press, 1993.

Sporns, O. Selectionist and instructionist ideas in neuroscience. International Review of Neurobiology, 37:3-26, 1994.

Sporns, O, & Edelman, GM. Solving Bernstein's problem: A proposal for the development of coordinated movement by selection. Child Development, 64:960-981, 1993.

Stengel, TJ. Assessing motor development in children. In Campbell, SK (Ed.), Pediatric Neurologic Physical Therapy, 2nd ed. New York: Churchill Livingstone, 1991, pp. 33-65.

Stengel, TJ, Attermeier, SM, Bly, L, & Heriza, CB. Evaluation of sensorimotor dysfunction. In Campbell, SK (Ed.), Pediatric Neurologic Physical Therapy. New York: Churchill Livingstone, 1984, pp. 13-87.

Stokes, NA, Deitz, JL, & Crowe, TK. The Peabody Developmental Fine Motor Scale: An interrater reliability study. American Journal of Occupational Therapy, 44:334-340, 1990.

Strick, PL, & Preston, JB. Two representations of the hand in area 4 of a primate. I. Motor output organization. Journal of Neurophysiology, 48:139-149, 1982a.

Strick, PL, & Preston, JB. Two representations of the hand in area 4 of a primate. II. Somatosensory input organization. Journal of Neurophysiology, 48:150-159, 1982b.

Task Force on Standards for Measurement in Physical Therapy. Standards for tests and measurements in physical therapy practice. Physical Therapy, 71:589-622, 1991.

Thelen, E. Coupling perception and action in the development of skill: A dynamic approach. In Bloch, H, & Bertenthal, BI (Eds.), Sensory-Motor Organization and Development in Infancy and Early Childhood. Dordrecht, Netherlands: Kluwer Academic, 1990, pp. 39-56.

Thelen, E. Motor development. A new synthesis. American Psychologist, 50:79-95, 1995.

Thelen, E, & Adolph, KE. Arnold L. Gesell: The paradox of nature and nurture. Developmental Psychology, 28:368-380, 1992.

Thelen, E, & Corbetta, D. Exploration and selection in the early acquisition of skill. International Review of Neurobiology, 37:75-102, 1994.

Thelen, E, Corbetta, D, Kamm, K, Spencer, JP, Schneider, K, & Zernicke, R. The transition to reaching: Mapping intention and intrinsic dynamics. Child Development, 64:1058-1098, 1993.

Thelen, E, Kelso, JAS, & Fogel, A. Self-organizing systems and infant motor development. Developmental Review, 7:39-65, 1987.

Thelen, E, & Ulrich, BD. Hidden skills: A dynamic systems analysis of treadmill stepping during the first year. Monographs of the Society for Research in Child Development. Serial No. 223, Vol. 56, No. 1. Chicago: University of Chicago Press, 1991.

Thelen, E, Ulrich, BD, & Jensen, JL. The developmental origins of locomotion. In Woollacott, MH, & Shumway-Cook, A (Eds.), Development of Posture and Gait across the Life Span. Columbia, SC: University of South Carolina Press, 1989, pp. 23-47.

Thorn, F, Gwiazda, J, Cruz, AA, Bauer, JA, & Held, R. The development of eye alignment, convergence, and sensory binocularity in young infants. Investigative Ophthalmology and Visual Science, 35:544-553, 1994.

Tscharnuter, I. A new therapy approach to movement organization. Physical and Occupational Therapy in Pediatrics, 13(2):19-40, 1993.

Ulrich, BD. Development of stepping patterns in human infants: A dynamical systems perspective. Journal of Motor Behavior, 21:329-408, 1989.

van Blankenstein, M, Welbergen, UR, & de Haas, JH. Le développement du nourrisson: Sa première année en 130 photographies. Paris: Presses Universitaires de France, 1962.

Vinter, A. Manual imitations and reaching behaviors: An illustration of action control in infancy. In Bard, C, Fleury, M, & Hay, L (Eds.), Development of Eye-Hand Coordination across the Life Span. Columbia, SC: University of South Carolina Press, 1990, pp. 157-187.

von Hofsten, C. Eye-hand coordination in the newborn. Developmental Psychology, 18:450-461, 1982.

Whitall, J, & Getchell, N. From walking to running: Applying a dynamical systems approach to the development of locomotor skills. Child Development, 66:1541-1553, 1995.

Williams, JR, & Scott, RB. Growth and development of Negro infants: Motor development and its relationship to child-rearing practices in two groups of Negro infants. Child Development, 24:103-121, 1953.

Wimmers, RH, Savelsbergh, GJP, Beek, PJ, & Hopkins, B. Evidence for a phase transition in the early development of prehension. Developmental Psychobiology, 32:235-248, 1998a.

Wimmers, RH, Savelsbergh, GJP, van der Kamp, J, & Hartelman, P. A developmental transition in prehension modeled as a cusp catastrophe. Developmental Psychobiology, 32:23-35, 1998b.

Zelazo, PR. The development of walking: New findings and old assumptions. Journal of Motor Behavior, 15:99-137, 1983.

Zelazo, PR, Zelazo, NA, & Kolb, S. "Walking" in the newborn. Science, 176:314-315, 1972.

CHAPTER

2

Motor Control: Developmental Aspects of Motor Control in Skill Acquisition

NINA S. BRADLEY, PT, PhD

What does it mean to say, "I use a motor control approach" in my clinical practice? The term "motor control" is now commonly used in both research and clinical arenas of physical therapy, perhaps too commonly so as to erode a clear understanding of its meaning. This chapter seeks to familiarize the clinician with the research field of motor control and, more specifically, how motor control applies to issues of development by addressing four objectives. The first objective of this chapter is to provide a brief discussion of some theories and hypotheses that have shaped the direction of research and current views on motor control. Research conducted to test theories and hypotheses of motor control, in turn, have led scientists to propose that physiologic, psychologic, and mechanical mechanisms or processes play select roles in the control of movement and can be studied under conditions of controlled observation. Thus the second objective of this chapter is to describe some of the processes that may control movement initiation or execution.

The third objective and emphasis of this chapter is to present the work of researchers that both describes motor skill acquisition and attempts to reveal the processes that drive or permit acquisition of skills such as posture, gait, reaching, and grasping. The fourth objective is to explore how a physical therapist might examine a child's movement problems employing current knowledge of motor control. If the four objectives are adequately addressed, perhaps the reader will ultimately share my view that the statement "I use a motor control approach . . . " is not really what the speaker intends to convey.

THEORIES, HYPOTHESES, AND MODELS

Defining the term *motor control* and describing many of the theoretic constructs common to the field are not easy tasks, in part because motor control is a multidisciplinary field of study drawing from a broad range of disciplines including anatomy, physiology, psychology, kinesiology, engineering, and physical therapy. Historically, theories of motor control typically emerged from within a field such as anatomy or psychology, whereas hypotheses and models often emerged from the integration of ideas across fields. One consequence of this cross-pollination is that theoretic constructs and terminology have taken on slightly different definitions from one disciplinary view to the next, often leaving resolution of the discrepancy in definitions to the persevering student. In this section we will briefly review some of the more well-known theories, hypotheses, and models of motor control to gain an understanding of the ideas commonly embraced or challenged.

Theories of motor control attempt to unite various observations and laws that emerge from scientific study to explain why they exist or how they relate to one another. Theories also provide the foundation for development of hypotheses, models, and new theories. Three distinctly different theoretic perspectives are currently encountered in motor control literature: maturational, learning, and dynamic-based views. In the discussion to follow, we will briefly consider each view. Hypotheses, in contrast, attempt to predict the relationship between observations and defined (or experimental) conditions. For example, the maturational-based theory of motor control proposes that emergence of behavior is primarily attributable to maturational changes in the nervous system. A hypothesis based on this theory is that independent finger movements emerge at 7 months of age because of specific physiologic changes occurring in the primary motor cortex, the corticospinal tract, or both just before 7 months. When experiments by a large number of scientists testing a hypothesis produce consistent findings, the hypothesis becomes a law. Thus laws define highly predictable relationships between variables, and in some instances these relationships can be mathematically specified. Fitts' law, for example, states that accuracy requirements and the distance over which a movement occurs can be used to predict movement time (Fitts, 1954). Models, in contrast to laws, are idealized constructs that incorporate a few select variables believed to be most powerful in explaining relationships between events, and are used by scientists to both visualize and test theories. A basic understanding of hypotheses and models is useful because they provide the rationale for most research designs and views currently found in motor control literature. For further elaboration on these topics, the reader is referred to discussions by Schmidt and Lee (1998) and Shumway-Cook and Woollacott (1995).

Historical Perspective

In the late 1800s the neurologist Ramón y Cajal discovered that Golgi silver stain could selectively label individual nerve cells. This advance led to the neuron doctrine and set the course for neurobiologic research and thinking in the twentieth century (Shepherd, 1991). The notion of "structure-function" and the maturational-based theory of motor control are two theoretic products of the neuron doctrine. Using silver stain, anatomists found that structural features distinguish subpopulations of neurons within and between regions of the nervous system and that morphologic changes occur during development. The array of morphologic findings led to the view that structural organization of the nervous system determines behavioral function (structure-function). Physiologists provided evidence for structure-function control of behavior by isolating portions of the nervous system (reduced preparations) that produced stereotypic movements such as the stretch reflex, the brisk contraction of a muscle in response to a quick elongation of the muscle and its proprioceptors. Based on his many studies of reflex function in the spinal cord of cats, dogs, and monkeys, Sherrington (1947 [original work published 1906]) espoused the view that behavior is hierarchically organized and the simple reflex (composed of a receptor, conductor, and effector organ) is the fundamental unit of neural integration. Furthermore, he proposed that motor behavior is the composite coordination of simple reflexes (e.g., reflex chaining) as excitatory and inhibitory actions are summated at the synapse.

Maturational-Based Theories

Sherrington's notion of reflex chaining so dominated the study of physiology in the first half of the twentieth century that physiologists gave little attention to other views of motor control in explanations of behavior (Gallistel, 1980). Structure-function organization and reflex chaining were commonly employed rationales in studies of motor development as evidenced by the temporal correlations commonly drawn between emerging stimulus-evoked behavior and anatomic changes in neural pathways (e.g., Humphrey, 1964). Thus early studies identified the neuroanatomic changes occurring around the time a new behavior emerged without considering whether other variables contributed to the behavioral change. Consequently, scientists proposed that certain predictable changes during neural maturation are the causal determinants of behavioral development (Hooker, 1958; McGraw, 1945), establishing the foundation for maturational theories. Concurrent with these developments, hierarchic reflex chaining evolved to include the notion that reflex behaviors are expressions of an animal's phylogenetic origins (Humphrey, 1970). Such views merged into the notions that earliest movements are primitive behaviors controlled by phylogenetically older neural structures and earliest movements eventually disappear as older neural structures are inhibited by later differentiating neural structures that are phylogenetically more recent (Touwen, 1984). It appears there was little or no scientific challenge of these neuromaturational views, perhaps because students of development took little notice of other directions in neurobiologic research that were emerging at the time (Gallistel, 1980).

Learning-Based Theories

During this same time period, psychologists were also attempting to form theories of development. Behaviorism looked to the role of the environment in shaping behavior and sought to determine what attributes of the environment trigger or shape behavior. Response chaining, for example, proposed that feedback becomes more strongly associated with action over practice, automating the sequences of action executed by the nervous system (Rosenbaum, 1991). According to response chaining, the environment is the controller of the automating process. Response chaining, like reflex chaining, explains the ordering of movements as the consequence of feedback from one movement that in turn activates the next movement. Thorndike extended the notion of response chaining to address how motor skills are learned, and in the law of effect he proposed that skills emerge as we repeat actions that are rewarded (Schmidt & Lee, 1998).

The law of effect and emphasis on feedback can also be identified in contemporary theories and models of motor learning such as Adams' closed-loop theory (Adams, 1971) and more recently in a theoretic construct put forward by Sporns and Edelman (1993). Adams proposed that we develop a perceptual memory trace for what a correct movement should feel like (expected sensory consequences) based on intrinsic feedback generated during movement implementation. The perceptual trace evaluates the actual sensory consequences (feedback) of a movement each time it is executed and selects the movement attributes that are compatible with the perceptual memory trace to establish a memory trace for movement execution parameters. According to Adam's learning-based theory, feedback during movement is required to learn a movement, but subsequent research indicated that we do not need to monitor ongoing movements in order to reinforce desirable movement parameters (Taub & Berman,

1968). This inconsistency between experimental results and theoretic prediction was subsequently addressed by Schmidt's schema theory (Schmidt, 1975), discussed later in this chapter.

As theories are tested, the outcomes reveal their shortcomings, clarify the boundaries of our understanding, and raise a new generation of questions. For example, tests of response chaining raised questions such as how we learn or execute movements when we cannot constantly monitor movement-dependent feedback, or how we manage to execute an apparently endless variety of new and varied movements with minimal difficulty. Cognitive and developmental psychologists sought to explain the development of new skills as either the determinants or the consequences of increasing cognitive abilities. For example, Piaget proposed that early motor skill acquisition is the outcome of preverbal learning processes incorporating sensorimotor experiences to form early notions of causation that are stored to later serve as an internal reference during the development of language and concrete cognitive operations. According to Piagetian theory, preverbal learning and motor skill acquisition are maturational processes that permit concrete and abstract learning to take place (Keogh & Sugden, 1985). Furthermore, a recent theoretic proposal suggests that over evolutionary time, actions or observed actions such as reaching to grasp may have driven language specialization in the human brain (Rizzolatti & Arbib, 1998). In contrast to maturationist theories, learning-based theories suggest that development of motor skill is the consequence of learning by trial and error to master and sequence units of action that in their rudimentary form are genetically determined. Connolly (1977) proposed, for example, that genetics endow the infant with the equivalent of computer hardware (neurologic and biomechanical features) and the infant's cognitive activities, equivalent to computer software, function to modify and adapt rudimentary units of movement into skilled action.

One of the most widely embraced of the learning theories, schema theory, proposes that motor development is a function of learning rules to evaluate, correct, and update memory traces for a given class of movements (Schmidt, 1975). Schema theory assumes the presence of three constructs: general motor programs and two types of memory traces, recall schema and recognition schema. In schema theory, general motor programs are loosely defined as sets of instructions that are responsible for organizing the invariant or fundamental components of a movement. Recall schemas are defined as memories of relationships between past movement parameters, past initial conditions, and the movement outcomes they produced. Recognition schemas are defined as memories of relationships between past movement parameters, past initial conditions, and the sensory consequences they produced. It is theorized that recall schemas function to establish rules regarding the relationship between movement parameters of a general motor program, such as force or velocity, and movement outcome for a given set of initial conditions that can be used to plan similar movements under anticipated conditions. Recognition schema, in turn, are proposed to compare sensory consequences with movement outcome in light of initial conditions to form a second set of rules that can be used to predict the expected sensory consequences for similar movement outcomes during anticipated initial conditions. The expected sensory consequences are proposed to serve as a perceptual memory trace for evaluating new movements. When movements are generated too quickly (ballistically) to be corrected by feedback as they are executed (i.e., open loop), it is theorized that intrinsic feedback, an efferent copy of the motor command, can be compared with the expected sensory consequences to evaluate the movements during execution or after they are completed. It is theorized that the schema are established and refined as a function of practice. See Chapter 6 by Larin for further discussion of motor learning theories.

Schema theory does not attempt to explain the establishment of motor programs, nor does it attempt to ascribe them to specific neural structures. The term "motor program" is employed in a variety of ways by researchers from a variety of disciplinary backgrounds, which may help explain why there is no consensus as to what constitutes a motor program (Rosenbaum, 1991). In motor learning literature, motor programs are commonly invoked to explain the stereotypic attributes of a complex movement pattern that persist as movement parameters or context is altered. For example, it has been suggested that we have a general motor program for writing our name and its instructions are recognized in the features common to signing our name under different conditions with different tools, different parameters of movement, even different sets of muscles (Raibert, 1977). Motor learning literature also ascribes to motor programs the ability to generate complex movements without benefit of concurrent feedback, such as reaching for a target after administration of a local anesthetic or tourniquet, as well as ballistic movements that may be completed before feedback can contribute to the movement (Schmidt & Lee, 1998). In each of these instances, motor programs are viewed as learned sets of instructions. In neurobiology, however, motor programs are also called pattern generators and are viewed as ge-

netically inherited sets of instructions that control the stereotypic features of innate behaviors such as mating, defense, and locomotion (Kupfermann, 1991). Some of the strongest arguments in neurobiology for the existence of general motor programs refer to the many examples of an animal's ability to execute functional movements in the absence of feedback (Lashley, 1917; Polit & Bizzi, 1979; Taub & Berman, 1968). Where the movement instructions are stored is yet to be determined, but some investigators implicate the sensorimotor cortex (Asanuma & Keller, 1991) and cerebellum (Sanes et al., 1990) in motor learning or the prefrontal association cortex in motor memory and planning (Kupfermann, 1991).

Dynamic-Based Theories

A more recent theory receiving broad interest in recent years, established to explain the development of motor control, is the dynamic systems theory proposed by Thelen and her colleagues (Thelen & Smith, 1994; Thelen & Ulrich, 1991). The theory seeks to address what drives skill acquisition and a particular problem poorly handled by previous theories: how does a child move from one developmental stage of skill to another? A fundamental hypothesis of the theory is that there are multiple identifiable variables, such as muscle power, body mass, arousal, neural networks, motivation, and environmental forces (e.g., gravity and friction), that establish a context for movement initiation and execution. A second fundamental hypothesis is that the relationship (interaction) among these variables is in constant flux and therefore shapes the features of a movement as it unfolds. Thus dynamic systems theory proposes that developmental changes in motor behavior and skill performance can be explained in terms of dynamics common to physical, biologic, and computational systems. Developmental stages are viewed as attractor states that are governed by a set of variables, and transitions in behavior are viewed as flips between attractor states powered by change in one or more of the variables. For example, an animal may be capable of producing coordinated limb movements for stepping but incapable of locomoting until related postural skills are sufficient (Bradley, 1992). Or the pattern of limb movements may abruptly vary with changes in movement parameters such as velocity (Thelen & Smith, 1994). Behavioral solutions are thus the composite solution of neural, biomechanical, and environmental forces acting in concert (Swinnen et al., 1994).

Recent theoretic work by Sporns and Edelman (1993) has extended dynamic theory by developing the notion of dynamic selection. Rather than assuming the existence of genetically predetermined motor programs, they hypothesize that motor skills emerge from an interaction between development-related changes in movement dynamics and brain structure-function. Given that musculoskeletal anatomy and related biomechanics change dramatically over the course of development, the theory is primarily concerned with how the brain's circuitry can readily change to match or accommodate these changes. The theory incorporates three key hypotheses: a developing organism is genetically endowed with spontaneously generated behaviors that make up the basic movement repertoire; it is also endowed with a sensory system capable of detecting and recognizing movements having adaptive value; and the developing organism can select movements having adaptive value by varying synaptic strengths within and between brain circuits such that successive event selections will progressively modify the movement repertoire. In essence the theory proposes that there is a "handshaking" relationship between evolving movement mechanics and ongoing maturation of brain circuits, all of which is edited or biased by the adaptive value of a movement experienced. Recognizing the value of a movement experience will strengthen the probability of repetition, strengthening a behavior; failure to recognize its value will reduce the probability of repetition, thereby weakening the behavior. Thus this latter theory embraces attributes of maturational, learning, and dynamic theories to explain motor control development.

Current Hypotheses of Motor Control

Rather than proposing some unifying theory, many current hypotheses of motor control attempt to identify controlling variables for specific types of movement. Central pattern generators (CPGs) are proposed to account for the basic neural organization and function required to execute coordinated, rhythmic movements, such as locomotion, chewing, grooming (e.g., scratching), and respiration. CPGs are commonly defined as interneuronal networks, located in either the spinal cord or brainstem, that can order the selection and sequencing of motoneurons independent of descending or peripheral afferent neural input. Neural input from select supraspinal regions, such as the brainstem reticular nuclei, activate central pattern generators, and peripheral afferents, propriospinal regions, and other supraspinal regions modulate the output of central pattern generators and adapt the behavior to the movement context. Work in invertebrate species suggests that pattern generators can even alter their own configurations (i.e., intrinsic modulation) to produce more than one pattern associated with the same or differ-

ent behaviors (Katz & Frost, 1996). CPGs can also modulate the inputs they receive, gating potentially disruptive reflex actions such as nociceptive activation of the flexor withdrawal reflex when a limb is fully loaded during the stance phase of locomotion (for further review of pattern generators, see Grillner, 1996; Levitan & Kaczmarek, 1997; Rossignol, 1996). Until recently, the early presence of orderly or coordinated motor patterns at the onset of embryonic movement appeared to suggest that CPGs, including those for locomotion, are established during initial differentiation of the nervous system (Bradley & Bekoff, 1989). However, recent cellular studies appear to indicate that embryonic behaviors are the product of transient neural networks (discussed later in this chapter) that may have little or no participation in mature pattern-generating networks (O'Donovan & Chub, 1997).

A number of hypotheses of motor control specifically attempt to explain how we control discrete arm movements. According to the equilibrium-point hypothesis, also called the mass-spring hypothesis, the nervous system strives to control joint position in space, and every position can be defined by a unique combination of agonist and antagonist muscle forces that result in a net stiffness (Feldman, 1986). It is argued that muscles function like springs, and once a motor program is sufficiently established, it activates the appropriate muscles to contract and move a limb segment until the segment reaches the point in space where all active and passive muscle forces are in equilibrium. The equilibrium points composing a trajectory or end point of movement are achieved as a function of neural commands that regulate coactivation of alpha and gamma motoneurons (Feldman, 1986). Experimental evidence for the latter point is found in studies of spinal-transected frogs indicating that spinal neurons code for spatial equilibrium points of the leg during grooming (Bizzi et al., 1991); however, recent experimental studies using human subjects suggest that end point knowledge is insufficient and that the brain must also have some knowledge of the movement dynamics (Gomi & Kawato, 1996). Other hypotheses attempt to distinguish whether we learn to control movement with respect to intrinsic body coordinates of joint position, referred to as joint space, or with respect to extrinsic coordinates, referred to as hand space in the case of reaching (Kalaska & Crammond, 1992; Scott & Kalaska, 1995). Finally, some hypotheses attempt to determine which parameters, such as time, distance, or force, are controlled during movement initiation before correction. Most notable among these, the impulse-variability model proposes that the nervous system controls movement by planning the phasing and duration of muscle contractions (for review see Meyer et al., 1990). For further discussions on hypotheses of motor control, the reader is referred to additional sources (Jeannerod, 1990; Schmidt & Lee, 1998; Swinnen et al., 1994).

Researchers are also investigating the use of models for motor control based on developments in the fields of robotics and neural networks. Both approaches seek to incorporate perception and action to explain control of movement. Robotic models are based on the physics of perception and movement, assigning mathematic values to known neural and biomechanical relationships to explain movement outcome. Currently, in the area of autonomous robotics there is interest in simulating principles of dynamic systems using a new method called computational neuroethology. The method attempts to account not only for the neural and biomechanical elements of a robot but also for environmental context and the new phenomena that may emerge during action within that environment (Chiel & Beer, 1997). Neural network models are based on the assumption that no simplistic, predictable relationship exists among nerve cells to explain movement, but rather it is the phenomenon of their complex interactions that is believed to explain the movement outcome. Thus neural networks focus primarily on specifying the array of cellular and network properties that may govern how a population of neurons will self-assemble under a given set of conditions. For example, CPGs are typically modeled as discrete populations of neurons, but more recent studies examining rhythmic behaviors in invertebrates (Levitan & Kaczmarek, 1997) and chick embryos (O'Donovan & Chub, 1997) suggest that at least in some systems, the behavior emerges from the populational dynamics of neural interactions. In a neural network model, rhythmicity is attributed to reiterative functions as a consequence of recurrent connectivity within the neuron population, and populational behavior is chiefly attributed to various inhibitory relays (i.e., reciprocal inhibition) and select intracellular mechanisms (i.e., inhibitory rebound). During development, populational behavior may vary as a function of changing cellular properties; for example, some immature neurons have excessively negative resting membrane potentials such that inhibitory transmitters induce transient depolarizations and potentiate immature excitatory connections within a neural network producing spontaneous activity. Furthermore, the populational behavior of neural networks may flip between two or more stable states as a consequence of either intrinsic or extrinsic transmitter regulation (Katz & Frost, 1996). Models of motor control are in a sense an end point, the assimilation of data from experiments testing hypotheses derived from theories. Models can then, in turn, be used to test the extent to which we can generalize the findings of studies testing hypotheses and theories. As ideas are put through these tests, we can become more confident in estimating how they may be effectively applied in addressing practical and clinical problems of motor control.

MOTOR CONTROL VARIABLES

Characteristic of contemporary motor control research is the notion that multiple variables contribute to the initiation and execution of a movement. Thus it is generally assumed that to understand how movements are controlled, one must be able to identify which variables are important and determine how they interact during movement. In this section we will identify some possible variables and consider how investigators currently think these variables contribute to motor control. Borrowing from the ideas of Bernstein (1967), some investigators speak of motor control variables as systems or subsystems of control composed of many intrapersonal and extrapersonal variables (Thelen & Ulrich, 1991). In more eclectic terms, variables may be anything, be it physical, physiologic, or psychologic, that has an impact on movement planning or execution. Thus to identify the underlying processes that determine skill acquisition during development, one must know not only which variables are important at a given age, but also how each variable changes during development and the impact of that change on all the other variables involved. To successfully accomplish such a task requires an experimentalist's approach that controls as many variables as possible while methodically manipulating the one in question, a task that is rarely feasible in human studies. Furthermore, if a variable is dynamically context specific, even the experimental approach may be too artificial to truly understand its impact on motor control. Nonetheless, researchers are attempting to identify variables that are critical to skill acquisition. By nature, these variables are interactive, but for convenience we will refer to them here as being sensorimotor variables, mechanical variables, cognitive variables, and task requirements.

Sensorimotor Variables

Sensorimotor variables are those physiologic mechanisms or processes that reside within the nervous system. Central pattern generators are an example of a sensorimotor variable. By selecting and timing the activity of motoneurons, they play a key role in determining the pattern of muscle activity during movement (Grillner, 1996; Rossignol, 1996). For example, in the case of locomotion, central pattern generators determine which muscles are active in the stance phase of gait and which are active in swing. Central pattern generators can produce motor patterns or synergies similar to those produced during normal behavior even when deprived of afferent (sensory) information, but pattern generators are not the only determinants of the synergies that characterize rhythmic movements. When a cat rapidly shakes a paw to dislodge an irritant, for example, a novel combination of flexor and extensor activity is produced, referred to as a mixed synergy. The mixed synergy is partially determined by a spinal central pattern generator and partially determined by motion-dependent feedback from the leg (Koshland & Smith, 1989).

Movement synergies and neural mechanisms that alter or regulate them can also be viewed as sensorimotor variables controlling movement. A common view is that the formation of synergies for movement is the nervous system's solution to controlling the multiple degrees of freedom inherent in coordinating a multisegmented body (Bernstein, 1967). Although synergies, such as flexor and extensor synergies, have long been viewed as the stereotypic motoneuron patterns inherent in spinal neural circuitry, current views suggest that movement synergies are context specific and highly individualistic (Keshner, 1990). Supporting this view, anatomic and physiologic data in cats suggest that motoneuron pools for biarticular muscles of the leg are actually a collection of smaller pools that can be separately recruited in a task-specific manner (Pratt & Loeb, 1991). For example, portions or all of these pools may be recruited depending on movement parameters such as velocity or acceleration (Zernicke & Smith, 1996). Other studies suggest that synergies characterizing voluntary movement, particularly of the upper extremity, may be controlled by premotor cortical areas because specific patterns of corticoneuronal activity in these areas can be recorded before the onset of practiced movements (Georgopolous, 1990; Ghez, 1991). Sensorimotor variables that may contribute to regulation of muscle synergies to enhance performance include mechanisms controlling joint stiffness (Hasan, 1986), joint net torque (Horak & Macpherson, 1996), visuomotor and visuospatial processes (Lee et al., 1990; Schmidt & Lee, 1998), and in essence, all other perceptuomotor processes tuned to participate in planning or executing a movement. Developmental aspects of sensorimotor variables also include processes of change such as differentiation and refinement of neural networks, changes in sensory perception, neural conduction characteristics, changing motor unit properties, and force-producing capabilities. The latter two topics will be considered more fully with respect to musculoskeletal development in Chapter 4.

Mechanical Variables

Mechanical contributions to motor control are of particular interest in many disciplinary areas of research. Changes in total body mass and relative distribution of mass during development are accompanied by changes in length and center of mass per body segment. These changes, in turn, alter inertial forces due to gravity and friction during movement (Zernicke & Smith, 1996). In some instances these inertial forces may assist movement. In other instances they may oppose movement (Jensen et al., 1997). Together with other variables, they help shape movement (Chiel & Beer, 1997; Zernicke & Smith, 1996). Studies in animals and humans have demonstrated that motor skills are greatly affected by inertial forces (Hoy et al., 1985; Schneider et al., 1990) and that part of learning to perfect a skill is learning to anticipate and use these forces to execute a movement more efficiently (Schneider et al., 1989). The viscoelastic properties of musculoskeletal tissues are also an important mechanical variable in the control of movement (Tardieu et al., 1989). The passive elastic attributes of these tissues contribute to action by absorbing and releasing energy and have been suggested to reduce neural programming requirements for movement execution (Schneider et al., 1989; Zernicke & Smith, 1996).

Cognitive Variables

Cognitive variables may include variables that are dependent on conscious and subconscious processes such as reasoning, memory, or judgment to optimize performance. Such variables might include arousal, motivation, anticipatory or feedforward strategies, the selective use of feedback, practice, and memory. Variations in arousal can probably modify any other control variable, such as pattern generation (Thelen et al., 1982), or even whether a behavior is demonstrated (Bradley, 1992). Motivation may make multiple contributions to the control of movement. In some instances it may serve primarily to trigger activity, and in other instances motivation may determine the form of the consequent movement. For example, it has been suggested that hand path is straighter during reaches for a moving target than for a stationary one because the infant is more motivated to reach and make contact with a moving target (Hofsten, 1991). Cognitive-related variables likely emerge with and assist in skill mastery; toddlers as young as 13 to 14 months of age having only a few weeks of standing experience can selectively determine when to use manual assistance for maintaining postural control while standing on an array of support surfaces (Stoffregen et al., 1997). Cognitive processes associated with action are also important for acquiring spatial maps (memories) of the movement environment (McComas et al., 1997), are apparent in earliest anticipatory behaviors during infancy (such as the anticipatory head and eye turning during games of peekaboo), and may be delayed or differently configured in children with Down syndrome (Aruin & Almeida, 1997).

Anticipatory strategies, also called feedforward strategies, are a select form of anticipatory behavior characterized by movement adjustments time locked to voluntary movements (Massion, 1992). In the control of posture, anticipatory strategies minimize equilibrium disturbance. In other acts, anticipatory strategies minimize the amount of attention dedicated to monitoring feedback and making corrections after initial movement execution. Although anticipatory strategies are not usually conscious cognitive processes, they involve subconscious forecasting processes (Massion, 1992) that are essential for minimizing movement errors during perceptuomotor tasks (Viviani & Mounoud, 1990) and sometimes require considerable training such as the anticipatory postural adjustments observed in dancers (Mouchnino et al., 1990). Indeed, it is argued that anticipatory strategies are learned, that they are relatively fixed under stable conditions, but are adapted in less fixed situations only by learning from past movement experiences (Massion, 1992). Anticipatory strategies are observed in postural adjustments before the onset of whole body movements (Nashner & Forssberg, 1986), postural adjustments prior to onset of arm movements (Horak et al., 1984), shaping and orientation of the hand before contact with an object to be grasped (Jeannerod, 1984), and strategies to time body movements with timing demands of the environment (Viviani & Mounoud, 1990). Children, like adults, demonstrate anticipatory postural adjustments in trunk and leg muscles before lifting the arms (Riach & Hayes, 1990) or rising onto tiptoe (Haas et al., 1989) as early as 4 years of age. Anticipatory strategies during preparation to grasp, however, can be observed as early as 9 months of age (Forssberg et al., 1991; Hofsten & Rönnqvist, 1988) and appear to be present by 4 postnatal months, as evidenced by postural adjustments in neck and trunk musculature when infants are about to be pulled to sit or picked up from supine (Bayley, 1969) and adjustments in gaze as they anticipate an object's trajectory (van der Meer et al., 1994).

Whether all of these anticipatory strategies share some fundamental means of regulation has not been addressed experimentally, to my knowledge, but it is speculated that similarities may exist between feedforward strategies in postural and arm trajectory control (Massion, 1992). Nor is there any clear locus of control for any of the identified anticipatory strategies. It is generally thought that anticipatory postural adjustments are controlled by local spinal cord and brainstem networks, as well as by transcortical loops, including the motor and premotor cortices (Massion, 1992). Models of feedforward control hypothesize that the controller is likely to be a network that receives and compares afferent feedback and information about the desired movement (efferent copy) to set gain adjustments for modifying movement commands as they are executed (Massion, 1992). They may also function to reprogram postural responses (Horak & Nashner, 1986) or delay initiation of the voluntary command (Massion, 1992) when the command is destabilizing. Limited evidence to date suggests that feedforward strategies emerge subsequent to feedback strategies during development of a skill such as postural control in stance (Haas et al., 1989), that they are disrupted in children with cerebral palsy (Nashner et al., 1983), and that they are delayed or inadequate in children with Down syndrome (Sugden & Keogh, 1990).

The amount of attention dedicated to monitoring a movement is also viewed as a variable that can be modified to perfect a motor skill. It has been suggested that during development, children initially execute new movements in a ballistic manner, ignoring feedback, then swing to the opposite extreme attempting to process excessive amounts of feedback, before finally learning to selectively attend to feedback. An example of this transition proposed by Hay (1979) is described under *Reaching* later in this chapter. It is generally thought that once the child (or adult) learns to selectively attend to feedback, more attention (or mental processing) can be assigned to reading the environment and predicting the environmental changes and movement outcome as the movement is executed (Keogh & Sugden, 1985). Other cognitive variables related to learning, such as form and quantity of practice and the role of memory, are addressed within the context of motor learning in Chapter 6.

Task Requirements

Task requirements can also be considered distinct motor control variables. Task requirements may include any variable that can contribute to or in some way alter movement, including biomechanical requirements, meaningfulness, predictability, or any other variable associated with a given movement context. Physiologic recordings from several sensorimotor centers of the brain indicate that their participation in a task is context specific (Crutcher & Alexander, 1990; Ghez, 1991; Lemon, 1988). Task requirements shape motor strategies such as the response selection to postural perturbations—for example, recover a posture, step into a new posture, or execute protective extension (Horak & Nashner, 1986). Task requirements can also result in the gating of reflexes—for example, a noxious stimulus applied to the foot may produce a flexor withdrawal response if the leg is in the swing phase of gait, but an extensor "contact" response if the leg is in the stance phase (Rossignol & Drew, 1986). Similarly, task requirements may alter the strategy a child uses to reach for an object (Hofsten, 1991), and evidence suggests that the meaningfulness of the task may enhance or mask performance (van der Weel et al., 1991). The role of meaningfulness is demonstrated by comparing performance when a child is asked to perform a relatively abstract task (e.g., instructed to repetitively pronate and supine as far as possible) versus a concrete task (e.g., instructed to strike a tambourine, a task requiring repetitive pronation and supination). Children with cerebral palsy generate larger movement excursions following the concrete instructions than after the abstract instructions (van der Weel et al., 1991). In summary, task requirements, like all other variables we have considered, appear to play a crucial role in the control of movement. Control variables may add to or subtract from movement such that there may be multiple possible behavioral outcomes for a given set of centrally generated movement instructions.

For therapists interested in learning- or dynamic-based theories, thoughtful analyses of task requirements can generate both a deeper understanding of the minimal requirements for completing a task and an array of hypotheses as to why a client cannot complete the task. Analysis can also assist in determining how to modify and reduce task requirements so that a client can successfully complete the modified version of the task. For example, if biomechanical variables are rate limiting (i.e., the task requires more muscle force or rate of change in force than a patient can currently generate), the therapist may look for ways of scaling the amount of force required. If leg extensor muscles are too weak for a patient to rise from regular-height chairs, treatment may consist of standing from chairs of greater height, from chairs with armrests of varying height, or from an array of surfaces under varying degrees of buoyancy (in a pool). If cognitive variables are rate limiting and the task requires analysis of the environment or anticipatory planning, the therapist may

try to simplify the environment by reducing the number of distracting stimuli or range of possible choices that can be made and identify ways to enhance the interest in and focus on an essential cue for motor planning. For example, while initially working on eye-hand coordination, distracting stimuli may be removed from the room, the amount of effort (i.e., strength, coordination, or postural context) required to reach may be reduced, and the amount of spatiotemporal uncertainty may be minimal to none. The task would include elements known to be of significant interest to the child (e.g., favorite toys, cartoon characters, colors, textures, sounds). As success is achieved, the competing stimuli may be gradually returned, the amount of spatiotemporal uncertainty may be increased, the amount of effort required may be increased (strength, coordination, postural context), and effort may be made to expand the child's interests or attention. Applying learning-based theories, the objective would be to provide an array of movement conditions associated with an array of possible movement consequences from which the child can formulate rules of association. Applying dynamic-based theories, the objective would be to provide an array of movement contexts that would allow the child to discover his or her own movement solutions (see also discussions by Aruin & Almeida, 1997; Latash & Anson, 1996).

MOTOR SKILL ACQUISITION IN CHILDREN

This section examines specific areas of motor development in children and the variables currently viewed as critical to the process of skill acquisition. As will be demonstrated, many of the apparently key sensorimotor variables for control of a skill are already present in the earliest phases of postnatal development, suggesting that the basic neural substrate for orderly generation of skilled movement may be in place months to years before maturation of the nervous system is complete and adult behaviors are observed. Although neural maturation of sensorimotor variables for motor control is necessary to attain adult levels of skill, it is not sufficient to fully account for how or when skilled movement is achieved. Here we will consider some of the variables identified by researchers and how these variables may contribute to the control of four specific skill areas—postural control, locomotion, reaching, and grasping—during development.

Postural Control

Postural control is achieved via the cooperative interaction of multiple neural systems (e.g., visual, vestibular, and somatosensory systems) and cooperating musculoskeletal components so as to meet the behavioral goals of postural orientation and equilibrium (Horak & MacPherson, 1996). Although each of the three sensory systems is considered essential to optimal control of both static and dynamic posture, each system can compensate to some extent for the other two (Horak et al., 1990), and the relative importance of each system appears to vary with contextual demands (Horak et al., 1989; Horak & MacPherson, 1996). As we will see, acquiring skill to process and use the ensemble of sensory information in selecting a motor strategy may more fully account for the postnatal development of postural control than indices of physiologic maturation of any given sensory system. Achievement of postural control is often described in terms that emphasize the closed loop or sensory feedback aspects of balance correction; adaptive postural control, however, also employs open loop or anticipatory strategies. These anticipatory strategies function to minimize potential postural perturbations arising with movement initiation. Thus the process of establishing effective anticipatory strategies may also more fully account for the development of postural control than indices of postnatal changes in the closed loop attributes of any given sensory system or its impairment during development (Horak et al., 1988). In this section we will consider the contribution of sensorimotor variables, most notably the visual, vestibular, and somatosensory systems, and other variables contributing to the acquisition of postural control.

Visual System

Vision is perhaps the most powerful sensory system functioning to regulate posture, both for feedback correction and for selection of anticipatory postural strategies (Butterworth & Hicks, 1977; Lee & Aronson, 1974). The first to ascribe a proprioceptive function to vision, Gibson (1966) suggested that as light from the visual field strikes the retina, changes in light associated with movement create "optical flow patterns" interpreted by the brain to determine the position of the head and body with respect to the surrounding environment. It is argued that the large-amplitude postural sway observed in blind individuals is due to the absence of this optical flow information (Lee, 1980). Optical flow patterns can evoke dramatic postural responses in both children and adults. In a now classic set of studies, Lee and Lishman (1975) demonstrated that when an adult stands inside a closed space formed by three walls and a ceiling, a forward or backward movement of the wall facing the person (center wall, Fig. 2-1) will trigger a larger sway amplitude (S) than under static

visual conditions; the effect is greater if the postural task is made more difficult (e.g., standing on one leg). The effect of this visual stimulus is greatest if the visual stimulus moves along the anterior-posterior axis of vision (referred to as a looming visual stimulus, A) and least effective if it moves tangential (side to side, B) to the visual axis. In the latter case, extraocular muscle activity during visual tracking is thought to provide proprioceptive information used to discriminate between environment and body movements (Butterworth & Hicks, 1977; Lee & Lishman, 1975). In general, if the subject faces the center wall as it is slowly moved toward the subject, the subject will sway backward; if the wall is moved away from the subject, the subject will lean forward. If the entire enclosure is moved sideways from the subject's left to right (or vice versa), however, little or no change in posture is detected.

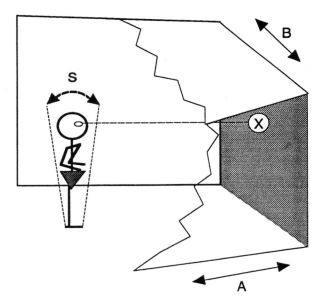

FIGURE 2-1. The subject is placed in the center of a partial room formed by three walls and a ceiling that can be slid along in direction A or B. When the subject is facing wall X, room motion in direction A creates a looming visual stimulus and triggers an increase in the magnitude of sway (S) in the anterior-posterior plane. Younger children are likely to sway closer to their limits of stability (noted by the dashed lines forming an inverted cone) when presented with a looming visual stimulus, but not when the visual stimulus moves side to side (direction B). (Adapted from Lee, DN, & Aronson, E. Visual proprioceptive control of standing in human infants. Perception & Psychophysics, 15:529–532, 1974.)

Children begin to demonstrate distinct postural responses to optical flow patterns early in development (Butterworth & Hicks, 1977; Lee & Aronson, 1974). When placed in the moving room, children 13 to 17 months old with 0.5 to 6.5 months of walking experience sway excessively and are apt to fall in response to a looming visual stimulus (Butterworth & Hicks, 1977). Postural responses to looming visual stimuli can be detected during stance as early as 5 months of age, preceding onset of independent stance (Foster et al., 1996). Forward-backward sway responses to looming visual stimuli are also observed during independent sitting in infants at 11 and 16 months (Butterworth & Hicks, 1977). The potential for visually triggered responses appears to be present by 2 postnatal months and perhaps as early as 6 postnatal days. For example, when a looming visual stimulus is presented to the infant supported in an infant seat, directionally appropriate neck muscle activity is observed; namely, approaching stimuli trigger neck extensor activity, and withdrawing stimuli trigger neck flexor activity (Yonas et al., 1977). Visual proprioception appears to play a dominant role in postural control during early childhood; if the eyes are closed during postural displacements in the anterior-posterior plane on a movable platform under conditions of normal vestibular and somatosensory information, the magnitude of sway for children 4 to 6 years of age is significantly greater than for children 7 to 10 years of age (Shumway-Cook & Woollacott, 1985a). By 7 to 10 years of age, children demonstrate responses similar to those in adults. Furthermore, it appears that if children lack visual information during development, they do not learn to minimize their postural sway to the same degree with increasing age as normally sighted children (Portfors-Yeomans & Riach, 1995).

Vestibular and Somatosensory Systems

The vestibular and somatosensory systems are also capable of generating directionally appropriate responses in the trunk and legs following anterior-posterior displacements in infants and toddlers in sitting (Harbourne et al., 1993; Hirschfeld & Forssberg, 1994) and in stance (Sveistrup & Woollacott, 1996). Commonly used testing methods and leg responses are illustrated in Figure 2–2. It is likely that vestibular and somatosensory systems participate in these postural tests during infancy because directionally appropriate muscle responses are generated even when infants are blindfolded (Woollacott et al., 1987). Directionally appropriate muscle responses are occasionally present during tests in sitting by 4 to 5 months of age (Harbourne et al., 1993). Directionally appropriate leg muscle responses are occasion-

ally present following the onset of mechanically induced sway by 7 to 9 months of age, as children master pull to stance and independent stance. Some infants can regain upright posture independently after the perturbation in stance and demonstrate directionally appropriate responses by 14 to 15 months, as they master independent walking (Haas et al., 1989; Shumway-Cook & Woollacott, 1985a; Sveistrup & Woollacott, 1996; Woollacott et al., 1987).

During the earliest phases of skill acquisition in sit and stance, activation of muscle responses tends to be slower and more variable than at subsequent phases of skill acquisition (Hadders-Algra et al., 1996; Shumway-Cook & Woollacott, 1985a; Sveistrup & Woollacott, 1996). As expected, latencies and consistency of response to tests of postural skill gradually approach adult levels of performance over childhood. It has been suggested that postural responses in infants and adults during sit and stance are produced by a central pattern generator (Hirschfeld & Forssberg, 1994). Argument for this view is that directionally appropriate responses to perturbations in sitting are generated as early as 4 to 5 months of age and before acquisition of independent sitting (Harbourne et al., 1993), suggesting that the response patterns are not acquired by learning (Hadders-Algra et al., 1996). Furthermore, according to this view, correct response selections are available in established central networks, but retrieval or activation of possible responses is variable because afferent and efferent neural components are immature. It is also possible that early responses are variable because young infants have not yet experienced and stored associations between the nuances of intertrial mechanical variability and best response. It is equally possible, borrowing from Sporns and Edelman's (1993) theoretic framework discussed earlier, that infants are inherently biased to produce a great array of responses so as to acquire sufficient memories for solving more challenging tasks at later ages. Variable responses also may be attributed to the availability of vision, for when vision is occluded infants produce more reliable vestibular and somatosensory-evoked neck responses following anterior-posterior displacements in sitting than when vision is available (Woollacott et al., 1987).

Intersensory Conflicts

Perhaps a more powerful account of initial limitations in postural control and progressive skill acquisition is set forth in studies that test a child's ability to manage intersensory conflict situations. Younger children find it nearly impossible to ignore visual information, even when it is grossly incorrect, as

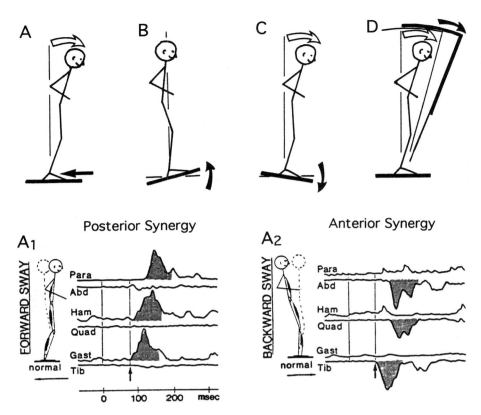

FIGURE 2–2. When a child is placed standing on a movable platform that is then displaced in the posterior direction at a fixed rate and duration (computer driven), the child sways forward and the posterior synergy is activated in a distal to proximal sequence over time to realign the head and trunk over the base of support (A_1). Conversely, displacement of the platform in the anterior direction produces a posterior sway that is corrected by activation of the anterior muscle synergy, also in a distal to proximal sequence (A_2). In both conditions illustrated, normal visual, vestibular, and somatosensory input are available. If the platform is rapidly rotated to produce ankle dorsiflexion (B) or plantarflexion (not shown), visual and vestibular inputs remain relatively stable throughout the perturbation, whereas somatosensory receptors register displacement. If, however, the platform is rapidly rotated in the same direction and synchronous with normal sway (C), somatosensory input remains relatively stable because the ankle angle changes little during the perturbation, whereas vestibular and visual receptors register the postural sway. Visual information regarding sway can be altered during testing by closing the eyes or by placing a dome around the head to provide a stable visual field (D). If vision is stabilized during platform translations, as in A, visual inputs will be in conflict with normal vestibular and somatosensory information. If vision is stabilized during platform rotations, as in B, both visual and vestibular inputs will be in conflict with somatosensory information. Finally, if vision is stabilized during platform rotations synchronized to normal sway (C), visual and somatosensory inputs will be in conflict with normal vestibular information. (Adapted from Nashner, LM, Shumway-Cook, A, & Marin, O. Stance posture control in select groups of children with cerebral palsy: Deficits in sensory organization and muscular coordination. Experimental Brain Research, 49:393–409, 1983, Fig. 1; and Horak, FB, & Nashner, LM. Central programming of postural movements: adaptation to altered support-surface configurations. Journal of Neurophysiology, 55:1369–1381, 1986, Fig. 2.)

underscored by the tendency of children to sway and fall when confronted by a looming visual stimulus (Butterworth & Hicks, 1977; Lee & Aronson, 1974). The looming stimulus presents a sensory conflict for the child; visual proprioception indicates that the relationship between posture and environment has changed, while vestibular information regarding the relationship between posture and gravity and somatosensory information regarding the relationship

between posture and support surface have not changed. Even in instances when visual and vestibular sensory information are reliable, conflicting somatosensory input, induced by rotation of the platform (see Fig. 2–2), will result in excessive sway or falls in 4- to 6-year-old children (Shumway-Cook & Woollacott, 1985a). However, a recent study using the moving room test (see Fig. 2–1) suggests that infants may start learning to reduce dependence on unreliable visual information shortly after they begin walking; the incidence of steps, staggers, or falls in response to room movement progressively declines with age after 3 or more months of walking experience (Foster et al., 1996). When children are presented with conflicting sensory information using computerized posturography tests that manipulate visual or somatosensory information (sensory organization testing, SOT) during stance on a movable platform, they are generally able to resolve the conflict and remain standing, but the magnitude of sway is increased from control levels, particularly in children 4 to 6 years of age. Postural responses during SOT approach adult levels of performance between 7 and 10 years of age (Rine et al., 1998; Shumway-Cook & Woollacott, 1985a).

Muscle Response Latencies

During stance perturbations, infants generate appropriate muscle responses even before they can sit or stand independently. When infants 4 to 5 months of age are manually supported in sitting and then briefly released, the lumbar paraspinals and hamstrings are recruited if the pelvis collapses anteriorly, whereas the paraspinals and quadriceps muscles are recruited if the pelvis collapses posteriorly (Harbourne et al., 1993). When infants 7 to 9 months of age stand with assistance on a moving platform, directionally appropriate responses may be observed in only one or two leg muscles. Muscle onset latencies under these conditions are greater and more variable than during independent stance at later ages (Hadders-Algra et al., 1996; Hirschfeld & Forssberg, 1994; Sveistrup & Woollacott, 1996). Children 4 to 6 years old often have muscle response latencies that are greater and more variable than children under 4 years of age. For example, when displaced in an anterior direction, children as young as 15 months of age sequentially activate the gastrocnemius and hamstrings, also referred to as the posterior synergy, at latencies within the ranges for children 7 to 10 years old; however, the average and range in temporal values for these parameters are considerably greater in 4- to 6-year-olds (Shumway-Cook & Woollacott, 1985a). It has been suggested that the greater variability observed in children 4 to 6 years old may reflect a period of transition as vision becomes less important and somatosensory information becomes more important in the control of posture (Shumway-Cook & Woollacott, 1985a). During this transition, children may be trying to process excessive amounts of information rather than selectively attending to the most pertinent sensory information, as has been suggested for other types of motor skill acquisition (Hay, 1979). Children may attempt

to process excessive amounts of information as a strategy for coping with limited ability to anticipate change in the environment (Keogh & Sugden, 1985). Yet another possible explanation for the variations in children's muscle response patterns may be found in variations in the biomechanics during testing (Harbourne et al., 1993; Hirschfeld & Forssberg, 1994).

Anticipatory Strategies

Cognitive processes for predicting the postural requirements and selecting timely anticipatory strategies in a given environment and movement context are also potential rate-limiting variables in postural control development. Typically, as we become expert in a movement task, we learn to recognize those sensory cues most reliable for predicting how the environment may change during movement execution, and we can learn to ignore less useful cues. Simultaneously, we learn to predict how our movements will change our relationship with respect to a more or less predictable environment and therefore determine the postural requirements for the task. In the adult, for example, when asked to rise onto tiptoes (from a plantigrade to digitigrade posture), ankle dorsiflexors are activated nearly 200 ms before ankle plantar flexors, apparently to shift the center of pressure at the foot-floor interface a sufficient amount forward before onset of postural elevation (Haas et al., 1989). Similar responses can be observed in some children as young as 4 years of age, the youngest children thus far cooperative in such laboratory recordings, whereas some children are unable to achieve digitigrade stance even by 10 years of age. The latter children exhibit insufficient anticipatory forward shifts in center of pressure before onset of postural elevation, with dorsiflexor to plantar flexor muscle onset latencies of less than 60 ms (Haas et al., 1989). Similar anterior shifts in center of pressure are present before raising an arm while standing at 4 years, the youngest age tested (Riach & Hayes, 1990), and activation of directionally appropriate leg muscle synergies is initiated before voluntary arm push-pull tasks at 7 to 9 years, the youngest age tested (Nashner et al., 1983). The overlap in refinements of feedback (perturbation-triggered corrections) and feedforward postural control in children between 4 and 10 years of age suggests that they are two distinct processes that emerge in parallel during development. Furthermore, it is suggested that children begin to learn anticipatory postural strategies to coordinate posture and locomotion with the onset of voluntary movements to sit and crawl (Haas et al., 1989). A recent study of rapid arm raising in stance suggests that anticipatory activation of trunk muscles is appropriate but delayed and center of pressure shifts at the feet are larger in individuals with Down syndrome than in age-matched control subjects (Aruin & Almeida, 1997), underscoring the potential importance of cognitive-related processes in postural control.

Biomechanical Constraints

In children under 4 years of age, it appears that some key rate-limiting variables are biomechanical in nature. Most notably, in the first postnatal year, the center of mass is proportionately higher than at any other age because of the combination of a large head and short limbs, requiring large force generation and regulation by neck and upper trunk musculature to counter the inertial forces created by displacements of the head. Second, in young walkers, the actual distance between floor contact and the center of mass is very small and results in much higher frequencies of postural sway with relatively larger arcs of motion than at later ages (Hayes & Riach, 1989; Usui et al., 1995). Consequently, younger children sway faster and closer to their limits of stability than older children and adults. Also, center of pressure along the anterior-posterior axis of the foot is more posterior at younger ages (Usui et al., 1995). Although younger children can produce adultlike muscle synergies for postural correction at latencies similar to adult values, given the aforementioned biomechanical constraints, adultlike responses may be too slow for regaining upright posture. Some developmental studies have also reported that the biomechanics associated with head position and pelvic rotation during perturbation trials can be notably variable (Harbourne et al., 1993; Hirschfeld & Forssberg, 1994). Thus it is likely that some trends in available postural data, such as the greater variability observed at younger ages, may be the consequence of small variations in postural alignment at onset of data collection trials rather than solely the consequence of an immature neural control system. That is to say, variable responses also may be the consequences of postural variations associated with behavioral variables such as restlessness, fatigue, apprehension, and novelty during laboratory testing.

Postural Response Strategies

Some mention should be made regarding the failure of researchers to find distinct sequences of development in postural responses (Perham et al., 1987). This probably reflects the fact that complex neuromuscular responses are available early in development, but that a child's ability to select the most favorable strategy and the immediate context in question are critical determinants. It is noteworthy that children with Down syndrome can produce correct neuromuscular patterns (i.e., posterior synergy with a distal to proximal activation of leg and thigh muscles) in response to postural perturbations in stance but the patterns are initiated at a greater latency than in other children of similar chronologic age (Shumway-Cook & Woollacott, 1985b). Thus, in children with Down syndrome, motor patterns for postural control appear to be available and similar to those in normal children, but may not be adequately timed to effectively regain upright posture before reaching the boundaries of stability in stance. Protective responses, however, appear to emerge before righting and equilibrium responses in children with Down syndrome (Haley, 1987), providing a highly effective strategy for limiting injury and a reasonably adaptive strategy if one cannot rely on other postural strategies.

Collectively, these findings and previous points of discussion suggest at least one possible hypothesis regarding the emergence of postural skills. Namely, children may possess the potential to produce a particular postural response despite the inability to evoke it under given testing conditions, but the postural response may be masked or overridden by more reliable strategies for a given context. The context specificity of a response is further underscored by the gradual changes in strategy observed over repeated trials when the postural perturbation is modified (Forssberg & Nashner, 1982). When children 4 to 6 years of age are subjected to repeated mechanical rotations of the ankle (into dorsiflexion) in stance, the posterior synergy is gradually suppressed because, under this context, activation of the synergy is potentially destabilizing (Shumway-Cook & Woollacott, 1985a). Furthermore, it appears that children begin to either consciously or subconsciously select a postural strategy from an array of possibilities (e.g., step, squat, reach for support pole) based on context as early as 13 to 14 months of age (Stoffregen et al., 1997).

Locomotion

The locomotor capabilities of the neonate and young infant have been vigorously explored in recent years. The theoretic bases and experimental designs for these studies were drawn from more than three decades of study into the control of locomotion in animals. Studies of locomotion and other rhythmic behaviors in animals have been important because they enabled investigations of motor control to move from a focus on classic reflex paradigms to the broader domain of natural, spontaneous motor behavior and the development of new research methods to study both naturally occurring behavior and corresponding physiologic systems under behaviorally restricted conditions. In particular, because locomotion is a rhythmic behavior with many kinematic and electromyographic (EMG) features that are repeated across cycles in predictable patterns under stable conditions, studies typically focus on the production of these features to test specific hypotheses of locomotor control and theories of motor control more generally. Because animal studies have contributed significantly to both the knowledge of and methods used to study locomotion in humans, and because they continue to influence clinical studies, such as the assisted weight support paradigms for treadmill locomotion, some animal studies on the control of locomotion will be considered briefly (for more details see Rossignol, 1996). Detailed discussion on the refinement of locomotion during childhood is presented in Chapter 3.

Development of Locomotion in Animals

Animal studies demonstrate the potential to produce either locomotion or potentially related forms of rhythmic limb movements during embryonic or neonatal development (Bradley & Bekoff, 1989). Newborn kittens, when separated from their mothers during feeding, take a few very hypermetric and awkward steps to return to their mother's teats, often falling in the process (Bradley & Smith, 1988). During these efforts, steps are occasionally characterized by the stereotypic features of reciprocal flexor-extensor EMG patterns similar to those occurring during adult locomotion. Adultlike muscle patterns are most readily apparent, however, when kittens are posturally supported while stepping on the moving belt of a treadmill or making stepping motions midair (airstepping). Typically, steps over ground are accompanied by extensive coactivation of antagonists at the ankle, suggesting that coactivation of ankle antagonists may be a functional strategy for increasing joint stiffness to compensate for limitations in postural control or muscle force production (Bradley & Smith, 1988). The appearance of adult features for locomotion in muscle activity of newborn kittens suggests that the neural networks for locomotion are established in the prenatal period. Studies of embryonic motility in chicks generally support this view because repetitive limb movements are characterized by orderly patterns of alternating flexor-extensor muscle activity (Bradley & Bekoff, 1990) and kinematics (Chambers et al.,

1995) across limb segments. However, the relationship between initial neural circuitry for embryonic motility and eventual locomotion has yet to be established (Bradley, 1999).

Parallels between Developing Animals and Humans

Several parallels can be drawn between studies of embryonic and neonatal animals and studies of rhythmic, locomotor-like leg movements in human infants. When supported on the treadmill, infants perform repetitive leg movements characterized by several kinematic features similar to adult locomotor behavior (Thelen & Ulrich, 1991; Ulrich et al., 1994; Yang et al., 1998b). Although infants 6 to 12 months of age become more reliable in producing a sustained pattern of alternating steps that is timed to the treadmill belt speed, even infants as young as 10 days of age occasionally demonstrate these features (Yang et al., 1998b). Neonatal infant stepping shares many features with early treadmill stepping. Most notably, hip, knee, and ankle joints are synchronously flexed during the swing phase and synchronously extended during the extensor phase; the excursions are accompanied by nonspecific EMG patterns; and there is an absence of both heel strike and push-off at the transitions between swing and stance (Forssberg, 1985). These features are also characteristic of infant kicking within the first 1 to 3 postnatal months (Jensen et al., 1994, 1995), suggesting that some of the mechanisms controlling treadmill stepping, and therefore locomotion, are already functional at birth.

The presence of some potential for locomotion at birth raises the question of whether that potential is established early in fetal development. Here again a parallel may be drawn with animal studies. Ultrasound studies of human fetal movement indicate that isolated kicks are initiated during the ninth embryonic week and alternating leg movements, reported to resemble neonatal stepping, are initiated with postural changes ("backward somersaults") in utero during the fourteenth embryonic week (de Vries et al., 1982). Thus human fetuses appear to exhibit stepping during the first half of the gestational period, about the same portion of the embryonic period when chicks exhibit organized EMG and kinematic features during spontaneous motility (Bradley & Bekoff, 1990; Chambers & Bradley, 1995). Given that low-risk preterm infants born at 34 weeks of gestational age demonstrate orderly kinematic patterns similar to those of full-term newborns, and that those features differing from full-term infants appear to be attributable to dynamic interactions emerging during movement (Heriza, 1988), the parallel between human fetuses and chick embryos appears reasonable (Fig. 2–3). In other words, the neural foundations for locomotion in humans may be assembled during neurogenesis, as they appear to be in other animals (Bradley & Bekoff, 1989).

Development of Locomotor Muscle Patterns in Humans

Until recently, it was believed that infant locomotion lacked adultlike features typically observed in EMG recordings. Failure to observe adultlike EMG patterns was often attributed to late myelinization of descending paths at caudal spinal levels (Sutherland et al., 1980), late maturation of cortical structures (Forssberg, 1992), or late myelination of peripheral nerves (Sutherland et al., 1988). However, in a recent study of treadmill locomotion, infants as young as 10 days of age occasionally produced steps characterized by alternating activation of antagonist muscles, and the extent of coactivation decreased with practice (Yang et al., 1998b). Furthermore, the relative duration of flexor and extensor burst durations varied with treadmill speed in a manner similar to that in adults. The failure to observe adultlike EMG patterns for locomotion in previous studies of prewalkers and early walkers may have been the result of adaptive strategies that masked this potential. For example, infants may have coactivated antagonist muscles to increase joint stiffness and stabilize limb posture as a compensation for insufficient postural control or control of force generation for supporting and transporting body mass (Bradley & Smith, 1988). Also, testing conditions may have masked the potential to generate adultlike locomotor EMG patterns; that is, support in stance or movement against gravity in supine likely altered the task requirements (Ulrich et al., 1994), necessitating a different EMG pattern. Conversely, the testing conditions may have lacked key features for expressing locomotor EMG patterns. For instance, in cats, the velocity of limb movements contributes to the generation of certain EMG patterns (Zernike & Smith, 1996).

Although there is wide support for the view that basic features of locomotion are spinally mediated, some argue that uniquely human features of gait emerge as spinal neural networks are transformed with maturation of higher neural centers (Forssberg, 1992). Specifically, it is argued that the basic patterns of alternating flexion and extension observed during neonatal stepping persist with development of locomotion, but that maturing sensorimotor input suppresses activation of ankle extensor motoneurons to permit heel contact at the onset of stance. As further support for this view, it is argued that the absence of heel strike in children with cerebral palsy is because cerebral injury impairs development of higher-center control over spinal neural networks for locomotion (Forssberg, 1985). Conversely, some researchers speculate that attributes of gait, such as heel strike, need not be specifically dictated by higher neural centers because they may emerge from the inertial interactions and associated feedback between body segments during movement (Thelen & Ulrich, 1991; Zernicke & Smith, 1996). For example, when cats walk at relatively fast speeds, the sartorius muscle produces a two-burst pattern, one during late stance and one during late swing, but the second burst does not consistently occur at slower walking speeds. Kinematic and kinetic analyses suggest that the burst in late swing functions to counteract extensor forces at the knee during faster walking speeds, but it is not required and therefore not recruited at slower speeds because viscoelastic properties of knee flexors are sufficient to counter these forces. Whether the muscle activity associated with heel strike is due to centrally organized commands or is the result of motion-dependent feedback has yet to be tested. Thus, to further explore neural versus cortical control of heel strike, one may experimentally test whether ankle angles during gait are velocity dependent. For example, do controlled increases in walking velocity produce larger dorsiflexion angles during swing? Perhaps the absolute velocities typically achieved during early locomotion are insufficient to express adultlike ankle control in the step cycle, or perhaps the rate of change in velocity is insufficient.

Biomechanical Variables

The emergence of locomotion during development is also determined by the interactive aspects of anatomy and environment during movement. Typically, infant stepping is not readily elicited beyond the first to second postnatal month under standard testing conditions, and it was long argued that the behavior disappears as a consequence of encephalization processes (the taking over of control) by maturing higher motor centers (McGraw, 1940). However, the postnatal decreases in rate of stepping temporally correlate with rapid weight gain, suggesting that morphologic changes in body mass may contribute to the "disappearance" of infant stepping. Two lines of evidence support this hypothesis. One, when infants are submerged in water up to chest level, both stepping rate and amplitude increase in comparison with stepping out of water (Thelen et al., 1984). Two, if weights equivalent to the weight gains at 5 and 6 postnatal weeks are added to the ankles of infants at 4 postnatal weeks, both stepping rate and amplitude decrease in comparison with stepping without ankle weights (Thelen

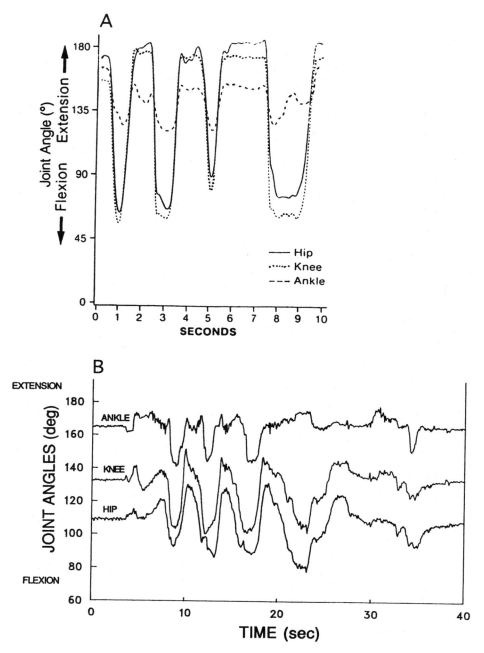

FIGURE 2-3. Kinematic analyses indicate that lower extremity movements are organized very early in development. When preterm infants initiate a sequence of several kicks at 40 weeks of gestational age, the alternation of flexion and extension at the hip is synchronous with motions of the knee and ankle in the same direction *(A)* and is similar to kicking movements during spontaneous motility in chick embryos in ovo at 9 embryonic days of age *(B)*. *(A,* Adapted from Heriza, CB. Comparison of leg movements in preterm infants at term with healthy full-term infants. Physical Therapy, *68*:1687–1693, 1988, Fig. 2.)

et al., 1984). Thus buoyancy appears to diminish the dampening effect of body mass and gravitational interactions, whereas added weight appears to augment the effect of these interactions. Results of animal studies underscore the notion that morphologic features of the organism interact with the environment to either express or mask potential abilities. Fetal rat pups, for example, exhibit interlimb coordination during spontaneous movements under buoyant conditions several days before testing under nonbuoyant conditions (Bekoff & Lau, 1980). Frog tadpoles exhibit coordinated leg movements several stages earlier in development if they can push off a mesh surface placed in an aquatic tank (Stehouwer & Farel, 1984). The latter point invites reconsideration of the discussion regarding heel contact in gait: heel strike may not be observed until independent walking is established because of immature morphologic characteristics of the infant foot interacting with a support surface. Given the considerable structural change the foot undergoes during the first postnatal year or more, it is conceivable that initial biomechanical features of the foot do not readily afford initiation of heel strike or push-off in the young infant.

Variables under Investigation

There is a growing interest in the relative contributions of mechanical and neural variables underlying control of leg movements in infants as methods for study of kinematic and kinetic methods become more affordable and less labor intensive. A collection of studies, for example, suggests that intersegmental dynamics are the critical determinants of leg coordination during kicking (Jensen et al., 1994, 1995; Schneider et al., 1990) and treadmill locomotion (Ulrich et al., 1994). During both kicking and supported treadmill locomotion, active muscle forces are used to initiate hip flexion against gravity, but it appears that gravity and passive (inertial) forces largely determine the spatiotemporal patterns of corresponding knee and ankle excursions. Furthermore, the extent of synchrony between leg joint rotations during kicking varies with the infant's posture and appears to be greater when the infant is supported upright than supine. The greater synchrony between leg joints in an upright posture may be due to the greater gravitation-related forces and therefore muscle force (and recruitment effort) required to overcome gravitational forces (Jensen et al., 1994). Conversely, the lesser synchrony between leg joints during supine kicking may be due to the more variable effects of gravity on the hip and ankle during the supine kick cycle. When the hip and ankle are positioned between 0 and 90°, gravity assists extension, whereas gravity assists flexion as joint position

exceeds 90° (Schneider et al., 1990). During both kicking and treadmill locomotion, the swing phase appears attributable to active flexor (muscle) forces at the hip, whereas the extensor phase is primarily attributable to gravity and passive (inertial) forces and, to a lesser extent, active flexor (muscle) forces as hip flexor muscles lengthen (Fig. 2–4).

Animal studies continue to offer insights and a source of inspiration for probing variables underlying development of locomotor control in human infants. Paradigms developed to study spinal control of interlimb coordination have been adapted to determine whether similar mechanisms may control reciprocal stepping in human infants. For example, when infants are supported on a treadmill and one leg is blocked during swing phase, the stance phase of the contralateral leg is lengthened, as in adult cats and humans (Yang et al., 1998a). Responses vary with extent of loading in the stance limb (e.g., increases in load result in lengthening of extensor burst duration and delay in onset of swing), which indicates that human infants as young as 3 months of age possess mechanisms for adaptive stepping observed in cats and kittens and attributed to spinal circuitry (Yang et al., 1998a). Nonetheless, studies in cats show that cortical centers normally play an important role in these adjustments, indicating that perception and planning are important neural contributions to control of locomotion (Drew, 1993). Animal studies also indicate that experience-based learning is important for refining rudimentary locomotor skills. For example, findings from a kinetic study of locomotion in neonatal chicks suggest that practice is required to acquire efficient energy absorption strategies for yield in stance (Muir et al., 1996).

Reaching

The past 20 years have seen dramatic demonstrations and reappraisals of the reaching abilities of newborn and young infants. In commonly employed static testing situations with the infant placed supine, reaching for a dangling, stationary target, such as a red ring, is initiated at approximately 3 to 4 postnatal months. Yet investigators have demonstrated that if newborns are adequately supported in an inclined posture and presented with a moving target, rudimentary eye-hand coordination can be distinguished from random hand movements within days after birth. By 4 months of age, infants are adept at contacting a moving object, and by 9 months they demonstrate adultlike reaching patterns as they catch a moving object. In this section, features characterizing the development of reaching and tracking skills will be described. For additional

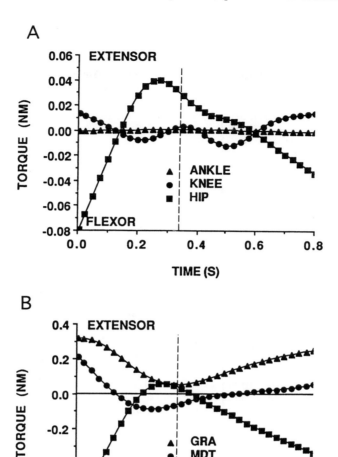

FIGURE 2–4. Motions of adjacent limb segments during kicking may arise from active forces due to muscle activity and passive forces due to gravity and inertia of the limb segments. For example, in the data presented here, an infant initiates a kick cycle starting from a semiextended position of 125° and achieves a peak flexion of 80° at 0.32 second (vertical dashed line) before the hip returns to the extended position. The motion into flexion is attributable primarily to an initial hip (HIP) flexor force or torque that is maximal at the outset (0.0 s) and begins to drop off as the hip moves into flexion *(A)*. The hip flexor force is due to active muscle force (MUS) during the first 0.2 second *(B)*. An extensor force develops between 0.2 and 0.3 second *(A)* as active hip flexor force decreases to 0 newton-meter *(B)* and serves to slow and reverse the hip motion into extension (0.32 s). Throughout the extension of the hip, there are small passive extensor forces due to gravity (GRA) and inertia (MDT) and a growing active hip flexor force (MUS) to lower the leg (B). (Adapted from Schneider, K, Zernicke, RF, Ulrich, BD, Jensen, JL, & Thelen, E. Understanding movement control in infants through the analysis of limb intersegmental dynamics. Journal of Motor Behavior, *22*:493–520, 1990, Fig. 3.)

discussion on the control of reaching, the reader may wish to refer to more comprehensive texts (Swinnen et al., 1994; Thelen & Smith, 1994).

Rudimentary Reaching Skills

A growing body of work suggests that arm movements of the neonate, like kicking movements, are rudimentary expressions of skilled reaching that emerges during the first postnatal year. Even arm movements of newborns appear to be purposeful (van der Meer et al., 1995) and spatiotemporally structured (Hofsten & Rönnqvist, 1993). It is generally held that reaching in the neonatal period is visually triggered and that hand trajectories are directed actions. For example, the number of arm movements is significantly greater when 3-day-old infants visually fixate on an object than when they do not (Hofsten, 1982). Similarly, when presented with a ball, a picture of a ball, or a blank card, infants 8 to 16 days old make more directed arm movements when presented with the ball or picture than the blank card (Rader & Stern, 1982). The directness of neonatal reaches was quantified in a study of 3-day-old newborns supported in a reclining infant seat and presented with a stimulus moving in an arc 12 cm from the eyes (Hofsten, 1982). Measurements for every hand movement exceeding 5 cm indicated that forward-extending arm movements were aimed much closer to the target (32° off target) while infants visually fixated on a target than while they looked elsewhere (52° off target) or closed their eyes (54° off target). Presentation of an object in the visual field elicited longer horizontal and vertical hand paths during arm movements than when no stimulus was present (Bergmeier, 1992). The directness of early reaching may indicate that there is a genetically established neural coordinate system that links the trajectories of the hand with the face and visually fixated objects within reach (Hofsten, 1982). Furthermore, ultrasound evidence of hand-to-face contact by 10 weeks of gestation (de Vries et al., 1982) suggests that there is a basic, genetically scripted neural network linking hand space with body space by the end of the first trimester of fetal development. Alternatively, early hand trajectory may be an emergent product of biomechanical variables rather than the product of detailed neural commands (Corbetta & Thelen, 1994; Fetters & Todd, 1987).

Infants 1 to 19 weeks of age, when presented with a slowly moving object, continue to display interest in the object, but during the weeks that neonatal reaching is transformed into functional reaching, the role of vision appears to change somewhat, and there are periods when reaching is less readily observed. Age-dependent declines in reaching responses are reported to occur between 8 and 16 postnatal days (Rader & Stern, 1982) and in the seventh postnatal week (Hofsten, 1984). Because neonatal reaching was initially viewed as a primitive, reflex-like behavior, the age-dependent decline was attributed to maturation of descending neural inputs, an argument similar to that for the "disappearance" of infant stepping (Connolly, 1977). It has also been suggested that the decline in reaching may occur because object contact, and therefore behavioral reinforcement, is rare, or because the infant does not have sufficient optimal opportunities (e.g., postural context) to practice during this time period (Bower, 1979). Alternatively, as infants become more interested in looking at objects, visual attention may inadvertently extinguish neonatal reaching efforts (Bergmeier, 1992). In the neonatal period, the hand is typically open during forward extension of the arm (Hofsten, 1982), but around the seventh postnatal week, when the rate of reaching briefly decreases, infants seem more interested in looking at the object and the hand posture is more likely to be fisted (Hofsten, 1984). Around 12 postnatal weeks, however, the frequency of reaching increases, and the hand resumes an open posture during reaches (Hofsten, 1984). During this time period, infants appear to acquire some ability to visually determine realistic reaching distances because they rarely initiate effort to contact objects out of reach (Field, 1977). Between 12 and 16 weeks, infants acquire considerable skill in aiming their reaches (Hofsten & Rönnqvist, 1988). By 15 weeks, infants can contact a moving object in as much as 90% of trials, and between 15 and 18 weeks, contact shifts from just touching to catching the moving object (Hofsten, 1979). Vision functions to elicit reaching throughout the transition from neonatal to functional reaching, but it is not used to guide hand trajectory (Lasky, 1977; Wishart et al., 1978) or to orient the hand toward the object before initial contact during this transitional period in skill level (Lockman et al., 1984). In fact, infants do not appear to require vision of their hands for initiating reaching or contact and grasp of an object (Clifton et al., 1993). These findings seem to suggest that younger infants initiate reaching using a ballistic strategy to aim the hand toward the target and then switch to a feedback strategy (vision, proprioception, or both) to make corrective movements for grasping once the object is contacted (Clifton et al., 1993). At 4 to 5 months, reaches are as good with vision available during the reach as when vision is removed after onset of the reach (Clifton et al., 1993; Wishart et al., 1978), and infants begin to adjust their gaze, anticipating the future trajectory of an object (van der Meer et al., 1994).

Infant Reaching Strategies

During the period from 12 to 36 postnatal weeks, several major changes occur in the form of reaching that suggest the development of a new control strategy (Hofsten, 1991). To determine how reaching is perfected and to investigate strategies used to control reaching during development, the velocity and distance paths of hand transport are measured from video records of infant performances. Based on standard research methods used in studies of adult behavior, trajectories are dissected into movement units, each containing one acceleration phase and one deceleration phase. Adult reaches are characterized by 1 to 2 movement units; the first unit functions to transport the hand 70 to 80% of the distance to the target, and is relatively long in duration, and the second unit functions to home in on the object and is relatively short in duration (Jeannerod, 1981). Between 19 and 31 postnatal weeks, infants progressively restructure reaches for a moving object from an average of 4 movement units per reach to 2 movement units (Hofsten, 1991); yet even at 19 weeks, 22% of reaches contain only 1 or 2 movement units. The sequencing of movement units is also modified;

the transport unit is the first movement unit in half of the reaches at 19 weeks, extending an average distance of 80 cm, whereas at 31 weeks, it is the first unit in 84% of reaches and extends 137 cm. Finally, the hand path trajectory straightens with age (Fig. 2–5), suggesting that, by 31 weeks, improved spatial planning contributes to advances in aiming skill as the hand is now transported closer to the target in a more efficient manner during the first movement unit, requiring fewer subsequent units to correct for errors (Hofsten, 1991).

This pattern of control does not appear to apply, however, when infants 5 to 9 months of age reach to grasp a stationary object placed on a horizontal (table) surface (Fetters & Todd, 1987). Under these conditions, movement units tend to be similar in duration (200 ms) for all ages, reaching distances, and positions (or order) within a reach (Fig. 2–6). Furthermore, there may not be a decrease in the number of movement units within the path or a change in the straightness of hand path under these conditions between 5 and 9 months. Both hand path distance (equivalent to twice the shortest possible distance) and mean reaching duration (800 ms) also appear to

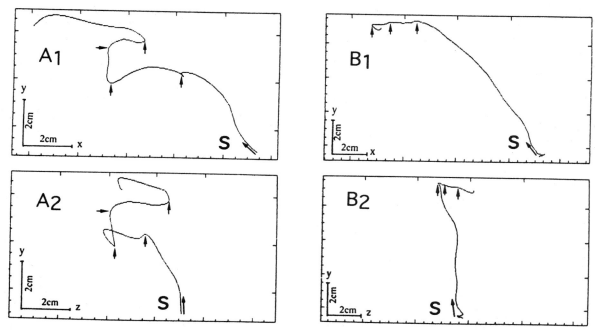

FIGURE 2–5. Hand paths become straighter and contain fewer movement units during the first postnatal year when reaching for a moving target. During a reach at 19 weeks of age *(A)*, 5 movement units are identified (by arrows) in views from the front *(A₁)* and the side *(A₂)*. Note that these movement units are similar in length. During a reach at 31 weeks of age in the same infant *(B)*, only 3 movement units are identified from the front *(B₁)* and side *(B₂)*. Note that most of the reaching distance is covered in the first movement unit. (Adapted from Hofsten, C von. Structuring of early reaching movements: A longitudinal study. Journal of Motor Behavior, 23:280–292, 1991, Figs. 3 and 4.)

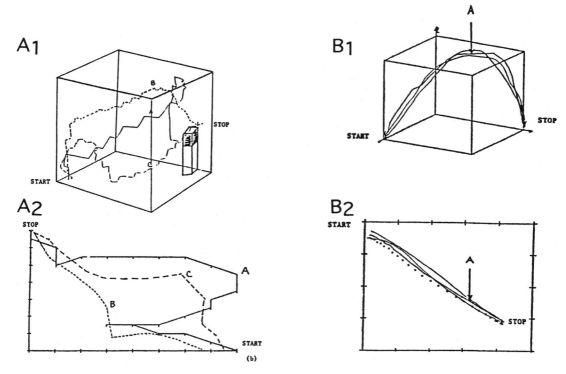

FIGURE 2–6. When reaching for a stationary object, infants exhibit reaches containing multiple movement units similar in duration. Three reaches are shown for a 9-month-old infant from a side view *(A₁)* and an overhead view *(A₂)*. Note the irregularities both within and between reaches as compared with adult performance from the side view *(B₁)* and overhead view *(B₂)*. (Adapted from Fetters, L, & Todd, J. Quantitative assessment of infant reaching movements. Journal of Motor Behavior, *19*:147–166, 1987, Figs. 4 and 5.)

be stable across ages and within adult limits, only more variable. These findings suggest that the movement speed and curvature of early functional reaching observed under stationary reaching conditions may be fundamental properties of both skilled and unskilled reaching controlled by biologic or physical constraints emerging from body-environment interactions (Fetters & Todd, 1987). These findings also point to the effect of task context on measurements used to explore control variables and the likelihood that control strategies vary with context (Hofsten, 1991). It has been suggested, for example, that hand path is straighter when reaching for a moving object than when reaching for a stationary one (Hofsten, 1979).

During the period from 5 to 9 months, infants begin to use visual information at the end of the reach as the hand approaches the target to correct for errors in hand path trajectory (Hofsten, 1979). Before 5 months of age, they take little notice of the hand during flight, but thereafter, if vision of the hand is blocked, as when infants reach for a virtual (mirror image) object, performance is frequently dis-

rupted (Lasky, 1977). Although infants continue to use a ballistic reaching strategy well into childhood, withdrawal of visual feedback begins to impair reaching skill at 6 to 7 months (Lasky, 1977; Wishart et al., 1978). To determine how reaching movements are controlled, investigators have explored parameters that characterize the straightness of the hand trajectory. In adults, the curved hand path during reaching is composed of straight line segments linked sequentially. The end of one segment and beginning of the next corresponds to a speed valley (deceleration and reacceleration) and a change in direction of the hand (Jeannerod, 1981). It is thought that each movement segment is ballistically generated and that corrections are made at these junctions between movement segments. To test whether path corrections are necessarily restricted to these speed valleys, Mathew and Cook (1990) examined the curved hand path in reaching trials of infants between 4 and 8 months old presented with a suspended object having some motion. Three-dimensional analyses of hand trajectories indicated that the initial movement segment is directed to-

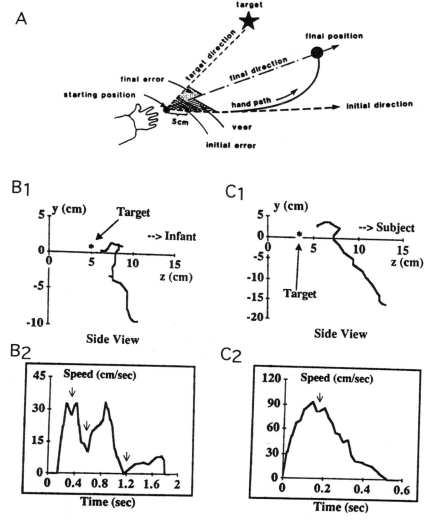

FIGURE 2-7. Analyses of hand path trajectories indicate that corrective movements occur throughout the reach even in young infants. Measurements of veering within a movement unit *(A)* indicate that initial hand trajectory is oriented toward the target and that correction in hand path is not limited exclusively to speed valleys (arrows in B_2 and C_2) adjoining consecutive movement units. Speed valleys, characteristic of adult reaching *(C_2)*, are also characteristic of infant reaching at as early as 6 postnatal months *(B_2)*, but are more numerous and greater in relative magnitude due to the greater number of irregularities in hand path *(B_1* versus *C_1)*. (Adapted from Mathew, A, & Cook, M. The control of reaching movements by young infants. Child Development, *61*:1238–1258, 1990, Figs. 1 and 2.)

ward the object at all ages tested and that changes in the path after reach onset tend to curve the hand toward the target to correct for error (Fig. 2–7). Also, measures of hand speed within a movement segment correlate with veering of the hand toward the target within the movement segment, suggesting that error correction occurs continuously rather than only at discrete intervals in hand transport. The relationship between veering within a movement unit and target location may indicate that when vision is available, reaching is not executed using a ballistic strategy. On the other hand, continuous veering within a movement unit may be the biomechanical consequence of projecting the arm through space, a notion that is consistent with the equilibrium point hypothesis for joint position in the mass-spring model of arm control (Hofsten, 1991; Polit & Bizzi, 1979).

During the first postnatal year, interlimb coordination of the arms and hands during reaching is characteristically variable. It has long been argued that early unilateral reaching is a consequence of asymmetric tonic neck reflexes, and bilateral reaching emerges as these reflex influences lessen (Fagard, 1994). Other possible explanations for variability in reaching strategies may be postural context during the reach and the characteristics of the target object (Fagard, 1994). In a longitudinal case study of one infant from 3 to 52 weeks of age, instances of bimanual reaching appeared to correlate with more variable kinetics, greater limb stiffness, and greater reaching velocities in the following arm as compared with the leading arm. These findings led the investigators to conclude that bimanual reaching predominates until infants learn to differentially control the following arm at approximately 6 to 7 months (Corbetta & Thelen, 1994). The degree of coupling between arms during reaching also appears to depend on the complexity of bimanual cooperation required, that is, whether one hand can remain relatively passive or must produce complementary movement patterns such as when holding a box lid up with one hand while extracting a toy with the other. Complementary bilateral reaching skill emerges at 9 to 10 months (Fagard & Pezé, 1997).

Reaching Strategies in School-Age Children

Studies in older children suggest that reaching strategies change very little from 9 months until approximately 7 years of age, at which time there appears to be a transitional period leading to an adult reaching strategy. When the visual field is displaced by a prism, children 5 years of age reach out to the apparent target location in 1 or 2 movement units before making corrective movements to move the hand to the actual target location (Hay, 1979). In contrast, 7-year-olds execute multiple small movement units (referred to as early braking), producing hand paths that begin to veer toward the actual target location early in the path, and 9- to 11-year-olds execute an initial movement unit that approaches the virtual target location but is then followed by a second, corrective unit (referred to as smooth braking) that alters the path before the hand reaches the virtual target location (Fig. 2–8). These findings suggest that 5-year-olds continue to use ballistic strategies much like those of older infants, whereas 7-year-olds constantly monitor their movements in a closed loop strategy to control their reaches. Between 9 and 11 years of age, children begin to combine these strategies to increase the efficiency of their movements and to reduce the amount of attention required (Hay, 1979; Keogh & Sugden, 1985). Consistent with these findings, a more recent study examining perceptual skill during an arm positioning task found that in the absence of vision, 8-year-olds produced greater errors in move-

ment amplitude than both 6- and 10-year-olds, yet at the end of a trial, using kinesthetic information, they were able to detect and reduce the magnitude of their end point error (Hay et al., 1994).

In a related vein, one current view of the clumsiness seen in children with mild to moderate movement dysfunction is that a sensory or attention problem hinders the ability of these children to identify or selectively attend to the most pertinent information during a reach (Schellekens et al., 1983). For example, study of hand paths during movement between two buttons in a repetitive tapping task in 8- to 10-year-olds with minimal neurologic dysfunction suggests that these children must constantly monitor and correct their actions. It is believed that using this closed loop strategy leaves little opportunity to attend to information for executing anticipatory adjustments and minimizing the amount of error correction required. In comparison with age-matched controls, children with minimal neurologic dysfunction appear to execute more movement units per reach. The first movement unit is less likely to be the longest unit or to achieve the greatest acceleration, and each unit tends to contain more acceleration irregularities (Schellekens et al., 1983). Not surprisingly, these children tend to have more difficulty maintaining task orientation. It is generally thought that children with these types of movement dysfunction tend to rely heavily on vision, when it is available, to assist manual tracking of a continuously moving stimulus (a coincident-timing task) with a predictable path. Once again, clumsy children (ages 6 and 11) are slower than age-matched controls (van der Meulen et al., 1991a). Their movement distance during an acceleration phase is more variable than that of control children, their tracking motions are more delayed, and they perform more trials with apparently suboptimal attention. When these children are presented with an unpredictable tracking task, they have greater difficulty attending to the task than age-matched controls, perhaps because they cannot identify a compensatory strategy (van der Meulen et al., 1991b). When presented with a predictable tracking task, however, 7-year-olds with minimal brain dysfunction give themselves more time to cope with less efficient reaching skills by planning a hand trajectory that will intercept a moving target further along its trajectory (Forsström & Hofsten, 1982). For discussion on the establishment of coincident-timing strategies, the reader is referred to a review by Goodgold-Edwards (1991).

In summary, the variables and processes that contribute to an emerging control of reaching skills during infancy and childhood are similar to variables contributing to those for posture and locomotion. In each instance, rudimentary aspects of control can

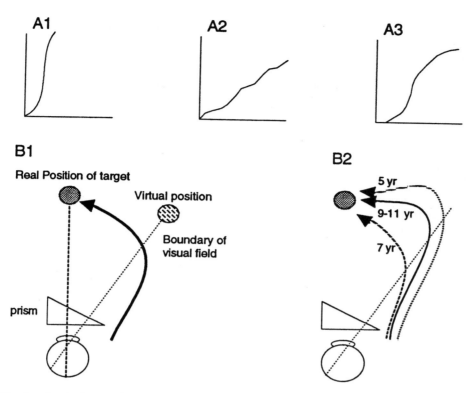

FIGURE 2–8. Hand paths during reaching to a stationary target correspond to the use of visual information to plan and control reaching. Ballistic reaches exhibit smooth trajectories with no distinct points of path correction, suggesting that they are preplanned and executed open loop *(A₁)*, whereas early braking reaches are executed closed loop, using vision to continuously monitor and correct error *(A₂)*. Late-braking reaches, in contrast, combine open loop and closed loop strategies to maximize reaching efficiency by preplanning 70 to 80% of the trajectory and then correcting trajectory error in the final approach to the target *(A₃)*. The use of these three strategies can be demonstrated by using a prism to displace the visual field *(B₁)*. Under these conditions, it is apparent that children 5 years of age use a ballistic reaching strategy, because they correct their hand path only after they have reached or surpassed the target's virtual position *(B₂)*. In contrast, 7-year-olds, using an early braking strategy, identify the discrepancy between real and virtual target position as soon as the hand enters the visual field, and 9- and 11-year-olds, using a late-braking strategy, almost reach the virtual target position before detecting the discrepancy. (Adapted from Hay, L. Spatial-temporal analysis of movements in children: motor programs versus feedback in the development of reaching. Journal of Motor Behavior, *11*:188–200, 1979, Figs. 1 and 4.)

be observed in very young infants if optimal conditions are provided, suggesting that some neural contributions to control of these skills are established in the fetal or neonatal period of development. In each instance, early skills appear to be more or less automatic; that is, they appear to be activated by relevant stimuli and shaped by contextual variables, such as the biomechanical interactions of moving body segments in space. Feedback does not appear to play an important role in controlling these early skills. Each of these early skills, however, undergoes important transformations as children learn to monitor their movements, predict the potential consequences of their actions for a given context, and develop anticipatory strategies for efficient movement execution.

As shown in the following section, these variables also contribute to the development of grasp control.

Grasping

Hand function has long been viewed as one of the key responsibilities of the motor cortex. Classical studies linked onset of fine motor milestones with myelination of the lateral precentral gyrus (Lawrence & Hopkins, 1976). Based originally on pyramidal lesion studies in monkeys (Lawrence & Kuypers, 1968), it is generally accepted that reaching and grasping are controlled by separate subcortical neural systems. Following lesion of the lateral brainstem, monkeys cannot control hand movements independently of arm movements, yet they can use the limbs for walking and climbing. After lesion of the ventrolateral path, in contrast, monkeys can no longer control the posture of the limb, but they can pick up food with their hands. Recent studies suggest that the potential for coordinated hand movements may be present earlier than previously appreciated and that anatomic changes in descending neural paths, although necessary, may not be sufficient to account for development of hand control. For example, ultrasound recordings indicate that human fetuses begin extending their fingers during isolated arm movements by 12 weeks of gestation (de Vries et al., 1982), long before myelination of the corticospinal tract can account for these rudimentary actions. Furthermore, observation of spontaneous hand movements in neonates indicates that the hand is not always in a stereotypic posture of flexion (closed fist) or extension (open). The hands continuously move between these extremes and, in so doing, they exhibit considerable variability, suggesting that the potential for independent finger control is present at birth. By 3 months, index finger forces can be clearly differentiated from those of other fingers during grasping (Lantz et al., 1996). If there is sufficient neural substrate to produce motor commands for independent finger actions at birth, why do fine motor milestones typically emerge several months later? In this section, the acquisition of grasp control and recent studies identifying variables that may help account for acquisition are reviewed.

Rudimentary Perceptual Control of Grasping

Although reaching and grasping skills are intimately related in a functional sense, control of grasping is distinguished from control of reaching by the different roles ascribed to the anatomic structures discussed above and by apparent differences in perceptuomotor control of these two skills (Hofsten, 1990). The initial trajectory of reaching (phase 1 reaching) is based on visual definition of the object's location in space and executed using a ballistic or open loop strategy, processes that do not appear to be linked with control of grasping. During execution of the reach (phase 2 reaching), visual feedback (Jeannerod, 1981) or proprioceptive feedback (Prablanc & Pélisson, 1990) may be used to define arm position as part of a closed loop strategy to correct for initial errors in trajectory. At the onset of phase 2 reaching, the hand is open maximally and then begins to close just before target contact, suggesting that anticipatory preparation for grasping is integrated with phase 2 reaching (Jeannerod, 1981).

Data indicate that before 2 months of age, infants execute only the ballistic phase of reaching, and

activity of the hand is not separately controlled from that of the limb to attempt grasping. The hand is typically open during neonatal reaching; however, hand posture is independent of the reach trajectory and does not vary with or without visual fixation of the target (Hofsten, 1984). Thus the prevailing view is that during reaching in the neonatal period, the arm and hand are synergistically coupled (Hofsten, 1990). This synergistic link between arm and hand is said to be functionally disconnected at approximately 2 postnatal months when the hand is more frequently fisted during arm movements into extension. By 3 months, the hand begins to open once again during reaching, but only when the infant visually fixates on the target (Hofsten, 1984). Such gains are typically attributed to anatomic changes in corticomotoneuronal connections (Lawrence & Hopkins, 1976), but another variable to consider at this age is the development of binocular coordination for depth perception (Hofsten, 1990). Acquisition of grasp control at this particular period of development may be primarily attributable to the emergence of adequate visual processing for learning how to implement closed loop (visually dominated) control of hand movements. By 4 months, infants can use vision to correct hand trajectory when it is displaced by a prism (McDonnell, 1975). By 5 to 6 months, infants expect to see their hand during a reach, but if vision of the hand is blocked, their performance is disturbed (Lasky, 1977). Furthermore, infants 5 to 6 months of age use visual information for adjusting grip configuration relative to object size (Newell et al., 1993). Around 6 postnatal months, infants can occasionally execute an adultlike (phase 1 and 2) reach-to-grasp movement pattern, and by 9 months, they can execute the pattern reliably (Hofsten, 1979). To briefly return to an earlier question regarding control of independent finger movements, we might hypothesize that independent finger movements and grasping skills emerge in the middle of the first year because the visual system is now sufficiently operational to employ and sculpture available corticomotoneuronal networks or because infants at this age have finally acquired a sufficient amount of initial visual experience of the hand to master control of the fingers. The extent of these visual experiences of the hands, in turn, may be limited initially by postural requirements (e.g., stabilizing both head and hand position to visualize the effects of self-initiated finger actions) such that postural control may be another rate-limiting variable in acquisition of independent finger movements. As suggested by others, the essential constraints on development of grasp control have yet to be determined (Newell et al., 1993).

Emergence of Anticipatory Control

With the onset of functional reaching, infants begin to develop perceptual abilities for reading the environment in such a way as to shape reaching and grasping skills. At the onset of functional reaching, they are not inclined to reach for objects that are placed at the perimeter of their reach (Fetters & Todd, 1987). At 5 months of age, they begin to orient their hand toward the object, either just before or at the beginning of the reach (Hofsten & Fazel-Zandy, 1984), as well as shape the hand in anticipation of object size constraints during manipulation (Newell et al., 1993). At this age, infants primarily rely on contact with the object to orient and successfully grasp the object, but over the next 3 months, infants begin to use visual information to both anticipate contact and orient their hand with respect to the object (Lockman et al., 1984). When adults reach to grasp an object, the distance between index finger and thumb is set with respect to object size at the onset of reaching (Jakobson & Goodale, 1991; Jeannerod, 1981). Anticipation of object size is similarly observed in the hand posture of 9- to 13-month-old infants during reaching (Hofsten & Rönnqvist, 1988), suggesting that young infants quickly learn to preprogram reaches for object size, location, and distance on the basis of visual information. The grasp of infants older than 9 months continues to exhibit some immature features, one being the relatively constrained range in hand opening when infants are presented with an assortment of objects varying in size. The hand may open in exaggerated postures, often considered residual retention of more primitive or yet undifferentiated manual behaviors due to corticomotoneuronal immaturity (Twitchell, 1970). Alternatively, infants may open the hand widely as a strategy to compensate for limited ability to estimate the task requirements for grasping an object (Hofsten, 1990); adults exhibit similar exaggerated hand postures when visual feedback is either withdrawn or its availability is unpredictable (Jakobson & Goodale, 1991). Anticipatory strategies are also apparent in control of precision grip and load forces, as discussed next.

Maturation of Precision Grip and Load Force Control

Once contact is initiated, the infant must coordinate normal (grip) and frictional (load) forces to grasp and lift an object (Johansson & Westling, 1988). Adults coordinate these forces synchronously, whereas infants and young children coordinate them sequentially (Forssberg et al., 1991). To quantitatively examine grip control, infants are encouraged to pick up a toy that is equipped with force transducers to measure the grip forces of the opposing thumb and index finger and the load force necessary to lift the object off the table (Fig. 2–9). During the preload phase (initial contact with the object), infants as young as 8 months of age contact the object with one finger before the other, creating a latency to onset of grip force that is significantly greater than in infants 18 months of age or older. Infants and young children also tend to press down on the object, creating a negative load force before reversing the direction of force to successfully lift the object off the table. Infants and young children generate a significant portion of the total grip force (often twice the magnitude of adult grasps) for grasping before initiating the load force, and during the load phase they typically exhibit multiple peaks in records for both of these forces. Adults, in contrast, scale the increases in grip and load forces in an economic, synchronous, and nearly linear manner with only a single peak near the middle of the load phase (Forssberg et al., 1991). These findings suggest that the smooth execution of an adult grasp is the consequence of anticipating the object's weight so as to select an appropriate target force magnitude and scaling over time (Johansson & Westling, 1988).

The recent studies on control of grasp (Forssberg et al., 1991, 1992, 1995) are consistent with a reoccurring theme of this chapter: infants appear to possess the neural substrate to execute skilled motor patterns early in development, but demonstration of this potential is unreliable. First, these studies indicate that by 8 months of age infants can produce each of the actions required for a precision grip, and by 12 months of age infants can occasionally assemble all the components to produce adult-like force patterns, but there is considerable variability in performance across trials. These studies also indicate that infants and young children use far more force than required, a common finding in studies of motor development (Keogh & Sugden, 1985). It has been suggested that the variability and excessive forces used in their strategies may be the consequence of immature corticospinal pathways or motor units (Forssberg et al., 1991). On the other hand, variable performance and use of excessive force may be compensatory strategies to cope with limited experience and one or more limited perceptuomotor abilities, such as the ability to extract sufficient information from visual input and limited ability to estimate the potential consequences of a motor action. Children as young as 2 years of age are able to adjust grip and load forces with respect to the degree of friction or potential slip during repeated lifts of the same object, but when the coefficient of friction is randomized over trials, they cannot adapt grip and load forces effectively. Thus with sufficient practice they

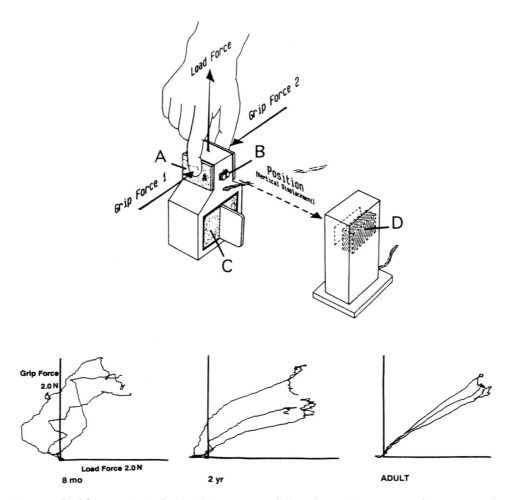

FIGURE 2–9. One method for quantitatively describing grasping skills and examining aspects of motor control is to measure the combination of grip and load forces over time. Precision grip force is the net normal force exerted by the index finger (Grip Force 1) and thumb (Grip Force 2), and load force is the tangential or friction force exerted when lifting the object against gravity (positive values) or pushing the object down into the table (negative force). The mass of the object can be varied by exchanging weights (C), and displacement of the object can be detected by infrared diodes (B) and a sensor (D). By 8 months of age, infants first press down on the object (negative X values), then increase grip force (positive Y values) before initiating a load (positive X values) to lift the object. By 2 years of age, positive load and grip forces are scaled in a synchronous, more linear fashion similar to that in adults, and negative loading force is less apparent. (Adapted from Forssberg, H, Eliasson, AC, Kinoshita, H, Johansson, RS, & Westling, G. Development of human precision grip. I. Basic coordination of force. Experimental Brain Research, 85:451–457, 1991, Figs. 1 and 4.)

can formulate rules for more adult-like performance, but if confronted with uncertainty, they do not know how to draw from limited previous experience.

Because it was assumed that the nervous system is hierarchically organized, it was widely held in the developmental literature that cortical control over reflexes determines when various forms of grasping emerge or disappear by dominating or inhibiting an action, or failing to accomplish either because of immature neural transmission (Twitchell, 1970). Such assumptions do not appear to be compatible,

however, with current electrophysiologic studies of the motor cortex. Although motor cortex and corticospinal inputs function to recruit hand muscles (Lemon & Mantel, 1989), motor cortex activity does not exhibit a consistent relationship with respect to either a movement or a movement-related activity in other areas of the brain. Such inconsistencies have led investigators to support a heterarchic rather than hierarchic view of motor control (Kalaska & Crammond, 1992). Recent studies on the control of the precision grasp in children with cerebral palsy also challenge these assumptions and demonstrate that maturation of the motor cortex and corticomotoneuronal pathways, although necessary, are not sufficient to account for the development of either normal or abnormal motor control (see also Newell et al., 1993). Variables such as anticipatory control and effective use of feedback information also must be considered if control of movements is to be more fully understood. When normal children 6 to 8 years of age are asked to grasp and lift a 200 g object repeatedly, they initiate nearly synchronous, linear increases in grip and load forces with a single peak in magnitude, as do adults. Children with cerebral palsy (diplegia or hemiplegia), in contrast, tend to initiate the forces sequentially, as do younger normal children (Eliasson et al., 1991). That is to say, at least some children with cerebral palsy can produce the requisite forces, but they have difficulty selecting or executing efficient grasp strategies. Available data indicate that these children have difficulty regulating the timing and magnitude of force during both dynamic and static phases, and they tend to bear down on the object before lifting it (Fig. 2–10). When these children are asked to grasp and lift objects of two different weights, presented in blocked and randomized trials, they also have difficulty scaling forces with respect to object weight during both nonrandom and random presentation of the two weights (Eliasson et al., 1992), but if they are given a sufficient number of practice trials, they can anticipate and scale grasp force parameters (Eliasson et al., 1995; Steenbergen et al., 1998). Children with cerebral palsy may also have difficulty stabilizing their gaze so that they can effectively use the available visual information (Lee et al., 1990). Given that the normal acquisition of grasp control has a protracted period of development (Forssberg et al., 1991, 1992, 1995), it is also possible that these children do not experience sufficient amounts and variety of practice to use available information for developing efficient strategies, an issue previously raised by Goodgold-Edwards (1991).

Refinements in the control of grasping continue to occur well into late childhood. Young children execute grasps characterized by multipeaked variations in grip and load forces and do not execute the smooth, coincident increases and decreases in these forces characteristic of adult grasping until approximately 8 years of age (Forssberg et al., 1991). Transitions to smooth, single-peak force patterns may in part be due to gradual improvements in anticipatory strategies. To test the use of anticipatory strategies, children 1 to 15 years of age lifted each of two different weights over 6 consecutive trials and then over 25 trials with the weights randomly presented (Forssberg et al., 1992). Results suggested that children as young as 1 to 2 years of age scale grip and load force based on information from the preceding lift of the object, and by 2 to 3 years of age, they can use this information to adjust the rate of increase in grip and load force for each weight. Furthermore, 2- to 3-year-olds can transfer weight information from lifts with one hand to modulate lifts with the other hand (Gordon et al., 1994). It appears that the scaling of grip and load force rates continues to change until approximately 8 to 15 years of age, depending on the order of presentation of the weights, suggesting that anticipatory skills do not achieve adult levels until some point in this age range. Children begin to use visual information (size of object to estimate its weight) to anticipate task requirements and scale grip and load forces by 3 to 4 years of age (Gordon et al., 1992). Data seem to suggest that by 5 to 6 years of age, children can make compensations for slip (Forssberg et al., 1995) and adjust lifts with one hand based on lifts with the other hand (Gordon et al., 1994) with skill approaching adult levels of performance but require more practice than adults to do so.

Collectively, the studies described in this section demonstrate that grasping is a complex skill involving many different aspects of sensorimotor control. Innate or rudimentary skills, biomechanics, experience, and other context-dependent variables probably contribute to the rapid changes in motor control observed in the first year of life. Even during earliest exercise of skill, infants are probably building a database of information for transforming their skills as they become increasingly more intent on shaping their experiences. Probably one of the views enjoying the greatest consensus among researchers in the field of motor control today is the view that all aspects of movement execution, including the basic physiology, biomechanics, perceptual processing, and development of strategies, must be closely examined under varying movement conditions to better understand the acquisition of motor control during normal development and when it goes awry.

MOTOR CONTROL RESEARCH: CLINICAL IMPLICATIONS

The implied assumption of motor control research is that it will advance clinical interventions to improve or restore motor function limited as a consequence of disease or injury. This is indeed an exciting time for those researchers and clinicians interested in building links between movement science and clinical rehabilitation practice to improve examination and treatment of movement problems. New ideas and approaches are emerging as scientists and clinicians test the generality of theory-driven find-

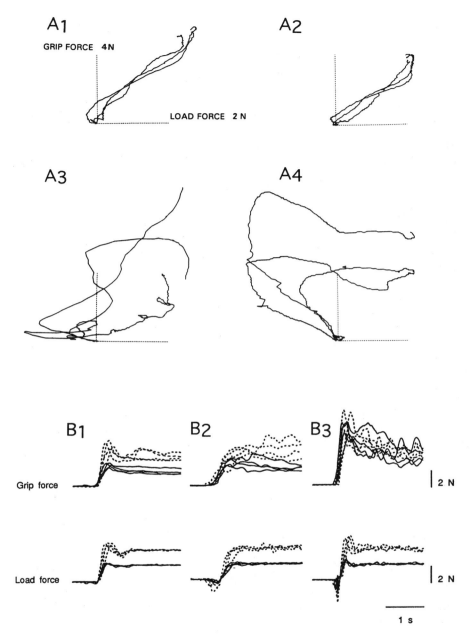

FIGURE 2–10. Children with cerebral palsy demonstrate some of the same force patterns during grasping to lift as those observed in younger normal children. Although age-matched (6 to 8 years old) normal children *(A₁)* exhibit synchronous scaling of grip and load forces, some children with diplegia *(A₃)* or hemiplegia *(A₄)* exhibit marked negative load force at the onset of a grasp, serial ordering of grip and positive loading forces, and grip force magnitudes twice that of normal children. However, children with less severely disabling cerebral palsy, such as one child with mild diplegia *(A₂)*, may exhibit more normal, age-appropriate grasp patterns. In addition to difficulty coordinating grip and load forces, children with hemiplegia *(B₂)* and diplegia *(B₃)* have greater difficulty scaling grip force with respect to object weight than normal children *(B₁)*. During lifts of a 400 g weight (dashed lines), normal children apply larger grip forces than for a 200 g weight (solid lines), and grip force quickly peaks and then drops to a stable level. Grip forces in children with cerebral palsy, in contrast, are slow to reach peak magnitude, are unstable during the static phase of the lift, and are not scaled reliably with respect to object weight. (*A,* Adapted from Eliasson, AC, Gordon, AM, & Forssberg, H. Basic co-ordination of manipulative forces of children with cerebral palsy. *Developmental Medicine and Child Neurology, 33*:661–670, 1991, Fig. 4. *B,* Adapted from Eliasson, AC, Gordon, AM, & Forssberg, H. Impaired anticipatory control of isometric forces during grasping by children with cerebral palsy. *Developmental Medicine and Child Neurology, 34*:216–225, 1992, Fig. 3.)

ings applied to various patient populations. It will take well-designed studies addressing specific links between science and practice, however, to know precisely the implications of motor control studies for specific problems encountered in rehabilitation practice. In this section, some possible implications of movement science for clinical practice are briefly discussed with respect to examination and treatment of motor control problems.

Clinical Assessment Tools

The vast majority of tools currently available for examination of motor control are based on neural maturation or learning theories, but more recently developed tools appear to reflect changing views of development, such as that espoused by the dynamic systems theory. Maturational-based tools can be readily identified by an emphasis on reflex testing (Palisano, 1993). Such tools focus on reflex, or evoked, behaviors because it is assumed that expression of these behaviors indicates the level of neural integration and function achieved (Touwen, 1984). In many of these tests, little or no consideration is given to other variables that may enhance, depress, or otherwise alter expression of the evoked behaviors. Even some maturational-based tools are beginning to consider broader views of motor development, however, as variables such as state behavior (e.g., level of arousal) are included in testing protocols or grading of responses. In many cases, the theoretic underpinnings of a given assessment tool are not so clear. For instance, some motor assessment tools are composed of tests to determine milestone achievements and may be viewed as indicators of the extent of neural maturation and corticospinal control, as posed by McGraw (1940, 1945), or as behavioral indicators of cognitive maturation, as originally posed by Piaget (Keogh & Sugden, 1985). In other instances, examinations are composed of milestones solely because they appear to display statistical or diagnostic significance (Hopkins & Prechtl, 1984). Tools incorporating a dynamic-based view of development attempt to examine spontaneous, self-produced movements under more naturalistic conditions, recognizing that multiple variables contribute to movement (Hadders-Algra & Prechtl, 1992). All motor assessment tools provide some indication of ability or extent of control, but we have yet to realize tests that tell us precisely how and why control is limited or has broken down, and this is one of the greatest barriers in our efforts to bridge the gap between the research lab and the clinic. In this section, the following tools for examination of motor skill acquisition will be briefly reviewed with respect to some of the motor control issues discussed in this

chapter: General Movement Assessment, Dubowitz Neurological Assessment, Movement Assessment of Infants, Gross Motor Performance Measure, Miller Assessment for Preschoolers, Sensory Integration and Praxis Tests, and Assessment of Motor and Process Skills.

General Movement Assessment

A quality of General Movement Assessment (GMA) examines the spontaneous movements of preterm and term newborns and young infants (Einspieler et al., 1997). The GMA has been broadly applied to term and preterm infants with an array of clinical diagnoses in recent years, suggesting that it is an effective tool for predicting neurologic outcome at 2 years of age, cerebral palsy in particular (Prechtl, 1997). The examination consists of observation and classification of spontaneous movements while the infant lies in the supine position. Only movements generated while the infant is in an awake, noncrying state are analyzed and classified by movement quality. Classifications include writhing, fidgety, wiggling-oscillating, saccadic, and swatting, and classification definitions distinguish frequency, amplitude, power, speed, flow, irregularity, and abruptness of the movements. Based on ethologic methods, the design of the GMA reflects a theoretic view that maturation is not a fixed sequence of differentiation, but rather a continuous transformation of behavior (Hopkins and Prechtl, 1984). The theoretic framework of the GMA also incorporates the views that general spontaneous movement is a distinct, coordinated pattern of activity in the healthy newborn and that self-organizing neural networks, extrinsic factors, and endogenous maturational processes are likely contributors to the emergence of the different movement qualities (Hadders-Algra & Prechtl, 1992).

Recent applications of the GMA tool suggest that it is reliable, is valid, and has strong predictive potential for examining the neurologic status of a preterm, term, or young infant. Intertester agreement appears to be good to strong, sensitivity is strong across age groups from preterm to 3 months corrected age, and specificity is strong by 3 months of age (Einspieler et al., 1997). Low specificity at earlier ages is attributed to spontaneous resolution of early dysfunction. The GMA appears to exhibit greater sensitivity and specificity than neurologic examination in brain-damaged preterm and term infants between 26 weeks of gestational age and 6 months corrected age (Cioni et al., 1997a, 1997b). Movements that are disorganized, excessively monotonous, cramped, or stereotypic are highly correlated with neural malformations or severe brain lesions (Albers & Jorch 1994;

Bos et al., 1998; Ferrari et al., 1997). It is interesting to note that GMA scores do not appear to correlate with neurologic examinations consisting of commonly elicited reflexes and behaviors or muscle tone (Geerdink & Hopkins, 1993; Hadders-Algra & Prechtl, 1992).

Dubowitz Neurological Assessment

The Dubowitz Neurological Assessment of the Preterm and Full-Term Newborn Infant is an example of a tool based on traditional, neuromaturational views of development, designed to examine preterm and full-term infants soon after birth and during the neonatal period for the purpose of detecting deviations or resolutions of neurologic problems (Dubowitz & Dubowitz, 1981). It consists of 32 items evaluating four areas: response decrement to repeated stimuli, movement and tone, reflexes, and behavior. Using a five-point scale, scoring of each item is criteria referenced and criteria are ordered according to expected changes with increasing gestational age. The infant's state of arousal is considered in the interpretation of findings. Selection and design of the test items for the Dubowitz Neurological Assessment were based on four criteria: expected findings for full-term infants at 3 days of age; good agreement between observers; some measure of higher neurologic function; usefulness for examining ill infants. Test items are examiner-evoked responses with the exception of one item for describing the quality of spontaneous body movements and another for identifying the presence of specific abnormal movement or posture. The authors report that a cluster of abnormal scores, such as the presence of asymmetries or increased tone and diminished leg mobility, may indicate that an intraventricular hemorrhage has occurred (Dubowitz & Dubowitz, 1981) and motor abnormalities may eventually emerge (Dubowitz et al., 1984). They also suggest that an abnormal score during initial examination may be of less prognostic significance than milder but more persisting signs. From the findings, it may be suggested that these examiner-evoked movements provide very little information on the control of movement or its development, except when viewed collectively, and even then the primary information seems to be an indication of general neural intactness, not of the specific motor pathologic processes likely to unfold. The lack of sensitivity to specific motor function or dysfunction in these types of examinations may be because the test procedures only superficially screen brain function, but reasons for dysfunction can be varied and even multifactorial. Nonetheless, recent study of the tool suggests that scores correlate with perinatal risk rating,

ultrasonography findings, and neurologic status at 1 year, leading investigators to suggest that the Dubowitz Neurological Assessment is a valid tool and may be used to develop management protocols in the neonatal intensive care unit (Campbell, 1999; Molteno et al., 1995).

Movement Assessment of Infants

The Movement Assessment of Infants (MAI) is a tool designed for the purposes of identifying motor dysfunction, changes in the status of motor dysfunction, and establishment of an intervention program for infants from birth to 1 year of age (Chandler et al., 1980). The MAI is a criterion-referenced examination composed of 65 items selected to evaluate four areas: muscle tone, reflexes, automatic reactions, and volitional movement. Each item is scored on a scale of 0 to 4 or 0 to 6 points and checked for asymmetric or rostrocaudal variations to obtain an "at-risk score" for motor dysfunction. Like other maturational-based assessment tools, the current version of the MAI contains many examiner-evoked test procedures and it does not attempt to control for contextual variables such as state of arousal. It does include, however, items to examine spontaneous motor features such as self-initiated postures and behaviors commonly identified in milestone schedules of development that are scored for quality or level of proficiency. Theoretic justification for items of the MAI has not been specified, but it would appear that each is included for its statistical potential to discriminate abnormal deviations in motor development.

Unlike many assessment tools currently available, the test properties of the MAI have been studied by several investigators and the findings reviewed (Palisano, 1993). In general, studies seem to indicate that reliability is weakest for items requiring handling of the infant by the examiner and greatest for those not requiring handling (Haley et al., 1986). Studies also appear to indicate that the MAI is sensitive, readily identifying deviations in motor development that may predict motor dysfunction at later ages, but that it exhibits poor specificity because it also identifies some normal infants (Schneider et al., 1988) and infants with transient medical problems as being at risk for later motor dysfunction (Harris, 1987; Swanson et al., 1992). It appears that the most consistently reliable and predictive portion of the MAI is the section on volitional movement, because it is the only section to exhibit a strong relationship with outcome (at 18 months) at both the 4-month and 8-month examinations (Swanson et al., 1992). To date, there does not appear to be any data to suggest that the MAI can predict the types or cause of motor dysfunction likely to emerge during development, nor is there evidence that the MAI effectively addresses the tasks (treatment and change in status) for which it was also designed. Investigators indicate that there is continued effort to improve the MAI (Swanson et al., 1992).

Gross Motor Performance Measure

The Gross Motor Function Measure (GMFM) (see Chapter 1) and its companion, the Gross Motor Performance Measure (GMPM), were specifically designed to examine the status and change in status of motor proficiency due to therapeutic interventions in children with cerebral palsy (Boyce et al., 1991; Russell et al., 1989). The theoretic basis for design of the GMFM was the measurement property of responsiveness, or ability to show change in motor function, in a population of children from 5 months to 12 years of age and having cerebral palsy. Studies suggest that the GMFM is both a responsive (Russell et al., 1989) and valid (Bjornson et al., 1997) measurement tool. The GMPM consists of 20 motor skills commonly performed by normal children less than 5 years of age derived from the GMFM that measure proficiency in eight areas of motor function: activities in supine, prone, four-point, sitting, kneeling, and standing positions and during walking and climbing. Each item is scored for three attributes using a criterion-referenced scale to indicate the postural alignment, selective control and coordination, and stabilization of weight during the task. Most items involve either movements requiring a change in posture, such as during progression (crawling or walking) or action while maintaining a posture (extending an arm while in sitting or four-point position). The GMPM was designed to examine qualities of movement believed by therapists to be problematic but amenable to intervention in children with cerebral palsy. The use of physical aids or orthoses is noted on the score sheet, but use of these is not reflected in scoring and no other possible variables affecting motor control are considered. The GMPM does not examine qualities of performance such as speed, effort, or efficiency, nor can it specify the underlying cause of dysfunction in control. Study of GMPM measurement properties by the authors suggests that reliability is excellent but construct validity is uncertain (Boyce et al., 1995). There appears to be moderate agreement between GMPM and GMFM scores for children with cerebral palsy and age-matched controls, but poor agreement between GMPM scores and therapists' ratings of performance. Nevertheless, there appears to be good agreement between changes in GMPM scores and therapists' indications of improvement in children with cerebral palsy, suggesting that the GMPM is a responsive motor performance assessment tool (Boyce et al., 1995).

Miller Assessment for Preschoolers

The Miller Assessment for Preschoolers (MAP) was designed as a screening tool to identify mild or moderate delays in development of children between approximately 3 and 6 years of age at risk for future school-related problems and to refer them for more in-depth examinations (Miller, 1982). The current version of the MAP consists of 27 core items to address sensory, motor, cognitive, and combined abilities, drawn from previously existing tools based on statistical support, time required to execute an item, and extent of equipment required. Sensorimotor items include tests of position and movement sense, stereognosis, postural stability, mobility, and coordination (fine motor, gross motor, and oral motor). Unlike most available motor assessment tools, some sensorimotor items are specifically treated as cognitive dependent, such as the ability to sequence or imitate movements. The assessment also considers the role of behavior (e.g., concentration, need for reward, social interaction) in examining performance. To date there have been only a few studies of limited scope evaluating MAP measurement properties and the test's usefulness (Daniels & Bressler, 1990; Miller, 1988; Schneider et al., 1995). As in other tests available, the MAP can describe motor abilities and limitations, but the assessment does not delineate precisely why or how motor control has broken down.

Sensory Integration and Praxis Tests

The Sensory Integration and Praxis Tests (SIPT), formerly known as the Southern California Sensory Integration Tests, are sensorimotor assessment tools for children between the ages of 4 and 9 years having mild to moderate learning impairment in the absence of frank organic disease, mental retardation, and primary sensory deficit (Ayres, 1989). Unlike many assessment tools, the theoretic basis for design, sensory integration theory, is precise and composed of three primary postulates: (1) learning is dependent on the intake and processing of sensory experiences from movement and the environment; (2) deficits in sensory processing can lead to deficits in motor planning and execution; and (3) active participation in meaningful tasks can improve sensory integrative processes and motor learning (Fisher & Bundy, 1992). The assessment tool consists of 17 tests. Initial portions of the SIPT examining balance, proprioceptive and tactile sensation, and control of specific movements are used to identify whether there is a sensory processing disorder in one of three areas, vestibular-proprioception, tactile discrimination, or sensory modulation, that may be indicative of integrative dysfunction. If a cluster of scores suggests dysfunction in one of these areas, subsequent portions of the SIPT are used to identify a disorder in bilateral integration and sequencing praxis, somatodyspraxia, or sensory modulation. Although the SIPT seeks to identify only sensory processing problems, it examines motor performance across a broad range of tasks that include tests for tactile discrimination, movement planning, tactile defensiveness, perception of form and space, and visuomotor coordination. Like most formalized examinations of sensorimotor abilities, the SIPT is standardized; however, the SIPT is scored by computer (at Western Psychological Services in the United States). Because the SIPT is a relatively new test, there are as yet few studies available on measurement properties and test usefulness (Cermack & Murray, 1991; Kimball, 1990; Mulligan, 1996).

Assessment of Motor and Process Skills

The Assessment of Motor and Process Skills (AMPS) is a new tool developed to evaluate motor skills and series of actions (called process skills) leading to completion of a task (Fisher, 1994). Design of the AMPS is based on sensory integration theory for the purpose of evaluating the behavioral manifestation of sensory integrative dysfunction in children (Bundy & Fisher, 1992) and adults (Fisher, 1994). Selection of specific items in the AMPS is based on the assumption that the items collectively represent the abilities underlying performance of common tasks and therefore can be used to estimate overall function and to identify specific deficits limiting function for use in planning therapeutic intervention. The AMPS contains 15 motor skills items to examine strength, posture, mobility, fine motor capabilities, and subtle postural adjustment capabilities, plus 20 process skills to measure attentional, conceptual, organizational, and adaptive capabilities. To evaluate these skills, the subject selects a common activity, such as fixing a sandwich, from a range of 30 possible activities listed in the AMPS manual. Each of the skills is then scored on a four-point scale describing levels of competence displayed while the subject completes the activity. Scores for each of the motor skills are then adjusted for the level of task difficulty so that performance can be related to a continuum of performance capacity to compare and predict performance for tasks of lesser or greater difficulty. Findings for a preliminary study of some AMPS test properties are available (Fisher,

1994). Although children were included in studies during early development of the AMPS, all studies published thus far have looked only at adult populations; however, these studies suggest that AMPS is a valid tool across cultures (Goto et al., 1996) and gender (Duran & Fisher, 1996).

In summary, there are a number of motor assessment tools currently available, and only a small representative sample of more general, comprehensive tools is reviewed here. As efforts are made to extend research in motor control to issues of assessment, greater attention to theoretic framework and purpose of test design is required to determine whether an assessment tool exhibits not only good measurement properties, but also yields measures consistent with current knowledge of the processes and mechanisms of motor control. Many assessment tools commonly used in rehabilitation are based primarily on maturational-based theories (Palisano, 1993) and possess few if any properties reflecting current views of motor control. It is likely that as rehabilitation specialists take more interest in research supporting dynamic-based theories, a new generation of assessment tools will reflect this view as well. By way of example, a study in young children with hemiplegia caused by cerebral palsy nicely demonstrates how one variable alone, task specificity, can alter the results of a simple measurement such as joint angle (van der Weel et al., 1991). Additionally, there are new tools under development that borrow directly from current research methods in motor control, suggesting that in the future there may be a new generation of standardized, selective motor control assessment tools for children, more akin to specific laboratory tests. Examples of this selective motor assessment approach are the Melbourne Assessment of Unilateral Upper Limb Function (Johnson et al., 1994), measurement of prehensile movements (Steenbergen et al., 1998), and an array of postural assessments adapted to children (Westcott et al., 1997).

Implications for Treatment

It seems reasonable to start from the acknowledged assumption that issues regarding application of contemporary research in motor control to clinical assessment also pertain to application of the same research to treatment. Conceptualization begins with understanding the theoretic basis for why a certain action is taken and specifying the expected consequences predicted by the theory enlisted. Excellent reviews of the theoretic bases and expected consequences enlisted by physical therapists during much of this century are available (Gordon, 1987; Horak, 1991, 1992) and will only be highlighted here. Some examples of possible implications for treatment drawn from motor control research will complete this section and chapter.

Evolving Bases for Treatment

Most neurotherapeutic approaches used in physical therapy were originally based on reflex and hierarchic models of motor control (Gordon, 1987; Horak, 1991). Treatment approaches based on maturational-based theory typically ascribed to a hierarchic model of motor skill acquisition and enlisted a facilitation model of treatment. In practical terms, it was assumed that motor development in the child progressed in a specific sequence of reflexes, movement patterns, and milestones, and that a child had to experience each facet of this sequence to acquire normal, age-appropriate motor control. Based on the facilitation model of treatment, it was assumed that externally driven sensory experience of these sequences, such as the passive and guided movements generated by a therapist or caregiver, could alter the damaged nervous system in such a way that the child with motor impairment might acquire more normal-functioning motor pathways. Conversely, the facilitation model also assumed that abnormal or undesirable movement experiences could reinforce pathologic pathways, severely limiting ultimate gains in motor control. Such logic can be found in various forms of treatment adapted from theoretic neurorehabilitation models developed by (but not limited to) the Bobaths (Bobath & Bobath, 1984), Brunnstrom (1970), Knott (1966), and Vojta (Aufschnaiter, 1992). Typically, maturational-based treatment approaches have emphasized inhibiting abnormal postural muscle tone and primitive reflexes, breaking up abnormal movement patterns, and providing movement experiences in prescribed sequences to acquire motor skills (e.g., proximal to distal progression of body control and hierarchically ordered motor milestones). Documented dissatisfactions with this approach include poor carryover to functional activities, insufficient active movement by the patient, lack of attention to movement-related variables that are extrinsic to the nervous system, and failure to produce normal movement patterns once abnormal muscle tone or primitive reflexes were inhibited (Horak, 1991).

As dissatisfaction with maturational-based approaches to treatment and other related therapies has grown, aspects of each have been combined and modified to incorporate more recent motor control research. One approach, developed by Carr and Shepard (1987), is organized around goal-directed, functional behaviors and considers the importance of both peripheral and central neural function as

well as the environment in learning to accomplish specific functional goals. The goal-oriented approach is based on the systems model of motor control, first proposed by Bernstein (1967). According to this model, function of each contributing system and interaction among systems is dictated by the demands of task goals during a given movement (Fig. 2–11, A). Thus, unlike other approaches, the goal-directed approach assumes that movement patterns will vary according to the goal and systems contributing to a given movement. Similarly, the goal-directed approach assumes that there may be multiple satisfactory movement pattern solutions for achieving a goal; therefore a patient is encouraged to find multiple strategies for accomplishing a goal. Active, self-initiated movement is encouraged and principles of motor learning are used to enhance practice and learning of new movement strategies. Because it is relatively new, there are aspects of this approach that are yet undeveloped, such as methods for more precisely specifying the quality of movement and how to enhance motor learning processes (Horak, 1991). Thus far, the approach also does not address whether the learner has limited or vast movement experience (i.e., a young child versus an adult), and the approach is not coupled with a specified assessment methodology. Nevertheless, this goal-directed treatment approach is the closest approximation to a dynamic theory-based (or systems) model of rehabilitation currently found in clinical practice.

Horak (1992) has proposed the development of a goal-oriented approach that more precisely reflects the systems model of Bernstein. In this model of rehabilitation, Horak draws together each of the systems identified in motor control research as contributors to a class of goals, such as postural stability (Fig. 2–11, B). Starting from the upper right corner of the model, the musculoskeletal system contributes the net biomechanical forces for postural control resulting from active contractile forces, passive elastic forces, and displacements of multilinked body segments. The central set provides anticipatory strategies based on past experience to minimize the potential for postural instability as it emerges during movement. Environmental adaptation provides a means for using both feedforward and feedback control to adapt postural strategies to a particular task or environment. Based on somatosensory, vestibular, and visual information, perception of orientation determines the postural orientation goal for the task at hand. Sensory interaction provides a means for adjusting the relative dominance of all sensory inputs based on current postural context, previous postural experience, and postural expectations. Finally, sensorimotor strategies provide a collection of innate and learned movement strategies (that can be adapted by the actions of all other systems) to simplify planning of an action and effectively meet the postural goal. A similar but more simplified model has been offered by Shumway-Cook and Woollacott (1995), emphasizing the interaction of three spheres, the individual, the task, and the environment.

Hypothetical Applications

With the close of this chapter, a few hypothetical examples of how the systems model for rehabilitation might be used are provided for the reader to ponder. First, consider a new walker eagerly attempt-

ing to reach for a bright shiny toy with one hand while standing and holding on to a small piece of furniture with the other hand. Employing the model in Figure 2–11, *B*, the goal is to remain standing while reaching for the toy. The musculoskeletal system will contribute biomechanical variables such as a relatively high center of gravity resulting in a greater sway frequency (see the section on posture) and produce responses limited by a small and relatively undeveloped lever system at the leg-ankle-foot for generating force against the floor. Because the infant is a new walker and has little experience, the central set will have limited predictive capacity and few anticipatory strategies from which to generate a plan for

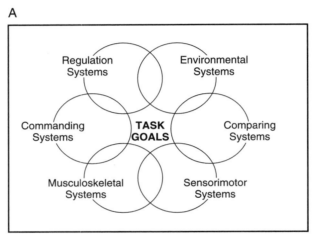

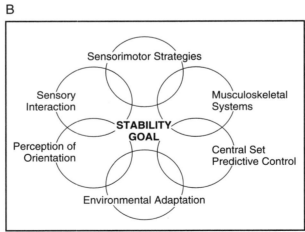

FIGURE 2–11. The Systems Model of Motor Control *(A)* and Systems Model of Rehabilitation *(B)* specify a collection of systems as contributing to the control of movement. The organization of these systems is heterarchic rather than hierarchic, suggesting that control shifts among the contributing systems as a function of the goal for a given task. (*A*, Adapted from Horak, FB. Assumptions underlying motor control for neurologic rehabilitation. In Lister, MJ [Ed.], Contemporary Management of Motor Control Problems, Proceedings of the II Step Conference. Alexandria, VA: Foundation for Physical Therapy, 1991, pp. 11–28, Fig. 4–7. *B*, Adapted from Horak, FB. Motor control models underlying neurologic rehabilitation. In Forssberg, H, & Hirschfeld, H [Eds.], Movement Disorders in Children, Medicine and Sport Science, Vol. 36. Basel: Karger, 1992, pp. 21–30, Fig. 2.)

minimizing a shift in center of gravity as the reach is initiated. Thus the central set may be viewed as a limiting system in this task. Given limited predictive skills, environmental adaptations may only generate feedback strategies for correcting postural perturbations creating demands on attention that reduce the infant's attention to other tasks or interests. Because the infant has several months of experience in a gravitational environment, perception of orientation is not likely to be a limiting system in this task. The infant will likely rely almost exclusively on vision to control his or her posture because sensory interaction, also a limiting system, will not yet have determined how to adjust the relative dominance of each contributing sensory system. Because of biomechanical variables (faster sway and shorter distance to the limits of stability) and a dependence on feedback rather than feedforward correction strategies, the timing or sequencing of ankle (sensorimotor) strategies may not be sufficiently effective or reliable to correct posture before the infant sways to the limits of stability. In this case, sensorimotor strategies may select to stabilize posture by increasing stiffness about the ankle (e.g., co-contracting antagonist ankle muscles) or to prepare to break a fall by selecting a directionally appropriate protective extension response.

In contrast to hypothetical interpretations, immature motor skills or actions have typically been viewed as indicative of a nervous system not yet able to execute adaptive, coordinated motor commands. If one embraces multifactorial assumptions of motor control, however, immature motor actions may also be viewed as adaptive strategies to cope with inherent immaturity in one or more contributing systems. The failure to see a motor pattern associated with more mature responses need not mean that it cannot be produced by sensorimotor strategies; rather, the pattern may be potentially available, but not seen because other contributing systems cannot support it. Immature motor actions may also be the emergent consequences of biomechanical or other environmental constraints and affordances that contribute forces or cues and shape the movement differently as it is executed through a physical space or movement context. Studies by Thelen and colleagues provide a wide range of examples describing how infant kicking is altered with changes in biomechanics and environment (Thelen & Smith, 1994).

If a neural lesion is added to the systems model, consideration must also be given to the various direct and indirect effects of the lesion, including disuse, on each contributing system. Because each system's participation is viewed as being organized around a specific task, even abnormal or atypical motor behaviors can be interpreted as being the patient's current solution for attempting to achieve a goal (see also Latash & Anson, 1996). Returning to the new walker's attempt to reach, as described previously, consider the presence of mild spastic diplegia. Attempting to reach for the toy, the infant rises up on his or her toes, the heels seldom in contact with the ground, reducing the effectiveness of an ankle strategy and increasing the likelihood of a hip strategy for correcting postural sway. In this instance, in addition to the contributions of normal rate-limiting systems, weakness and changes in compliance of leg muscles further diminish the effectiveness of the postural lever system. Given the state of other systems, sensorimotor strategies may select to activate extensor muscles excessively in an effort to control posture for a number of possible reasons. For example, the extensor posture may keep the center of mass forward within a new cone of stability that is biomechanically more advantageous than if the center of mass shifts posteriorly; if the center of mass shifts posteriorly, strength or timing of the anterior postural synergy may not be sufficient to make a correcting anterior adjustment in posture. Another possible reason for selection of the extensor synergy may be to reduce the number of degrees of freedom and enhance stiffness where phasing or force generation of muscle is insufficient. According to the systems model, each contributing system is also influenced by the function of all other systems. Thus another implication of the model is that if function of one or more systems is altered by a pathologic process, other systems will be altered as well. Similarly, if these systems have not fully matured at the time a pathologic process occurs, maturational processes of any or all systems may be seriously altered. Another implication for rehabilitation is the need to anticipate both the direct and indirect effects of a pathologic process on each contributing system. For example, a lesion affecting the musculoskeletal system may result in a significantly reduced level of activity, practice, and variety of experiences necessary for maturation of the central set or any other contributing systems. The reader is encouraged to develop hypothetical examples that may be meaningful to a clinical problem at hand.

As one becomes discontent with the current state of knowledge, experience, or practice, it is difficult to not be overly frustrated and critical. Criticism of accepted practices may take on a life of its own, creating the impression that the current state of affairs, in this case clinical practice, is in a sorry state. Such is not necessarily the case or necessarily the view of those generating the criticism. As discussed previously in this chapter, maturational-based views and approaches to practice have experienced considerable criticism. However, as research in motor control began to take hold in recent years, maturational-based approaches to treatment were also undergoing modification by their creators (Bobath & Bobath, 1984), a point not always appreciated by either the practitioners or critics of maturational-based views (Mayston, 1992). Future motor control research and efforts to link it with practice may even lead to preservation of some treatment approaches currently under scrutiny, but advances in knowledge may also suggest different reasons or different expected outcomes from those previously proposed. A uniquely specified "motor control theory" does not exist, and thus it is illogical to say there is a motor control approach to examination or treatment. There is, however, a dynamic disciplinary field of motor control research that offers opportunities to develop, test, and thoughtfully critique assumptions underlying physical therapy practice.

References

Adams, JA. A closed-loop theory of motor learning. Journal of Motor Behavior, 3:111–149, 1971.

Albers, S, & Jorch, G. Prognostic significance of spontaneous motility in very immature preterm infants under intensive care treatment. Biology of the Neonate, 66:182–187, 1994.

Aruin, AS, & Almeida, GL. A coactivation strategy in anticipatory postural adjustments in persons with Down syndrome. Motor Control, 1:178–191, 1997.

Asanuma, H, & Keller, A. Neuronal mechanisms of motor learning in mammals. Neuroreport, 2:217–224, 1991.

Aufschnaiter, D von. Vojta: a neurophysiological treatment. In Forssberg, H, & Hirschfeld, H (Eds.), Movement Disorders in Children, Medicine and Sport Science, Vol. 36. Basel: Karger, 1992, pp. 7–15.

Ayres, AJ. Sensory Integration and Praxis Tests. Los Angeles: Western Psychological Services, 1989.

Bayley, N. Bayley Scales of Infant Development. New York: Psychological Corporation, 1969.

Bekoff, A, & Lau, B. Interlimb coordination in 20-day rat fetuses. Journal of Experimental Zoology, 214:173–175, 1980.

Bergmeier, SA. An investigation of reaching in the neonate. Pediatric Physical Therapy, 4:3–11, 1992.

Bernstein, N. The Coordination and Regulation of Movements. London: Pergamon, 1967.

Bizzi, E, Mussa-Ivaldi, FA, & Gisler, S. Computations underlying the execution of movement: A biological perspective. Science, 253:287–291, 1991.

Bjornson, KF, Graubert, CS, Buford, VL, & McLaughlin, J. Validity of the Gross Motor Function Measure. Pediatric Physical Therapy, 10:43–47, 1997.

Bobath, K, & Bobath, B. The neuro-developmental treatment. Clinics in Developmental Medicine, 90:6–18, 1984.

Bos, AF, Martijn, A, Okken, A, & Prechtl, HF. Quality of general movements in preterm infants with transient periventricular echodensities. Acta Paediatrica, 87:328–335, 1998.

Bower, TGR. Human Development. San Francisco: Freeman, 1979.

Boyce, W, Gowland, C, Hardy, S, Rosenbaum, P, Lane, M, Plews, N, Goldsmith, C, & Russell, D. Development of a quality of movement measure for children with cerebral palsy. Physical Therapy, 71:820–832, 1991.

Boyce, W, Gowland, C, Rosenbaum, PL, Lane, M, Plews, N, Goldsmith, CH, Russell, DJ, Wright, V, Potter, S, & Harding, D. The Gross Motor Performance Measure: validity and responsiveness of a measure of quality of movement. Physical Therapy, 75:603–613, 1995.

Bradley, NS. What are the principles of motor development? In Forssberg, H, & Hirschfeld, H (Eds.), Movement Disorders in Children, Medicine and Sport Science, Vol. 36. Basel: Karger, 1992, pp. 41–49.

Bradley, NS. Transformations in embryonic motility in chick: kinematic correlates of type I and II motility at E9 and E12. Journal of Neurophysiology, 81:1486–1494, 1999.

Bradley, NS, & Bekoff, A. Development of locomotion: animal models. In Woollacott, M, & Shumway-Cook, A (Eds.), The Development of Posture and Gait Across the Lifespan. Columbia: University of South Carolina Press, 1989, pp. 48–73.

Bradley, NS, & Bekoff, A. Development of coordinated movement in chicks: I. Temporal analysis of hindlimb muscle synergies at embryonic days 9 and 10. Developmental Psychobiology, 23:763–782, 1990.

Bradley, NS, & Smith, JL. Neuromuscular patterns of stereotypic hindlimb behaviors in the first two postnatal months. I. Stepping in normal kittens. Developmental Brain Research, 38:37–52, 1988.

Brunnstrom, S. Movement Therapy in Hemiplegia. New York: Harper & Row, 1970.

Bundy, AC, & Fisher, AG. Evaluation of sensory integration dysfunction. In Forssberg, H, & Hirschfeld, H (Eds.), Movement Disorders in Children, Medicine and Sport Science (Vol. 36). Basel: Karger, 1992, pp. 272–277.

Butterworth, G, & Hicks, L. Visual proprioception and postural stability in infancy. A developmental study. Perception, 6:255–262, 1977.

Campbell, SK. The infant at risk for developmental disability. In Campbell, SK (Ed.), Decision Making in Pediatric Neurologic Physical Therapy. Philadelphia: Churchill Livingstone, 1999, pp. 260–332.

Carr, JH, & Shepherd, RB. Assumptions underlying physical therapy intervention: theoretical and historical perspectives. In Carr, JH, & Shepherd, RB (Eds.), Movement Science Foundations for Physical Therapy in Rehabilitation. Rockville, MD: Aspen, 1987, pp. 31–92.

Cermack, SA, & Murray, EA. The validity of the constructional subtests of the Sensory Integration and Praxis Tests. American Journal of Occupational Therapy, 45:539–543, 1991.

Chambers, SH, Bradley, NS, & Orosz, MD. Kinematic analysis of wing and leg movements for type I motility in E9 chick embryos. Experimental Brain Research, 103:218–226, 1995.

Chandler, LS, Andrews, MS, & Swanson, MW. Movement Assessment of Infants. Rolling Bay, WA: Chandler, Andrews, & Swanson, 1980.

Chiel, H, & Beer, AR. The brain has a body: adaptive behavior emerges from interactions of nervous system, body and environment. Trends in Neuroscience, 20:553–557, 1997.

Cioni, G, Ferrari, F, Einspieler, C, Paolicelli, PB, Barbani, MT, & Prechtl, HF. Comparison between observation of spontaneous movements and neurological examination in preterm infants. Journal of Pediatrics, 130:704–711, 1997a.

Cioni, G, Prechtl, HF, Ferrari, F, Paolicelli, PB, Einspieler, C, & Roversi, MF. Which better predicts later outcome in full-term infants: quality of general movements or neurological examination? Early Human Development, 50:71–85, 1997b.

Clifton, RK, Muir, DW, Ashmead, DH, & Clarkson, MG. Is visually guided reaching in early infancy a myth? Child Development, 64:1099–1110, 1993.

Connolly, K. The nature of motor skill development. Journal of Human Movement Studies, 3:128–143, 1977.

Corbetta, D, & Thelen, E. Shifting patterns of interlimb coordination in infants' reaching: a case study. In Swinnen, SP, Heuer, H, Massion, J, & Casaer, P (Eds.), Interlimb Coordination: Neural, Dynamical, and Cognitive Constraints. San Diego: Academic Press, 1994, pp. 413–438.

Crutcher, MD, & Alexander, GE. Movement-related neuronal activity selectively coding either direction or muscle pattern in 3 motor areas of the monkey. Journal of Neurophysiology, 64:151–163, 1990.

Daniels, LE, & Bressler, S. The Miller Assessment for Preschoolers: clinical use with children with developmental delay. American Journal of Occupational Therapy, 44:48–53, 1990.

de Vries, JIP, Visser, GHA, & Prechtl, HFR. The emergence of fetal behavior: I. Qualitative aspects. Early Human Development, 7:301–322, 1982.

Drew, T. Motor cortical activity during voluntary gait modifications in the cat. I. Cells related to the forelimbs. Journal of Neurophysiology, 66:919–938, 1993.

Dubowitz, L, & Dubowitz, V. The Neurological Assessment of the Preterm and Full-term Newborn Infant. Clinics in Developmental Medicine, 79:1–103, 1981.

Dubowitz, LMS, Dubowitz, V, Palmer, PG, Miller, G, Fawer, CL, & Levine, MI. Correlation of neurologic assessment in the preterm newborn infant with outcome at 1 year. Journal of Pediatrics, 105:452–456, 1984.

Duran, LJ, & Fisher, AG. Male and female performance on the Assessment of Motor Process Skills. Archives of Physical Medicine and Rehabilitation, 77:1019–1024, 1996.

Einspieler, C, Prechtl, HF, Ferrari, F, Cioni, G, & Bos, AF. The qualitative assessment of general movements in preterm, term and young infants—Review of the methodology. Early Human Development, 50:47–60, 1997.

Eliasson, AC, Gordon, AM, & Forssberg, H. Basic co-ordination of manipulative forces of children with cerebral palsy. Developmental Medicine and Child Neurology, 33:661–670, 1991.

Eliasson, AC, Gordon, AM, & Forssberg, H. Impaired anticipatory control of isometric forces during grasping by children with cerebral palsy. Developmental Medicine and Child Neurology, 34:216–225, 1992.

Eliasson, AC, Gordon, AM, & Forssberg, H. Tactile control of isometric fingertip forces during grasping in children with cerebral palsy. Developmental Medicine and Child Neurology, 37:72–84, 1995.

Fagard, J. Manual strategies and interlimb coordination during reaching, grasping, and manipulating throughout the first year of life. In Swinnen, SP, Heuer, H, Massion, J, & Casaer, P (Eds.), Interlimb Coordination: Neural, Dynamical, and Cognitive Constraints. San Diego: Academic Press, 1994, pp. 439–460.

Fagard, J, & Pezé, A. Age changes in interlimb coupling and the development of bimanual coordination. Journal of Motor Behavior, 29:199–208, 1997.

Feldman, AG. Once more on the Equilibrium-Point Hypothesis (l model) for motor control. Journal of Motor Behavior, 18:17–54, 1986.

Ferrari, F, Prechtl, HF, Cioni, G, Roversi, MF, Einspieler, C, Gallo, C, Paolicelli, PB, & Cavazzuti, GB. Posture, spontaneous movements, and behavioral state organization in infants affected by brain malformations. Early Human Development, 50:87–113, 1997.

Fetters, L, & Todd, J. Quantitative assessment of infant reaching movements. Journal of Motor Behavior, 19:147–166, 1987.

Field, J. Coordination of vision and prehension in young infants. Child Development, 48:97–103, 1977.

Fisher, AG. Development of a functional assessment that adjusts ability measures for task simplicity and rater leniency. In Wilson M (Ed.), Objective Measurement: Theory Into Practice, Vol. 2. Norwood: Ablex, 1994, pp. 145–175.

Fisher, AG, & Bundy, AC. (1992). Sensory integration theory. In Forssberg, H, & Hirschfeld, H (Eds.), Movement Disorders in Children, Medicine and Sport Science, Vol. 36. Basel: Karger, 1992, pp. 16–20.

Fitts, PM. The information capacity of the human motor system in controlling the amplitude of movement. Journal of Experimental Psychology, 47:381–391, 1954.

Forssberg, H. Ontogeny of human locomotor control. I. Infant stepping, supported locomotion and transition to independent locomotion. Experimental Brain Research, 57:480–493, 1985.

Forssberg, H. Evolution of plantigrade gait: Is there a neuronal correlate? Developmental Medicine and Child Neurology, 34:920–925, 1992.

Forssberg, H, Eliasson, AC, Kinoshita, H, Johansson, RS, & Westling, G. Development of human precision grip. I. Basic coordination of force. Experimental Brain Research, 85:451–457, 1991.

Forssberg, H, Eliasson, AC, Kinoshita, H, Westling, G, & Johansson, RS. Development of human precision grip. IV. Tactile adaptation of isometric finger forces to the frictional condition. Experimental Brain Research, 104:323–330, 1995.

Forssberg, H, Kinoshita, H, Eliasson, AC, Johansson, RS, Westling, G, & Gordon, AM. Development of human precision grip. II. Anticipatory control of isometric forces targeted for object's weight. Experimental Brain Research, 90:393–398, 1992.

Forssberg, H, & Nashner, LM. Ontogenetic development of postural control in man: adaptation to altered support and visual conditions during stance. Journal of Neuroscience, 2:545–552, 1982.

Forsström, A, & Hofsten, C von. Visually directed reaching of children with motor impairments. Developmental Medicine and Child Neurology, 24:653–661, 1982.

Foster, EC, Sveistrup, H, & Woollacott, MH. Transitions in visual proprioception: a cross-sectional developmental study of the effect of visual flow on postural control. Journal of Motor Behavior, 28:101–112, 1996.

Gallistel, CR. The Organization of Action: A New Synthesis. Hillsdale, NJ: Lawrence Erlbaum Associates, 1980.

Geerdink, JJ, & Hopkins, B. Qualitative changes in general movements and their prognostic value in preterm infants. European Journal of Pediatrics, 152:362–367, 1993.

Georgopolous, AP. Neurophysiology of reaching. In Jeannerod, M (Ed.), Attention and Performance XIII. Hillsdale, NJ: Lawrence Erlbaum Associates, 1990, pp. 227–263.

Ghez, C. Voluntary movements. In Kandel, ER, Schwartz, JH, & Jessell, TM (Eds.), Principles of Neuroscience, 3rd ed. New York: Elsevier, 1991, pp. 609–625.

Gibson, JJ. The Senses Considered as Perceptual Systems. Boston: Houghton Mifflin, 1966.

Gomi, H, & Kawato, M. Equilibrium-point control hypothesis examined by measured arm stiffness during multijoint movement. Science, 272:117–120, 1996.

Goodgold-Edwards, SA. Cognitive strategies during coincident timing tasks. Physical Therapy, 71:236–243, 1991.

Goto, S, Fisher, AG, & Mayberry, WL. The Assessment of Motor and Process Skills applied cross-culturally to the Japanese. American Journal of Occupational Therapy, 50:798–806, 1996.

Gordon, AM, Forssberg, H, & Iwasaki, N. Formation and lateralization of internal representations underlying motor commands during precision grip. Neuropsychologia, 32:555–568, 1994.

Gordon, AM, Forssberg, H, Johansson, RS, Eliasson, AC, & Westling, G. Development of human precision grip. III Integration of visual cues during the programming of isometric forces. Experimental Brain Research, 90:399–403, 1992.

Gordon, J. Assumptions underlying physical therapy intervention: theoretical and historical perspectives. In Carr, JH, & Shepherd, RB (Eds.), Movement Science Foundations for Physical Therapy in Rehabilitation. Rockville, MD: Aspen, 1987, pp. 1–30.

Grillner, S. Neural networks for vertebrate locomotion. Scientific American, 274:64–69, 1996.

Haas, G, Diener, HC, Rapp, H, & Dichgans, J. Development of feedback and feedforward control of upright stance. Developmental Medicine and Child Neurology, 31:481–488, 1989.

Hadders-Algra, M, Brogren, E, & Forssberg, H. Ontogeny of postural adjustments during sitting in infancy: variation, selection and modulation. Journal of Physiology, 493:273–288, 1996.

Hadders-Algra, M, & Prechtl, HFR. Developmental course of general movements in early infancy. I. Descriptive analysis of change in form. Early Human Development, 28:201–213, 1992.

Haley, S. Sequence of development of postural reactions by infants with Down syndrome. Developmental Medicine and Child Neurology, 29:674–679, 1987.

Haley, SM, Harris, SR, Tada, WL, et al. Item reliability of the Movement Assessment of Infants. Physical and Occupational Therapy in Pediatrics, 6(1):21–39, 1986.

Harbourne, RT, Giuliani, C, & Mac Neela, J. A kinematic and electromyographic analysis of the development of sitting posture in infants. Developmental Psychobiology, 26:51–64, 1993.

Harris, SR. Early detection of cerebral palsy: sensitivity and specificity of two motor assessment tools. Journal of Perinatology, 7:11–15, 1987.

Hasan, Z. Optimized movement trajectories and joint stiffness in unperturbed, inertially loaded movements. Biological Cybernetics, 53:373–382, 1986.

Hay, L. Spatial-temporal analysis of movements in children: motor programs versus feedback in the development of reaching. Journal of Motor Behavior, 11:188–200, 1979.

Hay, L, Fleury, M, Bard, C, & Teasdale, N. Resolving power of the perceptual and sensorimotor systems in 6- to 10-year-old children. Journal of Motor Behavior, 26:36–42, 1994.

Hayes, KC, & Riach, CL. Preparatory postural adjustments and postural sway in young children. In Woollacott, M, & Shumway-Cook, A (Eds.), The Development of Posture and Gait Across the Lifespan. Columbia: University of South Carolina Press, 1989, pp. 97–127.

Heriza, CB. Comparison of leg movements in preterm infants at term with healthy full-term infants. Physical Therapy, 68:1687–1693, 1988.

Hirschfeld, H, & Forssberg, H. Epigenetic development of postural responses for sitting during infancy. Experimental Brain Research, 97:528–540, 1994.

Hofsten, C von. Development of visually guided reaching: The approach phase. Journal of Human Movement Studies, 5:160–178, 1979.

Hofsten, C von. Eye-hand coordination in the newborn. Developmental Psychology, 18:450–461, 1982.

Hofsten, C von. Developmental changes in the organization of prereaching movements. Developmental Psychology, 20:378–388, 1984.

Hofsten, C von. A perception-action perspective on the development of manual movements. In Jeannerod, M (Ed.), Attention and Performance XIII. Hillsdale, NJ: Lawerence Erlbaum Associates, 1990, pp. 739–762.

Hofsten, C von. Structuring of early reaching movements: A longitudinal study. Journal of Motor Behavior, 23:280–292, 1991.

Hofsten, C von, & Fazel-Zandy, S. Development of visually guided hand orientation in reaching. Journal of Experimental Child Psychology, 38:208–219, 1984.

Hofsten, C von, & Rönnqvist, L. Preparation for grasping an object: A developmental study. Journal of Experimental Psychology: Human Perception and Performance, 14:610–621, 1988.

Hofsten, C von, & Rönnqvist, L. The structuring of neonatal arm movements. Child Development, 64:1046–1057, 1993.

Hooker, D. Evidence of prenatal function of the central nervous system in man. New York: American Museum of Natural History, 1958.

Hopkins, B, & Prechtl, HFR. A quantitative approach to the development of movements during early infancy. Clinics in Developmental Medicine, 94:179–197, 1984.

Horak, FB. Assumptions underlying motor control for neurologic rehabilitation. In Lister, MJ (Ed.), Contemporary Management of Motor Control Problems, Proceedings of the II Step Conference. Alexandria, VA: Foundation for Physical Therapy, 1991, pp. 11–28.

Horak, FB. Motor control models underlying neurologic rehabilitation. In Forssberg, H, & Hirschfeld, H (Eds.), Movement Disorders in Children, Medicine and Sport Science, Vol. 36. Basel: Karger, 1992, pp. 21–30.

Horak, FB, Diener, HC, & Nashner, LM. Influence of central set on human postural responses. Journal of Neurophysiology, 62:841–853, 1989.

Horak, FB, Esselman, P, Anderson ME, & Lynch, MK. The effects of movement velocity, mass displaced, and task certainty on associated postural adjustments made by normal and hemiplegic individuals. Journal of Neurology, Neurosurgery and Psychiatry, 47:1020–1028, 1984.

Horak, FB, & MacPherson, JM. Postural orientation and equilibrium. In Rowell, LB, & Sheperd, JT (Eds.), Handbook of Physiology, Section 12, Exercise: Regulation and Integration of Multiple Systems. New York: Oxford University Press, 1996, pp. 255–292.

Horak, FB, & Nashner, LM. Central programming of postural movements: adaptation to altered support-surface configurations. Journal of Neurophysiology, 55:1369–1381, 1986.

Horak, FB, Nashner, LM, & Diener, HC. Postural strategies associated with somatosensory and vestibular loss. Experimental Brain Research, 82:167–177, 1990.

Horak, FB, Shumway-Cook, A, Crowe, TK, & Black, FO. Vestibular function and motor proficiency of children with impaired hearing, or with learning disability and motor impairments. Developmental Medicine and Child Neurology, 30:64–79, 1988.

Hoy, MG, Zernicke, RF, & Smith, JL. Contrasting roles of inertial and muscle moments at the knee and ankle during paw-shake response. Journal of Neurophysiology, 54:1282–1294, 1985.

Humphrey, T. Some correlations between the appearance of human reflexes and the development of the nervous system. Progress in Brain Research, 4:93–135, 1964.

Humphrey, T. The development of human fetal activity and its relation to postnatal behavior. Advances in Child Development and Behavior, 5:1–57, 1970.

Jakobson, LS, & Goodale, MA. Factors affecting higher-order movement planning—A kinematic analysis of human prehension. Experimental Brain Research, 86:199–208, 1991.

Jeannerod, M. Intersegmental coordination during reaching at natural visual objects in infancy. In Long, J, & Baddeley, A (Eds.), Attention and Performance IX. Hillsdale, NJ: Lawrence Erlbaum Associates, 1981, pp. 153–168.

Jeannerod, M. The timing of natural prehension movement. Journal of Motor Behavior, 26:235–254, 1984.

Jeannerod, M (Ed.). Attention and Performance XIII: Motor Representation and Control. Hillsdale, NJ: Lawrence Erlbaum Associates, 1990.

Jensen, JL, Ulrich, BD, Thelen, E, Schneider, K, & Zernicke, RF. Adaptive dynamics of the leg movement patterns of human infants: I. The effects of posture on spontaneous kicking. Journal of Motor Behavior, 26: 303–312, 1994.

Jensen, JL, Thelen, E, Ulrich, BD, Schneider, K, & Zernicke, RF. Adaptive dynamics of the leg movement patterns of human infants: III. Age-related differences in limb control. Journal of Motor Behavior, 27: 366–374, 1995.

Jensen, RK, Sun, H, Treitz, T, & Parker, HE. Gravity constraints in infant motor development. Journal of Motor Behavior, 29:64–71, 1997.

Johansson, RS, & Westling, G. Coordinated isometric muscle commands adequately and erroneously programmed for the weight during lifting task with precision grip. Experimental Brain Research, 71:59–71, 1988.

Johnson, LM, Randall, MJ, Reddihough, DS, Oke, LE, Byrt, TA, & Bach, TM. Development of a clinical assessment of quality of movement for unilateral upper-limb function. Developmental Medicine and Child Neurology, 36:965–973, 1994.

Kalaska, JF, & Crammond, DJ. Cerebral cortical mechanisms of reaching movements. Science, 255:1517–1523, 1992.

Katz, PS, & Frost, WN. Intrinsic neuromodulation: Altering neuronal circuits from within. Trends in Neuroscience, 19:54–61, 1996.

Keogh, J, & Sugden, D. Movement Skill Development. New York: Macmillan, 1985.

Keshner, EA. Equilibrium and automatic postural reactions as indicators and facilitators in the treatment of balance disorders. In Touch: Topics in Pediatrics (Lesson 4). Alexandria, VA: American Physical Therapy Association, 1990, pp. 1–17.

Kimball, JG. Using the Sensory Integration and Praxis Tests to measure change: a pilot study. American Journal of Occupational Therapy, 44:603–608, 1990.

Knott, M. Neuromuscular facilitation in the child with central nervous system deficit. Journal of the American Physical Therapy Association, 7:721–724, 1966.

Koshland, GF, & Smith, JL. Paw-shake responses with joint immobilization—EMG changes with atypical feedback. Experimental Brain Research, 77:361–373, 1989.

Kupfermann, I. Localization of higher cognitive and affective functions: the association cortices. In Kandel, ER, Schwartz, JH, & Jessell, TM (Eds.), Principles of Neuroscience, 3rd ed. New York: Elsevier, 1991, pp. 823–838.

Lantz, C, Melén, K, & Forssberg, H. Early infant grasping involves radial fingers. Developmental Medicine and Child Neurology, 38: 668–674, 1996.

Lashley, KS. The accuracy of movement in the absence of excitation from the moving organ. American Journal of Physiology, 43:169–194, 1917.

Lasky, RE. The effect of visual feedback of the hand on the reaching and retrieval behavior of young infants. Child Development, 48: 112–117, 1977.

Latash, LM, & Anson, JG. What are normal movements in atypical populations? Behavioral and Brain Sciences, 19:55–106, 1996.

Lawrence, DG, & Hopkins, DA. The development of the motor control in the rhesus monkey: evidence concerning the role of corticomotorneuronal connections. Brain, 99:235–254, 1976.

Lawerence, DG, & Kuypers, HGJ. The functional organization of the motor system in the monkey: I. The effects of bilateral pyramidal lesions. Brain, 91:1–14, 1968.

Lee, DN. The optic flow-field: The foundation of vision. Philosophical Transactions of the Royal Society of London B, 290:169–179, 1980.

Lee, DN, & Aronson, E. Visual proprioceptive control of standing in human infants. Perception & Psychophysics, 15:529–532, 1974.

Lee, DN, Daniel, BM, Turnbull, J, & Cook, ML. Basic perceptuo-motor dysfunctions in cerebral palsy. In Jeannerod, M (Ed.), Attention and Performance XIII. Hillsdale, NJ: Lawrence Erlbaum Associates, 1990, pp. 583–603.

Lee, DN, & Lishman, JR. Visual proprioceptive control of stance. Journal of Human Movement Studies, 1:87–95, 1975.

Lemon, R. The output map of the primate motor cortex. Trends in Neuroscience, 11:501–506, 1988.

Lemon, R, & Mantel, GWH. The influence of changes in discharge frequency of corticospinal neurones on hand muscles in the monkey. Journal of Physiology, 413:351–378, 1989.

Levitan, IB, & Kaczmarek, LK. Neural networks and behavior. In The Neuron. Cell and Molecular Biology. New York: Oxford, 1997, pp. 451–474.

Lockman, JJ, Ashmead, DH, & Bushnell, EW. The development of anticipatory hand orientation during infancy. Journal of Experimental Child Psychology, 37:176–186, 1984.

Massion, J. Movement, posture and equilibrium—Interaction and coordination. Progress in Neurobiology, 38:35–56, 1992.

Mathew, A, & Cook, M. The control of reaching movements by young infants. Child Development, 61:1238–1258, 1990.

Mayston, MJ. The Bobath concept—Evolution and application. In Forssberg, H, & Hirschfeld, H (Eds.), Movement Disorders in Children, Medicine and Sport Science, Vol. 36. Basel: Karger, 1992, pp. 1–6.

McComas, J, Dulberg, C, & Latter, J. Children's memory for locations visited: Importance of movement and choice. Journal of Motor Behavior, 29:223–229, 1997.

McDonnell, P. The development of visually guided reaching. Perception & Psychophysics, 18:181–185, 1975.

McGraw, MB. Neuromuscular development of the human infant as exemplified in the achievement of erect locomotion. Journal of Pediatrics, 17:747–771, 1940.

McGraw, MB. The Neuromuscular Maturation of the Human Infant. New York: Hafner Press, 1945.

Meyer, DE, Smith, JEK, Kornblum, S, Abrams, RA, & Wright, CE. Speed-accuracy tradeoffs in aimed movements: Toward a theory of rapid voluntary action. In Jeannerod, M (Ed.), Attention and Performance XIII. Hillsdale, NJ: Lawrence Erlbaum Associates, 1990, pp. 173–226.

Miller, LJ. Miller Assessment of Preschoolers. Littleton, CO: Foundation for Knowledge in Development, 1982.

Miller, LJ. Longitudinal validity of the Miller Assessment for Preschoolers: study II. Perceptual Motor Skills, 66:811–814, 1988.

Molteno, C, Grosz, P, Wallace, P, & Jones, M. Neurological examination of the preterm and full-term infant at risk for developmental disabilities using the Dubowitz Neurological Assessment. Early Human Development, 41:167–176, 1995.

Mouchnino, L, Aurenty, R, Massion, J, & Pedotti, A. Coordinated control of posture and equilibrium during leg movement. In Brandt, T, Paulus, W, Bles, W, Dieterich, M, Krafczyk, S, & Straube, A (Eds.), Disorders of Posture and Gait. Stuttgart: Georg Thieme, 1990, pp. 68–71.

Muir, GD, Gosline, JM, & Steeves, JD. Ontogeny of bipedal locomotion: Walking and running in the chick. Journal of Physiology, 493:589–601, 1996.

Mulligan, S. An analysis of score patterns of children with attention disorders on the Sensory Integration and Praxis Tests. American Journal of Occupational Therapy, 50:647–654, 1996.

Nashner, LM, & Forssberg, H. Phase-dependent organization of postural adjustments associated with arm movements while walking. Journal of Neurophysiology, 55:1382–1394, 1986.

Nashner, LM, Shumway-Cook, A, & Marin, O. Stance posture control in select groups of children with cerebral palsy: Deficits in sensory organization and muscular coordination. Experimental Brain Research, 49:393–409, 1983.

Newell, KM, McDonald, PV, & Baillargeon, R. Body scale and infant grip configurations. Developmental Psychobiology, 26:195–205, 1993.

O'Donovan, MJ, & Chub, N. Population behavior and self-organization in the genesis of spontaneous rhythmic activity by developing spinal networks. Seminars in Cell and Developmental Biology, 8:21–28, 1997.

Palisano, RJ. Neuromotor and developmental assessment. In Wilhelm, IJ (Ed.), Physical Therapy Assessment in Early Infancy. New York: Churchill Livingstone, 1993, pp. 173–224.

Perham, H, Smick, JE, Hallum, A, & Nordstrom, T. Development of the lateral equilibrium reaction in stance. Developmental Medicine and Child Neurology, 29:758–765, 1987.

Polit, A, & Bizzi, E. Characteristics of motor programs underlying arm movements in monkeys. Journal of Neurophysiology, 42:183–194, 1979.

Portfors-Yeomans, CV, & Riach, CL. Frequency characteristics of postural control of children with and without visual impairment. Developmental Medicine and Child Neurology, 37:456–463, 1995.

Prablanc, C, & Pélisson, D. Gaze saccade orienting and hand pointing are locked to their goal by quick internal loops. In Jeannerod, M. (Ed.), Attention and Performance XIII. Hillsdale, NJ: Lawrence Erlbaum Associates, 1990, pp. 653–676.

Pratt, CA, & Loeb, GE. Functionally complex muscles of the cat hindlimb. 1. Patterns of activation across sartorius. Experimental Brain Research, 85:243–256, 1991.

Prechtl, HF. State of the art of a new functional assessment of the young nervous system. An early predictor of cerebral palsy. Early Human Development, 50:1–11, 1997.

Rader, N, & Stern, JD. Visually elicited reaching in neonates. Child Development, 53:1004–1007, 1982.

Raibert, MH. Motor control and learning by the state-space. Tech. Rep. AI-TR-439. Cambridge, MA: Massachusetts Institute of Technology, Artificial Intelligence Laboratory, 1977.

Riach, CL, & Hayes, KC. Anticipatory postural control in children. Journal of Motor Behavior, 22:250–266, 1990.

Rine, RM, Rubish, K, & Feeney, C. Measurement of sensory system effectiveness and maturational changes in postural control in young children. Pediatric Physical Therapy, 10:16–22, 1998.

Rizzolatti, G, & Arbib, MA. Language within our grasp. Trends in Neuroscience, 21:188–194, 1998.

Rosenbaum, DA. Human Motor Control. San Diego: Academic Press, 1991.

Rossignol, S. Neural control of stereotypic limb movements. In Rowell, LB, & Sheperd, JT (Eds.), Handbook of Physiology, Section 12, Exercise: Regulation and Integration of Multiple Systems. New York: Oxford University Press, 1996, pp. 173–216.

Rossignol, S, & Drew, T. Phasic modulation of reflexes during rhythmic activity. In Grillner, S, Stein, PSG, Stuart, DG, Forssberg, H, & Herman, RM (Eds.), Neurobiology of Vertebrate Locomotion. London: Macmillan Press Ltd., 1986, pp. 517–534.

Russell, DJ, Rosenbaum, PL, Cadman, DT, Gowland, C, Hardy S, & Jarvis, S. The Gross Motor Function Measure: a means to evaluate the effects of physical therapy. Developmental Medicine and Child Neurology, 31:341–353, 1989.

Sanes, JN, Dimitrov, B, & Hallett, M. Motor learning in patients with cerebellar dysfunction. Brain, 113:103–120, 1990.

Schellekens, JMH, Scholten, CA, & Kalverboer, AF. Visually guided hand movements in children with minor neurological dysfunction: response time and movement organization. Journal of Child Psychology and Psychiatry, 24:89–102, 1983.

Schmidt, RA. A schema theory of discrete motor skill learning. Psychological Review, 82:225–260, 1975.

Schmidt, RA, & Lee, TD. Motor Control and Learning: A Behavioral Emphasis, 3rd ed. Champaign, IL: Human Kinetics, 1998.

Schneider, E, Parush, S, Katz, N, & Miller, LJ. Performance of Israeli versus U.S. preschool children on the Miller Assessment for Preschoolers. American Journal of Occupational Therapy, 49:19–23, 1995.

Schneider, JW, Lee, W, & Chasnoff, IJ. Field testing of the Movement Assessment of Infants. Physical Therapy, 68:321–327, 1988.

Schneider, K, Zernicke, RF, Schmidt, RA, & Hart, TJ. Changes in limb dynamics during the practice of rapid arm movements. Journal of Biomechanics, 22:805–817, 1989.

Schneider, K, Zernicke, RF, Ulrich, BD, Jensen, JL, & Thelen, E. Understanding movement control in infants through the analysis of limb intersegmental dynamics. Journal of Motor Behavior, 22:493–520, 1990.

Scott, SH, & Kalaska, JF. Changes in motor cortex activity during reaching movements with similar hand paths but different arm postures. Journal of Neurophysiology, 73:2563–2567, 1995.

Shepherd, GM. Foundations of the Neuron Doctrine. New York: Oxford University Press, 1991.

Sherrington, CS. The Integrative Action of the Nervous System. New Haven: Yale University Press, 1947. (Original work published 1906.)

Shumway-Cook, A, & Woollacott, M. The growth of stability: postural control from a development perspective. Journal of Motor Behavior, 17:131–147, 1985a.

Shumway-Cook, A, & Woollacott, M. Dynamics of postural control in the child with Down syndrome. Physical Therapy, 9:1315–1322, 1985b.

Shumway-Cook, A, & Woollacott, M. Motor Control Theory and Practical Applications. Baltimore: Williams & Wilkins, 1995.

Sporns, O, & Edelman, GM. Solving Bernstein's problem: a proposal for the development of coordinated movement by selection. Child Development, 64:960–981, 1993.

Steenbergen, B, Hulstijn, W, Lemmens, IHL, & Meulenbroek, RGJ. The timing of prehensile movements in subjects with cerebral palsy. Developmental Medicine and Child Neurology, 40:108–114, 1998.

Stehouwer, DJ, & Farel, PB. Development of hindlimb locomotor behavior in the frog. Developmental Psychobiology, 17:217–232, 1984.

Stoffregen, TA, Adolph, K, Thelen, E, Gorday, KM, & Sheng, YY. Toddlers' postural adaptations to different support surfaces. Motor Control, 1:119–137, 1997.

Sugden, DA, & Keogh, JF. Problems in Movement Skill Development. Columbia: University of South Carolina Press, 1990.

Sutherland, DH, Olshen, RA, Biden, EN, & Wyatt, MP. The development of mature walking. Clinics in Developmental Medicine, 104/105:1–227, 1988.

Sutherland, DH, Olshen, R, Cooper, L, & Woo, SL. The development of mature gait. Journal of Bone and Joint Surgery, 62:336–353, 1980.

Sveistrup, H, & Woollacott, MH. Longitudinal development of the automatic postural response in infants. Journal of Motor Behavior, 28:58–70, 1996.

Swanson, MW, Bennet, FC, Shy, KK, & Whitfield, MF. Identification of neurodevelopmental abnormality at four and eight months by the Movement Assessment of Infants. Developmental Medicine and Child Neurology, 34:321–337, 1992.

Swinnen, SP, Heuer, H, Massion, J, & Casaer, P (Eds.). Interlimb Coordination: Neural, Dynamical, and Cognitive Constraints. San Diego: Academic Press, 1994.

Tardieu, C, Laspargot, A, Tabary, C, & Bret, M. Toe-walking in children with cerebral palsy: contributions of contracture and excessive contraction of triceps surae muscle. Physical Therapy, 69:656–662, 1989.

Taub, E, & Berman, AJ. Movement and learning in the absence of sensory feedback. In Freedman, SJ (Ed.), The Neuropsychology of Spatially Oriented Behavior. Homewood, IL: Dorsey Press, 1968.

Thelen, E, Fisher, DM, & Ridley-Johnson, R. The relationship between physical growth and a newborn reflex. Infant Behavior and Development, 7:479–493, 1984.

Thelen, E, Fisher, DM, Ridley-Johnson, R, & Griffin, NJ. Effects of body build and arousal on newborn infant stepping. Developmental Psychobiology, 15:447–453, 1982.

Thelen, E, & Smith, LB. A Dynamic Systems Approach to the Development of Cognition and Action. Cambridge, MA: MIT Press, 1994.

Thelen, E, & Ulrich, BD. Hidden skills: A dynamic systems analysis of treadmill stepping during the first year. Monographs of the Society for Research in Child Development, 56:1–98, 1991.

Touwen, BCL. Primitive reflexes—conceptual or semantic problem? Clinics in Developmental Medicine, 94:115–125, 1984.

Twitchell, TE. Reflex mechanisms and the development of prehension. In Connolly, K (Ed.), Mechanisms of Motor Skill Development. London: Academic Press, 1970, pp. 25–37.

Ulrich, BD, Jensen, JL, Thelen, E, Schneider, K, & Zernicke, RF. Adaptive dynamics of the leg movement patterns of human infants: II. Treadmill stepping in infants and adults. Journal of Motor Behavior, 26: 313–324, 1994.

Usui, N, Maekawa, K, & Hirasawa, Y. Development of the upright postural sway of children. Developmental Medicine and Child Neurology, 37:985–996, 1995.

van der Meer, ALH, van der Weel, FR, & Lee, DN. Prospective control in catching by infants. Perception, 23:287–302, 1994.

van der Meer, ALH, van der Weel, FR, & Lee, DN. The functional significance of arm movements in neonates. Science, 267:693–695, 1995.

van der Meulen, JHP, Vandergon, JJD, Gielen, CCA, Gooskens, RHJ, & Willemse, J. Visuomotor performance of normal and clumsy children. 1. Fast goal-directed arm-movements with and without visual feedback. Developmental Medicine and Child Neurology, 33: 40–54, 1991a.

van der Meulen, JHP, Vandergon, JJD, Gielen, CCA, Gooskens, RHJ, & Willemse, J. Visuomotor performance of normal and clumsy children. 2. Arm-tracking with and without visual feedback. Developmental Medicine and Child Neurology, 33:118–129, 1991b.

van der Weel, FR, van der Meer, ALH, & Lee, DH. Effect of task on movement control in cerebral palsy: implications for assessment and therapy. Developmental Medicine and Child Neurology, 33: 419–426, 1991.

Viviani, P, & Mounoud, P. Perceptuomotor compatibility in pursuit tracking of two-dimensional movements. Journal of Motor Behavior, 22:407–443, 1990.

Westcott, SL, Lowes, LP, & Richardson, PK. Evaluation of postural stability in children: current theories and assessment tools. Physical Therapy, *77*:629–645, 1997.

Wishart, JG, Bower, TGR, & Dunked, J. Reaching in the dark. Perception, *7*:507–512, 1978.

Woollacott, M, Debu, B, & Mowatt, M. Neuromuscular control of posture in the infant and child. Journal of Motor Behavior, *19*:167–186, 1987.

Yang, JF, Stephens, MJ, & Vishram, R. Transient disturbances to one limb produce coordinated, bilateral responses during infant stepping. Journal of Neurophysiology, *79*:2329–2337, 1998a.

Yang, JF, Stephens, MJ, & Vishram, R. Infant stepping: a method to study the sensory control of human walking. Journal of Physiology, *507*:927–937, 1998b.

Yonas, A, Bechtold, AG, Frankel, D, Gordon, FR, McRoberts, G, Norcia, A, & Sternfels, S. Development of sensitivity to information for impending collision. Perception and Psychophysics, *21*:97–104, 1977.

Zernicke, RF, & Smith, JS. Biomechanical insights into neural control of movement. In Rowell, LB, & Sheperd, JT (Eds.), Handbook of Physiology, Section 12, Exercise: Regulation and Integration of Multiple Systems. New York: Oxford University Press, 1996, pp. 293–330.

CHAPTER
3

Gait: Development and Analysis

JEAN L. STOUT, PT, MS

One of the first questions asked by many parents whose child has recently been diagnosed as having a motor impairment, or whose child has suffered an injury that affects movement is, "Will my child walk?" or "Will my child walk again?" The reason for emphasis on the task of walking apart from many other abilities (which are sometimes more functional), I believe, is the measure of independence and social acceptance with which the task of walking is associated. The ultimate goal for families, and sometimes pediatric therapists as well, becomes independent walking for the child. Although the variables that contribute to this important ability are numerous and complex, a child is usually able to stand and walk by 9 to 15 months of age (see Chapter 1). Normative data from the Alberta Infant Motor Scale (AIMS) indicate that 50% of infants will achieve independent standing by the age of 10.5 months, take first steps by 11 months, and walk independently by the age of 11.5 months (Piper & Darrah, 1994). Furthermore, the pattern is mature by the age of 3.5 years (Sutherland et al., 1980), all without instruc-

tion. The complexity of the task has been studied extensively since the days of Saunders (1953) and Murray (1964), and study continues today. Improved computerized techniques and new theories of motor control and balance contribute to better understanding of the components of walking. Understanding how we walk was once required only for those in the fields of child development and rehabilitation. Today walking is studied by many disciplines, including engineering. The extent and duration of the research in the area is a statement of its continued importance.

The purpose of this chapter is to provide an overview of the aspects of gait important to physical therapists treating children. These include the development of gait and its refinement in childhood, the normal components of walking as identified by gait analysis, and a description of some of the common abnormalities in gait found in children with physical disabilities. Guidelines for when a computerized gait analysis is desirable will also be addressed. Those interested in more extensive information are referred to a number of excellent resources on the topic (Gage, 1991; Inman et al., 1981; Ounpuu et al., 1991; Perry, 1992; Rose et al., 1991; Stout et al., 1993, 1994; Sutherland, 1984; Sutherland et al., 1980, 1988; Winter, 1979, 1983, 1987, 1990).

DEVELOPMENT OF GAIT

Gage (1991) suggests that normal walking has five major attributes: (1) stability in stance, (2) sufficient foot clearance in swing, (3) appropriate prepositioning of the foot for initial contact, (4) adequate step length, and (5) energy conservation. When independent ambulation begins in the toddler only the prerequisites for these attributes are present. The prerequisites, however, are likely to be more important to the attainment of walking than the attributes themselves. The attributes develop over time with normal growth, maturation, and refinement of the skill. Scales of motor development illustrate that even during the time period between first steps and independent walking important balance abilities are achieved (Bly, 1994; Piper & Darrah, 1994). Loss of the five attributes occurs in pathologic gait because of a loss or failure to achieve the prerequisites. The prerequisites related to the development and skill of locomotion have already been suggested in Chapter 1 during the review of the eight subsystems proposed on the basis of the dynamic systems theory (Heriza, 1991). These include adequate motor control and central nervous system (CNS) maturation (implying an intact neurologic system), adequate range of motion (ROM), strength, appropriate bone structure and composition, and intact sensation (proprioception). As suggested by Campbell, the development of a motor pattern (in this case walking) "depends on a combination of mechanical [including structural], neurologic, cognitive, and perceptual factors." A brief description of the biomechanical and neurologic factors that contribute to the development and refinement of walking follows.

Neurologic Factors

Campbell (Chapter 1) and Bradley (Chapter 2) have discussed the primary neurologic factors related to walking and other motor tasks. To briefly review, the basic neural organization and function used to execute locomotion is thought to be controlled by a central pattern generator located either in the spinal cord or in the brainstem (Connelly & Forssberg, 1997; Grillner, 1981). Descending neural input activates the central pattern generator (Jordan, 1986), and descending and peripheral input (Armstrong, 1986; Loeb, 1986) modify the output to adapt the execution to stability requirements and the

demands of the specific task and environment. The central pattern generator is believed to organize the activation and firing sequence of muscles during gait. The parallels between developing animals and humans, and the parallels between the sequencing and timing of infant stepping, kicking, and locomotion in both disabled and nondisabled infants (Forssberg, 1985; Thelen, 1986; Thelen & Cooke, 1987; Thelen & Ulrich, 1991; Ulrich & Ulrich, 1995; Zelazo, 1983), have led individuals to suggest that the neural foundations for locomotion are present at a very early stage in prenatal development (Bradley & Bekoff, 1989). Postnatally, the major periods of accelerated brain growth in relation to body growth occur between 3 and 10 months of age (Epstein, 1979), and the myelination that develops during this time probably contributes to the neural organization required for independent locomotion.

Mechanical Factors

Adequate ROM, strength, appropriate bone structure and composition, and body composition also affect the emergence of locomotion and its refinement. These variables have significant ramifications as mechanical factors in the development of walking. ROM, strength, bony structure, and the ability to manage gravitational and inertial forces of the lower extremities affect the early patterns of walking. In the presence of normal motor control and maturation, constraints in any of these mechanical variables change patterns; as the constraints change, so do the movement and the muscle activity involved in motor control. Kugler and colleagues (1982) suggest that changes seen in the development of many skills may be the result of critical dimension changes in the body of the growing child. This is also reflected in more recent work, which indicates that infants often have to physically grow into the body dimensions needed for optimal functioning and develop adequate conduction time for activation of central pattern generators (Connelly & Forssberg, 1997; Jensen & Bothner, 1998). Gajdosik and Gajdosik present an extensive review of musculoskeletal development and adaptation in Chapter 4.

Determinants of Walking

Sutherland and colleagues (1980) identified five important determinants of mature walking. The determinants distinguish walking that is considered "mature" (age 3 years and older) from walking that is "immature" (age 2.5 years and younger). The most important of the 13 variables analyzed were the duration of single-limb stance, walking velocity, cadence, step length, and the ratio of pelvic span to ankle spread. The variable with the least discriminating power was the presence or absence of a heel strike at initial contact.

The duration of single-limb stance is, as the name implies, the length of time during which only one foot is on the ground during stance phase. As a child's walking pattern matures the duration of single-limb stance increases, implying a measure of increasing stability and increasing control. The most rapid change occurs between ages 1.5 and 3.5 years.

Step length is defined as the longitudinal distance between the two feet. It is a parameter closely related to changes in height and leg length. Step length increases throughout childhood until growth is complete. A linear relationship between step length and leg length is present from age 1 to age 7. A linear relationship between step length and age exists from age 1 to age 4.

Walking velocity increases with age from age 1 to age 7, although the rate of change decreases from age 4 to age 7. A child and an adult may walk at a similar velocity if the child has an increased cadence or takes more steps per minute than the adult. Cadence gradually decreases with age throughout childhood. The most rapid reduction in cadence occurs between the ages of 1 and 2 years.

The changes with respect to age in these and other determinants are outlined in Table 3–1. These determinants will be discussed as the refinement of walking is described at various ages.

Refinement of Gait by Age

Birth to Age 9 Months

The disproportionate contribution of fat content to overall increases in body mass over the first 8 months of postnatal life causes infants to be relatively weak during a time when they are developing the motor control and coordination skills to progress toward independent ambulation (Thelen et al., 1982, 1984). Studies suggest that bigger, fatter infants achieve locomotor milestones later than their smaller peers for this reason (Adolph, 1997). From birth to 6 months of age, the body fat of the infant rises from 12% to 25% of body mass (Spady, 1989). Adipose tissue is a major component of weight gain during the first 4 months of postnatal life, with increases in lipids accounting for more than 40% of total weight gain during this time (Fomon, 1967). Between 4 and 12 months of age increased lipid content accounts for approximately 20% of increased weight. With increasing age and mobility, fat content drops and muscle mass increases.

Not only mass but also body proportions change as infants grow. During the first few months of life,

the fastest rate of growth occurs in the extremities as opposed to the head and trunk. Inertial characteristics of body segments change with growth and the effects of gravity. It has been demonstrated that the resistance to motion in limb segments (segment moments of inertia) more than doubles and triples during the first 6 months of life (Jensen & Bothner, 1998; Sun & Jensen, 1994).

The body structure of infants as they develop the ability to stand upright with support and to cruise independently affects their posture and movement patterns. Flexion "contractures" are present at the hips, and range of external rotation is slightly greater than range of internal rotation. Range of hip abduction is slightly increased at 8 to 9 months of age but has been slowly decreasing since birth (Coon et al., 1975; Haas et al., 1973; Phelps et al., 1985; Sutherland et al., 1988; Walker, 1991). Femoral anteversion* (a forward or anterior orientation of the head and neck with respect to the frontal plane) and femoral antetorsion (a twist of the bone in its longitudinal axis) of the hips are both present (Bleck, 1982, 1987; Cusick & Stuberg, 1992; Engel & Staheli, 1974; Fabray et al., 1973). The magnitude of the femoral torsion is 40 to 50°.

Structurally, the knees in the frontal plane exhibit genu varum, or bowing in the tibiofemoral angle (Fig. 3–1) (Salenius & Vankka, 1975; Tachdjian, 1990). The tibia and fibula exhibit neutral alignment about the longitudinal axis, which represents slight internal torsion relative to adult values (Staheli & Engel, 1972; Staheli et al., 1985). A medial inclination of the talotibial articulation is present in the infant, producing an everted talocrural mortise (Bernhardt, 1988; Root et al., 1971; Tachdjian, 1985; Valmassy, 1984). The medial inclination of the joint is manifested in an everted heel position in weight bearing. Supported walking at this age is characterized by wide abduction, external rotation, and flexion at the hips (Bly, 1994), bowed legs, and an everted heel position.

The postural control and development of antigravity muscle strength that are gained over the first 9 months of life are important precursors to the development of independent ambulation. The frequency and the amount of practice of activities such as kicking have been shown to affect the age of onset of ambulation, both in disabled and nondisabled infants (Adolph, 1997; Ulrich & Ulrich, 1995). Antigravity strength of the hip flexors in the lower ex-

---

*Femoral anteversion and femoral antetorsion are often used as synonymous terms in orthopedic literature to refer to the torsion or the medial twist between the axis of the head and neck of the femur and the axis of the femoral condyles.

TABLE 3–1. Changes in Typical Time and Distance Parameters at Selected Ages from the Onset of Walking through Age 7

Time and Distance Parameters	Age			
	1 year	1.5 years	3 years	7 years
Opposite toe-off (% cycle)	17	18	16	12
Opposite foot-strike (% cycle)	49	50	50	50
Single stance (% cycle)	32	32	35	38
Toe-off (% cycle)	67	68	66	62
Step length (cm)	22	25	33	48
Stride length (cm)	43	50	67	97
Cycle time (s)	0.68	0.70	0.77	0.83
Cadence (steps/min)	176	171	154	144
Walking velocity (cm/s)	64	71	86	114
Walking velocity (m/min)	38.4	42.6	51.6	68.4

Modified from Sutherland, DH, Olshen, RA, Biden, EN, & Wyatt, MP. The Development of Mature Walking. London: Mac Keith Press, 1988.

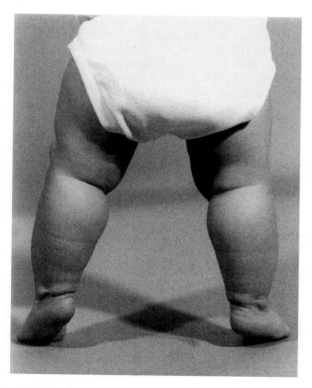

FIGURE 3–1. An 8-month-old infant with physiologic varus in the tibiofemoral angle.

tremities is built early on in the developmental process by kicking from the supine position. Hip extensor strength in both concentric and eccentric types of muscle contractions similar to those used in ambulation begins from activities in the prone position but gradually builds as the infant begins creeping and kneeling activities. Bly describes infants of 8 months of age exhibiting the ability to rise from a kneeling to standing position, which requires closed chain hip and knee extension. Cruising along furniture builds strength of the hip abductors (Bly, 1994).

By 8 months of age, the visual, proprioceptive, and vestibular systems work together to consistently bring the center of mass back to a stable position after perturbation in a seated position (Woollacott et al., 1989). Needed postural corrections in response to visual flow for a particular skill often predate the development of that skill (Adolph, 1997; Butterworth & Hicks, 1977; Hirschfield & Forssberg, 1994; Woollacott et al., 1989). For example, Butterworth and Hicks (1977) demonstrated that infants who could sit alone but could not stand independently exhibited the same appropriate postural adjustments to visual information that simulated movement as did infants who were able to walk independently.

Age 9 to 15 Months

Lower extremity alignment and body structure at the onset of ambulation are characterized by a standing posture with a wide base of support and the hips in abduction, flexion, and slight external rotation. The tibias display mild internal torsion, and varus is still present in the tibiofemoral angle; the heel position in weight bearing remains everted because of the inclination of the mortise joint. The child's center of mass is proportionately closer to the head and upper trunk (at the lower thoracic level) than in an older child, whose center of mass is located at midlumbar level, or in an adult, whose center of mass is located at the sacral level (Palmer, 1944). Although differential growth rates are allowing the head to become relatively smaller than the rest of the body, the head is still proportionately large. The ratio of body fat to muscle mass is still high, contributing to weakness relative to the demands of upright posture. Coming upright against the force of gravity puts new demands on muscle strength. Muscles (particularly the abdominals, hip flexors, knee extensors, and ankle dorsiflexors) must work in new antigravity positions, which further increases functional weakness. Despite the structural limitations, infants exhibit the necessary postural responses to compensate for visual and support-surface perturbations that are inherent in the task of upright locomotion (Berger et al., 1985; Butterworth & Hicks, 1977; Shumway-Cook & Woollacott, 1985; Thelen et al., 1989; Woollacott et al., 1989).

The base of support in an infant at the onset of ambulation is wide for both structural and stability reasons. Mediolateral (side to side) stability is achieved, but anteroposterior stability is limited. Progression takes place in the sagittal plane; if the head moves outside the limits of stability at the base of support, balance is lost.

The rate-limiting factors associated with the ability to demonstrate upright locomotion are (1) sufficient extensor muscle strength to support the body's weight on a single-limb base of support, (2) dynamic balance, and (3) postural control (Connelly & Forssberg, 1997; Thelen et al., 1989). The critical dimension of the body to be controlled is the head within the limits of stability of the base of support. The pattern displayed by a beginning walker is similar to that of an experienced walker on a slippery surface (i.e., small steps, a widened base of support, and maintenance of the body and limbs very upright in an extended, stiff position). The work of Sutherland and colleagues (1988) characterizes infant ambulation as consisting of a wide base of support, increased hip and knee flexion, full foot initial contact in plantar flexion, a short stride, increased cadence, and a relative footdrop in swing phase.

Motorically, the initial pattern and execution of the first steps are thought to be related to the patterns used in stepping and kicking during early infancy (Thelen & Cooke, 1987) and may be constrained by this pattern. That is, just as the structural makeup of the body drives the initial posture, so may the primitive generator for kicking and stepping drive the muscle activity for early walking. The reduced frequency of kicking in children with Down syndrome has been shown to be correlated with a later age of walking than in typically developing infants (Ulrich & Ulrich, 1995). Both kicking and stepping are alternating reciprocal patterns of movement between the limbs. Each has a flexion phase (in gait, analogous to swing) and an extension phase (in gait, analogous to stance). Thelen and colleagues (1989) suggest that the ability to generate steplike patterns is continuous from the newborn period through in-

dependent locomotion and that the pattern demonstrated in beginning upright ambulation is a modified, more flexible version of the earlier pattern that has been modified by changes in strength, neurologic maturation, and the mechanics of upright posture.

The electromyographic (EMG) patterns of activity at the onset of independent ambulation demonstrate significant co-contraction across antagonistic muscle groups—the anterior tibialis and gastrocnemius during swing phase and the quadriceps and hamstrings muscles during stance phase (Kazai et al., 1976; Okamoto & Kumamoto, 1972; Sutherland et al., 1980, 1988; Thelen & Cooke, 1987). Coactivation patterns result from the need for stability.

As stated previously, Thelen and colleagues suggest that it is not the pattern-generating capabilities or motor control postural abilities that constrain the onset of independent locomotion. Development of sufficient extensor strength is believed to be the critical variable (Thelen et al., 1989). This belief is consistent with other views for the requirements of walking, including stance phase stability (Gage, 1991) and the need to maintain a net extensor muscle support moment as described by Winter (1987, 1990).

Age 18 to 24 Months

As the child grows, body structure changes, increases in strength, neurologic maturation, and walking experience all play a part in altering the walking pattern. By 18 months of age, the varus angulation of the tibiofemoral angle in the frontal plane has resolved and the limb is straight (Fig. 3–2) (Tachdjian, 1990; see also Chapter 4). No change is noted in excessive femoral antetorsion, although limitation in hip extension ROM is reduced to an average of 4°, indicating that remodeling is underway (Fabray et al., 1973; Phelps et al., 1985). Range of hip abduction is no longer excessive. Because of decreased abduction and improved stability, the base of support has decreased. Dynamic balance and strength have also improved. A heel strike has not consistently emerged in the 18-month-old child (Sutherland et al., 1980, 1988), but the lessened base of support allows for more anterior-posterior movement over the planted foot. Heel position remains everted (Root et al., 1971; Valmassy, 1984). The viscoelastic and inertial properties of the stretched stance limb begin to be exploited to propel the leg in swing (Thelen & Cooke, 1987). A knee flexion wave begins to emerge during initial stance phase as a heel strike develops and knee extensor contraction absorbs some of the impact of floor contact (Sutherland et al., 1980, 1988). The duration of stance phase re-

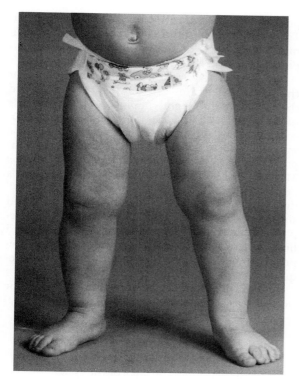

FIGURE 3–2. Standing posture of an 18-month-old toddler. The varus in the tibiofemoral angle has resolved, and the limb is straight.

mains prolonged, and cadence is increased relative to mature gait (see Table 3–1).

The efficiency of locomotion slowly improves during the period from 18 to 24 months of age as the center of mass descends from a position high above the lower extremities to one in close proximity to the chief motor power in the legs. Stability of any body is inversely related to the distance of its center of mass from its base of support. Between the first and second years of life, the legs are growing proportionately longer, becoming the most rapidly increasing dimension of the body. These events bring the center of mass closer to the proximal end of the lower limbs (Palmer, 1944).

Controversy exists over whether heel strike develops as a result of neurologic maturation or gradual changes in body structure, base of support, improved strength, and improved stability (Forssberg, 1985, 1992; Thelen & Cooke, 1987; Thelen et al., 1989). It is likely that each variable is important. A consistent heel strike develops by 24 months of age (Sutherland et al., 1980, 1988). Requirements include refined motor control, strength, and dynamic balance to sustain stability on a small area of contact (the heel). Children with impaired walking ability

lack a heel strike at initial contact. This may be caused by either lack of motor control or the inherent choice of maintaining stability by use of a larger area of initial contact (Gage, 1991).

The EMG patterns at this age show decreasing co-contraction in antagonistic muscle groups, implying increased control and stability. The primary changes occur in the duration of stance phase activity (Okamoto & Kumamoto, 1972; Sutherland et al., 1980, 1988). The durations of stance phase quadriceps, medial hamstring, and anterior tibialis muscle activity are all decreased in the 18- to 24-month-old as compared with those seen in the 12-month-old. By age 2, the late swing phase–early stance phase EMG activity monitored in the gastroc-soleus complex of the 12- to 18-month-old child has disappeared (Sutherland et al., 1980, 1988).

Age 3 to 3.5 Years

Between the ages of 3 and 3.5 years, the joint angles associated with walking mature into the adult pattern (Sutherland et al., 1980, 1988). Structurally, the tibiofemoral angle, which was neutral at 18 months of age, now shows maximum valgus alignment (Salenius & Vankka, 1975) (Fig. 3–3). Femoral antetorsion of the hip is decreasing but remains increased in relation to that measured in an adult. The center of mass is closer to the extremities as the rate of lower extremity growth stabilizes (Palmer, 1944). Heel eversion in weight bearing can still be observed but is decreasing. Measurement by motion analysis demonstrates that a heel strike is consistently present in conjunction with a knee flexion wave in early stance (Sutherland et al., 1980, 1988). EMG activity has a mature pattern by this age.

Age 6 to 7 Years

By age 7, the gait patterns by standards of movement or motion are fully mature. Minimal changes are noted when compared with the adult pattern, although time and distance variables continue to vary with age and stature (Sutherland et al., 1980, 1988). Balance and postural control demonstrate renewed stability after a period of disequilibrium often seen between ages 4 and 6 years (Shumway-Cook & Woollacott, 1985; Woollacott et al., 1989). Structurally, the tibiofemoral angle has returned to neutral (Tachdjian, 1990), and femoral antetorsion is largely resolved but still slightly higher than that measured in the adult (Bleck, 1987; Fabray et al., 1973). The inclination of the talotibial joint is no longer present, and heel position is neutral by age 7 (Valmassy, 1984). A period of disproportionate growth with respect to body dimensions has also passed. The center

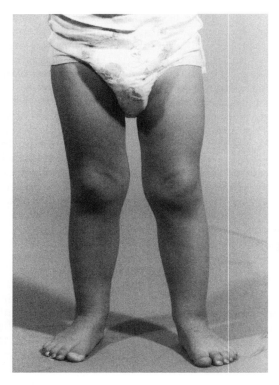

FIGURE 3–3. The tibiofemoral alignment of a 3-year-old showing maximum physiologic valgus.

of mass is still slightly higher than in the adult, at the level of the third lumbar vertebra (Palmer, 1944).

COMPONENTS OF NORMAL GAIT AS MEASURED BY GAIT ANALYSIS

As stated previously, extensive research has been done and continues to be done in the area of gait. Numerous textbooks and basic research articles have been written on the topic (Gage, 1991; Inman et al., 1981; Ounpuu et al., 1991; Perry, 1992; Rose et al., 1991, 1993; Sepulveda et al., 1993; Stout et al., 1993; Sutherland, 1984; Sutherland et al., 1980, 1988; Winter, 1979, 1983, 1987, 1990; Zajac & Gordon, 1989). This section describes the normal components of mature walking as identified by three-dimensional computerized analysis of movement and forces, electromyography, and energy expenditure in a functional context.

One complete gait cycle refers to a single stride that begins when one foot strikes the ground and ends when the same foot strikes the ground again. The gait cycle is divided into two major phases—stance and swing. Stance phase is associated with the period of time when the foot is on the ground; swing phase is the period of time when the foot is in the air. The stance phase of the gait cycle occupies approximately 60% of the cycle, and the swing phase occupies approximately 40%.

Perry (1992) developed a generic terminology for the functional phases of gait that further divided the gait cycle into eight subphases. Each subphase has a functional objective that assists in the accomplishment of one of three basic tasks of the walking cycle: weight acceptance, single-limb support, and limb advancement (Rancho Los Amigos Medical Center, 1989). The basic tasks that Perry's group described are similar to the "attributes" discussed by Gage (1991): weight acceptance and single-limb support (stability in stance and prepositioning of the foot for initial contact) and limb advancement (foot clearance in swing, prepositioning of the foot for initial contact, and adequate step length).

Stance phase is divided into five subphases or instantaneous events (Fig. 3–4):

1. Initial contact (0–2% of the cycle)
2. Loading response (0–10% of the cycle)
3. Midstance (10–30% of the cycle)
4. Terminal stance (30–50% of the cycle)
5. Preswing (50–60% of the cycle)

Opposite leg toe-off and opposite initial contact occur at 10% and 50% of the gait cycle, respectively. Thus there are two periods of double support during the walking cycle when both feet are on the ground. These occur during loading response (just after initial contact) and preswing (just before toe-off). Each occupies approximately 10% of the gait cycle.

Swing phase begins at toe-off and occurs during the period of single support of the stance limb. Three subphases are identified (see Fig. 3–4):

1. Initial swing (60–73% of the cycle)
2. Midswing (73–87% of the cycle)
3. Terminal swing (87–100% of the cycle)

Temporal Measurement Definitions and Common Terms

The following definitions will be helpful in the description of walking as used in gait analysis:

Cadence: The frequency of steps taken in a given amount of time, usually measured in steps per minute.

Concentric muscle contraction: A shortening contraction that produces acceleration. Positive work results and power generation occurs.

Eccentric muscle contraction: A lengthening contrac-

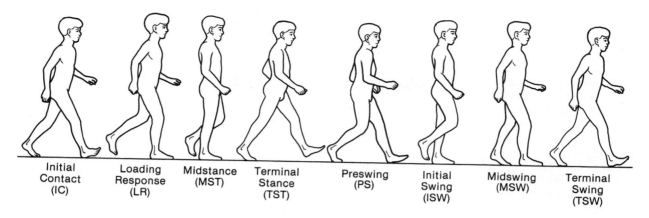

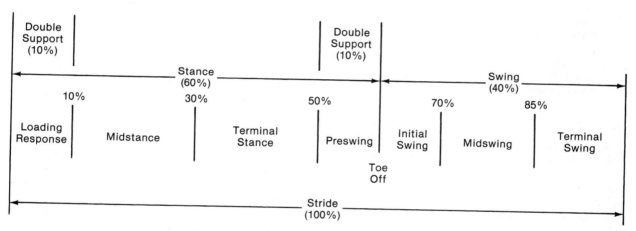

FIGURE 3–4. One complete gait cycle depicting stance phase and swing phase. The cycle begins with initial contact of the right foot. Stance phase has five subphases; swing phase has three subphases. Initial contact and toe-off are instantaneous events. (Adapted from Gage, JR. An overview of normal walking. In Greene, WB [Ed.], Instructional Course Lectures, Vol. 39. Park Ridge, IL: American Academy of Orthopaedic Surgeons, 1990.)

tion that produces deceleration. Negative work results and power absorption occurs. The efficiency of negative work or power absorption by a muscle is 3 to 9 times higher than that of positive work (Inman et al., 1981).

External load: Ground reaction forces, inertial forces, and gravitational forces that affect joint motion.

Isometric muscle contraction: A stabilizing contraction that produces no net power. Force is produced without length change in the muscle.

Joint moment: A force acting at a distance from an axis causing a rotation about that axis is called a torque or moment (moment equals force times perpendicular distance). In the body, moments are produced external to the body by ground reaction forces, forces

related to gravity, and inertial forces. Moments internal to the body are produced by muscle forces, ligamentous forces, or forces produced by joint capsules. Joint moments in this chapter will represent the physiologic response of the body generated in response to an external load in accordance with the definition used by Ounpuu and colleagues (Ounpuu et al., 1991).

Joint power: The net rate of energy absorption or generation. *Mechanical power* is defined as the work performed per unit of time. *Joint power* is defined as the product of the net joint moment and the joint angular velocity. Muscles are the primary internal power producers in the body. Muscles can also be internal power absorbers. Ligaments usually absorb power.

Kinematics: The parameters used to describe motion without regard to forces. These include linear or angular displacements, velocities, and accelerations.

Kinetics: The parameters that describe the causes of the movement. These include external and internal forces such as gravitational forces, ground reaction forces, inertial forces, muscle or ligament forces, joint moments, and joint powers.

Step length: The longitudinal distance between the two feet. Right step length is measured from the first point of contact of the left foot to the first point of contact of the right foot.

Stride length: The longitudinal distance between the initial contact of one foot and the next initial contact of the same foot. It is the sum of the right and left step lengths and represents the distance traversed in one complete gait cycle.

Walking velocity: The rate of walking or the distance traversed in a specified length of time. Velocity can be expressed as stride length divided by cycle time or the product of step length and cadence.

Kinematics

Kinematics in gait analysis can be collected in either two or three dimensions. Common to all types of computerized motion analysis is a reference system such as the use of markers or targets placed on the body and aligned with respect to specific anatomic landmarks. Two-dimensional motion systems provide joint angles that are a direct measure of the motion of the marker set placed on the skin. Three-dimensional systems reference the marker coordinate system to an internal coordinate system based on an estimation of the locations of the anatomic joint centers. The outputs, regardless of two- or three-dimensional technique, are displayed as a series of graphs of a single gait cycle for each joint in a given plane of motion. Figure 3–5 gives an example of three-dimensional motion data from Gillette Children's Specialty Healthcare.

Kinetics

Kinetics represent the parameters that describe the causes of the movement. These include external and internal forces such as gravitational forces, ground reaction forces, inertial forces, muscle or ligament forces, joint moments, and joint powers. Kinetic data as part of two- or three-dimensional gait analysis are obtained from a combination of force plate and kinematic information and are displayed as joint moments and joint powers. The force plate provides information regarding the ground reaction force, and the kinematics provide information regarding the joint angular velocities. Anthropometric measurements of the body are also required. The method commonly used to calculate joint moments and powers is called "inverse dynamics" and is based on a linked segment model approach (Winter, 1990). A ground reaction force method is another method sometimes used (Winter, 1990).

A moment or torque is a force acting at a distance that causes an object to rotate. A joint moment represents the physiologic response of the body generated in response to an external load (Ounpuu et al., 1991). In my laboratory, what is displayed on the graphs is the net joint moment, which represents the sum of all internal joint moments in a particular plane at a particular joint. The moments refer primarily to the muscle forces that are acting to control segment rotation, but internal joint moments can be generated by ligaments, joint capsules, and fascia as well. The net joint moment depicts which muscle group is dominant but does not denote the relative contributions of muscle groups on either side of the joint. For example, in the sagittal plane, a net extensor moment at the hip during stance phase implies that the hip extensors are dominant. Hip flexors may or may not contribute, but the overall moment is an extensor moment. The hip extensor muscles are active to counteract an external moment created by the ground reaction force that is tending to flex the hip (Fig. 3–6). The ground reaction force tends to flex the hip because it is anterior to the joint center.

Power, in mechanical terms, is defined as the rate of doing work. *Joint power* is defined as the net joint moment multiplied by the joint angular velocity. Muscles are the primary internal power producers in the body. A muscle's ability to produce power is affected by its cross-sectional area. Other factors that affect power include fiber type, the length-tension ratio, and the degree of fatigue (see Chapter 4). Muscles can also be internal power absorbers. Ligaments usually absorb power. The power graphs display whether power is generated (positive work) or absorbed (negative work). Concentric muscle action is associated with power generation, and eccentric muscle action is associated with power absorption. In the previous example of the hip, the hip is extending in the presence of a net extensor moment; therefore power generation occurs (Fig. 3–7). Normal sagittal plane kinematics and kinetics can be found in Figure 3–8.

Electromyography

The electrical signal associated with the neuromuscular activation of a muscle is measured by elec-

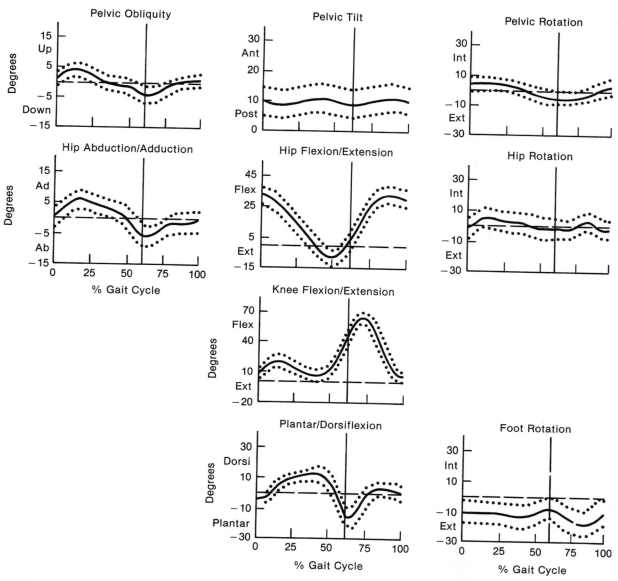

FIGURE 3-5. Representative normal three-dimensional motion data from Gillette Children's Specialty Healthcare. In this and subsequent normative figures, one complete gait cycle is depicted and is normalized to 100% of the stride. The mean *(solid line)* and one standard deviation *(dashed line)* are displayed of composite data collected from children ages 4 to 19 years. Stance phase is separated from swing phase in each graph by the vertical line. Each graph represents the same walking cycle. Each row displays a different joint: from top to bottom are pelvis, hip, knee, and ankle. Each column displays the movements of a different joint in the same plane of motion; from left to right are the coronal plane—front view, sagittal plane—side view, and transverse plane—rotational view. *Note:* The pelvis is measured with respect to laboratory coordinates, the hip with respect to the pelvis, and the knee with respect to the thigh. Foot rotation graph represents foot progression angle, not rotation of the foot with respect to the tibia.

tromyography (Basmajian & DeLuca, 1985; Winter, 1990). It represents the pattern of motor unit activation. Electromyographic data can provide information about the timing of muscle activity and, in some cases, about the intensity of muscle con-

traction. Under some conditions EMG amplitude has been shown to be related to force (Komi, 1973; Vredenbregt & Rau, 1973), but the usefulness of this aspect for assessment of walking is limited because the relationship is valid only under isometric condi-

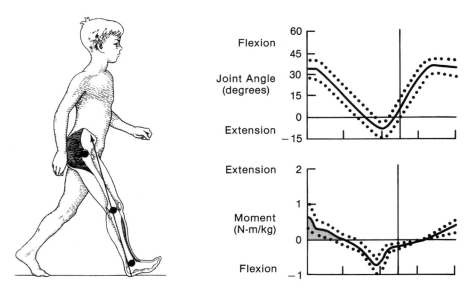

FIGURE 3–6. An example of an internal joint moment produced at the right hip. Because the ground reaction force falls anterior to the hip joint, the joint would flex without internally produced resistance. The joint moment graph demonstrates a net extensor moment at the hip *(shaded)* as the body's internal resistance to the external force. The internal moment is produced by dominant action of the hip extensor muscles. (Adapted in part from Gage, JR. Gait Analysis in Cerebral Palsy. London: Mac Keith Press, 1991.)

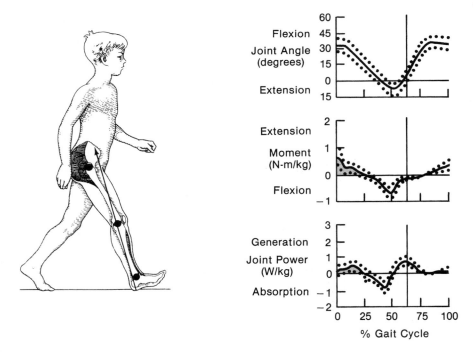

FIGURE 3–7. An example of power generation at the right hip. Because the hip is extending and a net extensor moment is present, power generation *(shaded)* occurs. The units for power are watts per kilogram. By convention, power generation is represented by positive deflection on the graph; power absorption is negative. (Adapted in part from Gage, JR. Gait Analysis in Cerebral Palsy. London: Mac Keith Press, 1991.)

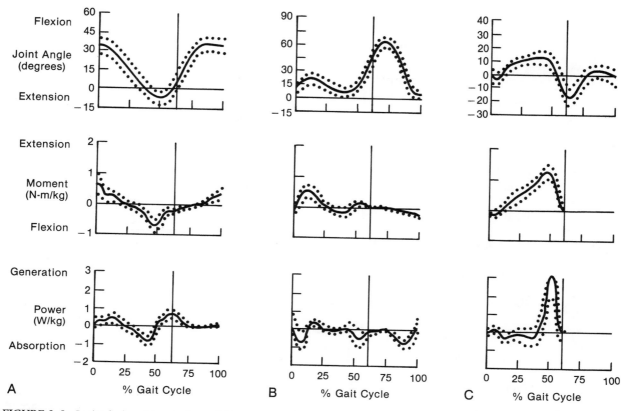

FIGURE 3–8. Sagittal plane kinematics and kinetics of the hip *(A)*, knee *(B)*, and ankle *(C)*. Each graph represents the same walking cycle, with the mean *(solid line)* and one standard deviation *(dashed line)*. The top row shows the kinematic graphs; the middle row, the joint moments; and the bottom row, the joint powers. Units for the kinematics are degrees. The units for joint moments (newton-meters/kilogram) and powers (watts/kilogram) are standardized for body weight.

tions and when no coactivation is occurring. The amplitude of an EMG signal is affected by the rate of motor unit firing and the number of motor units active at any given time. The type and proportion of different motor units firing also affects amplitude. In addition, many external factors, including electrode location, type of electrode used, interelectrode distance, skin temperature, and amount of subcutaneous fat, also affect the amplitude of the signal (Basmajian & DeLuca, 1985). Comparing EMG amplitudes across muscles, or within or between subjects, should be done with caution and adequate understanding of the complexity involved in interpretation. Current research focuses on understanding the relationship of muscle activity and force with joint kinematics and kinetics using engineering principles (Zajac & Gordon, 1989). Combining engineering principles with neural network representations is advancing the understanding of the effects of EMG activity even further (Sepulveda et al., 1993).

Each muscle has a particular time during the walking cycle when activity is present or absent and a particular pattern of increasing or decreasing motor unit activity. These timings have been documented for both children and adults (Ounpuu et al., 1991; Perry, 1992; Sutherland et al., 1988; Winter & Yack, 1987). An example can be found in Figure 3–9. EMG data can be collected using surface or fine wire (indwelling) electrodes. Reviews on the advantages and disadvantages of each have been published (Kadaba et al., 1985).

KINEMATICS, KINETICS, AND ELECTROMYOGRAPHY IN NORMAL GAIT

A detailed description of activity in the lower extremities during each phase of the gait cycle is presented in this section, including a summary of hip, knee, and ankle kinematics and kinetics with associ-

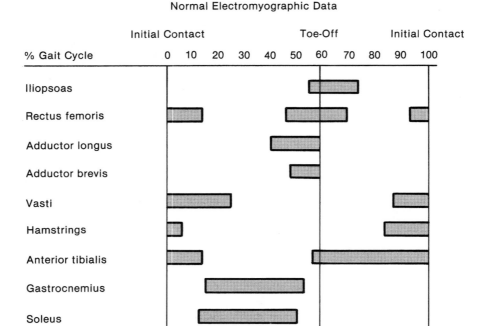

FIGURE 3–9. The phasic (on/off) EMG activity of the major muscles used during walking. (Adapted from Ounpuu, S, Gage, JR, & Davis, RB. Three-dimensional lower extremity joint kinetics in normal pediatric gait. Journal of Pediatric Orthopaedics, *11*:341–349, 1991, p. 344.)

ated muscle activity. Sagittal plane events are emphasized. The reader should refer to the kinematic and kinetic plots.

Sagittal Plane

At *initial contact* (0% of the gait cycle) the ankle is in a position of neutral dorsiflexion, the knee is in minimal flexion, and the hip is in approximately 35° of flexion. The objective of this event is appropriate pre-positioning of the foot to begin the gait cycle. The ground reaction force at initial contact is passing through the heel and is anterior to both the knee and the hip. The gluteus maximus and hamstrings muscles are active to control the external flexor moment at the hip. The hamstrings also assist in preventing knee hyperextension. Anterior tibialis and quadriceps activity initiates the loading response (Fig. 3–10).

Loading response (Fig. 3–11) is a period of acceptance of body weight while maintaining stability and progression. The purpose of loading response is to cushion or absorb the impact of the body's moment of inertia. It is the first period of double support and occurs between 0 and 10% of the gait cycle, beginning after initial contact and ending when the entire foot is in contact with the floor. The ankle is plantar flexing at this time under controlled eccentric contraction of the anterior tibialis muscle. The dominant internal moment at the ankle is a dorsiflexor moment because the dorsiflexor muscles are dominant. The power curve depicts absorption because the anterior tibialis muscle is contracting eccentrically. Gage (1991) and Perry (1992) refer to loading response as the first "rocker" of ankle stance phase.

The knee undergoes an initial phase of flexion to approximately 15° (average value). Both hamstring activity and quadriceps muscle activity are present. Because the quadriceps muscles are acting eccentrically to decelerate knee flexion, the power graph depicts absorption. Whenever the joint movement and the joint moment are opposite each other, power absorption is occurring.

The hip during loading response is extending by concentric action of the hip extensor muscles (gluteus maximus, gluteus minimus, and hamstrings).

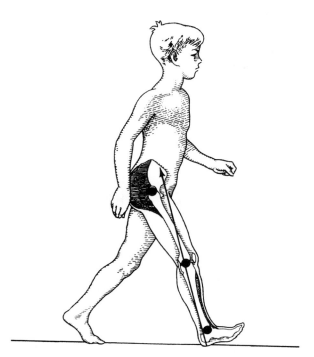

FIGURE 3–10. Initial contact of the gait cycle. (From Gage, JR. Gait Analysis in Cerebral Palsy. London: Mac Keith Press, 1991.)

The hamstrings are able to work as hip extensors because knee motion is stabilized by the single joint muscles of the quadriceps. The internal moment is extensor, and the power graph depicts generation. Because the external ground reaction force falls anterior to the hip joint, without the action of the hip extensors the joint would collapse into flexion.

Midstance (Fig. 3–12) is the beginning of the single-support phase of the gait cycle and extends from the period of 10 to 30% of the cycle. The goal during midstance is to maintain trunk and limb stability and allow smooth progression over a stationary foot when the entire plantar surface is in contact with the floor. The ankle is in a period of increasing dorsiflexion that is controlled by eccentric contraction of the soleus muscle. The moment graph demonstrates a dominant plantar flexor moment and the power graph a period of absorption. The second rocker of ankle stance phase occurs during midstance (Gage, 1991).

The knee extends during midstance. The vastus medialis, vastus intermedius, and vastus lateralis muscles work initially to stabilize the knee until the ground reaction force passes anterior to the knee joint. Once the ground reaction force is anterior to the knee, extension is passive. The joint moment at the knee is an extensor moment. The power graph

shows initial decreasing absorption followed by generation. This period of power generation is the only one produced at the knee during the entire gait cycle.

The hip is also extending during midstance. The joint moment is extensor, and power is generated, implicating concentric action of the hip extensor muscles. The internal extension moment, however, is decreasing during this time. When the ground reaction force becomes posterior to the hip joint, a transition occurs from a concentric (power generation) extensor moment to an eccentric (power absorption) flexor moment.

Terminal stance (Fig. 3–13) is the second half of the single-support phase and occurs from 30 to 50% of the gait cycle. This period begins when the ground reaction force passes anterior to the knee and posterior to the hip and often occurs with heel rise. During this phase of the gait cycle, forward progression of the tibia is arrested and further increase in dorsiflexion is limited. The ankle begins a period of decreasing dorsiflexion by concentric contraction of the gastrocnemius and soleus muscles, producing power generation. One of the primary power productions that propels an individual through the walking cycle is generated at the ankle during terminal stance (36% of the total power generation produced during the walking cycle) (Ounpuu et al., 1991; Winter, 1987). Heel rise marks the period of the third rocker of ankle stance phase (Gage, 1991).

The knee moves from relative extension to increasing flexion during terminal stance. An internal flexor moment is dominant because the ground reaction force falls in front of the knee. Power is absorbed. The internal flexor moment is produced by a combination of ligamentous resistance and flexor activity of the gastrocnemius muscle.

The hip continues to extend during terminal stance. Because the ground reaction force is posterior to the joint center, extension is resisted by an internal flexor moment. Power is absorbed, suggesting that the flexor moment is produced by tension force of the iliofemoral ligament.

Preswing (Fig. 3–14) is the second period of double support during the walking cycle and occurs at 50 to 60% of the cycle. The function of preswing is to advance the limb into swing; preswing ends at toe-off. The stance phase extremity is unweighted as weight is accepted on the opposite limb. The ankle is now in true plantar flexion, and the plantar flexor moment remains dominant. The magnitude of the moment is rapidly decreasing, however, and power generation falls rapidly to zero.

The knee joint is flexing during preswing and reaches approximately 45° (average value) at toe-off. The internal muscle moment is extensor, and power is absorbed. Activity of the rectus femoris muscle is

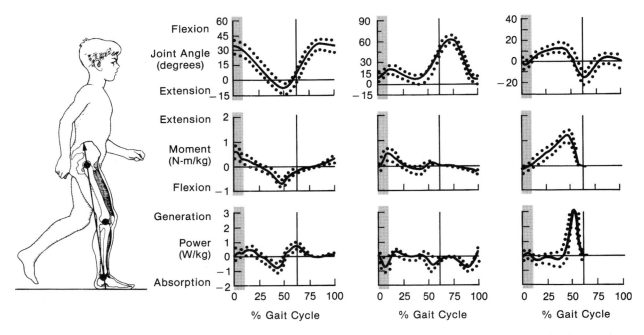

FIGURE 3–11. Loading response (0–10% of the gait cycle). (Adapted from Gage, JR. Gait Analysis in Cerebral Palsy. London: Mac Keith Press, 1991.)

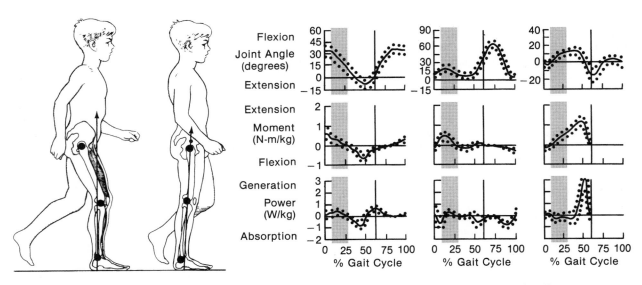

FIGURE 3–12. Midstance (at 10–30% of the gait cycle). (Adapted from Gage, JR. An overview of normal walking. In Greene, WB [Ed.], Instructional Course Lectures, Vol. 39. Park Ridge, IL: American Academy of Orthopaedic Surgeons, 1990.)

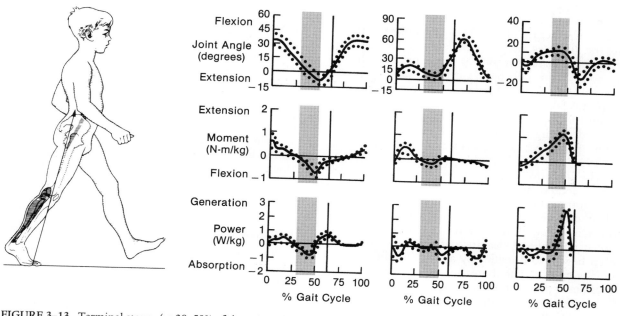

FIGURE 3–13. Terminal stance (at 30–50% of the gait cycle). (Adapted from Gage, JR. Gait Analysis in Cerebral Palsy. London: Mac Keith Press, 1991.)

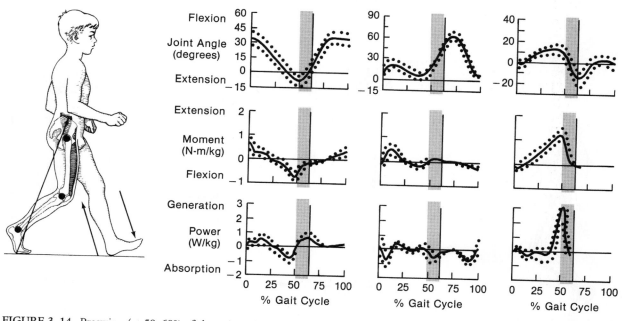

FIGURE 3–14. Preswing (at 50–60% of the gait cycle). (Adapted from Gage, JR. Gait Analysis in Cerebral Palsy. London: Mac Keith Press, 1991.)

probably responsible for this activity and assists the deceleration of the moment of inertia of the shank.

The hip begins to flex in preswing. The dominant moment is a flexor moment, and power is generated. Concentric action of the hip flexor muscles, primarily the iliopsoas, produces the activity. Occasionally the rectus femoris muscle is active to augment hip flexion. This usually occurs at faster walking speeds. Peak flexor power of the hip is generated at toe-off. Hip musculature (both extensors and flexors) is responsible for the majority of positive work performed during the walking cycle (56%), with most being produced during stance phase (Ounpuu et al., 1991).

The objective of *initial swing* (Fig. 3–15) is foot clearance and limb advancement. Initial swing occurs from 60 to 73% of the gait cycle. Maximum plantar flexion occurs at the ankle in initial swing. At the same time, peak knee flexion occurs, uniquely timed for optimal clearance of the foot. The ankle then begins to dorsiflex by activity of the anterior tibialis muscle. The dominant muscle moment is a dorsiflexor moment. Power output is negligible.

The hip flexes during initial swing, which also assists foot clearance. A flexor moment remains dominant, and power generation is occurring by concentric activity of the hip flexors.

The goals of *midswing* (Fig. 3–16) remain foot clearance and limb advancement, and it occurs between 73 and 87% of the gait cycle. The ankle is dorsiflexing during this time by concentric action of the anterior tibialis muscle. The knee is extending by inertial forces without muscle activity. The hip is flexing.

The primary purpose of *terminal swing* (Fig. 3–17) is pre-positioning of the limb for weight acceptance. This phase occupies the period between 87 and 100% of the gait cycle. The ankle begins to plantar flex by eccentric action of the anterior tibialis muscle to position the ankle in neutral. A flexor moment is dominant at the knee with power absorption as knee extension is controlled by eccentric action of the hamstrings to decelerate the forward swing of the thigh. The quadriceps muscles also become active to assist with control of the knee. Minimal movement is noted at the hip at this time.

Coronal Plane

The function of hip and pelvis motion in the coronal plane is to optimize the vertical excursion of the center of mass (Figs. 3–5 and 3–18). At initial contact the pelvis in the coronal plane is level and the hip is in neutral abduction and adduction. The stance side of the pelvis rises 5° at the beginning of loading response in conjunction with adduction of the stance limb. The dropping of the pelvis on the unsupported limb is caused by the ground reaction

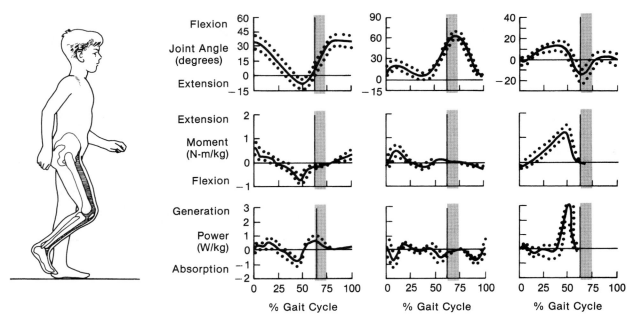

FIGURE 3–15. Initial swing (at 60–73% of the gait cycle). (Adapted from Gage, JR. An overview of normal walking. In Greene, WB [Ed.], Instructional Course Lectures, Vol. 39. Park Ridge, IL: American Academy of Orthopaedic Surgeons, 1990.)

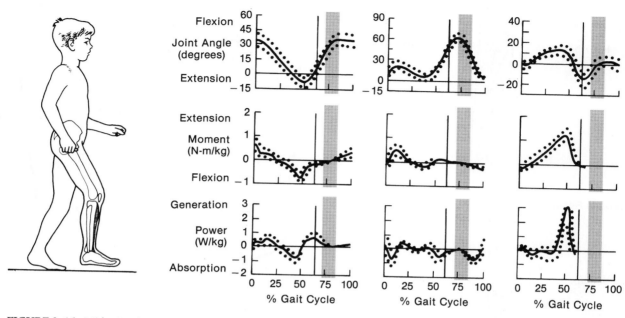

FIGURE 3–16. Midswing (at 73–87% of the gait cycle). (Adapted from Gage, JR. An overview of normal walking. In Greene, WB [Ed.], Instructional Course Lectures, Vol. 39. Park Ridge, IL: American Academy of Orthopaedic Surgeons, 1990.)

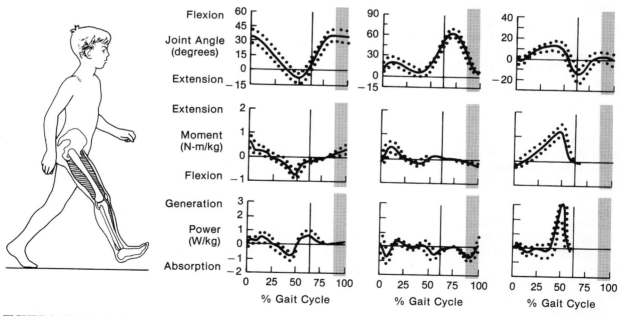

FIGURE 3–17. Terminal swing (at 87–100% of the gait cycle). (Adapted from Gage, JR. An overview of normal walking. In Greene, WB [Ed.], Instructional Course Lectures, Vol. 39. Park Ridge, IL: American Academy of Orthopaedic Surgeons, 1990.)

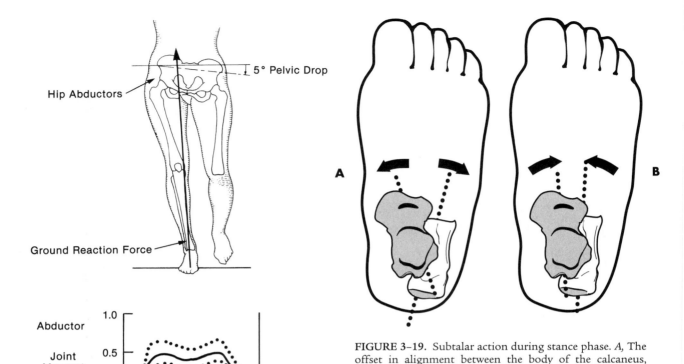

FIGURE 3–18. Coronal plane hip joint kinetics. (From Gage, JR. Gait Analysis in Cerebral Palsy. London: Mac Keith Press, 1991.)

FIGURE 3–19. Subtalar action during stance phase. *A,* The offset in alignment between the body of the calcaneus, which accepts floor contact, and the tibia, which transmits body weight, causes the calcaneus to evert on the talus. The long axis of the calcaneus and the long axis of the talus diverge from each other as the talus rotates inward. *B,* Subtalar joint inversion during terminal stance repositions the calcaneus under the talus, and the long axis of the bones converge but are not parallel.

force on the supported limb, which produces an external adduction moment at hip, knee, and ankle. The external adduction moment is resisted by eccentric control of the hip abductors. This allows the stance side of the pelvis to rise and the unsupported side to drop.

The pelvis and hip motion reverses in midstance as concentric control by the hip abductors of the stance limb acts to raise the pelvis. This action assists clearance on the swing side. During preswing the hip on the stance side goes into abduction in preparation for toe-off.

Ankle and foot motion in the coronal plane is complex, but it is also very important to efficient gait. It is not routinely measured during full body gait analysis because of inadequate multisegment foot models. The literature is confusing because of variations in the terms used to describe motions occurring in the foot. The following de-

scription is consistent with nomenclature used by Perry (1992).

At initial contact, as stated earlier, an external adduction moment is present at the ankle and foot. The position of the anatomic body of the calcaneus, which accepts floor contact, is lateral to the tibia, which transmits body weight onto the talus from above. This causes the calcaneus to evert on the talus and reduces the support the calcaneus provides the talus (Fig. 3–19, *A*). The eversion of the calcaneus on the talus occurs during the initial part of the gait cycle (loading response and early midstance). It is controlled by ligaments surrounding the subtalar joint, as well as eccentric muscle action of the anterior tibialis and posterior tibialis muscles. Maximum eversion occurs at the onset of single-leg stance (15% of the gait cycle). Motion reverses during the remainder of midstance under muscular action of the posterior tibialis and the soleus and the gradual shift of weight bearing to the forefoot. Subtalar joint neutral is reached by 40% of the gait cycle—the midpoint of terminal stance. Inversion locks the midtarsal joint and provides increased stability of the foot during weight bearing on the forefoot. It also moves the calcaneus back under the talus (Fig. 3–19, B). Peak inversion occurs at the end of terminal stance when ankle power generation is at its peak. Excessive inversion is avoided by co-contraction of the peroneal muscles (peroneus longus and peroneus brevis) during terminal stance and preswing. The subtalar joint is typically in a neutral position during swing phase until slight inversion begins again during the last 20% of the gait cycle.

Transverse Plane

The end result of transverse plane motion is stride elongation (see Fig. 3–5). This is accomplished by internal pelvis and hip rotation under the control of the adductor magnus muscle. During the first half of stance phase internal rotation occurs at the pelvis and hip that reverses in the last half of stance. The pelvis is at its maximum posterior position at toe-off. The foot is positioned 5 to 10° (average value) external to the line of progression throughout the entire walking cycle. Subtalar joint action produces rotations of the tibia as part of the closed chain mortise joint. The reader is referred to other texts for explanation of the transverse plane motions at the ankle and knee (Inman et al., 1981; Perry, 1992).

Energy Expenditure

The purpose of many of the events in the walking cycle in all three planes of motion is to optimize energy expenditure or reduce the vertical translation of the center of mass. Gage (1991) includes energy conservation as one of the five attributes of normal gait and states that variation in this attribute encompasses the deviations of the other four attributes.

The mechanisms that the body uses to conserve energy are optimizing the excursion of the center of mass, control of momentum, and active or passive transfer of energy between body segments. The vertical and horizontal displacements of the center of mass are almost sinusoidal and are equal and opposite during typical walking (Winter, 1987). The body accomplishes this through the three pelvic rotations (rotation, tilt, and obliquity) and coordinated knee and ankle motion. Inman and colleagues (1981) demonstrated that without pelvic rotation and with stiff limbs, the center of mass of the body would be lifted approximately 9.5 cm with each step. Normal vertical excursion of the body averages approximately 4.5 cm.

Determination of energy expenditure in gait has been a topic of research since the 1950s (Coates & Meade, 1960; Passmore & Durnin, 1955; Ralston, 1958). Ralston (1958) hypothesized that individuals naturally select a speed of walking that allows a minimum of energy expenditure. If true, this has direct implications for the child with a motor impairment. His research suggested that energy expenditure during walking is directly proportional to the square of velocity.

Research by Waters and associates (1988) includes information on energy expenditure in children. A linear relationship between velocity and rate of oxygen consumption is described, but the data fail to include velocities below 40 meters per minute or a reference (zero velocity) data collection. Data collected at my laboratory are consistent with Ralston's research and demonstrate that the rate of oxygen consumption varies with the square of velocity (Koop, SE, & Stout, JL, 1991, unpublished data). These data include standing zero velocity resting values and data collected at walking velocities below 40 meters per minute (Fig. 3–20, A). Preschool children are found to be less efficient than either school-age children or teenagers (Fig. 3–20, B).

An alternative to the use of measuring oxygen consumption to estimate energy expenditure involves calculation of the mechanical work required for walking. Kinematic measurements, anthropometric measurements, and kinetic analyses of internal and external loads are required for use of this method (Olney et al., 1990; Winter, 1990). The advantage of mechanical energy estimation is that the energy requirements of individual joints can be calculated. One of the disadvantages, particularly in the assessment of pathologic gait, is that the use of external loads to judge the work associated with walking does not measure the body's ability to efficiently respond to the external loads. Co-contraction associated with spasticity is unaccounted for (Rose SA et al., 1991).

Heart rate is often used as a substitute clinical measure for oxygen uptake and therefore metabolic energy expenditure because of the linear relationship of heart rate to oxygen uptake (Rose J et al., 1989, 1990). Low mechanical efficiency, however, creates disproportionately high submaximal heart rates in individuals with cerebral palsy (CP), making submaximal heart rate a poor predictor of aerobic capacity in this group (Bar-Or, 1983). I have observed high and inconsistent heart rate in relation to oxygen uptake in various clinical populations including CP. Caution should be taken if consideration is being given to this method of estimation of energy expenditure. See Chapter 5 for more information on aerobic capacity.

USE OF GAIT ANALYSIS IN ASSESSING PATHOLOGY

Gait analysis is a useful tool in examining walking pathology in children with physical disabilities because it provides objective measurement of the

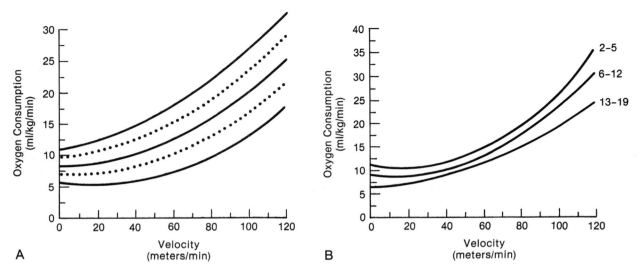

FIGURE 3–20. *A*, Normative values of the rate of metabolic oxygen onsumption versus velocity for 150 children 2 to 19 years of age. The units for oxygen consumption are standardized for body weight. The mean and 2 standard deviations are displayed. *B*, Mean values for three age groups: 2- to 5-year-olds, 6- to 12-year-olds, and 13- to 19-year-olds. (Unpublished data collected at Gillette Children's Specialty Healthcare.)

magnitude of deviations. It also allows the interpreter to analyze data from all planes of motion for a single gait cycle. Just as computed tomography has improved on radiography, gait analysis improves on the evaluator's clinical examination and visual observation. Gait analysis data in the hands of a critical evaluator will never be used in isolation. Clinical examination by a physician, physical therapist, or trained kinesiologist is a vital part of the evaluation. The family's goals for treatment are important as well.

Guidelines for Referral

Guidelines for determining when formal gait analysis should be recommended in the plan of care for a child with a walking disability depend on many factors. The child's age, diagnosis, progress in physical therapy, and goals of intervention are all taken into consideration. Analysis is best when the child's gait pattern is mature, but waiting for a mature walking pattern is not always possible. One key to remember is that current gait analysis techniques provide a single "snapshot" in time. Even if a gait pattern is consistent from cycle to cycle on a given day, if it is not consistent from one week or one month to the next, the value of that single snapshot for decision making is more limited. For this reason, children, adolescents, or adults who are making rapid progress in rehabilitation are not ideal candidates for gait analysis.

Typically, the impetus for referral for gait analysis is a change in treatment. That change in treatment may or may not be surgical in nature. Bracing or prosthetic changes, or medication changes that may affect balance or walking, can be indicators as well. Unless the treatment program specifically affects the child's walking, a three-dimensional gait analysis may not be the best measurement tool for assessing results of changes in a therapy program.

Children under age 3 are not candidates for three-dimensional gait analysis because of their small physical size, their reluctance to cooperate for the duration of the required testing, and their immature gait patterns. Children between 3 and 5 years of age can be tested in the laboratory if their size, behavior, and walking are adequate for the testing process. Because their age and maturity of gait pattern are not ideal, analysis is usually reserved for use as a baseline before surgical intervention. In this age range, interventions such as selective dorsal rhizotomy have increased the number of children who have a gait analysis before the age of 5 years.

The optimal age for a formal three-dimensional gait analysis is typically from age 6 onward. Changes in treatment, whether they are bracing or prosthetic changes, medication changes, or surgical interventions, can all be evaluated. Analysis before a treatment change provides a baseline to assist in the decision-making process of what those specific changes should be. Sometimes no specific treatment changes are recommended. Analysis after treatment provides evaluation of the effects of that treatment. Many people do not appreciate the importance of posttreatment evaluation. What they fail to realize is that effective change and improvements in treatment techniques cannot occur without posttreatment evaluation. The combined knowledge of previous posttreatment evaluations plays an important part in the ability to accurately identify problems and solutions to pretreatment problems.

Assessing Gait Pathology

A gait analysis laboratory should be considered a measurement tool. Information from a gait laboratory can assist in differentiation of primary impairments from secondary compensations. Primary impairments are those abnormalities that are a direct result of CNS injury; secondary compensations refer to the mechanisms used by the individual to circumvent the primary abnormalities. In addition to use in treatment of conditions such as CP and myelomeningocele, gait data can also be used to assess the effects on walking of orthotic devices in various populations or of different prosthetic devices in individuals with amputations. Gait analysis at repetitive intervals can assist in the examination of the progression of a particular deformity or condition or the effects of a particular controlled treatment regimen (including surgery, medication, or physical therapy).

Specific physical therapy recommendations are often difficult to determine with gait laboratory data alone. Evaluation during a gait analysis typically includes only a limited documentation of physical findings and is not a complete physical therapy examination. The EMG information from most gait laboratories does not provide information about strength of muscle contraction and cannot be used to determine which muscles are to be strengthened and how. A thorough knowledge of muscle mechanics and normal gait combined with manual muscle testing allows the therapist to answer these questions. EMG activity can, however, determine whether muscle activity is present or absent and the timing of that muscle activity, which can be useful to determine whether a particular muscle is available for strengthening and to conjecture about what the consequences of that strengthening might be. Kinetic analysis provides joint moment and power information that is sometimes useful for this purpose. In summary, the gait laboratory can be an objective measuring tool for the physical therapist.

Returning to the prerequisites for development of any skill, gait pathology can be created by abnormal motor control, spasticity, loss of ROM, decreased strength, loss of sensation, and bony deformity. Each can result in primary impairments and secondary compensatory mechanisms used to produce or to maintain useful function. Gait analysis can be used to distinguish between the two. It can be used to identify areas of bony abnormality and loss of functional ROM and to document areas of relative weakness or spasticity. The information is always used in conjunction with a clinical examination. The use of gait analysis in assessment of impairments in CP is discussed here as an example of how information is used and interpreted. Limitations of gait analysis are also discussed. Gait analysis is in no way limited to examination of CP or any one gait pathology.

Common Gait Abnormalities in Cerebral Palsy

Bony Deformity

Bony deformities are assessed best by clinical examination and radiography. Gait analysis data measure the functional effect of the bony deformity on the child's walking. Bony deformities are examples of secondary impairments because they are not caused directly by the CNS lesion. They can result from failure of physiologic bone remodeling, the effects of spasticity and muscle imbalance, disuse, attempts at function, or any combination of these factors. These deformities (except for leg length discrepancies) are best assessed in the transverse plane data. Once they have occurred they become a primary focus for orthopedic treatment because they cannot be corrected by conservative management. True bony deformity cannot be corrected by physical therapy. Three common bony abnormalities seen in children with CP are internal femoral torsion, external tibial torsion, and subtalar joint subluxation.

INTERNAL FEMORAL TORSION (FEMORAL ANTETORSION)

Visually, internal femoral torsion appears as internal rotation of the femurs during walking and is measured as such on kinematic analysis. Antetorsion (forward torsion) is a true structural twist deformity of the long axis of the femur. The cause is a combination of (1) persistent physiologic antetorsion in the infant because of delayed weight bearing and (2) abnormal muscle forces created by spasticity (Bleck, 1987; Gage, 1991). Femoral antetorsion is not synonymous with valgus angulation of the femoral neck–shaft angle (coxa valga) or the anterior or forward position of the head and neck of the femur relative to the frontal plane (anteversion). Antetorsion can be clinically measured as the degree of internal femoral rotation in the prone position required to position the greater trochanter most "lateral" or parallel to the supporting surface (Ryder & Crane, 1953).

Usually, in the presence of internal femoral torsion there is loss of passive external rotation range and the range of internal rotation is excessive; often the ratio of internal to external rotation is equal to or greater than 3:1 (Fig. 3–21). Femoral antetorsion and the degree of internal rotation measured on kinematic data are correlated, but they are different measurements.

EXTERNAL TIBIAL TORSION

External tibial torsion is an external rotation or torsion of the long axis of the tibia. It is measured most appropriately by physical examination of the transmalleolar axis or thigh-foot axis and not by gait analysis, unless the system used measures the rotation of the foot with respect to the tibia. External tibial torsion is a true bony deformity that often

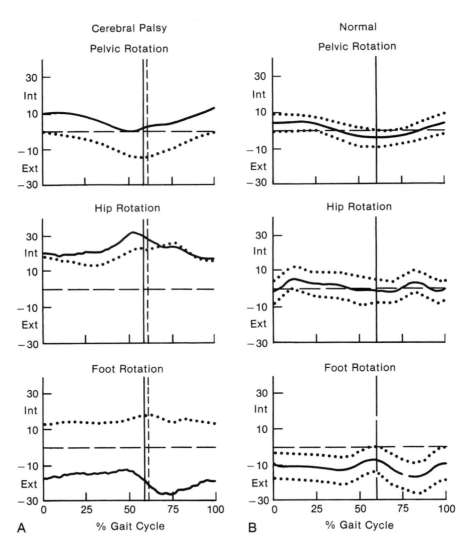

FIGURE 3–21. An example of kinematic graphs from *(A)* a 10-year-old child with spastic diplegic cerebral palsy compared with *(B)* normative data for pelvic and hip rotation and foot progression. Results of bony deformity are often seen in the transverse or rotational plane. Graphs for the child with cerebral palsy depict the right side *(solid line)* and the left side *(dashed line)* for a representative gait cycle. The normative graphs display the mean *(solid line)* and one standard deviation *(dashed line)*. The hip rotation graph in the child with cerebral palsy shows bilateral internal hip rotation. The foot rotation graph displays an appropriate external foot progression on the right side *(solid line)* despite internal hip rotation on the right side. This could result from either subtalar joint subluxation or external tibial torsion, or a combination of both. By physical examination this child has bilateral femoral antetorsion and a right external tibial torsion.

develops as a secondary impairment to internal femoral torsion. Limited knee motion that results in repetitive dragging of the foot in an externally rotated posture for clearance can also result in the deformity. In the presence of femoral antetorsion, external tibial torsion is difficult to observe visually because the foot progression angle may not appear abnormal. The knee sometimes has a valgus appearance, but it is not a coronal plane abnormality (Fig. 3–22). The internal torsion of the femur is compensated by external torsion of the tibia so that the foot remains in the direction of progression (see Figs. 3–21 and 3–22).

PES VALGUS (SUBTALAR JOINT SUBLUXATION)

Pes valgus is most common in children with spastic diplegic or spastic quadriplegic types of CP and less often occurs in children with spastic hemiplegia. Caused by a relative subluxation of the talus on the os calcis, it usually develops because of muscle imbalance and a combination of tightness and weakness. Visually, the calcaneus is positioned in eversion. Kinematic data do not identify subtalar joint subluxation. The effect of the deformity is measured in the plantar flexion–dorsiflexion and foot rotation graphs. Physical and radiographic examination is required.

Inadequate Range of Motion and Spasticity

Gage (1991) often refers to CP as a condition that preferentially affects two joint muscles because it is

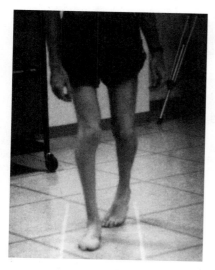

FIGURE 3–22. A 30-year-old adult with spastic diplegic cerebral palsy. Note the internal hip position on the right side (knee in) and the foot progression angle that is neutral to the line of progression. This individual has an external tibial torsion on the right side.

primarily in the two-joint muscles that spasticity contributes to the abnormalities associated with walking. Most two-joint muscles are predominantly fast-twitch muscles used for rapid force production. Loss of ROM creates static contracture; spasticity imposes loss of ROM in dynamic situations because of resistance to stretch (Kruger & Gage, 1986; Rose SA et al., 1993). The effects of inadequate ROM and spasticity can be measured in all three planes of motion but are most prevalently seen in the sagittal plane. Examples measured by gait analysis are an abnormal plantar flexion–knee extension couple, crouch gait, and limited swing-phase knee motion.

ABNORMAL PLANTAR FLEXION–KNEE EXTENSION COUPLE

During normal walking, the plantar flexion–knee extension couple is a force couple whereby the soleus and the gastrocnemius muscles control forward momentum and the forward progression of the ground reaction force by eccentric contraction. Children with CP often enter the walking cycle with a footflat initial contact, which rapidly places the gastrocnemius under premature tension at both ends of the muscle. Gage (1991) postulated that in response to the stretch, spasticity is elicited that can restrict tibial advancement, produce knee extension (hyperextension), and reduce the extent of dorsiflexion (plantar flexion). The spastic response is revealed in a biphasic pattern during stance phase of increasing dorsiflexion and then decreasing dorsiflexion in the kinematics and by an abnormal plantar flexor power generation coincident in time with the first decrease of dorsiflexion in the cycle in the kinetics. Occasionally, the EMG activity is biphasic as well (Fig. 3–23). The abnormal power generation elevates the body's center of mass and functionally increases energy expenditure.

CROUCHED POSTURE

Caused by hip flexion contractures or tightness, knee flexion contractures or tightness, excessive plantar flexor muscle weakness, or any combination of these conditions, increased flexion is seen at all joints in the sagittal plane in crouched gait (Fig. 3–24).

LIMITED SWING-PHASE KNEE MOTION

Limitation of motion at the knee in swing phase usually begins in preswing, where motion is also inadequate. Momentum for swing phase in normal gait is generated by the acceleration force of the gastrocnemius muscle that drives the ground reaction force behind the knee. When the gastrocnemius force generation is reduced, as is often the case in CP, the hip flexors supply the momentum to clear the

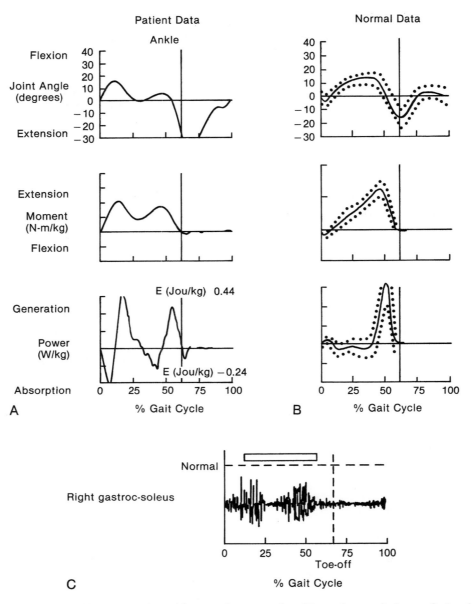

FIGURE 3–23. Kinematics and kinetics at the ankle joint demonstrating (A) an abnormal plantar flexion–knee extension couple in a child with cerebral palsy compared with (B) normal. The ankle kinematics of the patient display a biphasic pattern in stance phase—increasing dorsiflexion–decreasing dorsiflexion—that repeats itself. This results in a biphasic plantar flexor moment as well, and an inappropriate midstance power generation. C, Surface EMG record from the gastroc-soleus complex also exhibits two bursts of activity coinciding with the power generation.

extremity. The rectus femoris is often recruited as a hip flexor. If this muscle is spastic it maintains its action as a knee extensor. The already diminished knee flexion in preswing is further inhibited by spastic restraint that does not allow further knee flexion (see Fig. 3–24).

Weakness

Weakness cannot be measured directly by gait analysis. The type of electromyography used does not provide information regarding strength. Kinematic data measure only the effects; it is up to the clinician to interpret whether the pattern is present

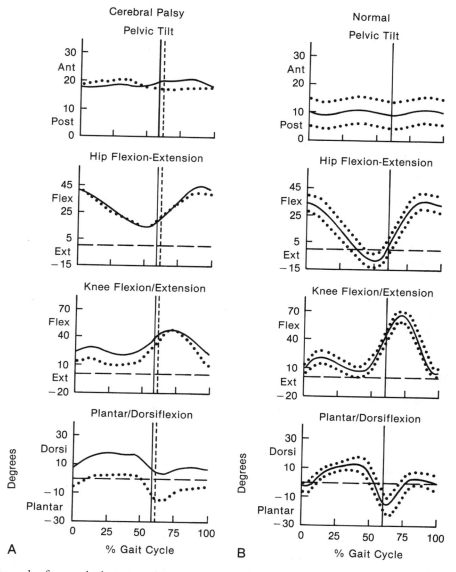

FIGURE 3–24. Example of a crouched posture of increased hip and knee flexion in the sagittal plane of a 10-year-old child with cerebral palsy *(A)* as compared with normal *(B)*. Patient data compare the child's right side *(solid line)* with the left *(dashed line)*. The posture at the knee is asymmetric, with increased knee flexion during stance phase on the right side. Swing-phase knee flexion is also decreased.

as the result of weakness or tightness. Kinetic data do provide a limited measure of weakness if full ROM is available at the joint. Power can be produced only if joint movement is present. The best measure of strength is by physical examination, although this is complicated by the presence of spasticity.

HIP ABDUCTOR WEAKNESS

Weakness of the hip abductor muscles in CP, as in any other type of gait disorder, produces an uncon-trolled pelvic drop on the swing side and lateral trunk shift over the stance limb. The ground reaction force in the coronal plane produces an external adduction moment at all joints of the stance limb. If abductor strength is insufficient, the lateral trunk shift positions the ground reaction force through the hip joint center so no abductor moment is needed. Hip abductor muscle weakness is frequently (but not necessarily) seen in children with femoral antetorsion because the torsion creates an inadequate lever arm over which the gluteus medius muscle is able to act, imposing functional weakness. On kinematic graphs hip abductor weakness is displayed as increased adduction. Differentiation between hip abductor muscle weakness and hip adductor tightness cannot be done solely using kinematic data.

GASTROCNEMIUS-SOLEUS WEAKNESS

Plantar flexor muscle weakness primarily affects terminal stance and preswing phases of the gait cycle, but midstance is also affected. During midstance, the soleus is not able to control the progression of the ground reaction force that is anterior to the ankle, and excessive dorsiflexion results. Heel rise is delayed in terminal stance because gastrocnemius power may also be insufficient. Excessive dorsiflexion can drive the knees into flexion as well. Quadriceps muscle activity may be required to maintain an upright posture if the trunk is vertical, resulting in increased energy expense. Clearance is achieved by the proximal hip flexors because the plantar flexor muscles alone are insufficient. This results in an insufficient acceleration force in terminal stance and imposes a slower gait velocity.

CONCLUSION

The prerequisites for any motor function, including gait, develop as the CNS matures and the body grows, producing physiologic changes in the mechanics and the neurophysiology of the system. The attributes of normal gait are lost in pathologic conditions such as CP because of the primary impairments of loss of selective motor control and balance, abnormal tone and sensation, muscle weakness, and secondary impairments such as bony deformity and loss of ROM.

This chapter was designed to provide an overview of the refinement of gait in childhood, the components of normal gait as measured by gait analysis, and a brief introduction to the use of gait analysis in examination of gait pathology. A gait laboratory is only a measuring tool and is a supplement, not a substitute, for other tools used to assess gait pathology.

Research in the area of gait continues to be a topic of great interest. As measurement techniques improve, our knowledge of walking and its development becomes more refined. With a clear understanding of normal gait, we can better understand the mechanisms of pathologic gait. Here the science of physical therapy melds into the art of physical therapy practice for the children we treat.

ACKNOWLEDGMENTS

I would like to thank Dr. Jim Gage and Dr. Steven Koop, whose philosophy and understanding of normal gait and treatment of children with gait pathologies are significant contributions to this chapter. I am privileged to work with both of them.

References

Adolph, K. Learning in the development of infant locomotion. Monographs of the Society for Research in Child Development. Serial #251, Vol. 62:3. Chicago: University of Chicago Press, 1997.

Armstrong, DM. The motor cortex and locomotion in the cat. In Grillner, S, Stein, PSG, Stuart, DG, Forssberg H, Herman, RM, & Wallen, P (Eds.), Neurobiology of Vertebrate Locomotion. London: Macmillan, 1986, pp. 121–137.

Bar-Or, O. Neuromuscular diseases. In Bar-Or, O, Pediatric Sports Medicine for the Practitioner. New York: Springer-Verlag, 1983, pp. 227–249.

Basmajian, JV, & DeLuca, CJ. Muscles Alive: Their Functions Revealed by Electromyography, 5th ed. Baltimore: Williams & Wilkins, 1985.

Berger, W, Quintern, J, & Dietz, V. Stance and gait perturbations in children: Developmental aspects of compensatory mechanisms. Electroencephalography and Clinical Neurophysiology, 61:385–395, 1985.

Bernhardt, DB. Prenatal and postnatal growth and development of the foot and ankle. Physical Therapy, 68:1831–1839, 1988.

Bleck, EE. Developmental orthopaedics: III. Toddlers. Developmental Medicine and Child Neurology, 24:533–555, 1982.

Bleck, EE. Orthopaedic Management in Cerebral Palsy. London: Mac Keith Press, 1987, pp. 323–328.

Bly, L. Motor Skills Acquisition in the First Year: An Illustrated Guide to Normal Development. Tucson, AZ: Therapy Skill Builders, 1994.

Bradley, NS, & Bekoff, A. Development of locomotion: Animal models. In Woollacott, MH, & Shumway-Cook, A (Eds.), Development of Posture and Gait Across the Lifespan. Columbia, SC: University of South Carolina Press, 1989, pp. 48–73.

Butterworth, G, & Hicks, L. Visual proprioception and postural stability in infancy: A developmental study. Perception, 6:255–262, 1977.

Coates, JE, & Meade, F. The energy demand and mechanical energy demand in walking. Ergonomics, 3:97–119, 1960.

Coon, V, Donato, G, Houser, C, & Bleck, EE. Normal ranges of hip motion in infants six weeks, three months, and six months of age. Clinical Orthopaedics and Related Research, 110:256–260, 1975.

Connelly, KJ, & Forssberg, H (Eds.). Neurophysiology and Neuropsychology of Motor Development. London: Mac Keith Press, 1997.

Cusick, BD, & Stuberg, WA. Assessment of lower-extremity alignment in the transverse plane: Implications for management of children with neuromotor dysfunction. Physical Therapy, 72:3–15, 1992.

Engel, GM, & Staheli, LT. The natural history of torsion and other factors influencing gait in childhood: A study of the angle of gait, tibial torsion, knee angle, hip rotation, and the development of the arch in normal children. Clinical Orthopaedics, 99:12–17, 1974.

Epstein, HT. Correlated brain and intelligence development in humans. In Hahn, ME, Jensen, C, & Dudek, BC (Eds.), Development and Evolution of Brain Size: Behavioral Implications. New York: Academic Press, 1979, pp. 111–131.

Fabray, G, MacEwen, GD, & Shands, AR. Torsion of the femur: A study in normal and pathological conditions. Journal of Bone and Joint Surgery (American), 55:1726–1738, 1973.

Fomon, SJ. Body composition of the male referenced infant during the first year of life. Pediatrics, 40:863–867, 1967.

Forssberg, H. Ontogeny of human locomotor control: I. Infant stepping, supported locomotion and transition to independent locomotion. Experimental Brain Research, 57:480–493, 1985.

Forssberg, H. Evolution of plantigrade gait: Is there a neuronal correlate? Developmental Medicine and Child Neurology, 34:916–925, 1992.

Gage, JR. Gait Analysis in Cerebral Palsy. London: Mac Keith Press, 1991.

Grillner, S. Control of locomotion in bipeds, tetrapods, and fish. In Geiger, SR (Ed.), Handbook of Physiology, Vol. 2. Bethesda, MD: American Physiological Society, 1981, pp. 1179–1236.

Haas, SS, Epps, CH, Jr, & Adams, JP. Normal ranges of hip motion in the newborn. Clinical Orthopaedics, 91:114–118, 1973.

Heriza, C. Motor development: Traditional and contemporary theories. In Lister, MJ (Ed.), Contemporary Management of Motor Control Problems: Proceedings of the II STEP Conference. Alexandria, VA: Foundation for Physical Therapy, 1991, pp. 99–126.

Hirschfield, H, & Forssberg, H. Epigenetic development of postural responses for sitting during infancy. Experimental Brain Research, 97:528–540, 1994.

Inman, VT, Ralston, HJ, & Todd, F. Human Walking. Baltimore: Williams & Wilkins, 1981.

Jensen, JL, & Bothner, KA. Infant motor development: The biomechanics of change. In van Praagh, E (Ed.), Pediatric Anaerobic Performance. Champaign, IL: Human Kinetics, 1998, pp. 23–43.

Jordan, LM. Initiation of locomotion from the mammalian brainstem. In Grillner, S, Stein, PSG, Stuart, DG, Forssberg, H, Herman, RM, & Wallen, P (Eds.), Neurobiology of Vertebrate Locomotion. London: Macmillan Press, 1986, pp. 21–37.

Kadaba, MP, Wooten, ME, & Gainery, J. Repeatability of phasic muscle activity: Performance of surface and intramuscular electrodes. Journal of Orthopedic Research, 3:350–359, 1985.

Kazai, N, Okamoto, T, & Kumamoto, M. Electromyographic study of supported walking of infants in the initial period of learning to walk. In Komi, PV (Ed.), Biomechanics V: Proceedings of the Fifth International Congress on Biomechanics. Baltimore: University Park Press, 1976, pp. 311–318.

Komi, PV. Relationship between muscle tension, EMG, and velocity of contraction under concentric and eccentric work. In Desmedt, JE (Ed.), New Developments in Electromyography and Clinical Neurophysiology. Basel, Switzerland: S Karger AG, Medical and Scientific Publishers, 1973, pp. 596–606.

Kruger, MP, & Gage, JR. Stance phase foot rocker problems in spastic diplegia. Developmental Medicine and Child Neurology, 28(suppl 53):4, 1986.

Kugler, PN, Kelso, JA, & Turvey, MT. On the control and coordination of naturally developing systems. In Kelso, JAS, & Clark, JE (Eds.), The Development of Movement Control and Coordination. New York: John Wiley & Sons, 1982, pp. 79–93.

Loeb, GE. Kinematic factors in the generation and role of sensory feedback during locomotion. In Grillner, S, Stein, PSG, Stuart, DG, Forssberg, H, Herman, RM, & Wallen, P (Eds.), Neurobiology of Vertebrate Locomotion. London: Macmillan Press, 1986, pp. 547–561.

Murray, MP, Drought, AB, & Kory, RC. Walking patterns of normal men. Journal of Bone and Joint Surgery (American), 46:355–360, 1964.

Okamoto, T, & Kumamoto, M. Electromyographic study of the learning process of walking in infants. Electromyography, 12:149–158, 1972.

Olney, SJ, MacPhail, HEA, Hedden, DM, & Boyce, WF. Work and power in hemiplegic cerebral palsy gait. Physical Therapy, 70:431–438, 1990.

Ounpuu, S, Gage, JR, & Davis, RB, III. Three-dimensional lower extremity joint kinetics in normal pediatric gait. Journal of Pediatric Orthopedics, 11:341–349, 1991.

Palmer, CE. Studies of the center of gravity in the human body. Child Development, 15:99–180, 1944.

Passmore, R, & Durnin, GA. Human energy expenditure. Physiological Reviews, 35:801–839, 1955.

Perry, J. Gait Analysis: Normal and Pathological Function. Thorofare, NJ: Slack, 1992.

Phelps, E, Smith, LJ, & Hallum, A. Normal ranges of hip motion of infants between 9 and 24 months of age. Developmental Medicine and Child Neurology, 27:785–793, 1985.

Piper, MC, & Darrah, J. Motor Assessment of the Developing Infant. Philadelphia: WB Saunders, 1994.

Ralston, HJ. Energy-speed relation and optimal speed during level walking. Internationale Zeitschrift fur Angewandte Physiologie, 17:277–283, 1958.

Rancho Los Amigos Medical Center, Pathokinesiology Department, Physical Therapy Department. Observational Gait Analysis Handbook. Downey, CA: The Professional Staff Association of Rancho Los Amigos Medical Center, 1989.

Root, ML, Orien, WP, Weed, JH, & Hughes, RJ. Biomechanical Examination of the Foot, Vol. 1. Los Angeles: Clinical Biomechanics, 1971.

Rose, J, Gamble, JG, Burgos, A, Medeiros, J, & Haskell, WL. Energy expenditure index of walking for normal children and children with cerebral palsy. Developmental Medicine and Child Neurology, 32:333–340, 1990.

Rose, J, Gamble, JG, Medeiros, J, Burgos, A, & Haskell, WL. Energy cost of walking in normal children and in those with cerebral palsy: Comparison of heart rate and oxygen uptake. Pediatric Orthopedics, 9:276–279, 1989.

Rose, SA, DeLuca, PA, Davis, RB, III, Ounpuu, S, & Gage, JR. Kinematic and kinetic evaluation of the ankle following lengthening of the gastrocnemius fascia in children with cerebral palsy. Journal of Pediatric Orthopedics. 13:727–732, 1993.

Rose, SA, Ounpuu, S, & DeLuca, PA. Strategies for the assessment of pediatric gait in the clinical setting. Physical Therapy, 71:961–980, 1991.

Ryder, CT, & Crane, L: Measuring femoral anteversion: The problem and a method. Journal of Bone and Joint Surgery (American), 35: 321–328, 1953.

Salenius, P, & Vankka, E. The development of the tibiofemoral angle in children. Journal of Bone and Joint Surgery (American), 57:259–261, 1975.

Saunders, JB, Inman, VT, & Eberhart, HD. The major determinants in normal and pathological gait. Journal of Bone and Joint Surgery (American), 35:543–559, 1953.

Sepulveda, F, Wells, DM, & Vaughan, CL. A neural network representation of electromyography and joint dynamics in human gait. Journal of Biomechanics, 26:101–109, 1993.

Shumway-Cook, A, & Woollacott, MH. The growth of stability: Postural control from a developmental perspective. Journal of Motor Behavior, 17:131–147, 1985.

Spady, DW. Normal body composition of infants and children. Ross Conference on Pediatric Research, Ross Laboratories, Columbus, Ohio, 98:67–73, 1989.

Staheli, LT, Corbett, M, Wyss, C, & King, H. Lower extremity rotational problems in children. Journal of Bone and Joint Surgery (American), 67:39–47, 1985.

Staheli, LT, & Engel, GM. Tibial torsion: A method of assessment and a survey of normal children. Clinical Orthopaedics, 86:183–186, 1972.

Stout, JL, Hagen, BT, & Gage, JR. Normal Walking: An Overview Based on Gait Analysis. Hagen, BT, & Stout, JL (Producers). St. Paul, MN: Gillette Children's Specialty Healthcare and Meditech Communications, 1993 (Videotape).

Stout, JL, Hagen, BT, & Gage, JR. Principles of Pathologic Gait in Cerebral Palsy. Hagen, BT, & Stout, JL (Producers). St. Paul, MN: Gillette Children's Specialty Healthcare and Meditech Communications, 1994 (Videotape).

Sun, H, & Jensen, R. Body segment growth during infancy. Journal of Biomechanics, 27:265–275, 1994.

Sutherland, DH. Gait Disorders in Childhood and Adolescence. Baltimore: Williams & Wilkins, 1984.

Sutherland, DH, Olshen, RA, Biden, EN, & Wyatt, MP. The Development of Mature Walking. London: Mac Keith Press, 1988.

Sutherland, DH, Olshen, RA, Cooper, L, & Woo, S. The development of mature gait. Journal of Bone and Joint Surgery (American), 62:336–353, 1980.

Tachdjian, MO. The Child's Foot. Philadelphia: WB Saunders, 1985.

Tachdjian, MO. Pediatric Orthopaedics, Vol. 4, 2nd ed. Philadelphia: WB Saunders, 1990, pp. 2820–2835.

Thelen, E. Treadmill elicited stepping in seven-month-old infants. Child Development, 57:1498–1506, 1986.

Thelen, E, & Cooke, DW. Relationship between newborn stepping and later walking: A new interpretation. Developmental Medicine and Child Neurology, 29:380–393, 1987.

Thelen, E, Fisher, DM, & Ridley-Johnson, R. The relationship between physical growth and a newborn reflex. Infant Behavior and Development, 7:479–493, 1984.

Thelen, E, Fisher, DM, Ridley-Johnson, R, & Griffin, NJ. Effects of body build and arousal on newborn infant stepping. Developmental Psychobiology, 15:447–453, 1982.

Thelen, E, & Ulrich, BD. Hidden skills: A dynamic systems analysis of treadmill stepping during the first year. Monographs of the Society for Research in Child Development, 56:1–98, 1991.

Thelen, E, Ulrich, BD, & Jensen, JL. The developmental origins of locomotion. In Woollacott, MH, & Shumway-Cook, A (Eds.), Development of Posture and Gait Across the Lifespan. Columbia, SC: University of South Carolina Press, 1989, pp. 25–47.

Ulrich, BD, & Ulrich, DA. Spontaneous leg movements of infants with Down syndrome and nondisabled infants. Child Development, 66:1844–1849, 1995.

Valmassy, RL. Biomechanical evaluation of child. In Ganley, JV (Ed.), Symposium on Podopediatrics. Philadelphia: WB Saunders, 1984, pp. 563–579.

Vredenbregt, J, & Rau, G. Surface electromyography in relation to force, muscle length, and endurance. In Desmedt, JE (Ed.), New Developments in Electromyography and Clinical Neurophysiology. Basel, Switzerland: S Karger AG, Medical and Scientific Publishers, 1973, pp. 607–622.

Walker, JM. Musculoskeletal development: A review. Physical Therapy, 71:878–889, 1991.

Waters, RL, Lunsford, BR, Perry, J, & Byrd, R. Energy-speed relationship of walking: Standard tables. Journal of Orthopaedic Research, 6:215–222, 1988.

Winter, DA. The Biomechanics of Human Movement. New York: John Wiley & Sons, 1979.

Winter, DA. Biomechanical motor patterns in normal walking. Journal of Motor Behavior, 15:302–330, 1983.

Winter, DA. The Biomechanics of Motor Control and Human Gait. Waterloo, Ontario: University of Waterloo Press, 1987.

Winter, DA. Biomechanics and Motor Control of Normal Human Movement, 2nd ed. New York: John Wiley & Sons, 1990.

Winter, DA, & Yack, HJ. EMG profiles during normal human walking: Stride to stride and intersubject variability. Electroencephalography and Clinical Neurophysiology, 67:402–411, 1987.

Woollacott, MH, Shumway-Cook, A, & Williams, HG. The development of posture and balance control in children. In Woollacott, MH, & Shumway-Cook, A (Eds.), Development of Posture and Gait Across the Lifespan. Columbia, SC: University of South Carolina Press, 1989, pp. 77–96.

Zajac, FE, & Gordon, ME. Determining muscle's force and action in multiarticular movement. Exercise Science and Sports Sciences Reviews, 17:187–231, 1989.

Zelazo, PR. The development of walking: New findings and old assumptions. Journal of Motor Behavior, 15:99–137, 1983.

CHAPTER

4

Musculoskeletal Development and Adaptation

CARRIE G. GAJDOSIK, PT, MS
RICHARD L. GAJDOSIK, PT, PhD

Pediatric physical therapists routinely address clinical conditions that influence the growth and development of the musculoskeletal system, either directly or indirectly. Therapeutic interventions are often designed to promote musculoskeletal adaptations in an effort to prevent or correct physical impairments with the hope of enhancing function. Accordingly, knowledge of normal growth and development and of the principles of adaptation of the musculoskeletal system is essential for understanding the efficacy of interventions. The purposes of this chapter are to (1) describe the growth and development of muscle and bone and (2) describe the adaptation of muscle and bone, including the effects of various interventions designed to promote desired adaptations.

MUSCULOSKELETAL DEVELOPMENT

Muscle Tissue

The embryologic development of muscle has been well described in many texts and articles, and few controversies exist regarding the sequence of gross

anatomic changes during the embryologic period (Davis & Dobbing, 1974; Moore KL, 1988; Owen et al., 1980). Embryonic myoblasts arise from mesodermal cells and eventually differentiate to form myotubes. These immature, multinucleate tubular structures, which develop from two distinct lineages, are labeled either "primary" or "secondary." The primary myotubes are first observed at approximately 5 weeks of gestational age and are known to develop and differentiate without neural influence. The secondary myotubes are seen several weeks later. The growth and development of these myotubes are more heavily dependent on neural input, without which they may be smaller, fewer in number, or malformed (Grove, 1989; Mastaglia, 1974; Miller, 1991; Sanes, 1987). By 20 weeks of gestational age, most myotubes have fused to form muscle fibers and many of the fibers have a microscopic content similar to that of adult fibers.

The motor unit, which consists of a motoneuron and the muscle fibers it innervates, begins its formation with the development of the neuromuscular junction. By 8 weeks of gestation, acetylcholine

117

receptors are found around the circumference of the myotubular membrane (Hesselmans et al., 1993). This timing corresponds to the earliest fetal movement, which is observed in the intercostal muscles. The presence of motor activity indicates that a viable connection between the neuromuscular junction and the motor axon has occurred. Several motor axons originating from different somites innervate the newly formed end plates. This polyneuronal innervation results in motor units that are much larger than those found in adults. During the prenatal and first years of life, synaptic elimination results in each neuromuscular junction receiving innervation by only one axon (Gramsbergen et al., 1997). This adult pattern of one axon per muscle fiber permits a reproducible and predictable increase of force during performance of a task (Purves & Lichtman, 1980; Thompson, 1986). Why fetal muscles are innervated initially by several axons and later undergo the elimination of all but one axon is not well established. It does not appear that the reason is to ensure that every muscle fiber is innervated. In partially denervated muscles of animals, the few remaining muscle fibers still undergo synaptic elimination, thus reducing the size of the motor unit (Brown et al., 1976; Thompson & Jansen, 1977). During the last half of gestational growth, the number and size of muscle fibers increase rapidly so that most of the skeletal muscle has developed by birth. Through the first year of life, muscle fibers continue to increase in number from either the division of existing cells or the differentiation of myoblasts into secondary myotubes (Mastaglia, 1974). During the growing years, muscle fibers increase in length and cross-sectional area by the addition of sarcomeres (Kitiyakara & Angevine, 1963). Their final size is dependent on many factors, including blood supply, innervation, nutrition, gender, genetics, and exercise.

During fetal development, differentiation of the myotubes into the different types of muscle fibers (type I [slow twitch] and type II [fast twitch]) is directed by intrinsic genetic programs (Miller, 1991; Slaton, 1981). Two basic theories have been proposed to explain how fetal muscle fibers differentiate. From the 1960s to the early 1980s, it was widely accepted that the fiber type of developing undifferentiated myotubes was determined by the innervating motoneurons (Buller et al., 1960; Kamieniecka, 1968). Later studies, however, supported a second proposal that fetal muscle fibers can differentiate without neuronal input (Butler et al., 1982; Sanes, 1987; Thompson et al., 1990). Both theories are now accepted because myotubes are known to develop from two distinct lineages. Muscle tissue derived from primary myotubes differentiates into the two basic fiber types predominantly without the influence of the motoneuron, whereas muscle tissue derived from the secondary myotubes is mostly dependent on innervation for differentiation into muscle fiber types (Butler et al., 1982; Grinnell, 1995; Grove, 1989; Miller, 1991). When the muscle tissue is initially innervated, most of the motor axons innervate the primary myotubes before the secondary. Because most primary myotubes eventually differentiate into type I fibers, these fibers are the first to appear in the fetus. Type II fibers, which mostly develop from the secondary myotubes, are observed at about 30 weeks of gestation (Colling-Saltin, 1978; Grinnell, 1995). In adults, the expression of muscle fiber types is dependent on neuronal input, regardless of whether the muscle was derived from primary or secondary myotubes. Fiber type preference is also strongly influenced by disease, the function of the muscle, type of physical activity, and electrical stimulation.

Skeletal and Articular Structures

Like muscle tissue, both the skeletal and articular tissues arise from the mesodermal layer of the embryo. Mesenchymal cells condense to form templates of the skeleton. From this point, two distinct processes of bone formation take place: (1) endochondral ossification and (2) intramembranous ossification. All bones, with the exception of the clavicle, mandible, and skull, are formed by endochondral ossification (also called intracartilaginous ossification) (Moore KL, 1988; Royer, 1974; Walker, 1991). During the early embryonic period, collagenous and elastic fibers are deposited on the mesenchymal models and form cartilaginous models. Bone minerals are deposited on these new models and gradually replace the cartilage via the process of ossification. Intramembranous ossification occurs directly in the mesenchymal model. Mesenchymal cells differentiate into osteoblasts that deposit a matrix called osteoid tissue. This tissue is organized into bone as calcium phosphate is deposited.

Ossification at the primary ossification centers, typically in the center of the diaphysis or body of the bone, commences at the end of the embryonic period (eighth fetal week). By the time of birth, the diaphyses are almost ossified, whereas the epiphyses, or distal ends of the bone, remain cartilaginous. During early childhood, the secondary ossification centers appear in the epiphyses, and ossification proceeds in this section of the bone. The timing of complete ossification varies with each particular bone. Most bones are fully ossified by 20 years of age, but for a few bones the process can continue into adulthood (Moore KL, 1988). After birth, long bones grow in length at the epiphyseal plate, which is between the diaphysis and the epiphysis. This cartilaginous plate rapidly proliferates on the diaphyseal side of the bone. The resultant chondrocytes, arranged in parallel columns, become enlarged and are then converted into bone by endochondral ossification (McKibbin, 1980; Rodriguez et al., 1992). Eventually the epiphyseal plate is ossified, the diaphyses and epiphyses are joined, and the growth of the bone in length is considered complete.

Bone also increases in size through appositional growth, which is the accumulation of new bone on the bone surfaces. This results in an increase in thickness and density of the diaphysis. The most rapid period of bone growth is prenatal. A marked decrease in the rate of growth is noted at birth, but throughout childhood the decline is more gradual. A midgrowth spurt occurs at age 7 and again at puberty (Gasser et al., 1991).

Joint formation begins about the time that the cartilaginous models are formed. In a specialized area between these models, the interzonal mesenchyma differentiates to form the joint. The basic structures of the joint are formed during the sixth to eighth week of gestation, but the final shape develops throughout early childhood under the influence of the forces of movement and compression (Drachman & Sokoloff, 1966). The hip is a good example of how a joint changes shape during the fetal period. At 12 weeks of gestational age, the acetabulum is extremely deep and the head of the femur, which is quite round, is well covered (Fig. 4–1) (Ralis & McKibbin, 1973). As the fetus increases in age, the relative depth of the acetabulum decreases as the head of the femur becomes more hemispheric. At birth, the acetabulum is so shallow that it covers less than one half of the femoral head, and this results in a relatively unstable hip. This change is thought to allow for easier passage through the vaginal canal. During postnatal growth, the forces of compression and movement contribute to an increase in the depth of the acetabulum. The head of the femur becomes rounder, but it never achieves the roundness that it had during the early fetal period.

ADAPTATIONS OF MUSCLE AND BONE

The musculoskeletal system demonstrates a remarkable ability to adapt to the physical demands, or lack of physical demands, placed on the system. The presence of a pathologic condition may adversely influence the structure and function of any component of the system, and this process may result in impairments. For example, congenital deformities, disease processes, or abnormal growth of bone may lead to strength and length adaptations that cause impairments of the muscle-tendon unit

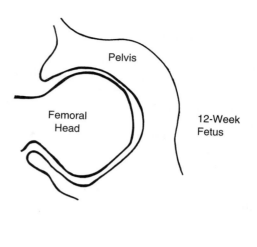

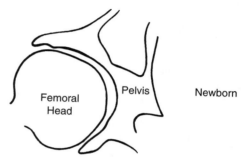

FIGURE 4–1. A schematic diagram of the fetal and newborn hip joint illustrating the change in acetabular coverage of the femoral head. The coverage is extensive in the 12-week fetus, but reduced in the newborn.

(MTU). Congenital or acquired central nervous system deficits, such as cerebral palsy (CP), bring about sensorimotor changes that may promote unwanted shortening adaptations and length impairments of the MTU. These changes may ultimately compromise the structural and functional integrity of the joints and bone, leading to secondary impairments. Pathologic conditions of the MTU itself, for example, muscular dystrophies, may also lead to secondary, unwanted adaptations and impairments of the joints and bone. The normal process of adaptation can either enhance function or lead to impairment, functional limitations, and disability.

Changes in Muscle Fiber Types

Muscle fiber types are susceptible to both internal and external influences. In normal muscle, fiber types are randomly distributed to form a mosaic pattern and there is little variation in fiber size. In the presence of disease or dysfunction, this pattern is altered. One fiber type can become predominant, fiber size can change (due to hypertrophy or atrophy), or the mosaic pattern can be lost when similar fiber types clump together. These changes have been useful in the diagnosis of certain pathologic conditions of muscle. Less information is available on changes in fiber types for children with disabilities than for adults, and there may be some differences between the two age groups (Brooke & Engel, 1969; Tanabe & Nonaka, 1987). Selective atrophy of type II fibers is commonly seen in individuals with muscle disease, especially when muscle strength is compromised by disuse. Adults with steroid-induced strength deficits have selective type II atrophy (Rothstein & Rose, 1982). This same pattern may be observed in children who receive steroids to treat such diseases as juvenile rheumatoid arthritis. Denervated muscles show atrophy of both major types of fibers, but type II fibers show more atrophy than type I fibers. This pattern is probably true for children with myelodysplasia, although it has not been documented. Malnourished children are at risk for a loss of type II fibers, which are thought to be converted to type I fibers (Ward & Stickland, 1991). Selective atrophy of type I fibers is less common but is observed in children with hypotonia (Brooke & Engel, 1969) and in children with congenital myotonic dystrophy (Farkas-Bargeton et al., 1988). An immobilized limb has been reported to show a greater atrophy of type I fibers than of type II fibers, although this change appears to be variable and dependent on the presence or absence of pain, the length of time the limb was immobilized, or the particular muscle that was immobilized (Rose & Rothstein, 1982).

Predominance of either fiber type may occur in the presence of disease. Type I predominance is typically found in myopathic conditions such as Duchenne muscular dystrophy (Brooke & Engel, 1969), whereas type II predominance is associated with motoneuron diseases such as spinal muscular atrophy type 3 (Kugelberg-Welander disease) (Brooke, 1986).

In children with spastic CP, a consistent picture of muscle histopathology has not been reported, probably because of the limited number of investigative studies. Although it has been reported that a predominance of type II fiber atrophy is found in spastic muscles (Brooke & Engel, 1969), this has not been entirely supported in the more recent literature. Varying degrees of atrophy and hypertrophy of type I and type II fibers have been reported and appear to be dependent on muscle group, severity of CP, and age of the child (Castle et al., 1979; Ito et al., 1996; Romanini et al., 1989; Rose et al., 1994). Ito and colleagues (1996) reported a type I fiber predominance and a type IIB fiber deficiency in the gastrocnemius muscle of children with diplegic or hemiplegic CP. They also noted a greater variation in fiber size, particularly in type I fibers, in the older children or the more severely involved limb. In contrast, Rose and associates (1994) reported no difference in the distribution of type I fibers in children with spastic CP when compared with a control group of typically developing children. Unfortunately, the biopsies from the control group and the CP group were not from the same muscles. In this same study, 6 of the 10 children with CP had no evidence of atrophied fibers. Of the remaining four subjects, two had marked atrophy of type II fibers and two had significant atrophy of type I fibers.

Why do pediatric physical therapists need to know about muscle fiber types and their responses to outside influences? This question is difficult to answer because the clinical significance is not well understood. Rose and colleagues (1994) found that children with CP-spastic diplegia who had a predominance of type I fibers (in total area when compared with type II) expended more energy and had more prolonged electromyograph (EMG) activity during walking than children with CP and a predominance of type II fibers. Both Rose and colleagues (1994) and Ito and associates (1996) speculated that spasticity may produce structural changes within the developing muscle. If so, controlling the spasticity in the very young child may be a method for promoting more normal muscle development, which in turn may allow for more efficient expenditure of energy and better function. Rose and Rothstein (1982) speculated that the loss of fast-twitch fibers (type II) could affect the muscle's ability to protect joints during periods of sudden weight loading, whereas the person with a small number of slow-twitch fibers may not be able to preserve the joint integrity when endurance is required. Over time, either of these scenarios could lead to degenerative joint changes. Joint pain, a common complaint of adults with CP (Murphy et al., 1995; Turk et al., 1997), might be related to atypic fiber type distribution, but many factors can affect this secondary problem, such as obesity, abnormal control of movement, and excessive joint movement.

Although some children with CP have atrophy of type II fibers and have difficulty with ballistic movement, whether a causal relationship exists is unknown. How does the disorganization of movement affect atrophy of fibers? Working on ballistic exercises may increase the size of the type II fibers, but the important issue is whether this type of exercise influences function. Further studies of atypic fiber type distribution and its effect on function are needed. In the meantime, physical therapists should be aware that the two basic types of muscle fibers are influenced by exercise differently; that is, the effects of exercise on muscle fibers are training specific. Endurance training enhances the performance of type I fibers, whereas strength training enhances performance of type II fibers.

Structure and Function of the Normal Muscle-Tendon Unit

The normal MTU comprises skeletal muscle tissue proper (muscle fibers with actin and myosin protein filaments); two cytoskeletal systems within the muscle fibers (exosarcomeric and endosarcomeric); the supportive connective tissues within and around the muscle belly (endomysium, perimysium, and epimysium); and the dense regular connective tissues of the tendons that secure the MTU to bone. The total muscle force production is influenced by many factors, including the size of the muscle fibers, the firing rate of motor unit action potentials, the recruitment and derecruitment patterns, the muscle's architecture, the angle of pull, the lever arm, and the changes in the muscle's length.

The total muscle force is produced by the active and passive components of the MTU (Fig. 4-2), both of which are influenced by the MTU's length. To determine the active force produced by the MTU, the passive force is subtracted from the total force (see Fig. 4-2). The force produced by the active component depends primarily on the amount of overlap of the actin and myosin filaments. The maximum iso-

metric force is produced near the resting length of an isolated muscle, and the isometric force decreases as the muscle is either lengthened or shortened relative to the resting length. This change in force in relation to the change in length forms the basis of the sliding filament theory of muscle contraction (Gordon et al., 1966; Huxley & Peachey, 1961). The isometric force is nearly maximal at the resting length because the actin and myosin filaments are in a position of optimal overlap (Figs. 4-3 and 4-4). The force generated by the active component of the MTU depends on the integrity of the central and peripheral nervous systems, the excitation-contraction coupling mechanism, and the cross-sectional area of the skeletal muscle tissues. In a completely relaxed skeletal muscle (i.e., when the central nervous system is not intact or when there is no artificial stimulation), no active tension exists.

When resting muscle is passively stretched, the force produced by the passive component of the MTU is thought to be brought about by three mechanisms: (1) by stretching stable cross-links between the actin and myosin filaments, (2) by stretching proteins within the exosarcomeric and endosarcomeric cytoskeleton (series elastic component), and (3) by deformation of the connective tissues of the muscle (parallel elastic component). The passive component accounts for the resistance felt during passive stretch of a fully relaxed muscle. The passive tension that arises from the stretching of the stable interactions or cross-links between the actin and myosin filaments is the basis of the so-called filamentary resting tension hypothesis of passive tension (Hill, 1968, 1970a, 1970b). The stable bonds were believed to impart a stiffness because the actin-myosin cross-bridges stretch a short distance from the stable position before the contacts slip and reattach at other binding sites. Based on the results of more recent research methodologies, however, this theory is being revised. Recent studies have indicated that much of the stiffness of a stretched relaxed muscle actually comes from filamentous connections between the thick myosin filaments and the Z-disks of the sarcomere (Magid & Law, 1985), particularly when the sarcomere is stretched beyond the actin and myosin overlap (Granzier & Pollack, 1985) (Fig. 4-5). These filamentous connections consist of large, thin filaments of a giant protein that has been named "titin" (also called "connectin"). The titin protein attaches into the M-line region, or center of the myosin filament, courses longitudinally, and attaches into the Z-disks at the ends of the sarcomere. The titin protein forms a major component of the endosarcomeric cytoskeleton. This protein is now believed to be the major subcellular component that resists passive lengthening of a relaxed muscle, thus

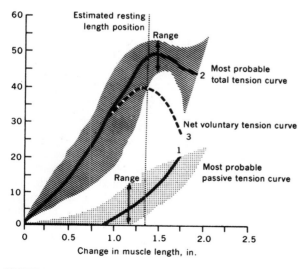

FIGURE 4-2. Classic length-tension curves for skeletal muscle. Net voluntary active tension is predicted by subtracting passive tension from total tension. (With permission from Astrand, P, & Rodahl, K. Textbook of Work Physiology, 2nd ed. New York: McGraw-Hill, 1977, p. 102.)

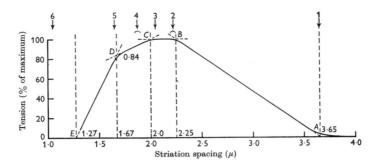

FIGURE 4–3. Schematic summary of tension changes in relation to sarcomere length changes. Arrows along the top are placed opposite the striation spacings for critical stages of actin and myosin filament overlap (see Fig. 4–4). (From Gordon, AM, Huxley, AF, & Julian, FJ. The variation in isometric tension with sarcomere length in vertebrate muscle fibers. Journal of Physiology, *184*:185, 1966.)

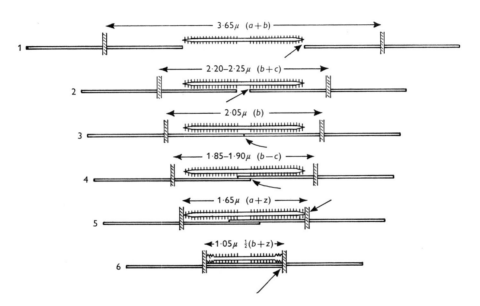

FIGURE 4–4. Critical stages in the increase of overlap between actin and myosin filaments as a sarcomere shortens. Numbers correspond to numbers in Fig. 4–3. (From Gordon, AM, Huxley, AF, & Julian, FJ. The variation in isometric tension with sarcomere length in vertebrate muscle fibers. Journal of Physiology, *184*:186, 1966.)

contributing to passive stiffness (Linke et al., 1996; Trombitas et al., 1998; Wang et al., 1993; Waterman-Storer, 1991). Nebulin is another giant protein that forms part of the endosarcomeric cytoskeleton. Nebulin is associated only with actin filaments within the I-band and is thought to provide structural support to actin's lattice array (see Fig. 4–5) (Waterman-Storer, 1991). Nebulin, however, is not thought to contribute to passive muscle stiffness.

In addition to titin's contribution to passive muscle stiffness, an intermediate-sized protein of the exosarcomeric cytoskeleton also is thought to contribute to passive muscle stiffness. This protein is known as "desmin" (also called "skeletin") (Tokuyasu et al., 1983; Wang & Ramirez-Mitchell, 1983). Desmin is the major subunit of the intermediate protein filaments forming the Z-disks (Wang & Ramirez-Mitchell, 1983). It serves to interconnect Z-disks transversely and to connect Z-disks with organelles (e.g., mitochondria), but not with the T-tubule system (Tokuyasu et al., 1983) (see Fig. 4–5). Moreover, desmin extends longitudinally from Z-disk to Z-disk outside of the sarcomere (Wang & Ramirez-Mitchell, 1983). Because of this longitudinal orientation between Z-disks outside of the sarcomere, the protein will lengthen as the sarcomere is stretched. Thus

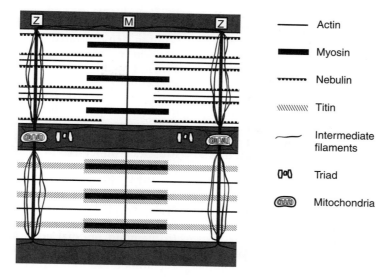

FIGURE 4–5. A schematic diagram of the proposed arrangement of cytoskeletal elements in and around the sarcomere. Both sarcomeres show the arrangement of intermediate filaments, composed mainly of the protein desmin, linking neighboring myofibrils both transversely and longitudinally at the Z-disk, and encircling the Z-disk. The upper sarcomere shows the arrangement of nebulin, running parallel to actin within the I-band. The lower sarcomere depicts titin's proposed location, stretching the full length of the half sarcomere, and attaching to myosin within the A-band. (Modified from Waterman-Storer CM. The cytoskeleton of skeletal muscle: Is it affected by exercise? A brief review. Medicine and Science in Sports and Exercise, *23*[11]:1243, 1991.)

desmin's elasticity is also thought to contribute to the passive stiffness of a stretched muscle. In summary, the potential contribution of the "resting filamentary tension" and the titin and desmin proteins indicate that multiple subcellular components contained within the muscle fibers contribute to the passive resistance one feels when stretching a relaxed, nonactivated muscle.

In addition to the subcellular components that contribute to this exponential increase in resistance, increased passive resistance is also influenced by lengthening of the connective tissues of the endomysium, perimysium, and epimysium of the muscle belly. Support for the influence of the connective tissues of skeletal muscles on resistance to passive stretch has been provided by studies of the normal structure of these tissues. The perimysium has a well-ordered crisscross array of crimped collagen fibers (Rowe, 1974, 1981). Because of this organization, the perimysium is considered tissue that is a major contributor to extracellular passive resistance (Borg & Caulfield, 1980). Examination of the perimysium with light microscopy (Rowe, 1974) and scanning electron microscopy (EM) (Williams & Goldspink, 1984) revealed that the orientation of the crimped collagen changes as the length of the muscle changes. The crimped arrangement of the perimysium, a system of sheets with a three-dimensional

weave surrounding muscle fasciculi, becomes uncrimped as the muscle is lengthened. This change, combined with mechanical realignment of the perimysium, contributes to the exponentially increased resistance, particularly near the end of maximal passive muscle lengthening. In contrast, tendons, which are composed of dense regular connective tissues, present very high stiffness (low passive compliance). Thus the length of tendons can generally be considered constant and noncontributory to the overall passive length-tension relationships of the stretched MTU (Halar et al., 1978; Stolov & Weilepp, 1966; Tardieu et al., 1982b).

Knowledge of the basic structures contributing to passive length-tension relationships of muscles is important clinically. The increasing resistance that a therapist feels as a normal relaxed muscle is stretched stems from lengthening subcellular proteins and extracellular connective tissues. The resistance a pediatric therapist feels at the end of the range of a lengthened muscle with spasticity may result from the resistance borne by these subcellular proteins and the extracellular connective tissues, and not from an activation of spasticity.

Although some resistance to passive lengthening is probably present at most functional muscle lengths, passive resistance increases exponentially (curvilinearly) as the muscle is lengthened beyond its resting length; passive resistance is the equivalent of resting muscle tone. As stated earlier, passive stiffness is the resistance one feels when passively stretching a relaxed muscle. Passive compliance is the reciprocal of passive stiffness; thus passive compliance is the "ease" with which the muscle lengthens. Although passive compliance can be represented as the ratio of change in muscle length to change in muscle force (Botelho et al., 1954), and passive stiffness can be represented as its reciprocal, to arrive at these measurements normally requires invasive research methods that are usually not possible in humans. Instead, passive compliance in humans is usually measured by the ratio of the change in the size of the joint angle to the change in the amount of passive torque (Gajdosik, 1991a; Gajdosik et al., 1990; Tardieu et al., 1982a; Tardieu et al., 1982). Passive stiffness can be represented by the ratio of the change in passive torque to a change in the joint angle.

Force and Length Adaptations in the Muscle-Tendon Unit

Animal Studies

Numerous experimental animal models have shown that anatomic and physiologic length adaptations of the MTU can be induced by immobilization, denervation, local contraction by artificial stimulation, or a combination of these methods. Researchers have used the length-tension curves to provide information about changes in the length and passive compliance of muscles in light of histologic and histochemical changes in the muscles. A passive length-tension curve is developed based on muscle tension that is produced as the muscle is stretched from its resting length to its maximal length. The initial take-up part of the curve (left part of the curve) represents the resting length and the end point of the curve (right part of the curve) represents the maximal length. Following intervention, the position and steepness of the curve may change, indicating a change in muscle length or stiffness. For example, a shift of the curve to the left indicates a shorter muscle, and a shift to the right indicates a longer muscle. A steeper curve indicates that the muscle is less compliant (stiffer).

When muscles were immobilized in shortened positions they showed a decrease in total force production, resulting from decreases in both the active force and the passive force (Alder et al., 1959; Williams & Goldspink, 1978). Muscle length also decreases (Alder et al., 1959; Stolov et al., 1971), a change brought about by a reduction in the number of sarcomeres (Goldspink et al., 1974; Tabary et al.,

1972; Williams & Goldspink, 1978). The soleus muscles of young mice immobilized in the shortened position demonstrated a decrease in the postnatal addition of sarcomeres (Williams & Goldspink, 1973). Protein synthesis and protein breakdown studies have demonstrated that muscles immobilized in shortened positions showed significant loss of tissue protein because of decreased synthesis and increased degradation (Williams & Goldspink, 1971), primarily at the ends of the muscle fibers. Muscles immobilized in the shortened position also presented a decreased resting length (Goldspink et al., 1974), and a reduced maximal length with decreased passive compliance (increased stiffness) (Tabary et al., 1972; Tardieu C et al., 1982b; Williams & Goldspink, 1978). The sarcomeres adapt in length to maintain optimal actin and myosin overlap in response to the loss in number of sarcomeres. When the immobilization is discontinued, the muscles readapt to gain their original sarcomere number and length characteristics.

Although changes in the resting lengths have been attributed to a loss of sarcomeres, the changes in passive compliance, demonstrated by changes in the steepness of the length-tension curves, have been attributed to changes in the connective tissues of the muscles (Tabary et al., 1972; Williams & Goldspink, 1978). Muscles immobilized in the shortened position demonstrated a greater abundance (Tabary et al., 1972; Williams & Goldspink, 1984) and remodeling (Williams & Goldspink, 1984) of connective tissues in the early stages of immobilization. Greater abundance of connective tissue has been assessed by determining the relative concentration of hydroxyproline in relation to the total volume of the muscle (Williams & Goldspink, 1984). Muscle fibers, however, atrophy without a decrease in their number (Cardenas et al., 1977); thus whether the absolute amount of connective tissue increases remains controversial. Evidence for remodeling was provided by scanning EM of the soleus muscles of mice immobilized in the shortened position for 2 weeks (Williams & Goldspink, 1984). The collagen fibers of the perimysium were oriented at more acute angles to the muscle fiber axis than were the collagen fibers of nonimmobilized muscles fixed in the same position. This collagen fiber arrangement at the immobilized shortened length resembled the arrangement found in nonimmobilized muscles held in lengthened positions (Fig. 4–6). As a result of the remodeling, greater tension per unit of passive elongation produced decreased passive compliance (increased stiffness). The passive length-tension curves were shifted to the left and appeared steeper, indicating that the muscles were shorter and stiffer after immobilization in the shortened position. The length-tension curves for

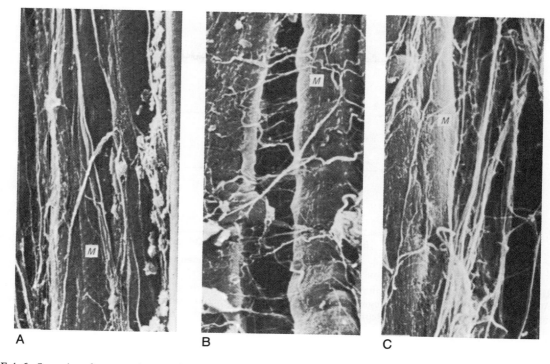

FIGURE 4–6. Scanning electron micrographs of collagen fibers in the perimysium. *A,* Normal muscle fixed in the lengthened position. *B,* Normal muscle fixed in the shortened position. *C,* Muscle immobilized for 2 weeks in the shortened position and then fixed in the same position. *M* = muscle fiber, ×1300. (From Williams, PE, & Goldspink, G. Connective tissue changes in immobilized muscle. Journal of Anatomy [London], *138*[2]:347, 1984. Reprinted with the permission of Cambridge University Press.)

young muscles (Fig. 4–7) and adult muscles were similar. Although the increased steepness of the curves for the muscles immobilized in the shortened position was explained by changes in the connective tissues, the decrease in the maximal passive force was probably influenced by a decrease in muscle mass because of muscle atrophy. Decreased muscle mass would result in the loss of subcellular proteins (myosin, actin, titin, and desmin), and this change would decrease both the maximal active and passive forces. The interrelationship of changes in the connective tissues and muscle proteins in light of changes in the form and position of length-tension curves is worthy of further study. Furthermore, applying the results of these studies with animals to explain the changes observed in human muscles must be done cautiously because the experimental conditions in the animal studies are usually not possible in humans.

Immobilization of muscles in lengthened positions has caused an increase in muscle length because of increases in the number of sarcomeres (Tabary et al., 1972; Williams & Goldspink, 1973, 1978), particularly at the ends of the muscle fibers. Similar results have been reported during normal postnatal growth of skeletal muscle fibers in young animals (Kitiyakara & Angevine, 1963; Williams & Goldspink, 1971). The addition of sarcomeres was accompanied by weight gain and increased protein synthesis after immobilization (Goldspink DF, 1977). The increased number of sarcomeres was not so great (19% increase) as the loss of sarcomeres in muscles immobilized in the shortened position (40% loss) (Tabary et al., 1972).

The active and passive length-tension curves for adult muscles that were immobilized in the lengthened position were shifted to the right (indicating that they were lengthened) compared with those of adult controls (i.e., nonimmobilized muscle). In young muscles immobilized in the lengthened position, however, the muscle belly length was decreased, so the curves of the experimental muscles were shifted to the left (Williams & Goldspink, 1978) (Fig. 4–8). Evidence suggests that a tendon elongates more readily in young, growing animals than in adult animals. In young mice with muscles immobilized in either the shortened or lengthened position, the overall muscle length was decreased, with a concomitant increase in tendon length (Williams &

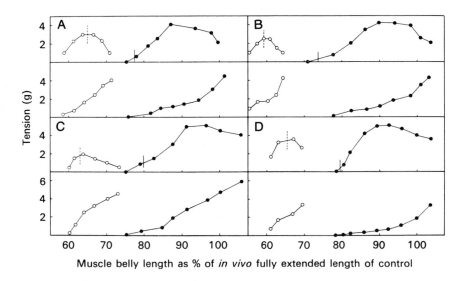

FIGURE 4–7. Length-tension curves for young muscles *(A–D)* immobilized in the shortened position (o) and their controls (●). (From Williams, PE, & Goldspink, G. Changes in sarcomere length and physiological properties in immobilized muscle. Journal of Anatomy [London], *127*[3]:464, 1978. Reprinted with the permission of Cambridge University Press.)

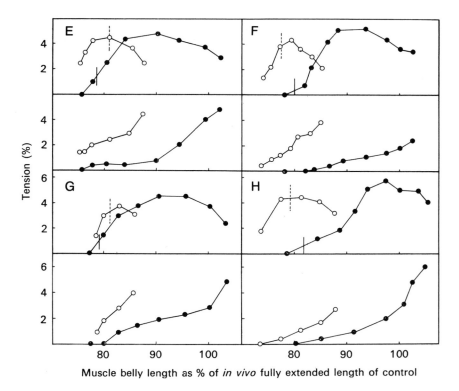

FIGURE 4–8. Length-tension curves for young animals *(E–H)* immobilized in the lengthened position (o) and their controls (●). (From Williams, PE, & Goldspink, G. Changes in sarcomere length and physiological properties in immobilized muscle. Journal of Anatomy [London], *127*[3]:464, 1978. Reprinted with the permission of Cambridge University Press.)

Goldspink, 1978). Thus in young animals a shorter muscle belly may result in strength deficits that are independent of the length of the MTU during immobilization. As with muscles immobilized in the shortened position, the sarcomere length adapts to maintain optimal actin and myosin overlap. Muscles immobilized in the lengthened position readapted to their original lengths when the immobilization was discontinued.

Studies of peripheral denervation of skeletal muscles have revealed obvious loss of the ability of the animal to generate voluntary active tension. After denervation, the passive length-tension relationship showed gradual changes over a period of weeks, with steeper length-tension curves and limited extensibility between their resting lengths and their maximal lengths compared with those of controls (Stolov et al., 1970; Thomson, 1955). Studies have also revealed that length adaptations may result from myogenic—but not neurogenic—responses to the immobilized length of muscles. In adult rats, denervated muscles immobilized in shortened positions showed muscle belly shortening after 8 weeks (Stolov et al., 1971), and a similar change was observed in adult cats after 4 weeks, with loss of up to 35% of the sarcomeres (Goldspink et al., 1974). The muscle belly shortening and decreased passive compliance were essentially the same as those observed in innervated muscles immobilized in shortened positions.

The reports that muscle length and associated physiologic changes may be independent of neuronal control were supported by studies of muscles stimulated with tetanus toxin (Huet de la Tour et al., 1979a, 1979b) or electrical stimulation (Tabary et al., 1981). Local injection of tetanus toxin into the soleus muscles of guinea pigs produced a shift in the passive length-tension curve toward the left, indicating a decrease in passive compliance (increased stiffness), and a 45% decrease in sarcomere number (Huet de la Tour et al., 1979b). The shortening adaptations were similar to those found after the muscles of cats were immobilized in shortened positions (Tabary et al., 1972). Analysis of the changes in sarcomere numbers in the soleus muscles of guinea pigs after length and tension were varied independently indicated that the length of muscles, not the tension, appeared to be the determining factor in sarcomere regulation (Huet de la Tour et al., 1979a). Contraction of a shortened muscle, however, may hasten sarcomere loss: electric stimulation of the sciatic nerve induced a 25% decrease in sarcomere numbers and decreased passive compliance within 12 hours (Tabary et al., 1981), whereas 5 days of shortening by immobilization in plaster casts alone was required to produce similar changes (Huet de la Tour et al., 1979b). The longitudinal growth rate of young, hypertonic muscles is also decreased. Spastic gastrocnemius muscles in very young mice have been shown to grow in length at only 55% of the rate of growing bone, whereas the rate of growth of normal gastrocnemius muscles was 100% of the rate of growing bone (Ziv et al., 1984).

Human Studies and Clinical Evidence

Studies of the length and passive compliance adaptations of the MTU in humans are less common than such studies in animals. Limited attempts to investigate the length and passive compliance responses to imposed changes in muscle length of children with neurologic impairments have been reported. Studies of children with CP and hypoextensible triceps surae muscles showed that they have muscle shortening and decreased passive compliance (increased stiffness) compared with findings in children with typical development (Tardieu C et al., 1982a). In another study, nine children with hypoextensible triceps surae muscles were casted for 3 weeks with these muscles placed in the lengthened position (Tardieu C et al., 1979). Four children showed passive length-tension curves that were shifted to the right with decreased slopes, indicating longer muscles with increased passive compliance, whereas five children had curves that were shifted to the right without a change in steepness (no change in passive compliance). In the same study, five children with hyperextensible triceps surae muscles were casted in a shortened position. The passive length-tension curves shifted to the left with increased slopes, indicating decreased passive compliance, in four of the five children.

In a follow-up study, children with CP and hypoextensible triceps surae muscles but no evidence of prolonged sustained contractions (group 1) were compared with children with CP and hypoextensible triceps surae muscles caused by an imbalance between triceps surae and dorsiflexion contractions (group 2) (Tardieu G et al., 1982). Both groups were treated with progressive casting to lengthen the muscles. Group 1 showed a shift to the right of the passive length-tension curve without a change in the slope of the curve. Group 2 presented curves that were shifted to the right with decreased slopes, showing increased passive compliance (decreased stiffness) (Fig. 4–9). The authors suggested that the children in group 2 showed normal muscle adaptation because of the passive compliance adaptation. These findings suggest that human muscles undergo adaptations that may be similar to those that have been reported for animals. This assumption is based on the association of the passive curves of animal and of human muscles, measured by noninvasive methods,

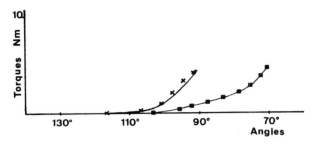

FIGURE 4-9. Results of successful progressive casting in child from group 2. × = passive torque curve before treatment, ■ = passive torque curve after treatment. The curve shifted to the right with increased passive compliance. (From Tardieu, G, Tardieu, C, Colbeau-Justin, P, & Lespargot, A. Muscle hypoextensibility in children with cerebral palsy: II. Therapeutic implications. Archives of Physical Medicine and Rehabilitation, 63:106, 1982.)

with the histologic and histochemical adaptations in animal muscles. The results of the study also elucidate the variability that can be expected in humans, particularly with regard to the possibility of different pathologic mechanisms underlying the adaptability of hypoextensible muscles in selected patient populations, such as children with CP (Tardieu et al., 1982).

Clinical observations clearly provide evidence that the musculoskeletal system of humans undergoes adaptations in response to immobilization, disuse, postural disturbances, and muscle imbalances in relation to specific pathologic disorders. It is well known that the skeletal muscles of a limb that is immobilized and not used will atrophy as a result of protein degradation (Sargeant et al., 1977). It is equally well known that normal muscle fibers respond to increased force and endurance demands by adaptive responses in structural, physiologic, and biochemical characteristics (Salmons & Hendriksson, 1981). The presence of pathologic conditions that alter skeletal muscles directly (e.g., muscular dystrophy) or indirectly from changes in the neurologic activity to the skeletal muscles (e.g., hypotonia or hypertonia) may lead to postural contractures and deformities from muscle imbalances and chronic positioning (Bunch, 1977; Sharrard, 1967; Tardieu et al., 1982a; Tardieu et al., 1982).

Many of the clinical manifestations of musculoskeletal disorders correlate well with the pathophysiologic conditions of the MTU described from experimental animal models. Abnormal shape in the structures of the vertebral column (e.g., hemivertebra) are associated with adaptations of the MTU and other soft tissues of the back. If the lower limbs of a child with flaccid paralysis are held in a specific pos-

ture for an extended period (e.g., hip flexion, abduction, and lateral rotation), the limbs adopt the characteristic position of the posture (Sharrard, 1967).

Long-term conservative interventions, such as stretching and casting, may facilitate desired adaptations of the MTU and enhance function, but much research is needed to examine these possibilities objectively. By contrast, surgical lengthening of the tendons of the triceps surae muscle group (Reimers, 1990a) and the hamstring muscle group (Damron et al., 1991; Lespargot et al., 1989; Reimers, 1990b) in children with CP has demonstrated enhanced function. Studies that examine the combined influence of both conservative and surgical interventions are clearly needed to determine the most efficacious methods of improving function.

Bone deformities and alterations in the MTU may result from abnormal skeletal growth, or both MTU and bone adaptations may be associated with abnormalities in muscle tonicity and muscle imbalances found with conditions such as CP. Numerous developmental changes in the musculoskeletal system have been associated with CP, and the changes correlate well with the presence of spasticity and imbalances in muscle force and muscle length. These include changes in the femur and acetabulum resulting in medial femoral torsion and hip disorders (Beals, 1969; Lewis et al., 1964), hip adduction contractures and knee flexion contractures in spastic adductor and hamstring muscles (Reimers, 1974), and severe equinus deformity because of spasticity and shortening adaptations of the calf musculature (Tardieu et al., 1982).

Skeletal Adaptations

The growth and resultant shape of the skeleton are affected by genetic coding, nutrition, and the combination of various mechanical forces that are imposed over time. The mass, girth, thickness, curvature, and trabecular arrangement of bone change as the forces of heredity and the environment play their roles. When examining skeletal adaptation, mechanical forces, such as muscle pull and weight bearing, are of interest to the pediatric physical therapist. Martin and McCulloch (1987) reported a case study of a child with congenital absence of a left tibia. At birth the left fibula was larger than the right fibula. This was thought to result from the forces of movement in utero. When the child reached 2 years of age, the fibula was surgically centered in relation to the femur to act as a tibia. Sixteen months later, the fibula looked like a tibia in shape, size, and strength. The authors believed that the mechanical stresses delivered in a functional weight-bearing manner induced the changes in the bone. Mechanical forces affect the shape of the maturing skeleton, which in turn affects the biomechanical function of the musculoskeletal system. Deformations of the skeletal system can lead to abnormalities in movement and impedance of function.

Effects of Forces on Skeletal Growth

From the time the cartilaginous template is formed, the basic shape of the skeletal system does not change. Each bone grows in length, width, and girth, but its relative form remains unchanged. Natural and atypic angular changes occur from compressive and shear forces at the epiphyseal plate. Compressive forces are perpendicular to the plate. Normal intermittent compressive forces, such as those produced by weight bearing or muscle pull, stimulate lengthening of bone (Arkin & Katz, 1956). If these forces are too great, the rate of growth is diminished.

Asymmetric forces affect the shape of the bone by stimulating growth in noncompressed areas while inhibiting bone development in areas of compression (Arkin & Katz, 1956). Although the bone appears to bend, it is actually growing asymmetrically as the epiphyseal plate realigns to the direction of the force. The clinical use of the effects of compression on the epiphyseal plate is exemplified by surgical stapling of the medial aspect of the epiphyseal plate of the proximal tibia to retard growth on that side to correct a genu valgum deformity (Mielke & Stevens, 1996). In children with unequal leg lengths, both sides of the plate on the longer leg are stapled to slow its growth until the shorter leg catches up (Edmonson & Crenshaw, 1980). Asymmetric proliferation of one or more epiphyseal growth plates located within a single bone can also lead to bone deformation. The spinal neural arch has six growth centers, three within each half of the arch. Chandraraj and Briggs (1991) speculated that uneven growth of either half of the neural arch may be a significant factor in the later development of idiopathic scoliosis.

Shear forces, which run parallel to the epiphyseal plate, can lead to torsional or twisting changes in the bone. The columns of chondrocytes around the periphery of the plate veer away from the shear forces in a twisting pattern (LeVeau & Bernhardt, 1984). The normal pull of muscles around a joint contributes to the shear forces, resulting in normal torsional changes in the long bones. For example, at birth, the tibia has 5° of medial torsion. By adulthood, the longitudinal orientation of the tibia has changed to 23 to 25° of lateral torsion (Bernhardt, 1988). The combination of atypic shear and compressive forces can lead to skeletal deformities, such as vertebral wedging, femoral anteversion, femoral or tibial-fibular torsion, genu valgum or varum, and pes planovalgus. Abnormalities of the skeletal system can lead to secondary problems of pain and dysfunction.

The typically developing child demonstrates interesting changes in the position of the knee in the frontal plane (Cheng et al., 1991; Heath & Staheli, 1993; Salenius & Vankka, 1975). At birth, the infant's knees are bowlegged (genu varum), but they gradually straighten until they reach a neutral alignment between the first and second years. The knee angulation then progresses toward genu valgum, reaching its peak between the ages of 2 and 4 years. After this time, the angle of genu valgum gradually decreases (Fig. 4–10). The final knee angle may differ according to race and gender. Heath and Staheli (1993) reported that by the age of 11 years the mean knee angle of Caucasian boys and girls was 5.8° of valgus and no child demonstrated genu varus. In contrast, Cheng and associates (1991) found that Chinese children of both genders progressed to genu varus of less than 5° in the preteen years. Cahuzac and co-workers (1995) studied European children and determined that by the age of 16 years girls maintained a valgus knee position and boys had developed a genu varus of 4.4°. The pediatric therapist should be aware that the presence of genu varus between the ages of 2 and 11 years may be considered atypical in white children (Heath & Staheli, 1993), but caution should be used when interpreting this finding in children of other races.

The level of compressive forces also affects the thickness and density of the bone shaft (Martin & McCulloch, 1987; Royer, 1974). The bone thickens via appositional growth when excessive compressive forces are applied, whereas a less than normal amount of compression leads to bone atrophy (Bernhardt, 1988). An increase in bone thickness and density is found in athletes compared with nonathletes. Nonathletes can, however, increase bone density with regular physical activity (Martin & McCulloch, 1987). Increases in cortical thickness, cross-sectional area, and resulting bone strength occur in response to increasing muscular strength and use in the typically developing child (Schönau, 1998). Children who do not experience normal levels of movement, muscle strength, or weight bearing are at risk for osteopenia (reduced bone mass) and the resultant osteoporosis, as is observed in children with myelodysplasia (Quan et al., 1998), CP (Lin & Henderson, 1996), and juvenile rheumatoid arthritis (Hopp et al., 1991).

The formation, growth, and integrity of articular cartilage are stimulated by compressive forces and movement between the bone surfaces (Ralis &

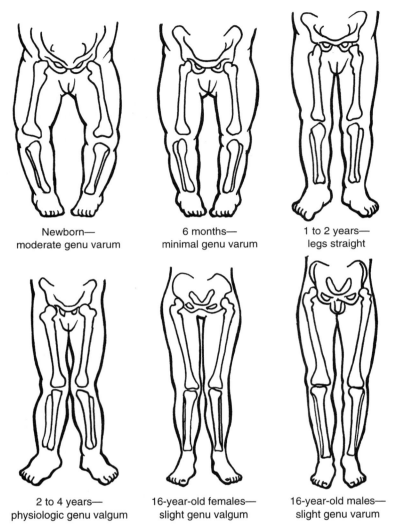

Newborn—
moderate genu varum

6 months—
minimal genu varum

1 to 2 years—
legs straight

2 to 4 years—
physiologic genu valgum

16-year-old females—
slight genu valgum

16-year-old males—
slight genu varum

FIGURE 4–10. Physiologic evolution of lower limb alignment at various ages in infancy and childhood. (Redrawn from Tachdjian, MO. Pediatric Orthopedics, 2nd ed. Philadelphia: WB Saunders, 1972, p. 1463.)

McKibbin, 1973). Intermittent joint loading leads to healthy, thick cartilage, but constant loading interrupts normal nutrition and the cartilage can eventually degenerate, leading to degenerative joint disease (Carter et al., 1987; Trueta, 1974). The role of movement in the development of joint shape and articular cartilage integrity is not clearly understood. In embryonic chicks, early joint formation occurred in the absence of mobility, but toward the end of the fetal period, cartilaginous bonds between the joint surfaces were present and the articular surfaces were flattened and misshaped (Drachman & Sokoloff, 1966). These changes have not been shown in hu-

mans. Movement may play a greater role in joint modeling after the joint is formed.

Skeletal deformities are common in children with muscle imbalances, spasticity, contractures, hypokinesis, and obesity, all of which apply abnormal mechanical forces to the growing skeleton. Although these deformities can occur throughout the growing period, the skeleton is most vulnerable during the first few years of life (prenatal and postnatal) when the rate of growth is greatest (Carter et al., 1987).

Fetal position has been related to various deformities, especially those that occur toward the end of the pregnancy. The incidence of tibial rotation and metatarsus adductus was reported to increase as the gestational age increased in preterm infants (Katz et al., 1990). Thus preterm infants born closer to term were more likely to have rotational deformities than were younger preterm infants. Many factors can cause prenatal deformities, including decreased amniotic fluid, the limited space in which the fetus can move in utero, multiple births, and external forces from tightly stretched uterine and abdominal walls. Some associated deformities are congenital torticollis, plagiocephaly (asymmetric head), and pelvic obliquity (Fulford & Brown, 1977; LeVeau & Bernhardt, 1984; Sherk et al., 1981). During the third trimester, the hip is especially vulnerable to dislocating forces because of its shallow acetabulum (Ralis & McKibbin, 1973; Sherk et al., 1981). Suzuki and Yamamuro (1986) reported that infants delivered in the single-breech position (i.e., hips flexed and knees extended) had a higher incidence of congenital hip dysplasia (CHD) than did infants born in cephalic, double-breech (i.e., both hips and knees flexed), or footling positions. It was postulated that, with extreme hip flexion combined with knee extension, the hamstrings pulled the head of the femur downward, thus stretching the compliant hip capsule. After birth, the femur was dislocated by the upward pull of the iliopsoas muscle when the infants were diapered and wrapped with the hips extended. This theory may explain why the incidence of CHD is higher among those Native American populations where newborns are strapped onto cradle boards or wrapped with the legs in adduction and extension (Coleman, 1968; Weinstein, 1987).

During normal postnatal growth, the depth of the acetabulum increases, progressively covering more of the femoral head until the age of 8 years, when the adult level of femoral head coverage is reached (Beals, 1969). Normal compressive forces through the hip help to form the acetabulum and the femoral head into their appropriate shapes. Atypic pressures, such as those caused by asymmetric pull by spastic muscles around the hip, deform the component parts of the hip and leave the child at risk for subluxation or dislocation (Gudjonsdottir & Mercer, 1997; Heinrich et al., 1991; Young et al., 1998).

Atypic changes in the shape of the acetabulum and femoral head have been reported in children with unstable or dislocated hips, such as children with congenitally dislocated hips, CP, or myelodysplasia. Buckley and colleagues (1991) examined 33 unstable hips in children with these disabilities and found that all had significantly more shallow acetabulae compared with those of a control group; the hip was most shallow in children with CP. The percentage of coverage of the head of the femur also was less for these children compared with that of control groups of children without disabilities. The children with disabilities had thinly developed articular surfaces and small, shallow acetabulae with poorly defined margins. Beals (1969) reported that the acetabulae of children with CP in his study had appeared normal after birth, but that they did not increase in depth as expected by the age of 2 years. Nevertheless, acetabular depth was comparable with that of the normal population when the children were 8 years old. All but 1 of the 40 children included in this study were walking at this age, suggesting that the dynamic compressive forces of walking contributed to increased depth of the acetabulum. Beals (1969) also supported use of a standing program to increase the depth of the hip joint.

The torsional changes of the bone observed in children with muscle imbalances or spasticity about the hip joint are good examples of the influence of the muscular system on the skeletal system. Femoral anteversion, or femoral torsion, is present when the proximal femur (i.e., head and neck) is rotated anteriorly in relation to the transcondylar axis of the femur. The greater trochanter is rotated to a more posterior location. At birth, the hip is in a position of about 30 degrees of femoral anteversion (Fabry et al., 1973). The femoral head, neck, and greater trochanteric areas are made of pliable cartilage and attached to the rigid osseus diaphysis. As the infant develops, normal torsional forces about this point of fixation cause a decrease in femoral anteversion. These torques are created by active lateral hip rotation and extension (Bleck, 1987). If these movements are lacking, as is frequently observed in children with CP, the infantile femoral anteversion does not decrease as it should. Excessive femoral anteversion has been associated with the in-toed gait of children with and without disabilities. Merchant (1965) explained this association by an alteration of gluteus medius muscle function in the presence of excessive femoral anteversion. The gluteus medius muscle is most effective in stabilizing the pelvis during the stance phase of gait when its insertion on the greater trochanter is in direct alignment with its origin. In excessive femoral anteversion, the greater trochanter is posterior to the midpoint of the ilium. To achieve maximal efficiency, the femur is rotated medially to align the insertion with the origin. The end result is an in-toed posture.

Changes in either the muscular or skeletal systems because of internal or external forces often have interactive effects. Understanding the influences of these two systems on the development and final outcome of each system and recognizing the period when these systems are most mutable assist the therapist in designing effective treatment programs, as well as in knowing when to discontinue treatment procedures.

Long-Term Effects of Atypical Musculoskeletal Development

Only recently have secondary disabilities in adults with developmental disabilities been the subject of investigation. A secondary condition occurs as a result of the primary condition and can cause further functional limitations and disability. Currently, researchers are primarily attempting to identify the secondary disabilities for various patient populations. No literature was found that investigated the actual structural changes in the musculoskeletal system that may result in or cause the secondary condition. Adults with CP have reported several problems that relate to the musculoskeletal system, including joint pain, skeletal deformities (e.g., scoliosis or hip dislocation), contractures, and fractures (Murphy et al., 1995; Turk et al., 1997). The lower extremities and the spine were the most common locations of pain.

Further study into the causes and prevention of secondary conditions is greatly needed to help guide the treatment of children with developmental disabilities. Pediatric therapists are appropriate professionals to educate parents and children about the lifelong attention that will need to be given to musculoskeletal problems, such as decreased strength and range of motion. Where appropriate, adolescents should be taught to be responsible for their physical and cardiopulmonary needs. Another role for pediatric therapists is educating their fellow orthopedic physical therapists who treat adults about the orthopedic problems in this neglected population of adults with CP, spina bifida, and other developmental disabilities. Campbell (1997) has written an excellent article on the issues surrounding secondary disabilities and how they can be addressed by pediatric therapists.

MEASUREMENT AND EFFECTS OF INTERVENTION

Fundamental goals of therapeutic intervention for physical disabilities include preventing or correcting the impairments that result from the underlying pathologic condition, or the normal physiologic adaptations superimposed on the pathologic condition. If impairments are prevented or corrected, presumably function will be enhanced and disability decreased. Impairments of the range of motion (ROM) available about a joint or multiple

joints and of the strength of the MTU are generally believed to bring about functional limitations and disability. Achieving maximal ROM by increasing the MTU length and achieving maximal strength are two fundamental goals of therapeutic intervention. Accurate assessments of ROM and strength are therefore important components of the physical therapy examination process.

Range-of-Motion Examination

A wide range of methods and instruments has been reported for examining the ROM about a joint or multiple joints, including simple visual estimation, use of various protractors and goniometers, measurements made from still photographs, and complex methods using computerized motion analysis systems. To most physical therapists, however, the universal goniometer (i.e., full-circle manual goniometer) remains the most versatile and widely used instrument in clinical practice. The design of the universal goniometer and the procedures for its use have been described in detail in numerous publications. The articles by M.L. Moore (1949a, 1949b) and the book by Norkin and White (1985) are particularly comprehensive and should be consulted for complete descriptions.

The reliability of goniometry is based on the reproducibility or stability of ROM measurements in relation to (1) the time intervals between comparable measurements or (2) the use of more than one rater. The ROM measurements must be reliable to be considered valid. Many factors influence the reliability and validity of goniometric measurements. These include consistency of the procedures applied, differences among joint actions and among the structure and function of body regions, passive versus active measurements, intrarater measurements (multiple measurements by one examiner) versus interrater measurements (multiple measurements by two or more examiners), normal day-to-day variations in ROM, and day-to-day variations in different pathologic conditions (Gajdosik & Bohannon, 1987).

Numerous studies have been reported on the ROM characteristics and the reliability of goniometry on adults, but reports on infants and children are more limited in number. Studies have demonstrated that full-term newborns present a limited range of hip and knee extension and greater dorsiflexion compared with measurements in adults (Drews et al., 1984; Waugh et al., 1983). These findings were attributed to the effects of intrauterine position and newborn flexor muscle tone. Consequently, clinicians should not use normal adult ROM values for comparisons with limb ROM measurements of the newborn. Studies with normal healthy children have indicated that ROM can probably be measured reliably (Haley et al., 1986), but studies of children with various pathologic conditions have shown that reliability varies with the number of raters and the pathologic problem. Pandya and colleagues (1985) studied seven upper and lower extremity joint limitations in 150 children with Duchenne muscular dystrophy and reported that intrarater reliability was high (intraclass correlation coefficient [ICC] range, .81–.91), but interrater reliability was lower, with a wide variation from joint to joint (ICC range, .25–.91). Stuberg and colleagues (1988) reported similar findings for children with CP.

Ashton and colleagues (1978) examined the day-to-day interrater reliability of measuring ROM of the hip in four children with spastic diplegia and found that the reliability tended to be lower for the two children with a moderate condition than for children with a mild condition. Harris and colleagues (1985) examined the goniometric reliability for a child with spastic quadriplegic CP and found that intrarater reliability exceeded interrater reliability, but both showed wide daily variations. The authors concluded that a variance of ± 10 to 15° in ROM over time does not signify a meaningful change in a child with spastic quadriplegic CP.

Bartlett and colleagues (1985) compared four methods of measuring hip extension (by prone extension, Thomas test, Mundale method, and pelvic-femoral angle) in 45 children, of whom 15 had spastic diplegia, 15 had meningomyelocele, and 15 had no known pathologic condition. They reported that the Thomas test was particularly difficult to apply to patients with spastic diplegia and that improved reliability for these children would most likely result by using one of the other methods. The least reliable test in the meningomyelocele group was that of Mundale, probably because of difficulty in identifying bony landmarks in the presence of obesity and deformities.

The results of these few studies clearly indicate that the reliability of ROM measurements is influenced by the specific patient problem. Additional research is needed to clarify the goniometric reliability among the many different types of patients treated by pediatric physical therapists. Moreover, studies are clearly needed to examine the effects of changes in ROM on function. In other words, can improved ROM predict improved function? In the meantime, therapists are encouraged to do their own reliability studies to establish confidence intervals for recognizing changes in ROM that are clinically significant. Because intrarater reliability has generally been shown to be acceptable, another alternative would be to have one therapist with demonstrated rating consistency perform all the goniometric measurements on one child.

Strength Examination

Accurate measurement of strength is important for identifying strength deficits and in documenting changes in strength as a result of interventions. Numerous methods of measuring strength are available, including the traditional procedures of manual muscle testing (Kendall & McCreary, 1983), use of various handheld force dynamometers (Bohannon & Andrews, 1987), and computerized isokinetic testing systems (Rothstein et al., 1987). Although manual muscle testing is probably the most versatile and widely used method, recent evidence indicates that handheld dynamometers may yield more precise measurements and are more sensitive to small changes in strength. Isokinetic systems are constructed primarily for use with adults, but they can be used with children who are large enough to fit the various components. The components could be modified, or smaller isokinetic devices could be developed to meet the special size requirements of children. Although strength deficits are a common impairment in many pediatric disabilities, the therapist must consider the reliability of the methods of measuring strength. Children must be able to understand the instructions and follow commands to produce accurate and reliable strength measurements. Children with typical development and as young as 6 years old have produced consistent force on an isokinetic machine for the movements of knee extension and dorsiflexion (Backman & Oberg, 1989; Merlini et al., 1995). The reliability of the strength measurements may also vary with the time of day, particularly for patients who are fatigued by the end of the day; with the level of the child's enthusiasm; with the testing environment; and with the testing clinician's rapport with the child. As with goniometry, standardization of testing procedures should improve the reliability of strength measurements.

Several authors have reported good consistency when testing the strength of children ranging in age from 5 years to 15 years and who had muscular dystrophy (e.g., Duchenne, limb-girdle, facioscapulohumeral, or myotonic muscular dystrophy). Strength was measured by manual muscle testing (Florence et al., 1984), isokinetic dynamometers (Sockolov et al., 1977), a handheld dynamometer (Stuberg & Metcalf, 1988), and an electronic string gauge (Brussock et al., 1992). Children between the ages of 9 and 17 years and with meningomyelocele yielded highly reliable results when their strength was measured with a handheld dynamometer (Effgen & Brown, 1992). In the past, the strength of spastic muscles was not tested because the hypertonicity was believed to confound and compromise objective measurements. In addition, strengthening a spastic muscle was contraindicated due to concerns of increasing muscle tone and encouraging abnormal movement patterns. Children with CP have since been found to have strength deficits (Wiley & Damiano, 1998), but the presence of spasticity appears to have some effect on the reliability. Van der Berg-Emons and associates (1996) examined the reliability of testing isokinetic muscle strength in 12 children with spastic CP and 39 children with typical development between the ages of 6 and 12 years. Using an isokinetic device, they measured quadriceps and hamstring muscle strength at three different speeds. The children with CP had lower levels of reliability than the comparison group, and as the speed increased the reliability decreased. The authors concluded that at 30°/s children with CP could produce consistent results, but at higher speeds the measurements were not repeatable. Further study of the reliability of strength testing in children with CP is needed, especially with the variety of methods of measuring strength that are available to the pediatric therapist today.

The impact of spasticity on the strength of antagonist muscle groups also warrants consideration. The importance of considering strength measurements of antagonists to spastic muscles was demonstrated by examination of the strength changes of the dorsiflexor muscles after surgical lengthening of the triceps surae muscle group (Reimers, 1990a) and of the quadriceps muscles after surgical lengthening of the hamstring muscle group (Reimers, 1990b) of children with CP. The strength of the dorsiflexors increased by 50% 4 weeks postoperatively and by more than 200% 14 months postoperatively (Reimers, 1990a). The strength of the quadriceps muscle group decreased by 70% 4 weeks postoperatively but was regained by 7 months, and by 13 months postoperatively the strength had increased by more than 50% (Reimers, 1990b). Taken together, these studies confirm the idea that antagonist muscle strength improves when the spastic agonist muscle group is lengthened. We encourage clinicians to examine methods of objectively measuring muscle strength in children with CP to study the changes in muscle strength resulting from both conservative and surgical interventions.

In addition to the possibility of objectively measuring the voluntary force produced in spastic muscles, a combination of technologies may now permit objective assessments of the degree of underlying hypertonicity. Isokinetic passive movements at different velocities, combined with the recording of EMG activity of the agonist and antagonist muscles, could permit quantification of hypertonicity because muscles with spasticity present a markedly increased velocity-dependent neuromuscular response to passive lengthening (Price et al., 1991). Rapid passive

lengthening of spastic calf muscles through a dorsiflexion range of motion can yield an increase in the amount of passive resistance and EMG activity. For example, Boiteau and colleagues (1995) passively stretched the calf muscles of 10 children with spastic CP at 10°/s and at 190°/s. They measured the resistance to the stretch at 10° of dorsiflexion and attributed the passive force at 10°/s stretch to nonreflex components. The force at the 190°/s stretch was much higher because it included reflex muscle activation from the spasticity (documented with EMG). The study demonstrated that the reflex and nonreflex components of spastic hypertonia can be measured reliably. If change in the passive resistive force caused by the reflex and the nonreflex components of spasticity can be assessed independently, the effects of specific therapeutic interventions that target each component can be determined and related to changes in function. These possibilities are particularly worthy of future study, and clinicians are encouraged to participate in research projects to help examine these possibilities.

Effects of Intervention on the Musculoskeletal System

Objective evidence of the effects of strengthening exercises for particular pediatric conditions is limited, but increasing. In the past, concerns about whether strengthening muscles of children with degenerative disorders would lead to a more rapid progression of the disorder have probably limited the application of strengthening programs. Some of the limited evidence available, however, indicates that submaximal exercise has no negative effect and may be of limited value in increasing strength in Duchenne muscular dystrophy (de Lateur & Giaconi, 1979). Several current studies with children with CP have shown that after participating in a resistive exercise program, the children improved their function during gait (Damiano & Abel, 1998; Damiano et al., 1995) and increased their scores on the Gross Motor Function Measure (Damiano & Abel, 1998; MacPhail & Kramer, 1995). In a study by O'Connell and Barnhart (1995), three children with CP and three with meningomyelocele participated in a progressive circuit muscular strength training program. After 8 weeks, these children propelled their wheelchairs significantly farther during a 12-minute test period when compared with the pretraining test results. Their speed, however, did not increase during a 50-meter dash. We encourage clinicians to continue to document the relationship of strength changes to changes in the functional abilities of the children.

Passive and active slow static stretching exercises are used routinely as accepted methods of addressing abnormally short MTUs. Static stretching is believed to promote lengthening adaptations of the MTU, represented clinically by increases in ROM. Given the difficulty of measuring the direct effects of stretching exercises on muscle and connective tissues in humans, the changes observed in the ROM in humans are assumed to be based on associated histologic, biochemical, anatomic, and physiologic changes similar to those observed directly in animal models. For example, evidence has indicated that static stretching of adult hamstring muscles brings about lengthening and passive resistance adaptations similar to the adaptations reported for animal muscles immobilized in the lengthened position (Gajdosik, 1991b). Even prolonged passive stretching of MTUs in a state of severe contracture from long-term hypertonicity and shortening may promote lengthening adaptations and increased ROM in children with CP (McPherson et al., 1984). Whether changes observed from the stretching regimens are brought about by decreased neurologic excitability (hypertonicity), by adaptations in the muscle and connective tissues of the MTU, or by both remains controversial and worthy of investigation.

Serial casting and inhibitive casting methods have also been used to promote lengthening adaptations of the MTU, especially for children with CP or head injuries. Serial casting employs the principles of lengthening and shortening adaptations within the MTU. As discussed earlier in this chapter, investigators have demonstrated that when hypoextensible, abnormally short muscles of children with CP were serially casted in lengthened positions, increased length and passive compliance adaptations were enhanced (Tardieu et al., 1979, 1982a; Tardieu et al., 1982). In other words, the muscles were longer and more compliant. The researchers indicated that the adaptations resulted directly from changes in the MTU, but changes in the neurologic excitability of the muscles were not reported.

Given the possibility that connective tissue adaptations (i.e., proliferation and remodeling) may contribute to the adaptations observed in the MTU, procedures such as soft tissue, joint, and myofascial mobilization could also contribute to the desired adaptations. As a result of increased attention in continuing education offerings, treatment of the connective tissues in children is increasing. Case reports and systematic research on these approaches are direly needed.

The differences in effect between serial casting and inhibitive casting are difficult to identify. In a review of casting principles and theories, Carlson (1984) indicated that proponents of inhibitive casting suggest that the casting procedures have a neuro-

physiologic influence on the motoneuron excitability that results in a reduction in spasticity. As stated earlier, the observed lengthening changes in the MTU may result from changes in the MTU directly or from changes in muscle activation patterns and not necessarily from changes in motoneuron excitability. The finding of enhanced strength and function of the antagonist muscle group after surgical lengthening of the agonist muscle groups (Reimers, 1990a, 1990b) supports the hypothesis that functional changes result from direct changes in muscle length, not from altered motoneuron excitability. This proposal was also supported by the finding that splinting spastic muscles of patients with brain damage changed ROM without altering the integrated EMG activity of the muscles when compared with the activity in muscles that were not splinted (Mills, 1984). A more recent study examined the effects of 3 weeks of dorsiflexion serial casting on the reflex characteristics of spastic calf muscles of children with CP ($n = 7$) (Brouwer et al., 1998). The authors reported that casting brought about increased dorsiflexion ROM and that the angle of reflex excitability elicited by a rapid dorsiflexion stretch also was shifted toward increased dorsiflexion. The soleus and tibialis anterior coactivation EMG tracings, however, did not change as a result of the casting. A major problem in interpreting the clinical reports of the effects of inhibitory casting is the confusing and variable definition of "tone." Is tone caused by central or peripheral influences or by both? Knowledge of the interrelationships among the length, tension, and passive compliance of the MTU and of the neurologic excitability of the muscles of children with neurologic impairment and how the interrelationships are influenced by therapeutic interventions remains sparse. Additional research is needed to explore the effects of many therapeutic methods on the active and passive characteristics of the MTU, including such methods as muscle strengthening and stretching, soft tissue mobilization, and casting. The application of passive isokinetic movements combined with recording of EMG, as described earlier in this chapter, could be used to examine the effects of these interventions on spastic muscles. In the meantime, clinicians should maintain objective records of strength and ROM and attempt to correlate these findings with specific therapeutic interventions and functional outcomes.

The shape and size of the skeletal system are most susceptible to alteration during periods of rapid growth; hence undesirable forces, as well as appropriate corrective forces, are most influential during childhood. Many deformities that occur during the fetal or early postnatal period are more easily corrected in the infant than in the older child. For example, congenitally dislocated hips often readily respond to bracing during the first year of life (Sherk et al., 1981). If, however, the dislocated hip is not diagnosed until after 12 months, surgery is often necessary. Bracing for idiopathic scoliosis is most effective for preventing worsening of the curve during the preteen and teenage years (Cassella & Hall, 1991). Once an individual has stopped growing, the external support is no longer needed.

The influence of orthoses on the growth of children has not been thoroughly investigated. Bleck (1987) reported that full-control hip-knee-ankle orthoses have not been successful in preventing structural deformities in children with CP. These children still developed dislocated hips or hip flexion contractures. In a study of 204 children, Lee (1982) reported that, regardless of the type of CP, the presence or absence of bracing did not influence the development of deformities. Bracing did not diminish the need for surgery to correct deformities, nor did it prevent recurrences of deformities after the surgery. Lee and Bleck (1980) reported a 9% recurrence rate of shortening after Achilles tendon lengthening in children with CP who did not wear night splints to maintain tendon length. This rate, however, was comparable with that reported in other studies of children who did wear night splints (Bleck, 1987). Preventing deformities via bracing may be more difficult in children with abnormal tone than in those with normal tone or paralysis. Or, perhaps, results are related to the specific type of bracing that is employed. Plastic total contact orthoses may be more effective at preventing deformities than the traditional metal braces.

Orthoses can also lead to the development of secondary deformities. Lusskin (1966) reported two case studies of children with lower extremity paralysis resulting from polio. Both children had marked tibial-fibular torsion and were braced in knee-ankle-foot orthoses with the knees and feet facing forward. As a result, a rotational force was placed at the ankle and foot, and these children developed severe metatarsus adductus and heel varus. Children who wear total contact ankle-foot orthoses for most of their growing years may be at risk for stunted growth of the foot and lower limb. The circumferential compressive forces and the restriction in active movement can interfere with normal musculoskeletal growth. Pediatric physical therapists have an important responsibility to understand the effects of external devices on the growing child. While trying to solve one problem, the therapist may inadvertently create another.

Weight-bearing activities are thought to retard the loss of bone mass and help shape the joint. In a preliminary study, Stuberg (1992) found that 60 minutes of standing 4 or 5 times a week increased the bone mineral density of nonambulatory children with severe to profound CP. When the standing program was discontinued, bone mineral density decreased. Standing programs may also help deepen the acetabulum. The contact between the femoral head and the acetabulum in weight bearing helps in the development of the normal shape of the acetabulum, which contributes to a stable hip socket (Beals, 1969; Harrison, 1961).

Movement has been reported to affect the formation and shape of joints in fetal animals (Drachman & Sokoloff, 1966; Murray & Drachman, 1969). Movement allows the compressive forces to be spread throughout the joint surface rather than be confined to a small area. Combining weight-bearing activities with movement would create more desirable forces for joint formation. Although no research has been reported on the effects on hip formation of stationary standing devices, such as prone boards or standing platforms, it appears reasonable to use caution when using these devices with very young children. Because remodeling of the bone and associated joints takes place most readily during the first few years of life and because the acetabular shape is fairly well defined by the age of 3 years (Ralis & McKibbin, 1973), early intervention with weight-bearing activities may have a substantial influence on the shape and function of the joint. To help shape the joint, chronologic age and not developmental age may be more important when determining when to begin weight-bearing activities. Although standing is important, the length of time the child stands during any one period may need to be controlled.

For the young child with severe delays in motor development in whom independent walking (with or without devices) is unlikely and hip dislocation is a risk, early and prolonged standing may be beneficial in developing a deeper hip joint. The shape of the acetabulum may not be appropriate for walking, but the hip may be more stable. Over time, this early standing may help prevent or decrease the severity of a dislocated hip. For children with milder delays, less stationary standing time and more weight bearing with movement may help develop a more normally shaped hip socket. This may contribute to an improved gait and a decrease in the risk of osteoarthritis in adulthood. More research in this area would give the pediatric physical therapist valuable information for designing intervention using programs with weight-bearing activities.

In summary, this chapter reviewed the normal growth and development of the musculoskeletal system, with emphasis on the adaptations of muscle and bone associated with pathologic conditions encountered by pediatric physical therapists. The microscopic and macroscopic structure and function of the normal MTU and the force and length adaptations to imposed physical changes, such as immobilization and denervation, have been well documented in nonhuman studies using invasive methods of investigation. The results of human studies using noninvasive methods of investigation indicate that the human MTU undergoes adaptations similar to those reported for animals. The clinical evidence for the musculoskeletal adaptations supports these research findings.

In the developing child, atypic changes in the MTU can exert forces on the skeletal system, resulting in bone deformities. Pediatric physical therapists routinely measure physical impairments and develop therapeutic interventions designed to promote musculoskeletal adaptations. To document therapeutic efficacy in relation to specific pediatric disorders, therapists are encouraged to use objective measures of ROM and strength during specific interventions for correlating changes in musculoskeletal impairments with functional outcomes. Additional research is needed to examine the efficacy of therapeutic strengthening and stretching programs and their interrelation with other interventions, such as surgical procedures. The application of new research technologies, such as isokinetic dynamometry and EMG, may now permit objective measurement of the impairments associated with neuromuscular disorders and the effects of interventions designed to influence these disorders. Further controlled studies will enhance the scientific basis for using physical therapy to promote improved functional outcomes.

References

Alder, AB, Crawford, GNC, & Edwards, GR. The effect of limitation of movement on longitudinal muscle growth. Proceedings of the Royal Society of London. Series B: Biological Sciences, 150:554–562, 1959.

Arkin, AM, & Katz, JF. The effects of pressure on epiphyseal growth. Journal of Bone and Joint Surgery (American), 38:1056–1076, 1956.

Ashton, BB, Pickles, B, & Roll, JW. Reliability of goniometric measurements of hip motion in spastic cerebral palsy. Developmental Medicine and Child Neurology, 20:87–94, 1978.

Backman, E, & Oberg, B. Isokinetic muscle torque in the dorsiflexors of the ankle of children 6–12 years of age. Scandinavian Journal of Rehabilitation Medicine, 21:97–103, 1989.

Bartlett, MD, Wolf, LS, Shurtleff, DB, & Staheli, LT. Hip flexion contractures: A comparison of measurement procedures. Archives of Physical Medicine and Rehabilitation, 66:620–625, 1985.

Beals, RK. Developmental changes in the femur and acetabulum in spastic paraplegia and diplegia. Developmental Medicine and Child Neurology, 11:303–313, 1969.

Bernhardt, DB. Prenatal and postnatal growth and development of the foot and ankle. Physical Therapy, 68:1831–1839, 1988.

Bleck, EE. Orthopedic Management in Cerebral Palsy. Philadelphia: JB Lippincott, 1987.

Bohannon, RW, & Andrews, AW. Inter-rater reliability of hand-held dynamometer. Physical Therapy, 67:931–933, 1987.

Boiteau, M, Malouin, F, & Richards, CL. Use of a hand-held dynamometer and the Kin-Com dynamometer for evaluating spastic hypertonia in children: A reliability study. Physical Therapy 75:796–802, 1995.

Borg, TK, & Caulfield, JB. Morphology of connective tissue in skeletal muscle. Tissue and Cell, 12:197–207, 1980.

Botelho, SY, Cander, L, & Guiti, N. Passive and active tension-length diagrams of intact skeletal muscle in normal women of different ages. Journal of Applied Physiology, 7:93–95, 1954.

Brooke, MH. A Clinician's View of Neuromuscular Disease. Baltimore: Williams & Wilkins, 1986.

Brooke, MH, & Engel, WK. The histographic analyses of human muscle biopsies with regard to fiber types: 4. Children's biopsies. Neurology, 19:591–605, 1969.

Brouwer, B, Wheeldon, RK, & Stradiotto-Parker, N. Reflex excitability and isometric force production in cerebral palsy: The effect of serial casting. Developmental Medicine and Child Neurology, 40:168–175, 1998.

Brown, MC, Jansen, JKS, & Van Essen, D. Polyneuronal innervation of skeletal muscle in newborn rats and its elimination during maturation. Journal of Physiology, 261:387–422, 1976.

Brussock, CM, Haley, SH, Munsat, TL, & Bernhardt, DB. Measurement of isometric force in children with and without Duchenne's muscular dystrophy. Physical Therapy, 72:105–114, 1992.

Buckley, SL, Sponseller, PD, & Maged, D. The acetabulum in congenital and neuromuscular hip instability. Journal of Pediatric Orthopedics, 11:498–501, 1991.

Buller, AJ, Eccles, JC, & Eccles, RM. Differentiation of fast and slow muscles in the cat hind limb. Journal of Physiology, 150:399–416, 1960.

Bunch, W. Origin and mechanism of postnatal deformities. Pediatric Clinics of North America, 24:679–684, 1977.

Butler, J, Cosmos, E, & Brienley, J. Differentiation of muscle fiber types in aneurogenic muscles of the chick embryo. Journal of Experimental Zoology, 224:65–80, 1982.

Cahuzac, J, Vardon, D, & Sales de Gauzy, J. Development of the clinical tibiofemoral angle in normal adolescents. Journal of Bone and Joint Surgery (British), 77:729–732, 1995.

Campbell, SK. Therapy programs for children that last a lifetime. Physical and Occupational Therapy in Pediatrics, 17(1):1–15, 1997.

Cardenas, DD, Stolov, WC, & Hardy, R. Muscle fiber number in immobilization atrophy. Archives of Physical Medicine and Rehabilitation, 58:423–426, 1977.

Carlson, SJ. A neurophysiological analysis of inhibitive casting. Physical and Occupational Therapy in Pediatrics, 4(4):31–42, 1984.

Carter, DR, Orr, TE, Fyhrie, DP, & Schurman, DJ. Influences of mechanical stress on prenatal and postnatal skeletal development. Clinical Orthopedics and Related Research, 219:237–250, 1987.

Cassella, MC, & Hall, JE. Current treatment approaches in the nonoperative and operative management of adolescent idiopathic scoliosis. Physical Therapy, 71:897–909, 1991.

Castle, ME, Reyman, TA, & Schneider, M. Pathology of spastic muscle in cerebral palsy. Clinical Orthopedics, 142:223–232, 1979.

Chandraraj, S, & Briggs, CA. Multiple growth cartilages in the neural arch. Anatomical Record, 230(1):114–120, 1991.

Cheng, JCY, Chan, PS, Chiang, SC, & Hui, PW. Angular and rotational profile of the lower limb in 2,630 Chinese children. Journal of Pediatric Orthopedics, 11:154–161, 1991.

Coleman, SS. Congenital dysplasia of the hip in the Navajo infant. Clinical Orthopedics and Related Research, 56:179–193, 1968.

Colling-Saltin, A. Enzyme histochemisty on skeletal muscle of the human fetus. Journal of Neurological Science, 39:169–185, 1978.

Damiano, DL, & Abel, MF. Functional outcomes of strength training in spastic cerebral palsy. Archives of Physical Medicine and Rehabilitation, 79:119–125, 1998.

Damiano, DL, Kelly, LE, & Vaughn, CL. Effects of quadriceps femoris muscle strengthening on crouch gait in children with spastic diplegia. Physical Therapy, 75:658–667, 1995.

Damron, T, Breed, AL, & Roecker, E. Hamstring tenotomies in cerebral palsy: Long-term retrospective analysis. Journal of Pediatric Orthopedics, *11*:514–519, 1991.

Davis, JA, & Dobbing, J (Eds.). Scientific Foundations of Paediatrics. Philadelphia: WB Saunders, 1974.

de Lateur, BJ, & Giaconi, RM. Effect on maximal strength of submaximal exercise in Duchenne muscular dystrophy. American Journal of Physical Medicine, *58*:26–36, 1979.

Drachman, DB, & Sokoloff, L. The role of movement in embryonic joint development. Developmental Biology, *14*:401–420, 1966.

Drews, JE, Vraciu, JK, & Pellino, G. Range of motion of the joints of the lower extremities of newborns. Physical and Occupational Therapy in Pediatrics, *4*(2):49–62, 1984.

Edmonson, AD, & Crenshaw, AH (Eds.). Campbell's Operative Orthopaedics, Vol. 2. St. Louis: Mosby, 1980.

Effgen, SK, & Brown, DA. Long-term stability of hand-held dynamometric measurements in children who have myelomeningocele. Physical Therapy, *72*:458–465, 1992.

Fabry, G, Belguim, L, MacEwen, GD, & Shands, AR. Torsion of the femur. The Journal of Bone and Joint Surgery (American), *55*: 1726–1738, 1973.

Farkas-Bargeton, E, Barbet, JP, Dancea, S, Wehrle, R, Checouri, A, & Dulac, O. Immaturity of muscle fibers in the congenital form of myotonic dystrophy: Its consequences and its origin. Journal of the Neurological Sciences, *83*(2–3):145–159, 1988.

Florence, JM, Pandya, S, King, WM, Robison, JD, Signore, LC, Wentzell, M, & Province, MA. Clinical trials in Duchenne dystrophy: Standardization and reliability of evaluation procedures. Physical Therapy, *64*:41–45, 1984.

Fulford, G, & Brown, J. Position as a cause of deformity in children with cerebral palsy. Developmental Medicine and Child Neurology, *18*:305–314, 1977.

Gajdosik, RL. Passive compliance and length of clinically short hamstring muscles of healthy men. Clinical Biomechanics, *6*:239–244, 1991a.

Gajdosik, RL. Effects of static stretching on the maximal length and resistance to passive stretch of short hamstring muscles. Journal of Orthopedic Sports and Physical Therapy, *14*:250–255, 1991b.

Gajdosik, RL, & Bohannon, RW. Clinical measurement of range of motion: Review of goniometry emphasizing reliability and validity. Physical Therapy, *67*:1867–1872, 1987.

Gajdosik, RL, Guiliani, CA, & Bohannon, RW. Passive compliance of the hamstring muscles of healthy men and women. Clinical Biomechanics, *5*:23–29, 1990.

Gasser, T, Kneip, A, Ziegler, P, Largo, R, Molinari, L, & Prader, A. The dynamics of growth of width in distance, velocity and acceleration. Annals of Human Biology, *18*(5):449–461, 1991.

Goldspink, DF. The influence of immobilization and stretch on protein turnover of rat skeletal muscle. Journal of Physiology, *64*:267–282, 1977.

Goldspink, G, Tabary, C, Tabary, JC, Tardieu, C, & Tardieu, G. Effect of denervation on the adaptation of sarcomere number and muscle extensibility to the functional length of the muscle. Journal of Physiology, *236*:733–742, 1974.

Gordon, AM, Huxley, AF, & Julian, FJ. The variation in isometric tension with sarcomere length in vertebrate muscle fibers. Journal of Physiology, *184*:170–192, 1966.

Gramsbergen, A, IJkema-Paassen, J, Nikkels, PGJ, & Hadders-Algra, M. Regression of polyneural innervation in the human psoas muscle. Early Human Development, *49*:49–61, 1997.

Granzier, HLM, & Pollack, GH. Stepwise shortening in unstimulated frog skeletal muscle fibers. Journal of Physiology, *362*:173–188, 1985.

Grinnell, AD. Dynamics of nerve-muscle interaction in developing and mature neuromuscular junctions. Physiological Reviews, *75*:789–834, 1995.

Grove, BK. Muscle differentiation and the origin of muscle fiber diversity. CRC Critical Reviews of Neurobiology, *4*(3):201–234, 1989.

Gudjonsdottir, B, & Mercer, VS. Hip and spine in children with cerebral palsy: Musculoskeletal development and clinical implications. Pediatric Physical Therapy, *9*:179–185, 1997.

Halar, EM, Stolov, WC, Venkatesh, B, Brozovivh, FV, & Harley, JD. Gastrocnemius muscle belly and tendon length in stroke patients and able-bodied persons. Archives of Physical Medicine and Rehabilitation, *59*:467–484, 1978.

Haley, SM, Tada, WL, & Carmichael, EM. Spinal mobility in young children: A normative study. Physical Therapy, *66*:1697–1703, 1986.

Harris, SR, Smith, LH, & Krukowski, L. Goniometric reliability for a child with spastic quadriplegia. Journal of Pediatric Orthopedics, *5*:348–351, 1985.

Harrison, TJ. The influence of the femoral head on pelvic growth and acetabular form in the rat. Journal of Anatomy (British), *95*:12–24, 1961.

Heath, CH, & Staheli, LT. Normal limits of knee angle in white children—genu varum and genu valgum. Journal of Pediatric Orthopedics, *13*:259–262, 1993.

Heinrich, SD, MacEwen, GD, & Zembo, MM. Hip dysplasia, subluxation, and dislocation in cerebral palsy: An arthrographic analysis. Journal of Pediatric Orthopedics, *11*:488–493, 1991.

Hesselmans, LFGM, Jennekens, FGI, Van Den Oord, CJM, Veldman, H, & Vincent, A. Development of innervation of skeletal muscle fibers in man: Relation to acetylcholine receptors. Anatomical Record, *236*:553–562, 1993.

Hill, DK. Tension due to interaction between sliding filaments in resting striated muscle: The effect of stimulation. Journal of Physiology, *199*:637–684, 1968.

Hill, DK. The effect of temperature in the range of 0–35° C on the resting tension of frog's muscle. Journal of Physiology, *208*:725–739, 1970a.

Hill, DK. The effect of temperature on the resting tension of frog's muscle in hypertonic solutions. Journal of Physiology, *208*:741–756, 1970b.

Hopp, R, Degan, J, Gallager, JC, & Cassidy, JT. Estimation of bone mineral density in children with juvenile rheumatoid arthritis. Journal of Rheumatology, *18*:1235–1239, 1991.

Huet de la Tour, E, Tabary, JC, Tabary, C, & Tardieu, C. The respective roles of muscle length and muscle tension in sarcomere number adaptation of guinea-pig soleus muscle. Journal de Physiologie, *75*:589–592, 1979a.

Huet de la Tour, E, Tardieu, C, Tabary, JC, & Tabary, C. Decreased muscle extensibility and reduction of sarcomere number in soleus muscle following local injection of tetanus toxin. Journal of the Neurological Sciences, *40*:123–131, 1979b.

Huxley, AF, & Peachey, LD. The maximum length for contraction in vertebrate striated muscle. Journal of Physiology, *156*:150–165, 1961.

Ito, J, Araki, A, Tanaka, H, Tasaki, T, Cho, K, & Yamazaki, R. Muscle histopathology in spastic cerebral palsy. Brain and Development, *18*:299–303, 1996.

Kamieniecka, L. The stages of development of human fetal muscles with reference to some muscular diseases. Journal of the Neurological Sciences, *7*:319–329, 1968.

Katz, K, Naor, N, Merlob, P, & Wielunsky, E. Rotational deformities of the tibia and foot in preterm infants. Journal of Pediatric Orthopedics, *10*:483–485, 1990.

Kendall, FP, & McCreary, EK. Muscles Testing and Function, 3rd ed. Baltimore: Williams & Wilkins, 1983.

Kitiyakara, A, & Angevine, DM. A study of the pattern of postembryonic growth of *M. gracilis* in mice. Developmental Biology, *8*:322–340, 1963.

Lee, CL. Role of lower extremity bracing in cerebral palsy (Abstract). Developmental Medicine and Child Neurology, *24*:250–251, 1982.

Lee, CL, & Bleck, EE. Surgical correction of equinus deformity in cerebral palsy. Developmental Medicine and Child Neurology, *22*: 287–292, 1980.

Lespargot, A, Tardieu, C, Bret, MD, Tabary, C, & Singh, B. Is tendon surgery for the knee flexors justified in cerebral palsy? French Journal of Orthopedic Surgery, 3(4):446–450, 1989.

LeVeau, BF, & Bernhardt, DB. Effects of forces on the growth, development, and maintenance of the human body. Physical Therapy, 64:1874–1882, 1984.

Lewis, FR, Samilson, RR, & Lucas, DB. Femoral torsion and coxa valga in cerebral palsy: A preliminary report. Developmental Medicine and Child Neurology, 6:591–597, 1964.

Lin, PP, & Henderson, RC. Bone mineralization in the affected extremities of children with spastic hemiplegia. Developmental Medicine and Child Neurology, 38:782–786, 1996.

Linke, WA, Ivemeyer, M, Olivieri, N, Lolmerer, B, Ruegg, JC, & Labeit, S. Towards a molecular understanding of the elasticity of titin. Journal of Molecular Biology, 261:62–71, 1996.

Lusskin, R. The influence of errors in bracing upon deformity of the lower extremity. Archives of Physical Medicine and Rehabilitation, 47:520–525, 1966.

MacPhail, HEA, & Kramer, JF. Effect of isokinetic strength-training on functional ability and walking efficiency in adolescents with cerebral palsy. Developmental Medicine and Child Neurology, 38:763–775, 1995.

Magid, A, & Law, DJ. Myofibrils bear most of the resting tension in frog skeletal muscle. Science, 230:1280–1282, 1985.

Martin, AD, & McCulloch, RG. Bone dynamics: Stress, strain, and fracture. Journal of Sports Sciences, 5:155–163, 1987.

Mastaglia, FL. The growth and development of the skeletal muscles. In Davis, JA, & Dobbing, J (Eds.), Scientific Foundations of Paediatrics. Philadelphia: WB Saunders, 1974, pp. 348–375.

McKibbin, B. The structure of the epiphysis. In Owen, R, Goodfellow, J, & Bullough, P (Eds.), Scientific Foundations of Orthopaedics and Traumatology. Philadelphia: WB Saunders, 1980.

McPherson, JJ, Arends, TG, Michaels, MJ, & Trettin, K. The range of motion of long term knee contractures of four spastic cerebral palsied children: A pilot study. Physical and Occupational Therapy in Pediatrics, 4(1):17–34, 1984.

Merchant, AJ. Hip abduction muscle force. Journal of Bone and Joint Surgery (American), 47:462–475, 1965.

Merlini, L, Dell'Accio, D, & Granata, C. Reliability of dynamic strength knee muscle testing in children. Journal of Sports Physical Therapy, 22:73–76, 1995.

Mielke, CH, & Stevens, PM. Hemiepiphyseal stapling for knee deformities in children younger than 10 years: A preliminary report. Journal of Pediatric Orthopaedics, 16:423–429, 1996.

Miller, JB. Review article: Myoblasts, myosins, MyoDs, and the diversification of muscle fibers. Neuromuscular Disorders, 1:7–17, 1991.

Mills, VM. Electromyographic results of inhibitory splinting. Physical Therapy, 64:190–193, 1984.

Moore, KL. The Developing Human: Clinically Oriented Embryology, 4th ed. Philadelphia: WB Saunders, 1988.

Moore, ML. The measurement of joint motion: Part I. Introductory review of the literature. Physical Therapy Review, 29:195–205, 1949a.

Moore, ML. The measurement of joint motion: Part II. The technique of goniometry. Physical Therapy Review, 29:256–264, 1949b.

Murphy, KP, Molnar, GE, & Lankasky, K. Medical and functional status of adults with cerebral palsy. Developmental Medicine and Child Neurology, 37:1075–1084, 1995.

Murray, PDF, & Drachman, DB. The role of movement in the development of joints and the related structures: The head and neck in the chick embryo. Journal of Embryology and Experimental Morphology, 22:349–371, 1969.

Norkin, CC, & White, DJ. Measurement of Joint Motion: A Guide to Goniometry. Philadelphia: FA Davis, 1985.

O'Connell, DG, & Barnhart, R. Improvement in wheelchair propulsion in pediatric wheelchair users through resistance training: A pilot study. Archives of Physical Medicine and Rehabilitation, 76:368–372, 1995.

Owen, R, Goodfellow, J, & Bullough, P (Eds.). Scientific Foundations of Orthopaedics and Traumatology. Philadelphia: WB Saunders, 1980.

Pandya, S, Florence, JM, King, WM, Robison, JD, Oxman, M, & Province, MA. Reliability of goniometric measurements in patients with Duchenne muscular dystrophy. Physical Therapy, 65:1339–1342, 1985.

Price, R, Bjornson, KF, Lehmann, JF, McLaughlin, JF, & Hays, RM. Quantitative measurement of spasticity in children with cerebral palsy. Developmental Medicine and Child Neurology, 33:585–595, 1991.

Purves, D, & Lichtman, JW. Elimination of synapses in the developing nervous system. Science, 210:153–157, 1980.

Quan, A, Adams, R, Ekmark, E, & Baum, M. Bone mineral density in children with myelomeningocele (Abstract). Pediatrics, 102:628, 1998.

Ralis, Z, & McKibbin, B. Changes in shape of the human hip joint during its development and their relation to stability. Journal of Bone and Joint Surgery (British), 55:780–785, 1973.

Reimers, J. Contracture of the hamstrings in spastic cerebral palsy: A study of three methods of operative correction. Journal of Bone and Joint Surgery (British), 56:102–109, 1974.

Reimers, J. Functional changes in the antagonists after lengthening the agonists in cerebral palsy: I. Triceps surae lengthening. Clinical Orthopedics and Related Research, 253:30–34, 1990a.

Reimers, J. Functional changes in the antagonists after lengthening the agonists in cerebral palsy: II. Quadriceps strength before and after distal hamstring lengthening. Clinical Orthopedics and Related Research, 253:35–37, 1990b.

Rodriguez, TI, Razquin, S, Palacios, T, & Rubio, V. Human growth plate development in the fetal and neonatal period. Journal of Orthopaedic Research, 10(1):62–71, 1992.

Romanini, L, Villani, C, Meloni, C, & Calvisi, V. Histological and morphological aspects of muscle in infantile cerebral palsy. Italian Journal of Orthopaedics and Traumatology, 15:87–93, 1989.

Rose, J, Haskell, WL, Gamble, JG, Hamilton, RL, Brown, DA, & Rinsky, L. Muscle pathology and clinical measures of disability in children with cerebral palsy. Journal of Orthopaedic Research, 12:758–768, 1994.

Rose, SJ, & Rothstein, JM. Muscle mutability: Part 1. General concepts and adaptation to altered patterns of use. Physical Therapy, 62:1773–1784, 1982.

Rothstein, JM, Lamb, RL, & Mayhew, TP. Clinical uses of isokinetic measurements: Critical issues. Physical Therapy, 67:1840–1844, 1987.

Rothstein, JM, & Rose, SJ. Muscle mutability. Part 2, Adaptation to drugs, metabolic factors, and aging. Physical Therapy, 62:1788–1798, 1982.

Rowe, RWD. Collagen fibre arrangement in intramuscular connective tissue. Changes associated with muscle shortening and their possible relevance to raw meat toughness measurements. Journal of Food Technology, 9:501–508, 1974.

Rowe, RWD. Morphology of perimysial and endomysial connective tissue in skeletal muscle. Tissue and Cell, 13:681–690, 1981.

Royer, P. Growth of bony tissue. In Davis, JA, & Dobbing, J (Eds.), Scientific Foundations of Paediatrics. Philadelphia: WB Saunders, 1974.

Salenius, P, & Vankka, E. The development of the tibiofemoral angle in children. Journal of Bone and Joint Surgery (American), 57:259–261, 1975.

Salmons, S, & Hendriksson, J. The adaptive response of skeletal muscle to increased use. Muscle and Nerve, 4:94–105, 1981.

Sanes, JR. Cell lineage and the origin of muscle fiber types. Trends in Neurosciences, 10(6):119–121, 1987.

Sargeant, AJ, Davies, CTM, Edwards, RHT, Maunder, C, & Young, A. Functional and structural changes after disuse of human muscle. Clinical Science and Molecular Medicine, 52:337–342, 1977.

Schönau, E. The development of the skeletal system in children and the influence of muscular strength. Hormone Research, 49:27-31, 1998.

Sharrard, WJW. Paralytic deformity in the lower limb. Journal of Bone and Joint Surgery (British), 49:731-747, 1967.

Sherk, HH, Pasquariello, PS, & Watters, WC. Congenital dislocation of the hip. Clinical Pediatrics, 20(8):513-520, 1981.

Slaton, D. Muscle fiber types and their development in the human fetus. Physical and Occupational Therapy in Pediatrics, 1(3):47-57, 1981.

Sockolov, R, Irwin, B, Dressendorfer, RH, & Bernauer, EM. Exercise performance in 6- to 11-year-old boys with Duchenne muscular dystrophy. Archives of Physical Medicine and Rehabilitation, 58:195-200, 1977.

Stolov, WC, Riddell, WM, & Shrier, KP. Effect of electrical stimulation on contracture of immobilized, innervated and denervated muscle (Abstract). Archives in Physical Medicine and Rehabilitation, 52:589, 1971.

Stolov, WC, & Weilepp, TG. Passive length-tension relationship of intact muscle, epimysium, and tendon in normal and denervated gastrocnemius of the rat. Archives in Physical Medicine and Rehabilitation, 47:612-620, 1966.

Stolov, WC, Weilepp, TB, Jr, & Riddell, WM. Passive length-tension relationship and hydroxyproline content of chronically denervated skeletal muscle. Archives in Physical Medicine and Rehabilitation, 51:517-525, 1970.

Stuberg, WA. Considerations related to weight-bearing programs in children with developmental disabilities. Physical Therapy, 72:35-40, 1992.

Stuberg, WA, Fuchs, RH, & Miedaner, JA. Reliability of goniometric measurements of children with cerebral palsy. Developmental Medicine and Child Neurology, 30:657-666, 1988a.

Stuberg, WA, Metcalf, WK. Reliability of quantitative muscle testing in healthy children and in children with Duchenne muscular dystrophy using a hand-held dynamometer. Physical Therapy, 68:977-982, 1988b.

Suzuki, S, & Yamamuro, T. Correction of fetal posture and congenital dislocation of hip. Acta Orthopaedica Scandinavica, 57:81-84, 1986.

Tabary, JC, Tabary, C, Tardieu, C, Tardieu, G, & Goldspink, G. Physiological and structural changes in the cat's soleus muscle due to immobilization at different lengths by plaster casts. Journal of Physiology, 224:231-244, 1972.

Tabary, JC, Tardieu, C, Tardieu, G, & Tabary, C. Experimental rapid sarcomere loss with concomitant hypoextensibility. Muscle and Nerve, 4:198-203, 1981.

Tanabe, Y, & Nonaka, I. Congenital myotonic dystrophy. Changes in muscle pathology with aging. Journal of the Neurological Sciences, 77:59-68, 1987.

Tardieu, C, Huet de la Tour, E, Bret, MD, & Tardieu, G. Muscle hypoextensibility in children with cerebral palsy: I. Clinical and experimental observations. Archives of Physical Medicine and Rehabilitation, 63:97-102, 1982a.

Tardieu, C, Tabary, JC, Tabary, C, & Tardieu, G. Adaptation of connective tissue length to immobilization in the lengthened and shortened positions in the cat soleus muscle. Journal de Physiologie, 78:214-220, 1982b.

Tardieu, C, Tardieu, G, Colbeau-Justin, P, & Huet de la Tour, E. Trophic muscle regulation in children with congenital cerebral lesions. Journal of the Neurological Sciences, 42:357-364, 1979.

Tardieu, G, Tardieu, C, Colbeau-Justin, P, & Lespargot, A. Muscle hypoextensibility in children with cerebral palsy: II. Therapeutic implications. Archives of Physical Medicine and Rehabilitation, 63:103-107, 1982.

Thompson, WJ. Changes in the innervation of mammalian skeletal muscle fibers during postnatal development. Trends in Neurosciences, 9:25-28, 1986.

Thompson, WJ, Condon, K, & Astrow, SH. The origin and selective innervation of early muscle fiber types in the rat. Journal of Neurobiology, 21(1):212-222, 1990.

Thompson, WJ, & Jansen, JKS. The extent of sprouting of remaining motor units in partly denervated immature and adult rat soleus muscle. Neuroscience, 2:523-535, 1977.

Thomson, JD. Mechanical characteristics of skeletal muscle undergoing atrophy of degeneration. American Journal of Physical Medicine, 34:606-611, 1955.

Tokuyasu, KT, Dutton, AH, & Singer, SJ. Immunoelectron microscopic studies of desmin (skeletin) localization and intermediate filament organization in chicken skeletal muscle. The Journal of Cell Biology, 96:1727-1735, 1983.

Trombitas, K, Greaser, M, Labeit, S, Jin, JP, Kellermayer, M, Helmes, M, & Granzier, H. Titin extensibility in situ: Entropic elasticity of permanently folded and permanently unfolded molecular segments. The Journal of Cell Biology, 140:853-859, 1998.

Trueta, T. The growth and development of bone and joints: Orthopedic aspects. In Davis, JA, & Dobbing, J (Eds.), Scientific Foundations of Paediatrics. Philadelphia: WB Saunders, 1974.

Turk, MA, Geremski, CA, & Rosenbaum, PF. Secondary Conditions of Adults with Cerebral Palsy: A Final Report. Syracuse, NY: State University of New York, 1997.

van der Berg-Emons, RJG, van Baak, MA, de Barbanson, DC, Speth, L, & Saris, WHM. Reliability of tests to determine peak aerobic power, anaerobic power and isokinetic muscle strength in children with spastic cerebral palsy. Developmental Medicine and Child Neurology, 38:1117-1125, 1996.

Walker, JM. Musculoskeletal development: A review. Physical Therapy, 71:878-889, 1991.

Ward, SS, & Stickland, NC. Why are slow and fast muscles differentially affected during prenatal under-nutrition? Muscle and Nerve, 14(3):259-267, 1991.

Wang, K, & Ramirez-Mitchell, R. A network of transverse and longitudinal intermediate filaments is associated with sarcomeres of adult vertebrate skeletal muscle. The Journal of Cell Biology, 96:562-570, 1983.

Wang, K, McCarter, R, Wright, J, Beverly, J, & Ramirez-Mitchell, R. Viscoelasticity of the sarcomere matrix of skeletal muscles: The titin-myosin composite filament is a dual-stage molecular spring. Biophysical Journal, 64:1161-1177, 1993.

Waterman-Storer, CM. The cytoskeleton of skeletal muscle: Is it affected by exercise? A brief review. Medicine and Science in Sports and Exercise, 23(11):1240-1249, 1991.

Waugh, KG, Minkel, JL, Parker, R, & Coon, VA. Measurement of selected hip, knee, and ankle joint motions in newborns. Physical Therapy, 63:1616-1621, 1983.

Weinstein, SL. Natural history of congenital hip dislocation (CDH) and hip dysplasia. Clinical Orthopedics and Related Research, 225:62-75, 1987.

Wiley, ME, & Damiano, DL. Lower-extremity strength profiles in spastic cerebral palsy. Developmental Medicine and Child Neurology, 40:100-107, 1998.

Williams, PE, & Goldspink, G. Longitudinal growth of striated muscle fibers. Journal of Cell Science, 9:751-767, 1971.

Williams, PE, & Goldspink, G. The effect of immobilization on the longitudinal growth of striated muscle fibers. Journal of Anatomy (London), 116:45-55, 1973.

Williams, PE, & Goldspink, G. Changes in sarcomere length and physiological properties in immobilized muscle. Journal of Anatomy (London), 127:459-468, 1978.

Williams, PE, & Goldspink, G. Connective tissue changes in immobilized muscle. Journal of Anatomy (London), 138:342-350, 1984.

Young, NL, Wright, JG, Lam, TP, Rajaratnam, K, Stephens, D, & Wedge, JH. Windswept hip deformity in spastic quadriplegic cerebral palsy. Pediatric Physical Therapy, 10:94-100, 1998.

Ziv, I, Blackburn, N, Rang, M, & Koreska, J. Muscle growth in normal and spastic mice. Developmental Medicine and Child Neurology, 26:94-99, 1984.

CHAPTER 5

Physical Fitness during Childhood and Adolescence

JEAN L. STOUT, PT, MS

The "Guide to Physical Therapist Practice" emphasizes primary prevention and risk reduction strategies as an important component of therapeutic intervention to "buffer the disablement process" (American Physical Therapy Association, 1997). According to the 1996 Surgeon General's report on physical activity and health, individuals with disabilities are less likely to engage in sustained or vigorous physical activity than are individuals without disabilities (United States Department of Health and Human Services, 1996). Ensuring physical fitness is one path to buffering the disablement process of a number of conditions. As clinicians who design exercise programs and treat children with disabilities, we have a unique responsibility to understand and promote physical fitness as an aspect of those programs. It is a unique responsibility because we can have a great impact on the exercise lifestyle that children develop and carry with them throughout their lives. It is a unique responsibility because we care for a group of children who might otherwise be physically inactive. Many believe that promotion of lifelong habits of physical activity in childhood will have direct and indirect effects on health and prevention of disease in adulthood (Blair et al., 1989; Haskell et al., 1985; Simons-Morton et al., 1987; Strong, 1990).

What defines "physical fitness" for able-bodied children? Are the criteria for physical fitness different in children with disabilities? How do we help children with physical disabilities incorporate physical fitness into the limitations of their disability? This chapter is designed to answer those questions and to provide the reader with an understanding of (1) physical fitness and the cardiopulmonary response to exercise in children of different ages who do not have disabling conditions; (2) the components of physical fitness (cardiorespiratory endurance, muscular strength and endurance, flexibility, and body composition) (Table 5–1); (3) the standards of fitness components consistent with good health; (4) the effects of training and conditioning on overall physical fitness; (5) the components of fitness in various special populations; and (6) guides for program planning. The chapter also includes a review of current physical fitness tests.

TABLE 5-1. Health-Related Fitness Components and the Rationale for Importance to Health Promotion and Disease Prevention

Component	Rationale
Cardiorespiratory endurance	Improved physical working capacity
	Reduced fatigue
	Reduced risk of coronary heart disease
	Optimal growth and development
Muscular strength and endurance	Improved functional capacity for lifting and carrying
	Reduced risk of lower back pain
	Optimal posture
	Optimal growth and development
Flexibility	Enhanced functional capacity for bending and twisting
	Reduced risk of lower back pain
	Optimal growth and development
Body composition	Reduced risk of hypertension
	Reduced risk of coronary heart disease
	Reduced risk of diabetes
	Optimal growth and development

Adapted from Pate, RR, & Shephard, RJ. Characteristics of physical fitness in youth. In Gisolfi, CV, & Lamb, DR (Eds.), Perspectives in Exercise Science and Sports Medicine, Vol. 2: Youth, Exercise, and Sport. Indianapolis, IN: Benchmark Press, 1989, pp. 1–45.

HEALTH, PHYSICAL ACTIVITY, AND PHYSICAL FITNESS

Physical fitness is difficult to define because it cannot be measured directly. Physical fitness is generally viewed as having two facets—health-related fitness and the more traditional motor fitness. Motor fitness generally includes physical abilities that relate to athletic performance, whereas health-related fitness includes abilities related to daily function and health maintenance. Physical activity is thought to be the path both to physical fitness and to good health, but they are not synonymous terms. Physical activity refers to the amount of exercise in which an individual engages. Studies suggest that a positive correlation exists between activity and fitness, but at least 80% of the variability in fitness measures cannot be explained (Pate et al., 1990; Ross & Gilbert, 1985; Ross & Pate, 1987). Physical activity may improve physical fitness and health at the same time, but the improvement in health may be caused by biologic changes different from those responsible for improvement in physical fitness (Haskell et al., 1985). Corbin (1987) suggested that some of the benefits from physical activity that are important to health have no relationship to what is defined as physical fitness per se. One example is the importance of regular exercise to a reduced risk of osteoporosis; osteoporosis is related to health but not to the components of physical fitness. We do not know how much physical activity is necessary for health and fitness in children.

The premise that physical activity is the path to both physical fitness and good health has become a primary focus in programs instituted by the United States Department of Health and Human Services. As early as 1985, the Centers for Disease Control put forth a specific activity plan for youth through old age to attain specific health fitness goals and achieve optimal health benefits. Developing lifelong physical activity patterns was one of the specific goals for children (Haskell et al., 1985). In 1990, *Healthy Children 2000* was introduced—a major federal planning document for health promotion and disease prevention for children (United States Department of Health and Human Services, 1990). Eight objectives were outlined to increase the physical activity and fitness levels of youth, with a target date of attainment by the year 2000 (Table 5-2). Altered targets have been incorporated into the draft objectives of *Healthy People 2010* (United States Department of Health and Human Services, 1998). Mid-decade evaluation of the original objectives as they relate to children has produced both encouraging and disappointing results. Many of the targets proposed for year 2000 have been retained for the 2010 objectives. One target (objective 4, Table 5-2) has been surpassed for youth in grades 9 through 12. Others (objectives 5, 6, and 7, Table 5-2) moved away from year 2000 targets. Another (objective 8, Table 5-2) no longer appears in the new objectives. Perhaps the greatest disappointment has been lack of data available for children younger than high school (grades K through 8) (United States Department of Health and Human Services, 1995). As a result, none of the targets proposed for 2010 objectives are directed toward elementary-age and junior high-age children.

Physical activity as the path to physical fitness is no less surprising than the relationship of physical activity to improved health and disease prevention. The content of the current nationwide objectives has been guided in part by the concept of health-related fitness. What is different may be the intensity of physical activity required to be physically fit compared with what is necessary to receive benefits to health. Regardless of intensity, both physical fitness and improved health begin with physical activity. If promotion of lifelong habits of physical activity in childhood has direct and indirect effects on fitness, health, and prevention of disease in adulthood (Blair et al., 1989; Haskell et al., 1985; Simons-Morton et al., 1987; Strong, 1990), this should be no less true for children with physical disabilities. The concept of physical fitness becomes more important because as

TABLE 5–2. Objectives for Improved Physical Activity and Fitness

Risk Reduction Objectives

1. Increase to at least 30% the proportion of people age 6 and older who engage regularly, preferably daily, in light to moderate physical activity for at least 30 minutes daily.
2. Increase to at least 20% the proportion of people age 18 and older and to at least 75% the proportion of children and adolescents age 6 through 17 who engage in vigorous physical activity that promotes the development and maintenance of cardiorespiratory fitness 3 or more days per week for 20 or more minutes per occasion.
3. Reduce to no more than 15% the proportion of people age 6 and older who engage in no leisure time physical activity.
4. Increase to at least 40% the proportion of people age 6 and older who regularly perform physical activities that enhance and maintain muscular strength, muscular endurance, and flexibility.
5. Increase to at least 50% the proportion of overweight people age 12 and older who have adopted sound dietary practices combined with regular physical activity to attain an appropriate body weight.

Service and Protection Objectives

6. Increase to at least 50% the proportion of children and adolescents in first through twelfth grade who participate in daily school physical education.
7. Increase to at least 50% the proportion of physical education class time that students spend being physically active, preferably engaged in lifetime physical activities.

Health Status Objective

8. Reduce overweight to a prevalence of no more than 20% among people age 20 and older and no more than 15% among adolescents age 12 through 19.

From United States Department of Health and Human Services. Healthy Children 2000: National Health Promotion and Disease Prevention Objectives Related to Mothers, Infants, Children, Adolescents, and Youth. Washington, DC: Public Health Service, 1990.

individuals become less active in adulthood, the decrease in activity level is more likely to result in loss of function, injury, or both.

Definition of Physical Fitness

As defined previously, health-related fitness is a state characterized by (1) an ability to perform daily activities with vigor and (2) traits and capacities that are associated with low risk of premature development of hypokinetic disease (i.e., physical inactivity) (Pate, 1983). Physical fitness is multidimensional. A combination of traits and capacities contributes to physical fitness, and the interaction among them creates true fitness. Each facet is a unique, independent characteristic or ability that is not highly correlated with other components. As the concept of health-related fitness has gained acceptance, four basic components have been identified: cardiorespiratory endurance, muscular strength and endurance, flexibility, and body composition. The rationale for the importance of these parameters in day-to-day functional capacity, health promotion, and disease prevention, and therefore physical fitness, is presented in Table 5–1. The relative independence of the components from one another has been verified by low correlations between components. Of the 60 possible correlation coefficients among test items for these components, only 6 were greater than .35 (Ross & Gilbert, 1985; Ross & Pate, 1987).

Cardiopulmonary response to exercise in the growing child is reviewed next. The remainder of this chapter is directed toward reviewing the components of health-related fitness and current physical fitness tests.

Cardiopulmonary Response to Exercise

As in adults, the response of a child to exercise (a single event or repeated exercise) includes physiologic changes in the cardiovascular and pulmonary systems, as well as metabolic effects. In children, however, differences in physiologic changes are seen as growth and development occur. Physiologic capacities depend on growth of the myocardium, skeleton, and skeletal muscle. Maturation and improved efficiency of the cardiovascular, pulmonary, metabolic, and musculoskeletal systems are also important. The physical work capacity of children increases approximately eightfold in absolute terms between the ages of 6 and 12 years, partially as a result of growth and maturation (Adams, 1973). The absolute exercise capacity of children may be less than that of adults, but relative exercise capacity is similar.

Any exercise, in a child or an adult, increases the energy expenditure of the body. The energy for muscle contraction and exercise depends on splitting of adenosine triphosphate (ATP) at the cellular level. ATP is available in small quantities in resting muscle, but once contraction starts, additional sources are required if contraction is to be maintained. Three sources of ATP are available: (1) creatine phosphate (CP), (2) glycolysis, and (3) the tricarboxylic acid or Krebs cycle. It is beyond the scope of this chapter to describe these mechanisms in detail. The reader is referred to a standard textbook of exercise physiology (Astrand & Rodahl, 1986).

CP and glycolysis as sources of ATP are referred to as anaerobic pathways because they do not require the presence of oxygen. CP is found in the sarcoplasm of the muscle cell. During breakdown it releases a high-energy phosphate bond that can be combined with adenosine diphosphate (ADP) to create ATP.

$$CP \rightarrow C + P_i + \text{Energy} \qquad [1]$$
$$ADP + P_i + \text{Energy} \rightarrow ATP \qquad [2]$$

CP breakdown together with ATP production provides enough energy for 10 to 15 seconds of exercise. Glycolysis, the other anaerobic pathway, breaks down glucose to produce pyruvic acid or lactic acid and ATP. This reaction takes place in the sarcoplasm of the cell. Together, glycolysis and CP breakdown are methods of anaerobic energy production that can sustain energy for muscle contraction for 40 to 50 seconds.

Energy production by the tricarboxylic acid cycle is called an aerobic pathway because it requires oxygen. A supply of oxygen is required for sustained exercise and depends on the aerobic pathway. Most, if not all, activities use both aerobic and anaerobic pathways for supply of ATP, but often tasks are more highly dependent on one type of pathway than the other.

Because aerobic pathways must be used to sustain exercise, an index of maximal aerobic power is used to reflect the highest metabolic rate made available by aerobic energy. The most common index is maximal oxygen uptake (Vo_2max), or the highest volume of oxygen that can be consumed per unit time. Oxygen supply to muscle is described by the Fick equation: oxygen uptake (Vo_2) is equal to cardiac output (CO) times the difference in oxygen content between arterial (Cao_2) and mixed venous (Cvo_2) blood, or

$$Vo_2 = CO \times (Cao_2 - Cvo_2)$$

Because CO is the product of heart rate and stroke volume, the following relationship is also true:

$$Vo_2 = \text{Heart rate} \times \text{Stroke volume} \times \text{Arteriovenous } O_2 \text{ difference}$$

For Vo_2 to increase, one or more of these factors must increase. During exercise, CO is elevated by increases in both heart rate and stroke volume. Elevated blood flow to the muscles increases the difference in oxygen content between arterial and venous blood.

Vo_2max increases throughout childhood from approximately 1 L/min at age 5 years to 3 to 4 L/min at puberty (Braden & Strong, 1990). These changes occur as a result of maturation of the cardiovascular, pulmonary, metabolic, and musculoskeletal systems. As a child grows, the cardiopulmonary and musculoskeletal systems are integrated so that oxygen flow during exercise optimally meets the energy demands of the muscle cells, regardless of body size (Cooper et al., 1984).

Cardiac Output

CO in children, as in adults, rises at the beginning of exercise or on transition from a lower to a higher level of exercise. CO increases by an increase in both stroke volume and heart rate. CO in children is similar to that in adults despite the fact that stroke volume in a 5-year-old is about 25% of the stroke volume in an adult (Godfrey, 1981). Stroke volume increases as total heart volume increases. At all levels of exercise, stroke volume in boys is somewhat higher than it is in girls (Bar-Or, 1983c). CO levels in children are similar to those in adults because of an increased heart rate throughout childhood. Maximal heart rates in children vary between 195 and 215 beats per minute and decrease by 0.7 to 0.8 beats per minute per year after maturity (Braden & Strong, 1990).

Arteriovenous Difference and Hemoglobin Concentration

At rest, the difference between arterial and mixed venous blood oxygen content is the same in children as in adults (Sproul & Simpson, 1964). Research suggests, however, that children have a higher blood flow to muscles after exercise than do young adults, resulting in a higher arteriovenous oxygen difference (Koch, 1974). Greater muscle blood flow facilitates increased oxygen transport to exercising muscles and thus a decrease in the oxygen content of the mixed venous blood.

Hemoglobin concentration is lower in children than in the average adult and thus affects the oxygen transport capacity of the blood in children (Krahenbuhl et al., 1985). Studies suggest that total hemoglobin concentration in 11- and 12-year-olds is approximately 78% of that in adults (Krahenbuhl et al., 1985).

Arterial Blood Pressure

Lower exercise blood pressure is seen in children than in adults, a finding consistent with a lower CO and stroke volume. Blood pressure may also be reduced because of lower peripheral vascular resistance secondary to shorter blood vessels (Bar-Or, 1983c).

Ventilation

Ventilation is the rate of exchange of air between the lungs and ambient air, measured in liters per minute. In absolute terms, ventilation increases with age. Ventilation normalized by body weight is the same for children and adults at maximal activity (Bar-Or, 1983c). At submaximal exercise levels, ventilation is higher in children and decreases with age, suggesting that children have a lower ventilatory reserve than do adults. Studies suggest that children have less efficient ventilation than do adults (i.e., more air is needed to supply 1 L of oxygen in a child than in an adult) (Bar-Or, 1983c).

Vital Capacity

Vital capacity in a 5-year-old child is about 20% of that in an adult and increases with age. It is highly correlated with body size, particularly height (Godfrey, 1981), and generally has not been found to be a limiting factor of exercise performance.

Respiratory Rate

Children have a higher respiratory rate than do adults during both maximal and submaximal exercise. A high rate of respiration compensates for decreased lung volume; respiratory rate decreases as lung volume increases (Bar-Or, 1983c).

Blood Lactate

Blood and muscle lactate levels are lower in children than in adults (Astrand, 1952; Ericksson et al., 1971, 1973). It has been suggested but not confirmed that lactate production is related to testosterone production and therefore to sexual maturity in boys. Low lactate production in children could limit glycolytic capacity and thus contribute to reduced anaerobic capacity.

Table 5–3 summarizes comparisons between children and adults for various cardiopulmonary variables. Growth and maturation play a vital part in determining the values of these variables. Despite size differences between adults and children (which might lead one to believe that oxygen transport in children is less efficient because they are smaller), optimal oxygen transport is maintained by highly integrated functions between the cardiopulmonary and musculoskeletal systems.

Review of Tests of Physical Fitness

Numerous physical fitness tests have been developed and are in use in physical education curricula across the country. Five tests are worthy of review because of their nationwide use and the likelihood that they will constitute the standards for future testing of youth and children. One of these tests, the National Children and Youth Fitness Study Tests I and II (Ross & Gilbert, 1985; Ross & Pate, 1987), was used as the basis for current levels of fitness across the country by the United States Department of Health and Human Services (1990) in drafting objectives for *Healthy Children 2000*. Each test reviewed in this chapter emphasizes health-related fitness com-

TABLE 5–3. Cardiopulmonary Function Variables and Response to Exercise in Children

Function	Child vs. Adult Response	Sex Differences
Heart rate (max, submax)	Higher	M = F (max); F > M (submax)
Stroke volume (max, submax)	Lower	M > F
Cardiac output (max, submax)	Lower, similar	
Arteriovenous difference (submax)	Similar	
Blood flow to active muscle	Higher	M = F
Blood pressure	Lower	
Hemoglobin concentration	Lower	
Ventilation/kg body wt (max)	Similar	
Ventilation/kg body wt (submax)	Higher	
Respiratory rate (max, submax)	Higher	
Tidal volume and vital capacity (max)	Lower	
Tidal volume and vital capacity (submax)	Lower	
Blood lactate levels (max, submax)	Similar/lower	M > F after puberty
	Lower	

Adapted from Bar-Or, O. Pediatric Sports Medicine for the Practitioner. New York: Springer-Verlag, 1983, pp. 19, 31, 46.

max = maximal exercise; submax = submaximal exercise.

ponents. Most tests provide some information regarding interrater reliability, but none specifically includes information on the validity of individual test items. Most information on the validity of individual test items has been provided by separate investigators or published separately subsequent to the development of the test batteries (Cureton & Warren, 1990; Going, 1988; Jackson & Coleman, 1976; Jackson & Baker, 1986; Safrit, 1990). A comparison of the four tests and their components is presented in Table 5–4.

Current Tests

AAHPERD PHYSICAL BEST PROGRAM

This program, originally designed to be both a physical fitness measure and an educational program to promote health and prevent disease, was developed by the American Alliance for Health, Physical Education, Recreation, and Dance (AAHPERD) (1988). In 1993, AAPHERD adopted the Prudential

TABLE 5-4. **Review of Current Physical Fitness Tests**

Test	Component of Fitness	Test Items	Standard	Reliability/Validity
Chrysler–AAU Physical Fitness Program (1987)	Cardiorespiratory endurance Lower back flexibility Muscular strength/ endurance Upper body muscle strength/endurance	Endurance run V-sit and reach Bent knee sit-up Pull-up/flexed arm hang	Normative (for ages 6–16 yr) (not nationwide)	Not all data externally valid
Prudential FITNESSGRAM (Cooper Institute for Aerobics Research, 1987, 1993)	Cardiorespiratory endurance Lower back flexibility Upper body strength Abdominal strength Body composition Agility (K-3)	1-mile run Sit and reach Pull-up/flexed arm hang Sit-ups Skinfold measurement Shuttle run	Criterion	(Morrow et al., 1993) Partial work reported 1990 (Cureton & Warren, 1990)
National Child and Youth Fitness Study (Ross & Gilbert, 1985; Ross & Pate, 1987)	Cardiorespiratory endurance Lower back flexibility Upper body strength/ endurance Abdominal strength/ endurance Body composition	1-mile walk-run Half-mile walk-run Sit and reach Modified pull-up Bent knee sit-up Sum of skinfolds (triceps/sub-scapular/calf)	U.S. norms (for ages 6–18 yr)	(Ross, Katz, & Gilbert, 1985) (Ross et al., 1987)
Presidential Physical Fitness Program (President's Council, 1987)	Cardiorespiratory endurance Lower back flexibility Upper body strength/ endurance Abdominal strength/ endurance Ability/power	1-mile walk-run Sit and reach Pull-up Bent knee sit-up/ curl-up Shuttle run	U.S. norms (for ages 6–18 yr)	General terms of validity reported; no specifics

FITNESSGRAM (Morrow et al., 1993) to measure physical fitness status and no longer uses its original fitness battery. The Physical Best Program remains active in its educational component to promote youth fitness.

CHRYSLER FUND–AMATEUR ATHLETIC UNION PHYSICAL FITNESS PROGRAM

The Physical Fitness Program by Chrysler Fund–Amateur Athletic Union (1987) consists of four required items and one optional item. Although the test battery is norm referenced, it is referenced by test administrators. The sample therefore is not systematically representative of the nation. A critique of the test suggests that not all data are externally valid. Significant differences in mean values in test items were noted when compared with those of other tests and when compared with results among different test administrators (Safrit, 1990; Sodoma, 1986). The test items show some variation from other tests (see Table 5-4). The absence of a standard testing

protocol among test administrators raises questions about the reliability and thus the validity of the test.

PRUDENTIAL FITNESSGRAM PROGRAM

This test is a battery that uses criterion-referenced standards. The program was developed by the Cooper Institute for Aerobics Research (1987). In 1993, a revised version became known as the Prudential FITNESSGRAM Program (Morrow et al., 1993). Limited information is available on the reliability and validity of the specific standards in the test manual. Research on the validity and reliability of the cardiorespiratory endurance standards has been published separately (Cureton & Warren, 1990). Development of the standards was based on determining (1) the lowest level of the laboratory standard for cardiorespiratory endurance, (Vo_2max) consistent with minimal risk of disease and adequate functional capacity; (2) the timing standards of the mile walk-run, consistent with the minimal Vo_2max; and (3) a comparison of the standards with available national normative data to evaluate both consistency and accuracy. Standards using the Prudential FITNESSGRAM for individuals with disabilities are currently being developed (Seaman et al., 1995).

NATIONAL CHILDREN, YOUTH, AND FITNESS STUDY (NCYFS) I AND II

These tests were national studies undertaken to assess current levels of physical fitness of children and youth in the United States. Initiated by the United States Office of Disease Prevention and Health Promotion (Pate et al., 1987; Ross et al., 1985), the results have been used to set appropriate targets for improved health and fitness. The NCYFS I produced normative data by sex and age and sex and grade for children and youth age 10 to 18 years, and NCYFS II provided the same information for children age 6 to 9 years. Training procedures were developed for test administrators, and interrater reliability estimates were found to be .99 for body composition measurements. Concurrent validity for some test items had already been established (Jackson & Coleman, 1976).

PRESIDENTIAL PHYSICAL FITNESS PROGRAM

This is a norm-referenced test created by the President's Council on Physical Fitness and Sports (1987). Validity is not addressed, but some reliability information is provided.

Comparison of Tests

All the tests measure similar components of health-related fitness. Each includes items for testing cardiorespiratory endurance, muscular strength and endurance, and flexibility. Only two of the four tests measure body composition. The tests differ in the reference standard used. Tests are either norm-referenced (performance is compared with that of a national U.S. sample of children taking the same test) or criterion-referenced (performance is compared with a preset standard consistent with fitness). The criterion for each item is independent of the performance of other children on the same test. The Prudential FITNESSGRAM is the only criterion-referenced test.

Appropriate reliability and validity data are not available for any of the tests reviewed, and thus the tests do not meet standards for measurement required of scientific clinical tools (American Psychological Association, 1985). Users must be cautious in the interpretation of scores and their meaning. Strict and rigid interpretation of the test results would be incorrect and should be avoided until further evidence of reliability and validity is available. Procedures for evaluating reliability and validity of criterion-referenced tests are available (Safrit, 1989).

COMPONENTS OF PHYSICAL FITNESS

The components of health-related fitness, as mentioned earlier, are cardiorespiratory endurance, muscular strength and endurance, flexibility, and body composition. The following information will be reviewed for each component:

1. The criterion measure of the component
2. Laboratory measurement
3. Developmental aspects of the component and standards by age
4. Field measurement of the component and its validity in relation to the criterion measure
5. Standards by age as determined by the FITNESSGRAM program, a computer-scored fitness test with a health-related focus
6. Physical activities with high correlation to the particular fitness component
7. Response to training
8. Assessment of the component in children with disabilities

Cardiorespiratory Endurance

Criterion Measure

The most widely used criterion measure for cardiorespiratory endurance is directly measured Vo_2max, sometimes referred to as maximal aerobic power. This component measures the capabilities of the cardiovascular and pulmonary systems and is significant because oxygen supply to the tissues depends on the efficiency and capacity of these systems. Vo_2max is the highest rate of oxygen consumed by the body in a given time period during exercise of a significant portion of body muscle mass (Krahenbuhl et al., 1985). Cardiorespiratory endurance is so important to overall fitness that many people view physical fitness as being synonymous with cardiorespiratory endurance (Simons-Morton et al., 1987).

Laboratory Measurement

Laboratory measurement techniques include measurement of Vo_2max during progressive exercise to the point of exhaustion with the use of an ergometer. This method is referred to as direct determination of Vo_2max. Indirect determination methods predict Vo_2max from submaximal exercise.

DIRECT DETERMINATION

An ergometer is a device that measures the amount of work performed under controlled conditions. The two devices commonly available are a cycle ergometer and a treadmill. The cycle ergometer has the advantage of being relatively inexpensive and portable, but compared with the treadmill, it exercises a smaller total muscle mass. With the cycle ergometer, local fatigue develops (primarily in knee extensors), resulting in premature termination of the testing. Depending on the source, values of Vo_2max are reported to be 5 to 30% lower on a cycle ergometer than on a treadmill (Bar-Or, 1983a; Braden & Strong, 1990; Krahenbuhl et al., 1985). For children, the coordination and rhythm, or cadence, required on a cycle ergometer are sometimes difficult to achieve. Both the treadmill and the cycle ergometers present problems when used to test populations with disabilities, in particular those with impairments of balance or coordination.

A variety of protocols for direct determination can be used with children. The most common protocol is one in which resistance, inclination, speed, or height is increased every 1 to 3 minutes without interruption until the child can no longer maintain the activity. In interrupted protocols, which are sometimes used, there is an interruption between each successive increment of exercise. Examples of some common direct determination protocols are given in Table 5-5. The main criterion for indicating that Vo_2max has been achieved during a progressive protocol is that an increase in power load is not accompanied by an increased Vo_2 (usually 2 ml/kg/min or higher) (Krahenbuhl et al., 1985). Astrand (1952), however, reported that 5% of all children tested failed to reach a plateau in Vo_2, even though evidence from secondary criteria suggested that exhaustion had been reached.

Despite the difficulty of determining attainment of Vo_2max, studies suggest that the reliability of direct determination testing with children is high. Coefficients of variation of 3, 5, and 8% for Vo_2max determined by treadmill walk-jogging, running, and walking, respectively, have been reported (Paterson & Cunningham, 1978). A mean variation of 4.5% was reported for children exercising to exhaustion on a cycle ergometer on 12 different occasions (Cumming et al., 1967).

INDIRECT DETERMINATION

Indirect determination methods use submaximal exercise to indirectly predict Vo_2max. The child is not taken to his or her self-imposed maximum. Heart rate during one or more stages is the variable most commonly used to derive the index of Vo_2max. Step tests for children are usually submaximal tests, using recovery heart rate to predict Vo_2max. Evidence suggests that height-specific step tests can be reliable predictors of Vo_2max (Francis & Feinstein, 1991). Important limitations exist, however, in predicting Vo_2max from submaximal exercise data, and these should always be kept in mind (Wyndham,

TABLE 5-5. Direct Determination All-out Protocols

Bruce Treadmill Protocol			
Stage	Speed (mph)	Grade (%)	Duration (min)
1	1.7	10	3
2	2.5	12	3
3	3.4	14	3
4	4.2	16	3
5	5.0	18	3
6	5.5	20	3
7	6.0	22	3

McMaster Progressive Continuous Cycling Test			
Body Height (cm)	Initial Load (watts)	Increments (watts)	Duration (min)
<119.9	12.5	12.5	2
120–139.9	12.5	25.0	2
140–159.9	25.0	25.0	2
>160	25.0	25.0 (F) 50.0 (M)	2

Adapted from Bar-Or, O. Appendix II: Procedures for exercise testing in children. In Bar-Or, O, Pediatric Sports Medicine for the Practitioner. New York: Springer-Verlag, 1983, pp. 315–341.

Watts = joules per second.

1976). Examples of test protocols are presented in Table 5-6.

The W_{170} is an index used to predict mechanical power in a submaximal test. Two or more measurements of heart rate are obtained at different power or workloads, and heart rate is then extrapolated to 170 beats per minute. The corresponding power is W_{170}. This index, originally described by Wahlund (1948), is based on the assumption that heart rate is linearly related to power at 170 beats per minute or less. To minimize error, more than two heart rate measurements are taken, one of which is as close as possible to 170 beats per minute.

Developmental Aspects of Cardiorespiratory Endurance

Absolute maximal aerobic power, or Vo_2max, increases with age throughout childhood and is slightly higher in boys than in girls (Krahenbuhl et al., 1985; Rutenfranz et al., 1990; Shvartz & Reibold, 1990). Initial differences during early childhood are approximately 10%, increasing to 25% by age 14 years, and exceeding 50% by age 16 (Krahenbuhl et al., 1985). The development of a greater muscle mass in boys and increasing differences in the amount of time spent in vigorous physical exercise are the most commonly given explanations. Overall, the physical working capacity of children increases approxi-

TABLE 5–6. **Indirect Determination Protocols**

Adams Submaximal Progressive Continuous Cycling Test*

Body Weight (kg)	Stage 1 (watts)	Stage 2 (watts)	Stage 3 (watts)
30	16.5	33.0	50.0
30–39.9	16.5	50.0	83.0
40–59.9	16.5	50.0	100.0
>60	16.5	83.0	133.0

Stage duration = 6 min
Performance by W_{170}

Modified 3-Minute Step Test†

Stage	Duration (min)	Ascent Rate (ascents/min)
1	3	22
2	3	26
3	3	30

Step height dependent on height
Performance by recovery heart rate

*Adapted from Bar-Or, O. Appendix II: Procedures for exercise testing in children. In Bar-Or, O. Pediatric Sports Medicine for the Practitioner. New York: Springer-Verlag, 1983, pp. 315–341.

†Adapted and reprinted by permission from Francis, K, & Culpepper, M. Height adjusted, rate specific, single stage, step test for predicting maximal oxygen consumption. Southern Medical Journal, 82:602–606, 1989.

mately eightfold between the ages of 6 and 12 years. Few data are available on Vo_2max for children younger than age 6 (Adams, 1973).

Relative to body weight, only a 1% change in Vo_2max is noted between the ages of 6 and 16 years for boys (52.8 ml/kg/min at age 6; 53.5 ml/kg/min at age 16), whereas girls display a 12% reduction between the same ages (52.0 ml/kg/min at age 6; 40.5 ml/kg/min at age 16) (Krahenbuhl et al., 1985; Shvartz & Reibold, 1990). Vo_2max is highly correlated with lean body mass. The decline in Vo_2max in girls begins around age 10, when changes in body composition occur as girls develop a relatively increased amount of subcutaneous fat. When Vo_2max is measured with reference to lean body mass, the difference in values between the sexes disappears (Braden & Strong, 1990).

Increases in body dimensions, however, do not account for all changes in Vo_2max that occur with growth. When comparing same-sex adolescents of different ages with identical body weight or body height, the positive relationship with age remains (Sprynarova & Reisenauer, 1978). Functional changes in cardiovascular, pulmonary, and musculoskeletal systems resulting in improved efficiency with maturity may play a role. Cooper and colleagues (1984), however, suggested that the functional com-

ponents of body systems are integrated so that aerobic capacity is optimized throughout the growth process.

Measurement in the Field

The most common measure of cardiorespiratory fitness in the field is a long-distance run of various structures or lengths. All the physical fitness batteries reviewed previously have a distance run test, commonly a 1-mile run. Test-retest reliability of Vo_2max during field testing has been shown to be between .60 and .95 (Cunningham et al., 1977; Safrit, 1990). Jackson and Coleman (1976) studied the construct validity of various distance run tests and the concurrent validity of the 9- and 12-minute run tests in elementary schoolchildren. Results suggested that both the 9- and 12-minute distance runs were valid measures of the construct and displayed concurrent validity with Vo_2max. Safrit (1990) suggested that a 9-minute run is a distance of at least 1 mile. Both the 1200- and 1600-meter runs were significantly related to Vo_2max, but only the 1600-meter run had correlation coefficients above .60, which is generally accepted as the lower limit for a useful fitness test (Krahenbuhl et al., 1978; Mathews, 1973). Validation values in the range of .40 to .80 between corresponding performance and weight-relative Vo_2max have been reported (Safrit, 1990).

Standards by Age

Standards of performance are determined by ranking a child's performance in relation to the performance of a group of children tested on the same test (norm-referenced standard) or against an established criterion found to be consistent with good health (criterion-referenced standard). One advantage of criterion-referenced standards is that they are independent of the proportion of the population that meets the standards. A ranking by a norm-referenced standard does not necessarily represent a desirable level of fitness or performance. The limitation of criterion-referenced standards, however, is that they are somewhat arbitrary and that the criteria used in the current physical fitness tests differ from one another (Cureton & Warren, 1990). Establishing the validity of criterion-referenced standards for performance is in progress.

Cureton and Warren (1990) described the procedures for development of criterion standards for the FITNESSGRAM Program. Validity coefficients for the FITNESSGRAM Program range from .73 to 1.00 when compared with the criterion standard of Vo_2max. The actual percentage of Vo_2max that is used during the walk-run test, however, is unknown,

TABLE 5-7. **One-Mile Walk-Run Standards**

Age (yr)	Criterion* Standard		FITNESSGRAM† Field Standard		NCYFS I, II‡ Percentiles	
	M	F	M	F	M	F
5	42.0	40.0	16:00	17:00	—	—
6	42.0	40.0	15:00	16:00	—	—
7	42.0	40.0	14:00	15:00	—	—
8	42.0	40.0	13:00	14:30	15	15
9	42.0	40.0	12:00	13:00	20	20
10	42.0	39.0	11:00	12:00	25	35
11	42.0	38.0	11:00	12:00	20	40
12	42.0	37.0	10:00	11:30	30	30
13	42.0	36.0	9:30	10:30	20	35
14	42.0	35.0	8:30	10:30	35	50
15	42.0	35.0	8:30	10:30	25	55
16	42.0	35.0	8:30	10:30	20	50
17	42.0	35.0	8:30	10:30	30	50

Adapted from Cureton, KJ, & Warren, GL. Criterion-referenced standards for youth health related fitness tests: A tutorial. Research Quarterly for Exercise and Sport, 61:7-19, 1990; Ross, JG, Dotson, CO, Gilbert, CG, & Katz, SJ. The national youth and fitness study I: New standards for fitness measurement. Journal of Physical Education, Recreation and Dance, 56:62-66, 1985; Ross, JG, Delpy, LA, Christenson, GM, Gold, RS, & Damberg, CL. The national youth and fitness study II: Study procedures and quality control. Journal of Physical Education, Recreation and Dance, 58:57-62, 1987.

Criterion standard as set by FITNESSGRAM in ml/kg/min of oxygen uptake.
†Minutes required to complete a 1-mile walk-run.
‡Percentile rank of children performing this standard in National Children, Youth, and Fitness Study (NCYFS) I, II.

which makes evaluation of any or all values difficult. A comparison of walk-run standards by age is provided in Table 5-7.

Physical Activities

Activities that are highly correlated with development of cardiorespiratory endurance are boxing, running, rowing, swimming, cross-country skiing, and bicycling. The common component among these activities is a prolonged, sustained demand on the cardiorespiratory system that requires general stamina.

Response to Training

Debate exists over whether maximal aerobic power of prepubescents is a component that can be affected by training. Research results are equivocal. Those studies that report improvement in aerobic power with training suggest that the principles of training of prepubescents, that is, frequency, intensity, and duration, are similar to those for adults (Simons-Morton et al., 1987). The functional results of conditioning on the cardiorespiratory system include decreased heart rate, increased stroke volume, improved respiratory muscular endurance, and decreased respiration rate (Bar-Or, 1983c; Braden & Strong, 1990). A more specific focus on conditioning and training will be found later in this chapter.

Assessment of Cardiorespiratory Endurance in Children with Disabilities

Children with disabilities often exhibit decreased or limited exercise capacity relative to their nondisabled peers. This can result from either their limited participation in exercise, which leads to deconditioning, or the specific pathologic factors of their disability that limit exercise-related functions. Regardless of the cause, children with disabilities often enter a cycle of decreased activity that precipitates a loss of fitness and further decreases in activity levels.

Pathophysiologic factors that may limit cardiorespiratory endurance can sometimes be separated by the specific component of the Fick equation that they affect. This provides a convenient way to categorize conditions or diseases by the fitness components they affect most (Bar-Or, 1983c, 1986) (Fig. 5-1). Studies suggest that maximal aerobic uptake is limited not only by central mechanisms of the cardiopulmonary system but also by peripheral mechanisms controlling blood flow, excitation processes in the muscle fiber, local fatigue, and enzyme availability (Green & Patla, 1992; Saltin & Strange, 1992; Sutton, 1992). When considering the limitations or reductions in Vo_2max in children with disabilities, both central and peripheral limitations must be considered.

CEREBRAL PALSY

Directly measured maximal aerobic capacity of children and adolescents with cerebral palsy is 10 to

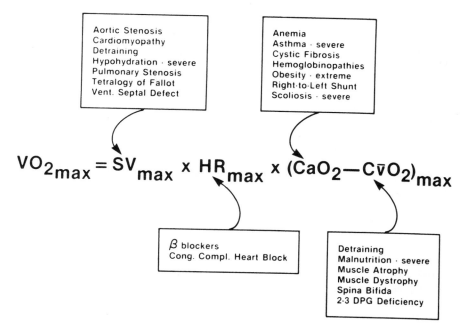

FIGURE 5–1. Maximal aerobic power (Vo_2max) and pathology. The Fick equation and specific pathologic conditions that affect its variables and reduce Vo_2max are shown. (From Bar-Or, O. Exercise as a diagnostic tool in pediatrics. In Bar-Or, O., Pediatric Sports Medicine for the Practitioner. New York: Springer-Verlag, 1983, p. 72.)

30% less than that of controls (Bar-Or et al., 1976; Lundberg, 1978; Lundberg et al., 1967). It would seem that peripheral mechanisms related to the neuromuscular disorder itself are more likely to contribute to decreased capacity than are central cardiopulmonary mechanisms, although this has not been studied. When indirectly assessed from submaximal heart rate, aerobic capacity of adolescents was found to be reduced by 50% (Lundberg et al., 1967). Low mechanical efficiency creates disproportionately high submaximal heart rates in individuals with cerebral palsy, making submaximal heart rate a poor predictor of maximal aerobic power (Bar-Or, 1983b). Submaximal exercise tests, in general, underestimate aerobic capacity in poorly trained individuals (Astrand & Rodahl, 1986; Wyndham, 1976). Numerous studies suggest that heart rate is a good predictor or an appropriate substitute clinical measure of Vo_2 because of its linear relationship to heart rate (Rose et al., 1989, 1990). It is not a measure of maximal aerobic capacity, however, and therefore it is not an alternative measure of cardiorespiratory fitness.

An increase in blood flow to exercising muscles after conditioning is a response observed in children with cerebral palsy but not seen in able-bodied children (Lundberg & Pernow, 1970). Spastic muscles of individuals with adult-onset brain damage exhibit subnormal blood flow during exercise (Landin et al., 1977). (Whether the rate of blood flow changes after conditioning in individuals with adult-onset brain injury is not known.) One hypothesis to explain the increase in blood flow in conditioned individuals with cerebral palsy is that it results from a decrease in spasticity. More rapid deterioration of maximal aerobic uptake is seen after discontinuation of training in children with cerebral palsy than in able-bodied children (Bar-Or, 1983b).

Functional assessments that relate to the cardiorespiratory fitness of children with various disabilities are becoming more commonplace. The Pediatric Orthopedic Society of North America recently developed a functional outcomes questionnaire directed toward assessment of pediatric musculoskeletal conditions (Daltroy et al., 1998). Within this questionnaire are questions regarding a child's ability to complete a 1-mile and a 3-mile run. As more institutions caring for children with disabilities incorporate this assessment and others like it in daily practice, insight will be gained that may assist in determination of cardiorespiratory fitness. Standards for field testing aerobic capacity in individuals with cerebral palsy using a long-distance run have been previously published for children age 10 to 17 years (Winnick & Short, 1985). Seaman and colleagues (1995) present a review of alternative test items that can be used to assess aerobic capacity in children with various disabilities, including cerebral palsy.

JUVENILE RHEUMATOID ARTHRITIS

Maximal aerobic capacity measured by cycle ergometry in children with juvenile rheumatoid arthritis has been reported to be 15 to 30% lower than in their peers matched by age, sex, and body surface area (Giannini & Protas, 1991, 1992). No correlation was found between severity of articular disease and aerobic capacity, however. Children with juvenile rheumatoid arthritis have a shorter duration of exercise before exhaustion, which occurs at a lower than normal work rate with a lower peak heart rate. Deficient oxygen extraction from exercising muscles or low blood flow to exercising muscles has been postulated to occur in this population as a result of decreased activity levels (Bar-Or, 1983b, 1986).

SCOLIOSIS

Chest deformity, decreased lung size, and decreased physical activity are believed to contribute to the lower maximal aerobic capacity of children with advanced scoliosis. No functional or exercise-related deficits are found in children with minor or moderate scoliosis (Bar-Or, 1983b). For those with advanced scoliosis, limitations of 50 to 70% in Vo_2max have been reported. Vo_2 and minute ventilation are decreased and pulmonary artery pressure increased at maximal exercise relative to able-bodied standards. Some improvements are seen with conditioning.

MENTAL RETARDATION

Most studies indicate that individuals with mental retardation display lower Vo_2max scores than do their nondisabled peers (Lavay et al., 1990); however, significant variability has been reported among individuals with the same level of disability. Technical problems associated with testing individuals with mental retardation are encountered that create difficulties in establishing reliable and valid information. Treadmill testing appears to be the most reliable form of testing. Field test standards and alternative test items for aerobic capacity in individuals with both mild and moderate metal retardation are available (Seaman et al., 1995).

Muscular Strength and Endurance

The second component of physical fitness is muscular strength and endurance. Strength is required for movement and has a direct impact on effective performance. Strength is also important for optimal posture and reduced risk of lower back pain. Muscular strength, muscular endurance, and muscular power are not synonymous terms. Muscular strength refers to maximal contractile force. Muscular endurance is the ability of muscles to perform work and

assumes some component of muscular strength. Muscular power refers to the ability to release maximal muscular force within a specified time. As velocity increases or time decreases (for maximal muscular force to be obtained), power increases. Because muscular endurance and muscular power have their basis in muscular strength, strength will be the primary point of this discussion.

Laboratory Measurement

The laboratory standard for muscular strength is strength measured by dynamometry. Tests include isometric dynamometry, isokinetic dynamometry, and single-repetition maximal isotonic dynamometry. Most measurements are made on specific, selected muscles, and then results are extrapolated to give "whole body" strength. Unfortunately, a limitation for setting standards of strength is that force measurements depend on the type of dynamometer used (Blimkie, 1989). The most commonly selected measures are hand grip, elbow flexion and extension, knee flexion and extension, and plantar flexion strength.

Isokinetic strength testing during childhood and adolescence is a relatively new area of study. The reliability of isokinetic testing in children presents unique issues because of the variability of muscle coordination and neuromuscular maturation. Coefficients of variation from 5 to 11% have been reported (Blimkie, 1989). Children demonstrate the capacity to perform consistent maximal voluntary contraction under controlled conditions by age 6 to 7 years. The limited amount of research and available data do not allow definite conclusions on the effects of age and gender differences on isokinetic strength development. However, body weight and muscle cross-sectional area appear to correlate positively with isokinetic strength. Gender differences are minimal between ages 7 and 11. After age 13, boys tend to have greater isokinetic strength for the muscles tested (Baltzopoulos & Kellis, 1998; Gaul, 1996).

DEVELOPMENTAL ASPECTS AND STANDARDS BY AGE

GRIP STRENGTH. Grip strength is the most commonly reported upper extremity strength measure in children. Absolute strength scores, however, are highly sensitive to the type of dynamometer used and to its positioning, making the results of studies difficult to compare. In general, single-hand grip strength increases from an average of approximately 5 kg for children at age 3 years to 45 kg for boys at age 17 and 30 kg for girls at age 17. Bilateral grip strength has been measured at a mean of 25 kg for children at age 7 years, increasing to an average of

95 kg for boys and 50 kg for girls by age 17 years (Blimkie, 1989). The rate of increase in strength for boys rises dramatically at puberty.

ELBOW FLEXION AND EXTENSION. Isometric elbow flexion strength is greater than isometric elbow extension strength throughout childhood and adolescence, and the difference between them increases with increasing age (Fowler & Gardner, 1967). The extension/flexion strength ratio for boys is approximately 0.76 at the age of 7.5 years and decreases to 0.57 during late adolescence. No data are available for girls.

SHOULDER FLEXION AND EXTENSION. A single study has addressed isokinetic strength values for shoulder flexion and extension in children (Brodie et al., 1986). Twenty-four untrained, prepubescent boys with an average age of 11.7 years were tested on a Cybex II (Ronkonkoma, NY) at 6 different velocities. Mean values for peak torque for shoulder extension were relatively constant at speeds of between 60 and 150 degrees per second (13.2 and 13.7 newton-meters); mean values for shoulder flexion increased as speed increased (12.5–24.3 newton-meters).

KNEE FLEXION AND EXTENSION. Isokinetic knee flexion strength and knee extension strength also increase throughout childhood. Results from Alexander and Molnar (1973) and Molnar and Alexander (1973) indicated that knee extension strength exceeds knee flexion strength for both sexes at all ages. Average knee flexion strength varies from 30 to 50% of average knee extension strength for girls and 28 to 65% for boys. Boys have slightly greater strength than do girls before puberty but consistently greater strength from the age of 10 years onward.

TRUNK FLEXION AND EXTENSION. Few data are available for laboratory dynamometry standards for trunk strength in children. Clinical data have been collected for the ability of children to sustain isometric trunk flexion (actually a test of muscular endurance) between the ages of 3 and 7 years (Lefkof, 1986). An isotonic test of the number of hook-lying sit-ups performed was also included in the study. Both the endurance for isometric trunk flexion and the ability to perform sit-ups improved with age. The greatest improvement occurred between the ages of 5 and 6 years, when average performance at least doubled. These results are important because the typical field test for muscular strength and endurance is performance of sit-ups.

COMPOSITE STRENGTH. Composite strength provides a measure of overall or general strength and consists of a total strength score from several muscle groups. Usually, grip strength, thrust strength (shoulder girdle), and shoulder pull measures are included in composite strength scores (Carron & Bailey, 1974; Faust, 1977). Unfortunately, I can find no measures of composite strength that include lower extremity or trunk strength. The pattern of increase in composite strength during childhood is similar to that of grip strength.

EVOKED RESPONSES

A second method for muscular function assessment in the laboratory is by evoked responses from electrical stimulation. Muscle contractile characteristics are studied with this methodology, including force production. Few data are available for children (Blimkie, 1989; Blimkie & Sale, 1998).

Developmental Aspects of Muscular Strength and Endurance

Gajdosik and Gajdosik describe the development of the musculoskeletal system in Chapter 4 of this volume. Development of strength depends on the development of force production and is influenced by numerous factors, for example, the muscle's cross-sectional area (Malina, 1986). Muscular strength in absolute terms increases linearly with chronologic age from early childhood in both sexes to approximately age 13 to 14 years. Increases in strength are closely related to increases in muscle mass during growth. Boys have greater strength than do girls at all ages (seen as early as age 3 years) and have larger absolute and relative amounts of muscle (kilogram of muscle per kilogram of body weight) (Blimkie, 1989; Malina, 1986). The sex difference in relative strength (per kilogram of body mass) before puberty is at least in part caused by a higher proportion of body fat in girls from midchildhood onward, a difference similar to the trend in cardiorespiratory endurance (Faust, 1977; Malina, 1986). Rarick and Thompson (1956) suggested that boys are 11 to 13% stronger than girls during childhood. This value reaches 20% by adulthood for strength per cross-sectional area of muscle (Maughan et al., 1983). Correlates and determinants of strength are thought to include age, body size, muscle size, muscle fiber type and size, muscle contractile properties, and biomechanical influences.

During adolescence, there is a marked acceleration in development of strength, particularly in boys. Boys between the ages of 10 and 16 years who were followed longitudinally showed a 23% increase in strength per year. Peak growth in muscle mass occurred during and after peak weight gain, but maximal strength development occurred after peak velocity of growth in height and weight, suggesting that muscle tissue increases first in mass and then in strength (Carron & Bailey, 1974; Malina, 1986). Girls generally show peak strength development before peak weight gain (Faust, 1977). Overall muscle mass increases more than 5 times in males from childhood to adulthood; the increase in females is 3.5 times.

Differentiation in strength between the sexes at puberty is, at least in part, caused by differences in hormonal concentrations, particularly testosterone. Hormones other than the male sex steroids also make an important contribution (Florini, 1987). Unfortunately, no pediatric studies to date have correlated age-associated changes in endocrinologic function with muscle size and muscular strength.

Measurement in the Field

Field measurements of muscular strength usually entail movement of part or all of the body mass against gravity. The two common tests for muscular strength are the flexed arm hang and the sit-up. All the fitness tests previously reviewed include a sit-up test and a pull-up or flexed arm hang test. The correlation between abdominal strength and endurance and shoulder girdle strength as measures of absolute strength for physical fitness is not well established. Although strength is considered an important part of physical fitness, the standards to meet minimal fitness requirements in this area are the least clear. This may result from lack of quantitative research in this area.

SIT-UPS. The exact relationship between sit-up performance and abdominal strength and endurance is unclear. How abdominal strength is related to a given number of sit-ups is unknown. Test-retest reliability estimates for sit-ups measured for 11- to 14-year-olds range from .64 to .94 for both boys and girls (Safrit & Wood, 1987).

Standards of performance as determined by the FITNESSGRAM battery are listed in Table 5-8. The percentage of children who achieved criterion ranged from 80% at age 7 years to 62% at age 16 to 17 years (Blair et al., 1989). These results are slightly different from those attained on the NCYFS I and II (Ross & Gilbert, 1985; Ross & Pate, 1987).

CHIN-UPS AND FLEXED ARM HANG. The validity of chin-ups and the flexed arm hang as measures of upper body strength is questionable. Berger and Medlin (1969) suggested that the number of chin-ups as a measure of absolute strength is not valid because body weight is inversely related to the number of chin-ups performed. Considine (1973) demonstrated that pull-ups do not provide an indicator of shoulder girdle strength. The NCYFS II developed a modified pull-up test for 6- to 9-year-olds to overcome the problems associated with body weight (Pate et al., 1987).

STANDARDS BY AGE

The standards of performance for the FITNESSGRAM Program are listed in Table 5-8. No data

TABLE 5-8. **Field Standards for Strength**

Age (yr)	FITNESSGRAM* Sit-ups		FITNESSGRAM Pull-ups		FITNESSGRAM Flexed Arm Hang		NCYFS I, II† Sit-ups	
	F	M	F	M	F	M	F	M
5	20	20	1	1	5	5	—	—
6	20	20	1	1	5	5	60	60
7	20	20	1	1	5	5	35–40	35–40
8	25	25	1	1	8	10	45–50	45–50
9	25	25	1	1	8	10	45–50	35–40
10	30	30	1	1	8	10	30–40	30–40
11	30	30	1	1	8	10	25–30	25–30
12	30	35	1	1	8	10	30	40
13	30	35	1	2	12	10	40	30
14	35	40	1	3	12	15	50	50
15	35	40	1	5	12	25	50	40
16	35	40	1	5	12	25	50	40

Data from Blair, SN, Clark, DG, Cureton, KJ, & Powell, KE. Exercise and fitness in childhood: Implications for a lifetime of health. In Gisolfi, CV, & Lamb, DR (Eds.), Perspectives in Exercise Science and Sports Medicine, Vol. 2: Youth, Exercise, and Sport. Indianapolis, IN: Benchmark Press, 1989, pp. 401–430; Ross, JG, Delpy, LA, Cristenson, GM, Gold, RS, & Damberg, CL. The national youth and fitness study II: Study procedures and quality control. Journal of Physical Education, Recreation and Dance, *58*:57–62, 1987; and Ross, JG, Dotson, CO, Gilbert, GG, & Katz, SJ. The national youth and fitness study I: New standards for fitness measurement. Journal of Physical Education, Recreation and Dance, *56*:62–66, 1985.

*Number of sit-ups performed in 1 min.

†Percentile rank of children performing FITNESSGRAM standards from National Children, Youth, and Fitness Study (NCYFS) I, II.

are available on the validity or reliability of these standards.

Branta and colleagues (1984) assessed the performance of children on the flexed arm hang as part of a longitudinal study of age changes in motor skills during childhood and adolescence. The minimum standards for fitness on the flexed arm hang set by the FITNESSGRAM Program are less than the measured performance for children at each age in this study. A general increase in the mean performance was noted throughout childhood in both sexes. The greatest gains occurred between the ages of 5 and 6 years and 12 and 13 years for girls and between 5 and 6, 7 and 8, and 13 and 14 years for boys. Both groups showed substantial improvements in performance at puberty. Sex differences were apparent by age 8 years. Relative gains across the age span were substantially higher for boys than for girls.

Physical Activities

Activities that have a high correlation with muscular strength are gymnastics, jumping, sprinting, weight lifting, and wrestling. Local muscular endurance is affected by cycling, figure skating, and middle-distance running.

Response to Training

Training-induced increases in strength can be influenced by numerous factors, including enhancement of motivation, improvement in coordination, increase in number of contractile proteins per cross-sectional area of muscle, and hypertrophy of muscle (Mersch & Stoboy, 1989). Gains in strength and muscle mass can be achieved by children with training at or after puberty. Prepubescent children also show improvements in force output with training but appear to have difficulty in increasing muscle mass (Bar-Or, 1983c; Sale, 1989). Strength improvements in prepubescent children have thus been attributed to neurologic adaptations to training and improved motor unit activation rather than to increased cross-sectional area of muscle (Blimkie et al., 1989; Komi, 1986; Weltman et al., 1986). Direct evidence for the role of neurologic adaptation during strength training has been documented by increases in integrated electromyograph amplitudes and maximal isokinetic strength following an 8-week strength program (Ozmun et al., 1994). Because the magnitude of changes in neuromuscular activation is generally smaller than the observed increases in strength, it has been postulated that improved movement coordination is a contributor to strength gains—particularly in complex multijoint exercises

(Blimkie & Sale, 1998). Neuromuscular maturation in the prepubescent child is therefore an important contributor to strength and should not be underestimated.

Assessment of Muscular Strength and Endurance in Children with Disabilities

Muscular strength and endurance are crucial fitness components for walking, lifting, and performing most daily functions. Deficits of muscular strength in children with disabilities are a primary focus for the clinician in an attempt to improve (or maintain) maximum function. It is important to keep in mind, however, that strength as measured clinically is not simply the ability of a muscle to generate force. Strength as measured clinically is the effectiveness of the muscle force to produce movement of the joint. This encompasses both the ability of the muscle to generate force and appropriate skeletal alignment on which the muscles act. In children with disabilities, strength deficits result from either the muscles' inability to generate force or malalignment of the skeleton or a combination of both.

MUSCULAR DYSTROPHY

Strength measurements by dynamometry in children with muscular dystrophy (MD) exhibit progressive deterioration as compared with healthy children (Fowler & Gardner, 1967). A failure of muscular strength to increase with growth is seen. The result is that the absolute strength in a child with MD at the age of 16 years is similar to that of a healthy 5-year-old.

Serial longitudinal measurements indicate that muscle strength decreases linearly with age approximately .25 manual muscle testing units per year from ages 5 to 13 years. Typically, by the time strength declined to grade 4 (manual muscle testing units), isometric strength measures are 40 to 50% of normal control values (Kilmer et al., 1993; McDonald et al., 1995).

Muscular endurance, the ability to sustain static or rhythmic contraction for long periods, is also affected in children with MD. Ninety-two percent of the children tested by Hosking and colleagues (1976) scored below the 5th percentile for strength in holding the head 45° off the ground. Measurement on the Wingate anaerobic cycling test indicates that both peak muscular power and mean muscular power output are significantly less than normal (Bar-Or, 1986). The test-retest reliability of this test for various neuromuscular and muscular disease conditions has been established (Tirosh et al., 1990).

CEREBRAL PALSY

Strength deficits in children with cerebral palsy are common. Whether voluntary strength can be accurately measured in the presence of spasticity and abnormal motor control is controversial. Strength profiles for lower extremity muscle groups in children with spastic cerebral palsy have recently become available (Wiley & Damiano, 1998). Children with spastic diplegia demonstrated strength values ranging from 16 to 71% of same-age peers depending on the muscle tested. The gluteus maximus and soleus muscles showed the greatest strength deficits. The involved side of children with hemiplegia exhibited values from 22 to 79% of strength values of same-age peers. The gluteus maximus and the anterior tibialis were the weakest muscles.

Inadequate joint moment and power production as measured by computerized gait analysis are seen in children with cerebral palsy (Gage, 1991; Olney et al., 1988). These measures provide indirect evidence in a functional context of decreased strength, because strength is a prerequisite for moment and power production. Power production by the ankle plantar flexor muscles in terminal stance phase provides a key source of power for forward motion during the normal walking cycle. Power production in terminal stance phase is often reduced in children with cerebral palsy. Occasionally, inappropriately timed power production results in excessive, but nonproductive, energy expenditure during gait (Gage, 1991) (Fig. 5–2).

Muscular endurance is also decreased in cerebral palsy. Performance on the Wingate anaerobic test in a group of children with cerebral palsy resulted in averages that were 2 to 4 standard deviations below the mean (Bar-Or, 1986).

Little information is available regarding modification of lower extremity strength field test items in children with cerebral palsy. Limited grip strength and flexed arm hang standards are available for upper extremity strength (Seaman et al., 1995). The United Cerebral Palsy Athletic Association uses functional abilities, including strength, to classify athletes for competition (United Cerebral Palsy Athletic Association, 1996).

Flexibility

The importance of flexibility as a component of health-related fitness is related to prevention of orthopedic impairments later in life, especially lower back pain (United States Department of Health and Human Services, 1990, 1998). Flexibility of the lower back, legs, and shoulders contributes to reduction of injury (Haskell et al., 1985). Limitations in spinal mobility can interfere with activities of daily living, such as dressing, turning, and driving. Restrictions in back mobility can also contribute to abnormalities in walking.

Criterion Measure

Joint range of motion (ROM) is the criterion used for standards of flexibility. Although the ROM measures for adults are well established and can be found in various textbooks (Norkin & White, 1985), ROM information for the pediatric population correlated with changes in stature is limited. Upper extremity ROM data for children are not well documented. The typical measurement tool is the universal goniometer. Gajdosik and Gajdosik review the reliability of goniometry in Chapter 4 of this volume.

FIGURE 5–2. Sagittal plane joint rotation (kinematic), joint moment, and power (kinetics) of a child with cerebral palsy versus a normal child. The child's joint moment is biphasic, and the power graph indicates two distinct bursts of power generation instead of one. The first burst is abnormal and functions to drive the center of gravity upward, not forward, which is nonproductive energy expenditure. (From Gage, JR. Gait Analysis in Cerebral Palsy. London: Mac Keith Press, 1991, p. 145.)

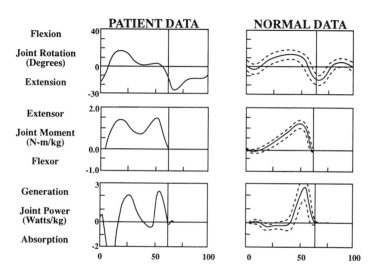

Laboratory Measurement and Developmental Aspects of Flexibility

EXTREMITY RANGE OF MOTION

Lower extremity passive ROM measurements have been described in the newborn, infant, and toddler (Drews et al., 1984; Phelps et al., 1985; Waugh et al., 1983). Newborn infants exhibit hypoextensibility of both hip and knee flexor muscles and increased popliteal angles consistent with the flexed posture in utero. Range increases in the first months of life. Ranges of hip abduction and rotations also differ from adult values.

Little to no information has been reported for ROM during childhood. Unpublished data from my laboratory on lower extremity ROM measurements in 140 children between the ages of 2 and 18 years suggest variation in some joints throughout childhood and relative stability in others (Stout JL, Phelps JA, Koop SE, unpublished data, 1991) (Table 5–9). Test-retest reliability is .95; interrater reliability is .90. Results suggested age and sex differences, with females exhibiting a trend toward more flexibility at all ages. Greater flexibility of the hamstring muscles in females is especially apparent during the teenage years in straight leg raising and popliteal angle measurements.

POSTURE AND SPINAL MOBILITY

Spinal mobility has been measured in both young children and adolescents (Haley et al., 1986; Moran et al., 1979). The technique of measurement of back mobility uses tape measure distance changes in bony landmark relationships before and after a standardized spinal movement. The concurrent validity of this measurement technique has been established (Moll & Wright, 1971; Moran et al., 1979). Anterior spinal flexion appears to remain relatively stable throughout childhood and adolescence, but lateral flexion increases linearly with age through adolescence and into early adulthood. Girls were significantly more flexible than boys in both anterior flexion and lateral flexion in the 5- to 9-year-old age group (Haley et al., 1986).

The relationship of posture to physical fitness is not often addressed in today's emphasis on health-related fitness. Previous research discussing the relationship of posture to fitness included the importance of posture to trunk strength and the potential for imbalance, back pain, headaches, foot pain, and orthopedic deformities (Clarke, 1979; Kendall & Kendall, 1952). Each aspect of posture may be important to mobility and cosmesis in children but becomes of greater importance in adulthood when impairment can lead to further deformity and loss of function.

THE NEW YORK STATE PHYSICAL FITNESS TEST. This test includes a posture assessment method consisting of three profiles of 13 posture areas. The test is used for children in grades 4 through 12. The 13 areas include head, shoulder, spine, hips, feet, and arches in the coronal plane and neck, chest, shoulders, upper back, trunk, abdomen, and lower back in the sagittal plane. The 50th percentile requires good posture scores on more than half the posture items (Clarke & Clarke, 1987).

THE ASSESSMENT OF BEHAVIORAL COMPONENTS. This scale, like the posture portion of the New York State Physical Fitness Test, includes a series of criterion-referenced postures in children. The scale rates the postures on degree of asymmetry and joint alignment (Hardy et al., 1988).

THE ADAMS FORWARD BENDING TEST. This test is a commonly used screening test for scoliosis. The back is viewed as the individual bends the trunk forward to 90°. The classic sign of scoliosis is the presence of a posterior rib hump during this motion (Bleck, 1991). Although children with scoliosis often develop lack of spinal mobility if the scoliosis becomes

TABLE 5–9. Selected Range-of-Motion Measurements during Childhood

Range-of-Motion Measure	2–5 Years		6–12 Years		13–19 Years	
	M	F	M	F	M	F
Straight leg raise	70	75	65	75	60	70
Popliteal angle (unilateral)*	15	10	30	25	40	25
Abduction†	60	60	50	55	45	50
Internal rotation‡	45	50	50	55	45	45
Femoral antetorsion§	10	15	7	7	0	0

*Supine position.
†Measured with hip extension.
‡Prone position.
§Prone position by lateral placement of the greater trochanter.
Note: All measurements in degrees.

severe, the Adams Forward Bending Test is not a test of trunk flexibility per se. Posture is often assessed in children with scoliosis for the presence of lordosis to assess hip flexibility; the presence of pelvic obliquity to assess flexibility of the adductors, abductors, and tensor fasciae latae; and the presence of a posterior pelvic tilt to assess hamstring flexibility. For more information on scoliosis, see Chapter 10.

GROSS MOTOR PERFORMANCE MEASURE. This instrument, designed as a quality-of-movement companion instrument to the Gross Motor Function Measure, includes postural alignment as one of its performance attributes. A five-point scale of quality is used for assessment of the attribute. This instrument was developed specifically as an examination tool for children with cerebral palsy (Boyce et al., 1991, 1995; Gowland et al., 1995).

Measurement in the Field

The field test for measurement of flexibility in tests of physical fitness is the sit and reach test, a measure of hamstring muscle and lower back flexibility. All physical fitness batteries used in the United States include a sit and reach test. The test-retest reliability of the sit and reach test has been found to be high; coefficients between .94 and .99 have been reported (Flint & Gudgell, 1966; Jackson & Baker, 1986; Macrae & Wright, 1969). Jackson and Baker (1986) assessed the criterion-related validity of the sit and reach test both for hamstring flexibility and for lower, upper, and total back flexibility. A moderate correlation was found with hamstring flexibility (.64) and a low correlation with lower back flexibility (.28). Upper back flexibility and total back flexibility were not correlated with the sit and reach scores.

Branta and colleagues (1984) found sex differences in the performance on the sit and reach test in children between 5 and 14 years of age, with girls showing better flexibility than boys at all ages. Girls showed little variability in flexibility from the ages of 5 to 11 years. Boys experienced a net loss of flexibility between the ages of 5 and 15. This is consistent with the goniometric measures of hamstring flexibility noted in my laboratory (Stout, JL, Phelps, JA, & Koop, SE, unpublished data, 1991).

Standards by Age

The criterion standard of performance on the FITNESSGRAM Program for the sit and reach test is 10 inches from the ages of 5 to 16 years. No variability with age or sex is allowed by the criterion. The FITNESSGRAM Program criterion is well below the average score obtained on the NCYFS I and II (Ross et al., 1985, 1987).

Physical Activities

Activities that require a high degree of flexibility include figure skating, gymnastics, jumping (track and field), and judo. Stretching is an important part of any exercise program for general warm-up before vigorous activity and to reduce the potential for injury. Possible physiologic mechanisms for the benefits of stretching include increased blood flow to muscles, increased mechanical efficiency of muscle and tendon, and reduction of viscosity within the muscle (Bar-Or, 1983c). Decreased resistance to extension of connective tissue leads to increased efficiency and power output by muscles. Much of this research has studied the adult population, but the same principles are believed to apply to children (Bar-Or, 1983c; Kuland & Tottossy, 1985; Yamashita et al., 1992).

Assessment of Flexibility in Children with Disabilities

For clinicians involved in the rehabilitation (or "habilitation") of children with musculoskeletal disorders, maintenance of flexibility or joint ROM is often a primary concern. Almost any musculoskeletal or neuromuscular disorder for which physical therapy is recommended includes treatment for loss of flexibility. Conditions such as cerebral palsy, juvenile rheumatoid arthritis, MD, or long bone fracture are common examples.

In Chapter 4, Gajdosik and Gajdosik addressed both the measurement and the effects of intervention on improving joint ROM in children. The interrater reliability of joint ROM measurements in children with spasticity has been found to be within the range of .50 to .85 (Ashton et al., 1978; Harris et al., 1985). Similar results have been found in adults (Boone et al., 1978; Ekstrand et al., 1982). Because maintenance of flexibility is an important component of most physical therapy programs for children with disabilities, methods for more reliable assessment of joint ROM are needed.

Field test standards for the sit and reach test and suggested modifications for test administration have been published for children with visual impairments, mental retardation, and Down syndrome (Seaman et al., 1995; Winnick & Short, 1985).

Body Composition

The term "body composition" is understood to mean total body content of water, protein, fat, and minerals (Dell, 1989). In reference to health-related fitness, body composition is used as a measure of body fatness or obesity. Attainment of appropriate body weight for overweight individuals was an explicit objective of *Healthy Children 2000* that has actually moved away from its target (United States Department of Health and Human Services, 1990, 1995). Because of the clustering effects of obesity with other risk factors for coronary artery disease, the relevance of obesity to a child's present and future health cannot be overemphasized. It has been suggested that regional distribution of abdominal fat is an important predictor of mortality, stroke, heart disease, and diabetes (Bray & Bouchard, 1988). Obesity rates for juveniles range between 10 and 25% in North America and appear to be increasing (Bar-Or, 1987; Ross & Gilbert, 1985; Ross & Pate, 1987).

Laboratory Measurement

The purposes of body composition measurement, whether in the laboratory or in the field, is to obtain a measure of fat-free or lean body mass. Chemical analysis is the only direct method to measure body composition (Klish, 1989). Because this is expensive and impractical, even laboratory standards of measurement are from indirect assessment. Most standards rely on formulas and models of composition that assume fat and lean body mass are constant. Because infants and children exhibit variable, not constant, body composition throughout childhood (Boileau et al., 1988; Haschke, 1989; Lohman, 1986; Spady, 1989), numerous problems in determining body composition in children are encountered. Use of adult standards leads to overestimation or underestimation of body fatness, depending on the technique (Boileau et al., 1988). All methods presented have some limitations for use with children, but all have been used. There is no one "gold standard" for children.

DENSITOMETRY

More commonly referred to as underwater or hydrostatic weighing, densitometry determines the density of an individual by dividing actual body weight by the decrease in weight when the person is completely submerged in water. The densities of fat and lean body mass are assumed to be constant and can be calculated for an individual when the density of the whole body is known. Although it is considered the gold standard for measurement of body composition in adults, it has limited applicability to young children.

TOTAL BODY WATER

The measurement of total body water is used as a means of estimating the nonfat portion of the body because neutral fat does not bind water. Stable isotopes of hydrogen or oxygen are administered orally and then measured to determine the amount of dilution in a body fluid.

BIOELECTRIC IMPEDANCE ANALYSIS

This method is based on the principle that impedance to electrical flow varies in proportion to the amount of lean tissue present. A weak electric current is passed through the body, and its impedance is measured.

Developmental Aspects of Body Composition

From birth through adolescence, body composition is constantly changing. Part of this change is caused by chemical maturation as a result of increasing mineral mass and hydration of adipose tissue (Spady, 1989). Chemical maturation occurs after adolescence, when the constants relating one component of body composition to another stabilize, until the last decades of life (Boileau et al., 1984, 1988; Lohman, 1986; Slaughter et al., 1984).

The four major components of body composition are water, protein, fat, and mineral. Reference models describe the body composition of these components in the child at various ages (Fomon, 1967; Fomon et al., 1982; Haschke, 1989; Haschke et al., 1981; Ziegler et al., 1976). A composite of these reference models and changes with growth in males appears in Figure 5–3.

Fat is the most variable component of body composition during infancy and childhood. Increases begin in utero when fat content changes from 2.5% at 1 kg of body weight to 12% at term gestation (Spady,

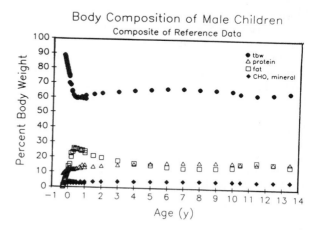

FIGURE 5–3. The normal body composition of male children as it changes with age. Data derived from data found in the descriptions of the reference fetus, infant, male child at 9 years, children from birth to 10 years, and the adolescent male. CHO = carbohydrate; tbw = total body water. (From Spady, DW. Normal body composition of infants and children. 98th Ross Laboratories Conference on Pediatric Research, 98:67–73, 1989. Used with permission of Ross Products Division, Abbott Laboratories, Columbus, OH 43216. © 1989 Ross Products Division, Abbott Laboratories.)

1989). The proportion of body fat rises from 12% to an average of 25% from birth to 6 months of age. Fat content decreases during early childhood as muscle mass increases. Sex differences are noted early in childhood; girls exhibit a greater percentage of fat content than do boys. At 6 to 8 years of age, the average fat content for boys is 13 to 15% and for girls, 16 to 18% (Lohman, 1987). During adolescence, fat content increases in girls so that between the ages of 14 and 16 years the mean percentage of fat content is 21 to 23%.

Water content of the body is approximately 89% of body weight at 24 weeks of gestation and drops to 75% at 40 weeks (Spady, 1989). By 4 months of age, water content stabilizes at approximately 60 to 65% and remains at that level until puberty. Protein content as a proportion of body weight increases from approximately 13% at birth to 15 to 17% at age 10 years. Mineral content of the body rises from 3% at birth to 5% at age 18 years.

Differences between the sexes exist in each major component of body composition throughout childhood and are magnified at adolescence. The major changes during adolescence in both sexes are a decrease in the percentage of water and an increase in the percentage of osseous minerals (Haschke, 1989; Lohman et al., 1984).

Measurement in the Field

Examination of body composition in the field is by measurement of skinfold thickness. The validity of this measure is suspect, just as the validity of laboratory methods is in question. The major problem is that skinfold measurement is based on the assumption that body surface measures and body density relationships are stable throughout childhood (Lohman, 1982). Two other threats to the validity of this measurement are (1) that use of skinfold thickness implies that the subcutaneous fat layer reflects the total amount of fat in the body and (2) that selected measurement sites reflect average thickness. These assumptions may not be true (Klish, 1989); however, Lohman and colleagues (1984) and Slaughter and colleagues (1984) did not find large deviations in skinfold distribution.

Despite this controversy, measurement of body composition is an important part of almost all health-related fitness tests. Concurrent validity has been demonstrated consistently with moderately high correlations of .70 to .85 between measurements of skinfolds and densitometry or potassium spectrometry (Going, 1988).

The typical sites for measurement of skinfold thickness are over the triceps brachii, subscapular area, and calf. Usually these areas are measured in some combination. Lohman (1987) has designed a series of charts for easy evaluation of skinfold thickness and percent body fatness based on either triceps and subscapular or triceps and calf skinfold measures. The method of estimation of percent body fatness from skinfold measurements involves estimating density from skinfold measurements and then converting density to percent body fatness. The reader is referred to other sources for more detailed information (Lohman, 1982, 1986; Slaughter et al., 1984). A 3 to 5% error is reported for adults when estimating body fatness from skinfold measurements (Lohman, 1982).

Standards by Age

The criterion values for ranges of body fatness conducive to optimal health in children are 10 to 25% for boys and 15 to 25% for girls (Lohman, 1987). Values higher than 25% in boys and 30% in girls are considered to place the child at risk for associated morbidity. This standard is consistent with the cutoffs at body composition of 32% for females and 25% for males set by the FITNESSGRAM Program (Blair et al., 1989). Results from the NCYFS I and II studies suggest that children within the 40th to 50th percentiles on the test items fall within the optimal ranges described earlier (Ross et al., 1985, 1987).

Response to Training

Conditioning and training programs may or may not affect body composition. If changes are to occur, the type of exercise must entail high-energy expenditure of high or intense effort. Appropriate activities include swimming, running, and weight training. Evidence of program effects on body composition is inconclusive in adults. Little information is available on children, but what is available indicates that percentage of body fatness can be reduced during training for specific sports but rises again when programs are discontinued (Parizkova, 1977; VonDobelin et al., 1972). General physical activity is associated with reduced body fatness as compared with physically inactive peers (Parizkova, 1974). Evidence is inconclusive as to whether obese children are less physically active than nonobese children.

Assessment of Body Composition in Children with Disabilities

PREMATURE INFANTS

Clinicians treat many children with disabilities who were born prematurely. Premature birth has been shown to affect body composition (Spady et al., 1987). Compared with a "reference" fetus of similar weight, the premature infant has a higher total fat content and lower total body water content. These differences in composition are probably the result of living outside the womb and being faced with the necessity of increasing body fat for temperature regulation. The implications of this altered body composition during growth have not been studied, nor has body composition been studied in premature infants who experience neonatal complications. They may or may not have effects on composition throughout childhood and into adulthood.

CEREBRAL PALSY

Few studies have been conducted on body composition of individuals with cerebral palsy (Bandini et al., 1991; Berg & Isaksson, 1970; van den Berg–Emons et al., 1998). All reported that adolescents with cerebral palsy are shorter and typically weigh less than their age-matched peers. Resting metabolic rate was found to be lower than the norm in all studies. However, contradictory findings were noted among the studies, which may or may not be related to differences in methodology. Results of the two older studies suggested that total body water as a percentage of body weight was higher in individuals with cerebral palsy than in controls (Bandini et al., 1991; Berg & Isaksson, 1970). Findings in the later studies indicated the opposite, suggesting an increased percentage of body fat (van den Berg–Emons et al., 1998). Van den Berg–Emons and colleagues postulated that children with cerebral palsy may have proportionately more subcutaneous fat in the lower extremity skinfold sites because of disuse. Thus using skinfold measurements as an estimation of body fat may not be appropriate in this population. The samples were relatively small and included children with a variety of types of cerebral palsy and of functional levels. Both type of cerebral palsy and functional level are likely to be important variables affecting body composition, but the conflicting results of the two studies cannot be resolved without further research.

MYELODYSPLASIA

The study by Bandini and colleagues (1991) also included individuals with myelodysplasia. This group, on average, showed decreased stature, reduced fat-free mass, and increased percentage of body fat as compared with able-bodied peers. The percentage of body fat was above the 95th percentile for all subjects with myelodysplasia. A significant correlation was not found between skinfold thickness and body composition, which suggests that fat distribution may be altered because of the type of paralysis. A previous study had also suggested that skinfold measurements and fat distribution may

be altered in myelodysplasia (Hayes-Allen & Tring, 1973). Both studies indicate that children with myelodysplasia are at risk for obesity.

CONDITIONING AND TRAINING

Whether the components of physical fitness can be affected by training programs is an important question, especially to clinicians who are designing programs for children with disabilities. Bar-Or (in 1983c) differentiated between the terms *conditioning* and *training*, which are often used interchangeably. *Physical conditioning* is defined as the process by which exercise, repeated over a specified duration, induces morphologic and functional changes in body systems and tissues. The tissues and systems can include skeletal muscles, the myocardium, adipose tissue, bones, tendons, ligaments, the central nervous system, and the endocrine system. Bar-Or (1983c) considered conditioning to consist of general exercise for overall physical fitness. *Training*, by contrast, is specific exercise designed to promote changes in performance of a particular type of activity. In the context of this chapter, training will be discussed in relation to specific fitness components, but overall conditioning will be discussed in reference to children with disabilities.

Fitness Components and Training in Children

Many of the physiologic changes that result from training and conditioning in adults also take place during the process of growth and maturation in childhood. These naturally occurring changes make it difficult to study the specific effects of conditioning and training. The primary components of physical fitness of interest to trainers are cardiorespiratory endurance and physical strength.

Cardiorespiratory Endurance

Some controversy exists over whether maximal aerobic power or Vo_2max can be increased by cardiorespiratory training in children (Bar-Or, 1983c; Krahenbuhl et al., 1985). Besides the improvements seen to occur naturally during growth and maturation, other problems in assessing the effects of training include seasonal differences in activity, difficulty in ensuring that a true Vo_2max has been reached during the testing process, and the already high level of physical activity in young children.

Krahenbuhl and colleagues (1985), in a review of training programs, concluded that maximal aerobic power can be significantly increased after regular intensive training in children of 8 to 14 years of age.

Endurance exercise appeared more effective than intermittent exercise. General physical education programs alone were not effective in improving Vo$_2$max. Effective activities included running, cycle ergometry, and swimming. Increases of 8 to 10% were measured in effective programs. Some studies reported little or no change in Vo$_2$max despite improved long-distance running performance after training programs lasting 1 to 9 weeks (Bar-Or, 1983c; Cumming et al., 1967).

Less controversy exists over whether training is effective in improving cardiorespiratory endurance in adolescence. The effects of training in adolescents appear to be similar to those in adults. The functional and morphologic changes of the cardiovascular and pulmonary systems that take place as a result of training are listed in Table 5-10. Training effects usually include increases in myocardial mass, stroke volume, ventilation, and respiratory muscular endurance.

Muscular Strength and Endurance

Muscular strength is a component of fitness that can be affected by training, especially in children at or after puberty. Resistance strength training refers to training for improved muscular strength by repeatedly overcoming heavy resistance. The practice of resistance strength training is problematic in preadolescent children because controversy exists regarding (1) whether children can make gains in strength and muscle mass, (2) whether gains improve athletic performance, and particularly (3) whether children are more susceptible to injury when participating in such training. Despite the controversy, resistance strength training has been shown to increase voluntary force production at all ages and may reduce the risk of injury during athletic participation (Blimkie & Sale, 1998; Sale, 1989).

In a review of strength training studies, Sale (1989) concluded that children can increase voluntary strength as a result of training, and, furthermore, children show a greater increase in strength than do adults when training-induced strength improvements are expressed as a percentage of change. During maximal voluntary contraction, children can develop the same force per unit of muscle cross-sectional area as adults despite differences in absolute strength and muscle size.

As previously described, the strength increases associated with growth are closely related to increases in muscle mass, including an increase in the number of both sarcomeres and fibrils per muscle fiber (Malina, 1986). The enhancement of muscular strength caused by growth is estimated to be approximately 1.5 kg per year from the age of 6 to 14 years (Mersch & Stoboy, 1989). In conjunction with

TABLE 5-10. Cardiorespiratory Function Variables and Response to Training in Children

Function Variable	Change with Training
Heart volume	Increase
Blood volume	Increase
Total hemoglobin	Slight increase
Stroke volume (max, submax)	Increase
Cardiac output (max, submax)	Increase, no change, or decrease
Arteriovenous difference (submax)	No change
Blood flow to active muscle	No change
Ventilation/kg body wt (max)	Increase
Ventilation/kg body wt (submax)	Decrease
Respiratory rate (submax)	Decrease
Tidal volume (max)	Increase
Respiratory muscle endurance	Increase

Adapted from Bar-Or, O. Physiologic responses to exercise in healthy children. In Bar-Or, O., Pediatric Sports Medicine for the Practitioner. New York: Springer-Verlag, 1983, p. 49.

max = maximal exercise; submax = submaximal exercise.

"muscular" adaptations, neural adaptations associated with improved coordination and motor learning may also play a role. For example, the increases in voluntary strength noted with training in prepubescent children have been found to be independent of increased muscle mass or hypertrophy such as that seen in postpubescent children or adults (Blimkie et al., 1989; Sale, 1989; Weltman et al., 1986). Improved motor unit activation and neural adaptations (including more appropriate co-contraction of synergist muscles and inhibition of antagonist muscles, as well as improvements in motor unit recruitment order and firing frequency within the prime movers) are believed to play a role in producing training effects in both adults and children (Komi, 1986; Moritani & DeVries, 1979). It has been suggested that, during the early stages of training, neural adaptation predominates in producing altered performance. Muscular adaptation contributes in the later stages of training (Blimkie & Sale, 1998; Sale, 1989) (Fig. 5-4).

Principles of Training

The principles of an effective training program include specificity, as well as guidelines for intensity, frequency, and duration of exercise. Rules for children are essentially the same as those for adults.

Specificity

The changes that take place in the body as a result of training are specific to the type of exercise performed and to the tissue involved. Myocardial tissue,

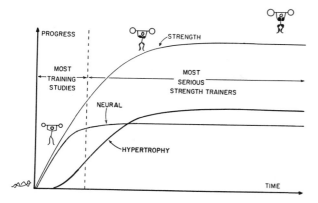

FIGURE 5–4. Relative roles of neural and muscular adaptation in strength training. Neural adaptation plays the biggest role in the early phase of training, which can last up to several weeks. Muscular adaptation predominates later and is limited by the extent that muscles can hypertrophy. (From Sale, DG. Strength training in children. In Gisolfi, CV, & Lamb, DR [Eds.], Perspectives in Exercise Science and Sports Medicine, Vol. 2: Youth, Exercise, and Sport. Indianapolis, IN: Benchmark Press, 1989, p. 180.)

for example, is affected by long-distance running but not by resistance strength training. The type of contraction (concentric, eccentric, or isometric), the number of repetitions performed, the velocity of muscle contraction, and the particular muscles exercised all influence the results of a strength training program. Different sports develop different components of fitness.

Intensity

Activity at a certain intensity is required to achieve conditioning or training effects. Intensity should be determined as a percentage of the individual's maximum because the same amount of activity can represent two entirely different levels of intensity for two different individuals. For example, a child with cerebral palsy who walks at the same velocity as an able-bodied child may consume twice as much oxygen, so walking as a form of exercise for the child with cerebral palsy is more intense. Although Vo_2 depends on the square of velocity, an average 6- to 12-year-old walking at an average velocity consumes about 25% of Vo_2max; for a child with cerebral palsy, Vo_2 can be as high as 75 to 90% of Vo_2max (personal observation, 1998).

Intensity threshold refers to the intensity of exercise below which few or no training or conditioning effects are observed (Bar-Or, 1983c). The intensity threshold of maximal aerobic power in adults required to produce a training effect is 60 to 70% of Vo_2max. The threshold for strength is approximately 60 to 65% of maximal voluntary contraction. The principle of overload in strength training is in part related to the intensity threshold of exercise. Overload refers to a task that requires considerable voluntary effort to complete. No specific data are available for intensity thresholds for children, but they are thought to be at least equal to those of adults. Whether intensity thresholds for children with various disabilities are the same as those for able-bodied children is also unknown.

Frequency

The optimal frequency of training depends on the type of program, and frequency is interrelated with intensity and duration. Two or three times per week is a general rule of thumb (Bar-Or, 1983c).

Duration

Any program, whether a therapeutic program or a fitness program, requires a minimum implementation time before benefits are seen. Most effective conditioning programs last at least 6 to 8 weeks. The optimal duration of an exercise session depends on the type of program. In general, the session should consist of a warm-up phase of 10 minutes, an exercise phase above the exercise threshold for 15 to 30 minutes, and a 5- to 7-minute cool-down period. The warm-up phase has been shown to be important for increasing performance of both aerobic and anaerobic tasks in children (Bar-Or, 1983c). The warm-up period should include (1) activities to raise core body temperature, (2) stretching exercises, and (3) activities specific to the exercise task. The American Academy of Pediatrics (1983) recommends that strength-training regimens for children include activities to provide strength training for all parts of the body to ensure balanced development.

The duration of the exercise phase in strength training is sometimes associated with the goal of achieving maximal overload. This is usually done in one of two ways—either by repeating brief maximal contractions or by repeating submaximal contractions to the point of fatigue.

Progression

A conditioning or training program must be progressive in its demands for continued improvement. The intensity threshold, the duration of exercise sessions, the number of repetitions performed during a session, or the frequency of exercise sessions may need to be increased. All contribute individually and collectively to the progression of the exercise program.

Conditioning in Children with Disabilities

Cerebral Palsy

As children with cerebral palsy approach and move through adolescence, an important aspect of function is the ability to maintain ambulation. Vo_2 during ambulation in preadolescent children with cerebral palsy (ages 6 to 12 years) is more than twice that of able-bodied children walking at the same velocity (Koop et al., 1989). If body weight and adiposity increase in adolescence without an increase in muscular strength, maximal aerobic capacity decreases, and the task of walking becomes more and more difficult. Growth in mass is a cubic function (volume), and growth in strength is a function of the square (cross-sectional muscle area). As previously mentioned, muscles increase in mass first, then in strength (Malina, 1986). During the adolescent growth spurt, mass increases at a faster rate than does strength. For able-bodied children, this process occurs without noticeable deficit or loss of function, but for children with cerebral palsy, loss of function sometimes occurs because the rate of increase in strength is inadequate to support the rate of increase in muscle mass. A major goal of physical therapy for adolescents with cerebral palsy is maintenance of the ability to ambulate throughout the growth spurt. If a child has maximal strength and aerobic capacity on entering the growth spurt, function is also likely to be at maximal capacity. Conditioning in a child with cerebral palsy could play a vital role in the process of maximizing the potential not only of the adolescent but of the preadolescent as well.

The ultimate goal of conditioning programs for children with cerebral palsy is to retard or reverse the deterioration of capacity expected during adolescence. In a longitudinal study of adolescents with cerebral palsy, Lundberg (1973) found that heart rate at a given power load increased an average of 10 beats per minute per year, implying decreasing efficiency. Studies have demonstrated that conditioning effects in the population of children and adolescents with cerebral palsy are similar to those of children without disability (Bar-Or et al., 1976; Berg, 1970b; Lundberg & Pernow, 1970; Lundberg et al., 1967). Increased strength, ROM, and functional endurance have also been reported as a result of a strengthening program (Horvat, 1987). Greater attention is now given to the benefits of strengthening in both children and adolescents with cerebral palsy. Damiano and colleagues report strength gains after a resistive exercise training program. Functional improvements in both gait and Gross Motor Function Measure scores are noted, as well as decreases in spasticity (Damiano & Abel, 1998; Damiano et al., 1995a, 1995b).

One study that addressed the issue of changes in body composition as a result of conditioning showed no change in the percentage of body fat after a 4-month program (Berg, 1970a). A conditioning response unique to individuals with cerebral palsy is an increase in blood flow to exercising muscles (Lundberg & Pernow, 1970). This may reflect a physiologic mechanism in which conditioning and strengthening decrease the effects of spasticity.

Evidence suggests that neither regular physical education classes nor habitual activities are sufficient to induce conditioning changes in children with cerebral palsy (Berg, 1970b; Dresen, 1985). The program must increase intensity beyond habitual exercise levels. The duration of the overall program should be longer than 6 weeks; results of 6-week training programs are equivocal (Ekblom & Lundberg, 1968). Target heart rate was typically maintained for 15 to 30 minutes in most studies. Activities in accordance with the child's ability were used; examples are cycle ergometry, swimming, running, and jogging.

Cystic Fibrosis

Cystic fibrosis is a hereditary disease affecting the exocrine glands. The lungs, gastrointestinal tract, and sweat glands produce excessive secretion. Airway obstruction, infection, and respiratory failure result from excess viscous mucus in the respiratory tract. Results of studies emphasizing aerobic conditioning for 3 to 5 months suggest that Vo_2max, endurance of respiratory muscles, and pulmonary function all show improvement (Jankowski, 1986; Orenstein et al., 1981; Zach et al., 1982). Jogging, cycling, swimming, weight lifting, and calisthenics of various durations and combinations were used.

In addition to the positive effects of conditioning on physical fitness, clinical benefits in the management of the disease are also reported (Bar-Or, 1985). Increased coughing and mucous clearance may reduce the need for chest therapy to manage secretions (Zach et al., 1982).

The effects of exercise on children with cystic fibrosis and other clinical populations must be closely monitored to reduce or avoid potential detrimental effects. Particular concerns in the population with cystic fibrosis are dehydration (especially in high heat) and oxygen desaturation (Bar-Or, 1985).

Muscular Dystrophy

The effects of conditioning patients with MD have been evaluated in numerous studies, which produced equivocal results (Abrahamson & Rogoff, 1952; DeLateur & Giaconi, 1979; Fowler et al., 1965;

Vignos & Watkins, 1966). Evaluation of the results must take into account that many of the studies were inadequately controlled for threats to internal validity. Results suggest that modest gains in strength can be made or the rate of deterioration retarded. In one study, DeLateur and Giaconi found no significant change in strength of the quadriceps femoris muscle after 6 weeks of a 6-month conditioning program of submaximal exercise. A modest, but not significant, increase in strength was found after 6 months. Each subject served as his or her own control. No deleterious effects of a strengthening program were found. Despite the lack of statistically significant effects, the increase in strength may be enough to deter future deterioration.

CONCLUSION

This chapter was designed to provide information on physical fitness and conditioning in the able-bodied child for promoting health and preventing disease. The components of fitness, how they are tested, and how they contribute to health were reviewed. An understanding of physical fitness, physical activity, and conditioning is valuable for appreciating the impact of disabling conditions on these variables. Health-related physical fitness is important for reducing future health risks in every child, regardless of the presence or absence of disability. Preadolescent fitness may be especially important to the child with a disability because of the effects the particular disability may have on the child as he or she enters puberty and adulthood. The design of exercise programs (their intensity, frequency, and duration) should encompass the minimal requirements for physical fitness, as well as incorporate therapeutic goals. Exercise programs should be designed so that the energy requirements for accomplishing day-to-day activities through the growth period are met. Meeting this goal is likely to require additional exercise beyond current therapy or physical education. One of our goals as pediatric therapists should be to ensure, to whatever extent possible, that our clients end their childhood with a fitness level suitable to a healthy adulthood. Research is needed to document the extent to which this goal can be met for specific populations and levels of disability.

Much research remains to be done in the able-bodied population as well. Reliability and validity studies must continue on criterion-based measures now being used to determine minimal fitness levels. Research must establish reliable, valid, and universal criteria, both in the laboratory and in the field. Continued identification of the relationship between childhood physical activity and fitness and health in adulthood is vital to our overall understanding of health-related fitness.

Research to benefit populations with disabilities or children with special needs has barely begun. With the inadequate base of research in children without disability, developing standards of fitness for specific disabled populations begins at a disadvantage. A question that remains to be answered is whether the fitness performance criteria for children without disabilities are valid for children with disabilities or special needs. Experience with development of testing and measurement tools for other purposes would suggest they are not. Are children with disabilities such as cerebral palsy more fit because they expend in walking an amount of energy equivalent to that of an able-bodied person walking up and down stairs all day long? Are the thresholds and target zones for fitness improvement the same for children with a variety of disabilities as for able-bodied children? How are conditioning and training programs best designed for children with disabilities? Do conditioning programs initiated before the onset of puberty help maintain fitness during and after puberty? What are the physiologic and behavioral factors that limit a child's capacity to improve fitness variables or to exercise? How much exercise is detrimental? How do presurgical strengthening programs affect the recovery of strength after surgery? Questions such as these are only the beginning of our quest for understanding. The journey has just begun.

References

Abrahamson, AS, & Rogoff, J. Physical treatment in muscular dystrophy (Abstract). In Proceedings of the 2nd Medical Conference. Muscular Dystrophy Association, 1952, pp. 123–124.

Adams, FH. Factors affecting the working capacity of children and adolescents. In Rarick, GL (Ed.), Physical Activity: Human Growth and Development. New York: Academic Press, 1973, pp. 89–90.

Alexander, J, & Molnar, GE. Muscular strength in children: Preliminary report on objective standards. Archives of Physical Medicine and Rehabilitation, 54:424–427, 1973.

American Academy of Pediatrics. Weight training and weightlifting: Information for the pediatrician. Physician and Sports Medicine, 11(3):157–161, 1983.

American Alliance for Health, Physical Education, Recreation, and Dance. The AAHPERD Physical Best Program. Reston, VA: American Alliance for Health Physical Education, Recreation, and Dance, 1988.

American Physical Therapy Association. Guide to physical therapist practice. Physical Therapy, 77:1163–1650, 1997.

American Psychological Association. Standards for Educational and Psychological Testing. Washington, DC: American Psychological Association, 1985.

Ashton BB, Pickles, B, & Roll, JW. Reliability of goniometric measurements of hip motion in spastic cerebral palsy. Developmental Medicine and Child Neurology, 20:87–94, 1978.

Astrand PO. Experimental Studies of Physical Working Capacity in Relation to Sex and Age. Copenhagen: Ejnar Munksgaard, 1952.

Astrand, PO, & Rodahl, K (Eds.). Textbook of Work Physiology: Physiological Bases of Exercise. New York: McGraw-Hill, 1986.

Baltzopoulos, V, & Kellis, E: Isokinetic strength during childhood and adolescence. In Van Praagh, E (Ed.), Pediatric Anaerobic Performance. Champaign, IL: Human Kinetics, 1998, pp. 225–240.

Bandini, LG, Schoeller, DA, Fukagawa, NK, Wykes, LJ, & Dietz, WH. Body composition and energy expenditure in adolescents with cerebral palsy or myelodysplasia. Pediatric Research, 29:70–77, 1991.

Bar-Or, O. Appendix II: Procedures for exercise testing in children. In Bar-Or, O, Pediatric Sports Medicine for the Practitioner. New York: Springer-Verlag, 1983a, pp. 315–341.

Bar-Or, O. Neuromuscular diseases. In Bar-Or, O, Pediatric Sports Medicine for the Practitioner. New York: Springer-Verlag, 1983b, pp. 227–249.

Bar-Or, O. Physiologic responses to exercise in healthy children. In Bar-Or, O, Pediatric Sports Medicine for the Practitioner. New York: Springer-Verlag, 1983c, pp. 1–65.

Bar-Or, O. Physical conditioning in children with cardiorespiratory disease. Exercise and Sport Sciences Reviews, 13:305–334, 1985.

Bar-Or, O. Pathophysiological factors which limit the exercise capacity of the sick child. Medicine and Science in Sports and Exercise, 18:276–282, 1986.

Bar-Or, O. A commentary to children and fitness: A public health perspective. Research Quarterly for Exercise and Sport, 58:304–307, 1987.

Bar-Or, O, Inbar, O, & Spira, R. Physiological effects of a sports rehabilitation program on cerebral palsied and poliomyelitic adolescents. Medicine and Science in Sports, 8:157–161, 1976.

Berg, K. Effect of physical activation and improved nutrition on the body composition of school children with cerebral palsy. Acta Paediatrica Supplement, 204:53–69, 1970a.

Berg, K. Effect of physical training of school children with cerebral palsy. Acta Paediatrica Supplement, 204:27–33, 1970b.

Berg, K, & Isaksson, B. Body composition and nutrition of school children with cerebral palsy. Acta Paediatrica Supplement, 204:41–52, 1970.

Berger, RA, & Medlin, RL. Evaluation of Berger's 1-RM chin test for junior high school mates. Research Quarterly, 40:460–463, 1969.

Blair, SN, Clark, DG, Cureton, KJ, & Powell, KE. Exercise and fitness in childhood: Implications for a lifetime of health. In Gisolfi, CV, & Lamb, DR (Eds.), Perspectives in Exercise Science and Sports Medicine, Vol. 2: Youth, Exercise, and Sport. Indianapolis, IN: Benchmark Press, 1989, pp. 401–430.

Bleck, E. Adolescent idiopathic scoliosis. Developmental Medicine and Child Neurology, 33:167–173, 1991.

Blimkie, CJR. Age and sex associated variation in strength during childhood: Anthropometric, morphologic, neurologic, biomechanical, endocrinologic, genetic, and physical activity correlates. In Gisolfi, CV, & Lamb, DR (Eds.), Perspectives in Exercise Science and Sports Medicine, Vol. 2: Youth, Exercise, and Sport. Indianapolis, IN: Benchmark Press, 1989, pp. 99–163.

Blimkie, CJR, Ramsay, J, Sale, D, MacDougall, D, Smith, K, & Garner, K. Effects of 10 weeks of resistance training on strength development in prepubertal boys. In Osteid, S, & Carlsen, KH (Eds.), Children and Exercise XIII. Champaign, IL: Human Kinetics, 1989, pp. 183–197.

Blimkie, CJR, & Sale, DG: Strength development and trainability during childhood. In Van Praagh, E (Ed.), Pediatric Anaerobic Performance. Champaign, IL: Human Kinetics, 1998, pp. 193–224.

Boileau, RA, Lohman, TG, & Slaughter, MH. Exercise and body composition in children and youth. Scandinavian Journal of Sport Sciences, 7:7–17, 1985.

Boileau, RA, Lohman, TG, Slaughter, MH, Ball, TE, Going, SB, & Hendrix, MK. Hydration of the fat-free body in children during maturation. Human Biology, 56:651–666, 1984.

Boileau, RA, Lohman, TG, Slaughter, MH, Horswill, CA, & Stillman, RJ. Problems associated with determining body composition in maturing youngsters. In Brown, EW, & Branta, CF (Eds.), Competitive Sports for Children and Youth: An Overview of Research and Issues. Champaign, IL: Human Kinetics, 1988, pp. 3–16.

Boone, DC, Azen, SP, Lin, CM, Spense, C, Baron, C, & Lee, L. Reliability of goniometric measurements. Physical Therapy, 58:1355–1360, 1978.

Boyce, WF, Gowland, C, Hardy, S, Rosenbaum, PL, Lane, M, Plews, N, Goldsmith C, & Russell, DJ. Development of a quality-of-movement measure for children with cerebral palsy. Physical Therapy, 71:820–828, 1991.

Boyce, WF, Gowland, C, Rosenbaum, PL, Lane, M, Plews, N, Goldsmith, CH, Russell, DJ, Wright, V, Potter, S, & Harding, D. The Gross Motor Performance Measure: Validity and responsiveness of a measure of quality of movement. Physical Therapy, 75:603–613, 1995.

Braden, DS, & Strong, WB. Cardiovascular responses to exercise in childhood. American Journal of Diseases of Children, 144:1255–1260, 1990.

Branta, C, Haubenstricker, J, & Seefeldt, V. Age changes in motor skills during childhood and adolescence. Exercise and Sport Sciences Reviews, 12:467–520, 1984.

Bray, GA, & Bouchard, C. Role of fat distribution during growth and its relationship to health. American Journal of Clinical Nutrition, 47:551–552, 1988.

Brodie, DA, Burnie, J, Eston, RG, & Royce, JA. Isokinetic strength and flexibility characteristics in preadolescent boys. In Rutenfranz, J, Mocellin, R, & Klimt, F (Eds.), Children and Exercise XII. Champaign, IL: Human Kinetics, 1986, pp. 309–319.

Carron, AV, & Bailey, DA. Strength development in boys from 10–16 years. Monographs of the Society for Research in Child Development, 39:1–37, 1974.

Chrysler Fund–Amateur Athletic Union. Physical Fitness Program. Bloomington, IN: Chrysler Fund–Amateur Athletic Union, 1987.

Clarke, HH. Posture. Physical Fitness Research Digest, 9:1–23, 1979.

Clarke, HH, & Clarke, DH. Application of Measurement in Physical Education. Englewood Cliffs, NJ: Prentice-Hall, 1987, pp. 93–99.

Considine, WJ. An Analysis of Selected Upper Body Tasks as Measures of Strength (Abstract). American Association of Health, Physical Education and Recreation, 25:74, 1973.

Cooper, DM, Weiler-Ravell, D, Whipp, BJ, & Wasserman, K. Growth-related changes in oxygen uptake and heart rate during progressive exercise in children. Pediatric Research, 18:845–851, 1984.

Corbin CB. Youth fitness, exercise and health: There is much to be done. Research Quarterly for Exercise and Sport, 58:308–314, 1987.

Cumming, GR, Goodwin, A, Baggley, G, & Antel, J. Repeated measurements of aerobic capacity during a week of intensive training at a youth track camp. Canadian Journal of Physiology and Pharmacology, 45:805–811, 1967.

Cunningham, DA, MacFarlane-VanWaterschoot, B, Paterson, DH, Lefcoe, M, & Sangal, SP. Reliability and reproducibility of maximal oxygen uptake in children. Medicine and Science in Sports, 9:104–108, 1977.

Cureton, KJ, & Warren, GL. Criterion-referenced standards for youth health-related fitness tests: A tutorial. Research Quarterly for Exercise and Sport, 61:7–19, 1990.

Daltroy, LH, Liang, MH, & Fossel, AH. The POSNA pediatric musculoskeletal functional health questionnaire: Report on reliability, validity, and sensitivity to change. Journal of Pediatric Orthopaedics, 18:561–571, 1998.

Damiano, DL, & Abel, MF. Functional outcomes of strength training in spastic cerebral palsy. Archives of Physical Medicine and Rehabilitation, 79:119–125, 1998.

Damiano, DL, Kelly, LE, & Vaughan, CL. Effects of quadriceps muscle strengthening on crouch gait in children with spastic diplegia. Physical Therapy, 75:668–671, 1995a.

Damiano, DL, Vaughan, CL, & Abel, MF. Muscle response to heavy resistance exercise in children with spastic cerebral palsy. Developmental Medicine and Child Neurology, 37:731–739, 1995b.

DeLateur, BJ, & Giaconi, RM. Effect on maximal strength of submaximal exercise in Duchenne muscular dystrophy. American Journal of Physical Medicine, 58:26–36, 1979.

Dell, RB. Comparison of densitometric methods applicable to infants and small children for studying body composition. Ross Laboratories Conference on Pediatric Research, *98*:22–30, 1989.

Dresen, MHW. Physical and psychological effects of training on handicapped children. In Binkhorst, RA, Kemper, HCG, & Saris, WHM (Eds.), Children and Exercise XI. Champaign, IL: Human Kinetics, 1985, pp. 203–209.

Drews, J, Vraciu, JK, & Pellino, G. Range of motion of the joints of the lower extremities of newborns. Physical and Occupational Therapy in Pediatrics, *4*(2):49–62, 1984.

Ekblom, B, & Lundberg, A. Effect of training on adolescents with severe motor handicaps. Acta Paediatrica Scandinavica, *57*:17–23, 1968.

Ekstrand, J, Wiktorsson, M, Oberg, B, & Gillquist, J. Lower extremity goniometric measurements: A study to determine their reliability. Archives of Physical Medicine and Rehabilitation, *63*:171–175, 1982.

Eriksson, BO, Gollnick, PD, & Saltin, B. Muscle metabolism and enzyme activities after training in boys 11–13 years old. Acta Physiologica Scandinavica, *87*:485–487, 1973.

Eriksson, BO, Karlsson, J, & Saltin, B. Muscle metabolites during exercise in pubertal boys. Acta Paediatrica Scandinavica Supplement, *217*:154–157, 1971.

Faust, MS. Somatic development of adolescent girls. Society for Research in Child Development, *42*:1–90, 1977.

Flint, MM, & Gudgell, J. Electromyographic study of abdominal muscular activity during exercise. Research Quarterly, *36*:29–37, 1966.

Florini, JR. Hormonal control of muscle growth. Muscle and Nerve, *10*:577–598, 1987.

Fomon, SJ. Body composition of the male reference infant during the first year of life. Pediatrics, *40*:863–867, 1967.

Fomon, SJ, Haschke, F, Ziegler, EE, & Nelson, SE. Body composition of reference children from birth to age 10 years. American Journal of Clinical Nutrition, *35*:1169–1173, 1982.

Fowler, WM, & Gardner, GW. Quantitative strength measurements in muscular dystrophy. Archives of Physical Medicine and Rehabilitation, *48*:629–644, 1967.

Fowler, WM, Pearson, CM, Egstrom, GH, & Gardner, GW. Ineffective treatment of muscular dystrophy with an anabolic steroid and other measures. New England Journal of Medicine, *272*:875–882, 1965.

Francis, K, & Feinstein, R. A simple height-specific and rate-specific step test for children. Southern Medical Journal, *84*:169–174, 1991.

Gage, JR. Gait Analysis in Cerebral Palsy. London: Mac Keith Press, 1991.

Gaul, C. Muscular strength and endurance. In Docherty, D (Ed.), Measurement in Pediatric Exercise Science. Champaign, IL: Human Kinetics, 1996, pp. 225–228.

Giannini, MJ, & Protas, EJ. Aerobic capacity in juvenile rheumatoid arthritis patients and healthy children. Arthritis Care and Research, *4*:131–135, 1991.

Giannini, MJ, & Protas, EJ. Exercise response in children with and without juvenile rheumatoid arthritis: A comparison study. Physical Therapy, *72*:365–372, 1992.

Godfrey, S. Growth and development of the cardiopulmonary response to exercise. In Davis, JA, & Dobbing, J (Eds.), Scientific Foundations in Paediatrics. London: William Heinemann Medical Books, 1981, pp. 450–460.

Going, S. Physical best: Body composition in the assessment of youth fitness. Journal of Physical Education, Recreation and Dance, *59*(9):32–36, 1988.

Gowland, C, Boyce, WF, Wright, V, Russell, DJ, Goldsmith, CH, & Rosenbaum, PL. Reliability of the Gross Motor Performance Measure. Physical Therapy, *75*:597–602, 1995.

Green, HJ, & Patla, AE. Maximal aerobic power: Neuromuscular and metabolic considerations. Medicine and Science in Sports and Exercise, *24*:38–46, 1992.

Haley, SM, Tada, WL, & Carmichael, EM. Spinal mobility in young children: A normative study. Physical Therapy, *66*:1697–1703, 1986.

Harris, SR, Smith, LH, & Krukowski, L. Goniometric reliability for a child with spastic quadriplegia. Journal of Pediatric Orthopedics, *5*:348–351, 1985.

Haschke, F. Body composition during adolescence. Ross Laboratories Conference on Pediatric Research, *98*:76–82, 1989.

Haschke, F, Fomon, SJ, & Ziegler, EE. Body composition of a nine year old reference boy. Pediatric Research, *15*:847–850, 1981.

Haskell, WL, Montoye, HJ, & Orenstein, D. Physical activity and exercise to achieve health-related fitness components. Public Health Reports, *100*:202–212, 1985.

Hayes-Allen, MC, & Tring, FC. Obesity: Another hazard for spina bifida children. British Journal of Preventive and Social Medicine, *27*:192–196, 1973.

Horvat, M. Effects of a progressive resistance training program on an individual with spastic cerebral palsy. American Corrective Therapy Journal, *41*:7–10, 1987.

Hosking, GP, Bhat, US, Dubowitz, V, & Edwards, HT. Measurement of muscle strength and performance in children with normal and diseased muscle. Archives of Disease in Childhood, *51*:957–963, 1976.

Institute for Aerobics Research. FITNESSGRAM Users Manual. Dallas, TX: Institute for Aerobics Research, 1987.

Jackson, AS, & Coleman, AE. Validation of distance run tests for elementary school children. Research Quarterly, *47*:86–94, 1976.

Jackson, AW, & Baker, AA. The relationship of the sit and reach test to criterion measures of hamstring and back flexibility in young females. Research Quarterly for Exercise and Sport, *57*:183–186, 1986.

Jankowski, JW. Exercise testing and exercise prescription for individuals with cystic fibrosis. In Skinner, JS (Ed.), Testing and Exercise Prescription for Special Cases. Philadelphia: Lea & Febiger, 1986.

Kendall, HO, & Kendall, FP. Posture and Pain. Baltimore: Williams & Wilkins, 1952, p. 104.

Kilmer, DD, Abresch, RT, & Fowler, WM. Serial manual muscle testing in Duchenne muscular dystrophy. Archives of Physical Medicine and Rehabilitation, *74*:1168–1171, 1993.

Klish, WJ. The "gold standard." Ross Laboratories Conference on Pediatric Research, *98*:4–7, 1989.

Koch, G. Muscle blood flow after ischemic work during bicycle ergometer work in boys aged 12. Acta Pediatrica Belgica Supplement, *28*:29–39, 1974.

Komi, PV. Training muscle strength and power: Interaction of neuromotoric, hypertrophic, and mechanical factors. International Journal of Sports Medicine, *7*(suppl):10–15, 1986.

Koop, SE, Stout, JL, Drinken, WH, & Starr, RC. Energy cost of walking in children with cerebral palsy (Abstract). Physical Therapy, *69*:386, 1989.

Krahenbuhl, GS, Pangrazi, RP, Peterson, GW, Burkett, LN, & Schneider, MJ. Field testing of cardiorespiratory fitness in primary school children. Medicine and Science in Sports, *10*:208–213, 1978.

Krahenbuhl, GS, Skinner, JS, & Kohrt, WM. Developmental aspects of maximal aerobic power in children. Exercise and Sport Sciences Reviews, *13*:503–538, 1985.

Kuland, DN, & Tottossy, M. Warm-up strength and power. Clinics in Sports Medicine, *4*:137–158, 1985.

Landin, S, Hagenfeldt, L, Saltin, B, & Wahren, J. Muscle metabolism during exercise in hemiparetic patients. Clinical Science and Molecular Medicine, *53*:257–269, 1977.

Lavay, B, Reid, G, & Cressler-Chaviz, M. Measuring the cardiovascular endurance of persons with mental retardation: A critical review. Exercise and Sport Sciences Reviews, *18*:263–290, 1990.

Lefkof, MB. Trunk flexion in healthy children aged 3 to 7 years. Physical Therapy, *66*:39–44, 1986.

Lohman, TG. Measurement of body composition in children. Journal of Physical Education, Recreation and Dance, 53(7):67–70, 1982.

Lohman, TG. Applicability of body composition techniques and constants for children and youth. Exercise and Sport Sciences Reviews, 14:325–357, 1986.

Lohman, TG. The use of skinfold to estimate body fatness on children and youth. Journal of Physical Education, Recreation and Dance, 58(9):98–102, 1987.

Lohman, TG, Slaughter, MH, Boileau, RA, Bunt, J, & Lussier, L. Bone mineral measurements and their relation to body density in children, youth, and adults. Human Biology, 56:667–679, 1984.

Lundberg, A. Changes in the working pulse during the school year in adolescents with cerebral palsy. Scandinavian Journal of Rehabilitation Medicine, 5:12–17, 1973.

Lundberg, A. Maximal aerobic capacity in young people with spastic cerebral palsy. Developmental Medicine and Child Neurology, 20:205–210, 1978.

Lundberg, A, Ovenfors, CO, & Saltin, B. The effect of physical training on school children with cerebral palsy. Acta Paediatrica Scandinavica, 56:182–188, 1967.

Lundberg, A, & Pernow, B. The effect of physical training on oxygen utilization and lactate formation in the exercising muscle of adolescents with motor handicaps. Scandinavian Journal of Clinical and Laboratory Investigation, 26:89–96, 1970.

Macrae, I, & Wright, V. Measurement of back movement. Annals of the Rheumatic Diseases, 52:584–589, 1969.

Malina, RM. Growth of muscle and muscle mass. In Falkner, F, & Tanner, JM (Eds.), Human Growth: A Comprehensive Treatise, Vol. 2: Postnatal Growth. New York: Plenum Press, 1986, pp. 77–99.

Mathews, DK. Measurement in Physical Education, 4th ed. Philadelphia: WB Saunders, 1973, pp. 28–29.

Maughan, RJ, Watson, JS, & Weir, J. Strength and cross-sectional area of human skeletal muscle. Journal of Physiology, 338:37–49, 1983.

McDonald, CM, Abresch, RT, Carter, GT, Fowler, W, Jr., Johnson, ER, & Kilmer, DD. Profiles of neuromuscular diseases: Duchenne muscular dystrophy. American Journal of Physical Medicine and Rehabilitation, 74:S70–92, 1995.

Mersch, F, & Stoboy, H. Strength training and muscle hypertrophy in children. In Osteid, S, & Carlsen, KH (Eds.), Children and Exercise XIII. Champaign, IL: Human Kinetics, 1989, pp. 165–182.

Moll, JMH, & Wright, V. Normal range of spinal mobility: An objective clinical study. Annals of the Rheumatic Diseases, 30:381–386, 1971.

Molnar, GE, & Alexander, J. Objective, quantitative muscle testing in children: A pilot study. Archives of Physical Medicine and Rehabilitation, 54:224–228, 1973.

Moran, HM, Hall, MA, Barr, A, & Ansell, B. Spinal mobility of the adolescent. Rheumatology Rehabilitation, 18:181–185, 1979.

Moritani, T, & DeVries, HA. Neural factors versus hypertrophy in the time course of muscle strength gain. American Journal of Physical Medicine, 58:115–130, 1979.

Morris, JN, Heady, JA, Raffle, PAB, Roberts, CG, & Parks, JW. Coronary heart disease and physical activity of work. Lancet, 2:1053–1057, 1953.

Morrow, JR, Jr., Falls, HB, & Kohl, HW, III (Eds.). The Prudential FITNESSGRAM Technical Manual. Dallas, TX: The Cooper Institute for Aerobic Research, 1993.

Norkin, CC, & White, DJ. Measurement of Joint Motion: A Guide to Goniometry. Philadelphia: FA Davis, 1985.

Olney, SJ, Boyce, WF, & Wright, M. Lower extremity work patterns in gait of diplegic CP children (Abstract). Physical Therapy, 68:847, 1988.

Orenstein, DM, Franklin, BA, Doershuk, HK, Hellerstein, KJ, Germann, KJ, Horowitz, JG, & Stern, RC. Exercise conditioning and cardiopulmonary physical fitness in cystic fibrosis. The effects of a three-month supervised running program. Chest, 80:392–398, 1981.

Ozmun, JC, Mikesky, AE, Surburg, PR: Neuromuscular adaptations following prepubescent strength training. Medicine and Science in Sports and Exercise, 26:510–514, 1994.

Parizkova, J. Interrelationships between body size, body composition and function. Advances in Experimental Medicine and Biology, 49:119–123, 1974.

Parizkova, J. Body Fat and Physical Fitness: Body Composition and Lipid Metabolism in Different Regimens of Physical Activity. The Hague: Martinus Nijhoff, 1977, pp. 152–156.

Pate, RR. A new definition of youth fitness. Physician and Sports Medicine, 11:77–83, 1983.

Pate, RR, Dowda, MD, & Ross, JG. Associations between physical activity and physical fitness in American children. American Journal of Diseases of Children, 144:1123–1129, 1990.

Pate RR, Ross, JG, Baumgartner, TA, & Sparks, RE. The national children and youth fitness study II: The modified pull-up test. Journal of Physical Education, Recreation and Dance, 58:71–73, 1987.

Pate, RR, & Shephard, RJ. Characteristics of physical fitness in youth. In Gisolfi, CV, & Lamb, DR (Eds.), Perspectives in Exercise Science and Sports Medicine, Vol. 2: Youth, Exercise, and Sport. Indianapolis, IN: Benchmark Press, 1989, pp. 1–45.

Paterson, DH, & Cunningham, DA. Maximal oxygen uptake in children: Comparison of treadmill protocols at various speeds. Canadian Journal of Applied Sport Sciences, 3:188, 1978.

Phelps, E, Smith, LJ, & Hallum, A. Normal ranges of hip motion of infants between 9 and 24 months of age. Developmental Medicine and Child Neurology, 27:785–792, 1985.

President's Council on Physical Fitness and Sports. The Presidential Physical Fitness Program. Washington, DC: President's Council on Physical Fitness and Sports, 1987.

Rarick, GL, & Thompson, JAJ. Roentgenographic measures of leg size and ankle extensor strength of 7 year old children. Research Quarterly, 27:321–332, 1956.

Rose, J, Gamble, JG, Burgos, A, Medeiros, J, & Haskell, WL. Energy expenditure index of walking for normal children and children with cerebral palsy. Developmental Medicine and Child Neurology, 32:333–340, 1990.

Rose, J, Gamble, JG, Medeiros, J, Burgos, A, & Haskell, WL. Energy cost of walking in normal children and in those with cerebral palsy: Comparison of heart rate and oxygen uptake. Paediatric Orthopaedics, 9:276–279, 1989.

Ross, JG, Delpy, LA, Christenson, GM, Gold, RS, & Damberg, CL. The national youth and fitness study II: Study procedures and quality control. Journal of Physical Education, Recreation and Dance, 58:57–62, 1987.

Ross, JG, Dotson, CO, Gilbert, GG, & Katz, SJ. The national youth and fitness study I: New standards for fitness measurement. Journal of Physical Education, Recreation and Dance, 56:62–66, 1985.

Ross, JG, & Gilbert, GG. The national children and youth fitness study: A summary of findings. Journal of Physical Education, Recreation and Dance, 56:45–50, 1985.

Ross, JG, Katz, SJ, & Gilbert, GG: The national youth and fitness study I: Quality control. Journal of Physical Education, Recreation and Dance, 56:57–61, 1985.

Ross, JG, & Pate, RR. The national children and youth fitness study II: A summary of findings. Journal of Physical Education, Recreation and Dance, 58:51–56, 1987.

Ross, JG, Pate, RR, Delpy, LA, Gold, RS, & Svilar, M. The national children and youth fitness study II: New health related fitness norms. Journal of Physical Education, Recreation and Dance, 58:66–70, 1987.

Rutenfranz, J, Macek, M, Lange-Anderson, A, Bell, RD, Vavra, J, Radvansky, J, Klimmer, F, & Kylian, H. The relationship between changing body height and growth related changes in maximal aerobic power. European Journal of Applied Physiology, 60:282–287, 1990.

Safrit, MJ. Criterion-referenced measurement: Validity. In Safrit, MJ, & Wood, TM (Eds.), Measurement Concepts in Physical Education and Exercise Science. Champaign, IL: Human Kinetics, 1989, pp. 119–135.

Safrit, MJ. The validity and reliability of fitness tests for children: A review. Pediatric Exercise Science, 2:9–28, 1990.

Safrit, MJ, & Wood, TM: The test battery reliability of the health-related physical fitness test. Research Quarterly for Exercise and Sport, 58:160–167, 1987.

Sale, DG. Strength training in children. In Gisolfi, CV, & Lamb, DR (Eds.), Perspectives in Exercise Science and Sports Medicine, Vol. 2: Youth, Exercise, and Sport. Indianapolis IN: Benchmark Press, 1989, pp. 165–222.

Saltin, B, & Strange, S. Maximal oxygen uptake: Old and new arguments for a cardiovascular limitation. Medicine and Science in Sports and Exercise, 24:30–37, 1992.

Seaman, JA, & California Adapted Fitness Task Force. Test items and standards. In Seaman JA (Ed.), Physical Best and Individuals with Disabilities: A Handbook for Inclusion in Fitness Programs. Reston, VA: The American Alliance for Health, Physical Education, Recreation, and Dance, 1995, pp. 41–54.

Shvartz, E, & Reibold, RC. Aerobic fitness norms for males and females aged 6 to 75 years: A review. Aviation Space and Environmental Medicine, 61:3–11, 1990.

Simons-Morton, BG, O'Hara, NM, Simons-Morton, DG, & Parcel, GS. Children and fitness: A public health perspective. Research Quarterly for Exercise and Sport, 58:295–302, 1987.

Slaughter, MH, Lohman, TG, Boileau, RA, Stillman, RJ, VanLoan, M, Horswill, CA, & Wilmore, JH. Influence of maturation on relationship of skinfolds to body density: A cross-sectional study. Human Biology, 56:681–689, 1984.

Sodoma, CJ. Amateur Athlete Union physical fitness program validity for selected age group test results. Bloomington: Indiana University, 1986. Thesis.

Spady, DW. Normal body composition of infants and children. Ross Laboratories Conference on Pediatric Research, 98:67–73, 1989.

Spady, DW, Schiff, D, & Szymanski, WA. A description of the changing composition of the growing premature infant. Journal of Pediatric Gastroenterology and Nutrition, 6:730–738, 1987.

Sproul, A, & Simpson, E. Stroke volume and related hemodynamic data in normal children. Pediatrics, 33:912–916, 1964.

Sprynarova, S, & Reisenauer, R. Body dimensions and physiological indicators of physical fitness during adolescence. In Shephard, RJ, & Lavallee, H (Eds.), Physical Fitness Assessment. Springfield, IL: Charles C Thomas, 1978, pp. 32–37.

Strong, WB. Physical activity and children. Circulation, 81:1697–1701, 1990.

Sutton, JR. Vo₂max—New concepts on an old theme. Medicine and Science in Sports and Exercise, 24:26–29, 1992.

Tirosh, E, Bar-Or, O, & Rosenbaum, P. New muscle power test in neuromuscular disease. American Journal of Diseases of Children, 144:1083–1087, 1990.

United Cerebral Palsy Athletic Association. Classification System for Athletes. New Jersey, 1996.

United States Department of Health and Human Services. Healthy Children 2000: National Health Promotion and Disease Prevention Objectives Related to Mothers, Infants, Children, Adolescents, and Youth. Washington, DC: Public Health Service, 1990.

United States Department of Health and Human Services. Healthy People 2000: Progress Report for Physical Activity and Fitness. Washington, DC: Public Health Service, 1995.

United States Department of Health and Human Services. Physical Activity and Health: A Report of the Surgeon General. Atlanta, GA: United States Department of Health and Human Services, Centers for Disease Control and Prevention, National Center for Chronic Disease Prevention and Health Promotion, 1996.

United States Department of Health and Human Services. Healthy People 2010 Objectives: Draft for Public Comment. Washington, DC: United States Department of Health and Human Services, 1998.

van den Berg-Emos, RJG, van Baak, MA, & Westerterp, KR. Are skinfold measurements suitable to compare body fat between children with spastic cerebral palsy and healthy controls? Developmental Medicine and Child Neurology, 40:335–339, 1998.

Vignos, PJ, & Watkins, MP. The effect of exercise in muscular dystrophy. Journal of the American Medical Association, 197:843–848, 1966.

VonDobelin, W, & Eriksson, BO. Physical training, maximal oxygen uptake and dimensions of the oxygen transporting and metabolizing organs in boys 11–13 years of age. Acta Paediatrica Scandinavica, 61:653–657, 1972.

Wahlund, H. Determination of the physical working capacity. Acta Medica Scandinavica Supplement, 215:5–108, 1948.

Waugh, KG, Minkel, JL, Parker, R, & Coon, VA. Measurement of hip, knee, and ankle joints in newborns. Physical Therapy, 63:1616–1621, 1983.

Weltman, A, Janny, C, Rians, CB, Strand, K, Berg, B, Tippitt, S, Wise, J, Cahill, BR, & Katch, FI. The effects of hydraulic resistance strength training in pre-pubertal males. Medicine and Science in Sports and Exercise, 18:629–638, 1986.

Wiley, ME, & Damiano, DL. Lower extremity strength profiles in spastic cerebral palsy. Developmental Medicine and Child Neurology, 40:100–107, 1998.

Winnick, JP, & Short, FX: Physical Fitness Testing of the Disabled: Project UNIQUE. Champaign, IL: Human Kinetics, 1985, pp. 101–104.

Wyndham, C. Submaximal test for estimating maximal oxygen intake. Canadian Medical Association Journal, 96:736–742, 1976.

Yamashita, T, Seiichi, I, & Isao, O. Effect of muscle stretching on the activity of neuromuscular transmission. Medicine and Science in Sports and Exercise, 24:80–84, 1992.

Zach, MS, Oberwalder, J, & Hausler, F. Cystic fibrosis: Physical exercise vs chest physiotherapy. Archives of Disease in Childhood, 57:587–589, 1982.

Ziegler, EE, O'Donnell, AM, Nelson, SE, & Fomon, SJ. Body composition of the reference fetus. Growth, 40:329–334, 1976.

CHAPTER
6

Motor Learning: Theories and Strategies for the Practitioner

HÉLÈNE M. LARIN, PT, PhD

Learning or relearning motor tasks is a significant element of the rehabilitation process for a child with a neurologic or orthopedic impairment. Physical therapists continue to search for a better understanding and application to rehabilitation of the phenomenon of motor learning. The recent development of models for analyzing tasks and structuring instruction to promote motor learning may provide a helpful perspective for the pediatric physical therapist. Such models offer a means to systematically organize knowledge of movement, skill acquisition, and development.

In the past 100 years, researchers from various fields have investigated aspects of motor learning. At the cellular level, from animal studies, the "system [underlying learning is said] to consist of many parallel, redundant and possibly interacting compo-

nents" (Newell & Corcos, 1993). Researchers conducted in vivo studies primarily with persons without disabilities, with adults more than with children, and in laboratories more than in naturalistic environments, and they addressed isolated performance or learning behaviors. Despite working in these somewhat restricted milieux, researchers developed theories and models representing the body of knowledge of their time and also proposed a series of related instructional strategies. Through the years and even more today, physical therapists have had the difficult task of integrating the latest findings from research on motor learning into their working knowledge.

In my 1992 study on the use of motor learning principles in therapy, the review of videotapes of pediatric physical therapists during individual treatment sessions of preschool children with cerebral palsy (moderate spastic diplegia) revealed that they implemented most of the recognized strategies for motor learning and teaching (Larin, 1992). Throughout the sessions, therapists kept the children active, emphasized mobility over stability activities, and took periodic breaks. To a high degree, they maintained a stimulating environment related to the task at hand. The frequency of use for each instructional strategy, as assessed with the Motor Teaching Strategy Coding Measure (MTSCM-1), however, varied among therapists; the level of experience with neurologically impaired individuals was a factor in some cases. In a content analysis of recordings during two subsequent interviews, therapists demonstrated varying degrees of awareness or, sometimes, implicit knowledge of particular motor learning strategies. For example, the use of active mode, stimulating environmental conditions, waiting periods, assisted types of movements, and positive feedback received greater acknowledgment than the use of movement goals, specific task descriptions, or quantitative types of feedback to the child.

The relationship between clinicians' practice and implicit professional knowledge presented a mixed pattern that appeared to vary according to the characteristics of the (self-selected) tasks performed and the therapists' cognition of the motor learning strategies (Larin, 1992). Overall, therapists were aware of scientific knowledge of diverse origins, including some in motor learning, but were particularly cognizant of ecologic, motivational, and developmental theories. Thus a greater awareness and understanding of the contemporary body of knowledge on motor learning may help practitioners to maximize therapeutic opportunities. It may help therapists to 1) engage in self-analysis of their practice and identification of new or less exploited strategies; 2) adapt the information to their individual needs; 3) plan and perform examination and intervention sessions from a new perspective; and 4) engage in research documenting the applicability of principles of motor learning to intervention with children with disabilities.

To these ends, literature on concepts and strategies of motor learning and teaching is reviewed in the three main sections of this chapter; throughout, research findings on the learning process of children are highlighted. In the first section, a brief historical summary of the development of motor control and motor learning theories is presented. In the second, motor learning models from three authors who attempted to bridge the gap between theory and practice are briefly introduced. These models form the basis for the third section, in which a variety of instructional strategies are reviewed along with presentation of examples from pediatric clinical practice.

MOTOR CONTROL AND MOTOR LEARNING THEORIES: A HISTORICAL PERSPECTIVE

How does a person learn to control a new movement? How does one account for the complexity and variety of motor behavior in the process? These are some of the major questions theorists in motor control and motor learning have attempted to answer. The evolution of these concepts has gradually come to influence the body of knowledge, as well as the practice, of physical therapy.

Theoretic Groundwork

According to early views on the subject, motor learning was a process of "habit" formation (James, 1890); recently more sophisticated approaches have dealt with motor control and motor learning in terms of information processing theories and ecologic theories. The development of information processing theories can be related to the study of both slow and fast movements. The closed loop theories of movement control (Adams, 1971) emphasized the need for sensory input, sensory feedback, and rewards during repetition of movements that are slow and self-paced, the goal being to augment the intrinsic feedback and develop a perceptual memory trace of movements. These instructional strategies were considered necessary as event reinforcers.

In contrast, theorists who studied quickly executed movements discovered the existence of a structured, linear, hierarchic organization within the central nervous system (CNS) (Sheridan, 1984) and minimized the importance of the role of feedback. "Open loop" or "motor program" theories attributed skill acquisition to a central, executive motor program responsible for producing and executing selected, sequential subroutines in a top-down fashion for short, fixed, repeatable, automatic sequences of movements (Marteniuk, 1976). Consequently, step-by-step instructional strategies were promoted following systematic, developmental stages, with elicited movements prevailing over spontaneous movements and a preference for reflex activity over self-initiated activity. In a third point of view, McCulloch (1945), among others, proposed a "heterarchic" view of information processing: different levels of control interact, cooperate, and transfer control according to the need at hand rather than being subservient to an executive (Sheridan, 1984).

Schema Theories and Sensorimotor Theories

Another concept, *schema,* was to become significant in our understanding of information processing. In 1899, Woodworth and followers had enunciated the concept of schema as a set of rules serving as instructions for producing unique sequences of motor commands applicable to a variety of similar actions, referred to as a movement class. In 1975, Schmidt revived and expanded this concept in a schema theory. Schmidt emphasized the role of memory in motor learning and proposed the notion of two states of memory: recall and recognition schemas "stored" or programmed in the CNS as sets of rules. In the case of rapid, ballistic movements, motor experiences and memories would activate the recall schema (rule for movement production) and recognition schema (rule for establishing the relation between knowledge of the initial conditions, the environmental outcomes, and the expected sensory consequences for the purpose of response evaluation), resulting in the formation of motor learning structures.

From the original schema theory of Schmidt, certain predictions relating to motor learning have emerged: (1) practice variability promotes the building of a schema, especially for children; (2) after varied practice, novel responses in open-skills situations can be produced about as accurately as they can be after repeated practice (more so in children); and (3) the capability for error detection should exist mostly after fast movement and not after slow movement. In the latter case the recognition schema is said to be used to govern the ongoing production of the movement, leaving no more error detection capability after a slow movement (Schmidt, 1988).

To account for the great adaptability of the CNS, theorists attempted to combine the previous positions to develop what may be referred to as sensorimotor theories (Abbs et al., 1984; Marteniuk et al., 1988; Schmidt, 1991). They maintained the concepts of *heterarchy, schema,* a form of *motor program,* and added an *ecologic element* (from evolving behavioral theories mentioned later). Concepts such as *feedforward* and *feedback* processes within the CNS were also included.

Feedforward processes involve preparation of the system for anticipated consequences of movements that, in part, provide a postural set. Feedback regarding what is happening (or has happened) makes possible changes or midcourse correction of movement to bring about convergence to a goal. If the movement occurs too quickly for feedback to be used effectively for correction during the course of a movement, feedback information can be used as instructional information in the planning of a more refined set of commands the next time.

A sensorimotor integration termed *multimovement coordination* is also argued (Abbs et al., 1984; Marteniuk et al., 1988). It is proposed that sensory events are coded in efferent terms, specific to each learned task, and have the function of modifying the central storage of information. Among other issues, contemporary theorists have attempted to resolve the problem of storage of large amounts of information in the CNS and the problem of coping with the immense and complex variability of parameters in movement production, referred to as degrees of freedom. To solve this problem, Asatryan and Feldman (1965) advanced the mass-spring model, which hypothesizes that equilibrium points between the torques of agonist and antagonist muscles are programmed for efficiency. In 1967, Bernstein revived the original Ferrier concept of *synergy,* a phenomenon in which groups of muscles and joints are coupled with a common pool of afferent and efferent information to produce coordinated patterns of movement. See Chapter 2 for further discussion of these concepts.

The development of instructional strategies paralleled the expansion of these integrative theories of motor control and motor learning. Emphasis on the role of memory outlined the significance of the cognitive element in motor learning. The constructs of schema and motor program reinforced the need for repetition to enhance motor learning. Finally, the concepts of coordinating multiple degrees of freedom and synergy brought a greater focus on action specificity in practice.

Ecologic Approaches

Parallel to these developments and in reaction to the "habit" theory and information processing motor theories, Gibson (1966) and others (e.g., Turvey & Carello, 1986) proposed action systems or environment-related theories of motor control. For example, the direct perception theory (Michaels & Carello, 1981), a pure ecologic approach, considers the learning environment as specific to the child who actively and continuously explores and "picks up" the information "afforded" by the environment. Information is not presumed to be "processed" through memory or cognitive representation. Instead, according to the measure of attraction to the child, the biologic systems are said to "resonate" with the information the environment "broadcasts." According to this theory, perception and action form a closed unity; functional and relevant contexts for movement are therefore essential to promote motor learning.

Another aspect of this approach proposes that muscle groups and joints act as units, termed *muscle collectives* or *coordinative structures;* consequently, movements are said to be closely connected to the dynamic, mechanical properties of coordinative structures (e.g., length-tension and force-velocity relations), as opposed to a central representation. The formulation of these concepts has pointed toward more specific intervention strategies, such as (1) choosing or adapting individual, attractive sensorimotor environments; (2) respecting the child's interest in the selection of functional activities; and (3) promoting opportunities for muscle strengthening in particular needed ranges of movement, varied speeds, or coordinated movement patterns.

Dynamic Systems Theory

In the past decade, further "action systems" have been proposed, but the latest theory developed, elaborated, and promoted is the dynamic pattern theory of Kelso and colleagues (Kelso, 1991; Scholz, 1990; Thelen et al., 1987), also referred to as the dynamical systems approach (Kamm et al., 1990). According to this theory, motor behavior is said to emerge from the dynamic cooperation of all subsystems within the context of a specific task: CNS, biomechanical, psychologic, and social-environmental components. Each component is perceived as necessary but insufficient to explain movement changes. Patterns of movement are portrayed not as rigidly fixed or programmed in the CNS but as flexible, adaptable, and dynamic, yet having "preferred" paths. Functional movement synergies are self-assembled according to the interaction between the environment and the individual's intention. Dynamic systems theory emphasizes function more than instruction as the driving force for motor behavior (motor learning) and stresses the study of movement pattern transitions ("phasing" phenomena) rather than regular, repetitive occurrences.

The identification of critical variables leading to motor changes or motor learning becomes the focus of dynamic systems theory. The provision of specific instructional strategies (verbal and nonverbal) to the learner is dependent on a detailed assessment, which includes (1) observable collective variables called *order parameters,* such as temporal and spatial phasing between limbs and interjoint relationships; and (2) the dynamics of variables called *control parameters,* such as speed, loudness of voice, or surface (Heriza, 1991; Scholz, 1990). A task-oriented approach is emphasized. Further work on these and other variables will continue to expand our knowledge of motor learning and guide, to some extent, our therapeutic interventions by providing instructional models.

FROM MOTOR LEARNING TO MOTOR TEACHING MODELS

Learning or relearning motor skills and improving the performance of motor skills are two main effects of practice of particular interest to physical therapists. Learning occurs through an interaction of external and internal factors that influence the ability to process information (Toglia, 1991), and motor learning is a set of processes associated with practice that lead to relatively permanent changes in performance capability (Schmidt & Lee, 1999). That is, temporarily improved *performance* observed immediately following practice does not automatically equate to motor *learning* or necessarily imply that learning has occurred. Motor learning may be measured by the degree of long-term retention of performance capability, or the amount of transfer to different settings (near transfer), or to some different activity (far transfer). In therapeutic intervention, therefore, a conscious choice must be made between promoting motor learning and promoting performance; this choice determines the selection of instructional strategies. Systems for guidance in the selection and organization of relevant strategies in a comprehensive, coherent, and practical way have resulted from the development of models of motor teaching.

Models of motor teaching based on models of motor learning are few and relatively recent. They aim at improving the impact of motor teaching on persons with and without disabilities. The models have followed earlier work in the cognitive, educational domain. Orme's General Model of Teacher Behavior in Instruction (1978), including his series of practical teaching strategies, is one such source. Within this teaching model, the "teaching act" is described in six phases that are held to be necessary to elicit learning: (1) motivation, (2) presentation, (3) response guidance, (4) practice, (5) feedback, and (6) transfer. To be effective, these phases must be combined with arresting stimuli, including surprise, novelty, conflict, complexity, intensity, uncertainty, duration, and repetition. A close relationship exists between these cognitive concepts and those of the psychomotor-teaching models proposed by Gentile (1972, 1987), Marteniuk (1976, 1979), and Schmidt (1991).

The Gentile (1987) model for acquisition of motor skills is based on the proposition that skill learning takes place in two stages: initial and late. In the initial stage of learning of motor skills, the learner discovers a reasonably effective approach to desired movement patterns. In the later stage, the learner concentrates on achieving *skilled* performance (i.e., goal attainment and economy of effort). The latter processes are said to be task dependent, changing according to the environmental context and the function of the action. It follows that instructional interventions should be based on the structure of the task and on the environmental context in which it is to be performed while assisting the learner in moving from the initial stage of motor learning to the stage of skill acquisition.

The information processes involved in Gentile's initial stage are also reflected in the Marteniuk model of motor teaching based on his description of information processes of motor skill acquisition in the Human Perceptual-Motor Performance Model (Marteniuk, 1976). Figure 6–1 depicts the main elements of a motor teaching model. Marteniuk recognizes attention (alertness) and anticipation (expectation) as being of utmost importance for CNS preparation to receive and process perceptual information. Preparation includes potential factors affecting arousal for the therapeutic instruction such as stimulus intensity, variety, complexity, uncertainty, and meaningfulness; induced muscle tension; and physical exertion. Thus perception, decision, and action form the three basic components of the model. The perceptual mechanisms include information detection, comparison and recognition of kinesthetic information, selective attention (through meaningfulness) and short-term memory (assisted by knowledge of performance [KP]), knowledge of result (KR), noninterference, motor sequencing, cod-

ing and "chunking," and rehearsal, all concepts that are discussed later in this chapter. The second component, the decision mechanism, is influenced by certain information characteristics and measured by the reaction time (RT), which is the interval of time between the presentation of an unanticipated stimulus and the initiation of a motor response. RT decreases with increased anticipation and with decreased temporal and spatial (event) uncertainty, amount of information, number of possible alternative movements, movement precision demand (e.g., target size), and directional accuracy demand (Schmidt, 1991; Sideway, 1991). Other influential factors in decreasing RT are increased level of cognitive processes in mediating environmental stimuli and action (Weeks & Proctor, 1990), increased consistent practice, increased compatibility of information, and successively presented signals. Finally, the effector mechanism is said to contain a large number of motor commands; it organizes these commands to produce movement by activating muscles in correct sequential and temporal order.

Finally, Schmidt's Conceptual Model of Human Performance forms the basis for a series of comprehensive instructional strategies offered as guidelines (for able-bodied individuals) (Schmidt, 1991). Three main areas are proposed for consideration in composing instructional strategies: (1) preparation and design of practice, (2) organization and scheduling of practice, and (3) feedback for skill learning. Relevant instructional strategies should be adapted to the learner's stage of learning, in this case, as defined by Fitts and Posner (1967): verbal-cognitive, motor, and autonomous stages.

A concise survey follows of the suggested, theoretically based strategies that have been studied with different populations by various investigators. The applicability of these strategies to the pediatric population has been tested in some cases, but in other cases is assumed and remains to be verified. Overall, there is a high degree of consensus about the appropriate use of strategies of motor teaching among the promoters of these strategies; minor conflicts exist in certain instances.

MOTOR LEARNING AND TEACHING STRATEGIES IN PEDIATRICS

During a therapeutic session, each activity trial of the child becomes a unit of potential motor learning for which the therapist must decide on appropriate strategies. The selection of instructional strategies should reflect the *stage of learning* of the child (earlier or verbal-cognitive, later or motor, autonomous) for the motor task practiced. In addition, the potentially dichotomous goals of practice should be clear to the

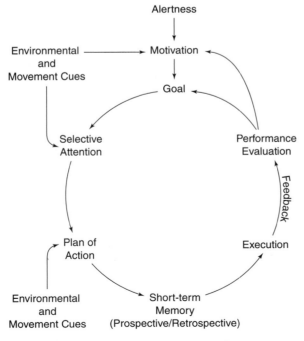

FIGURE 6–1. Motor teaching model: information processes in motor learning.

therapist: to optimize the child's *motor learning* (long-term retention and transfer to other tasks or settings) *or* the child's *motor performance* (greater ability within a task) during the treatment session. The specific goal of practice must be clear because instructional strategies effective in promoting retention of particular tasks, near transfer to a similar task, or far transfer to different activities will not necessarily lead to better performance during practice (Schmidt, 1991). In addition, the therapist must consider three potential sensitive periods for instructional intervention: before, during, and after the execution of *each* activity trial, whether the activity is static or dynamic.

Context

Before and during a treatment session, the overall *context* must be set and remain adequate and conducive to the child's learning. To a high degree, therapists have been found to maintain a stimulating environment and to motivate the child through verbal and visual stimuli during a treatment session (Carter, 1989; Larin, 1992).

First, the physical aspects of the environment must be considered. "Children learn more rapidly in stimulating and varied physical environments which meet basic human needs," including health and safety function, psychologic comfort, and aesthetic satisfaction, according to the "habitability" framework (Taylor & Gousie, 1988, p. 23). Because the physical aspects of the environment may be potential stressors on the child, more or less noise, light, color, and space cannot be ignored and may exert a direct effect on the child's level of motivation during a treatment session. Understanding of the child's attentional abilities and level of sensory processing and organization, as well as the influence of the environmental changes on movement production, is also crucial in enabling the therapist to modify and adapt the environment appropriately and individually for each child (Cook Merrill et al., 1990).

Both children and adults have been found to respond positively to a multicontext treatment approach. In this approach, the individual is required to apply the newly learned skill to multiple situations (Toglia, 1991). Consequently, one goal is to bring the child to a "context-independent state," decreasing the likelihood of association between a particular piece of information and a particular context. For example, individuals with severely limited physical and cognitive abilities who have demonstrated an increased level of goal attainment in a one-to-one therapy setting did not transfer the gains to their recess or home settings (Brown et al., 1998). In some clinical settings, an appropriate response has been the renovation of the traditional, contained treatment room with its standard equipment into various playground or household simulation contexts. Therapy may not begin and end at the threshold of a treatment room or even a treatment mat. The interaction milieu of home, school, and community remains the child's most functional context where varied practice and learning for transfer are most likely to occur.

Direct therapeutic intervention and program management ought to reflect this reality. For example, sitting in the waiting room, sitting for fine motor tasks or self-help, and sitting to pedal a tricycle become linked and provide real contexts for varied practice leading to motor learning of postural body control under a variety of conditions. Similarly, the same principle may be applied to climbing a bed, a chair, a step, or someone's lap. Another outcome in using the "multicontext treatment approach" is to enhance movement that is of interest to the child. Engaging in social interaction with puppets, other children, or adults may modify a child's level of participation in an activity (positively or negatively, depending on interest level).

Second, the socioculturoeducational aspect of the context that pertains to the quality of the instructor-learner interaction also affects the child's learning with respect to the amount and type of information transmitted (Simpson & Galbo, 1986). Effective *learning contexts* are those that promote initiations by the learner, reciprocity and shared control over the interaction between the less skilled (child) and the more skilled (therapist) party, and provision of responsive or content feedback rather than simply corrective feedback to the learner. In such contexts, children, whether mildly or moderately disabled, may gain more control over their own learning and reduce their level of dependence on adult control (Glynn, 1985).

The therapist seeks an integration and a balance between the dichotomous roles of playmate and instructor in his or her therapeutic intervention with the child. The playmate's role must feel genuine and pleasing to the child, and the instructor's role denotes supportive, confident, and effective guidance toward improved capabilities with a shared control of decision making. Therapeutic power is real and must be used with prudence. For example, the therapist may offer predetermined choices of activities to the child or take turns with the child in the decision-making process in an obvious, concrete, fair manner; above all the therapist should address the child within the "higher-order thinking skills" of the child (Ritson, 1987) and incorporate risk-taking behaviors (Cintas, 1992). In a treatment session, this may translate into the therapist's setting a challenging game, verbalizing the action or movement goal, and providing some timely, explicit feedback to the child, in spite of the child's minimal or delayed verbal and nonverbal communication skills and while being acutely attentive to the child's level of active participation.

Motivation and Prior Knowledge

In the pretask execution period, the child should gain *motivation* and clear, purposeful *prior knowledge* of the activity through auditory, visual, or proprioceptive signals (Higgins, 1991). The instructional strategies that relate to motivation include, for instance, action goal setting, preferably by or in conjunction with the child; selective attention (e.g., instructions, demonstration-modeling, and interference); and rehearsal (e.g., mental practice or describing the actions to be done).

Motivated learning is intentional learning for improvement. The learner must have (1) the perception of a skill as meaningful, useful, desirable, and having personal implications; (2) the experience of satisfaction from executing a movement; and (3) encouragement toward higher, achievable goals after task execution. The therapist may indirectly but positively influence the child's personal goals, self-perceptions, and cognitive-affective experiences through verbal and nonverbal communication. For example, counting out loud (with a meaningful tone of voice) the seconds spent in stride-standing, moving back and forth to place a basketball in the basket, marking points, and raising the basket or stepping back a step are ways to further challenge the child. Such strategies, however, may not be successful in motivating all children in spite of similar cognitive levels.

Motivated learning is an individual process. According to Ratner and Foley (1994), to facilitate children's "activity memory" (an integrated part of learning), emphasis must be placed on the individual's goals within a person-based perspective. All four features of the activities should be considered: outcomes, relational structure (between the activity and the learner), prospective processes (characteristics of anticipation and planning), and retrospective activation (repetition). To optimize this process of motivation leading to activity memory and motor learning, further insight is necessary into the learner's individual motivational variables relevant to physical skills; movement behavior in different contexts; and personal strategies, thoughts, and emotional responses during the learning process (Pohl et al., 1992). Therapists need to evaluate patients' motivation efficiently. Yet, until a valid and reliable tool is developed, therapists will continue to rely on general discussion, observation of conduct and actions, and information from others to evaluate motivation (Carlson, 1997).

Creative Behavior

Besides altering context, encouraging creative behaviors is a powerful means of enhancing the child's motivation. These primarily include fluency (e.g., movement variability); flexibility (e.g., movement independence); originality (e.g., in movement sequences); and elaboration. To gain fluency, the child needs to solve the same movement problem or goal through a number of different organizational approaches (i.e., motor equivalence). For example, the practice of going up the stairs for a child who has not yet mastered this skill may involve supervised creeping on hands and knees, hands and feet, sideways cruising up while holding onto the rail, and forward walking up with assistance (a device or manually). Promoting flexibility in therapy could entail allowing and acknowledging a child's independent thinking and creative movement response. Providing some basic movement information to the child, such as "Let's find a way to twist your shoulders," may support this behavior as well as allow originality in the child's movement sequences and may result in the production of a completely novel response. Such an approach is supported by Gibson's (1988) concept of "exploration" described as an active process with a perceptual, cognitive, and motor aspect.

Asking appropriate questions that require the child to think at his or her cognitive level and to perform the results of that thought process may lead to the fourth factor of movement creativity—elaboration. Such motor instructional strategies that go beyond the command style and promote process-oriented rather than product-oriented approaches constitute in themselves sources of motivation and enhance the desired, perceived internal control of the child (Ritson, 1987).

Goal Setting

Setting goals is another major, motivational, and knowledge-based instructional strategy available for use during a therapy session. First the therapist must consider the child's social influences, such as gender, age, cultural background, and personal socialization experiences, because these factors have been found to modify the learning of fundamental motor skills in young children (Garcia, 1994). For example, knowing that children up to the age of approximately 11 tend to hold "mastery goals" may guide the therapist in providing self-referenced achievement tasks rather than social comparison. In addition, the therapist's assessment of the child's cognitive ability to understand the task or goal will have a direct impact on potential learning of motor skills. Realizing that immediate social environmental conditions can override some preexisting goals of the child, the therapist may choose to provide a goal. Two types of goals may be provided: the goal may be related to the action (e.g., "Let's go slide") or to the movement itself, in this case, climbing the steps leading to the slide (e.g., "Let's see you bring one foot up very high and quickly"). As observed in Larin's (1992) study, therapists offered a verbal goal in 44 to 88% (average, 75%) of the activity trials during treatment sessions; the action goal accounted for 43% and the movement goal made up 47% of the verbal goals.

It is recommended that either type of goal be specific, consistent, attainable, and short in duration and that the standards be high enough to foster improved performance but not so high as to provoke discouragement by repeated failure (Edwards, 1988; Jones & Cale, 1997). Error awareness is a necessary element of the learning process. To ensure a successful learning experience, however, the therapist should guide the learner to make a decision on (evaluate) the environmental goal or related movement in a systematic, comparative fashion. Gentile (1972) suggests such an approach:

If a goal and movement are successful, use repetition.

If a goal is unsuccessful in spite of apparent good movement, help the learner in identifying relevant environmental conditions.

If a goal is successful but the movement produced a surprise success, describe the movement to the learner.

If both the goal and the movement are unsuccessful, encourage the learner and analyze further the task at hand.

Overall, the therapist should continue to explore movement options with the learner until repeated success in both movement and goal attainment are achieved. The use of movement scripts (i.e., chunks of typical patterns associated with specific movement functions and dysfunctions) may assist physical therapists to focus the intervention and assist the learner to successfully reach the goals and learn the intended movements (Embrey & Hylton, 1996).

Another useful tactic of the therapist is to ask the learner to set the goal. Movements "preselected" by the child result in greater goal clarity, increased energy production, and success, as well as superior reproduction of movements as compared with "constrained" movements selected by the instructor (Lewthwaite, 1990; Runnings & Diewert, 1982; Sage, 1984; Schempp, 1983; Schmidt, 1988). Preselection by the child has been found to be especially effec-

tive for children with low ability (Goldberger & Gerney, 1990). Once again, the experience of personal "locus of control" during an instructional session is of great importance for motor learning (Coster & Jaffe, 1991).

Instructions

The therapist's instructions before practice are critical for motivational purposes but also as feedforward input to convey information about the task requirements. This information should include a description of the task based on the learner's competencies, as well as on relevant environmental elements. The information may be verbally presented, nonverbally modeled, or both (Schmidt, 1991). The therapist's verbal instructions have the potential to bring the child's attention to different levels of information about a movement task. This information is closely associated with feedback information and with the environment. Examples include the following (Newell et al., 1990):

1. Intrinsic, sensorimotor information may address precise muscle-response organization (e.g., "Feel the muscles of your toes and legs pushing hard as you reach up").

2. Movement patterns or performance direction such as segmental body organization may be provided (e.g., "Bring your arm up, elbow straight, and open your hands to reach up").

3. The end result in the form of the action goal (e.g., "Let's decorate the top of the mirror") may activate the desired pattern of movement of reaching up.

4. Environmental information related to the action may guide the child's visual and auditory attentiveness (e.g., "The mirror is taller than you and is on wheels; the decorations are sticky and a bit heavy").

Appropriate instruction can enhance the child's selective attention and foster his or her ability to separate task-relevant information from task-irrelevant information, an integral part of the motor learning process based on Gibson's (1969) processes of perceptual learning: abstraction, filtering of irrelevant variables, and selective attention. With regard to the developmental, restrictive scanning strategies of younger children (Vurpillot, 1968), Stratton (1978) believes that lack of training and experience rather than processing capacity is the cause of children's deficits in information processing and attention capability. Children deserve to be given a chance to acquire strategies for improved selective attention.

Along with instruction, distractions may be provided. Interferences, such as people talking or walking or the therapist referring to other activities, may be presented to the child; these distractions simulate a real-world environment. Random practice, which will be discussed later, can also be considered as another source of contextual interference. Introducing this strategy early in the learning situation appears to produce the best results in improved ability to deal with irrelevant information (Stratton, 1978). Children with neurologic impairment, however, may display sensorivisual loss and cognitive deficits in the selective attentional system (Hood & Atkinson, 1990). Such a tactic, of course, must be used carefully with these children, for whom the addition of extraneous information may be overwhelming and counterproductive.

Verbal instructions about the motor activity (prior knowledge) should be offered, first, about the entire movement, describing the same speed and accuracy required in the desired skill (Gentile, 1987). According to the child's level of selective attention and capability of processing information, the therapist has the option to break down the verbal instructions, with an initial emphasis on only one or two essential elements of the skill; brevity and meaningfulness are important in this case. Minimal guidance from research is available because only limited data have been gathered on individual needs and the complexity and distribution of instructions appropriate for different age groups.

A combination of distance and location information, however, has been found to allow greater accuracy of movement reproduction, whether the movement practiced is active or passive (Runnings & Diewert, 1982). Furthermore, initial, specific information can be long-lasting: emphasis on accuracy leads to improved accuracy, and emphasis on speed leads to improved speed (Schmidt & Lee, 1999). Allowing further trial-and-error (no prompting) attempts before providing feedback or further instructions has also been reported to be superior to use of a guiding stimulus (prompting) exclusively. Children with learning disorders (cognitive and motor) may benefit from the same opportunity. However, children with cerebral palsy have been reported to respond with greater movement excursions (forearm pronation or supination) to concrete instructions (e.g., "Bang the drums"), rather than abstract instructions (e.g., "Turn the handle back and forth as far as possible") when compared with nondisabled children, who showed no difference between tasks (van der Weel et al., 1991). Verbal prompting is a useful strategy but should not be provided in proportion to the learning difficulty (Koegel & Rincover, 1976).

Nonverbal prompting should also be considered. Particularly for motor skill acquisition and retention of task processing occurring in the non-dominant hemisphere, facilitating attention with a combination of verbal and nonverbal strategies to the skill has been found to bring higher outcomes. A rationale is proposed: interhemispherical transfer promotes motor learning (Fairweather & Sidaway, 1994).

Demonstration or Modeling

Demonstration or modeling may complement or replace verbal instructions. Children tend to be more visually dependent than adults, who rely more on a combination of proprioceptive and visual input (Shumway-Cook & Woollacott, 1985). Observational motor learning is thus an effective strategy for developing the perceptual skills necessary for children to selectively attend to environmental cues (Arend, 1980). In addition, observational motor learning is said to improve performance, learning, and self-confidence (Weiss et al., 1993). Modeling is task specific and may be enhanced by verbal labeling (including spatial and temporal information [Schmidt & Lee, 1999]), rehearsal, temporal spacing of demonstrations, and verbal pretraining (i.e., the child verbally cueing himself or herself about movement demands) (Gould & Roberts, 1982). With low-skilled subjects, however, peer modeling (i.e., watching an unskilled person learning a motor skill) has been found to be more effective than instructor modeling (Schmidt & Lee, 1999). Effective use of modeling is said to include an initial demonstration followed by further demonstration throughout practice (Williams, 1993).

Therapists were observed to use demonstrations minimally in the treatment of preschool children with a diagnosis of cerebral palsy, although they claimed greater use with children 6 years of age and older (Larin, 1992). Coordinating therapy sessions among therapists with similar patients to encourage reciprocal peer modeling should be recognized as a potentially valuable tool of motor teaching (see Group Therapy later in this chapter).

Purposeful Tasks

"Given appropriate tasks and sufficiently guided practice, gross motor skill learning in young children can be effectively enhanced through planned instruction" (Haubenstricker & Seefeldt, 1986, p. 65). Purposeful tasks are more appropriate than reflexive or passive behaviors (Bernstein, 1967). Purposeful tasks are active, voluntarily regulated (from initiation to termination), goal directed (Croce & DePaepe, 1989), and meaningful to the learner (Ratner & Foley, 1994; van der Weel et al., 1991). Heart rates and perceived exertion ratings are significantly lower during purposeful tasks than during nonpurposeful activities (Bakshi et al., 1991). In addition, the individual's freely chosen work rate (preferred rhythm) has been found to be the most efficient for performance across a variety of tasks (Fetters, 1991; Sparrow, 1983), particularly for 5-year-old children (Williams, 1985). Purposeful tasks of individuals with neuromotor disorders, however, do not necessarily lead to the same level of movement efficiency achieved by nondisabled individuals. Gait studies in children with cerebral palsy, for example, have revealed reduced muscle activity, uneven kinetic energy patterns, and mechanical energy cost above normal values (Olney, 1989). Similar findings were also reported in a study of the kinematics and kinetics of running in children with cerebral palsy (Davids et al., 1998).

The "will to act" on the part of the learner builds up over a long time before a movement begins (120 ms); in fact it is longer than reaction time to a stimulus (30 to 80 ms) (Kelso, 1991). Hence, the pretask period is important for information processing, decision making, and response programming. The ability to rapidly process information increases progressively up to 18 years of age, reducing response latency (Clark, 1982); this phenomenon has been found to be more prevalent in males than females (Thomas et al., 1981). In addition, the speed of the reaction time is related to a series of factors as previously mentioned. Both children's and adults' most accurate anticipations, when confronted with velocity problems, are made when they experience them in the context of their daily activities (Wade, 1980), a natural phenomenon referred to as stimulus-response compatibility (Schmidt, 1991). Functional, ecological, relevant goals elicit faster and smoother movements than nonfunctional goals (Lin et al., 1998). Certain biomechanical parameters have also been identified as decisive in achieving optimum anticipatory postural adjustments and motor outcome, for example, configuration of the base of support before moving (Brenière et al., 1987) or in regaining balance (Tarantola et al., 1997). Moreover, feedback anticipation seems to emerge from feedback experiences (Haas et al., 1989). Individuals with verbal-motor performance deficits, however, take longer to organize and initiate movements (Elliot et al., 1991). Children with cerebral palsy show deficits in the sensorimotor organization and muscular coordination of their anticipatory activities (Duff & Gordon, 1998; Nashner et al., 1983); they tend to compensate with early onset of force production and overall high force outputs (Eliasson et al., 1991, 1992).

Based on this research, the therapist would do well to promote practice of relevant, functional, purposeful tasks; to use spatial and temporal anticipation strategies to increase the readiness of the child to respond (i.e., informing the child of what will occur [and when]); and to use routine rather than random activities to influence reaction time and facilitate anticipation skills (Schmidt, 1991) necessary for the development of activity memory (Ratner & Foley, 1994). Permitting information processing to occur requires a "waiting" period on the part of the therapist. Therapists have been observed waiting for the child's action or reaction in an average of 66% of activity trials in a treatment session (range, 48–93%). Most therapists (85% of the sample) were aware of their use of this strategy, but various rationales were offered (Larin, 1992).

Task Sequencing and Related Issues

Information processing demands vary with the type of task, making task classification taxonomies useful as an adjunct to planning a developmentally appropriate motor learning program. Purposeful tasks have been classified as continuous, serial, or discrete; open or closed; and complex or simple (Schmidt, 1988, 1991) (Table 6–1).

The sequencing of tasks plays an important role in motor learning and teaching. Different paradigms exist for sequencing tasks and instructions effectively. Gentile's (1987, 1992) taxonomy of tasks is one guide for the examination of a child's functional abilities and response to task demands, for the selection of functionally appropriate activities, and for planning therapeutic interventions. Progression may require modifications of the activities in several directions on the taxonomy template. Table 6–2 provides a series of examples in which both body status and environmental context are considered. Knowledge of movement scripts (i.e., chunks of typical patterns of movement) may further assist physical therapists in performing these complex tasks (Embrey & Hylton, 1996).

Other systems also exist to assist practitioners in the sequencing of motor skill learning. Bressan and Woollacott (1982) proposed a paradigm in which skill construction, stabilization, and differentiation represent phases in the progressive control of the muscle synergies' program for motor skill acquisition. Wickstrom (1977) and Roberton and Halverson (1977) broke down skills into components of movement (intratask) and determinants of movement sequences relevant to other tasks (intertask), the former leading to the latter. More recently, Davis and Burton (1991) proposed an ecologic task analysis system based on the dynamic relationship between task environmental and performer factors. They suggested four instructional guidelines: (1) identify the task in terms of function (rather than

TABLE 6-1. Task Classification: Types, Characteristics, and Implications

Type	Continuous	Discrete	Serial	Open	Closed	Complex	Simple
Characteristics	Series of ongoing modifications No recognizable beginning or end Longer movement time Fatiguing Example: swim, run	Minimal feedback information effect Recognizable beginning and end Shorter movement time Minimal fatigue Example: kick, write signature	Combination of continuous and discrete	Constant unpredictable and uncertain environment Needs to adapt behavior to changing environment Cannot effectively plan the response (on the spot decisions) Example: walk and step over obstacle	Stable predictable environment Allow advance organization of movement Can plan in advance Can learn with practice Example: put hat on	Requires more coordination or more body parts Requires longer time to initiate	Requires less coordination and fewer body parts Requires less time to initiate
Practical, instructional implications	Focus = sensory information and how to modify More time for rest between trials Error detection *during* movement	Focus = pre-planning and production No attempt to modify during movement Less time for rest Increased number of trials Develop error detection through own response-produced feedback *after* movement		Focus = nature of environment (try to learn irregularities) Variable practice Flexibility	Focus = generation of pre-programmed actions Stability and consistency	Focus: keep arousal level fairly low More attention to describe and demonstrate Provide more feedback Budget more time	Focus: bring up arousal level More direct practice repetitions Provide less feedback

TABLE 6–2. **Gentile's Taxonomy of Tasks: Examples of Therapeutic Activities**

Environmental Context	Body Stability		Body in Motion	
	No Manipulation	With Manipulation	No Manipulation	With Manipulation
Stationary and no trial variability				
Stationary and trial variability				
Motion and no trial variability				
Motion and trial variability				

perfection), (2) allow the learner choices and freedom to use movements, (3) identify and manipulate the relevant and critical task dimensions and performer's variables, and (4) provide direct instruction on the movement pattern using performer-scaled or intrinsic units of measure (e.g., ratio, rather than comparative, normative units).

Overall task sequencing has been considered according to various dimensions: general or specific, more or less complex, blocked or random, and part or whole. Schema theory supports the approach of developing a general base of motor activities before developing specific skilled activities (Kerr, 1978) for both open and closed skills. Referring to developmentally delayed children, Croce and DePaepe (1989) have suggested teaching sequentially less complex patterns before more complex skills. Winstein (1991b), however, has cautioned against reducing the difficulty of a task to the point where the inherent nature of the task is altered. Such a practice could be detrimental to transfer of motor learning to the intended task. For example, emphasizing weight shift in standing as a subtask of locomotion did not achieve improved gait in adults with hemiparesis (Winstein et al., 1989), nor did a sitting activity heel-up heel-down rhythm task modify gait (Seitz & Wilson, 1987). In pediatrics, the use of infant walkers was not found to accelerate the onset or the quality of children's walking patterns (Kauffman & Ridenour, 1977).

One might extrapolate that children may not learn to kick in a standing position from practicing kicking in a sitting position or even performing pendular movements of the lower extremity in one-leg standing. Research results, however, are not entirely consistent with this view. Weight-bearing activities of the upper extremities have been reported to improve target-throwing skills in children 5 to 7 years of age with sensory integration disorders (Jarus & Gol, 1995). Using a specially designed tricycle to encourage hip extension resulted in improved gait in children with cerebral palsy (King et al., 1993). Choosing and sequencing tasks in a therapy session remains a complex yet important determinant of a child's motor learning. Clearly, more research is indicated.

In general, therapists have been reported to adhere, more or less consciously, to the concepts of general or specific and more or less complex task sequencing based on maturational and developmental theories (Larin, 1992). For example, a therapist may promote gross mobility before specific gait activities (e.g., initial heel contact), practice walking while holding onto a ball before free walking, or practice forward directional progression before changes of direction.

Contextual Interference: Blocked vs. Random

Task sequencing may also be "blocked," that is, practiced in drill-type repetition where all trials of a given task are completed before another task is undertaken (intratask processing), or in "random" sequence (i.e., mixed repetition of various tasks [intertask processing]). In the early, verbal-cognitive stage of motor learning, blocked practice is slightly more effective than random practice. Random sequencing, however, has proven more beneficial than blocked sequencing for motor learning, as measured on retention tests of motor skills. Random sequencing requires a greater number of trials, however, and typically degrades performance during the practice session; hence the acquisition-retention paradox known as the contextual interference effect (Fineman & Gentile, 1998; Schmidt & Lee, 1999). The facilitative effect of high contextual interference has been related to an increase in task difficulty during practice that requires a higher level of attention (see earlier section on instructions) (Smith, 1997).

Furthermore, repetitions lead to the acquisition of a motor skill if they occur under conditions that most closely resemble those normally encountered during the performance of that skill. Through repetition children have shown considerable improvement, as compared with older individuals, in learning a demanding movement (Nicolson, 1982). Three-month-old infants learned to kick and activate a mobile (Ohr et al., 1989) and infants 5 to 10 months old accelerated the development of their sitting postural responses with training (Hadders-Algra et al., 1996). Children with motor delay and children with a diagnosis of cerebral palsy have yielded similar findings from intensive, individual physical therapy sessions (Bower & McLellan, 1992; Mayo, 1991). Furthermore, in Horn and colleagues' (1995) study, young children with severe cerebral palsy demonstrated gains in the acquisition of specific movement components of treated and untreated skills, as well as in the generalization of skills to a different environment.

One may conclude that, during a treatment session, it is important for the therapist to regard repetition as a means to (1) explore movement options until there are one or more occurrences of total success (Gentile, 1987) and (2) practice several skills, rotating among them. The therapist should explain the paradoxical phenomenon to the child or caregiver (i.e., the trade-off between poorer, immediate performance versus long-term learning and retention performance as it is likely to affect motivation and motor learning). In general, however, therapists who stress the importance of repetition and claim to use this strategy have been observed to practice, on average, only four repetitions per activity, whether in a blocked or random sequencing (Larin, 1992). The principle of variety appears independent from and of higher order than the principle of repetition; this may be related to a misunderstanding of the criteria associated with effective random sequencing, in which a large number of trials is necessary.

Part vs. Whole

The sequence of the components of a task may also be presented in "parts" or as a "whole," depending on the nature of the skill. For rapid, discrete skills of short duration (less than 1 second), practice of the whole task from the outset leads to the best results. If the learner has the prerequisite skills to master the new skill in its entirety, or if the degree of cognitive processing is minimal, the "whole" method is reported to be far superior to one based on "parts" (Croce & DePaepe, 1989). The same approach applies to slower, serial, and continuous skills of long duration (more than 10 seconds). For very complex tasks, the most time-efficient approach is to first practice the most troublesome parts of the task. *Progressive part practice* follows to gradually integrate the parts as acquired into the whole task so as to minimize transfer problems between the two (Schmidt & Lee, 1999). According to the *specificity of learning hypothesis,* intertask transfer between two tasks does not happen or is very small if the two tasks are different in only very minor ways. It is therefore essential to use correct techniques during practice to master a motor skill (Ashy et al., 1988). To do so, it seems imperative for the therapist to differentiate skill characteristics and adopt the use of a taxonomy to guide practice.

Mental Practice

Practice is usually thought of as being physical (i.e., execution of a task with one's body); however, both physical and mental practice are useful strategies of motor teaching. Furthermore, a combination of mental and physical practice seems to be the most productive. Mental practice, also called *cognitive rehearsal* or *imagery practice,* is imagining one's correct performance of a motor task without any associated overt movement. This strategy has been mainly designated as an end result of practice, but it may be used in the pretask or posttask execution period, or between physical trials to enhance performance over motor learning. Using 3 to 5 minutes of mental practice, beginners and highly skilled performers have been reported to benefit from this type of practice, particularly in correcting errors in execution, increasing concentration, and strategy rehearsal.

Random imagery practice has been found to facilitate retention better than blocked imagery (Gabriele et al., 1989). Alternating actual practice and imagery practice has also been found to facilitate motor learning more than alternating actual practice and rest (Kohl et al., 1992).

Mental practice may also increase speed (Rawlings et al., 1972, in Maring, 1990), balance (Fansler et al., 1985), and accuracy and efficiency (Maring, 1990). A group of adolescents with mild cognitive impairments performed with significantly greater accuracy and less variability when combining physical practice with imagery rather than using physical practice alone (Poretta & Surburg, 1995; Surburg et al., 1995). Mental practice can also be left to the learner to use outside of coaching sessions. Despite the usefulness of mental practice, however, the emphasis should be on physical practice during a session (Feltz & Landers, 1983). The features of the activities (i.e., outcome, relation to learner, anticipation, and repetition) remain crucial to regulate and reflect the execution and interpretation of an act (Ratner & Foley, 1994) and to promote motor learning.

Therapists generally do not use much mental practice in intervention. Having a child anticipate a movement through mental practice is not considered a concrete enough activity for children younger than 5 years of age. When employed, however, therapists have reported using it occasionally with older children in practicing specific gross motor tasks, such as wheelchair transfers (Larin, 1992). Fazio (1992) presented an overview of "guided affective imagery" as an adjunct to a stimulating treatment approach. Given that planning a movement is, in itself, beneficial to motor learning, therapists may find that mental practice (adapted to the child's cognitive level) may be particularly effective in early practice, as findings with young adults have indicated (Schmidt & Lee, 1999). For example, the therapist might say "Let's think how it feels when you . . . , first you . . . , then you . . . ," or "Try to imagine you watch yourself on television," or "Pretend you are doing it like in a dream, close your eyes . . . " For brief periods of time, in a random fashion, children should be given the chance to experience and learn from mental practice.

Physical Practice: Determinants of Effectiveness

Physical practice remains essential to motor learning. Previously discussed aspects of such practice include the selected criterion (goal), task classification and dimensions, sequencing of tasks, and repetition. In addition, scheduling of practice and fatigue effects, degree of variability, physical guidance, and concurrent feedback also play important roles.

Scheduling

Scheduling of practice trials remains somewhat controversial. In general, "distributed" practice (i.e., when the amount of rest between trials equals or exceeds the amount of time in a trial) has been found to improve performance; and "massed" practice (i.e., when the amount of practice time in a trial is greater than the amount of rest between trials) enhances learning, in spite of fatigue (Gentile, 1987). Schmidt and Lee (1999), however, indicated that distributed practice facilitates both performance and learning more than massed practice for continuous tasks. More specifically, massed practice is advocated for discrete tasks, in which the skill level of the learner is higher and in which peak performance on a well-learned skill is needed. For continuous tasks, however, only slight negative effects of massed practice on learning are reported. In this case, distributed practice over a long time period is most beneficial because the tasks require greater energy expenditures. The same is true for complex tasks and in the presence of a lower level of motivation from the learner (Sage, 1984).

Realistically, motor activities are usually performed under gradually increasing amounts of fatigue; Schmidt (1991) suggested that, to be effective, practice must be somewhat difficult and effortful. For children with cerebral palsy, increased fatigue caused by repetition of activities has been found to be associated with progress toward certain motor goals (Bower & McLellan, 1992). One concludes that some degree of fatigue is a necessary element in motor learning and should be explained to the child and caregiver. Therapists must ensure that the child's nutritional status, particularly the iron level, is adequate to sustain the physical performance and endurance required (Lozoff, 1989), that treatment sessions contain sufficient rest to remain energizing and challenging for the child, and, most important, that treatment sessions are safe, avoiding accidents.

In therapy sessions as in sport training, practice periods tend to be fixed in length; no single, optimal practice/rest ratio has been determined to be most effective in maximizing learning in all types of tasks. Each task must therefore be analyzed, and the analysis used to guide decisions about practice scheduling. "The issue of practice distribution and total practice involves *trade-off*. Distributed practice results in the most learning per time in training but requires the most total time to complete. Massed practice results in reduced benefits per time in training but requires the least total time" (Schmidt & Lee, 1999, p. 297).

Variability

Another determinant of motor learning is the amount of variability—rehearsal of many variations of the same movement class. Actions within a movement class are said to share a particular relative timing and similar sequences of movements (Schmidt, 1991): for example, clapping hands and making music, banging objects together or altering a parameter or a part of an action such as throwing (e.g., higher, faster, longer). The conditions under which a task is learned affect the ability to navigate in error fields; the more "noise," the more rapid the learning of a new task with similar error structure (Newell & Corcos, 1993). There are two main purposes for using variability: first, to enhance generalizability and adaptability when one task-practice contributes to the performance of another in the same class of movement; and, second, to establish competence throughout a dimension (i.e., altering either distance, speed, direction, or timing) while maintaining the same fundamental pattern.

Use of variability as teaching strategy has been more effective for children and female subjects than for male adults (Sage, 1984; Schmidt & Lee, 1999). Overall, low-variable practice (overlearning through practice of the same task) translates into greater performance on the practiced task; this outcome has also been found to apply to individuals with learning disabilities performing a serial-type motor skill (Heitman et al., 1997). High-variable practice yields high performance on task transfer within a similar movement class (Carson & Wiegand, 1979; Shea & Kohl, 1990) and better retention of learning when skill variations are from different classes of movement (Hall & Magill, 1995), as long as the tasks are similar to (and "surrounded by") the criterion task. Furthermore, high-variable practice leads to more generalizability, adaptability, and competence throughout a dimension (i.e., distance, speed, direction, or timing) while maintaining the same fundamental pattern. A caveat is that "similar" may mean different things at different ages (van Rossum, 1980); the breadth of a class of "similar" movements under a given motor program remains equivocal (Schmidt, 1977). For example, slowing down a movement too much might destroy its essential dynamics (Fetters, 1991; VanSant, 1990). Yet Horn and colleagues (1995) found that children 21 to 34 months old were able to generalize movement components to an untreated, related skill from a skill gained during sessions in which neuromotor and behavioral approaches were used.

Optimum variability of practice for open or closed motor skills also differs. For open tasks, practice should be diversified, providing the learner with variations encountered in the habitual environment. However, Eidson and Stadulis (1991) reported no significant effect from the type of practice for an open skill in children with a moderate mental handicap; variable practice, however, reduced error in a closed skill. In general, practice for closed tasks should be consistent, enabling the learner to refine the movement pattern (i.e., decrease the variability of the movement trajectory [Darling & Cooke, 1987]), particularly after the acquisition phase during the later stages of motor learning (Gentile, 1987). In early learning, for example, therapists may slow down the activity somewhat while practicing small blocks of several trials of an activity (open or closed). Soon after, one must shift to random practice of two or more movement classes with variable practice on each (Sage, 1984). Random and variable practice generally leads to greater retention and error detection, at least for spatial performance (Sherwood, 1996). Besides undertaking variable tasks, the learner must apply the newly learned skill to multiple situations or environments; both children and adults respond positively to a multicontext treatment approach (Toglia, 1991). To provide the optimum variability of practice, physical therapists should perform rapid procedural changes in harmony with the learner's motor behavior. Embrey and Adams (1996) revealed that experienced clinicians make smooth changes of procedures approximately every 46 seconds compared with the more abrupt changes of procedures by novices with a mean of every 86 seconds. Further insight into clinical decision making is necessary to assess fully the impact of procedure changes on the learner.

Guidance

Guidance from the instructor or from mechanical equipment (e.g., metronome) is an effective method to restrict movement errors during the performance of a task. Physical or verbal guidance techniques assist the learner, in varying degrees, through the proper movements of the task. The use of rhythmic auditory stimulation (RAS) was shown to improve the gait patterns of children with mild to moderate spastic diplegia (Thaut et al., 1998). Physical or verbal guidance or both, often referred to as "facilitation" in the therapeutic milieu, has traditionally been a major strategy used by therapists in neurorehabilitation. Carter's (1989) findings, however, indicated that therapists spend more time in handling behaviors (facilitation, stimulation, inhibition, passive movements, and other maneuvers) than in using verbal behaviors (instructions, praise, criticism). Therapists have also been observed to provide physical guidance during 78% of the activity trials in a treatment session while spending 11% on passive, task-related activities and 11% on allowing independent movements (Larin, 1992).

Providing a relative frequency of guidance (i.e., for a certain percentage of trials during practice) contributes more to learning than use of continuous input (Salmoni et al., 1984; Winstein, 1994), as will relative frequency rather than continuous feedback (Lee et al., 1990). Some guidance can be beneficial when interspersed with active practice trials. Moreover, with able-bodied individuals, guidance has been found most effective 1) in early practice of unfamiliar tasks, 2) for slower rather than rapid and ballistic tasks, and 3) in the prevention of injury and reduction of fear (Schmidt & Lee, 1999). For intervention with children with physical disabilities, Tscharnuter (1993) provides experiential guidelines in her approach on the grading and direction of therapeutic handling input (guidance) to provide proprioceptive, tactile, and kinesthetic experiential information relevant to tasks. These guidelines emphasize the stability aspect through activation from the support surface contact or base of support to achieve self-initiated movements.

Guidance has a considerable positive effect on performance during the trials of the practiced task (i.e., in the acquisition phase) but not on learning. It modifies the feel of the task, and the learner relies too strongly on it, developing a dependency (Salmoni and colleagues' guidance hypothesis, 1984). Continuous guidance alters the task, greatly reducing its specificity and transfer potential. Trial-and-error, or "discovery," procedures, however, result in learning (i.e., more effective retention and transfer performance). "Forced use" may be an adjunct strategy to promote such experience (Crocker et al., 1997).

Given that response time decreases with increasing age, the therapist should provide adequate time for a child to respond before intervening to initiate a motor sequence (Steyer David, 1985). The therapist should generally aim at reducing the use of guidance while increasing independent practice; this goal was noted to be predominant in therapists' current professional knowledge base (Larin, 1992). When needed, the therapist should provide a "relative frequency" of guidance rather than continuous input and possibly alternate between trial and error, independent movements, and guided movements. Reduced guidance in therapy may progress from firm physical handling with verbal input to a lesser, modified physical contact and verbal input, to minimal verbal input with supervision, to nonverbal, nonphysical guidance. Such characteristics of physical guidance are contained in the contemporary neurodevelopmental treatment (NDT)/Bobath concept and in practice using facilitation techniques: guiding and grading physical, direct input toward and away from the base of support to facilitate stability and mobility, respectively. NDT emphasizes "gradual withdrawal of the therapist's direct input" and now promotes a "less hands-on" approach than was used in the past (Mayston, 1992; NDTA, 1997).

Feedback

Some form of feedback is essential for motor learning. Feedback may occur before, during (concurrent), or after (terminal) and be immediate or delayed, with respect to the task execution. Terminal feedback has been studied the most (Salmoni et al., 1984) and is the most frequently used in therapy (Larin, 1992).

Two Types of Feedback

Two types of feedback are recognized: intrinsic and extrinsic. Intrinsic feedback is related to the child's inherent, rich, and varied sensory channels involved in practicing a task, provided the CNS is intact. Intrinsic feedback may be augmented by information concerning the movement or the degree of goal attainment (Holding, 1965). Extrinsic feedback, also called augmented or enhanced feedback, speeds up the learning rate, whereas no feedback and irrelevant feedback conditions do not result in learning. Any feedback has the potential to generate rapid and permanent motor learning if it adds essential information to the task-intrinsic feedback of the learner, but it is not needed in all learning tasks. Certain skills provide sufficient task-intrinsic feedback to enable the learner to improve performance. In some cases, augmented feedback can even hinder skill learning (Magill, 1994).

Feedback may be provided verbally or nonverbally. The latter refers to sensory feedback, such as proprioceptive, auditory, visual, tactile, and electromyographic inputs, through the use of manual "handling" devices or media (Hartveld & Hegarty, 1996). Extrinsic feedback may be of several types: qualitative (e.g., "good," "right," "no") or quantitative feedback related to distance or magnitude of error (e.g., "three more steps"). It may trigger motivation and provide reinforcement. One purpose of extrinsic feedback is to give the child information (success or error) on the environmental outcome and on his or her movement patterns. Therapists, however, tend to provide primarily positive, qualitative verbal feedback (in Larin's study, 47% of activity trials com-

pared with 6% of negative reinforcement and 9% of quantitative feedback). Furthermore, according to Carter's (1989) findings, therapists' "praise" may reinforce abnormal as much as normal movements and their "criticism" may act as punishment for abnormal movements.

Outcome information is termed *knowledge of result* (KR) and refers to direction and magnitude (Schmidt, 1991) or superficial movement features such as topology, timing (duration and speed), direction, amplitude or distance, or forcefulness (Gentile, 1987). Information on kinetics and kinematics is termed *knowledge of performance* (KP). Kinematic feedback is information on positions, time, velocities, patterns of coordination, or movement patterning; kinetic measures are descriptors of the forces that produce the kinematic variables (Schmidt, 1988). For Gentile (1987), kinematic feedback is mainly information on fundamental movement patterns such as timing or sequencing information.

There are inconsistencies between authors in their definitions of KR and KP, but they generally agree that KR information about goal achievement does not always ensure learning enhancement and that KP information about movement pattern is the most powerful form of feedback for motor learning and the most useful in motor teaching (Gentile, 1987; Schmidt & Lee, 1999) depending on the skill learned (Magill, 1994). Overall, a combination of KP and KR is superior to one or the other form of feedback alone for both open and closed skills. KP is particularly suggested for closed skills, and KR plus KP, including information on anticipatory functions, for open skills (Gentile, 1987).

Accuracy of Feedback

The accuracy of augmented feedback is important. Erroneous feedback will diminish performance and learning, particularly when provided continuously. Periodic erroneous KR is less disruptive (Schmidt & Lee, 1999). Adolescents with a diagnosis of cerebral palsy have shown improvement in the accuracy of their performance of a simple arm movement when provided with feedback on their actual time of movement, as have nondisabled individuals (Harbourne, 1991). Therefore, the therapist should (1) evaluate the skill (i.e., sensory-motor feedback, novelty, and difficulty level); (2) evaluate augmented feedback characteristics; and (3) evaluate the meaningfulness of the augmented feedback for the learner (Magill, 1994). At any time, feedback should focus on only one or two movement features and should be easily understood by the learner (e.g., "I like your quick reaching up above your head to catch the butterfly," or "It is good to push hard with your feet on the floor and keep a tall, straight back") and accompanied by nonverbal cueing.

Precision of Feedback

More precise, more frequent, and more immediate feedback during practice facilitates performance, but each has been found to be detrimental to learning and to produce dependency in the same way as physical guidance (see Salmoni and colleagues' guidance hypothesis, 1984). Increased precision of feedback content may lead to increased learning, but the precision level of the verbal feedback must be adapted to the learner's level (i.e., less precision earlier, somewhat more precision later). An optimal level of precision has been hypothesized. If feedback is more or less precise than the optimum, subsequent performance is less accurate.

The optimal level of precision has been shown to increase with age. Young children naturally tend to ignore relevant information and respond immediately without using feedback (Barclay & Newell, 1980). Children, however, *can* use feedback to improve their learning, when required. Between the ages of 3.5 and 5 years, they have been reported to make fewer errors when provided with more precise feedback (Shapiro, 1977). Increasingly precise feedback, however, tends to result in more error for younger children (grade 2) but in more accuracy for older children (grade 4).The choice of wording and the format of presentation are critical. Verbal feedback should be presented in key words and short phrases whether it is about the environmental goal (e.g., "It is great that you put your hat on") or about the movement itself (e.g., "Your feet are nice and straight and no kissing knees," "It is very good holding your arms out with elbows straight like an airplane; let's count to twenty moving your wings up and down," "This was too fast and your chin was poking out").

Timing of Feedback

Frequent feedback distracts and interferes with the information-processing activities leading to learning (retention); frequent feedback produces excessive response variability in skill acquisition (Wulf & Schmidt, 1994). Concurrent feedback and terminal, continuous feedback (after each trial), although more effective for performance during practice and for guiding directly to the environmental goal, maximize dependency. The use of "relative" frequency is advocated over continuous feedback (Schmidt & Lee, 1999); for example, providing 50% relative feedback resulted in significantly better learning as measured by retention than providing 100% frequency

feedback and concurrent feedback (Vander Linden et al., 1993; Wulf et al., 1994).

In a one-to-one learning situation (such as a therapy session), reducing the relative frequency of feedback (i.e., increasing the number of no-feedback trials [blank trials]) not only increases learning but also helps the learner to develop an error-detection mechanism and to become more active in problem solving. In addition, asking the child to guess the performance *before* feedback is given helps him or her to focus attention on the task and its sensory qualities (Gentile, 1987). The optimum frequency appears to vary in direct proportion to the complexity of the task. Various methods exist to use a relative frequency of feedback in practice. Intermittent (occasional) feedback may be provided in several different, systematic ways. In *summary* feedback, feedback is withheld for a predetermined number of trials (e.g., 15 to 16 trials during a simple task or in the early part of practice or 5 trials during a complex task or as proficiency increases) (Gable et al., 1991). Then feedback is provided about each trial in a series of trials but only after the series is completed. In the practice of a complex perceptuomotor skill, however, adults have been found to learn equally well when summary feedback ranged between 1 and 20 trials (Christensen et al., 1992). In *average* feedback, an average score is provided after a series of trials is completed (e.g., "The last five times, you sat down slowly and gently all throughout with no flop"). Both summary and average feedback have been reported to promote similar acquisition and retention performance (Weeks & Sherwood, 1994).

In using feedback, the goals are improved learning and performance without feedback, with the child being capable of detecting his or her own errors. One approach consists of a *fading* procedure in which feedback usage is arbitrarily decreased, on an individual basis, from higher to lower relative frequency during the practice session, leading finally to a complete withdrawal. Still another approach is *bandwidth* corrective feedback, which is particularly useful in the earlier stage of learning. Informative feedback is provided only when the learner performs outside a preset band of accuracy (motivational feedback may be used within the bandwidth). For example, a therapist may decide to provide quantitative feedback (KR or KP) only when the child rotates the head less than 45° to look to the right and left sides. This procedure allows for a certain margin of error, and the absence of informative feedback helps reinforce the learner to execute repetitions. For movement tasks, bandwidth feedback has been reported to enhance accuracy and stability better than a pure, relative frequency condition (Winstein, 1991a). Bandwidth KR conditions facilitate learning regardless of the specificity of the movement goal (Lee & Maraj, 1994). Recent studies on *learner-determined* presentation of feedback (KR) indicate that retention is facilitated for subjects who choose when to receive KR compared with subjects who received experimenter-determined KR (Schmidt & Lee, 1999).

Finally, the temporal aspect of extrinsic feedback is another factor influencing learning. Random KR is more beneficial than blocked KR (Schmidt & Lee, 1999). Delayed feedback plus the patient's estimation of outcome error have been reported to improve both performance and retention (motor learning) (Liu & Wrisberg, 1997). After a trial, three distinct periods of time may be considered: *feedback delay, postfeedback delay,* and *intertrial interval.* Extrinsic feedback provided immediately after a trial (a frequent schedule in physical therapy) is actually detrimental to learning, whereas feedback delayed by several seconds to several minutes has no significant negative effect on learning. Learning happens as long as competing events do not occur and interfere during the delay interval. Feedback delay allows the child to engage in the appropriate information processing and retention learning. The postfeedback delay interval (time between the provision of feedback and the next trial) does not appear as a powerful factor in learning as long as the interval is longer than approximately 5 seconds, allowing for planning the next movement. Extremely short (less than 5 seconds) or long (days or weeks) postfeedback delay intervals were reported to have a detrimental effect on performance accuracy, more so in children than in adults. A 12-second processing time, however, reduced performance variability, thereby increasing performance stability in children and adults (Schmidt & Lee, 1999). In addition, postresponse feedback tends to improve retention learning in young adults (Winstein et al., 1996). Other motor activities (interferences) performed during this interval also have a negative effect on the next performance but, in contrast to a feedback-delay interval, do not affect learning negatively and may even produce retention learning (Lee & Magill, 1985).

The effects of the intertrial interval, that is, the time between two trials (the sum of the feedback delay and postfeedback delay intervals), have been the subject of controversy. If too short, inputs conducive to learning may not be processed; if too long, forgetting may occur. Practically, as long as the interval is not too short, this does not appear to affect motor learning adversely (Schmidt, 1988). Therapists, therefore, might optimally delay their intermittent feedback several seconds to several minutes and wait about 12 seconds before engaging the child in the next trial of activity.

Session Length and Frequency

Some considerations are now presented regarding the length (duration) and frequency of the whole therapeutic (practice) session from a motor learning perspective. Length and frequency may vary for three main reasons: (1) the level of demands of the task and related fatigue of the child (i.e., physical, attention, processing, and performance in general); (2) the skill level of the child (i.e., beginner, intermediate, advanced); and (3) the nature of the skill. For beginners, sessions that are demanding should generally be short at first, gradually increasing with the skill level, but frequent and spaced over a long period of time. The intensity of intervention should be purposefully determined. Treatment goals should be functionally oriented and consequently require numerous hours of practice based on sound motor control and pedagogic principles (Croce & DePaepe, 1989; Singer, 1990). Findings from a study on the delivery mode of physical therapists in Ontario treatment centers indicated that individual therapy sessions for preschool children with moderate spastic diplegia last an average of 48 minutes, including 20% (about 10 minutes) of rest; they have an average frequency of 1.4 sessions per week (Larin, 1992).

Determining treatment intensity tends to be the privilege of institutional policy makers and individual therapists. In spite of tools such as the Pediatric Screening manual (Taylor et al., 1983) to assist in this task, therapists stated rationales for intervention frequency and duration that appeared to be primarily based on economic, logistic, and experiential factors (Larin, 1992). Variations in the intensity of therapeutic intervention have been related to therapist availability and severity of infant motor delay; that is, infants with more delayed development tend to receive a greater amount of individual therapy time (Haley, 1988).

Recent meta-analyses have suggested that a high level of intensity and duration may have a positive effect on the efficacy of early intervention, particularly for populations with disabilities (Casto, 1985; Innocenti, 1991). More specifically, in neuropediatrics, Mayo (1991), Bower and McLellan (1992), Horn and colleagues (1995), and Bower and associates (1996) provided evidence that increasing the intensity, duration, and frequency of individual therapy sessions produced substantial change in children's motor development and accelerated acquisition of motor skills. In Mayo's study, infants younger than 18 months of age with delayed or abnormal motor behavior who received weekly, individual, neurodevelopmental therapy for 1 hour over a period of 6 months showed greater changes in their motor development than those who received monthly, individual, 1-hour periods of intervention. In Bower and McLellan's study, children 2 to 12 years old with a diagnosis of cerebral palsy of various types and learning difficulties were involved in individual, 1-hour therapy sessions each school day for 3 weeks; these children demonstrated accelerated acquisition of motor skills during the intervention period compared with before and after.

In a more recent study from Bower and associates (1996), 44 children with spastic quadriplegia of ages 3 to 11 years participated in four groups combining conventional versus intensive physical therapy, and generalized goals vs specific measurable goals. Over the 2-week period, intensive physical therapy produced a slightly greater effect as measured by the Gross Motor Function Measure (GMFM). However, the factor more strongly associated with increased motor skill acquisition was the use of specific measurable goals. Finally, in Horn and colleagues' (1995) study, children with severe cerebral palsy, between 21 and 34 months old, who participated in a neurobehavioral intervention four times per week for 6 to 8 months, demonstrated gains in the acquisition of specific movement components of a treated exemplar skill and of an untreated exemplar skill (requiring the targeted movement components). The children also demonstrated generalization of the trained exemplar skill by performing the skill in a different environment.

Individual intensive direct intervention cannot be excluded from a child's management program. Benefits and constraints must be carefully weighed in making decisions regarding the frequency and intensity of interventions to promote motor learning. Periods of time when movement patterns are in transition during the child's development may potentially emerge as sensitive periods for intervention (Heriza, 1991). Indicators of prognosis found in the "Guide to Physical Therapist Practice" (American Physical Therapy Association, 1997), however, "dictate" the extent of therapeutic sessions per episode of care and do not sufficiently consider the individual needs of the children from a motor-learning perspective. Such guidelines pose serious limitations on physical therapy practice and service delivery. Although the fewer, direct sessions may be optimized with a motor learning framework and specific goals attainment, group therapy and caregiver education and training are increasingly integrated in the therapeutic intervention to meet the challenge.

Group Therapy

Group treatment sessions have been reported to be used by 68% of physical therapists in educational settings (Effgen & Klepper, 1994); 50% of therapists

working with infants and young children provided combinations of individual and group treatment (Lawlor & Henderson, 1989). Yet limited information is available on the logistics and effectiveness of the approach in pediatrics.

Most therapy groups are informal—patients work on individual tasks or several patients are treated at the same time. Documentation is usually maintained on an individual rather than a group basis (Duncombe & Howe, 1995). Therapeutic factors that influence the outcome of group treatments have been identified in occupational therapy for patients with psychosocial disabilities (Falk-Kessler et al., 1991) but have not been fully investigated for clients with physical disabilities. Two small groups of preschool children with developmental delay demonstrated similar increases in both fine and gross motor skills from participating in either individual/direct therapy or group/consultation physical and occupational therapies (Davis & Gavin, 1994). School-age children with learning disabilities, however, were found to benefit significantly more from the large group and consultation intervention than from a combination of small and large group, therapist-directed intervention as measured by change on the Bruininks-Oseretsky Test of Motor Proficiency. Yet when the progress within each group was examined, both methods of service delivery were reported as effective for the particular group of students served (Palisano, 1989). In the adult population, the effectiveness of group education programs for low-back pain has yet to be demonstrated (Cohen et al., 1994), but group therapy has been found to be effective for individuals with hemiplegia, Parkinson disease and multiple sclerosis (Duncombe & Howe, 1995). Clients in group therapy achieved their maximum goal earlier than individually treated clients and maintained their functional status; group therapy was also found to be more cost-effective (Duncombe & Howe, 1995; Trahey, 1991). Appropriate motor learning strategies must be considered in the delivery of group intervention design. Further investigations are needed on delivery models, functional outcomes, and cost-effectiveness of group therapy for children with physical disabilities.

Caregiver Education and Training

Type and frequency of intervention should never be limited to direct, individual, 30-minute to 1-hour treatment sessions or group sessions. The daily activities of the child offer numerous occasions for intervention and should be viewed as an indispensable part of the child's total plan of care. In these instances, the child's motor learning and motor performance may be enhanced or impaired. It is of utmost importance that the instructions provided to the parents or caregivers for addressing the child's functional motor activities reflect motor learning principles and employ relevant motor teaching strategies. The therapeutic and teaching process in caregiver education and training should include both behavioral and reflective orientations and aim at increased caregiver confidence. Behavioral, goal-directed, structured approaches appear more likely to produce change in skills, particularly when modeling, role-play, and feedback are used (van Hasselt et al., 1987). Approaches that include a broad range of relevant skills, such as problem-solving strategies, family interactions, and support, appear to be more effective (with the likelihood of maintenance and generalization) than those concentrating on a limited set of techniques or tasks (Cunningham, 1985).

The involvement of caregivers in planning and applying intervention is embodied in the notion of parent-professional partnership (Mittler & Mittler, 1983) and the family-centered approach (Rosenbaum et al., 1998), as well as in governmental mandates. Although no single approach can respond to the needs of all caregivers, guidelines on some specific strategies are available.

1. Responsiveness to caregiver needs is more important than the location or format of the program. Home and school or center-based approaches should be considered (Gardner & Chapman, 1993).

2. Educational and training programs should lead to long-lasting intrinsic motivation rather than short-lasting extrinsic motivation. Caregiver education should focus on observation, recognition, and acceptance of subtle displays of improvement in the child's development because these have been found to be effective in motivating caregivers to participate in the implementation of home programs for their children (Moxley-Haegert & Serbin, 1983).

3. Mothers benefit from observing and interacting with therapists, often adopting and extrapolating some of the therapeutic activities into their daily routine (Hinjosa & Anderson, 1991).

4. Caregivers are not simply a vehicle for professionals' well-intentioned programs. What we ask of caregivers must make sense in terms of their individual goals, energies, living style and philosophy (McConachie, 1991).

CLINICAL EXAMPLE

In an attempt to unify the various theoretic and instructional concepts presented in this chapter, clinical scenarios intended to foster motor learning and motor performance are now presented. Therapists are encouraged to develop other scenarios based on their clinical experience, reinforcing certain aspects of their professional knowledge and practice and modifying and improving others.

A pediatric physical therapist is engaged in an individual, 1-hour, direct intervention session with a 5-year-old child of average cognitive ability who has a movement dysfunction (diagnosis: moderate spastic diplegia). Without underestimating other potential biomechanical or physiologic needs pertinent to the management of this child, the following functional goal is selected for its potentially broad application in daily activities: following 6 months of intensive therapy and management, the child will be able to walk with a posterior walker the length of the corridor from the classroom to the gym (approximately 50 feet) together with other classmates (nondisabled children) with improved efficiency as measured by a 25% increase in step length and speed (distance per minute), a 25% decrease in cadence (steps per minute), and a decreased heart rate (beats per minute).

The therapist's associated, movement-oriented therapeutic goal, in this case, is to obtain greater selective control (dissociation) of the lower extremities during gait as related to (1) range of movement (i.e., hip and knee flexion and extension); (2) muscle activity (i.e., stability and mobility; stance and swing); and (3) compensatory movement patterns (i.e., upper trunk, upper extremity excess assistance). Improved endurance is also targeted.

The child is functioning at the early stage or verbal-cognitive to motor stages of motor learning in which he or she needs to discover a reasonable, effective approach to the desired movement pattern of walking. Walking is a dynamic, continuous, complex, open-type, functional activity. The objectives are, in one scenario, to gain a short- and long-term skilled "performance" and, in a second scenario, to "learn" the multiple facets of gait. First, the similarities of therapeutic, instructional strategies used in the two scenarios are presented, followed by their respective differences.

Similarities

In both scenarios, the therapist pays attention to the physical aspect of intervention, planning and preparing the different functional areas to ensure security, fun, and appropriateness for the child's motivational level, attentional abilities, and sensory processing status. To this end, the playroom (treatment room) is organized into three ecologically valid stations entailing use of upright movement: cafeteria, library, and dance floor. The corridor leading to the washroom and classroom is also selected as a therapeutic environment.

In a friendly, respectful, and "partnership" manner, the therapist presents in an exciting and genuine way (verbal and nonverbal) the various predetermined, novel play areas. First, the therapist asks the child what he or she would like to do in each area, with more rather than fewer details (promoting preselected goals). On the child's response, the therapist encourages the child through verbal guidance, for about 3 to 5 minutes, to imagine himself or herself doing the chosen activity. The activity may be repeated before moving to the next station (mixing actual and imaginary practice). Then, as necessary, the therapist describes some of the possible movement activities in each (using modeling and verbal labeling) (e.g., "You may reach up or down for your preferred books, going up and down the stool," or "You may dance with slow or fast music, rocking"). The therapist adds his or her choice to the list, incorporating certain risk-taking behaviors (e.g., "I would really like ballet dancing, on one foot, like that!"), and then negotiates, takes turns in the decision making, and gradually fades out the directives to the child.

The therapist's instructions to the child throughout the session incorporate elements of arresting stimuli (e.g., surprise or uncertainty) and are often presented in "chunks." These instructions relate to the child's preselected environmental goals (e.g., "Let's go get your Sesame Street book from the top shelf") but also, if not more, to increasing the child's awareness of certain aspects of the movement pattern. The therapist questions the child (e.g., "How do you reach it so high?" [climbing up on bench with one foot], "What do you do not to fall?" [keep feet apart and stay up straight], or "How does it feel to go so fast?").

Alternating with questions, the therapist also provides relevant information directly about the skill of walking to increase the child's selective attention to critical features. At times this information is about aspects of the environment affecting gait (e.g., "The floor is hard, let's walk on the carpet, it feels soft," or "Watch for the door, which may open quickly; walk more to the side"). At other times, it is about the whole movement (e.g., "Let's walk nice and straight") and, as necessary, about one or two aspects of the movement practiced (e.g., "Keep your feet straight pointing toward Big Bird [touching them] and three fingers further [showing on one's hand]," or "Arms down and knees up straight").

Apart from providing a combination of these two forms of information (environment and movement), the therapist fosters the child's self-correction in different ways. The therapist asks the child: "Tell me what you need to remember and be attentive to before you begin walking" (verbal pretraining). The therapist models some of the correct or incorrect

movements and labels certain important features (e.g., "Look, my toes are all stretched out"). At times, without physical prompting, the therapist asks the child to correct his or her posture or movement (e.g., "Tell me what you need to change"). At other times, the therapist points out to the child how his or her friend performs certain aspects of gait when meeting the friend in the corridor or when in the same playroom area.

In addition, functional selective attention is enhanced by introducing distractions early on and randomly in the treatment session, according, of course, to the child's response (level of confusion and attentiveness) and also to the objective of the practice session (i.e., performance or learning). These might be people walking by, talking, playing, or singing (opened window or door or shared playroom) or using a combination of activities, such as entertaining a conversation or singing while walking. First distractions are gradually introduced (i.e., the child can anticipate them), but as soon as possible they are randomly presented (i.e., unanticipated) to promote greater adaptability and function.

Different activities are practiced in a random fashion, and each one is repeated several times, maintaining a reasonably high level of complexity. Such a sequence might comprise the following: the child sits at the edge of a small rocking chair, one foot slightly in front of the other, stands up and climbs up and down a stool several times to reach different books, coming down through half kneel, and reaching down to give them to a puppet sitting nearby; then the child stands up the same way, picks up a baton and walks forward, sideways, and then backward to the dance floor where ballet starts. Because the child may not be performing optimally during the session, the paradox of performance and learning is explained (in age-appropriate terms) and encouragement given to the child.

Most activities are generated voluntarily with particular attention to the initiation of the movements for the purpose of attaining shorter reaction times and decreased use of compensatory synergies. In addition to setting relative daily living contexts, the therapist instructs the child (with and without the use of modeling) on how to prepare for movement, with an emphasis on adequate base of support and postural, biomechanical alignment (e.g., "One foot behind, one in front, and lean forward to stand up," or "Hip up and straight to bring other foot up on stool and climb," "Pretty tall back to walk backward"). Acknowledging the latency period of the child's reactions, the therapist waits for the child's voluntary initiation of movement. Then the therapist gradually reduces the anticipatory input to the child (fading process) and requests more accuracy and speed in performing the activities, increasing the child's adaptability through use of a greater level of uncertainty (random activities).

Walking and related activities are complex skills to practice. In spite of this, when possible, each activity sequence is practiced in its entirety from the beginning (e.g., kneel to half kneel to stride standing, climbing up and down, walking in different directions). However, if an activity is too complex for the child and totally unsuccessful (goal and movement), the most troublesome parts of the activity are practiced individually, alternating regularly with practice of the whole activity (with physical guidance) for gradual integration and function (progressive part practice). For example, working toward climbing up could involve practicing sustaining weight transfer on one leg for short periods of time, maintaining an erect trunk while bringing the other leg up and down at different heights, transferring weight onto the other leg while placing a foot on the stool and swinging back and forth, and trunk leaning forward over a leg using momentum to climb up. In addition, mental practice is interspersed among the physical trials.

Differences

The practice of walking and related activities for the alternative purposes of performance or learning requires different practice scheduling, degrees of variability, application of physical guidance, and provision of feedback to the child. The differences particular to the two motor teaching scenarios follow.

In the scenario aiming at short- and long-term performance, the therapist chooses a distributed scheduling of practice in which the amount of rest between trials equals or exceeds the amount of time in a trial; hence, fatigue building to the point of impairing performance during the treatment session is avoided. Overlearning an activity becomes the goal; therefore, the therapist does not vary greatly among activities, and, in this case, the time spent walking forward predominates in the treatment session.

In the early stage of motor performance, the therapist uses a high degree of verbal and physical guidance to correct most of the child's movement errors and to obtain an immediate performance. Precise, extrinsic feedback is offered frequently and immediately to the child during (concurrent) and after (continuous terminal) activity trials. The therapist praises the child's success, referring to the goal or movement, and indicates mistakes in a corrective and encouraging manner. In addition, the therapist supplies KR and KP focused on one or two movement features (including anticipatory function) easily understood by the child (e.g., "Great, you kept your hip straight and moved your foot gently up," reinforced by facial expression, or "Oh! What a little step that was; let's stand nicely up tall on this [touch] leg to help take a bigger step to dance with the Sesame Street music!"). Another tactic used might be asking the child to "guess" the level of his or her performance before providing feedback. The feedback is not offered immediately after the performance but rather is delayed several seconds to several minutes and the next trial initiated another 5 to 12 seconds after the feedback. Another tactic would be to ask the child when he or she wants to obtain feedback. At all times interferences (distractions) are minimized to strengthen the performance. In the later stage of refined motor performance, however, practice is associated primarily with intrinsic feedback and minimal therapist input.

In the scenario aiming at learning, the therapist first chooses a massed scheduling of practice in which the amount of practice time in a trial is greater than the amount of rest between trials, in spite of fatigue building up and the likelihood that performance will deteriorate during the treatment session. Distributed scheduling, however, is also advantageous in the practice of complex, continuous activities such as walking. The therapist then begins using a distributed practice schedule and gradually increases the intensity of practice with repetitions; the practice remains somewhat difficult and effortful and generates fatigue.

High-variable practice leads to learning for retention and transfer, particularly in the case of open skills such as walking. The therapist diversifies the activities in two ways: (1) the practice of different but similar actions (intertask with the same movement class) (e.g., marching, standing up from half kneeling, climbing up a stool or even stairs [if one concedes that they all require various types of dissociation]); and (2) the practice of the same task altering one characteristic such as distance, speed, direction, or timing of the movement pattern (intratask), for example, walking a moderate and long distance, at moderate and fast speeds (not too slow), forward, sideways, and backward and on varied surfaces. In the early learning of an activity, the therapist may reduce somewhat the speed and sequence of practice into small blocks of several trials, breaking down the activity; soon after, the therapist shifts to random, variable practice, using the same speed and accuracy of the entire, desired, age-appropriate gait and practicing in different situations and environments.

In practice for learning, the therapist uses the least possible amount of verbal and physical guidance (relative frequency) in a fading manner. A combination of trial-and-error, guided, and independent movements is incorporated in the child's practice session. When guidance is used, the degree and the timing are adjusted to the child's need at the different periods of a task practice (i.e., preset anticipatory postural adjustments, movement initiation, sustained control, or termination) and to the child's need to gain stability and mobility. In the early stage of practice, however, when movements are somewhat slower and activities unfamiliar (e.g., half kneeling or walking backward) and the child is more fearful and at risk of injury, the therapist employs a greater amount of guidance while attempting to gradually reduce it as much as possible. This is achieved by offering less manual support or more distal assistance or by using a medium between the therapist and the child (e.g., baton, ball, book, walker).

Extrinsic feedback provided for learning purposes is of the same types as for performance (i.e., qualitative and quantitative [KR + KP]); the level of precision and frequency, however, differs. Earlier in practice, the precision of the feedback is minimal, offered in key words or short sentences, and then increased as the child progresses. The therapist presents feedback in a relative frequency during the treatment session; the higher the task complexity for the child, the more feedback is provided. The therapist chooses among five ways to determine this relative frequency: (1) fading (i.e., gradually reducing to no feedback); (2) average (e.g., after every fifth trial, giving feedback about that trial); (3) summary (e.g., after a predetermined number of five trials, giving feedback about all the previous trials); (4) bandwidth technique (i.e., only after trials in which performance is outside a predetermined acceptable range, allowing for a margin of error); or (5) learner-determined presentation of feedback (in age-appropriate terms). The timing of the feedback for learning remains the same as for performance purposes (i.e., several seconds to several minutes after a trial with a delay of 5 to 12 seconds before the next trial). Finally, to heighten learning, the therapist introduces other motor activities or distractors (interferences) at a higher rate than in the performance scenario.

CONCLUSION

Future Research

Clinical and laboratory research is required to further document the factors of critical importance to motor learning of children. Normative data are greatly needed on information processing, particularly during the early stage of skill acquisition in young children. Comparative and single-subject data banks on the motor learning processes of children with motor impairment would assist the practitioner and researcher in their respective and collaborative activities. Instructional strategies for motor learning and performance must be tested on large populations of children at varied ages with different motor, cognitive, and social levels of functioning.

Clinical research is also required to further understand therapists' practice and knowledge (explicit and implicit) of the motor learning framework. The study of groups of therapists treating various populations of children with neurologic and orthopedic impairment would reveal a more comprehensive picture of motor teaching patterns used in pediatric physical therapy. More specifically, investigation may address how therapists formulate goals (action or movement) for treatment sessions as a whole, as well as for each task practiced, with regard to emphasis on performance versus motor learning, function, or neuromuscular needs. Further insight into the therapists' taxonomy of tasks is necessary to ascertain the appropriateness and sequencing of strategies and optimal types of scheduling practice. Through research with control and experimental groups, the optimal proportions of strategies for different populations could be determined.

Implications

The motor learning framework has direct implications for the physical therapist as clinical educator interacting with the child, the child's parents or caregivers, colleagues, and students. In the learning-teaching relationship, guidelines from models are useful to provide sound principles for adapting tested strategies to the learner. A motor learning approach is pertinent to each of these interactions.

Motor learning theories have been transposed into motor teaching models, and numerous instructional strategies have been suggested. Therapists already use many of the strategies with varying degrees of conscious selection and competency. Their professional working knowledge, however, does not usually incorporate all of the important elements of the theoretic motor learning framework. The professional challenge is to continuously relate new theories to knowledge derived from practice. This chapter on motor learning may provide pediatric physical therapists with useful information for such a process. It may also offer a means to guide therapists' systematic reflection on their practice and to foster renewed energy in therapy.

References

Abbs, JH, Gracco, VL, & Cole, KJ. Control of multimovement coordination: Sensorimotor mechanisms in speech motor programming. Journal of Motor Behavior, 16:195-231, 1984.

Adams, JA. A closed-loop theory of motor learning. Journal of Motor Behavior, 3:111-149, 1971.

American Physical Therapy Association. Guide to Physical Therapist Practice. Physical Therapy, 77:1163-1650, 1997.

Arend, S. Developing perceptual skills prior to motor performance. Motor Skills: Theory into Practice, 4:11–17, 1980.

Asatryan, DG, & Feldman, AG. Biophysics of complex systems and mathematical models. Biophysics, 10:925–935, 1965.

Ashy, MH, Lee, AM, & Landin, DK. Relationship of practice using correct technique to achievement in a motor skill. Journal of Teaching in Physical Education, 7:115–120, 1988.

Bakshi, R, Bhambhani, Y, & Madill, H. The effects of task preference during purposeful and nonpurposeful activities. American Journal of Occupational Therapy, 45:912–916, 1991.

Barclay, C, & Newell, K. Children's processing of information in motor skill acquisition. Journal of Experimental Child Psychology, 30:98–108, 1980.

Bernstein, N. The Co-ordination and Regulation of Movements. Oxford: Pergamon Press, 1967.

Bower, E, & McLellan, DL. Effect of increased exposure to physiotherapy on skill acquisition of children with cerebral palsy. Developmental Medicine and Child Neurology, 34:25–39, 1992.

Bower E, McLellan, DL, Arney, J, & Campbell, MJ. A randomised controlled trial of different intensities of physiotherapy and different goal-setting procedures in 44 children with cerebral palsy. Developmental Medicine and Child Neurology, 38:226–237, 1996.

Brenière, Y, Cuong Do, M, & Bouisset, S. Are dynamic phenomena prior to stepping essential to walking? Journal of Motor Behavior, 19:62–76, 1987.

Bressan, ES, & Woollacott, MH. A prescriptive paradigm for sequencing instruction in physical education. Human Movement Science, 1:155–175, 1982.

Brown, DA, Effgen, SK, & Palisano, RJ. Performance following ability-focussed physical therapy intervention in individuals with severely limited physical and cognitive abilities. Physical Therapy, 78:934–950, 1998.

Carlson, JL. Evaluating patient motivation in physical disabilities practice settings. The American Journal of Occupational Therapy, 51:347–351, 1997.

Carson, LM, & Wiegand, RL. Motor schema formation and retention in young children: A test of Schmidt's schema theory. Journal of Motor Behavior, 11:247–251, 1979.

Carter, RE. A Behavioral Analysis of Interactions between Physical Therapists and Children with Cerebral Palsy during Treatment. Unpublished doctoral dissertation, Northern Illinois University, 1989.

Casto, G. The Relationships between Program Intensity and Efficacy in Early Intervention. Unpublished manuscript, Utah State University, Early Intervention Research Institute, Logan, Utah, 1985.

Christensen, S, Fitch, N, & Winstein, C. Acquisition and retention of a partial weight bearing skill: Effect of practice with summary knowledge of results (Abstract). Physical Therapy, 72(suppl 6):S51–S52, 1992.

Cintas, HM. The relationship of motor skill level and risk-taking during exploration in toddlers. Pediatric Physical Therapy, 4:165–170, 1992.

Clark, JE. Developmental differences in response processing. Journal of Motor Behavior, 14:247-254, 1982.

Cohen, JE, Goel, V, Frank, JW, Bombardier, C, Peloso, P, & Guillemin, F. Group education interventions for people with low back pain. Spine, 19:1214–1222, 1994.

Cook Merrill, S, Slavik, B, Holloway, E, Richter, E, & David, S. Environment: Implications for Occupational Therapy Practice. Rockville, MD: American Occupational Therapy Association, 1990.

Coster, WJ, & Jaffe, LE. Current concepts of children's perceptions of control. American Journal of Occupational Therapy, 45:19–25, 1991.

Croce, R, & DePaepe, J. A critique of therapeutic intervention programming with reference to an alternative approach based on motor learning theory. Physical and Occupational Therapy in Pediatrics, 9(3):5–33, 1989.

Crocker, MD, MacKay-Lyons, M, & McDonnell, E. Forced use of the upper extremity in cerebral palsy: A single-case design. The American Journal of Occupational Therapy, 51:824–833, 1997.

Cunningham, C. Training and education approaches for parents of children with special needs. British Journal of Medical Psychology, 58:285–305, 1985.

Darling, WG, & Cooke, JD. Changes in the variability of movement trajectories with practice. Journal of Motor Behavior, 19:291-309, 1987.

Davids, JR, Bagley, AM, & Bryan, M. Kinematic and kinetic analysis of running in children with cerebral palsy. Developmental Medicine and Child Neurology, 40:528–535, 1998.

Davis, PL, & Gavin, WJ. Comparison of individual group/consultation treatment methods for preschool children with developmental delays. American Journal of Occupational Therapy, 48:155–161, 1994.

Davis, WE, & Burton, AW. Ecological task analysis: Translating movement behavior theory into practice. Adapted Physical Activity Quarterly, 8:154–177, 1991.

Duff, SV, & Gordon, AM. Sensorimotor control of the hand in children with hemiplegic cerebral palsy: Use of tactile and proprioceptive information (Abstract). Physical Therapy, 78:S37, 1998.

Duncombe, LW, & Howe, MC. Group treatment: Goals, tasks, and economic implications. American Journal of Occupational Therapy, 49:199–205, 1995.

Edwards, R. The effects of performance standards on behavior patterns and motor skill achievement in children. Journal of Teaching in Physical Education, 7:90–102, 1988.

Effgen, SK, & Klepper, SE. Survey of physical therapy practice in educational settings. Pediatric Physical Therapy, 6:15–21, 1994.

Eidson, TA, & Stadulis, RE. Effects of variability of practice on the transfer and performance of open and closed motor skills. Adapted Physical Activity Quarterly, 8:342–356, 1991.

Eliasson, A, Gordon, AM, & Forssberg, H. Basic co-ordination of manipulative forces of children with cerebral palsy. Developmental Medicine and Child Neurology, 33:661–670, 1991.

Eliasson, A, Gordon, AM, & Forssberg, H. Impaired anticipatory control of isometric forces during grasping by children with cerebral palsy. Developmental Medicine and Child Neurology, 34:216–225, 1992.

Elliot, D, Gray, S, & Weeks, DJ. Verbal cuing and motor skill acquisition for adults with Down syndrome. Adapted Physical Activity Quarterly, 8:210–220, 1991.

Embrey, DG, & Adams, LS. Clinical applications of procedural changes by experienced and novice pediatric physical therapists. Pediatric Physical Therapy, 8:122–132, 1996.

Embrey, DG, & Hylton, N. Clinical applications of movement scripts by experienced and novice pediatric physical therapists. Pediatric Physical Therapy, 8:3–14, 1996.

Fairweather, MM, & Sidaway, B. Hemispheric teaching strategies in the acquisition and retention of a motor skill. Research Quarterly for Exercise and Sport, 65:40–47, 1994.

Falk-Kessler, J, Momich, C, and Perel, S. Therapeutic factors in occupational therapy groups. American Journal of Occupational Therapy, 45:59–66, 1991.

Fansler, CL, Poff, CL, & Shepard, KF. Effects of mental practice on balance in elderly women. Physical Therapy, 65:1332–1338, 1985.

Fazio, LS. Tell me a story: The therapeutic metaphor in the practice of pediatric occupational therapy. American Journal of Occupational Therapy, 46:112–119, 1992.

Feltz, DL, & Landers, DM. The effects of mental practice on motor skill learning and performance: A meta-analysis. Journal of Sport Psychology, 5:25–57, 1983.

Fetters, L: Cerebral palsy: Contemporary treatment concepts. In Lister, MJ (Ed.), Contemporary Management of Motor Control Problems: Proceedings of the II Step Conference. Alexandria, VA: Foundation for Physical Therapy, 1991, pp. 219-224.

Fineman, JB, & Gentile, AM. Variability of practice and transfer of training (Abstract). Physical Therapy, 78:S42, 1998.

Fitts, PM, & Posner, MI. Human Performance. Belmont, CA: Brooks/Cole, 1967.

Gable, CD, Shea, CH, & Wright, DL. Summary knowledge of results. Research Quarterly for Exercise and Sport, 62:285–292, 1991.

Gabriele, TE, Hall, CR, & Buckolz, EE. Practice schedule effects on the acquisition and retention of a motor skill. Human Movement Science, 6:1–16, 1987.

Garcia, C. Gender differences in young children's interactions when learning fundamental motor skills. Research Quarterly for Exercise and Sport, 65:213–225, 1994.

Gardner, JF, & Chapman, MS. Developing Staff Competence for Supporting People with Developmental Disabilities. Baltimore: Paul H. Brookes, 1993.

Gentile, AM. A working model of skill acquisition with application to teaching. Quest, 44:3–23, 1972.

Gentile, AM. Skill acquisition: Action, movement, and neuromotor processes. In Carr, JA, & Shepherd, RB (Eds.), Movement Science: Foundations for Physical Therapy in Rehabilitation. Rockville, MD: Aspen, 1987, pp. 93–154.

Gentile, AM. The nature of skill acquisition: Therapeutic implications for children with movement disorders. Medicine and Sport Science, 36:31–40, 1992.

Gibson, EJ. Principles of Perceptual Learning and Development. New York: Appleton-Century-Crofts, 1969.

Gibson, EJ. Exploratory behavior in the development of perceiving, acting, and the acquiring of knowledge. Annual Review of Psychology, 39:1–41, 1988.

Gibson, JJ. The senses considered as perceptual systems. Boston: Houghton-Miffin, 1966.

Glynn, T. Contexts for learning: Implications for mildly and moderately handicapped children. Australian and New Zealand Journal of Developmental Disabilities, 10:257–263, 1985.

Goldberger, M, & Gerney, P. Effects of learner use of practice time on skill acquisition of fifth grade children. Journal of Teaching in Physical Education, 10:84–95, 1990.

Gould, DR, & Roberts, GC. Modeling and motor skill acquisition. Quest, 33:214–230, 1982.

Haas, G, Diener, HC, Rapp, H, & Dichgans, J. Development of feedback and feedforward control of upright stance. Developmental Medicine and Child Neurology, 31:481–488, 1989.

Hadders-Algra, M, Brogen, E, & Forssberg, H. Training affects the development of postural adjustments in sitting infants. Journal of Physiology, 493:289–298, 1996.

Haley, SM. Patterns of physical and occupational therapy implementation in early motor intervention. Topics in Early Childhood Special Education, 7:46–63, 1988.

Hall, KG, & Magill, RA. Variability of practice and contextual interference in motor skill learning. Journal of Motor Behavior, 27:299–309, 1995.

Harbourne, RT. Error detection skills in cerebral palsy (Abstract). Physical Therapy, 71(suppl 6):S9, 1991.

Hartveld, A, & Hegarty, JR. Augmented feedback and physiotherapy practice. Physiotherapy, 82:480–490, 1996.

Haubenstricker, J, & Seefeldt, V. Acquisition of motor skills during childhood. In Seefeldt, V. (Ed.), Physical Activity and Well Being. Reston, VA: American Alliance for Health, Physical Education, Recreation and Dance, 1986, pp. 41–104.

Heitman, R, Erdmann, J, Gurchiek, L, Kovaleski, J, & Gilley, W. From the field. Constant versus variable practice in learning a motor task using individuals with learning disabilities. Clinical Kinesiology, 51:62–65, 1997.

Heriza, CB. Implications of a dynamical systems approach to understanding infant kicking behavior. Physical Therapy, 71:222–235, 1991.

Higgins, S. Motor skill acquisition. Physical Therapy, 71:123–139, 1991.

Hinjosa, J, & Anderson, J. Mother's perceptions of home treatment programs for their preschool children with cerebral palsy. American Journal of Occupational Therapy, 45:273–279, 1991.

Holding, DH. Principles of Training. Oxford, England: Pergamon Press, 1965.

Hood, B, & Atkinson, J. Sensory visual loss and cognitive deficits in the selective attentional system of normal infants and neurologically impaired children. Developmental Medicine and Child Neurology, 32:1067–1077, 1990.

Horn, EM, Warren, SF, & Jones, HA. An experimental analysis of neurobehavioral motor intervention. Developmental Medicine and Child Neurology, 37:697–714, 1995.

Innocenti, MS. More or less: A review of intensity as a program variable in early intervention. Paper presented at the meeting of the Society for Research in Child Development, Seattle, WA, April 1991.

James, W. The Principles of Psychology, Vol. 1. New York: Holt, 1890.

Jarus, T, & Gol, D. The effect of kinesthetic stimulation on the acquisition and retention of a gross motor skill by children with and without sensory integration disorders. Physical and Occupational Therapy in Pediatrics, 14(3/4):59–73, 1995.

Jones, G, & Cale, A. Goal difficulty, anxiety and performance. Ergonomics, 40:319–333, 1997.

Kamm, K, Thelen, E, & Jensen, JL. A dynamical systems approach to motor development. Physical Therapy, 70:763–775, 1990.

Kauffman, IB, & Ridenour, M. Influence of an infant walker on onset and quality of walking pattern of locomotion: An electromyographic investigation. Perceptual and Motor Skills, 45:1323–1329, 1977.

Kelso, JAS. Anticipatory dynamical systems, intrinsic pattern dynamics and skill learning. Human Movement Science, 10:93–111, 1991.

Kerr, R. Schema theory applied to skill acquisition. Motor Skills: Theory into Practice, 3:15–20, 1978.

King, EM, Gooch, JE, Howell, GH, Peters, ML, Bloswick, DS, & Brown, DR. Evaluation of the hip-extensor tricycle in improving gait in children with cerebral palsy. Developmental Medicine and Child Neurology, 35:1048–1054, 1993.

Koegel, RL, & Rincover, A. Some detrimental effects of using extra stimuli to guide learning in normal and autistic children. Journal of Abnormal Child Psychology, 4:59–71, 1976.

Kohl, RM, Ellis, SD, & Roenker, DL. Alternating actual and imagery practice: Preliminary theoretical considerations. Research Quarterly for Exercise and Sport, 63:162–170, 1992.

Larin, H. Knowledge in Practice: Motor Learning Theories in Pediatric Physiotherapy. Unpublished doctoral dissertation, University of Toronto, 1992.

Lawlor, MC, & Henderson, A. A descriptive study of the clinical patterns of occupational therapy working with infants and young children. American Journal of Occupational Therapy, 43:755–764, 1989.

Lee, TD, & Magill, RA. Can forgetting facilitate acquisition? In Goodman, D, Wilberg, RB, & Franks, IM (Eds.), Differing Perspectives in Motor Learning, Memory, and Control. North Holland: Elsevier Science, 1985, pp. 3–22.

Lee, TD, & Maraj, BK. Effects of bandwidth goals and bandwidth knowledge of results on motor learning. Research Quarterly for Exercise and Sport, 65:244–249, 1994.

Lee, TD, White, MA, & Carnaham, H. On the role of knowledge of results in motor learning: Exploring the guidance hypothesis. Journal of Motor Behavior, 22:191–208, 1990.

Lewthwaite, R. Motivational considerations in physical activity involvement. Physical Therapy, 70:808–819, 1990.

Lin, K, Wu, C, & Trombly, CA. Effects of task goal on movement kinematics and line bisection performance in adults without disabilities. American Journal of Occupational Therapy, 52:179–187, 1998.

Liu, J, & Wrisberg, CA. The effect of knowledge of results delay and the subjective estimation of movement on the acquisition and retention of a motor skill. Research Quarterly for Exercise and Sport, 68:145–151, 1997.

Lozoff, B. Iron and learning potential in childhood. Bulletin of the New York Academy of Medicine, 65:1050–1066, 1989.

Magill, RA. The influence of augmented feedback on skill learning depends on characteristics of the skill and the learner. Quest, 46:314–327, 1994.

Maring, JR. Effects of mental practice on rate of skill acquisition. Physical Therapy, 70:165–172, 1990.

Marteniuk, RG. Information Processing in Motor Skills. New York: Holt, Rinehart & Winston, 1976.

Marteniuk, RG. Motor skill performance and learning: Considerations for rehabilitation. Physiotherapy Canada, 31:187–202, 1979.

Marteniuk, RG, Mackenzie, CL, & Leavitt, JL. Representational and physical accounts of motor and learning: can they account for the data? In Colley, AM, & Beech, JR (Eds.): Cognition and Action in Skilled Behavior. North-Holland: Elsevier Science, 1988, pp. 173–190.

Mayo, NE. The effect of physical therapy for children with motor delay and cerebral palsy. American Journal of Physical Medicine and Rehabilitation, 70:258–267, 1991.

Mayston, MJ. The Bobath concept: Evolution and application. Medicine and Sport Science, 36:1–6, 1992.

McConachie, HR. Home-based teaching: What are we asking parents? Child: Care, Health and Development, 17:123–136, 1991.

McCulloch, WS. A heterarchy of values determined by the topology of nervous nets. Bulletin of Mathematical Biophysics, 7:89–95, 1945.

Michaels, CF, & Carello, C. Direct Perception. Englewood Cliffs, NJ: Prentice-Hall, 1981.

Mittler, PJ, & Mittler, H. Partnership with parents: An overview. In Mittler, P, & McConachie, H (Eds.), Parents, Professionals and Mentally Handicapped People: Approaches to Partnership. Beckenham: Croom Helm, 1983.

Moxley-Haegert, L, & Serbin, LA. Developmental education for parents of delayed infants: Effects on parental motivation and children's development. Child Development, 54:1324–1331, 1983.

Nashner, LM, Shumway-Cook, A, & Marin, O. Stance posture control in select groups of children with cerebral palsy: Deficits in sensory organization and muscular coordination. Experimental Brain Research, 49:393–409, 1983.

NDTA. Neuro-Developmental Treatment Association—Instructors Group Minutes. Chicago, IL: NDTA, 1997.

Newell, KM, Carlton, MJ, & Antoniou, A. The interaction of criterion and feedback information in learning a drawing task. Journal of Motor Behavior, 22:536–552, 1990.

Newell, KM, & Corcos, DM. Variability and Motor Control. Champaign, IL: Human Kinetics, 1993.

Nicolson, RI. Cognitive factors in simple reactions: A developmental study. Journal of Motor Behavior, 14:69–80, 1982.

Ohr, PS, Fagen, JW, Rovee-Collier, C, Hayne, H, & Vander Linde, E. Amount of training and retention by infants. Developmental Psychobiology, 22:69–80, 1989.

Olney, S. New developments in the biomechanics of gait in children with cerebral palsy. In Topics in Pediatrics: Lesson 1. Alexandria, VA: American Physical Therapy Association, 1989.

Orme, M. Teaching Strategies Kit. Toronto, Ontario: Ontario Institute for Studies in Education, 1978.

Palisano, RJ. Comparison of two methods of service delivery for students with learning disabilities. Physical and Occupational Therapy in Pediatrics, 9(3):79–100, 1989.

Pohl, PS, Winstein, C, & Lewthwaite, R. Processes underlying motor learning: A methodological perspective (Abstract). Physical Therapy, 72(suppl 6):S10, 1992.

Poretta, DL, & Surburg, PR. Imagery and physical practice in the acquisition of gross motor timing of coincidence by adolescents with mild mental retardation. Perceptual and Motor Skills, 80:1171–1183, 1995.

Ratner, HH, & Foley, MA. A unifying framework for the development of children's activity memory. Advances in Child Development, 25:33–105, 1994.

Ritson, RJ. Psychomotor skill teaching: Beyond the command style. Journal of Physical Education, Recreation, and Dance, 58:36–37, 1987.

Roberton, MA, & Halverson, LE. The developing child—His changing movement. In London, B (Ed.), Physical Education for Children: A Focus on the Teaching Process. Philadelphia: Lea & Febiger, 1977.

Rosenbaum, P, King, S, Law, M, King, G, & Evans J. Family-centered service: A conceptual framework and research review. Physical and Occupational Therapy in Pediatrics, 18(1):1–20, 1998.

Runnings, DW, & Diewert, GL. Movement cue reproduction under preselection. Journal of Motor Behavior, 14:213–227, 1982.

Sage, GH. Motor Learning and Control: A Neuropsychological Approach. Dubuque, IA: William C. Brown, 1984.

Salmoni, AW, Schmidt, RA, & Walter, CB. Knowledge of results and motor learning: A review and critical reappraisal. Psychological Bulletin, 95:355–386, 1984.

Schempp, PG. Enhancing creative thinking: A study of children making decisions in human movement programs. Human Movement Science, 2:91–104, 1983.

Schmidt, RA. A schema theory of discrete motor skill learning. Psychological Review, 82:225–260, 1975.

Schmidt, RA. Schema theory: Implications for movement education. Motor Skills: Theory into Practice, 2:36–48, 1977.

Schmidt, RA. Motor control and learning: A behavioral emphasis. Champaign, IL: Human Kinetics Publishers, 1988.

Schmidt, RA. Motor Learning and Performance. Champaign, IL: Human Kinetics Publishers, 1991.

Schmidt, RA, & Lee, TD. Motor Control and Learning: A Behavioral Emphasis. Champaign, IL: Human Kinetics, 1999.

Scholz, JP. Dynamic pattern theory: Some implications for therapeutics. Physical Therapy, 70:827–843, 1990.

Seitz, RH, & Wilson, CL. Effect on gait of motor task learning acquired in a sitting position. Physical Therapy, 67:1089–1094, 1987.

Shapiro, DC. Knowledge of results and motor learning in preschool children. Research Quarterly for Exercise and Sport, 48:154–158, 1977.

Shea, CH, & Kohl, RM. Specificity and variability of practice. Research Quarterly for Exercise and Sport, 61:169–177, 1990.

Sheridan, MR. Planning and controlling simple movements. In Smyth, MM, & Wing, AM (Eds.), The Psychology of Human Movement. London: Academic Press, 1984, pp. 47–82.

Sherwood, DE. The benefits of random variable practice for spatial accuracy and error detection in a rapid aiming task. Research Quarterly for Exercise and Sport, 67:35–43, 1996.

Shumway-Cook, A, & Woollacott, MH. The growth of stability: Postural control from a developmental perspective. Journal of Motor Behavior, 17:131–147, 1985.

Sideway, B. Motor programming as a function of constraints on movement initiation. Journal of Motor Behavior, 23:120–130, 1991.

Simpson, RL, & Galbo, JJ. Interaction and learning: Theorizing on the art of teaching. Interchange, 17:37–51, 1986.

Singer, RN. Motor learning research: Meaningful ways for physical educators or waste of time? Quest, 42:114–125, 1990.

Smith, PJ. Attention and the contextual interference effect for a continuous task. Perceptual and Motor Skills, 84:83–92, 1997.

Sparrow, WA. The efficiency of skilled performance. Journal of Motor Behavior, 15:237–261, 1983.

Steyer David, K. Motor sequencing strategies in school-aged children. Physical Therapy, 65:883–889, 1985.

Stratton, RK. Information processing deficits in children's motor performance: Implications for instruction. Motor Skills: Theory into Practice, 3:49–55, 1978.

Surburg, PR, Poretta, DL, & Sutlive, V. Use of imagery practice for improving a motor skill. Adapted Physical Activity Quarterly, 12: 217–227, 1995.

Tarantola, J, Nardone, A, Tacchini, E, & Schieppati, M. Human stance stability improves with the repetition of the task: Effect of foot position and visual condition. Neuroscience Letters, 228:75–78, 1997.

Taylor, A, & Gousie, G. The ecology of learning environments for children. CEFP Journal, July-August:23–28, 1988.

Taylor, D, Christopher, M, & Freshman, S. Pediatric Screening: A Tool for Occupational and Physical Therapists. Seattle: University of Washington, 1983.

Thaut, MH, Hurt, CP, Dragon, D, & McIntosh, GC. Rhythmic entrainment of gait patterns in children with cerebral palsy. AACPDM Abstracts, 40:15, 1998.

Thelen, E, Kelso, JAS, & Fogel, A. Self-organizing systems and infant motor development. Developmental Reviews, 7:39–65, 1987.

Thomas, JR, Gallagher, JD, & Purvis, GJ. Reaction time and anticipation time: Effects of development. Research Quarterly for Exercise and Sport, 52:359–367, 1981.

Toglia, JP. Generalization of treatment: A multicontext approach to cognitive perceptual impairment in adults with brain injury. American Journal of Occupational Therapy, 45:505–516, 1991.

Trahey PH. A comparison of cost-effectiveness of two types of occupational therapy services. American Journal of Occupational Therapy, 45:397–400, 1991.

Tscharnuter, I. A new therapy approach to movement organization. Physical and Occupational Therapy in Pediatrics, 13(2):19–40, 1993.

Turvey, MT, & Carello, C. The ecological approach to perceiving-acting: A pictorial essay. Acta Psychologica, 63:133–155, 1986.

Vander Linden, DW, Cauraugh, JH, & Green, TA. The effect of frequency of kinetic feedback on learning an isometric motor force production task in nondisabled subjects. Physical Therapy, 73:79–87, 1993.

van der Weel, FR, van der Meer, ALH, & Lee, DN. Effect of task on movement control in cerebral palsy: Implications for assessment and therapy. Developmental Medicine and Child Neurology, 33: 419–426, 1991.

Van Hasselt, VB, Sisson, LA, & Aach, SR. Parent training to increase compliance in a young multihandicapped child. Journal of Behavior Therapy and Experimental Psychiatry, 18:275–283, 1987.

van Rossum, JHA. The level of organization of the motor schema. Journal of Motor Behavior, 12:145–148, 1980.

VanSant, AF. Life-span development in functional tasks. Physical Therapy, 70:788–798, 1990.

Vurpillot, E. The development of scanning strategies and their relation to visual differentiation. Journal of Experimental Child Psychology, 6:632–650, 1968.

Wade, MG. Coincidence anticipation of young normal and handicapped children. Journal of Motor Behavior, 12:103–112, 1980.

Weeks, DL, & Sherwood, DE. A comparison of knowledge of results scheduling methods for promoting motor skill acquisition and retention. Research Quarterly for Exercise and Sport, 65:136–142, 1994.

Weiss, MR, Ebbeck, V, & Wiese-Bjornstal, DM. Developmental and psychological factors related to children's observational learning of physical skills. Pediatric Exercise Science, 5:301–317, 1993.

Wickstrom, RL. Fundamental Motor Patterns. Philadelphia: Lea & Febiger, 1977.

Williams, JG. Motoric modeling: Theory and research. Journal of Human Movement Studies, 24:237–279, 1993.

Williams, K. Age difference on a coincident anticipation task: Influence of stereotypic or "preferred" movement speed. Journal of Motor Behavior, 17:389–410, 1985.

Winstein, CJ. Knowledge of results and motor learning: Implications for physical therapy. Physical Therapy, 71:140–149, 1991a.

Winstein, CJ. Designing practice for motor learning: Clinical implications. In Lister, MJ (Ed.), Contemporary Management of Motor Control Problems. Proceedings of the II Step Conference. Alexandria, VA: Foundation for Physical Therapy, 1991b, pp. 65–76.

Winstein, CJ. Effects of physical guidance and knowledge of results on motor learning: Support for the guidance hypothesis. Research Quarterly for Exercise and Sport, 65:316–323, 1994.

Winstein, CJ, Gardner, ER, McNeal, DR, Barto, PT, & Nicholson, DE. Standing balance training: Effect on balance and locomotion in hemiparetic adults. Archives of Physical Medicine and Rehabilitation, 70:755–762, 1989.

Winstein, CJ, Pohl, PS, Cardinale, C, Green, A, Scholtz, L, & Sauber Waters, C. Learning a partial-weight-bearing skill: Effectiveness of two forms of feedback. Physical Therapy, 76:985–993, 1996.

Woodworth, RS. The accuracy of voluntary movement. Psychological Review, 3(suppl 2), 1899.

Wulf, G, Lee, TD, & Schmidt, RA. Reducing knowledge of results about relative versus absolute timing: Differential effects on learning. Journal of Motor Behavior, 26:362–369, 1994.

Wulf, G, & Schmidt, RA. Feedback-induced variability and the learning of generalized motor programs. Journal of Motor Behavior, 26:348–361, 1994.

Recommended References

Duncombe, LW, & Howe, MC. Group treatment: Goals, tasks, and economic implications. American Journal of Occupational Therapy, 49:199–205, 1995.

Horn, EM, Warren, SF, & Jones, HA. An experimental analysis of neurobehavioral motor intervention. Developmental Medicine & Child Neurology, 37:697–714, 1995.

Jones G, & Cale, A. Goal difficulty, anxiety and performance. Ergonomics, 40:319–333, 1997.

Magill, RA. The influence of augmented feedback on skill learning depends on characteristics of the skill and the learner. Quest, 46:314–327, 1994.

Schmidt, RA, & Lee, TD. Motor control and learning: A behavioral emphasis. Champaign, IL: Human Kinetics, 1999.

Winstein, CJ. Effects of physical guidance and knowledge of results on motor learning: Support for the guidance hypothesis. Research Quarterly for Exercise and Sport, 65:316–323, 1994.

CHAPTER
7

Decision Making
in Pediatric Physical Therapy

ROBERT J. PALISANO, PT, ScD
SUZANN K. CAMPBELL, PT, PhD, FAPTA
SUSAN R. HARRIS, PT, PhD, FAPTA

Every day, pediatric physical therapists must make decisions that affect the lives of children and their families. On what basis do we make these important decisions? Physical therapy has long used the empirical base of collective experience in clinical practice that is passed down from clinicians and educators to successive generations of new practitioners. Although this knowledge has served clinicians and their clients well throughout the brief history of our discipline, today's health care climate requires more. Increasingly, physicians and other health professionals, third-party payers, and the public expect that physical therapists will use scientific evidence and more valid and reliable decision methods as the basis for their practice. In managed care settings, cost efficiency and client satisfaction measures are expected as guides to what will be approved and reimbursed. Care principles enunciated by clients have entered the picture, too, as consumers became active advocates for best practice (Harrison, 1993).

In general, pediatric physical therapists make several types of decisions: (1) who needs intervention and why; (2) how children in need of intervention should be served, for example, which direct interventions should be applied, what types of home instruction should be provided, how should care be coordinated; (3) how outcomes of intervention and child and family satisfaction should be documented; (4) the number of visits required to achieve anticipated outcomes; and (5) how the overall clinical program should be evaluated for effectiveness and efficiency in achieving goals, attaining functional outcomes, promoting health, and preventing disability. The purpose of this chapter is to describe the problems inherent in making decisions and to review the methods that pediatric physical therapists have available to them for making different types of decisions.

Discussion of these topics can best be made from the perspective of evidence-based practice and the disabling process. Thus, before embarking on our task of analyzing decision making, we describe the conceptual framework for evidence-based practice and the disabling process.

EVIDENCE-BASED PRACTICE

Evidence-based practice refers to the use of the best available knowledge and research to guide clinical decision making within the context of the individual client (Sackett et al., 1996). The Evidence-Based Medicine Working Group (1992) proposes that an evidence-based approach to clinical decision making emphasizes findings from sound clinical research and deemphasizes intuition, unsystematic clinical experience, and explanations based on pathophysiology. Despite recognition of the importance of research findings to guide practice decisions, fewer than 20% of all medical practices are evidence based (Eddy, 1992). This finding is not consistent with the current health care climate in which providers are increasingly having to demonstrate the effectiveness of interventions, including the ability to provide quality care and a desirable cost/benefit ratio (Lansky, Butler, & Waller, 1992).

To what extent do pediatric physical therapists base their clinical decisions on the best available knowledge and research evidence? Therapists make decisions on complex issues related to examination, prognosis, plan of care, coordination of care, and anticipated outcomes on a daily basis. Yet the information on which decisions are based may be of variable quality. Some information may be obtained from published clinical research and review articles that summarize current knowledge. More often, however, therapists make decisions based on expert opinion, advice from a colleague, information from textbooks and continuing education courses, and personal experience, all of which may be subject to bias (Thomson-O'Brien & Moreland, 1998).

An evidence-based approach to decision making is predicated on the physical therapist's ability to analyze and apply information. This involves access to new information, appraisal of the level of evidence on which the information is based, and determination of the extent to which that information is applicable to individual children and their families. Harris (1996) and Golden (1980) pose several thought-provoking questions for professionals to ask themselves when analyzing the scientific merit of an intervention:

1. Is the theory on which the intervention is based consistent with current knowledge?
2. Is the population for whom the intervention is intended identified?
3. Are the goals and outcomes of intervention consistent with the needs of the intended population?
4. Are potential adverse effects of the intervention identified?
5. What is the level of evidence that supports the effectiveness of the intervention?

6. Are advocates of the intervention open to discussing limitations?

A negative response to one or more of these questions is a warning sign that an intervention lacks objective evidence. The reader is referred to a special series titled "Users' Guide to the Medical Literature" (1993, 1994) for detailed information on how to search for and critically appraise journal articles from an evidenced-based perspective.

Level of evidence is particularly germane to pediatric physical therapy where there is limited clinical research. Sackett and colleagues (1985) has proposed a system that relates the strength of the experimental design to recommendations for clinical practice. The results of randomized clinical trials provide the strongest evidence followed by nonrandomized studies of children who did and children who did not receive the intervention followed by single-subject designs. Single-subject research can be incorporated into clinical practice and is described later in this chapter. Although the results of research provide the strongest evidence for the effectiveness of an intervention, randomized clinical trials are difficult to design and conduct for many of the populations of children who receive physical therapy. Consequently, therapists must rely on other types of evidence to support clinical decision making. Such evidence includes consensus statements, review articles, practice guidelines, databases generated through systematic clinical documentation, program evaluation, expert opinion, and individual clinical experience. The use of practice guidelines, databases, and program evaluations in clinical decision making are discussed later in this chapter.

Consensus documents and review articles are important resources for evidence-based practice. Consensus documents are intended to generate statements regarding the effectiveness of an intervention. Conclusions are generally derived from research evidence and professional opinion. In 1990, the Section on Pediatrics of the American Physical Therapy Association sponsored a consensus conference on the effectiveness of physical therapy in the management of children with cerebral palsy (Campbell, 1990). The summary statements described interventions supported by some research evidence, interventions that lack supporting research, and interventions that lack supporting research but, based on the clinical experience of conference participants, were judged to warrant investigation.

Meta-analysis is a quantitative reviewing procedure that provides a method of comparing results of several studies and determining the mean intervention effect for all of the studies reviewed. The meta-analyses performed by Ottenbacher and associates on the effects of sensory integration therapy (1982) and neurodevelopmental treatment (1986) serve as a model of the type of evidence that should be made available to practicing clinicians. More recently, Boyd and colleagues (1994) evaluated the literature on the effectiveness of physical therapy in the management of children with cystic fibrosis based on Sackett's levels of evidence (see Chapter 26), and Darrah and associates (1997) reviewed the effects of progressive resisted muscle strengthening in children with cerebral palsy based on Sackett's levels of evidence and a group consensus exercise involving 17 therapists. Pediatric physical therapists, especially board-certified clinical specialists and those working in education and research settings, are encouraged to promote transfer of research findings into clinical practice through participation in consensus exercises and publication of review articles that summarize evidence for a particular intervention.

An evidence-based approach to clinical decision making should also encompass the perspectives of the child and family. Presentation of information to families in a useful and acceptable form encourages active participation in decision making. A consumer's guide to therapeutic services for families of children with disabilities was recently developed through the combined efforts of several professional and parent organizations (Human Services Research Unit, 1995). Included in the guide is a consumer checklist that consists of the following six questions:

1. Will achievement of goals make a real difference in the lives of the child and family?

2. Is there a formal process to discontinue or change the course of treatment if there is no progress?

3. Are treatments as much a part of the child's day-to-day life as possible?

4. Are parents, teachers, and other individuals present in the child's daily life as involved in the planning and provision of treatment as they could be?

5. Are the professionals involved in assessing the child and planning treatment experienced in serving children with similar disabilities?

6. Are sources of financial support sufficient for the cost of the planned treatment?

From the perspective of the child and family, the answer to all six questions should be yes.

Traditionally, physical therapists have assumed that it is the responsibility of the researchers in our profession to determine the effectiveness of interventions. We disagree with this perspective and support the viewpoint of Harris (1996) that "the responsibility to deliver evidence-based treatment rests with all members of a profession." Objective documentation of goals and outcomes and consideration of the factors that may have contributed to change provide therapists a basis for determining need for service, deciding on the most appropriate services, and evaluating the outcomes of intervention. Collaboration between researchers and clinicians is important to identify the research questions that are most relevant to pediatric physical therapy. All physical therapists are strongly encouraged to consider the levels of evidence that form the basis for their clinical decisions. In particular, the impact of decisions based on expert opinion and personal experience should be carefully monitored and alternatives considered should the outcome of the decision be less than desirable.

MODELING THE DISABLING PROCESS

The impact of an intervention can affect the performance of an individual in a variety of ways. For example, a child's ability to use ambulation in school might be improved by working on strength of leg muscles, but it also might be improved by helping the child to organize his or her learning materials better in order to have less to carry from one class to another. To understand how interventions affect functional performance, it is helpful to consider disabilities and interventions in the context of a conceptual framework. Two similar but complementary approaches exist for classifying functional performance in the presence of potentially disabling conditions. They are general conceptual models but can be elaborated for description of specific disorders. One is the World Health Organization's International Classification of Impairments, Disabilities, and Handicaps (Grimby et al., 1988; World Health Organization, 1980); the other is the four-dimensional classification of pathology, impairment, functional limitations, and disability developed by Nagi and elaborated by others (Guccione, 1991; Nagi, 1969, 1991, n.d.; Schenkman & Butler, 1989). These two models have been integrated by the National Center for Medical Rehabilitation Research (NCMRR) (National Institutes of Health, 1993) to form a five-dimensional model (Fig. 7–1). The five dimensions of the disabling process are pathophysiology, impairments, functional limitations, disabilities, and societal limitations. The focus of the classification is the person with a disabling condition, and the five dimensions interact in complex ways rather than form a simple hierarchy.

The five dimensions are defined here and then elaborated on in examples related to decision making in the sections that follow. The key concepts in the conceptual model are illustrated by means of two

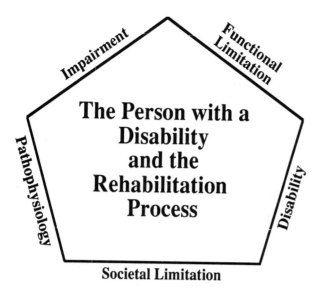

The Person with a Disability and the Rehabilitation Process

Impairment

Functional Limitation

Pathophysiology

Disability

Societal Limitation

FIGURE 7–1. Domains of science relevant to medical rehabilitation and the disabling process. (From National Institutes of Health. Research Plan for the National Center for Medical Rehabilitation Research. Bethesda, MD: National Institutes of Health, 1993, p. 34.)

examples: one, a condition that can be diagnosed at birth; the other, a condition in which diagnostic uncertainty may remain for many months. The examples used are the child with myelodysplasia and the child with spastic diplegia, emphasizing the motor dysfunction characteristic of these conditions (Molnar, 1992). The framework for classifying the disabling process, however, can be broadened to include all types of disability or multiple aspects of disability within any given condition.

The conceptual framework for understanding the disabling process begins with *pathophysiology,* the underlying medical or injury processes at the cellular and tissue levels that are primarily studied and managed by basic scientists or medical specialists, such as the neonatologist or the neurosurgeon. In the child with myelodysplasia, a failure of neural tube closure results in an open spine with neural tissues extruded into a myelomeningocele. In the child who will develop spastic diplegia, a white matter infarct in the periventricular areas caused by hypoxia is an example of a pathophysiologic condition leading to this particular type of cerebral palsy. Damage to the corticospinal tracts and other nervous system pathways traveling through the periventricular areas is a likely result of hypoxic effects on these areas. Primary prevention strategies at this level are currently aimed at understanding nutritional deficiencies that might cause neural tube defects and at discovering means

of preventing hypoxic-ischemic events that lead to cerebral palsy.

The complexity of modeling the disabling process can be appreciated if we remind ourselves that many children born prematurely who demonstrate pathologic findings on ultrasound examination of the periventricular area do not develop cerebral palsy. The challenge for clinical practitioners is to understand the signs and symptoms that verify a diagnosis of developmental impairment or to identify a child who is recovering from such a potentially disabling event. Similarly, for myelodysplasia, level of the lesion does not correlate perfectly with functional capabilities because of individual variations in nerve root innervation of muscles.

The second dimension of the model is *impairment.* Present at this level are the organ and system disorders that potentially will impair functioning at the organism or person level. Impairments are not necessarily recognized in the lesioned area (the brain and spinal cord in our examples) but result from it. In myelodysplasia, sensorimotor impairments include lack of sensation, total or partial denervation of muscles, and muscle atrophy, resulting in paralysis of the lower extremities. In spastic diplegia, sensorimotor impairments include decreased force and power output by the neuromuscular system, poor selective control of movements, and poor anticipatory regulation of postural set for movement, all well-known abnormalities resulting from periventricular damage to the corticospinal tracts or damage to the supplementary cortical motor areas involved in motor planning and coordination (Campbell, 1992). Impaired balance, efficiency, endurance, and coordination of movement are seen in both conditions. These impairments are known effects of cerebral palsy that all physical therapists can recognize once they are fully present; however, definitive diagnosis may not be apparent until some months after birth.

An important concept for therapists to understand is that of secondary prevention (Pope & Tarlov, 1991). Early in the course of a disabling condition, the pathophysiologic process results in identifiable impairments that may or may not be permanent or even affect function. The purpose of secondary prevention efforts is to limit impairment and thereby preserve as much function as possible. Parents of children with myelodysplasia must be taught proper handling and skin care to prevent fractures and skin breakdown. Scoliosis and decreased pulmonary function may be late-appearing secondary impairments that can seriously affect overall functional performance and quality of life. In the province of physical therapy, secondary prevention clearly involves the role of early intervention.

For children with spastic diplegia, it also involves education for parents that enables them to avoid allowing their child to fall into movement habits that may later impair function by leading to muscle hypoextensibility (e.g., W-sitting) and that provides them with advice about when to seek medical attention for developing problems, such as worsening contractures.

The combination of impairments in one or more systems may lead to *functional limitations,* the third dimension of the conceptual framework. Functional limitations involve whole body function, for example, slow and inefficient gait and tendency to lose one's sitting balance while using the arms for dressing. Functional limitations result from impairments and are typically assessed in a clinical setting but may or may not be remediable. By contrast, not all impairments result in limitations of function. For example, a slight contracture of a hamstring muscle does not cause obvious functional limitation; at some level, however, tight hamstrings begin to impair gait and other activities. The problems of children with various types of disabilities begin to become more similar at this level of the disabling process, although unique characteristics of both children and conditions dictate individualized treatment planning and intervention. For example, children with myelodysplasia must have individualized attention to deal with bowel and bladder functions. Functional limitations of gait in myelodysplasia and spastic diplegia may be relatively similar (poor endurance and balance, for example), yet because different impairments cause the functional limitations, children with these two conditions require different types of assistive devices and intervention strategies.

When functional limitations persist for long periods and are not remediable or cannot be compensated for by use of assistive devices or orthoses, *disabilities* result. At this level, children fail to fulfill normal life roles, such as participation in school, play, or family activities, and quality of life may be seriously affected for both children and their families. For children with myelodysplasia, social consequences of bowel and bladder dysfunction can be serious if not adequately handled, even resulting in anorexia in an individual's desperate attempt to decrease incontinence. For children with spastic diplegia, disabilities might include lack of independence in dressing or mobility, learning problems because of perceptual impairments, or inability to participate in sports with peers who are able-bodied. It is important to note that the degree of disability does not necessarily follow directly from functional limitations and shows high individual variability. Depression and low self-esteem, for example, if not recognized and treated, can impair social interaction and lead to decreased participation in activities that are functionally possible for the individual.

An example of assessment of impairments, functional limitations, and disabilities in a child with cerebral palsy is provided by Almeida and colleagues (1997) as a demonstration of multidimensional examination of the outcomes of use of intrathecally administered baclofen. Impairments were reduced initially but not always sustained over time, and improved independence reduced disability; effects on functional limitations were small.

The most severe dimension of dysfunction in the disabling process is called *handicap* in the World Health Organization's model (World Health Organization, 1980) or *societal limitations* in the NCMRR model (National Institutes of Health, 1993). Handicaps result when societal barriers prevent an individual from functioning at the highest level of which he or she is capable. Societal limitations might include architectural barriers to mobility, inability to attend a day care center because of rules that exclude children who are incontinent, or the need for special equipment that is prohibitively expensive or not covered by insurance. Problems such as these often fall outside the usual purview of rehabilitation specialists and must be addressed through problem identification and action at the community and societal level.

The International Classification of Impairments, Activities, and Participation (ICIDH-2) (World Health Organization, 1997), a revision of the International Classification of Impairments, Disabilities, and Handicaps (World Health Organization, 1980), is presently undergoing field trials. The ICIDH-2 incorporates biologic and social perspectives of disablement to more fully represent the impact of health conditions on individual life, including participation in society (Fig. 7–2). The ICIDH is being revised to (1) better describe the reciprocal relationships among impairment, disability, and handicap; (2) more adequately reflect the role of the social and physical environment in the disablement process; (3) increase awareness of the consequences of health conditions and people's right to participation; (4) represent dimensions and constructs in a neutral way to avoid negative connotations; and (5) create a multipurpose classification system that is applicable to many disciplines and sectors.

In the ICIDH-2, the dimension of *impairment* is expanded to include not only the loss or abnormality of body structure but also loss or abnormality of physiologic or psychologic function. The concept of functional limitation previously was regarded as being an element of disability. The dimension of *activity/activity limitation* (formerly *disability*) describes the nature and extent of functioning at the level of the

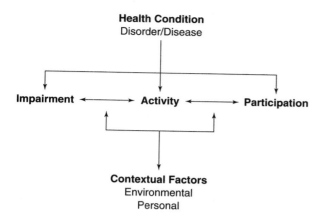

Health Condition
Disorder/Disease

Impairment ←→ Activity ←→ Participation

Contextual Factors
Environmental
Personal

FIGURE 7–2. Current understanding of interactions within the ICIDH-2 dimensions. (From WHO: International Classification of Impairments, Activities and Participation, Beta-1 draft for field trials, World Health Organization, June 1997.)

person. Activities range from simple tasks to complex skills. For example, holding objects is an elementary activity that is important for more complex activities such as feeding, dressing, work, or leisure. Activities may be carried out using assistive technology or the help of another person. Activity is limited when a person has difficulty in performance or is unable to perform at all (based on expectations for a person without disability). The dimension of *participation/participation restriction* (formerly *handicaps*) refers to the nature and extent of a person's involvement in life situations and represents the complex interactions of health condition, impairment, activity, and the context in which a person lives (physical, social, and attitudinal environment). Participation is classified into seven areas: personal maintenance; mobility; exchange of information; social relationships; education, work, leisure, and spirituality; economic life; and civic and community life. The impact of a person's impairment or activity limitation on participation may vary depending on environmental factors.

The example of a child with spastic diplegia will be used to illustrate the dimensions and classifications of the ICIDH-2. The child's impairments in *neuromusculoskeletal and movement-related functions* include reduced *muscular force, muscular endurance,* and *balance.* These impairments are thought to cause activity limitation. Activity limitations exist in *movement activities* and *moving around.* The child's specific activity limitations include difficulty with *moving on a sloping surface, moving amid immobile and moving objects,* and *climbing playground equipment.* The child demonstrates full *participation in home environment mobility. Participation in mobility outside the home* is re-

stricted. The child occasionally falls when walking from the bus to the classroom. Although the child has several friends and enjoys physical activity, participation in recess and physical education is restricted. Social and physical environmental factors that contribute to restricted participation include the following: teachers are concerned that the child will get injured; the child's classroom is at the end of the school most distant from the playground; the terrain of the school yard is uneven; and students are crowded on the playground equipment.

The dimensions of the disabling process encompassed by the practice of pediatric physical therapy are most likely to be those of impairment, functional limitation, and disability. In health-related interventions for children with disabilities, goals are often aimed at the impairment dimension; in public school settings, children's goals are more likely to address functional limitations and disability. These dimensions will be considered further when problems and processes for making diagnostic, prescriptive, outcome assessment, and program evaluation decisions are discussed.

PHYSICAL THERAPY DIAGNOSIS

Historically, answers to the question "Who needs treatment by a physical therapist and what for?" were simple to obtain. Physicians identified the problem—the medical diagnosis—and referred children to physical therapists, sometimes with a specific prescription, at other times for "evaluation and treatment" at the therapist's discretion. For many of the disorders treated by pediatric physical therapists, physicians remain the primary diagnosticians at the level of identification of pathophysiologic processes. Few standardized practice guidelines exist, however, to guide physicians in deciding who would benefit or when to refer children with developmental disabilities, and physicians' practices vary widely. For example, research on physicians' decisions regarding referral for physical therapy of children with suspected cerebral motor dysfunction indicates that the decision to refer is related to the physician's diagnostic certainty, perceived severity of the child's involvement, and belief in the value of physical therapy (Campbell & Gardner, 1992). The diagnostic certainty expressed by physicians in the study who reviewed a series of standardized videotaped cases varied widely. Furthermore, the probability of referral varied with physician specialty. Orthopedists were less likely and physiatrists more likely to refer a child younger than 2 years of age for physical therapy than were pediatricians or neurologists.

Under the current health care model and evolving state licensure laws, however, physical therapists increasingly serve as the point of entry into physical therapy services, either as independent practitioners, as part of a comprehensive diagnostic and intervention team, as related service providers in educational settings, or as practitioners in other venues. To be deemed worthy of such a powerful role, physical therapists need valid and reliable decision-making procedures that result in the provision of truly necessary services in the most cost-effective manner.

The diagnostic decisions that physical therapists make are typically in the realm of impairments and functional limitations. In the "Guide to Physical Therapist Practice" (American Physical Therapy Association, 1997), a diagnosis is defined as a cluster of signs, symptoms, syndromes, or categories whose purpose is to guide the physical therapist in determining the most appropriate intervention for a child and family. For example, therapists are best qualified to make decisions regarding whether a client has impairments of strength or passive range of motion, the presence of and degree to which a client has functional limitations of mobility, and the presence of developmental gross motor delay and the types of impairments contributing to that delay. Few diagnostic tests are available, however, with adequate sensitivity and specificity for identifying and defining the impairments and functional limitations we hope to diagnose. Aylward (1997) describes the need to evaluate tests further for both diagnostic classification accuracy and also relative risk, that is, the probability of a child later displaying a developmental problem if results of an earlier screening test were abnormal or suspect.

The Problem of Predictability

Most often, the decision regarding who needs treatment revolves around the diagnosis of developmental delay or the presence of signs of aberrant development, such as those seen in the motor control dysfunction associated with cerebral palsy. The most useful means for assessing delayed or aberrant development are likely to be standardized developmental scales that have been normed on large populations. The predictive validity of those tests that currently exist, however, has been problematic.

What do we know about prediction of outcomes from early assessment? The bulk of the literature on assessment in infancy suggests that little regarding outcome in later years can be successfully predicted for individual children and certainly little from typical developmental assessment scales (Harbst, 1990; Kopp, 1987; Piper et al., 1991; Rosenblith, 1992). For example, poor motor performance scores early in life have some capacity for identifying children at risk for developmental problems, but in a nonspecific

way. Poor motor scores may later be associated with cerebral palsy, mental retardation, or even blindness and behavioral problems (Campbell & Wilhelm, 1985; Ferrari et al., 1990; Nelson & Ellenberg, 1982). The process of recovery from early medical complications and the role of the environment a family provides for optimal recovery and facilitation of development also contribute to the difficulty in predicting developmental outcomes. Test scores at any single point in time may be inadequate for making a decision regarding whether a child's development is permanently impaired until the time for maximally effecting important long-term outcomes has already passed. A conceptual framework that encompasses the complexity involved in early brain lesions or abnormal development is needed. Aylward and Kenny (1979) and Gordon and Jens (1988) have suggested models for early identification of developmental disabilities (Campbell, 1993), and Campbell (1999) recently suggested a critical pathway for follow-up examination of infants at risk for developmental disabilities in the first year of life. A test that shows promise in the prediction of poor motor outcome, the Alberta Infant Motor Scale (Darrah et al., 1998), is included in the model. Models are also available from the work of other disciplines that, if fully implemented in clinical practice, might make decision making more systematic and more precise and accurate (Watts, 1985, 1989). These models can help us decide whom to treat and for what, can aid communication with other health professionals, and can explicitly allow for input from the child's family.

Clinical Decision Theory

One conceptual framework for developing new diagnostic procedures and measurement instruments is clinical decision theory (Dowie & Elstein, 1988). This theory assumes that clinical judgment encompasses such a complex set of tasks that mathematic algorithms and decision models incorporating the results of research on important clinical problems are likely to be more successful than is clinical judgment for making diagnostic and treatment decisions.

In decision theory, probabilities of various outcomes are assessed based on variables such as previous historical events or assessments, potential negative results of various decisions, and patient or family judgments regarding the value of various potential positive and negative outcomes. In the diagnostic area, for example, risk for cerebral palsy or motor developmental delay could be estimated based on a combination of findings such as ultrasound results at birth, general movement assessment, and tests of postural control and motor milestone achievement at successive ages. Bayesian statistical models allow the degree of risk calculated at earlier points in time to be incorporated as factors in an equation using current test results, thus establishing a cumulative risk probability that takes into account prior history as well as current functioning (Slovik & Lichtenstein, 1971). Studies of decision equations based on variables such as these have almost universally found that diagnostic decisions made with such algorithms are much more reliable than those based on clinicians' judgments (Dawes et al., 1989).

Decision models such as those just described do not currently exist for pediatric physical therapy, but it is entirely possible to develop them. What is needed is data from large research studies on the variables believed to be important that can then be developed into probability-of-outcome equations. The data needed may actually be available in the literature and in large clinical centers for several conditions, such as spastic diplegia. For this condition, many long-term follow-up studies using sophisticated imaging techniques and developmental examination have already been published. Longitudinal assessment records available in many large centers should help identify developmental test scores at particular ages that are likely to suggest ominous outcomes or significant milestones that can be used as markers of developmental progress in prediction equations. Even the imperfection of prediction that is likely to exist, given the data currently available, is likely to be better than current methods involving even more imperfect clinical judgment. Furthermore, deciding to try such a method will lead to the gradual development of a clinical database that will improve the methods used to make decisions.

Why have decision models proved to be better than experienced clinicians' judgments? As Goldberg (1991) suggested, rehabilitation specialists tend to base decisions on personal clinical experience, intuition, and hunches. Studies of clinical judgment suggest the many ways in which bias is introduced into the examination and decision-making process when operating in such a mode (Sackett et al., 1985). Practitioners are liable to make errors of both omission and commission in clinical examinations, and evaluative judgments made from data collected tend to be overly affected by recent experiences with other clients. Furthermore, the sensory perception of clinicians varies from time to time, owing to fatigue and other factors, including assumptions made from client history and from biased expectations. Studies have also revealed that practitioners immediately formulate hypotheses regarding what is wrong (or right) and then collect data to rule out or in the various hypotheses entertained (Dowie & Elstein,

1988). Obviously, if the true situation is not one of the entertained hypotheses, judgment is likely to go awry. Experienced clinicians tend to have a broader base of knowledge from which to generate appropriate hypotheses than do novices (Embry & Nirider, 1996; Embry et al., 1996); nevertheless, their clinical decisions can still be impaired by any of the various factors just mentioned. Use of standardized assessments, a systematic data-gathering protocol, and decision algorithms can guard against such unreliability in clinical judgment.

Classification of Impairment and Functional Limitation

Use of taxonomic classification systems for describing disability is another means to improve clinical decision making. All clinicians know that no two clients with the same disorder are exactly alike. Establishing taxonomies for the description of constellations of impairments or functional limitations occurring in children with particular conditions can lead to improved diagnosis and prognosis on which to base clinical decisions. Taxonomic classification is also useful in generating studies of differential intervention effects for subcategories of disability and studies of whether different types of interventions are most appropriate for different subcategories. But are there ways to identify the underlying impairments at the systems level, and are there clinically practical means for classification of children based on either impairment or functional limitation?

Work on developing diagnostic systems for classifying patients with low back pain is already well under way in physical therapy (Binkley et al., 1993). Recent research on neonates and young infants also suggests that we may, indeed, have the means for identifying the primary impairments in cerebral palsy at an early age (Prechtl et al., 1997). All clinicians know that children with cerebral palsy are characterized by stereotypic movement patterns and lack of selective control. Prechtl and colleagues have developed an assessment of general movement that characterizes the movement pattern in cerebral palsy as being one of "cramped synchrony," with a paucity of selective joint movements, especially in the rotational components (Ferrari et al., 1990). Their work has also demonstrated that clinical examination of children with known signs of brain pathophysiologic impairment can identify the effects of such lesions on movement, and that these effects can be qualitatively and quantitatively described longitudinally and used to predict recovery or nonrecovery from early nonoptimal medical conditions and events. The test is totally noninvasive because it involves observation of spontaneous movement from

15-minute to 1-hour videotapes (depending on age). Use of this general movement examination to diagnose high risk for cerebral palsy has the potential to eliminate the problem of late referral because of diagnostic uncertainty identified by Campbell and Gardner (1992).

Crenna and colleagues (1992) have demonstrated that cerebral palsy can also be described on the basis of a constellation of impairments, leading to a taxonomic classification system that differs greatly from traditional ways of classifying cerebral palsy by area of involvement and presence of spasticity or movement dysfunction. The impairments used for classification include spasticity, muscle coactivation, muscle hypoextensibility, and paresis. Categories of the taxonomy have been related to functional performance capabilities in children with hemiplegia.

Palisano and associates (1997) have developed the Gross Motor Function Classification System (GMFCS) for children with cerebral palsy that is based on the concepts of functional abilities and limitations. The GMFCS was developed for children with cerebral palsy who are 12 years of age and younger and is analogous to the staging and grading systems used in medicine. A classification is made by determining which of five levels best represents the child's present abilities and limitations in gross motor function in home, school, and community settings. The authors propose that classification based on functional abilities and limitations should enhance communication among professionals and families with respect to (1) efficient utilization of medical and rehabilitation services, (2) the creation of databases describing the development of children with cerebral palsy, and (3) comparing and generalizing the results of program evaluations and outcomes research. The terms *functional related groups, severity of disability, case-mix complexity,* and *risk adjustment* have been used to describe methods of grouping patients for evaluating internal quality standards or for comparative analysis of intervention outcomes across sites (benchmarking).

The GMFCS is intended to be quick and easy to use. Classification is based on the child's self-initiated movement with emphasis on sitting and walking. The title for each level represents the highest level of mobility that a child is expected to achieve between 6 and 12 years of age (Box 7–1). The description for each level is broad and not intended to describe all aspects of the motor function of individual children. For each level, separate descriptions are provided for children in the following age bands: less than 2 years, 2 to 4 years, 4 to 6 years, and 6 to 12 years. Distinctions among levels of gross motor function are based on functional limitations, the need for assistive mobility devices (walkers, crutches,

---

BOX 7–1. Summary of Level of Mobility That a Child is Expected to Achieve between 6 to 12 Years of Age for Each of the Five Levels of the Gross Motor Function Classification System

Level	Abilities and Limitations
I	Walks without restrictions; limitations in more advanced gross motor skills
II	Walks without assistive devices; limitations walking outdoors and in the community
III	Walks with assistive mobility devices; limitations walking outdoors and in the community
IV	Self-mobility with limitations; children are transported or use power mobility outdoors and in the community
V	Self-mobility is severely limited even with the use of assistive technology

---

canes), wheeled mobility, and to a lessor extent quality of movement. The scale is ordinal with no intent that the distances between levels be considered equal or that children with cerebral palsy are equally distributed among the five levels.

Nominal and Delphi surveys of consensus methods involving 48 experts were used to provide evidence of content validity, including whether the distinctions for each level represented differences in gross motor function that were clinically meaningful. Interrater reliability was examined by 51 physical therapists and occupational therapists who worked in pairs to independently classify the gross motor function of 77 children with cerebral palsy. Kappa was 0.55 for children less than 2 years of age (fair to good agreement beyond chance) and 0.75 for children 2 to 12 years of age (excellent agreement beyond chance), providing evidence that therapists are able to accurately classify a child's level of gross motor function, particularly for older children. The GMFCS is currently being used in a prospective longitudinal study involving 700 children with cerebral palsy whose purpose is to construct motor development curves for each of the five levels of the GMFCS (Rosenbaum et al., 1997).

The classification of impairments, functional limitations, and disabilities within the framework of the disabling process can be used to develop a comprehensive clinical examination protocol, either for determining whether a disabling condition exists or for developing intervention goals and outcomes appropriate for various levels of dysfunction. Tests at the level of impairment are likely to be the most discipline specific, whereas assessments of problems along the dimension of disability heavily involve the client and family and are most often interdisciplinary.

ESTABLISHING A PLAN OF CARE

Having identified the need for intervention for the presence of impairments or functional limitations, the therapist's next important decision is related to the plan of care. What procedures and techniques should be implemented, how often and for how long, and which goals and outcomes should be established?

Depending on the family's needs and goals and the child's age, overall developmental level, and specific problems and competencies identified by the physical therapist and other members of the assessment team, intervention goals and outcomes might focus on various aspects of the disabling process. For example, emphasis might be aimed at reducing impairment (emphasizing strength, endurance, muscle tone, postural control, or other factors), at overcoming functional limitations through practice of specific tasks or use of compensatory strategies for achieving functional performance, or at reducing or preventing disability through provision of assistive devices. Use of the conceptual model of the disabling process helps clarify which goals and outcomes are most appropriate for any developmental stage and disability and identify the methods of intervention.

Such decisions are frequently sources of professional conflict because members of each discipline view the disabling process from their unique perspectives and may develop entirely different outcomes and potential solutions for the same constellation of impairments, functional limitations, and disabilities. Even when clinicians agree on overall outcomes, priorities may differ (Butler, 1991). The resolution of such conflicts through the use of effective team consensus-building processes, however, can lead to elegant program plans that truly meet clients' needs. Both preventive and ameliorative approaches may be necessary; however, both stages of life and stages of the disease or condition affect the decision regarding which outcomes are the most important to attain in the limited time that is likely to be available (Campbell, 1997).

For example, if primary impairments can be limited by early therapy, some functional limitations that would otherwise result as a part of the natural history of a condition may be avoided. Thus, prevention at this level of the disabling process involves attempts to limit impairment resulting from the lesion and to promote developmentally appropriate functional capabilities. For example, most therapists believe that early intervention for children with spastic diplegia produces a more efficient gait later. Little research exists to document such effects, however. One of the few studies that suggests such a result is a comparison of early (before

9 months) versus late Vojta therapy that reported that children whose treatment began before 9 months of age walked earlier, on average, and with better postural alignment than did those treated later (Kanda et al., 1984). Theoretically, early intervention should also result in prevention or reduction of secondary impairments, such as contractures and deformities, that are not generally present as primary impairments in children. Rather, they develop later as a result of habitual movement using compensatory patterns or overactive muscles with paretic antagonists or as a result of overall poverty of movement and disuse. Until we develop tests that clearly separate elements of underlying impairment from functional limitations that may be primary or may result from use of compensatory strategies to enhance function, we will be unable to document the value of early or preventive intervention for cerebral palsy and other conditions present in early childhood. With appropriate measurement tools available, studies of the efficacy and effectiveness of early intervention at the impairment level will be possible. Until such time as this information is available, however, therapists will continue to come into conflict with physicians and other professionals (including other therapists) who believe that intervention does not need to begin early or can be carried out by parents, does not need to include hands-on treatment by therapists, and should be aimed at provision of compensatory strategies to increase function rather than at treatment of underlying impairment.

When functional limitations persist for long periods and are not remediable or cannot be compensated for, children may fail to succeed in normal life roles, such as participation in school, play, or family activities. Therapy planning should start with interdisciplinary assessment at the disability level when a condition that impairs developmental progress and functional capabilities is already well established. This involves asking which roles and skills are needed and appropriate for a specific child at his or her particular stage of life and must involve the family and teachers as full participants in the examination process. When disabilities are present or can be prevented, each discipline considers what contributions it has to make and plans further exploratory examination or intervention accordingly, again in concert with the family and other team members. In the case of our example of the child with spastic diplegia, a therapist may decide that independent locomotion is a future goal but that the child needs an assistive device at the moment to allow him or her to keep up with ambulatory peers. Other members of the rehabilitation team will have their own unique contributions to make to the solution of the problems of lack of mobility and other functional limitations. Giangreco (1995) emphasizes that *all* professionals should have the same goals rather than separate disciplinary goals when intervention takes place in a school setting.

The setting in which treatment is to be provided shapes the goals, outcomes, and intervention methods to be used. For example, care of children in educational settings is by law aimed at preventing disabilities in learning and educational attainment. Related services are provided in the nation's public schools solely for this purpose, so the outcomes of therapy must be targeted at disability-level problems and competencies. Therapists, teachers, families, and other professionals must all be clear regarding these priorities and realize that decision making for school therapy may not meet all of the needs for intervention that children with disabilities have. Impairments may not be treated at all in such settings, and only functional limitations that can be directly related to the prevention or alleviation of educational disabilities will be managed under the public law mandate.

Decision theory can again be helpful in making choices for intervention strategies. Specific models are available in the clinical literature for involving patients and their families in making decisions regarding which treatments should be applied (Watts, 1985, 1989; Weed & Zimny, 1989). These models incorporate both research-based knowledge regarding the possible costs and benefits of implementation of different approaches to the problem under consideration and also the values clients place on differing outcomes and the risks they are willing to incur, given the probabilities of both positive and negative outcomes. Such models have been discussed in the physical therapy literature for years, but little use has been made of such strategies for improving the decision-making process and involving clients more in deciding the course of their own treatment.

Although explicit conceptual models for describing various disabling conditions along with fully elaborated assessment and decision protocols are not currently available in pediatric physical therapy, provision of services must, of course, continue. To the extent that decision making in physical therapy is complex and that in many cases there is no single solution to a problem, decision models can be particularly helpful. The experienced therapist may find decision models of value in organizing and externalizing thought processes. Models are also of value in bridging the theory-practice gap in the clinical education of physical therapy students and recent graduates.

The Hypothesis-Oriented Algorithm for Clinicians (HOAC) was developed by Rothstein and Echternach (1986) to provide physical therapists with a systematic method for clinical decision making and patient care that is independent of methods of examination and intervention philosophy. An algorithm uses a branching approach to decision making, involving several steps that are intended to narrow the focus of the problem and direct the practitioner to the appropriate plan of action. Echternach and Rothstein (1989) stated that their interest in decision making was stimulated by observations that examinations performed by physical therapists did not always appear to have a direct bearing on the plan of care and that the use of treatment protocols in physical therapy seemed to replace the thought process associated with *individualizing* treatment to the patient's unique set of problems. The HOAC is not supported by a database, is not computer generated, and is not intended to provide specific guidelines for examination and intervention decisions. Rather, the HOAC provides a format to guide the physical therapist through the decision-making process.

The HOAC consists of two parts. The first part addresses assessment and treatment planning and consists of eight steps: (1) initial data collection, (2) problem statement and goals, (3) examination, (4) generation of a hypothesis, (5) plan reevaluation methodology, (6) plan treatment strategy, (7) plan treatment tactics, and (8) and implement treatment (Fig. 7–3). Step 4, in which the therapist formulates hypotheses (clinical impressions) about the cause of a patient's problem in motor function, is particularly important. Physical therapists frequently treat children who have several primary and secondary impairments that can cause limitations in function and disability. When using the HOAC, therefore, therapists are encouraged to consider all possible hypotheses, to prioritize multiple hypotheses, and to consider how each hypothesis relates to the others.

The second part is a branching program that consists of a series of questions that serve to direct the physical therapist in further problem solving when goals have not been achieved. Successful application of the HOAC lies in the ability of the physical therapist to define outcomes and to evaluate whether the outcomes have been achieved. Chapters in *Decision Making in Pediatric Neurologic Physical Therapy* (Campbell, 1999) provide examples of use of the HOAC to guide reflection on practice with children with neurologic dysfunction. The HOAC model is compatible with the elements of patient/client management in the "Guide to Physical Therapist Practice" (American Physical Therapy Association, 1997) described in the next section.

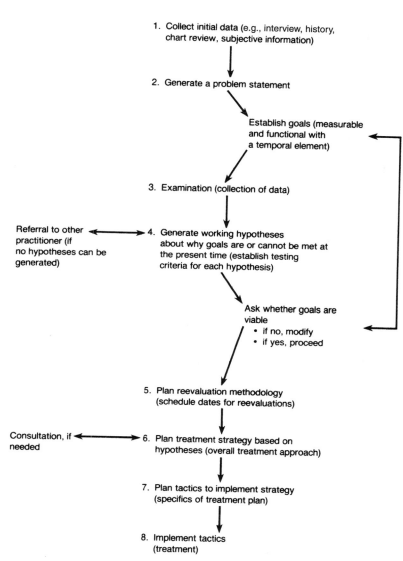

1. Collect initial data (e.g., interview, history, chart review, subjective information)

2. Generate a problem statement

Establish goals (measurable and functional with a temporal element)

3. Examination (collection of data)

Referral to other practitioner (if no hypotheses can be generated)

4. Generate working hypotheses about why goals are or cannot be met at the present time (establish testing criteria for each hypothesis)

Ask whether goals are viable
- if no, modify
- if yes, proceed

5. Plan reevaluation methodology (schedule dates for reevaluations)

Consultation, if needed

6. Plan treatment strategy based on hypotheses (overall treatment approach)

7. Plan tactics to implement strategy (specifics of treatment plan)

8. Implement tactics (treatment)

FIGURE 7–3. Hypothesis-Oriented Algorithm for Clinicians. Part One: Guidelines for evaluation and treatment planning. (From Rothstein, JM, & Echternach, JL. Hypothesis-oriented algorithm for clinicians: A method for evaluation and treatment planning. Physical Therapy, 66:1389, 1986. Reprinted from *Physical Therapy* with the permission of the American Physical Therapy Association.)

"Guide to Physical Therapist Practice"

The "Guide to Physical Therapist Practice" (American Physical Therapy Association, 1997) is a consensus document based on the opinions of more than 800 physical therapist clinicians. The guide was developed by the American Physical Therapy Association between 1995 and 1997 to (1) describe generally accepted physical therapist practice, (2) standardize terminology, and (3) delineate preferred practice patterns that describe common sets of management strategies used by physical therapists for selected patient/client diagnostic groups. The guide represents a first step in the development of practice guidelines (which are usually based on a comprehensive search of peer-reviewed literature) in that it classifies patients/clients and identifies the range of current options for care. A patient is an individual who receives physical therapy and direct intervention. A client is someone who is not necessarily sick or injured but could benefit from physical therapy. Clients are also businesses, school systems, and others to whom physical therapists offer services. The guide is not based on clinical research but is intended to promote outcomes research. The document is evolving and will be systematically revised as the knowledge base of physical therapy increases and examination and intervention strategies change.

The guide incorporates the model of the disabling process, presented earlier in this chapter, and the

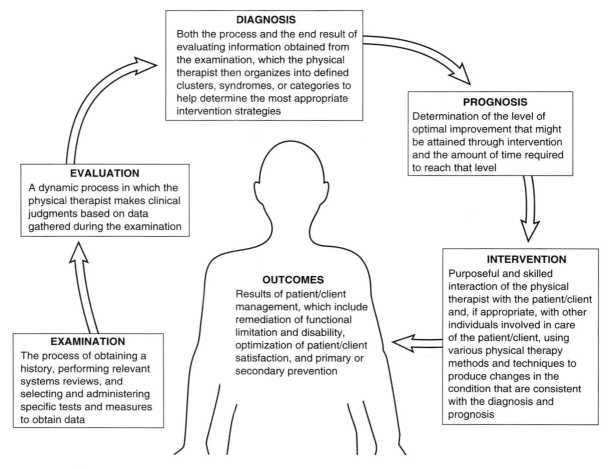

FIGURE 7–4. The elements of patient/client management leading to optimal outcomes. (Reprinted from "Guide to Physical Therapist Practice" with the permission of the American Physical Therapy Association.)

concepts of prevention and wellness. Part One describes the elements of patient/client management and explains the tests, measures, and interventions performed by physical therapists. Part Two includes the preferred practice patterns grouped into four areas: musculoskeletal, neuromuscular, cardiopulmonary, and integumentary. In addition to physical therapists, the guide was developed for use by health care policy makers, third-party payers, managed care providers, and other health care professionals. The guide is intended to do the following:

1. Enhance the quality of physical therapy
2. Enhance coordination of care among health care providers
3. Improve patient/client satisfaction with physical therapy services
4. Promote appropriate utilization of physical therapy services

5. Increase efficiency of and reimbursement for physical therapy services
6. Promote cost reduction through prevention and wellness initiatives

Model of Patient/Client Management

The guide is based on a model of patient/client management designed to maximize outcomes through a systematic and comprehensive approach to decision making. The model includes five elements: examination, evaluation, diagnosis, prognosis, and intervention. The relationship among the five elements is presented in Figure 7–4.

EXAMINATION

The physical therapist is required to perform an examination before any intervention. The examination consists of the history, systems review, and selected tests and measures. The history is an account of the child's past and current health status, which is obtained through an interview with the child and caregivers and review of medical and educational records. As part of the history, the physical therapist identifies the child and family expectations and desired outcomes of physical therapy. A useful means for documenting and quantifying family expectations is the Canadian Occupational Performance Measure (Law et al., 1991). The physical therapist then considers whether these expectations and outcomes are realistic in the context of examination and evaluation data.

The systems review is a brief screening that is intended to help focus the subsequent examination and identify possible health problems that require consultation with or referral to another health care provider. After analyzing information from the history and systems review, the physical therapist examines the child more closely, selecting tests and measures to obtain sufficient data to make an evaluation, establish a diagnosis and a prognosis, and select appropriate interventions.

EVALUATION

Evaluation refers to the physical therapist's analysis and synthesis of results of the examination and leads to a physical therapy diagnosis. Evaluation is a process in which the physical therapist makes judgments about the status of the child based on the information gathered from the examination. This includes judgment of the severity of impairment, functional limitation, and disability; system involvement; the living environment; and social supports. The definition of evaluation in the guide is more specific than what is common in clinical practice where evaluation is used interchangeably with assessment and examination.

DIAGNOSIS

The physical therapy diagnosis is a label encompassing a cluster of signs, syndromes, or categories. The diagnosis is reached through the evaluation process and is intended to guide the physical therapist in determining the most appropriate interventions for each child and family. Diagnosis as an element of physical therapy management does not refer to the medical diagnosis (disease or pathophysiology). Rather, the diagnosis represents patients/clients who are grouped by impairments of the musculoskeletal, neuromuscular, cardiopulmonary, or integumentary system. Diagnosis is associated with a preferred pattern of patient/client management that identifies the range of current options for care.

PROGNOSIS

Perhaps the greatest challenge to patient/client management is determination of the likely outcomes of intervention. Prognosis refers to the predicted optimal level of improvement in function and the amount of service needed to reach that level (frequency and duration of intervention). A trend in managed health care is periodic and episodic intervals of therapy services based on specific functional problems. This is a marked departure for children with developmental disabilities for whom ongoing services have traditionally been reimbursed based on medical diagnosis. Presently, therapists have limited evidence to guide decisions on level of service. At this point in the process of patient/client management, the physical therapist establishes a plan of care that includes the following:

1. Long-term and short-term goals and outcomes
2. Intervention procedures and techniques
3. Recommendations for duration and frequency of intervention
4. Discharge criteria

In the guide, *goals* refer to impairments and *outcomes* refer to a reduction in functional limitation, optimization of health status, prevention of disability, and optimization of patient/client satisfaction. The latter three areas have not been conventionally addressed with specific outcome measures in pediatric practice, and models for doing so are needed.

INTERVENTION

Intervention is the purposeful and skilled interaction of the physical therapist with the patient/client and, when appropriate, with other individuals involved in patient/client care. Various physical therapy procedures and techniques are used during intervention to enable the child and family to achieve goals and outcomes that are consistent with the child's diagnosis and prognosis. Physical therapy intervention has three components: (1) coordination, communication, and documentation; (2) patient/client-related instruction; and (3) direct intervention.

COORDINATION, COMMUNICATION, AND DOCUMENTATION. These services are provided for all children and their families to ensure appropriate, coordinated, comprehensive, and cost-effective services and efficient integration or reintegration to home, community, and work (job/school/play). Services may include (1) case management, (2) coordination of care with family and other professionals, (3) discharge planning, (4) education plans, (5) case conferences, and (6) documentation of all elements of patient/client management. Based on our experience in tailoring continuing education experiences for the needs of physical therapists, this is an area of particular challenge. Children with disabilities are managed in a variety of settings, from public schools to private offices or rehabilitation facilities to specialty clinics for orthotics, surgery, and assistive technology. Therapists in each of these settings complain of the lack of coordination of services among settings and the paucity of effective and timely information sharing among health professionals, teachers, and families.

PATIENT/CLIENT-RELATED INSTRUCTION. These services are provided for all families to educate them about the child's current condition, the plan of care, and future transition to home, work, or community roles. Methods of instruction include demonstration; modeling; verbal, written, or pictorial instruction; and periodic reexamination and reassessment of the home program. The educational backgrounds, needs, and learning styles of family members must be considered during this process.

DIRECT INTERVENTION. Direct interventions provided by physical therapists include (1) therapeutic exercise; (2) functional training in self-care and home management; (3) functional training in the community and at work (job/school/play); (4) manual therapy techniques; (5) prescription, application, and fabrication of devices and equipment; (6) airway clearance techniques; and (7) physical agents and mechanical modalities. The first three interventions listed form the core of most physical therapy plans of care.

OUTCOMES

At each step of patient/client management, the physical therapist considers the possible outcomes. The therapist also engages in outcome data collection and analysis. Outcomes include minimization of functional limitation, optimization of health status, prevention of disability, and optimization of patient/client satisfaction. Horn and colleagues (1997) recently introduced and tested an innovation in documenting outcomes of intervention, which therapists can use to show that treatment of impairments results in functional improvements that generalize to settings outside of the immediate treatment environment. Three domains that appear repeatedly in the research on interpersonal aspects of care are information exchange; respectful and supportive care; and partnership and enabling (King et al., 1996). Rosenbaum and associates (1998), in a review of research on family-centered service, conclude that parents of children with physical disabilities have positive perceptions of how services are provided to their children but are not as satisfied with information exchange.

PREFERRED PRACTICE PATTERNS

The preferred practice patterns are organized by the five elements of patient/client management. Most preferred practice patterns are applicable to both children and adults. Neuromuscular pattern A: Impaired Motor Function and Sensory Integrity Associated with Congenital or Acquired Disorders of the Central Nervous System in Infancy, Childhood, and Adolescence; and cardiopulmonary pattern J: Impaired Ventilation, Respiration, and Aerobic Capacity and Endurance Secondary to Respiratory Failure in the Neonate are the two patterns specific to pediatrics. The "Guide to Physical Therapist Practice" does not specifically address physical therapist practice in early intervention and in the public schools. Public laws and guidelines for physical therapist practice in these settings are presented in Chapters 31 and 32.

Clinical Reasoning

Although decision models can be helpful for physical therapy management, they do not eliminate the need for physical therapists to have a strong knowledge base, problem solve, and make sound clinical judgments. Indeed, research on problem solving has repeatedly confirmed that skill in problem solving is problem specific, indicating that one can solve problems better with a comprehensive base of knowledge about the problem. Clinical reasoning refers to the many ways a practitioner thinks about and interprets an idea or phenomenon and incorporates knowledge, experience, problem solving, judgment, and decision making (Fleming, 1991). Watts (1985) described decision making as both an art and a science. She suggested that many decisions are made with a degree of uncertainty and reflect intuitive thought processes. Magistro (1989) proposed that clinical decisions in physical therapy are derived from both theoretic knowledge and practice experiences that intelligently influence our courses of action. He discussed the role of intuition and suggested that practice decisions are not always apparent as rational thought processes. Magistro's perspective is consistent with Brenner's (1984) conceptualization of professional development. Brenner described the transition from novice to expert as involving a shift from the use of explicit, verbally based theoretic knowledge to the use of highly implicit and embodied practical knowledge.

Mattingly (1991) has proposed an interpretive or meaning-centered model of clinical reasoning in occupational therapy that emphasizes implicit and embodied knowledge. She conceptualized clinical reasoning as the process of deciding on the appropriate action for an individual patient at a particular time. Theoretic knowledge is viewed as a starting point but not as a strict plan for action. As part of the process of individualizing treatment, the therapist makes judgments and improvises in moving from general practice guidelines to the requirements of a specific situation. Mattingly suggested that the knowledge that guides judgment and improvisation is often embodied in the therapist's hands or eyes in a manner that is difficult to translate into words. Part of the therapist's expertise, therefore, is reflected in implicit thought processes that are translated into habitual ways of observing and interacting with patients. The perspective that clinical reasoning involves more than the ability to apply theory and learned technical skill may explain the frustration of physical therapy students when they first attempt to apply classroom material to the clinical setting.

Mattingly (1991) proposed that through experience therapists develop the implicit knowledge that is integral to clinical reasoning. The therapist learns to attend to relevant cues and modify therapeutic interventions in response to these cues. Furthermore, therapists are often not completely aware of how they use implicit knowledge to identify problems, develop treatment plans, and engage the patient in the therapeutic process. On the basis of the results of a study in which occupational therapists described their assessment practices (Rogers & Masagatani, 1982), Mattingly suggested that pediatric therapists incorporate a minimum of five domains of knowledge into their thought processes: (1) understanding of the child's motivation, commitments, and tolerances; (2) assessment of the environment in which the task is taking place; (3) knowledge of the child's physical and cognitive deficits and capacities; (4) perception of the therapeutic relationship; and (5) immediate and long-term goals. Effective clinical reasoning enables the occupational therapist to improvise treatment and address the unique meaning of disability as it relates to a particular patient.

Clinical reasoning by pediatric physical therapists has been examined during direct intervention with children who have cerebral palsy. Carter (1989) examined the behavioral interactions between physical therapists and children with cerebral palsy during a neurodevelopmental treatment (NDT) session. The behaviors of an experimental group of seven physical therapists who attended an 8-week NDT certification course were compared with those of a control group of six physical therapists who were not certified in NDT and seven physical therapists who were NDT course instructors. Therapists were videotaped before and after the NDT certification course. There were no statistically significant differences between the behavioral interactions of therapists in the experimental and control groups after the NDT course. Physical therapists in both groups employed facilitation procedures with little reinforcement of the children's responses, and inhibition procedures were followed by abnormal movement a significant number of times. In contrast, NDT instructors produced more normal movement responses from the children, and facilitation procedures were followed by normal movement a significant number of times. Furthermore, the NDT instructors anticipated abnormal movements before they were observed and responded with inhibition procedures. Carter (1989) concluded that the manner in which the NDT instructors used facilitation and inhibition procedures was in accordance with behavioral learning principles.

Although Carter (1989) did not formally assess clinical reasoning, his results support Brenner's distinction between novice and expert practitioners. Comments from the physical therapists in the experimental group suggested that after the NDT course, they were more concerned with their hand placement and the particulars of movement than with the response they obtained from the children. This implies that during treatment, the physical therapists in the experimental group focused their thought processes on explicit knowledge, which is characteristic of the novice practitioner. By contrast, the treatment behaviors of the NDT instructors suggested that they thought less about the psychomotor aspects of treatment and attended to relevant cues about the children's responses. The NDT instructors' ability to anticipate abnormal movement suggested that they used implicit knowledge to select treatment procedures, a characteristic of the expert practitioner.

In a second study, Larin (1992) investigated physical therapists' explicit and implicit knowledge of motor learning and the relationship between this knowledge and their practice. The subjects were 21 pediatric physical therapists who had between 8 months and 27 years of experience. The physical therapists were videotaped during individual treatment sessions with preschool-age children who had a diagnosis of spastic diplegia. After the treatment session, the therapists viewed the videotape and a stimulated-recall interview was held. During a second interview, the therapists were asked to comment on their ideas, beliefs, theories, and the sources of knowledge they had used in their treatment sessions.

The physical therapists were found to have implemented motor-learning strategies but to have done so in varying degrees. More-experienced therapists promoted more independent movements, whereas less-experienced therapists treated the children in a richer environment, employed more nonverbal cues, and more frequently assisted a child's self-initiated movement. A clear relationship between implicit professional knowledge and practice was not found. Qualitative analysis suggested that motor-learning strategies were frequently not organized in a consistent, effective framework of knowledge. This implies that many of the strategies were implemented incidentally and therefore did not represent meaningful integration of motor-learning strategies into pediatric physical therapy. In addition, the therapists provided an overwhelming impression that they did not routinely stop and think about what they were doing in their treatment sessions. The therapists indicated that their main sources of knowledge were clinical experience, continuing education, interaction with colleagues, and readings. Professional education was the source of knowledge that was least often mentioned.

Embrey and associates (Embrey & Adams, 1996; Embrey & Hylton, 1996; Embrey & Nirider, 1996; Embrey et al., 1996) used qualitative research methodology to describe the thought processes of three experienced (greater than 10 years of pediatric experience) and three novice (less than 2 years of pediatric experience) pediatric physical therapists while providing direct intervention to children with cerebral palsy. Therapists watched videotapes of the intervention sessions and were encouraged to "verbalize whatever comes to mind" following predetermined guidelines. The therapists' comments were transcribed and coded to identify and describe their decision-making processes. The experienced therapists verbalized changing their procedures every 46 seconds compared with every 86 seconds for the novice therapists. Experienced therapists verbalized sensitivity to the emotional and social needs of the children every 2 minutes; novice therapists verbalized psychosocial sensitivity every 3 minutes. Both groups of therapists verbalized self-monitoring (reflection on some aspect of their performance) during intervention about every 3 minutes. When verbalizing self-monitoring, experienced therapists made positive comments 81% of the time as compared with novice therapists' positive comments only 36% of the time. Self-monitoring was verbalized in conjunction with other characteristics of decision making 84% of the time by experienced therapists and 57% of the time by novice therapists. The experienced therapists appeared to make procedural changes and respond to the emotional and social needs of children with less interruption of the therapeutic process, whereas the novice therapists appeared to be limited in their clinical options when they perceived that therapy goals were not being achieved. The investigators suggest that within a treatment session, therapists make rapid, on-the-spot, clinical decisions based on improvisation and intuition.

A great deal remains to be learned about clinical reasoning in pediatric physical therapy. The results of the studies by Carter (1989), Larin (1992), and Embrey and co-workers (Embrey & Adams, 1996; Embrey & Hylton, 1996; Embrey & Nirider, 1996; Embrey et al., 1996) provide preliminary support for the concept that clinical reasoning involves the application not only of theory and psychomotor skill but also of intuitive or implicit thought processes. The results of Larin's study, however, suggest that a therapist's implicit knowledge may not be organized into an effective framework consistent with theory and that therapists have difficulty in explaining their thought processes during treatment. Pediatric physical therapists are encouraged to strive for better understanding of their thought processes not only to enhance their own professional development but also to serve their clients and educate physical therapy students more effectively. A better understanding of clinical reasoning is essential for the development of comprehensive decision models that reflect the broad scope of pediatric physical therapy.

ASSESSING INTERVENTION OUTCOMES

Physical therapists typically evaluate the effectiveness of an intervention by comparing patient performance with preset short- and long-term goals and outcomes developed on the basis of patient testing and observation. How can we guarantee, however, that the outcomes we identify are really the result of our intervention and not the effect of other interventions, of natural development, or of recovery? And how can we be sure that our interventions do not result in unintended negative consequences?

One clinical decision tool that has been used increasingly by pediatric physical therapists to assess the effectiveness of their interventions is the single-subject research design. The single-subject design is an experimental paradigm that is particularly useful for practicing clinicians who wish to study intensively the effects of intervention on individual patients within their caseload (Gonnella, 1989; Harris, 1993).

Nearly all pediatric physical therapists must develop individualized, measurable objectives for the children with whom they work as part of "best-practice" procedure, and the single-subject design represents a logical extension of this procedure. In developing individual behavioral objectives, therapists are required to specify patient outcomes that are expected to change as a result of introducing intervention. These behavioral objectives are analogous to outcome measures that are a form of *dependent variable,* a term that is universal to all types of experimental research designs.

A second major component of experimental research is selection of the independent variable or, in the case of physical therapy, the specific treatment technique that is being applied in an effort to effect positive change in the outcome variable. Obviously, careful treatment planning for the pediatric patient involves not only the selection of the outcome or target behavior, as represented in the individualized therapy objective, but also selection of a specific treatment technique that is designed to enhance change or facilitate improvement in the outcome behavior. In comparing the single-subject research design to physical therapy as it is typically provided in a clinical setting, Gonnella (1989) has stated that the first few steps are similar: the problem behavior is identified, baseline data are collected on the problem behavior, a treatment plan is developed and implemented, and changes in the problem behavior are assessed. However, several important differences exist between the single-subject design and the therapeutic model.

Whereas typically only one baseline assessment is taken in the therapeutic model, single-subject design mandates that a minimum of three data points must be collected on the outcome behavior before treatment is introduced (Barlow et al., 1984). A second criterion of single-subject research is that a very specific design should be implemented that involves sequential application and withdrawal of the intervention. Finally, performance must be measured repeatedly (and frequently) throughout each phase of the design. For a visual comparison of these two models as described and depicted by Gonnella (1989), see Figure 7–5.

Other important criteria of single-subject research designs are that the data collection procedures are both replicable and reliable (Ottenbacher, 1986). Percent agreement is typically used to assess consistency of scoring the behavioral objectives or outcome measures between two or more independent raters.

In his excellent text on single-subject designs for occupational and physical therapists, Ottenbacher (1986) has outlined six important steps for setting up such designs: (1) determining the setting in which the behavior or performance will be observed and recorded; (2) deciding on the method to collect data; (3) determining the length of time that the behavior will be observed and measured; (4) observing and recording client behavior; (5) recording and plotting the data collected; and (6) continuing measurement and recording procedures until requirements of the design have been satisfied. Pediatric physical therapists who wish to set up single-subject designs in their own clinical settings are advised to consult the Ottenbacher text, as well as other references in the physical therapy literature that describe this important clinical decision tool (Gonnella, 1989; Harris, 1993).

Since the early 1980s, pediatric physical and occupational therapists have used single-subject designs to examine the effects of "tone-reducing" (inhibitive) casts and orthoses in improving gait and standing

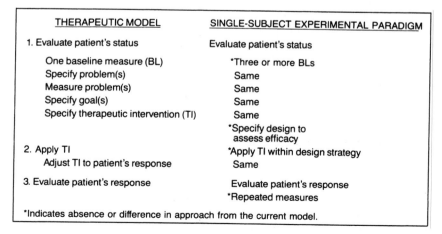

FIGURE 7–5. Comparison of therapeutic process with single-subject paradigm. (From Gonnella, C. Single-subject experimental paradigm as a clinical decision tool. Physical Therapy, *69*:603, 1989. Reprinted from *Physical Therapy* with the permission of the American Physical Therapy Association.)

balance in children with cerebral palsy (Harris & Riffle, 1986; Hinderer et al., 1988); to evaluate the influence of some specific well-defined NDT techniques on increasing heel contact (Laskas et al., 1985) and decreasing knee flexion during gait (Embrey et al., 1990) in children with cerebral palsy; to assess the effects of two different treatment approaches (behavior modification and a neurophysiologic approach) in reducing tongue protrusion in young children with Down syndrome (Purdy et al., 1987); and to examine the effects of different modes of mobility on school performance of children with myelodysplasia (Franks et al., 1991). These are but a sampling of the published reports that have used single-subject designs to examine treatment effectiveness.

In keeping with the pediatric examples outlined at the beginning of this chapter, two published single-subject studies will be described—one involving two children with spastic diplegia and the other involving three children with myelodysplasia. Reference will be made to the NCMRR model of the five dimensions of the disabling process in discussing the goals and outcomes of each of these studies.

In a single-subject study published in 1988, Hinderer and colleagues set out to evaluate the relative effects of tone-reducing casts and standard plaster casts on gait characteristics and functional locomotor activities in two young children with cerebral palsy. The first child (case 1) was a 3.5-year-old boy with mild spastic diplegia and mild mental retardation; spasticity was greater on the right. Some of the impairments noted in this child included gait deviations such as moderate in-toeing on the right, decreased stride length on the left, toe-dragging, forefoot weight-bearing, limited trunk rotation, and high-guard posture of the upper extremities. Functional limitations included the inability to walk up and down stairs without support and the inability to squat or rise to standing without support.

The second child (case 2) was a girl, age 5 years 9 months, with asymmetric spastic diplegia (greater involvement on the left), moderate ataxia, and normal intelligence quotient (IQ). Impairments included poor static and dynamic balance and unsteady gait with frequent falling. Specific gait deviations consisted of mild in-toeing on the left and difficulty with left toe clearance, limited trunk rotation, and a wide base of support. Functional limitations that resulted from these impairments included the inability to walk backward and balance on one leg and the need for upper extremity support to climb stairs and to move from squatting to standing.

An A-B-A-C crossover single-subject design was used in this study to evaluate the effects of the two different types of casts (the independent variables or specific intervention techniques). Tone-reducing casts were defined as those that "maintain the ankle at zero degrees and stabilize the toes and foot in neutral alignment by incorporating a footplate which supports the toes and the metatarsal, peroneal and longitudinal arches of the foot" (Hinderer et al., 1988, p. 371). Standard plaster casts held the ankle in neutral alignment but did not include a footplate.

The study began with both children in a baseline (A1) phase (no casts). In the second phase of the study, case 1 wore tone-reducing casts (B) and case 2 wore standard casts (C). Then the baseline condition (A2) was reinstituted for both subjects, after which the crossover of treatments occurred so that the design for case 1 was A1-B-A2-C and the design for case 2 was A1-C-A2-B.

Outcome measures (target behaviors) included footprint data used to analyze various gait parameters, specific developmentally appropriate fine motor tasks, and videotaped ratings by an interdisciplinary panel of experts on gait and functional motor activities. Data were collected two or three times per week for 19 weeks. The number of data points per phase ranged from 5 to 12. Interrater percent agreement for the gait measures was 96.1% and for the fine motor measures was 97.4%. Subjective impressions were also obtained from parents of the two children and their treating therapists.

One of the benefits of sequential application and withdrawal of interventions, as occurs in single-subject designs, is the ability to control for natural history, developmental maturation, and practice effects. Analysis of the fine motor data for the children in this study revealed that their performance continued to improve even during the baseline (no-cast) phases—thus suggesting that practice of these tasks was contributing more to their improvement than were the specific interventions. In a typical therapeutic model as described by Gonnella (1989) (see Fig. 7–5), such control is not possible and the treating therapist might assume that the improvements are due to the intervention itself whereas they may, in fact, be due to practicing the task or to other intervening variables such as developmental maturation.

Another benefit of this particular crossover design is the opportunity to compare two different interventions. Greater increases in stride length were noted for both children during the tone-reducing cast phases as compared with the standard cast condition. Blinded videotape analysis by the panel of experts revealed mild gait improvements for case 2 during the tone-reducing cast phase and functional improvements in standing balance, ability to walk backward, and ability to squat and return to upright. Owing to poor compliance by case 1, a standardized sequence of gait and functional motor activities was not obtained.

Although this study provided some limited support for the relative benefits of tone-reducing casts as compared with standard casts, the authors concluded their paper by making a plea for practitioners to document their own outcomes of tone-reducing casts and orthoses: "Single-subject research designs offer a clinically appropriate means for reliably studying their effectiveness, and are particularly indicated when studying a heterogeneous population, such as individuals with cerebral palsy, whose clinical presentation varies from day to day" (Hinderer et al., 1988, p. 375).

Another single-subject study compared the relative effects of assistive device ambulation (walker or crutches) and wheelchair mobility on three school performance measures for children with myelodysplasia (Franks et al., 1991). Subjects were students age 9, 10, and 15 years with L-4 or L-5 level myelomeningocele, all of whom had a physiologic cost index (an indicator of energy efficiency) of greater than 1.00 beat per meter when ambulating with assistive devices. The independent variables or specific interventions in this study were the assistive ambulation devices and the wheelchair. Outcomes assessed were reading fluency, visuomotor accuracy, and manual dexterity. A convincing rationale for this study was the frequent encouragement of ambulation for children with lumbar-level lesions in spite of the high energy costs (Waters & Lunsford, 1985).

In the case of these children with lumbar-level lesions, the pathophysiologic condition (myelodysplasia) led to impairments, including lower extremity paralysis, which had then resulted in functional limitations in gait and upright mobility. Basically, this study sought to examine whether secondary functional limitations that can result from ambulation, such as high energy cost, had a negative effect on school performance. If assisted ambulation does, in fact, result in greater energy costs, which in turn lead to poorer school performance, could such a decline in school performance actually lead to school failure, which might then be considered a long-term disability?

To examine these questions, an alternating condition single-subject design was used in which phase 1 was wheelchair propulsion, phase 2 was ambulation with crutches or walker, and phase 3 was again wheelchair propulsion. Each phase was 1 week in length (5 school days), with data collected daily on the three outcome measures: correct words per minute of a 100- to 200-word reading passage (reading fluency); visuomotor accuracy as assessed by the Motor Accuracy Test, Revised (Ayres, 1972); and manual dexterity as assessed on the Purdue Peg-board Assembly subtest (Tiffin, 1968). Although reading fluency was unaffected by the method of mobility and manual dexterity varied across the three subjects and the two treatment conditions, visuomotor accuracy scores were significantly lower for all three subjects during the assistive ambulation phase.

In an accompanying commentary on this article, Haley concluded that "implications of this study may cause us to step back from our often aggressive posture toward functional ambulation at all costs. If assisted ambulation is not energy efficient, time efficient, or safe or leads to an interruption in social, emotional, or cognitive growth, then alternate means of mobility must be considered. Is not the aim of the physical therapist to promote overall development rather than to promote ambulation at a significant cost? Is not efficient, independent mobility the real functional goal for children and their families?" (Haley, 1991, p. 578).

It is exactly these types of questions that we face daily in our clinical decision making as pediatric physical therapists. Using single-subject studies to examine effects of specific interventions systematically and replicating these studies across other subjects in other clinical settings will assist in allowing us to answer such questions. Therapists are encouraged to consult two recent references (Backman et al., 1997; Backman & Harris, 1999) that provide more information and examples of different types of single-subject designs commonly used in rehabilitation settings. It is the responsibility of all practicing therapists, be they clinicians, researchers, or educators, to provide ethically responsible and efficacious interventions for their clients. Systematic examination of intervention outcomes, through such strategies as the single-subject design, can assist us in attaining this goal.

PROGRAM EVALUATION

Although individual physical therapists frequently believe that they have done their professional jobs thoroughly when they have appropriately assessed outcomes in individual clients, professional practice requires additional evaluation of the overall impact and costs of physical therapy programs. Goldberg (1991), for example, suggested that therapeutic and surgical outcomes for children with cerebral palsy include technical outcomes of typical interventions, functional outcomes, parent and child satisfaction with both outcome and service delivery, and cost-effectiveness relative to other intervention approaches. Here, the tools include formal program evaluations and quality assurance programs involving evaluation of record keeping; monitoring of therapist adherence to program policies; assessment of interactions with clients, other providers, and third-party payers; and evaluation of client satisfaction and long-term outcomes.

Monitoring Services with a Database

Developments in the area of monitoring services and tracking outcomes include computerized approaches to creating a database on patients served that may also provide systematic, structured individual patient reports to guarantee uniform reporting of significant information across both therapists and types of patients (Jenkins, 1989; Lehmann et al., 1984; Shurtleff, 1991; Slagle & Gould, 1992). A database is a generalized set of computer programs that allows (1) entry of a variety of data by different authorized users; (2) organization of the data for storage; and (3) retrieval, updating, reorganization, and printing of output in the form of summary reports (Lehmann et al., 1984). Yearly statistics can be rapidly collated, care trends can be monitored across time, and data can be used for prospective or retrospective research (Slagle & Gould, 1992). Use of a database approach can guard against errors of both omission and commission by structuring therapists' reports and by automatically providing checks of entered data against a range of appropriate responses. When a database is developed along the lines of the conceptual framework of the disabling process, studies can be undertaken of how impairments or their alleviation affect functional limitations and whether disability in the patient's natural environment is reduced by the therapy provided. Such a system allows comparison of the performances of both patients and therapists across a range of functions and allows easy access to comparison of the processes and outcomes of contemporary patient care with that in historical populations. Development of national databases on specific client populations can form the basis for improving practice through comparison of institutional or regional differences in management strategies, identifying infrequent negative outcomes, and studying low-incidence conditions.

Slagle and Gould (1992) emphasized that only 27% of tertiary care neonatal units responding to a national survey of database use monitored the accuracy of their data, an essential element of a high-quality plan. Users liked their system best if it generated patient records, such as discharge summaries. In addition to these critical issues, Jenkins (1989) suggested that database developers should consider what aspects of care are likely to change over time in order to develop a system that is flexible in meeting long-term needs. Developers should consider how to collect enough data to be maximally useful for meeting such diverse needs as preparing annual reports and answering important research questions, while eliminating large amounts of data that are easy to collect but unlikely to be used (Slagle & Gould, 1992). In addition, a specific plan for maintaining overall quality of the database should be developed (Slagle & Gould, 1992).

In response to the growing trend for health care accountability, the Joint Commission on Accreditation of Healthcare Organizations (JCAHO) has begun to incorporate the use of outcomes and other performance measures into the accreditation process (Schyve, 1996). Effective in 1998, each accredited hospital must select an external data system vendor who will participate with the hospital in collecting data on two performance measures for up to 20% of its patient population. The JCAHO requirements focus on clinical performance measures designed to evaluate both the processes and outcomes of care. Processes of care include measures of patient satisfaction. The Measure of Processes of Caregiving (King et al., 1996), a parent report measure for use in programs serving children with developmental disabilities, is summarized in Chapter 31. Two pediatric outcome measures for which there is an external data system are the Functional Independence Measure for Children (Granger, 1987) through the Uniform Data System for Medical Rehabilitation, Buffalo, New York, and the Pediatric Evaluation of Disability Inventory (Haley et al., 1992) through the Center for Rehabilitation Effectiveness, Boston, Massachusetts.

Formal Program Evaluation

A more comprehensive approach to assessing program effectiveness is formal program evaluation (Shadish et al., 1991). (Note that in this section, in keeping with the research literature on the topic, the term *evaluation* is used to refer to assessment of overall program outcomes, not as used in the "Guide to Physical Therapist Practice" to refer to making judgments regarding patient examination data.) Although frequently using well-known social science methodology, formal evaluation practice since the 1960s has developed into a discipline in its own right. The explicit purpose of program evaluation is to assess the effects of programs in meeting their stated goals for the purpose of improving subsequent decision making about the program and, in a broader sense, for improving future program planning. Evaluation theory, although initially idealistic, has been expanded and revised based on the experience of program evaluators operating in the real world. These experiences have led to the recognition that (1) the achievement of stated goals may not be the only useful product of a social program; (2) there are many stakeholders involved in the typical program, some of whom are more concerned that the interests of their particular group are addressed than that program goals have been achieved; and (3) politics always act on programs in ways that may be difficult to identify but may mean that program evaluation results are not likely to change programs effectively in major ways. Because of these real-world complications, new evaluation theories have arisen, some complementary and some in more direct opposition to others.

"Theory connotes a body of knowledge that organizes, categorizes, describes, predicts, explains, and otherwise aids in understanding and controlling a topic" (Shadish et al., 1991, p. 30). Ideal evaluation theory describes and justifies why certain evaluation practices lead to particular types of results; clarifies the activities, processes, and goals of evaluation; explicates relationships among evaluative activities and the processes and goals they facilitate; and empirically tests propositions to identify and address those that conflict with research or other knowledge about evaluation (Shadish et al., 1991). The purpose of program evaluation theory is to specify the practices that are feasible for evaluators to use to garner evidence for the value of programs and to reduce identified problems of relevance to the program. Formulation of an appropriate methodology for evaluating a program depends on proper identification of the uses to which the evaluation results will be put. The prospective program evaluation planner needs to know who wants to know what and to what end.

The uses of evaluation results are usually considered to be of two major types: summative (outcomes or products) and formative (evaluation for the purpose of improving the program and understanding the processes by which the program operates). The former makes the supposition that an outcome of the evaluation itself might be abolition of the program; the latter generally assumes that the program will continue to exist and that better ways of improving the product or the provision of services are sought. Because studies of the uses to which evaluation results are put have generally shown that effects trickle down into new-generation programs, producing slow, incremental change rather than resulting in revolutions in thinking and implementation, recent theorists have emphasized that evaluation results may be most usefully thought of as being "enlightening," that is, having future use for program planners in thinking about issues, defining problems, and developing new perspectives and ideas. Those who formulate policy and implement programs seldom actively search for evidence, or if they do, tend to use

whatever fits with their current understanding of the problem under study. Information such as this has led to important studies of the uses of program evaluation and theoretic formulations regarding how information can be most usefully disseminated. In any case, whatever the purpose, program evaluation must be conducted based on the identified need for the program and how well it satisfies the needs identified, as well as meets the needs that might not have been previously identified but happen to be satisfied by the program. The best program evaluation designs also search for potential negative effects, such as those identified by the study of Franks and colleagues (1991) on mobility in children with myelodysplasia.

Arguments have arisen among program evaluation theorists regarding the value of quantitative versus qualitative evaluation methods. The randomized, controlled clinical trial remains, at least in medical areas, the most highly valued summative assessment of intervention outcomes, and it is especially valuable in studies of intervention with children because of the control needed to rule out the effects of maturation and other threats to internal validity (Norton & Strube, 1989; Shadish et al., 1991). Combined with causal modeling of the theoretically and empirically derived processes and factors influencing outcomes, clinical trials are most powerful in studies with large numbers of subjects or in studies seeking to identify low-incidence but potentially highly dangerous unintended negative effects. Qualitative methods, however, offer flexibility, a dynamic quality, and a unique ability to reflect the world from the perspective of multiple program stakeholders and participants. They are especially well suited for gathering answers to formative questions about the quality of program implementation and its meaning to participants. They may also be highly useful for studying the processes by which programs achieve useful outcomes in meeting needs of patients and society. Of most importance, however, are the use of methods appropriate to the level of development of the program (early development stage program, innovative demonstration project, established ongoing program), the problematic issues of concern to program stakeholders of various types, decisions under the control of the program to be made at a time when evaluation results will be available, and the level of uncertainty regarding critical program features. Methods tailored to these factors are most likely to result in effective use of program evaluation results.

Methods of program evaluation that emphasize the process of service delivery are well suited for examining the overall effectiveness of therapy programs. Wang and Ellett (1982) used the term *program validation* to describe a form of evaluative research useful in the development and refinement of innovative educational programs. The major purposes of program validation are to (1) obtain empirical evidence of the effectiveness of an innovative program, (2) identify aspects of the program that require improvement in order to achieve the intended outcomes, and (3) evaluate the feasibility of implementing the innovative program. Wolery and Bailey (1984) have proposed that a comprehensive evaluation of early intervention programs addresses the following questions:

1. Does the method of service delivery represent the best educational practice?

2. Is the intervention being implemented accurately and consistently?

3. Is an attempt being made to verify the effectiveness of the intervention objectively?

4. Does the program carefully monitor patient progress and demonstrate a sensitivity to points at which changes in service need to be made?

5. Does a system exist for determining the adequacy of patient progress and service delivery?

6. Is the program accomplishing its goals and objectives?

7. Does the service delivery system meet the needs and values of the community and clients it serves?

The questions proposed by Wolery and Bailey offer a framework for program evaluation of physical therapy services provided in a variety of settings, including the school system, acute care and rehabilitation hospitals for children, and private practices.

Three studies will serve to illustrate the scope of program evaluation and how questions are developed specific to particular programs. Haley and colleagues (1988) evaluated how physical therapy and occupational therapy services were implemented in six publicly funded early intervention programs in the greater Boston area. The authors examined the influences of infant, family, and program variables on the therapy services provided over a 6-month period. Dependent variables included intensity of individual therapy, intensity of group therapy, ratio of direct therapy to group therapy, ratio of home therapy to center therapy, and ratio of therapy time to total program time. Therapist availability predicted best whether an infant received individual therapy. Infants with more delayed motor development tended to receive more individual therapy and more total therapy. Infants received a higher proportion of therapy when (1) motor quotient was low and parent education was high, (2) infants were younger and therapist availability was high, and (3) infants were younger and parent education was high. Diagnostic risk factor and age did not predict type or intensity of therapy. Although the study was exploratory in nature and should not be generalized to other early intervention programs, the results contribute to the understanding of how infant characteristics and therapist availability influence the degree and types of intervention.

Holmes and colleagues (1987) evaluated the developmental progress of 64 of 203 infants who attended a publicly funded early intervention program in the Kansas City, Missouri, area during a 5-year period. The program included an intradisciplinary developmental assessment; development of an individualized educational and therapy program in conjunction with the parents; weekly or twice-weekly center-based physical therapy, speech therapy, and educational activities; monthly parent discussion groups; and home program activities planned by the staff and parents. The Early Intervention Developmental Profile (Rodgers et al., 1977), a multiple developmental domain curriculum-based assessment, was used to assess each infant. Infants were classified into five diagnostic groups to compare rates of development among infants receiving early intervention. Infants in the myelodysplasia, cerebral palsy, developmental delay, and multiple handicap diagnostic groups maintained their developmental rates during intervention, whereas the development quotient of infants in the Down syndrome group declined. Younger infants and infants with higher overall developmental quotients and higher developmental quotients in the cognitive domain on admission to the early intervention program demonstrated higher rates of developmental change. The authors concluded that although cause-and-effect relationships were not determined, the results suggested intervention efficacy for four of the groups. They recommended investigating the curricula for the infants with Down syndrome.

In the third study, Palisano (1989) evaluated two methods of therapy service delivery provided to students with learning disabilities who attended public school during the 1986–1987 school year. To serve adequately approximately 500 students receiving occupational and physical therapy, the therapy staff of the Delaware County, Pennsylvania, intermediate unit had instituted group and consultation methods of providing services to students with learning disabilities who met eligibility criteria. The therapists and teachers of students who participated in the study had worked together during the previous school year using the two methods of service delivery. Students in classrooms that received a combination of large group and small group therapy were compared with students in classrooms that received large group therapy and consultation. Methods of evaluation included student progress in motor, visuomotor, and visuoperceptual skills; the therapy needs of each group; teacher satisfaction; and use of available therapy resources. Both methods appeared to represent sound therapy practice. Interaction between the therapist and the teacher in establishing goals and planning group sessions was identified as integral to the success of both methods of service delivery. Recommendations for the following year included placing greater emphasis on achievement of functional goals, establishing group behavioral objectives, and examining similarities and differences between the services provided by occupational and physical therapy.

SUMMARY

Decision making is integral to determining who needs physical therapy and why, how cases should be managed, how outcomes should be documented, and what methods should be used for evaluating the effectiveness of clinical services. Pediatric physical therapists are increasingly becoming aware of the need to base their clinical decisions on the best available knowledge and research evidence. Clinical decision models for diagnosis, prediction of developmental or intervention outcome, and plans of care that are based on data from large research studies and statistical models have not been developed for pediatric physical therapy. Although models supported by a database are not currently available, conceptual models and objective methods of documentation and program evaluation can improve the decision-making process. In the "Guide to Physical Therapist Practice," the model of the disabling process and elements of patient/client management provide a conceptual framework for clinical decision making leading to optimal outcomes. The "Guide to Physical Therapist Practice" and the NCMRR model of the disabling process are applied in subsequent chapters on treatment of children with specific musculoskeletal, neurologic, and cardiopulmonary impairments. Although conceptual models are advantageous for organizing and externalizing thought processes, they do not eliminate the need for therapists to have a strong knowledge base, problem solve, and make sound clinical judgments. The limited research suggests that clinical reasoning involves the application not only of theory and psychomotor skill but also of intuitive or implicit thought processes.

Although physical therapists typically evaluate outcomes on the basis of whether children achieve short- and long-term goals or demonstrate improvement on standardized assessments of motor development and function, these methods do not indicate whether the outcomes were the result of intervention, because children are also expected to change as a result of maturational processes. Single-subject research designs are one clinical decision tool that enables pediatric physical therapists to evalu-

ate the effectiveness of their interventions for individual patients and to discover information of use in future research. In addition to evaluations of individual patient outcomes, professional practice requires evaluation of the overall effectiveness and costs of physical therapy programs. Monitoring of program inputs, implementation, and outputs is enhanced by computerized programs that allow the creation of databases on patient populations and provide a systematic, structured individual patient report. Formal methods of program evaluation provide information for assessing whether programs meet important consumer and societal needs, are properly implemented for maximal impact, and actually serve targeted populations. Use of formal experiments and data collection provides the opportunity to study cause-and-effect relationships among program inputs, interventions, and outcomes. Given the changing and complex nature of health care, pediatric physical therapists are challenged to enhance their use of more scientific evidence and more valid and reliable decision methods as the basis for their practice.

ACKNOWLEDGMENTS

The work reported in this chapter was partially supported by a grant to S.K. Campbell from the Agency for Health Care Policy and Research. Appreciation is expressed to Darl Vander Linden for his suggestions regarding classification of impairments, functional limitations, and disabilities in children with myelodysplasia.

Recommended Resources

Human Services Research Unit. Consumer's Guide: Therapeutic Services for Children with Disabilities, 1995. Copies may be obtained from the Publications Coordinator, Human Services Research Institute, 2336 Massachusetts Avenue, Cambridge, MA 02140. Phone: 617-876-0426.

References

Almeida, GL, Campbell, SK, Girolami, GL, Penn, RD, & Corcos, DM. Multi-dimensional assessment of motor function in a child with cerebral palsy following intrathecal administration of baclofen. Physical Therapy, 77:751–764, 1997.

American Physical Therapy Association. Guide to physical therapist practice. Physical Therapy, 77:1163–1650, 1997.

Aylward, GP. Conceptual issues in developmental screening and assessment. Developmental and Behavioral Pediatrics, 18:340–349, 1997.

Aylward, GP, & Kenny, TJ. Developmental follow-up: Inherent problems and a conceptual model. Journal of Pediatric Psychology, 4:331–343, 1979.

Ayres, AJ. Southern California Sensory Integration Tests. Los Angeles: Western Psychological Services, 1972.

Backman, CL, Harris, SR, Chisholm, JM, & Monette, AD. Single-subject research in rehabilitation: A review of studies using AB, withdrawal, multiple baseline, and alternating treatment designs. Archives of Physical Medicine and Rehabilitation, 78:1145–1153, 1997.

Backman, CL, & Harris, SR. Case studies, single subject research, and N of 1 randomized trials: Comparisons and contrasts. American Journal of Physical Medicine and Rehabilitation, *78*:170–176, 1999.

Barlow, DH, Hayes, SC, & Nelson, RO. The Scientist Practitioner: Research and Accountability in Clinical and Educational Settings. Emsford, NY: Pergamon Press, 1984.

Binkley, J, Finch, E, Hall, J, Black, T, & Gowland, C. Diagnostic classification of patients with low back pain: Report on a survey of physical therapy experts. Physical Therapy, *73*:138–155, 1993.

Boyd, S, Brooks, D, Agnew-Coughlin, J, & Ashwell, J. Evaluation of the literature on the effectiveness of physical therapy modalities in the management of children with cystic fibrosis. Pediatric Physical Therapy, *6*:70–74, 1994.

Brenner, P. From Novice to Expert: Excellence and Power in Clinical Nursing Practice. Reading, MA: Addison-Wesley, 1984.

Butler, C. Augmentative mobility: Why do it? Physical Medicine and Rehabilitation Clinics of North America, *2*:801–815, 1991.

Campbell, SK (Ed.). Proceedings of the consensus conference on the efficacy of physical therapy in the management of cerebral palsy. Pediatric Physical Therapy, *2*(3), 1990.

Campbell, SK. Measurement of motor performance in cerebral palsy. In Forrsberg, H, & Hirschfeld, H (Eds.), Movement Disorders in Children. Basel, Switzerland: Karger, 1992, pp. 264–271.

Campbell, SK. Future directions for physical therapy assessment in early infancy. In Wilhelm, IJ (Ed.), Physical Therapy Assessment in Early Infancy. New York: Churchill Livingstone, 1993, pp. 293–308.

Campbell, SK. Therapy programs for children that last a lifetime. Physical and Occupational Therapy in Pediatrics, *17*(1):1–15, 1997.

Campbell, SK. Models for decision making. In Campbell, SK (Ed.), Decision Making in Pediatric Neurologic Physical Therapy. Philadelphia: Churchill Livingstone, 1999, pp. 1–22.

Campbell, SK, & Gardner, HG. Physician Opinions on Referral of Children with Cerebral Palsy to Physical Therapy. Final Report of Grant R01 HS06429. Bethesda, MD: Agency for Health Care Policy and Research, 1992.

Campbell, SK, & Wilhelm, IJ. Development from birth to three years of fifteen children at high risk for central nervous system dysfunction. Physical Therapy, *65*:463–469, 1985.

Carter, RE. A behavioral analysis of interactions between physical therapists and children with cerebral palsy during treatment. Unpublished doctoral dissertation. Dekalb, IL: Northern Illinois University, 1989.

Crenna, P, Inverno, M, Frigo, C, Palmieri, R, & Fedrizzi, E. Pathophysiological profile of gait in children with cerebral palsy. In Forrsberg, H, & Hirschfeld, H (Eds.), Movement Disorders in Children. Basel, Switzerland: Karger, 1992, pp. 186–198.

Darrah, J, Fan, JSW, Chen, LC, Nunweiler, J, & Watkins, B. Review of the effects of progressive resisted muscle strengthening in children with cerebral palsy: A clinical consensus exercise. Pediatric Physical Therapy, *9*:12–17, 1997.

Darrah, J, Piper, M, & Watt, MJ. Assessment of gross motor skills of at-risk infants: Predictive validity of the Alberta Infant Motor Scale. Developmental Medicine and Child Neurology, *40*:485–491, 1998.

Dawes, RM, Faust, D, & Meehl, PE. Clinical versus actuarial judgment. Science, *243*:1668–1674, 1989.

Dowie, J, & Elstein, A (Eds.). Professional Judgment: A Reader in Clinical Decision Making. New York: Cambridge University Press, 1988.

Echternach, JL, & Rothstein, JM. Hypothesis-oriented algorithms. Physical Therapy, *69*:559–564, 1989.

Eddy, DM. Medicine, money, and mathematics. Bulletin of the American College of Surgeons, *77*:36–49, 1992.

Embrey, DG, & Adams, LS. Clinical applications of procedural changes by experienced and novice pediatric physical therapists. Pediatric Physical Therapy, *8*:122–132, 1996.

Embrey, DG, & Hylton, N. Clinical applications of movement scripts by experienced and novice pediatric physical therapists. Pediatric Physical Therapy, *8*:3–14, 1996.

Embrey, DG, & Nirider, B. Clinical applications of psychosocial sensitivity by experienced and novice pediatric physical therapists. Pediatric Physical Therapy, *8*:70–79, 1996.

Embrey, DG, Yates, L, & Mott, DH. Effects of neuro-developmental treatment and orthoses on knee flexion during gait: A single subject design. Physical Therapy, *70*:626–637, 1990.

Embrey, DG, Yates, L, Nirider, B, Hylton, N, & Adams, LS. Recommendations for pediatric physical therapists: Making clinical decisions for children with cerebral palsy. Pediatric Physical Therapy, *8*:165–170, 1996.

Evidence-Based Medicine Working Group. Evidence-based medicine: A new approach to teaching the practice of medicine. Journal of the American Medical Association, *268*(17):2420–2425, 1992.

Ferrari, F, Cioni, G, & Prechtl, HFR. Qualitative changes of general movements in preterm infants with brain lesions. Early Human Development, *23*:193–231, 1990.

Fleming, MH. Clinical reasoning in medicine compared to clinical reasoning in occupational therapy. American Journal of Occupational Therapy, *45*:988–996, 1991.

Franks, CA, Palisano, RJ, & Darbee, JC. The effect of walking with an assistive device and using a wheelchair on school performance in students with myelomeningocele. Physical Therapy, *71*:570–577, 1991.

Giangreco, MF. Related services decision-making: A foundational component of effective education for students with disabilities. Physical and Occupational Therapy in Pediatrics, *15*(2):47–67, 1995.

Goldberg, MJ. Commentary: Measuring outcomes in cerebral palsy. Journal of Pediatric Orthopedics, *11*:682–685, 1991.

Golden, GS. Nonstandard therapies in the developmental disabilities. American Journal of Diseases in Childhood, *134*:487–491, 1980.

Gonnella, C. Single-subject experimental paradigm as a clinical decision tool. Physical Therapy, *69*:601–609, 1989.

Gordon, BN, & Jens, KG. A conceptual model for tracking high-risk infants and making early service decisions. Journal of Developmental and Behavioral Pediatrics, *9*(5):279–286, 1988.

Granger, CV. Uniform Data System for Medical Rehabilitation: Guide for Functional Independence Measure. Buffalo: State University of New York, 1987.

Grimby, G, Finnstam, J, & Jette, AM. On the application of the WHO handicap classification in rehabilitation. Scandinavian Journal of Rehabilitation Medicine, *20*:93–98, 1988.

Guccione, AA. Physical therapy diagnosis and the relationship between impairments and function. Physical Therapy, *71*:499–503, 1991.

Haley, SM. Commentary on "The effect of walking with an assistive device and using a wheelchair on school performance in students with myelomeningocele." Physical Therapy, *71*:577–578, 1991.

Haley, SM, Coster, WJ, Ludlow, IH, Haltiwanger, JT, & Andrellos, P. Pediatric Evaluation of Disability Inventory. Boston: PEDI Research Group, 1992.

Haley, SM, Stephens, TE, & Larsen, AM. Patterns of physical and occupational therapy implementation in early motor intervention. Topics in Early Childhood Special Education, *7*(4):46–63, 1988.

Harbst, KB. Indicators of cerebral palsy 1985–1988. Physical and Occupational Therapy in Pediatrics, *10*(3):85–107, 1990.

Harris, SR. Research techniques for the clinician. In Connolly, BH, & Montgomery, PC (Eds.), Therapeutic Exercise in Developmental Disabilities, 2nd ed. Hixson, TN: Chattanooga Group, 1993, pp. 211–220.

Harris, SR. How should treatments be critiqued for scientific merit? Physical Therapy, *76*:175–181, 1996.

Harris, SR, & Riffle, K. Effects of inhibitive ankle-foot orthoses on standing balance in a child with cerebral palsy. Physical Therapy, *66*:663–667, 1986.

Harrison, H. The principles for family-centered neonatal care. Pediatrics, 92:643–650, 1993.

Hinderer, KA, Harris, SR, Purdy, AH, Chew, DE, Staheli, LT, McLaughlin, JF, & Jaffe, KM. Effects of "tone-reducing" vs. standard plaster casts on gait improvement of children with cerebral palsy. Developmental Medicine and Child Neurology, 30:370–377, 1988.

Holmes, GE, Britain, LA, Simpson, RL, & Hassanein, RS. Developmental progress of five groups of disabled children attending an early intervention program. Physical and Occupational Therapy in Pediatrics, 7(1):3–18, 1987.

Horn, EM, Warren, SF, & Jones, HA. An experimental analysis of neurobehavioral motor intervention. Developmental Medicine and Child Neurology, 37:697–714, 1997.

Human Services Research Unit. Consumer's Guide: Therapeutic Services for Children with Disabilities. Cambridge, MA: Human Services Research Institute, 1995.

Jenkins, D. A practical introduction to databases: Part 2. Biomedical Instrumentation and Technology, 23:109–112, 1989.

Kanda, T, Yuge, M, & Yamori, Y. Early physiotherapy in the treatment of spastic diplegia. Developmental Medicine and Child Neurology, 26:438–444, 1984.

King, GA, King, SM, & Rosenbaum, PL. Interpersonal aspects of caregiving and client outcomes: A review of the literature. Ambulatory and Child Health, 2:151–160, 1996.

Kopp, CB. Developmental risk: Historical reflections. In Osofsky, JD (Ed.), Handbook of Infant Development. New York: Wiley, 1987, pp. 881–912.

Lansky, D, Butler, JBV, & Waller, FT. Using health status measures in the hospital setting: From acute care to outcome management. Medical Care, 30(5 suppl):MS57–MS73, 1992.

Larin, HM. Knowledge in Practice: Motor Learning Theories in Pediatric Physiotherapy. Unpublished doctoral dissertation. University of Toronto, 1992.

Laskas, SA, Mullen, SL, Nelson, DL, & Willson-Broyles, M. Enhancement of two motor functions of the lower extremity in a child with spastic quadriplegia. Physical Therapy, 65:11–16, 1985.

Law, M, Baptiste, S, Carswell-Opzoomer, A, McColl, MA, Polatajko, H, & Pollack, N. Canadian Occupational Performance Measure Manual. Toronto, CA: CAOT Publications, 1991.

Lehmann, JF, Warren, CG, Smith, W, & Larson, J. Computerized data management as an aid to clinical decision making in rehabilitation medicine. Archives of Physical Medicine and Rehabilitation, 65:260–262, 1984.

Magistro, CM. Clinical decision making in physical therapy. Physical Therapy, 69:525–534, 1989.

Mattingly, C. What is clinical reasoning? American Journal of Occupational Therapy, 45:979–986, 1991.

Molnar, GE (Ed.). Pediatric Rehabilitation, 2nd ed. Baltimore: Williams & Wilkins, 1992.

Nagi, SZ. Disability and Rehabilitation. Columbus, OH: Ohio State University Press, 1969.

Nagi, SZ. Disability concepts revisited: Implications for prevention. In Pope, AN, & Tarlov, AR (Eds.), Disability in America: Toward a National Agenda for Prevention. Washington, DC: National Academy Press, 1991, pp. 309–327.

Nagi, SZ. Some conceptual issues in disability and rehabilitation. In Sussman, MB (Ed.), Sociology and Rehabilitation. New York: American Sociological Association, n.d., pp. 100–113.

National Institutes of Health. Research Plan for the National Center for Medical Rehabilitation Research. NIH Publication No. 93-3509. Bethesda, MD: National Institutes of Health, 1993.

Nelson, KB, & Ellenberg, JH. Children who "outgrew" cerebral palsy. Pediatrics, 69:529–536, 1982.

Norton, BJ, & Strube, MJ. Making decisions based on group designs and meta-analysis. Physical Therapy, 69:594–600, 1989.

Ottenbacher, K. Sensory integration therapy: Affect or effect. American Journal of Occupational Therapy, 36:571–577, 1982.

Ottenbacher, KJ. Evaluating Clinical Change: Strategies for Occupational and Physical Therapists. Baltimore: Williams & Wilkins, 1986.

Ottenbacher, KJ, Biocca, Z, DeCremer, G, Gevelinger, M, Jedlovec, KB, & Johnson, MB. Quantitative analysis of the effectiveness of pediatric physical therapy: Emphasis on the neurodevelopmental treatment approach. Physical Therapy, 66:1095–1101, 1986.

Palisano, R, Rosenbaum, P, Walter, S, Russell, D, Wood, E, & Galuppi, B. Development and reliability of a system to classify gross motor function of children with cerebral palsy. Developmental Medicine and Child Neurology, 39:214–223, 1997.

Palisano, RJ. Comparison of two methods of service delivery for students with learning disabilities. Physical and Occupational Therapy in Pediatrics, 9(3):79–100, 1989.

Piper, MC, Darrah, J, Pinnell, L, Watt, MJ, & Byrne, P. The consistency of sequential examinations in the early detection of neurological dysfunction. Physical and Occupational Therapy in Pediatrics, 11(3):27–44, 1991.

Pope, AN, & Tarlov, AR (Eds.). Disability in America: Toward a National Agenda for Prevention. Washington, DC: National Academy Press, 1991.

Prechtl, HFR, Einspieler, C, Cioni, G, Bos, AF, Ferrari, F, & Sontheimer, D. An early marker for neurological deficits after perinatal brain lesions. Lancet, 349:1361, 1997.

Purdy, AH, Deitz, JC, & Harris, SR. Efficacy of two treatment approaches to reduce tongue protrusion of children with Down syndrome. Developmental Medicine and Child Neurology, 29:469–476, 1987.

Rodgers, SJ, Donovon, CM, D'Eugenio, DB, Brown, SL, Lynch, EW, Moersch, MS, & Schafer, DS. Early intervention developmental profile. In Schafer, DS, & Moersch, MS (Eds.), Developmental Programming for Infants and Young Children, Vol. 2. Ann Arbor, MI: University of Michigan Press, 1977.

Rogers, J, & Masagatani, G. Clinical reasoning of occupational therapists during the initial assessment of physically disabled patients. Occupational Therapy Journal of Research, 2:195–219, 1982.

Rosenbaum, PL, King, S, Law, M, King, G, & Evans, J. Family-centered service: A conceptual framework and research review. Physical and Occupational Therapy in Pediatrics, 18(1):1–20, 1998.

Rosenbaum, PL, Palisano, RJ, Walter, S, & Russell, D. Motor growth curves in cerebral palsy: A guide for rehabilitation. Bethesda, MD: National Center for Medical Rehabilitation Research, National Institute for Child Health and Human Development, National Institutes of Health, 1997.

Rosenblith, JF. A singular career: Nancy Bayley. Developmental Psychology, 28:747–758, 1992.

Rothstein, JM, & Echternach, JL. Hypothesis-oriented algorithm for clinicians: A method for evaluation and treatment planning. Physical Therapy, 66:1388–1394, 1986.

Sackett, DL, Haynes, RB & Tugwell, P. Clinical Epidemiology: A Basic Science for Clinical Medicine. Boston: Little, Brown, 1985.

Sackett, DL, Rosenberg, WMC, Gray, JAM, Haynes, RB, & Richardson, WS. Evidence based medicine: What it is and what it isn't. British Medical Journal, 312:71–72, 1996.

Schenkman, M, & Butler, RB. A model for multisystem evaluation, interpretation, and treatment of individuals with neurologic dysfunction. Physical Therapy, 69:538–547, 1989.

Schyve, PM. The evolving role of the Joint Commission for the Accreditation of Health Care Organizations. Joint Commission Journal on Quality Improvement, 11:S54–S57, 1996.

Shadish, WR, Jr, Cook, TD, & Leviton, LC. Foundations of Program Evaluation: Theories of Practice. Newbury Park, CA: Sage, 1991.

Shurtleff, DB. Computer databases for pediatric disability: Clinical and research applications. Physical Medicine and Rehabilitation Clinics of North America, 2:665–687, 1991.

Slagle, TA, & Gould, JB. Database use in neonatal intensive care units: Success or failure. Pediatrics, 90:959–965, 1992.

Slovick, P, & Lichtenstein, S. Comparison of Bayesian and regression approaches to the study of information processing in judgment. Organizational Behavior and Human Performance, 6:649–744, 1971.

Thomson-O'Brien, MA, & Moreland, J. Evidence-based information circle. Physiotherapy Canada, Summer 1998, pp. 184–189.

Tiffin, J. Purdue Pegboard Examiner Manual. Chicago: Scientific Research Associates, 1968.

Users' guide to the medical literature. Journal of the American Medical Association, 270:2093–2097, 2598–2601, 1993; 271:59–63, 389–391, 703–707, 1615–1619, 1994.

Wang, MC, & Ellet, CD. Program validation: The state of the art. Topics in Early Childhood Special Education, 1(4):35–49, 1982.

Waters, RL, & Lunsford, BR. Energy cost of paraplegic locomotion. Journal of Bone and Joint Surgery (American), 67:1245–1250, 1985.

Watts, N. Decision analysis: A tool for improving physical therapy practice and education. In Wolf, SL (Ed.), Clinical Decision Making in Physical Therapy. Philadelphia: FA Davis, 1985, pp. 7–23.

Watts, N. Clinical decision analysis. Physical Therapy, 69:569–576, 1989.

Weed, LL, & Zimny, NJ. The problem-oriented system, problem-knowledge coupling, and clinical decision making. Physical Therapy, 69:565–568, 1989.

Wolery, M, & Bailey, DD. Alternatives to impact evaluation: Suggestions for program evaluation in early intervention. Journal of the Division for Early Childhood, 4:27–37, 1984.

World Health Organization. International Classification of Impairments, Disabilities, and Handicaps. Geneva: World Health Organization, 1980.

World Health Organization. ICIDH-2: International Classification of Impairments, Activities, and Participation. A Manual of Dimensions of Disablement and Functioning, Beta-1 Draft for Field Trials. Geneva: World Health Organization, 1997.

SECTION
II

MANAGEMENT OF MUSCULOSKELETAL IMPAIRMENT

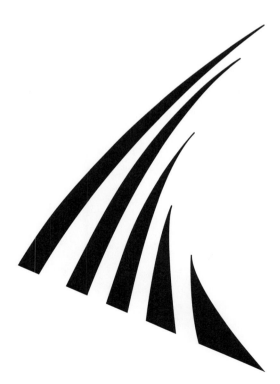

DARL W. VANDER LINDEN, PT, PhD

Section Editor

C H A P T E R
8

Juvenile Rheumatoid Arthritis

SHIRLEY ALBINSON SCULL, PT, MS

Chronic childhood arthritis can result from many different disorders, of which juvenile rheumatoid arthritis (JRA) is the most common. Other rheumatic diseases that cause joint pathology include systemic lupus erythematosus, Lyme disease, juvenile ankylosing spondylitis, scleroderma, and dermatomyositis. Juvenile rheumatoid arthritis causes musculoskeletal impairments such as joint contractures, weakness, postural deviations, and pain, which can result in limitations in functional mobility unless the medical and therapeutic management of the patient is optimal.

This chapter provides an overview of the child with juvenile rheumatoid arthritis and includes information on physical therapy examination and intervention strategies. Management of more complex episodes of care such as intervention after total joint replacement is discussed. A case history that describes the impact of the disease on a young child with JRA illustrates the role of the physical therapist and the impact on functional mobility.

ROLE OF THE THERAPIST

Physical therapists are essential members of the health care team that manages the musculoskeletal impairments of children with rheumatic disease, along with the pediatric rheumatologist, orthopedist, and occupational therapist. Other team members often include a nurse and social worker. Consultation may be obtained from psychologists, ophthalmologists, and cardiologists, depending on the child's needs (Rhodes, 1991).

On the basis of a comprehensive musculoskeletal examination, the therapist develops a problem list for each patient. Impairments such as loss of motion, weakness, postural deviations, and pain are analyzed for their impact on present function and their potential for creating future problems. Relationships between impairments and functional limitations are identified. Examples include muscle weakness secondary to disuse with an antalgic gait or knee flexion contracture secondary to leg length discrepancy. Part of the role of the physical therapist is early recognition of potential problems and development of a plan of care that involves prevention of secondary impairments.

Physical therapists instruct the child and parent in a home care program that includes splinting, exercises, positioning, joint conservation, activities of daily living (ADL), and advice regarding recreational activities. The interventions provided and treatment frequency will vary between rehabilitation centers (Hacket et al., 1996). Direct intervention is sometimes provided intensively during a short inpatient rehabilitation admission with the goals of improving functional skills and maximizing flexibility and strength. More often, children with JRA are treated regularly as outpatients. The rheumatology team must also communicate with personnel in the child's school in order to coordinate any needed modifications in the child's routine or environment.

The patient's goals and the family supports must be understood. The child's developmental age is used as a guideline to assist in determining appropriate functional goals and intervention methods. Guidance by the therapist may be necessary if the child's or the family's goals are unrealistic. Goals are prioritized so that the therapy program and home instructions are focused on those impairments and functional limitations that contribute most to current disabilities in daily life. Measurable goals that the patient understands and can monitor provide positive reinforcement.

INCIDENCE AND DIAGNOSTIC CLASSIFICATIONS

JRA is one of the more common chronic illnesses of childhood. A study in 1983 at the Mayo Clinic estimated the annual incidence to be 13.9 per 100,000. The prevalence was found to be 113.4 cases per 100,000 (Towner et al., 1983). There are 160,000 to 190,000 children with JRA in the United States (Cassidy & Petty, 1995).

The diagnostic criteria for JRA have been defined by the American College of Rheumatology (Cassidy & Petty, 1995). The age at onset is arbitrarily set at younger than 16 years to distinguish JRA from adult-onset disease. Arthritis is evidenced by joint swelling or effusion and the presence of two or more of the following signs: heat, limitation of range of motion (ROM), and tenderness or pain on motion. Symptoms must persist for a minimum of 6 weeks. Because no definitive laboratory tests are available to identify JRA, the diagnosis is made by exclusion of other rheumatic diseases or diagnoses such as joint infections, trauma, malignancies, or systemic illnesses, depending on the presenting symptoms.

Clinical signs during onset, defined as the first 6 months of the disease, are used to classify three distinct subtypes of JRA (Table 8–1) (Cassidy & Petty, 1995). Pauciarticular JRA is the most common subtype, affecting one to four joints, often a knee, ankle, or wrist. Patients with pauciarticular JRA have a 20% chance of developing inflammation of the iris and ciliary body known as anterior uveitis or iridocyclitis (Petty, 1987). Eye involvement is often asymptomatic, and therefore slit lamp biomicroscopy by an ophthalmologist is required at the time of diagnosis and periodically thereafter. Complications of iridocyclitis include synechiae, band keratopathy, and cataract. Functional blindness has been reported in 15 to 30% of eyes with uveitis, although routine screening and earlier diagnosis are improving these statistics (Cabral et al., 1992; Petty, 1987). Systemic or topical corticosteroids are prescribed to control inflammation and prevent blindness.

TABLE 8–1. **Classification of the Types of Onset of Juvenile Rheumatoid Arthritis**

Criterion	Polyarthritis	Oligoarthritis (Pauciarticular Disease)	Systemic Disease
Frequency of cases	40%	50%	10%
Number of joints involved	≥5	≤4	Variable
Age at onset	Throughout childhood; peak at 1–3 years	Early childhood; peak at 1–2 years	Throughout childhood; no peak
Sex ratio (F:M)	3:1	5:1	1:1
Systemic involvement	Moderate involvement	Not present	Prominent
Occurrence of chronic uveitis	5%	20%	Rare
Frequency of Seropositivity			
Rheumatoid factors	10% (increases with age)	Rare	Rare
Antinuclear antibodies	40–50%	75–85%*	10%
Prognosis	Guarded to moderately good	Excellent except for eyesight	Moderate to poor

From Cassidy, JT, & Petty, RE. Textbook of Pediatric Rheumatology, 3rd ed. Philadelphia: WB Saunders, 1995.
*In girls with uveitis.

Polyarticular disease onset (involving five or more joints) occurs in 40% of children with JRA. The number of joints involved can be 20 or more in some children. Joints commonly affected include the knees, ankles, elbows, wrists, cervical spine, and temporomandibular joint; a symmetric distribution is typical.

Systemic disease is the least common subtype, occurring in 10% of cases. As the name implies, systemic JRA is characterized by severe constitutional symptoms, including intermittent fevers to 39°C, rash (erythematous macules on the trunk and proximal extremities), hepatosplenomegaly, lymphadenopathy, pleuritis, and pericarditis. Onset of joint involvement may lag behind these systemic symptoms by months or, occasionally, 1 or 2 years.

The clinical course of the disease after 6 months may vary from the type of onset, such as pauciarticular onset with polyarticular course, further complicating the classification of these diseases.

ETIOLOGY AND PATHOPHYSIOLOGY

Multiple etiologies may be responsible for the various subtypes of diseases classified together as JRA, or a single cause may evolve into different clinical patterns as it interacts with the host (Cassidy & Petty, 1995). The etiology of JRA is unknown, although it is considered an autoimmune disorder and is probably multifactorial in origin. There are very few reports of cases of JRA in more than one member of the family. Studies of human leukocyte antigen types, however, show a high correlation between genetic predisposition to the disease and specific subtypes.

Often an environmental trigger such as infection or trauma precedes the onset of JRA, although the precise relationship between these events is not clear (Cassidy & Petty, 1995). Despite intensive efforts, no specific infectious agent has been identified in the blood or synovial tissue. Whatever the inciting event, joint inflammation is initiated and perpetuated by immunologic mechanisms.

The predominant cells in the joint fluid are neutrophils. These cells release a number of chemicals after ingesting immune complexes and cell debris. The chemicals cause pain, swelling, warmth, and effusion into the joint.

In the synovial membrane, the predominant cells are lymphocytes, mostly T cells. These cells are probably activated by the persistence of putative antigen. This, in turn, leads to production of antibodies by B cells and stimulation of macrophages. Cytokines produced by macrophages cause proliferation of fibroblasts, production of prostaglandins, and bone resorption. The inflammatory response causes the subsynovial tissues to become edematous and hyperemic. The synovium begins to proliferate, resulting in massive overgrowth called pannus. The pannus can actually invade the adjacent cartilage and bone, resulting in erosions.

Late joint changes include adhesions and osteophytes. Surrounding tissues such as tendons and ligaments undergo fibrosis, resulting in contracture. The underlying bone is scarred and damaged (Fig. 8–1), and the joint shape may become irregular. Subluxation can occur at the wrists and small joints of the hands and feet, or less commonly, there may be posterior subluxation of the tibia on the femur.

MEDICAL MANAGEMENT

A variety of medications are used to control joint inflammation (Fig. 8–2) (Cassidy & Petty, 1995). The first-line medication is a nonsteroidal anti-inflammatory drug such as naproxen, tolmetin, or ibuprofen. A slow-acting antirheumatic drug (SAARD) such as a gold salt, an antimalarial agent, D-penicillamine, or sulfasalazine may be added to the drug program. Glucocorticoids are potent and effective anti-inflammatory agents, but long-term use is avoided because of side effects such as growth retardation and Cushing's syndrome. Intra-articular injections of glucocorticoids may be used for several trials in monarticular disease or for target joints in polyarticular disease (Earley et al., 1988). Methotrexate has been shown to have a dramatic effect in controlling this disease provided liver enzyme studies are monitored to detect possible toxicity (Athreya & Cassidy, 1991; Giannini et al., 1992; Rose et al.,

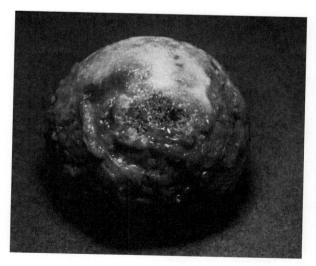

FIGURE 8–1. Synovial hypertrophy and destruction of cartilage and bone.

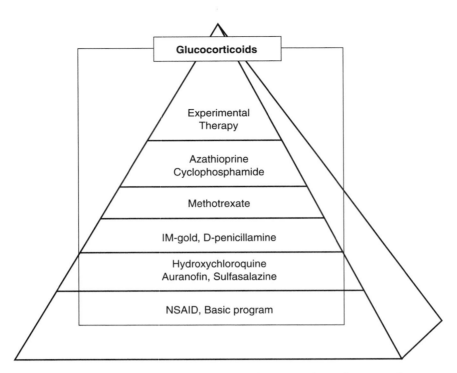

FIGURE 8–2. A pyramid of drugs may be introduced to control the disease. (Redrawn from Cassidy, JT, & Petty, RE. Textbook of Pediatric Rheumatology, 3rd ed. Philadelphia: WB Saunders, 1995.)

1990). Newer experimental approaches include other cytotoxic agents and immune modulators such as azathioprine and cyclophosphamide (Athreya & Cassidy, 1991).

PROGNOSIS

The number of children with JRA who enter into remission varies with the subtypes. Wallace and Levinson (1991) reviewed long-term outcome studies and discussed implications for early and aggressive medical management of inflammation before onset of joint destruction. Ten years after onset, 22 to 71% of children with pauciarticular JRA had active disease, 40 to 50% of children with polyarticular JRA had active disease, and 25 to 58% of children with systemic JRA had active disease. Ruperto and colleagues (1997) surveyed a cohort of American and Italian patients with JRA followed for longer than 5 years using assessments of functional status, pain, overall well-being, and quality of life. Long-term outcome was highly favorable for all variables. Children with polyarticular disease who are rheumatoid factor positive have the worst prognosis for unremitting arthritis with joint erosions (Schaller, 1983). Children with pauciarticular JRA do well functionally, except for possible complications related to

vision. Even children whose disease remits may have long-term musculoskeletal complications of contractures, postural deviations, and localized growth disturbances.

DISABILITIES

The type and degree of disability vary depending on the age of the child, the severity of the disease, and the family's coping strategies.

A nondisabled toddler or preschooler begins to achieve separation from the parent and some independence with ADL such as feeding, dressing, and toileting. A child with JRA who is in pain and refuses to cooperate, or one who gains attention because of his or her need for help, may cause difficulty with parent-child interactions. Parents may be frustrated, be tired, or feel guilty. Some parents adopt a style of being overprotective, discouraging their child's engagement in appropriate tasks such as playground activities with peers. Opportunities to master certain gross motor skills such as bike riding may be missed because of fear of injury.

The school-age child may have poor school attendance because of morning stiffness and time-consuming morning care. Some children are unable to walk on arising and must take a bath or do exercises to loosen up. Difficulty with mobility, such as needing to use an elevator instead of stairs, or inability to dress or toilet independently may lead to the child's rejection by other students. Postural deviations and other cosmetic differences have an impact on the child's self-esteem. Participation in physical education classes to the student's tolerance should be encouraged, but activities must be monitored to protect the joints (Scull & Athreya, 1995). Some children require a special, individualized education plan at school to address transportation, time requirements for examinations, adaptive physical education, or other related services. Physical therapists and occupational therapists in schools may provide direct services or consultation. Appropriate goals relate to attaining an optimal education by providing assistance with handwriting, mobility skills, physical education, or ADL (Whitehouse et al., 1989).

The adolescent's social roles in dating, driving, and entering the workforce are affected by functional impairments. Career selection must take into account the physical limitations of the individual. College plans may be complicated by the need for wheelchair accessibility and assistance from attendants. The ability to become fully independent from the family will be tested at this time.

The mature patient who becomes sexually active may require counseling to be comfortable during sexual activities. Pregnancy requires special consideration because of the effects on the arthritis. Medications may need to be altered because of the effects on the fetus. Delivery by cesarean section may be recommended.

MUSCULOSKELETAL IMPAIRMENTS

Joint Pathology

Joint pathology produces restricted ROM and, typically, flexion contractures, which should be assessed using a goniometer. Measurements of active ROM provide functional data but may be limited by joint pathology, weakness, or pain. Passive ROM provides a more accurate baseline for joint pathology and should be reliable for most joints to within ±5°. Additional examination of the joints should include ligamentous laxity and postural deficits, such as valgus or varus. Measurements of circumference can document swelling but are confusing in the presence of bony overgrowth. Synovial thickness, heat, or redness is also noted.

Inactivity stiffness can interfere with the ability to walk for up to 2 hours each morning. A warm tub bath is recommended on arising, with exercises performed in the water to decrease morning stiffness. The use of a small whirlpool may decrease pain be-

cause sensory receptors are stimulated that compete with pain signals (Michlovitz, 1996). In my experience, however, the primary benefits are the warmth and buoyancy of the water rather than its aeration. Other methods used to manage morning stiffness include resting night splints for the knees and a sleeping bag or blanket sleeper pajamas that provide neutral warmth (Scull et al., 1986).

Early radiographic changes include soft tissue swelling about the joints, widening of the joint space, osteoporosis near the joint, and periosteal new bone formation, especially in the phalanges, metacarpals, and metatarsals (Cassidy & Petty, 1995). After 2 or more years of active disease, radiographic changes may include marginal erosions and joint space narrowing secondary to loss of articular cartilage. Bony ankylosis may be seen, especially of the carpal or tarsal joints or cervical spine. Loose bodies that mechanically block joint motion may also be present.

Abnormalities of the hip occur in about 35% of cases. In young children, coxa valga may occur. Forces across the femoral epiphysis may cause widening of the femoral neck, resulting in restricted motion. Avascular necrosis can occur, sometimes as a complication of corticosteroid use, resulting in disabling hip pain and decreased function. Hip motion should be closely monitored because children with active hip disease often develop difficulty with ambulation.

Loss of normal flexibility can also be caused by muscle imbalance around a joint. This typically occurs in the hip flexors, adductors, hamstrings, and gastrocnemius of the lower extremities and in the wrist and finger flexors of the upper extremities. Tendon sheaths, which are lined with synovium, can develop tenosynovitis, typically manifested in the flexors and extensors extrinsic to the hand, resulting in loss of gliding motion.

Contractures

Contractures occur in a majority of cases of JRA. Minor contracture in joints of the lower extremities (less than 10°) may not have functional significance. However, if allowed to progress toward 15 to 20°, contractures can cause dysfunctional mobility or difficulty with daily living activities. Long-standing contractures may lead to growth abnormalities of the joint, the limb, or the spine, as secondary postural compensations are adopted because of abnormal alignment. Useful physical therapy techniques include exercise and splinting designed to lengthen the antagonist and strengthen the agonist (Scull, 1994). Later in the chapter, the indications for surgery for fixed contractures are discussed.

Exercise

Active ROM exercises are extremely important in the management of JRA. The patient should move all the joints through their full available ROM at least once a day. Combinations of movement patterns are taught for efficiency. Passive stretching exercises are avoided for acutely inflamed joints and for those that show signs of instability or mechanical derangement. Gentle, passive ROM exercise is indicated for contractures if joint inflammation is under medical control and if the restriction is believed to be at least partially muscular, with a stretchy feel at the end of the range of motion.

Flexion contractures of the hips and knees may be managed by gravity-assisted stretching in the prone position for 20 minutes per day, with feet suspended over the edge of the support (Fig. 8–3) (Scull et al., 1986). The weight of the lower leg drops the knee into extension. A sandbag may be placed over the buttocks for stabilization. If the patient lacks full neck rotation, a towel roll applied at the forehead may provide comfort.

Hand placement when passively stretching a knee flexion contracture must avoid use of a long lever arm because of the potential for posterior subluxation of the tibia on the femur. In addition, the patient may not tolerate hand placement over the patella.

If shoulder motion is available above 90°, exercise while in the supine position will allow gravity to assist the shoulder stretch. A baton held in both hands allows the patient to perform active assisted shoulder flexion. Proprioceptive neuromuscular facilitation patterns may also be taught.

At the neck, ROM should be assessed in both supine and sitting positions, with manual stabilization of the shoulders. A kyphotic sitting posture often interferes with optimal neck ROM. Apophyseal joint involvement may result in torticollis, with uni-lateral restriction of rotation, lateral flexion, and extension, and can proceed to fusion (Fried et al., 1983). Moist heat applied before the exercise program may be helpful in obtaining improved ROM (Emery & Bowyer, 1991). Clinicians must be mindful of the potential for atlantoaxial subluxation, which is a contraindication for exercise and should be identified by radiographs. In this instance, a cervical collar is recommended for car travel to avert deceleration injury in case of an impact.

Splinting

Slow prolonged stretch such as that provided by a dynamic splint is often more effective for reducing flexion contractures than exercise (Hepburn, 1987), although this has not yet been documented by clinical research for children with JRA. I have used dynamic splints (Fig. 8–4) successfully on elbow and knee flexion contractures for children age 2 years and older. The tension is set to patient tolerance and can be advanced as the contracture improves. Results should be measurable (greater than 10°) within 2

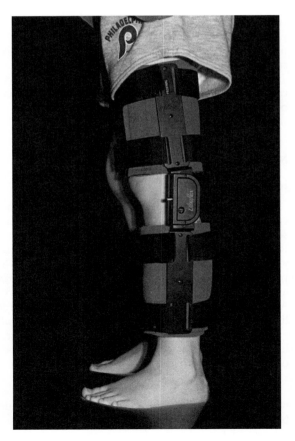

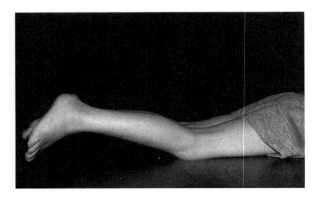

FIGURE 8–3. The prone position is used to stretch hip and knee flexion contractures.

FIGURE 8–4. Dynamic splinting is effective in stretching knee flexion contractures.

weeks. Some patients are able to tolerate splints during the hours of sleep, which gives maximum benefit. Others wear them two or three times a day for 1-hour periods. Traction may also be used to provide a prolonged stretch to flexion contractures but requires confinement to bed.

Serial casting or drop-out casts are used occasionally for knee flexion contractures that do not respond to exercise, positioning, or dynamic splinting (Melvin & Atwood, 1989). Because the patient is at risk for losing flexion when the joint is held in a cast, the cast should be bivalved for daily exercise or changed every 3 days. This intervention is typically selected as a last resort before surgery and would increase compliance for the patient who refused a home exercise program of exercise or splinting. Measurement of the ROM and an exercise program at the time of cast change maintains ROM and documents any improvement in motion.

Weakness

Secondary changes are seen in the muscles, especially atrophy resulting from disuse (Giannini & Protas, 1993). Examination should include dynamometry or manual muscle testing of key functional groups and may be done by isometric testing if resistance through the range increases discomfort (Scull, 1994). Strength ratings of less than 4 on a scale of 1 to 5 in lower extremity antigravity muscles may be expected to result in gait deviations and functional limitations, such as inability to climb stairs, although disease activity is also a good predictor of function (Fan et al., 1998). If the child is younger than 5 years of age, manual muscle testing may be difficult, and the ability to perform antigravity developmental patterns is a more useful way to test strength.

Strengthening exercises may be done isometrically if active exercise causes pain. Concentric and eccentric contractions are taught, if tolerated. Resisted exercises are restricted to weights less than a few pounds. Elastic bands are a useful product in pediatric treatment programs and can be progressed by choosing the next color of resistance. Play activities such as bicycle or tricycle riding are also useful for strengthening the lower extremities. Exercise in water can improve both strength and flexibility and reduce pain.

Growth Disturbances and Postural Abnormalities

JRA may affect posture and growth because the epiphyseal plates are open in children (White, 1990). Generalized growth retardation may be the result of the basic disease process or may be related to the side effects of use of corticosteroids. Small stature may be compounded by premature closure of the epiphyses. Proper attention to nutrition has to be incorporated into a management program (Henderson et al., 1992). Research protocols using growth hormone are in the process of being tested.

Local growth disturbances may result in leg length discrepancy. An increase in blood supply to the epiphysis because of inflammation results in overgrowth of the limb, especially with unilateral knee involvement. Posture should be assessed periodically and leg lengths measured for symmetry. A shoe lift can be added to correct leg length if it improves posture or gait.

Scoliosis, kyphosis, torticollis, and cervical lordosis may be the result of spinal involvement or habitual posture secondary to pain. Leg length discrepancy may also cause an oblique pelvis and secondary scoliosis. Early detection of postural abnormalities can prevent these secondary deformities.

Undergrowth of the mandible, called micrognathia, is seen in about 20% of cases of JRA, usually in children with polyarticular disease (White, 1990). Radiographic changes show shortening of the body and vertical rami of the mandible with widening of the mandibular notch. Orthodontic work may be required to correct for resultant malocclusion (Mayro et al., 1991).

Pain

Pain is assessed in children in a variety of ways, depending on the child's age (McGrath, 1990; Varni et al., 1987). One option is use of a visual analogue scale, which is a 10 cm line anchored at one end with the words "No pain" and at the other end with "Pain as bad as it could be." The child draws a line through the estimated amount of pain. Good correlation has been demonstrated between the child's, parent's, and physician's estimates of the present pain (Varni et al., 1987). A body outline can be given to the child to draw the location of pain (Fig. 8–5). Four developmentally appropriate labels of pain intensity are discussed, and the child selects a crayon color to represent each one. A list of pain descriptors has also been developed for pediatrics as part of the Pediatric Pain Questionnaire developed by Varni and associates (1987).

Because children with JRA are already taking one or more medications, the physician has few choices for ongoing management of chronic pain. Behavioral management techniques involving muscle relaxation, meditative breathing, and guided imagery can be taught to the child. Parents may also be instructed in appropriate behavior modification techniques that involve encouraging adaptive behaviors and discouraging maladaptive pain behaviors.

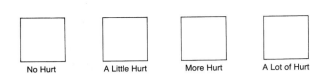

Pick the colors that mean *No Hurt, A Little Hurt, More Hurt,* and *A Lot of Hurt* to you and color in the boxes. Now, using those colors, color in the body to show how you feel. Where you have no hurt, use the *No Hurt* color to color in your body. If you have hurt or pain, use the color that tells how much hurt you have.

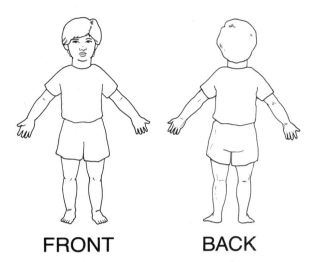

FIGURE 8–5. Pain may be assessed by allowing a child to color a body map. Intensity of pain is matched with four different colors.

FUNCTIONAL LIMITATIONS

The combination of pain, restricted ROM, muscle weakness, and skeletal deformities may result in significant functional limitations for the patient. The patient with mild involvement may show some gait deviations but be fully functional in the home and school environment. The patient with more severe involvement may require a wheelchair for community mobility and be dependent for many daily living activities. The American College of Rheumatology has proposed four categories of disabilities based on functional deficits (Hochberg et al., 1992):

Class I   Completely able to perform usual ADL (self-care, vocational, and avocational)

Class II   Able to perform usual self-care and vocational activities but limited in avocational activities

Class III   Able to perform usual self-care activities but limited in vocational and avocational activities

Class IV   Limited in ability to perform usual self-care, vocational, and avocational activities

These global functional categories have been studied in adults but not in children.

The Juvenile Arthritis Functional Assessment Scale (JAFAS) (Lovell et al., 1989) and the Childhood Health Assessment Questionnaire (CHAQ) (Singh et al., 1994) are specifically designed to assess the functional limitations for children with arthritis. The JAFAS is a list of 10 activities with accompanying criterion times (Fig. 8–6). A child is graded a 0

For each activity, please record how long the child took to perform the activity. If the activity was completed in less than or equal to the criterion time, then score the item as 0; if completed but requiring longer than the criterion time, score the item as 1; if unable to perform the activity, score the item as 2.

Activity	Criterion Time (seconds)	Observed Time (seconds)	Item Score 0	1	2
1. Button shirt/blouse	22.4	____	____	____	____
2. Pull shirt or sweater over head	14.6	____	____	____	____
3. Pull on both socks	27.2	____	____	____	____
4. Cut food with knife and fork	12.8	____	____	____	____
5. Get into bed	3.4	____	____	____	____
6. Get out of bed	2.9	____	____	____	____
7. Pick something up off of floor from standing position	2.4	____	____	____	____
8. From standing position sit on floor, then stand up	4.0	____	____	____	____
9. Walk 50 feet without assistance	15.1	____	____	____	____
10. Walk up flight of 5 steps	3.7	____	____	____	____
		TOTAL SCORE ____			

FIGURE 8–6. The Juvenile Arthritis Functional Assessment Scale (JAFAS) is a list of 10 functional activities that must be completed within the criterion time. (Reprinted with permission from Lovell, DJ, Howe, S, Shear, E, Hartner, S, McGirr, G, Schulte, M, & Levinson, J. Development of a disability measurement tool for juvenile rheumatoid arthritis: The Juvenile Arthritis Functional Assessment Scale. Arthritis and Rheumatism, *32*:1390–1395, 1989.)

when he or she meets or exceeds a criterion, 1 if he or she completes the activity slowly, and 2 if he or she is unable to perform. The test takes less than 10 minutes to complete and requires a minimum of simple equipment. A version is also designed to be scored by parental report and is called the Juvenile Arthritis Functional Assessment Report (JAFAR) (Howe et al., 1991).

The CHAQ (Fig. 8–7) covers dressing and grooming, arising, eating, walking, hygiene, reaching, gripping, and community mobility. The parent or child completes a checklist with four scoring choices:

1. Unable to do
2. Does with much difficulty
3. Does with some difficulty
4. Does without any difficulty

A list of aids or devices may be checked off to document which assistive devices are used.

Gait Abnormalities

Gait deviations are often the primary functional problem addressed by the physical therapist. Lechner and colleagues (1987) studied 30 children with JRA using the gait laboratory and described common deviations, such as decreased velocity, cadence, and stride length, as compared with controls. They also documented increased anterior pelvic tilt throughout the gait cycle, with decreased hip extension and decreased plantar flexion at toe-off (Fig. 8–8). Gait deviations may be caused by contractures, weakness, or pain. The clinician can develop hypotheses for interventions by analyzing the cause of the dysfunctional gait. Examination must also incorporate climbing activities such as ascending and descending stairs, ramps, and curbs.

Common foot deformities include loss of subtalar motion, such as a valgus hindfoot, combined with pronation (Fig. 8–9). Forefoot involvement is common and may be responsible for gait deviations such as lack of push-off, shortened stride length, and stiff-legged gait. The great toe may lose extension at the metatarsophalangeal joint or may deviate into a valgus position. The toes often develop a hammertoe posture.

Selecting comfortable yet supportive footwear is important for gait. Sneakers are generally the preferred footwear because they have a good arch support and cushioning throughout the sole. Special shoe modifications may need to be added, such as a metatarsal bar to provide a rocker-like surface to the sole of the forefoot, allowing a mechanical means to toe-off without requiring hyperextension of the toes (Fig. 8–10). Ankle-foot orthoses may be useful if the patient has pain in the ankles on weight bearing. Newer orthotic packages allow the therapist to experiment with a variety of custom-molded modifications to the shoes at a minimal cost.

A small percentage of children require an assistive device for ambulation. This may be indicated if lower extremity pain, contracture, or weakness prevents efficient weight bearing. Typically, such a child has polyarticular disease with significant upper extremity involvement necessitating the use of platform crutches (Lofstrand or axillary) or a wheeled walker with platform attachments to avoid weight bearing on the small joints of the wrist and hand.

Community Mobility

A few children who are unable to achieve independent community mobility may benefit from a wheelchair for outings. In this instance, lightweight wheelchairs are medically justifiable for joint conservation. In the preschool years, occasional use of a stroller may be necessary; a child's wagon and tricycle are other alternatives. By the time of entrance to high school, a power wheelchair can be considered for long distances. Patients with adequate lower extremity alignment and upper extremity strength may transfer with a stand-pivot-sit method, perhaps using an assistive device such as platform crutches.

Children with severe hand involvement may be unable to propel a manual wheelchair but may propel it by walking their feet on the floor or use a power wheelchair. Seat height from the floor has a critical effect on function, including propulsion and transfer. Posture in the chair should optimally be erect in order to prevent hip asymmetry or spinal deformity. Accessories such as brake extensions provide leverage for weak upper extremities. Swing-away or desk arms ensure close access to school desks.

The school or home should be examined for architectural barriers, and modifications should be recommended to facilitate mobility and transfers. A wheelchair-dependent child should have his or her living space on one floor, if possible. Electric-powered wheelchairs require ramps and a van for transportation, as well as a backup manual chair. Outings using a manually propelled chair must be planned in advance to allow for reasonable distances and frequent rests.

Self-Care Activities

Children's skills should be evaluated within the context of both the home and the school environments. Simple solutions such as a backpack for carrying books or asking the school to issue two sets of textbooks are well-accepted options. Other recommendations such as use of dressing aids may not be so readily accepted when they differ from the norm.

In this section, we are interested in learning how your child's illness affects his/her ability to function in daily life. Please feel free to add any comments on the back of this page. In the following questions, please check the one response that best describes your child's usual activities (averaged over an entire day) *OVER THE PAST WEEK*. If your child has difficulty in doing a certain activity or is unable to do it because he/she is too young but NOT because he/she is RESTRICTED BY ARTHRITIS, please mark it as "Not Applicable." ONLY NOTE THOSE DIFFICULTIES OR LIMITATIONS THAT ARE DUE TO ARTHRITIS.

	Without ANY Difficulty	With SOME Difficulty	With MUCH Difficulty	UNABLE To Do	Not Applicable
DRESSING & GROOMING Is your child able to:					
• Dress, including tying shoelaces and doing buttons?	_____	_____	_____	_____	_____
• Shampoo his/her hair?	_____	_____	_____	_____	_____
• Remove socks?	_____	_____	_____	_____	_____
• Cut fingernails/toenails?	_____	_____	_____	_____	_____
ARISING Is your child able to:					
• Stand up from a low chair or floor?	_____	_____	_____	_____	_____
• Get in and out of bed or stand up in crib?	_____	_____	_____	_____	_____
EATING Is your child able to:					
• Cut his/her own meat?	_____	_____	_____	_____	_____
• Lift a cup or glass to mouth?	_____	_____	_____	_____	_____
• Open a new cereal box?	_____	_____	_____	_____	_____
WALKING Is your child able to:					
• Walk outdoors on flat ground?	_____	_____	_____	_____	_____
• Climb up five steps?	_____	_____	_____	_____	_____

*Please check any AIDS or DEVICES that your child usually uses for any of the above activities.

_____Cane	_____Devices used for dressing (button hook, zipper pull, long-handled shoe horn, etc.)
_____Walker	_____Built-up pencil or special utensils
_____Crutches	_____Special or built-up chair
_____Wheelchair	_____Other (Specify:_____)

*Please check any categories for which your child usually needs help from another person BECAUSE OF ARTHRITIS:

_____Dressing and Grooming	_____Eating
_____Arising	_____Walking

	Without ANY Difficulty	With SOME Difficulty	With MUCH Difficulty	UNABLE To Do	Not Applicable
HYGIENE Is your child able to:					
• Wash and dry entire body?	_____	_____	_____	_____	_____
• Take a tub bath (get in and out of tub)?	_____	_____	_____	_____	_____
• Get on and off the toilet or potty chair?	_____	_____	_____	_____	_____
• Brush teeth?	_____	_____	_____	_____	_____
• Comb/brush hair?	_____	_____	_____	_____	_____
REACH Is your child able to:					
• Reach and get down a heavy object such as a large game or books from just above his/her head?	_____	_____	_____	_____	_____
• Bend down to pick up clothing or a piece of paper from the floor?	_____	_____	_____	_____	_____
• Pull on a sweater over his/her head?	_____	_____	_____	_____	_____
• Turn neck to look back over shoulder?	_____	_____	_____	_____	_____
GRIP Is your child able to:					
• Write or scribble with pen or pencil?	_____	_____	_____	_____	_____

FIGURE 8–7. The *Childhood Health Assessment Questionnaire* (CHAQ) is a checklist completed by the parent or child assessing functional activities. (Reprinted with permission from Singh, G, Athreya, B, Fries, JF, & Goldsmith, DP. Measurement of health status in children with JRA. Arthritis and Rheumatism, *37*:1761–1769, 1994.)

	Without ANY Difficulty	With SOME Difficulty	With MUCH Difficulty	UNABLE To Do	Not Applicable
GRIP (*Continued*)					
• Open car doors?	___	___	___	___	___
• Open jars that have been previously opened?	___	___	___	___	___
• Turn faucets on and off?	___	___	___	___	___
• Push open a door when he/she has to turn a door knob?	___	___	___	___	___
ACTIVITIES Is your child able to:					
• Run errands and shop?	___	___	___	___	___
• Get in and out of car or toy car or school bus?	___	___	___	___	___
• Ride bike or tricycle?	___	___	___	___	___
• Do household chores (e.g., wash dishes, take out trash, vacuuming, yardwork, make bed, clean room)?	___	___	___	___	___
• Run and play?	___	___	___	___	___

*Please check any AIDS or DEVICES that your child usually uses for any of the above activities:

_____ Raised toilet seat
_____ Bathtub seat
_____ Jar opener (for jars opened previously)

_____ Bathtub bar
_____ Long-handled appliances in reach
_____ Long-handled appliances in bathroom

*Please check any categories for which your child usually needs help from another person BECAUSE OF ARTHRITIS?

_____ Hygiene   _____ Gripping and Opening Things
_____ Reach   _____ Errands and Chores

We are also interested in learning whether your child has been affected by pain because of his or her illness.

*How much pain do you think your child has had because of his or her illness IN THE PAST WEEK?

Place a mark on the line below to indicate the severity of the pain.

No pain   Very severe pain
├───┤
0   100

HEALTH STATUS
1. Considering all the ways that arthritis affects your child, rate how your child is doing on the following scale by placing a mark on the line.

├───┤
0   100
Very well   Very poor
2. Is your child stiff in the morning?   _____ Yes   _____ No
   If YES, about how long does the stiffness usually last (in the past week)?
   Hours/Minutes _____

FIGURE 8–7, cont'd. For legend see opposite page.

Training in ADL can be time consuming, and counseling may be required to obtain the cooperation of the parent. Special devices for dressing may include a dressing stick to assist with reaching the feet to don pants or underwear, a zipper pull, a button hook, a sock aid, a long-handled shoehorn, or elastic shoelaces (Scull et al., 1986). Grooming the hair may require use of assistive devices as well.

Enlarging the handles of utensils and brushes makes gripping these objects easier. A variety of writing aids have enlarged diameters that improve writing endurance. In addition, the student may use a computer or a dictating device for many written tasks.

An area needing special attention is the bathroom. The tub may need to be equipped with a special seat and a grab bar to ensure safety. A long hose attached to the shower allows the child to bathe from a seated position. A long-handled sponge on a stick allows the child to reach more areas with ease. The toilet seat may need to be raised to a specific height to facilitate transfers. Sinks should be fitted with lever-type handles rather than knobs.

Principles of joint conservation are taught, including instruction on how to use the large joints of the body so as to avoid stress on the small joints of the wrists and hands. Books are carried in a backpack close to the center of gravity rather than in a

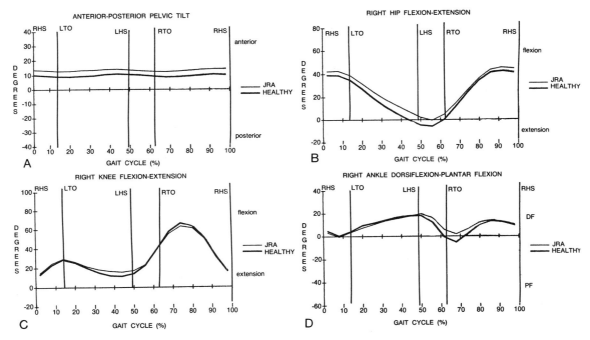

FIGURE 8–8. Gait studies have demonstrated common deviations in children with juvenile rheumatoid arthritis (JRA). *A,* Angle of anteroposterior pelvic tilt in the sagittal plane as a function of percentage of the gait cycle for both JRA group and healthy group subjects. *B,* Angle of right hip flexion-extension as a function of percentage of the gait cycle for both JRA group and healthy group subjects. *C,* Angle of right knee flexion-extension as a function of percentage of the gait cycle for both JRA group and healthy group subjects. *D,* Angle of right ankle dorsiflexion (DF) and plantar flexion (PF) as a function of percentage of the gait cycle for both JRA group and healthy group subjects. (From Lechner, DE, McCarthy, CF, & Holden, MK. Gait deviations in patients with juvenile rheumatoid arthritis. Physical Therapy, *67*:1335–1341, 1987. Reprinted from *Physical Therapy* with the permission of the American Physical Therapy Association.)

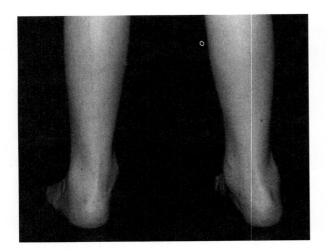

FIGURE 8–9. A common foot deformity is hindfoot valgus with pronation.

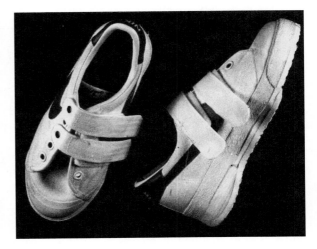

FIGURE 8–10. A metatarsal bar has been added to the sneaker to provide a rocker-like surface on the sole of the foot, allowing a mechanical means of toe-off.

briefcase. Some tasks can best be accomplished by increasing the lever arm, such as using a jar opener rather than twisting off a lid. Teaching patients to listen to their bodies and pace themselves is incorporated, as developmentally appropriate.

Avocational Activities

Because JRA interferes with normal mobility, the child does not have the usual opportunity to maintain cardiopulmonary endurance. Giannini and Protas (1992) studied 30 patients with JRA who were matched with controls for age, sex, and body surface area. An exercise tolerance test using cycle ergometry demonstrated deconditioning of the JRA group. Peak oxygen consumption, highest workload, exercise duration, and peak heart rate were all significantly lower in children with JRA as compared with controls. Surprisingly, the decreased aerobic capacity was unrelated to the severity of the articular disease as measured by the global articular disease severity score. This score is derived by summing all involved joints for swelling, pain on passive ROM, tenderness to palpation, and passive limitation of motion but is probably not specific enough to show correlation with endurance. Giannini and Protas (1992) concluded that aerobic conditioning programs should be recommended soon after diagnosis to prevent hypoactivity leading to deconditioning.

Klepper and colleagues (1992) corroborated the results of this study on 20 children with JRA, ages 6 to 11 years, using the Health-Related Physical Fitness Test. Klepper and colleagues (1996) went on to provide an 8-week program of low-impact aerobics to 25 children with chronic arthritis. Subjects improved in the 9-minute walk-run test as compared with study entry. A planned program of recreation such as swimming, cycling, or dance should achieve cardiopulmonary training effects if scheduled for 30 minutes three to five times per week (Klepper & Giannini, 1994).

Guided selection of recreational activities can also assist in reinforcing exercise goals, such as improving lower extremity ROM or strength. Young children enjoy upper extremity games such as "Simon Says." A special exercise videotape has been prepared by the Texas Scottish Rite Hospital (Carman, 1991) in which various ROM dances are performed to stories and music. Other home exercise programs are designed in a coloring book format, such as *Exercise with Kela* (Pediatric Arthritis Center of Hawaii, 1985), or as part of a parent information book, such as *We Can* (Arthritis Foundation, 1985).

School-age children are encouraged to participate in physical education classes to their tolerance. Certain activities are contraindicated, such as tumbling (especially headstands and somersaults), weight bearing on the upper extremities, contact sports, and high-impact activities such as jogging. Consultation between the physical therapist and the physical education teacher usually helps clarify the optimal exercise prescription for each child (Scull & Athreya, 1995).

SURGICAL PROCEDURES AND POSTSURGICAL REHABILITATION

Patients with mild involvement are managed by medication, splints, and therapy. Surgery may be considered, however, if conservative therapy fails to prevent joint contractures or if joint erosion is severe.

Soft tissue releases of the hip flexors, hamstrings, hip adductors, or heel cords are indicated for contractures that are resistant to conservative measures. Decompression of the joint and improved ROM also improve joint nutrition, and sometimes fibrocartilage is laid down (Swann, 1990). Occasionally, a simple manipulation under anesthesia is sufficient to regain motion, especially in a child who has been unwilling to cooperate with therapy.

Synovectomy may be performed arthroscopically, but the long-term effects may be disappointing (Jacobsen et al., 1985). It may be considered for a single joint, particularly the knee, which has active disease, effusion, and overgrowth of synovium in spite of adequate medical therapy. However, the degree of postoperative pain and muscle spasm often gives a poor outcome in children. A review of 41 procedures (Jacobsen et al., 1985) showed relief of swelling but no long-term changes in pain, ROM, or function.

Osteotomies are sometimes required to correct valgus or flexion contractures at the knee. Epiphysiodesis, or stapling of the growth plate, is occasionally used to correct limb length discrepancy or valgus deformity. Arthroplasty, or less frequently distal arthrodesis, may be required for the severely damaged joint that interferes with function and causes pain. Adolescents may be candidates for replacements of hips, knees, shoulders, elbows, or ankles. Wrist fusion or other types of hand surgery may improve ADL. Ankle fusion may be required to obtain a pain-free joint in neutral alignment.

Indications for arthroplasty include marked functional impairment, especially inability to ambulate, and disabling pain (Hyman & Gregg, 1991; Scott, 1990). Loss of motion, subluxation, and deformity are secondary reasons. Other selection criteria include ability to bear weight on the upper extremities with an assistive device and alignment of other lower extremity joints for weight bearing, both ipsilateral and contralateral. If multiple joints must

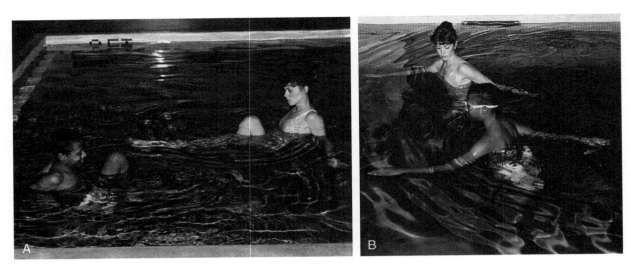

FIGURE 8–11. Aquatic therapy ideally includes therapeutic exercises for flexibility and strengthening *(A)*, as well as ambulation in deep water *(B)*.

be replaced, the hips are usually done before the knees. Rehabilitation is easier if the procedures are staged so that one joint is replaced at a time. The goals of rehabilitation are to achieve pain-free ROM and functional ambulation, usually with an assistive device.

Total hip prostheses are custom-designed in smaller sizes and ideally are porous allowing biologic fixation because cement may not last sufficiently long. Although skeletal maturity is desirable, children as young as 12 years of age have received total hip replacements (Hyman & Gregg, 1991).

The postoperative program includes passive ROM exercise with precautions to avoid hip flexion past 90°, adduction, and internal rotation. A foam abduction pillow is worn for 6 weeks, alternating with use of a continuous passive motion (CPM) machine. Isometric exercises are started early for strengthening of hip extensors and abductors and knee extensors. Gait training with an assistive device begins with weight bearing as tolerated during the first week. Stationary cycling may be attempted after several weeks if the seat height is set high and supervision is used to maintain hip precautions. Aquatic therapy consisting of exercises in sitting or standing position, and ambulation in chest-deep water is begun as soon as wound healing is complete and the staples are removed. Special pools with a movable floor allow gradual progression of the water depth to increase weight bearing (Fig. 8–11) (AFW of North America, Olean, NY).

Total knee arthroplasty is usually done with a cemented procedure and may be combined with re-lease of posterior structures, such as the hamstrings, the capsule, and the proximal gastrocnemius, if knee flexion contractures exist. The patella is routinely resurfaced with a plastic button cemented to the undersurface, and the lateral retinaculum is released to prevent further valgus deformity. The tibial tubercle must undergo osteotomy and fixation to gain exposure to the knee. Therefore early strengthening programs using isometric exercises and straight leg raises are tolerated better than short arc quadriceps exercises.

Patients are bearing full weight with a knee immobilizer on the second postoperative day. When the bulky dressing is removed by day 4, CPM is begun if sufficient wound healing is present. The ROM goal is 0 to 100° of knee motion. Ambulation aids are discontinued when the knee flexes to 90° and the quadriceps strength is grade 4/5 (good). Stationary cycling may be done if a range limiter is applied to the pedal to shorten the shank and allow the therapist to control the amount of knee flexion required during cycling (Fig. 8–12).

Complications of arthroplasty include loosening of components and infection. Wear of components is less problematic in this group because patients with JRA are typically small and have decreased activity levels. In a group of patients with a total of 72 hip replacements, 30% required revision after 10 years of follow-up (Swann, 1990). Nevertheless, keeping the patient ambulatory during the young-adult years was believed to be beneficial. The increased use of biologic fixation should improve these long-term results.

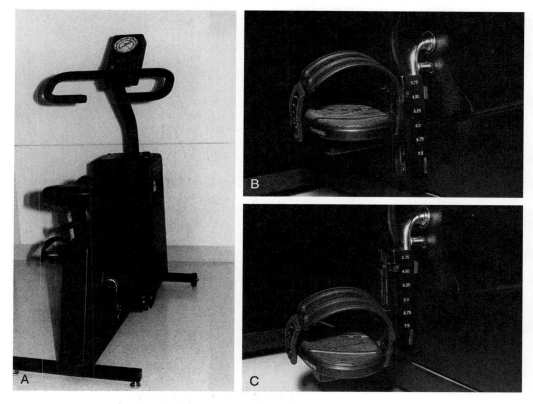

FIGURE 8–12. This ergometer *(A)* is equipped with a range limiter on the pedal *(B, C)*, which shortens the shank and allows the patient with limited knee flexion to cycle.

CONTINUOUS PASSIVE MOTION

CPM has been studied in animals as an alternative to rest and immobilization in the care of articular defects, fractures, septic arthritis, and tendon lacerations (Salter, 1989). Basic science studies have involved the creation of cartilaginous defects in rabbit joints and comparison of their gross and histologic differences following immobilization in a cast, intermittent active motion (cage activity), or CPM. The results show that CPM 1) is well tolerated by rabbits and seems to be pain free; 2) has a significant healing effect on cartilage, tendon, and ligamentous tissues; 3) prevents adhesions and joint stiffness; 4) does not interfere with healing incisions; and 5) is superior to rest for tissue healing. One week of immediate postoperative CPM at a slow speed was found to be as effective as 3 weeks of CPM.

Salter (1989) recommends early use of CPM following synovectomy, soft tissue releases, or arthroplasty. Units are available for the lower extremities, and CPM may be integrated with electrical stimulation of the quadriceps to facilitate full knee extension and prevent atrophy. Upper extremity units or universal joint units are also available to treat the shoulder and elbow.

Animal research is exploring the biologic resurfacing of joints in rabbits with periosteal grafts, including both autogenous grafts and allografts (Zarnett et al., 1987). Studies have demonstrated that articular cartilage can regenerate with CPM, with or without the additional periosteal grafts. Further study is needed before this approach is applied to humans, but the potential exists for future treatment of the young, active JRA patient who may wear out a prosthetic joint at an early age.

CASE HISTORY
AMANDA

Amanda is a 6-year-old girl with polyarticular JRA (Fig. 8-13). She has involvement of multiple joints, including the neck, temporomandibular joint, elbows, wrists, hands, knees, ankles, and toes. She is taking 14 mg per day of naproxen to control inflammation.

Impairments: She has 15° hip and knee flexion contractures bilaterally and is unable to extend the great

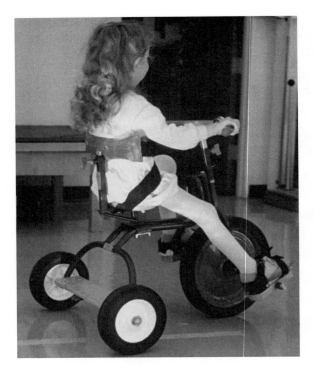

FIGURE 8–13. Amanda rides a tricycle adapted with foot sandals in order to increase the strength of lower extremity muscles.

toes, which are extremely painful. Cervical spine motion is limited in rotation and extension by 50%. Muscle strength grades are 4/5 (good) in the antigravity muscles of both lower extremities. Grip strength measured by a handheld dynamometer is 9 lb on the right and 8 lb on the left. Leg lengths are equal, and there are no postural deviations except a slightly forward head.

Functional limitations: Amanda ambulates independently, but her gait shows bilateral gluteus medius lurch, decreased hip extension at toe-off, decreased stride length, and poor push-off. She shifts her weight to the lateral borders of her feet.

Her ADL were assessed by the occupational therapist using the CHAQ. Amanda can complete all dressing in a reasonable amount of time except for donning her shoes and socks. Her mother shops carefully for clothing that is loose fitting with elastic rather than fasteners.

Disabilities: She is not able to keep up with the family on outings to the local mall. Amanda has significant stiffness following any period of inactivity. In the morning, she must be carried to the tub because she cannot walk for up to an hour. In class, she becomes stiff after sitting for circle time. She is unable to carry her tray in the cafeteria and often asks to be excused from recess.

Diagnosis no. 1: dysfunctional gait

Impairment 1-A. Metatarsophalangeal joint pain, especially during toe-off.

Goal: Improve gait, specifically increase stride length, increase push-off, decrease Trendelenburg sign.

Intervention:

1. Recommend sneakers for footwear.

2. Use cushioned insoles to decrease metatarsophalangeal pain.

3. Add metatarsal bar to shoe to allow rolling over forefoot.

Impairment 1-B. Weakness of lower extremity muscles.

Goal: Increase strength of antigravity muscles to 5/5 (normal).

Intervention:

1. Perform elastic band exercises for increased strength of gluteus medius, maximus, and quadriceps muscles.

2. Issue adaptive tricycle for use in school, especially during recess.

3. Encourage use of swings on school playground.

Impairment 1-C. Inactivity stiffness, especially on arising.

Goal: Decrease inactivity stiffness so that child will be able to ambulate on arising and move freely in classroom.

Intervention:

1. Wear posterior knee splints, of low temperature thermoplastics, at night, allowing the knees to rest in extension.

2. Take morning tub bath and perform active ROM exercises to decrease morning stiffness.

3. Encourage ambulating in the classroom every hour to avoid stiffness from inactivity.

Impairment 1-D. 15° hip and knee flexion contractures of both lower extremities.

Goal: Maintain or improve lower extremity ROM; hip and knee extension to minus 5°; great toe extension to 50°.

Intervention:

1. Recommend prone positioning for 20 minutes a day to decrease hip and knee flexion contractures.

2. Use passive ROM performed by mother after bath to increase metatarsophalangeal extension.

Diagnosis no. 2: dependent for ADL

Limitation 2-A. Dressing skills are not age appropriate.

Outcome: Develop ability to don and remove shoes and socks independently with a sock aid and elastic shoelaces.

Intervention:

1. Train for use of sock aid and shoe donning.

2. Provide dressing frame or doll as a toy to learn how to tie and lace shoes.

Continue to select clothes for ease of donning and doffing.

Impairment 2-A. Decreased grip strength.

Goal: Increase grip strength to 11 lb on the right and 9 lb on the left.

Intervention: Perform exercises with Play-Doh involving pinching and grasping.

Impairment 2-B. Daily activities can stress joints or cause postural deviations.

Goal: Prevent stress to involved joints and postural abnormalities.

Intervention:

1. Avoid tailor-sitting during circle time. Encourage use of a small stool.

2. Have occupational therapist make resting cock-up splint for wrists to be used during writing tasks.

3. Adapt pencils with soft buildup to increase diameter.

4. Recommend large-diameter crayons.

5. Provide patient-related instruction on joint conservation.

Diagnosis no. 3: psychosocial adjustment to disease

Societal Limitation 3-A. Potential for child to be excluded from children in peer group secondary to their lack of understanding of JRA.

Outcome: Integrate child into school setting for as normal a social experience as possible.

Intervention:

1. Communicate with teacher and school nurse about JRA.

2. Arrange for child to educate peers regarding JRA in appropriate method, such as show-and-tell session.

3. Provide written pamphlets from the Arthritis Foundation.

Reexamination of ROM, strength, and gait is done every other month at a rheumatology clinic where the child is seen by the rehabilitation team. If the knee flexion contractures do not improve with the home program, consideration will be given to prescribing a dynamic splint to be worn during the hours of sleep.

Amanda is still young and is not yet showing disabilities in carrying out her life roles at home and in school. The therapist should focus direct intervention on this child's impairments of ROM and strength to prevent further functional limitations in gait or ADL. Her foot pain and loss of toe motion suggest potential fixed deformity, which should be managed early with orthotics to decrease pain on weight bearing. Important outcomes such as Amanda's school attendance and her psychosocial interactions with peers and family should be monitored to prevent potential social isolation and to promote Amanda's full inclusion in school activities.

ACKNOWLEDGMENTS

With special thanks to Balu H. Athreya, MD, and Greg Keenan, MD, for their editorial assistance, and to Margi Ide for photography.

Recommended Resources

Arthritis Foundation
1330 West Peachtree Street
Atlanta, GA 30309
1-800-283-7800
http://www.arthritis.org
American Juvenile Arthritis Organization (AJAO), a council of the Arthritis Foundation

References

Arthritis Foundation. We Can: A Guide for Parents of Children with Arthritis. Atlanta: Arthritis Foundation, 1985.

Athreya, BH, & Cassidy, JT. Current status of the medical treatment of children with JRA. Rheumatic Disease Clinics of North America, 17:871–889, 1991.

Cabral, DA, Petty, RE, & Malleson, PN. Visual prognosis in children with chronic uveitis and arthritis. Arthritis and Rheumatism, 35: S229, 1992.

Carman, D. Where Are the Indians? An Exercise Video for Children. Dallas: Scottish Rite Hospital for Children, 1991 (Videotape).

Cassidy, JT, & Petty, RE. Textbook of Pediatric Rheumatology, 3rd ed. Philadelphia: WB Saunders, 1995.

Earley, A, Cuttica, RJ, McCullough, C, & Ansell, BM. Triamcinolone into the knee joint in juvenile chronic arthritis. Clinical Experiments in Rheumatology, 6:153–155, 1988.

Emery, HM, & Bowyer, S. Physical modalities of therapy in pediatric rheumatic diseases. Rheumatic Disease Clinics of North America, 17:1001–1014, 1991.

Fan, JS, Wessel, J, & Ellsworth, J. The relationship between strength and function in females with juvenile rheumatoid arthritis. Journal of Rheumatology, 25:1399–1405, 1998.

Fried, JA, Athreya, BH, Gregg, JR, Das, M, & Doughty, R. The cervical spine in juvenile rheumatoid arthritis. Clinical Orthopedics and Related Research, 179:102–106, 1983.

Giannini, EH, Brewer, EJ, Kuzmina, N, Shaikov, V, Maximov, A, Vorontsov, I, Fink, CW, Newman, AJ, Cassidy, JT, & Zemel, LS. Methotrexate in resistant juvenile rheumatoid arthritis: Results of the USA-USSR double-blind, placebo-controlled trial. New England Journal of Medicine, 326:1043–1049, 1992.

Giannini, MJ, & Protas, EJ. Exercise response in children with and without juvenile rheumatoid arthritis: A case comparison study. Physical Therapy, 72:365–372, 1992.

Giannini, MJ, & Protas, EJ. Comparison of peak isometric knee extensor torque in children with and without juvenile rheumatoid arthritis. Arthritis Care and Research, 6:82–87, 1993.

Hacket, J, Johnson, B, Parkin, A, & Southwood, T. Physiotherapy and occupational therapy for juvenile chronic arthritis: Custom and practice in five centres in the UK, USA and Canada. British Journal of Rheumatology, 35:695–699, 1996.

Henderson, CJ, Lovell, DJ, & Gregg, DJ. A nutritional screening test for use in children and adolescents with juvenile rheumatoid arthritis. Journal of Rheumatology, 19:1276–1281, 1992.

Hepburn, GR. Case studies: Contractures and stiff joint management with Dynasplint. Journal of Orthopedic and Sports Physical Therapy, 8:498–504, 1987.

Hochberg, MC, Chang, RW, Dwosh, F, Lindsey, S, Pincus, T, & Wolfe, F. The American College of Rheumatology 1991 revised criteria for the classification of global functional status in rheumatoid arthritis. Arthritis and Rheumatism, 35:498–502, 1992.

Howe, S, Levinson, J, Shear, E, Hartner, S, McGirr, G, Schulte, M, & Lovell, D. Development of a disability measurement tool for juvenile rheumatoid arthritis. The Juvenile Arthritis Functional Assessment Report for Children and Their Parents. Arthritis and Rheumatism, 34:873-880, 1991.

Hyman, BS, & Gregg, JR. Arthroplasty of the hip and knee in juvenile rheumatoid arthritis. Rheumatic Disease Clinics of North America, 17:971-983, 1991.

Jacobsen, ST, Levinson, JE, & Crawford, AH. Late results of synovectomy in juvenile rheumatoid arthritis. Journal of Bone and Joint Surgery (American), 67:8-15, 1985.

Klepper, S, Effgen, S, & Athreya, B. Effects of an 8 week physical conditioning program on the signs and symptoms of chronic arthritis in children. Arthritis and Rheumatism, 30:S1716, 1996.

Klepper, S, & Giannini, MJ. Physical conditioning in children with arthritis: Assessment and guidelines for exercise prescription. Arthritis Care and Research, 7:226-236, 1994.

Klepper, SE, Darbee, J, Effgen, SK, & Singsen, BH. Physical fitness levels in children with polyarticular juvenile rheumatoid arthritis. Arthritis Care and Research, 5:93-100, 1992.

Lechner, DE, McCarthy, CF, & Holden, MK. Gait deviations in patients with juvenile rheumatoid arthritis. Physical Therapy, 67:1335-1341, 1987.

Lovell, DJ, Howe, S, Shear, E, Hartner, S, McGirr, G, Schulte, M, & Levinson, J. Development of a disability measurement tool for juvenile rheumatoid arthritis: The Juvenile Arthritis Functional Assessment Scale. Arthritis and Rheumatism, 32:1390-1395, 1989.

Mayro, RF, DeLozier, JB, III, & Whitaker, LA. Facial reconstruction consideration in rheumatic diseases. Pediatric Rheumatology, 17:943-969, 1991.

McGrath, PA. Pain in Children: Nature, Assessment, Treatment. New York: Guilford Press, 1990.

Melvin, JL, & Atwood, M. Juvenile rheumatoid arthritis. In Melvin, JL (Ed.), Rheumatic Disease in the Adult and Child: Occupational Therapy and Rehabilitation, 3rd ed. Philadelphia: FA Davis, 1989.

Michlovitz, SL. Thermal Agents in Rehabilitation. Philadelphia: FA Davis, 1996.

Pediatric Arthritis Center of Hawaii. Exercise with Kela. Honolulu, HI: Kapio-lani Women's and Children's Medical Center, 1985.

Petty, RE. Current knowledge of the etiology and pathogenesis of chronic uveitis accompanying juvenile rheumatoid arthritis. Rheumatic Disease Clinics of North America, 13:19-31, 1987.

Rhodes, VJ. Physical therapy management of patients with juvenile rheumatoid arthritis. Physical Therapy, 71:910-919, 1991.

Rose, CD, Singsen, BH, Eichenfeld, AH, et al. Safety and efficacy of methotrexate therapy in juvenile rheumatoid arthritis. Journal of Pediatrics, 117:653, 1990.

Ruperto, N, Levinson, JE, Ravelli, A, Shear, ES, Tague, BL, Murray, K, Martini, A, & Ciannini, EH. Longterm health outcomes and quality of life in American and Italian inception cohorts of patients with juvenile rheumatoid arthritis. I. Outcome status. Journal of Rheumatology, 24:945-951, 1997.

Salter, RB. The biologic concept of continuous passive motion of synovial joints: The first 18 years of basic research and its clinical application. Clinical Orthopedics, 242:12-25, 1989.

Schaller, JG. Chronic arthritis in children. Clinical Orthopedics, 182:79-89, 1983.

Scott, RD. Total hip and knee arthroplasty in juvenile rheumatoid arthritis. Clinical Orthopedics and Related Research, 259:83-91, 1990.

Scull, SA. Juvenile rheumatoid arthritis. In Tecklin, JS (Ed.), Pediatric Physical Therapy, 2nd ed. Philadelphia: JB Lippincott, 1994.

Scull, SA, & Athreya, BH. Exercise and sports in childhood arthritis. In Goldberg, B (Ed.), Sports and Exercise for Chronically Ill Children. Champaign, IL: Human Kinetics, 1995.

Scull, SA, Dow, MB, & Athreya, BH. Physical and occupational therapy for children with rheumatic diseases. Pediatric Clinics of North America, 33:1053-1077, 1986.

Singh, G, Athreya, B, Fries, JF, & Goldsmith, DP. Measurement of health status in children with JRA. Arthritis and Rheumatism, 37:1761-1769, 1994.

Swann, MC. The surgery of juvenile chronic arthritis. Clinical Orthopedics and Related Research, 259:70-75, 1990.

Towner, SR, Michet, CJ, O'Fallon, WM, & Nelson, AM. The epidemiology of juvenile arthritis in Rochester, Minn. Arthritis and Rheumatism, 26:1208, 1983.

Varni, JW, Thompson, KL, & Hanson, V. The Varni/Thompson Pediatric Pain Questionnaire: I. Chronic musculoskeletal pain in juvenile rheumatoid arthritis. Pain, 28:27-38, 1987.

Wallace, CA, & Levinson, JE. Juvenile rheumatoid arthritis: Outcome and treatment for the 1990s. Rheumatic Disease Clinics of North America, 17:891-905, 1991.

White, PH. Growth abnormalities in children with juvenile rheumatoid arthritis. Clinical Orthopedics and Related Research, 259:46-50, 1990.

Whitehouse, R, Shope, JT, Sullivan, DB, & Kulik, CL. Children with juvenile rheumatoid arthritis at school. Clinical Pediatrics, 28:509-514, 1989.

Zarnett, R, Delaney, JR, O'Driscoll, SW, & Salter, RB. Cellular origin and evolution of neochondrogenesis in major full-thickness defects of a joint surface treated by free autogenous periosteal grafts and subjected to continuous passive motion in rabbits. Clinical Orthopedics, 222:267, 1987.

Juvenile Rheumatoid Arthritis
Practice Pattern

INTERVENTIONS

Coordination, Communication, and Documentation

Anticipated goals:

Care is coordinated with child, family, school, and other professionals.

Insurance payer understands needed rehabilitation services.

Need for modifications in school is determined.

Specific interventions:

Communication with community therapist

Prescriptions and letters of medical necessity to support rehabilitation needs

Individualized education plan (IEP)

Patient-Related Instruction

Anticipated goals:

Awareness and use of community resources is increased.

Behaviors that protect joints from secondary impairments are reduced.

Functional independence in ADL is increased.

Patient and family knowledge of the diagnosis, prognosis, interventions, and goals and outcomes is increased.

Interventions:

Home exercise program

Instruction regarding joint protection principles

Pamphlets from Arthritis Foundation regarding disease

Referrals to other community resources

DIRECT INTERVENTIONS

Therapeutic Exercise

Anticipated goals:

Ability to perform physical tasks related to self-care, home management, community and school integration, and leisure activities is increased.

Aerobic capacity is increased.

Gait is improved.

Joint and soft tissue swelling, inflammation, or restriction is reduced.

Joint integrity and mobility are improved.

Pain is decreased.

Postural control is improved.

Strength, power, and endurance are improved.

Interventions:

Aerobic activities

Aquatic exercise

Body mechanics training

Gait training

Postural training

Strengthening
    Active
    Active assistive

Modified from Impaired joint mobility, motor function, muscle performance, and range of motion associated with joint arthroplasty. Physical Therapy, 77:1327–1339, 1997.

Resistive—especially elastic resistance bands
Stretching

Passive range of motion
Therapeutic massage

Functional Training in Self-Care and Home Management

Anticipated goals:

Ability to perform physical tasks related to self-care and home management is increased.
Level of supervision required for task performance is decreased.

Interventions:

ADL training
Assistive and adaptive device or equipment training
Self-care or home management task adaptation
Leisure and play recommendations
Orthotic, protective, or supportive device or equipment training

Functional Training in Community and School Integration

Anticipated goals:

School attendance is improved.
Participation in peer groups for recreation and leisure activity is improved.
Architectural barriers to access home, school, and community resources are removed.

Interventions:

Appropriate transportation plan to school identified on IEP
Modifications to school instruction identified on IEP
ADL training
Assistive and adaptive device or equipment training
Adaptation of equipment to allow inclusion in recreation and leisure activity
Home and school site visit to plan for accommodation of any architectural barriers

Manual Therapy Techniques (Including Mobilization and Manipulation)

Anticipated goals:

Ability to perform motor skills is improved.
Joint integrity and mobility are improved.

Interventions:

Connective tissue massage

Prescription, Application, and Fabrication of Devices and Equipment

Anticipated goals:

Ability to perform physical tasks is increased.
Deformities are prevented.
Gait and locomotion are improved.
Joint stability is increased.
Optimal joint alignment is achieved.
Pain is decreased.
Protection of body parts is increased.

Interventions:

Adaptive devices or equipment
Assistive devices or equipment (ambulation aids, wheelchairs, ADL equipment)
Splints and orthotics (shoe inserts, resting splints, dynamic splints, braces)
Protective devices (splints, taping, elbow or knee pads)
Supportive devices (compression garments, cervical collars)

Electrotherapeutic Modalities

Anticipated goals:

Muscle performance is increased.
Pain is decreased.

Interventions:

Biofeedback
Transcutaneous electrical nerve stimulation (TENS)

Physical Agents and Mechanical Modalities

Anticipated goals:

Pain is decreased.
Soft tissue swelling, inflammation, or restriction is reduced.
Tolerance to positions and activities is increased.
Joint integrity and mobility are improved.

Interventions:

Cryotherapy (RICE—rest, ice, compression, elevation)
Hydrotherapy (aquatic therapy, whirlpool tanks)
Superficial thermal modalities (heat, paraffin baths, hot packs, fluidotherapy)
Continuous passive motion devices

CHAPTER
9

Hemophilia

SANDRA M. McGEE, PT

Hemophilia is the term used to collectively identify several X-linked disorders of blood coagulation. The most common of these are factor VIII deficiency, or hemophilia A, comprising 80 to 90% of the population with hemophilia, and factor IX deficiency, or hemophilia B. Hemophilia is present in approximately 1 in 10,000 males, and 60 to 65% of the patients will have a positive family history (Karayalcin, 1985).

Joint arthropathy from repeated hemarthroses is the most disabling consequence of the disorders. Recent advances in recombinant factor production and increased availability of factor replacement products in developed countries have resulted in more patients being treated prophylactically. This trend has greatly improved the quality of life of these patients and their families by reducing the incidence of joint hemorrhages and arthropathy. Unfortunately, easy access to factor replacement is not universally available and joint arthropathy continues to be the major cause of disability for thousands of people with hemophilia.

In this chapter the pathophysiology of hemarthrosis, medical management, primary impairments, functional limitations, and the role of physical therapy in examination and intervention are addressed. The case history presented at the conclusion of the chapter illustrates the physical therapy management (based on the American Physical Therapy Association's "Guide to Physical Therapist Practice") of one patient with hemophilia.

CLASSIFICATION

The severity of the disorder is determined by the amount of factor activity in the blood (Table 9–1). Over 60% of males with hemophilia A and 50% with hemophilia B have the severe form of the disorder. These patients are subject to recurrent hemorrhages that may occur spontaneously or as a result of minor trauma. Infants and toddlers may develop subcutaneous ecchymosis over bony prominences or large hematomas after intramuscular injections for vaccination against childhood diseases. By 3 to 4 years of age, bleeding into muscles and joints begins to present problems because of increased activity level, and it continues to be a major problem throughout childhood and adolescence.

In the moderate form of hemophilia A or B the patient may have spontaneous hemorrhages, but more frequently bleeding occurs as a result of trauma. The child with the mild form, however, will bleed only after severe trauma, and consequently hemophilia may not even be diagnosed in infancy or childhood (Buchanan, 1980).

Hemorrhages may occur anywhere in the body but most often are in the joint cavities. Muscles are the second most common site of bleeding, particularly in the iliopsoas, gastrocnemius, and forearm flexor muscle compartment. Hemorrhages within muscles can be dangerous owing to the risk of nerve compression from the hematoma. Patients with he-

mophilia may also be susceptible to hematuria, mucous membrane hemorrhages, and central nervous system hemorrhages. Fortunately, central nervous system hemorrhages are uncommon, developing in approximately 3% of the hemophilic population, but they are the major cause of death from these bleeding disorders (Buchanan, 1980).

HEMOPHILIC ARTHROPATHY

Pathophysiology

Hemarthrosis is the most clinically significant problem in hemophilia. It affects the hinge joints (knees, elbows, and ankles) most frequently because these joints have less muscular padding and a decreased ability to withstand lateral and rotary forces. When bleeding occurs into a joint, the joint becomes swollen, warm, and painful, and range of motion (ROM) is restricted (Corrigan, 1990). A single or infrequent bleeding episode will usually resolve without complication as the blood is resorbed. Recurrent hemarthroses, however, can lead to chronic synovitis and degenerative arthropathy. Although the mechanisms of recurrent bleeding leading to degenerative arthropathy are not well understood, Joist and Ameri (1990) have outlined a reasonable hypothesis (Fig. 9–1). Recurrent hemarthroses cause synovial hypertrophy with formation of villi, as well as pannus for-

TABLE 9–1. **Relation of Factor Levels to Severity of Clinical Manifestations of Hemophilia A and B**

Type	Factor Levels (VIII/IX) (Percent of Normal)	Type of Hemorrhage
Severe	<1	Spontaneous; hemarthroses and deep tissue hemorrhages
Moderate	1–5	Gross bleeding following mild to moderate trauma; some hemarthrosis; seldom spontaneous hemorrhage
Mild	5–25	Severe hemorrhage following moderate to severe trauma or surgery
High-risk carrier females	30–50	Gynecologic and obstetric hemorrhages

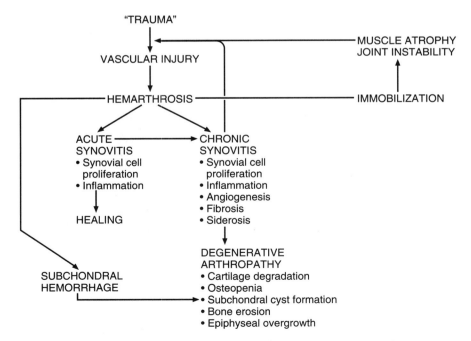

FIGURE 9–1. Joist and Ameri's concept of the pathogenesis of hemophilic arthropathy. (Redrawn from Joist, JH, & Ameri, A. Pathogenesis of hemophilic arthropathy. In Gilbert, MS, & Greene, WB [Eds.], Musculoskeletal Problems in Hemophilia. New York: National Hemophilia Foundation, 1990, pp. 20–25.)

mation on the joint cartilage. The hypertrophic, hyperemic synovium is more susceptible to mechanical trauma, leading to further bleeding. In addition, capsular stretching and muscle atrophy from immobilization and disuse increase joint instability, creating a vicious cycle that is difficult to break. The chronic synovitis and chemical reactions related to the breakdown of the blood in the joint eventually lead to cartilage damage, bone erosion, and bone remodeling.

Arnold and Hilgartner (1977) classified hemophilic arthropathy into five stages based on roentgenographic findings (Fig. 9–2). In stage 1, no

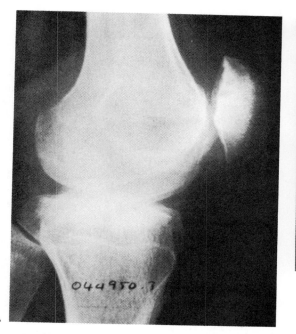

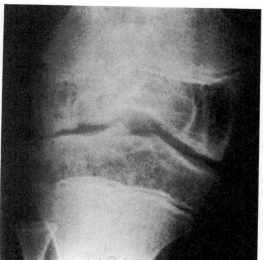

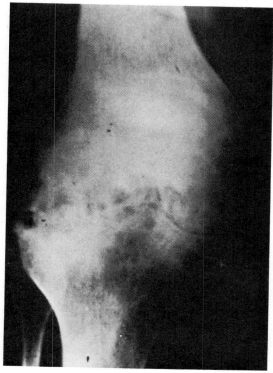

FIGURE 9–2. Hemophilic arthropathy. In stage 1, soft tissue swelling occurs without bony changes. Stage 2 consists of early osteoporosis and epiphyseal overgrowth. *A* to *C* illustrate stages 3 to 5. *A,* Stage 3: Joint disorganization, with patellar squaring and subchondral cysts but intact articular cartilage. *B,* Stage 4: Narrowing of joint space and damage to cartilage. *C,* Stage 5: Loss of joint space, fibrous joint contracture, and total destruction of cartilage. (From Arnold, WD, & Hilgartner, MW. Hemophilic arthropathy. Journal of Bone and Joint Surgery [American], *59*:288–305, 1977.)

bony abnormalities are seen but soft tissue swelling is present. Stage 2 is characterized by osteoporosis and overgrowth of the epiphyses, but the joint integrity is maintained. In stage 3, subchondral cysts are visible, squaring of the patella is evident when the knee is involved, and the intercondylar notch of the knee and the trochlear notch of the elbow are widened. The articular cartilage, however, is still intact. By stage 4, the joint space has narrowed and there is damage to the cartilage. In stage 5, there is fibrous joint contracture, loss of joint space, extensive enlargement of the epiphyses, and total destruction of the articular cartilage.

All children with moderate or severe hemophilia will suffer from hemarthroses. The aim of treatment is to slow down or halt the progression of joint destruction.

Medical Management

Bleeding episodes are managed medically by intravenous factor replacement, extracted from normal plasma or manufactured from recombinant DNA. Factor replacement should occur as soon as the patient feels stiffness or discomfort in a joint. These "prodromal" sensations can precede objective signs of bleeding by 4 to 6 hours. In an effort to control the bleeding as quickly as possible, many families are taught to perform infusions at home. Factor replacement may also be given before vigorous exercise, such as participation in intramural sports or intensive physical therapy. Some patients with frequent bleeding episodes may be placed on long-term prophylactic factor replacement (Corrigan, 1990).

In addition to factor replacement, hemarthroses are treated with rest, through immobilization and avoidance of weight bearing, until bleeding has resolved. Aspiration of the blood from the joints as a treatment modality has been reported in the literature after 1 to 2 decades of disuse (Corrigan, 1990; Gregosiewicz et al., 1989).

Orthopedic surgery may be indicated in patients with chronic synovitis or severe joint destruction. Synovectomy, both open and by arthroscopy, is frequently performed on knees and elbows in an effort to reduce bleeding episodes by removing fragile, hypertrophic synovium (Atkins et al., 1987). "Medical synovectomies" by intra-articular injection of radionucleotides are also being performed to ablate the synovium (Erken, 1991). Arthrodeses, osteotomies, and arthroplasties have been used when severe joint destruction causes intractable pain and disability.

Prognosis

Despite more aggressive and earlier home treatment of hemarthroses, severe joint arthropathy remains a major disabling consequence of hemophilia. Although the incidence of joint hemorrhages declines in late adolescence and early adulthood, joint destruction has already occurred in a large percentage of patients with severe hemophilia (Joist & Ameri, 1990).

The use of prophylaxis is changing this picture in developed countries. In Sweden, boys with severe hemophilia have been treated with prophylaxis since 1958. For the first 18 years of that program, factor was not always available on a regular basis, but for the next 15 years of the study, sufficient factor was available to maintain the level of the deficient factor in every boy at 1% or greater. All of the patients ($n = 15$) treated in the final 15 years of the study began treatment between 1 and 2 years of age and had virtually no bleeding episodes and normal joints by roentgenographic study (Nilsson et al., 1992). Unfortunately, factor supplies are not universally available and in developing countries may not be available even to treat major bleeding episodes.

The practice of primary prophylaxis is a controversial issue. Some of the arguments against its use include continued concern over exposure to viruses in blood products, long-term cost-benefit ratio, and the difficulty in obtaining regular venous access in young patients (Liesner et al., 1996).

In addition, between 10 and 15% of patients with hemophilia A develop antibodies (inhibitors) that are directed against the activity of factor VIII. Hemostasis is more difficult to achieve in patients with inhibitors. Immune tolerance therapy that provides daily exposure to factor concentrate may eliminate the inhibitor over time (Shopnick & Brettler, 1996).

Since the late 1970s, secondary complications of hemophilia have become a more significant health problem than the primary impairment. The child with severe hemophilia can use from 50,000 to 100,000 units of factor concentrate annually. (One unit is the amount of clotting activity in 1 ml of fresh pooled plasma.) The complications from receiving that amount of pooled human plasma are numerous (Corrigan, 1990). From 80 to 90% of all patients with severe hemophilia A and 55% of those with severe hemophilia B who received factor replacement between 1979 and 1984 test positive for human immunodeficiency virus (HIV) (Hilgartner, 1991). In addition, 80% of patients with severe hemophilia have hepatitis B surface antibodies and more than 50% have persistently elevated liver function test results that indicate chronic liver disease from hepatitis. Both the advent of a hepatitis B vaccine and the screening, heating, and pasteurization of blood products have diminished the incidence of hepatitis B and HIV infection as consequences of factor replacement therapy. No documented cases of HIV seroconversion in patients with hemophilia have been reported since 1985 (Corrigan, 1990). To further reduce the risks from factor replacement, factor VIII concentrate has been made in culture by recombinant DNA techniques and has been available since 1992; recombinant factor IX is also now available. These products are not entirely without risk, however, owing to their use of human albumin to stabilize the products (Shopnick & Brettler, 1996).

DISABILITIES

For the child with hemophilia, the degree and type of disability are similar to those of the child with juvenile rheumatoid arthritis and are dependent on the age of the child, on the severity of the disease, and often on the emotional support provided by the family.

The child with moderate or severe hemophilia is usually diagnosed shortly after birth or within the first few months of life. Parents are counseled to watch for signs of hemorrhages and to treat all head injuries as potentially life threatening. As the child begins to pull to stand, a lightweight protective helmet is usually prescribed, and parents may be advised to use knee and elbow pads to protect the joints of children who are learning how to walk. Understandably, parents may become overprotective and discourage peer group activities and playground play, such as swinging and sliding, that helps develop balance and coordination.

The child with severe hemophilia will begin to have more frequent joint and muscle hemorrhages by 3 years of age, as his activity level increases and he becomes physically able to run and jump, which may increase the incidence of direct trauma. Pain and frequent visits to the emergency department for factor replacement therapy may become the norm for many of these children and their families. Varied responses to their pain may cause differing disabilities. Some children may use their pain to maintain dependency on their parents by refusing to participate in normal activities of daily living (ADL). Other children may deny their pain because they know it means they will receive an intravenous injection and be immobilized. The young child may not understand that prompt treatment will relieve the pain and limit the need for more infusions (Holdredge & Cotta, 1989).

The school-age child with frequent hemorrhages may have poor school attendance because of time spent in emergency departments and the need to immobilize the joint. With the advent of home replacement therapy, time lost from school has become less of a problem, although special arrangements may need to be made for transporting the child on crutches. Children must be excused from physical education classes when acute hemarthroses occur and may need adaptive physical education programs if chronic arthropathy is present. Participation in organized sports is an important aspect of the school-age child's and adolescent's social life that may not be available for the child with hemophilia. Certain sports are absolutely contraindicated, and participation in other sports must be carefully evaluated by the entire medical team and family.

By late adolescence, many young men with severe hemophilia will have at least one arthropathic joint that causes chronic pain and stiffness, which may be disabling. The Musculoskeletal Committee of the World Federation of Hemophilia developed a scale for evaluating chronic pain using a 0 to 3 rating:

0   No pain; no functional deficit; no analgesic use needed (except for acute hemorrhage)

1   Mild pain; does not interfere with occupation or with ADL; may require occasional relief by a nonnarcotic analgesic

2   Moderate pain; causes partial or occasional interference with occupation or ADL; may require occasional narcotics for relief

3   Severe pain; interferes with performing occupation or carrying out ADL; requires frequent use of nonnarcotic or narcotic medication for relief (Holdredge & Cotta, 1989)

Many older adolescents and young adults not only face the aforementioned problems of the school-age child but also face peer and even community ostracism because of their HIV-positive status. At a time when peer acceptance and increasing independence are so important, they may face rejection and an increasing dependence on others as the HIV-related disease progresses.

Few published data exist on the degree of disability resulting from the musculoskeletal complications of hemophilia. Weissman (1977) reported on a study conducted by Ahlberg in 1966 on 250 boys and men with hemophilia. On a scale of 0 to 3, with 0 representing no disability and 3 representing severe arthropathy and wheelchair-dependent mobility, 50% scored 0 and less than 10% scored 3. As factor replacement products have become more available, the clinical impression is that the degree of disability has diminished. In my clinic, in which children with hemophilia are followed until their late teens, less than 5% of patients require assistive devices or orthoses for ambulation on a continuous basis and no patients are wheelchair dependent.

Primary Musculoskeletal Impairments

Atkins and colleagues (1987) reported that the prevalence of joint contracture in patients with the severe form of hemophilia is between 50 and 95%. These contractures are the result of recurrent hemarthroses and intramuscular bleeding episodes and most frequently involve knee and elbow flexion and ankle plantar flexion. Although recurrent intramuscular hemorrhages are rare, a single large hematoma can cause permanent joint contracture because the large volume of blood will cause localized necrosis; as the blood is reabsorbed the dead muscle fibers are replaced by fibrous tissue in a shortened position. This occurs in about 10% of all muscle hemorrhages and is most common in the plantar flexor and forearm muscles.

Contractures secondary to recurrent hemarthroses are related to a number of factors. Acute bleeding episodes are painful, and the patient is placed in a splint in the position of comfort, which at the knee and elbow is typically in flexion. Multiple hemorrhages, with frequent immobilization, can result in muscle shortening around a joint. As hemarthroses recur, with synovial hypertrophy and eventual articular cartilage destruction, bony changes, such as genu valgus, posterior subluxation of the tibia, and osteophytes, may occur. These changes may restrict ROM in a more permanent manner.

Muscle weakness is usually found around affected joints. In a study by Pietri and associates (1992), 10 patients (from 8 to 23 years of age) with unilateral knee involvement were strength tested on a Cybex 340 (Cybex, Division of Lumex, Ronkonkoma, NY) for knee strength (as measured by peak torque), total work, and average power output. The average number of knee hemarthroses per patient was seven, and minimal or no radiographic changes were seen in any patient. Peak torque at $60°/s$, total work, and average power were all significantly lower in the involved knee. The decreased muscle function was attributed to immobilization resulting in muscle atrophy, as well as reflex inhibition of the alpha motoneuron of the quadriceps muscle and facilitation of the hamstrings from slowly adapting capsular receptors sensitive to pressure and distention.

Another study by Strickler and Greene (1984) looked at isokinetic torque levels in the quadriceps and hamstrings muscles of males with hemophilia, ages 7 through adult. All their subjects demonstrated knee flexor and extensor strength deficits when compared with age-matched healthy subjects. Additionally, they found that as the degree of arthropathy and flexion deformities increased, muscle strength decreased, with a relatively greater decrease in extensor torque, resulting in a higher than normal flexor-extensor ratio. Normally, knee flexors are approximately 60% as strong as extensors. In the patients with hemophilia, flexor strength averaged 70% of extensors in those with no arthropathy and was greater than extensor strength in adolescents and adults with stage 4 arthropathy.

Peripheral nerve lesions are a potential consequence of large intramuscular hemorrhages, owing to compression on the nerve from the rapidly expanding hemorrhage. The highest incidence of lesions is to the femoral nerve after iliacus muscle hemorrhages. Fortunately, in the majority of cases, nerve function returns to normal within a few weeks or months, but the affected limb must be protected until full function returns (Houghton & Duthie, 1979).

Postural deviations may also be seen in the child with hemophilia. Leg length discrepancies can occur with epiphyseal overgrowth from hyperemia. Mechanical, or apparent, discrepancy can occur from a pelvic obliquity caused by psoas shortening after one or more hemorrhages. Whether real or apparent, this discrepancy may result in a postural scoliosis (Fernandez-Palazzi et al., 1990).

Hemarthroses, intramuscular hemorrhages, and hemophilic arthropathy are all sources of pain. The pain of an acute hemorrhage is usually relieved shortly after hemostasis is achieved by factor replacement. The chronic pain associated with a severely damaged joint is much more difficult to alleviate. Analgesics that contain aspirin or antihistamines must be avoided because they inhibit platelet function necessary for clotting. Narcotics may be necessary for severe, chronic pain but must be prescribed cautiously. Drug abuse among adolescents and adult males with hemophilia is a recognized problem, with one study finding that 21% of older patients with severe hemophilia abused drugs, including alcohol and prescribed painkillers, as well as illegal drugs (Jonas, 1989). Transcutaneous electrical nerve stimulation, biofeedback, relaxation, and guided imagery may be used for pain relief. Orthopedic surgery may be necessary to reduce unremitting pain by fusing a painful joint or replacing it (Corrigan, 1990).

Functional Limitations

The functional limitations for the child with hemophilia are dependent on the number of joints involved and the severity of the joint arthropathy. Gait deviations are seen most often and result from frequent immobilizations with subsequent weakness, joint changes, muscle shortening, and pain. Even mild gait deviations can create additional stress on joints and contribute to perpetuating the cycle of vulnerability to stress, recurrent hemarthrosis, synovitis, and further joint destruction. Weight bearing on a flexed knee not only increases the stress on the tibiofemoral and patellofemoral surfaces but also increases the quadriceps force required to maintain available extension against gravity. Despite the greater force required, Strickler and Greene (1984) found that subjects with arthropathy and knee flexion contractures demonstrated significantly reduced knee extension torque values.

Wheelchairs are usually not needed for children with hemophilia, except when acute hemorrhages in more than one joint prohibit the use of assistive devices for ambulation. As the child progresses to adulthood, more orthoses or ambulation aids may be used; but even in the adult population, less than 10% of persons with severe hemophilia need wheelchairs for mobility (Ahlberg, 1965).

Activities of daily living such as dressing, grooming, and hygiene may be problematic for the child with frequent elbow hemorrhages and decreased elbow extension and forearm pronation and supination. Carrying schoolbooks may stress the elbow joints and lead to bleeding. Although there are no functional assessment scales specific to the hemophilia population, evaluation using the Functional Independence Measure (FIM) or WeeFIM (for children younger than age 7) will provide a numerical score and an objective way to measure functional progress (State University of New York, 1991).

Cardiopulmonary endurance is frequently impaired in children with hemophilia. Koch and colleagues (1984) evaluated response to exercise in 11 boys with factor VIII deficiency, ranging in age from 8 to 15.5 years, according to a uniform bicycle protocol and compared their performances with data available for healthy children. All the boys had previously been encouraged to participate in the physical education program at school, as well as after-school activities. Although none of the patients had acute bleeding problems, pain, significant weakness, or orthopedic deformities, several had previously sustained lower extremity hemorrhages. Their performance on bicycle ergometry demonstrated that peak heart rate, minutes of exercise, physical working capacity (maximum workload per weight in kilograms), and mean power were all significantly lower than for a population of healthy children whose physical activities did not exceed age-appropriate recreation. The clinical implication stated by the authors was that physical education alone does not provide aerobic conditioning, so it is imperative to supplement physical education with an individualized exercise program for fitness.

The physical therapist may be involved in counseling the child and family about appropriate recreational activities to maintain cardiopulmonary and muscular fitness. Before beginning participation in any sport, a child should be evaluated for joint motion, muscle strength, flexibility, and ligament stability, with particular attention paid to those joints that are likely to be stressed by the chosen sport. Any deficiencies should be eliminated before participation in the sport begins. In addition, a sport-specific conditioning program should be implemented and appropriate protective wear discussed. (See Chapter 17 on sports injuries for additional relevant information.)

Participation in certain sports is contraindicated owing to the danger of traumatic hemorrhages. The National Hemophilia Foundation, in association with the American Red Cross, published a booklet in 1996 entitled *Hemophilia, Sports, and Exercise*. In this booklet, sports activities are divided into three categories: (1) recommended sports with minimal risks, such as swimming and cycling; (2) sports in which the physical, social, and psychologic benefits usually outweigh the risks; and (3) sports in which the risks outweigh the benefits. Contact sports, such as boxing, football, hockey, racquetball, and rugby, are in the highest risk category and not recommended for patients with hemophilia. Participation in most other sports can be considered, but the decision to participate should be made jointly by the child, his parents, and the members of a comprehensive hemophilia clinic team.

THE ROLE OF PHYSICAL THERAPY

Physical therapy for the child with hemophilia is aimed at maintaining strength and a good ROM in all joints and at preventing or diminishing disability. The majority of this therapy will occur in a clinic or outpatient setting with adjunctive home exercise programs. Unless the child has neurologic involvement from a central nervous system hemorrhage, his limitations rarely affect his educational abilities, so school physical therapy is not indicated.

Kasper and Dietrich (1985) recommend that a daily exercise program be followed from early childhood and encouraged with as much enthusiasm as other medical care. Clinical observations would suggest that strong muscles help support joints and decrease the frequency of hemorrhages, and several studies have demonstrated that participation in strengthening programs resulted in reduced bleeding episodes (Greene & Strickler, 1983; Koch et al., 1984; Timmermans, 1990). The specific type of strengthening program appears to be less important than daily participation. In the three case studies, a total of 64 patients participated in a wide variety of daily exercise programs for a period of 6 to 18 months. In all these studies, strength improved in all patients, and bleeding frequency decreased in all but two of Timmermans' patients.

Examination

Examination of the child with hemophilia should include gathering historical information about the location and frequency of bleeding episodes and the patient's normal activities. This information is essential in identifying the causative factors of hemorrhage and in designing a program to reduce the frequency and severity of hemorrhages. Objective data should include goniometric measurements of active and passive ROM and joint deformities, such as genu valgus. Valgus and varus stress tests and examination of calcaneal and subtalar mobility should be performed to determine ligamentous integrity.

Muscle strength is examined functionally in the child who is too young to participate in manual muscle testing; otherwise, manual muscle testing is performed. Isokinetic testing may be performed in the older child if more sensitive strength measures are desired, such as for postoperative rehabilitation or to determine readiness to participate in organized sports.

Leg lengths, both from the anterior-superior iliac spine to the medial malleolus and from the umbilicus to the medial malleolus, should be measured to rule out leg length discrepancy, either actual or apparent secondary to pelvic obliquity. Girth measurements at joints may reveal swelling, although they are more useful when done serially on one joint than in comparison with the contralateral limb, because repeated hemarthroses can cause bony overgrowth. Muscle girth measurements may be indicative of muscle atrophy.

In my clinic, gait is examined visually for gross abnormalities, including posture, stride length, stance time, and heel-toe progression. If a treadmill is available, increases in speed and elevation often reveal more subtle differences.

Balance and coordination can be screened quickly by observing stair climbing, single-limb stance, hopping, and skipping (if appropriate for age). Parental reports are usually accurate in identifying coordination problems, at which time more formal testing (e.g., with the Bruininks-Oseretsky Test of Motor Proficiency [Bruininks, 1978]) can be completed.

Gross motor development is examined annually in our clinic for the first few years of life using the Peabody Developmental Motor Scales (Folio & Fewell, 1983) if developmental problems are suspected. Otherwise, a simple screening tool such as the Denver II (Frankenburg et al., 1990) will give information about development in gross motor, fine motor, cognitive, and ADL skills.

Pain assessment must include the nature and severity of pain. The pain of an acute bleeding episode must be distinguished from the chronic pain of arthropathy. In the very young child who cannot verbalize his pain, the parents are instructed to watch for decreased use of a limb or changes in activity patterns or personality as signs of an acute bleeding episode. The chronic pain of arthropathy will not be evident until joint destruction has progressed to stage 4 or 5, which usually does not occur before the end of the first decade or into the second decade of life. For these preadolescent and older boys, visual analogue or numerical (0 to 10) scales can be used to measure pain (see Chapter 8).

Evaluation

Based on the examination findings and historical information provided by the patient, the physical therapist can determine the most appropriate intervention for the patient. Is this an acute or chronic problem? How does the patient's lifestyle affect his disease? How does the patient's disease affect his lifestyle? Goals and outcomes of treatment will be determined by the answers to these and other questions suggested by the examination findings.

Intervention

When hemostasis has been achieved after an acute hemorrhage, the child and family should be instructed in active exercises for ROM and strengthening. Koch and colleagues (1982) describe a physical therapy program for the knee with the following rules:

1. Passive ROM is contraindicated.
2. The isometric technique of alternating muscle contraction and relaxation is beneficial.
3. When the quadriceps muscle strength is in the fair range, the patient is encouraged to achieve full active knee extension in supine and sitting.
4. Active resistive exercises may be initiated when available knee flexion is at least 90° and there is less than a 15° flexion contracture.

During this subacute phase, factor replacement therapy is usually given before participation in physical therapy to minimize the risk of rebleeding and may be continued at regular intervals until the hemorrhage resolves. The exercise program must be individualized to progress from isometric to active-assistive, active, and finally resistive mode as the pain and swelling diminish and ROM and strength increase. Modalities such as ice, transcutaneous electrical nerve stimulation, and splints may be used to decrease joint pain and swelling, and hydrotherapy will allow for ROM, strengthening, and gait training activities to be performed with minimal stress to the joints.

Contracture Management

If the patient has recurrent hemarthroses without achieving full ROM and strength between bleeding episodes, a contracture will develop. Exercise alone may not be able to overcome the muscle shortening and intracapsular adhesions that may have formed. Timmermans (1989) has described a program using manual traction and mobilization techniques to relax the joint capsule, increase ROM, and decrease painful movements. Her method, as described below, is one way of approaching contracture management, although it has not been shown to be more effective than other methods.

Manual traction is applied in the position of comfort, taking care that there are no angular movements. With traction maintained, gentle manipulations may be performed to facilitate the restricted motion (e.g., anterior shifting of the tibia facilitates knee extension). Such techniques should only be used when the patient has received factor replacement and the therapist is experienced in both mobilization and management of hemophilia. They should never be used in the presence of severe instability or synovitis.

If full ROM cannot be achieved through exercise, several nonsurgical options are available. Although purely passive manual stretching is rarely indicated, slow stretching of joint contractures over relatively long periods has been shown to be effective (Weissman, 1977). Dynamic splints can provide a low-intensity, prolonged stretch and can be used in the patient's normal environment without difficulty. To reduce the risk of inducing a bleeding episode, tension on the dynamic splint is started at 0 or 0.5 and increased very slowly. If joint hemorrhage should occur, the dynamic splint is discontinued until the hemorrhage has resolved and then reapplied at a reduced tension. In one study, seven patients with chronic knee flexion contractures of greater than 15° were fitted with dynamic splints (Lang, 1990). The patients wore the dynamic splints at night for several months (range: 4–10), and all demonstrated ROM increases of at least 5°. Although three of these patients experienced knee hemarthroses during the study, each was able to resume use of the splint without restrictions. Despite modest increases in ROM, five of the seven patients reported decreased stiffness and subjective improvement in ambulation.

Dynamic sling traction has also been used to provide prolonged stretch but requires hospitalization and confinement to bed for an average of 2 weeks (Duthie, 1990). The Quengel cast-brace or Ilizarov device may be used when posterior subluxation of the tibia accompanies a knee flexion contracture. The cast brace has offset subluxation hinges that correct the subluxation while a toggle stick corrects the flexion contracture.

Serial casting and drop-out casts are another option for contracture management. My experience has been limited to use in patients who have severe gastrocnemius muscle hemorrhages with resultant decreased ROM. In one patient, a 70° knee flexion contracture present 1 month after hemorrhage was reduced to his prehemorrhage range of −15° of extension in 6 days by use of a drop-out cast and active knee extension exercises.

Orthotics

Splints and orthoses are commonly used in the management of joint and muscle hemorrhages, but their use must be carefully monitored to prevent overuse. The general rule is to use the least restrictive means necessary to protect the joints and to discontinue this use when the joint is strong enough to be without the extra protection, which is usually when strength and joint stability are in the good range. Therapists may be involved in the fabrication of splints to provide rest to a joint after a bleeding episode or surgery; to prevent or decrease the number of hemorrhages in a chronic joint, prevent or correct joint deformity, or improve function; or to provide support for weak or unstable joints (Holdredge, 1989). The splints are used as an adjunct to therapy and should not be used without a comprehensive program of strengthening exercises and joint stability, gait, and functional training.

Strengthening

Strengthening can be achieved through isometric, isotonic, or isokinetic exercise. The choice of type of exercise depends on the patient's ability to move the joint without pain, particularly after an acute hemarthrosis, or if there is need for immobilization. Isometric exercises are prescribed immediately after an acute hemarthrosis and continued until the joint is no longer tensely swollen and hot and can be moved without pain. Concentric exercises are then begun and progressed through active-assistive, active, and resistive modes. If the equipment is available, isokinetic exercises can be initiated when muscle strength is in the good range. If the equipment is unavailable, Greene and Strickler (1983) have described a "modified isokinetic" knee strengthening program that consists of using simultaneous contraction of the flexors of one leg against the extensors of the other leg. The patient is instructed to push with as much force as tolerated while allowing the legs to fully extend over a 5- to 10-second period and then to switch position of the legs. The benefit of isokinetic exercise is that resistance is accommodated to maintain maximum muscle tension throughout the full arc of motion, regardless of the relative strength of the muscle at any point along the arc.

Exercises prescribed should not jeopardize an unstable joint by overly stressing it and thereby increasing the risk of bleeding. For that reason, slow-speed isokinetics (150°/s and below) should be used cautiously or avoided. Progressive resistive exercise (isotonic or isokinetic) in the open chain provide both concentric and eccentric strengthening and are preferred initially to closed-chain eccentric exercise that could produce exercise-induced joint tissue damage from compressive forces. All exercise programs should be advanced slowly to allow for monitoring of effects on the joints (Pietri et al., 1992). Any signs of bleeding, such as increased swelling or pain or decreased ROM, will necessitate reducing the intensity of the exercise program and possibly exercising only under cover of factor replacement until supporting muscles are stronger.

Gait Training

Gait training focuses on correct positioning of the lower extremities and use of all joints and muscle groups. The patient should be taught a springy way of moving by pushing with the ankle and forefoot to allow the shock absorption of walking to be transferred to the muscles rather than the joints. Temporary use of crutches will transfer some of the weight bearing to the arms, which will decrease the load and pain on an affected lower extremity joint and allow for a more normal gait pattern to be simulated. Orthoses, such as the University of California Biomechanical Laboratory foot orthosis, are helpful when ankle laxity leads to hindfoot valgus, with weight bearing causing abnormal stresses all the way up the lower extremity (Timmermans, 1990).

Postsurgical Rehabilitation

Physical therapists in the pediatric setting will usually be involved only in rehabilitation after syn-

ovectomy in the child with hemophilia. Osteotomies and arthrodeses are performed for severe chronic arthropathy with marked deformity, instability, and pain, but there are no references in the literature to these procedures being performed on children. Similarly, arthroplasties of the hip and knee are being performed on adults with severe arthropathy but have not been reported in the pediatric literature.

CASE HISTORY
JIMMY

Jimmy is a 12-year-old boy with severe factor VIII deficiency. Two years ago, with a stage 3 arthropathy and 6-month history of chronic synovitis, he had arthroscopic synovectomy of the right knee with excellent results: ROM of 0 to 130°; quadriceps and hamstring muscle strength both 4+/5 (good +); and only two right knee hemorrhages, 6 months and 10 months earlier. He has been able to resume his favorite sport of tennis in the past year. He has noticed an increase in the incidence of left knee hemarthroses, and in the past month has had five knee bleeding episodes. He has been put on every-other-day factor replacement and referred to physical therapy for intensive rehabilitation.

Current examination reveals a boggy, swollen, but cool left knee. ROM is −30° of extension to 70° of flexion in the left knee. Within available range, quadriceps strength is 2/5 and hamstring strength is 3/5. Jimmy is ambulating with bilateral axillary crutches, with toe-touch weight bearing on the left. He scores a 6 of 7 (independent with assistive device) on all the mobility and transfer items on the FIM except tub transfers, which are scored a 4 (require moderate assistance). He denies resting pain but does have pain with motion.

Jimmy wants to be able to go to tennis camp in the summer, although his parents are not sure he should go because his left knee bleeding began when he started tennis lessons. They are afraid that the lessons three times per week may be causing too much stress on his knee joints.

Based on the history, the physical examination, Jimmy's goal of going to tennis camp, and his parent's concerns, the following intervention plan is established. For Jimmy to meet his goal and to address his parents' concerns, coordination with the hematology team regarding long-term prophylaxis and with the orthopedist regarding the extent of joint damage is imperative. If the orthopedist does not discourage tennis playing once both knees are rehabilitated, knee braces may need to be considered to reduce lateral stresses when Jimmy plays.

Jimmy also must agree to follow a conditioning program on a daily basis once his rehabilitation is completed as long as he is playing tennis. The conditioning program will include flexibility and strength training and aerobic conditioning to reduce the risk of injury.

Finally, the direct interventions chosen are aimed at first achieving full range of motion of both knees followed by strengthening, gait training, and conditioning.

Problem 1: 30° left knee flexion contracture

Goal: Improve ROM of both knees to 0 to 140°.
Plan:

1. Fabricate resting knee splint for hours of sleep to maintain maximum available extension at night. Revise splint as extension returns.

2. Use dynamic splinting during the day for prolonged stretch (Fig. 9–3).

3. Perform active ROM exercises.

Problem 2: decreased strength in both knees

Goal: Increase strength of quadriceps and hamstrings muscles of both legs to normal.
Plan:

1. For left knee, begin with isometric exercises and contract and relax techniques for ROM and strengthening. Begin active-assistive and active exercises when pain abates. When ROM is 15 to 90°, begin resistive exercises and advance slowly using low weights and high repetitions (Fig. 9–4).

2. For right knee, begin isokinetic strengthening at 180, 240, and 300° per second and joint stability activities, such as progressive resistive straight leg raises and single-limb minisquats.

3. For both lower extremities, begin strengthening and joint stability activities for hips and ankles (e.g., straight leg raises in prone and side-lying positions, heel raises, Biomechanical Ankle Platform System [BAPS] board [Camp, Jackson, MI]).

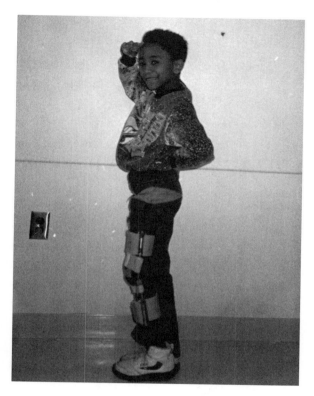

FIGURE 9–3. Dynamic splinting is used during the day to provide a prolonged stretch to the knee flexors.

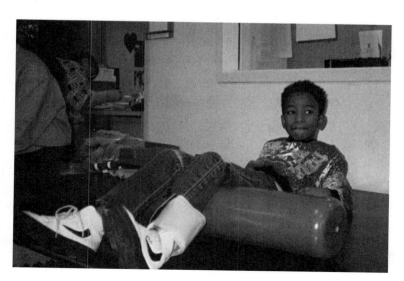

FIGURE 9–4. Resistive exercises with free weights are used for quadriceps strengthening. Later, isokinetic exercises will be added.

Problem 3: ambulation dysfunction: toe-touch weight bearing on left using bilateral axillary crutches

Outcome: Independent community ambulation without assistive devices.

Plan:

1. Maintain left weight bearing as tolerated in crutch ambulation until knee range is no less than 10 to 100° and quadriceps muscle strength is at least 3 + /5.

2. Practice gait training on the treadmill at slow speeds to encourage heel-toe gait pattern and equal stride and step lengths.

3. Progress to independent household ambulation and then community ambulation as ROM and strength improve.

Problem 4: inability to participate in physical education classes and other athletic functions with friends

Outcome: Maintain cardiovascular fitness and resume tennis.

Plan:

1. Participate in aquatic therapy and swimming, three times per week for 20 to 30 minutes.

2. Contact school physical education teacher and discuss alternatives to regular physical education program.

3. Consider taping or knee cage for both knees to reduce rotary forces while playing tennis, when able.

Jimmy will be seen three times a week in physical therapy until his ROM and strength return to normal and he is ambulating without an assistive device. He will also be given a home exercise program to supplement his physical therapy sessions. Because Jimmy's left knee flexion contracture is an acute problem, his range is expected to return quickly and he should be off crutches in 2 to 3 weeks. His strength will return more slowly, but if he is compliant with his home program he can be cut back to once-a-week physical therapy for monitoring progress and adjusting the home program. Current radiographs will be reviewed with the orthopedist to determine if playing tennis is an appropriate expectation; if so, Jimmy should be able to resume playing tennis within 3 months.

Recommended Resources

Buchanan, GR. Hemophilia. Pediatric Clinics of North America, *27*(2): 309–326, 1980.

Gilbert, MS, & Greene, WB (Eds.). Musculoskeletal Problems in Hemophilia. New York: National Hemophilia Foundation, 1990.

Hilgartner, MW, & Pochedly, C (Eds.). Hemophilia in the Child and Adult. New York: Raven Press, 1989.

National Hemophilia Foundation, 110 Greene Street, Suite 303, New York, NY 10012; Internet: www.infonhf.org.

National Hemophilia Foundation. Hemophilia, Sports, and Exercise. New York: National Hemophilia Foundation, 1996.

References

Ahlberg, A. Hemophilia in Sweden: VII. Incidence, treatment, and prophylaxis of arthropathy and other musculoskeletal manifestations of hemophilia A and B. Acta Orthopaedica Scandinavica, *77*:3–132, 1965.

Arnold, WD, & Hilgartner, MW. Hemophilic arthropathy. Journal of Bone and Joint Surgery (American), *59*:288–305, 1977.

Atkins, RM, Henderson, NJ, & Duthie, RB. Joint contractures in the hemophilias. Clinical Orthopedics and Related Research, *219*:97–105, 1987.

Bruininks, RH. Bruininks-Oseretsky Test of Motor Proficiency, Examiners Manual. Circle Pines, MN: American Guidance Service, 1978.

Buchanan, GR. Hemophilia. Pediatric clinics of North America, *27*(2): 309–326, 1980.

Corrigan, JJ. Coagulation disorders. In Miller, DR, & Bachner, RL (Eds.), Blood Disorders of Infancy and Childhood. St. Louis: Mosby, 1990, pp. 849–859.

Duthie, RB. Dynamic sling traction. In Gilbert, MS, & Greene, WB (Eds.), Musculoskeletal Problems in Hemophilia. New York: National Hemophilia Foundation, 1990, pp. 67–68.

Erkin, EHW. Radiocolloids in the management of hemophilic arthropathy in children and adolescents. Clinical Orthopedics and Related Research, *264*:129–134, 1991.

Fernandez-Palazzi, F, Rupcich, M, Rivas, S, & Bosch, N. Biomechanical alterations that impair evolution and prognosis of haemophilic arthropathy. In Gilbert, MS, & Greene, WB (Eds.), Musculoskeletal Problems in Hemophilia, 1990, pp. 34–44.

Folio, MR, & Fewell, RR. Peabody Developmental Motor Scales and Activity Cards. Allen, TX: DLM Teaching Resources, 1983.

Frankenburg, WK, Dodds, JB, Archer, P, Bresnick, B, Maschka, P, Edelman, N, & Shapiro, H. Denver II Screening Manual. Denver: Denver Developmental Materials, 1990.

Greene, WB, & Strickler, EM. A modified isokinetic strengthening program for patients with severe hemophilia. Developmental Medicine and Child Neurology, *25*:189–196, 1983.

Gregosiewicz, A, Wosko, I, & Kandzierski, G. Intraarticular bleeding in children with hemophilia: The prevention of arthropathy. Journal of Pediatric Orthopedics, *9*:182–185, 1989.

Hilgartner, MW. AIDS in the transfusion recipient. Pediatric Clinics of North America, *38*:121–129, 1991.

Holdredge, S. Thermoplastic splints. In Funk, S (Ed.), Rehabilitation in Hemophilia: Proceedings of a Conference. New York: National Hemophilia Foundation, 1989, pp. 38–44.

Holdredge, S, & Cotta, S. Physical therapy and rehabilitation in the care of the adult and child with hemophilia. In Hilgartner, MW, & Pochedly, C (Eds.), Hemophilia in the Child and Adult. New York: Raven Press, 1989, pp. 235–262.

Houghton, GR, & Duthie, RB. Orthopedic problems in hemophilia. Clinical Orthopedics and Related Research, *138*:197–216, 1979.

Joist, JH, & Ameri, A. Pathogenesis of hemophilic arthropathy. In Gilbert, MS, & Greene, WB (Eds.), Musculoskeletal Problems in Hemophilia. New York: National Hemophilia Foundation, 1990, pp. 20–25.

Jonas, DL. Drug abuse in hemophilia. In Hilgartner, MW, & Pochedly, C (Eds.), Hemophilia in the Child and Adult. New York: Raven Press, 1989, pp. 229–234.

Karayalcin, G. Current concepts in the management of hemophilia. Pediatric Annals, *14*:640–655, 1985.

Kasper, CK, & Dietrich, SL. Comprehensive management of hemophilia. Clinics in Haematology, *14*:491–492, 1985.

Koch, B, Cohen, S, Luban, NC, & Eng, G. Hemophiliac knee: Rehabilitation techniques. Archives of Physical Medicine and Rehabilitation, *63*:379–382, 1982.

Koch, B, Galioto, FM, Jr, Kelleher, J, & Goldstein, D. Physical fitness in children with hemophilia. Archives of Physical Medicine and Rehabilitation, *65*:324–326, 1984.

Lang, L. Dynasplint for knee flexion contractures in hemophilia. In Gilbert, MS, & Greene, WB (Eds.), Musculoskeletal Problems in Hemophilia. New York: National Hemophilia Foundation, 1990, pp. 83–86.

Liesner, RJ, Khair, K, & Hann, IM. The impact of prophylactic treatment on children with severe haemophilia. British Journal of Haematology, *92*:973–978, 1996.

Nilsson, IM, Berntorp, E, Lofqvist, T, & Pettersson, H. Twenty-five years' experience of prophylactic treatment in severe haemophilia A and B. Journal of Internal Medicine, *232*:25–32, 1992.

Pietri, MM, Frontera, WR, Pratts, IS, & Suarez, EL. Skeletal muscle function in patients with hemophilia A and unilateral hemarthroses of the knee. Archives of Physical Medicine and Rehabilitation, *73*:22–26, 1992.

Shopnick, RI, & Brettler, DB. Hemostasis. Clinical Orthopedics and Related Research, *328*:34–38. 1996.

State University of New York at Buffalo, Center for Functional Assessment Research, Department of Rehabilitation Medicine. Guide for the Use of the Uniform Data Set for Medical Rehabilitation Including the Functional Independence Measure for Children (WeeFIM). 1991.

Strickler, EM, & Greene, WB. Isokinetic torque levels in hemophiliac knee musculature. Archives of Physical Medicine and Rehabilitation, *65*:766–770, 1984.

Timmermans, H. Severe arthropathy of the hemophilic joint: a comprehensive rehabilitation program. In Funk, S (Ed.), Rehabilitation in Hemophilia: Proceedings of a Conference. New York: National Hemophilia Foundation, 1989, pp. 11–15.

Timmermans, H. The role of the physiotherapist. In Gilbert, MS, & Greene, WB (Eds.), Musculoskeletal Problems in Hemophilia. New York: National Hemophilia Foundation, 1990, pp. 115–121.

Weissman, J. Rehabilitation medicine and the hemophilic patient. Mt. Sinai Journal of Medicine, *44*:359–370, 1977.

CHAPTER
10

Spinal Conditions

CHERYL PATRICK, PT

The spine is the framework for our posture and our movement. It supports our cranium, extremities, and spinal cord; allows for trunk flexibility; acts as a shock absorber; and provides structural support for normal chest and respiratory development. Orthopedic concerns arise when spinal alignment is altered by congenital or progressive changes, producing scoliosis, kyphosis, or lordosis.

Each one or a combination of these conditions, if left untreated, can directly affect a child's pulmonary function, psychosocial well-being, potential for back pain, and life expectancy. We, as physical therapists, play a vital role in the detection and treatment of spinal conditions 2 to 3% of the population of school-age children (7–16 years) are at risk for adolescent idiopathic scoliosis, the most common form of scoliosis. The prevalence of other spinal conditions varies with the condition and underlying disease process (Bleck, 1991; Weinstein, 1989). This chapter addresses the prevalence and natural history, identification, examination, and treatment of these spinal conditions. Specific case histories are presented to discuss impairments, functional limitations, and disabilities of children with special conditions. Emphasis is on physical therapy intervention

with nonsurgical and surgical management of these spinal conditions.

Because pathologic spinal conditions are discussed in this chapter, it is necessary for the reader to have some knowledge of normal spinal development (Fig. 10–1). Therefore, a discussion of development in the embryologic, fetal, and childhood stages follows.

Fetal development is divided into three stages. The first 3 weeks after fertilization is termed the *pre-embryonic period*. The *embryonic period* is next, lasting from week 3 to week 8 of gestation; during this stage the organs of the body develop. The *fetal period* lasts from week 8 until term, and during this stage maturation and growth of all structures and organs occur (Moe et al., 1987).

Early development of the skeletal, muscular, and neural systems is related to the notochord. Cell proliferation occurs at approximately 3 weeks, forming a trilaminar structure with layers of ectoderm, mesoderm, and endoderm. Proliferation of the mesodermal tissue continues, forming 29 pairs of somites in the fourth week and the remainder (42–44 total) in the fifth week. Differentiation of the somites then occurs, producing 4 occipital, 8 cervical, 12 thoracic,

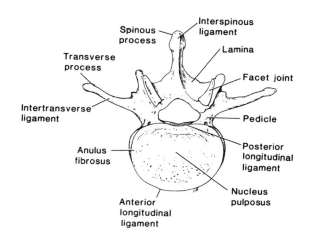

Spinous process
Interspinous ligament
Transverse process
Lamina
Facet joint
Intertransverse ligament
Pedicle
Anulus fibrosus
Posterior longitudinal ligament
Nucleus pulposus
Anterior longitudinal ligament

FIGURE 10–1. The L2 vertebra viewed from above. (From Moe, JH, Winter, RB, Bradford, DS, Ogilvie, JW, & Lonstein, JE. Scoliosis and Other Spinal Deformities, 2nd ed. Philadelphia: WB Saunders, 1987, p. 8.)

5 lumbar, 5 sacral, and 8 to 10 coccygeal somites. The occipital somites form a portion of the base of the skull and the articulation between the cranium and cervical vertebrae while the last 5 to 7 coccygeal somites disappear. Cervical, thoracic, lumbar, and sacral somites form the structures of the spine (Winter, 1983).

Proliferation of the somites occurs, developing three distinct areas. Dorsally the cells become dermatome, giving rise to the skin. Medially to the dermatome, cells migrate deep to give rise to skeletal muscle. The ventral and medial cells migrate toward the notochord and neural tube to form the sclerotome (Moe et al., 1987; Winter, 1983).

The sclerotomal cells proliferate and differentiate, giving rise to rudimentary vertebral structures, including rib buds. Chondrification begins at the cervicothoracic level, extending cranially and caudally. Centers of chondrification allow for formation of the solid cartilage model of a vertebra with no line of demarcation between body, neural arch, or rib rudiments (Moe et al., 1987).

Ossification occurs at primary and secondary centers. Ossification begins during the late fetal period and continues after birth. Primary centers of ossification extend to the spinous, transverse, and articular processes. Secondary ossification centers develop at the upper and lower portions of the vertebral body, at the tip of the spinous processes, and at each transverse process. These centers expand in late adolescence. Secondary ossification centers also develop in the ribs—one at the head of the rib and two in the tubercle. Ossification of the axis, atlas, and sacrum differs slightly from that of the other vertebrae. The atlas has two primary centers and one secondary

center of ossification, and the axis has five primary and two secondary centers of ossification. Ossification of the axis begins near the end of gestation with fusion of the two odontoid centers and is completed in the second decade of life with fusion of the odontoid and centrum. Fusion of the sacrum begins in adolescence and is completed in the third decade of life (Moe et al., 1987).

Spinal growth occurs throughout adolescence. A knowledge of spinal growth is essential in nonsurgical and surgical treatment of spinal deformities. Spinal growth does not proceed in a uniform linear pattern (Tanner et al., 1966; Tanner & Whitehouse, 1976). Two periods of rapid spinal growth occur: the first from birth to age 3 years and the second at the adolescent growth spurt. Between 3 years and the onset of puberty, growth is linear.

The spinal pubertal growth spurts occur at different chronologic and Tanner ages for females and males. In females, the growth spurt coincides with Tanner 2 or a chronologic age of 8 to 14 years, with the maximum growth occurring at a mean of 12 years of age. The spurt lasts 2.5 to 3 years (Calvo, 1957). The growth spurt occurs later in males, at Tanner 3 or chronologic age 11 to 16 years, with the maximum growth at age 14 years. These values are average values based on white Anglo-Saxon populations (Duval-Beaupere, 1972).

A fused area of the spine does not grow longitudinally, as documented by Moe and colleagues (1964). The surgeon, therefore, considers the information on spinal growth potential for each individual case.

SCOLIOSIS

Detection and Clinical Examination

Detection of scoliosis is primarily by identification of trunk, shoulder, or pelvic asymmetries. Children with asymmetries should be referred for a baseline evaluation to an orthopedic surgeon with an interest in and knowledge of scoliosis. Ideally, the surgeon should specialize in pediatrics or pediatric spines, be affiliated with a reputable medical center, and be part of a team that includes an orthotist, a nurse, and a physical therapist.

An examination begins with a complete patient history to obtain information regarding curve detection, familial conditions, general health, and physical maturity. The physical examination includes assessment of the deformity, general alignment, shoulder and pelvic symmetry, spinal alignment by forward bend test, trunk compensation using a plumb line, and leg length measurement. The examiner also evaluates signs and symptoms of any underlying disease and neurologic status. Rotation of the spine is quantified using a scoliometer with the forward bend test (Moe et al., 1987). This instrument works like a level placed astride the spinous processes to measure rotation of a rib hump or prominent lumbar paraspinal musculature.

Radiographs (initially two views: lateral and anterior-posterior) are used to determine location, type, and magnitude of the curve, as well as skeletal age. Skeletal maturity is determined using the Risser sign, which quantifies the amount of ossification of the iliac crest, using grades 0 to 5. Grades 1 to 4 are excursions from 25 to 100%, starting at the anterior-superior iliac spine. Grade 5 categorizes fusion of the iliac crest with the ileum (Zaouss & James, 1958). Grade 0 represents absence of ossification. Grades 0, 1, and 2 correlate with skeletal immaturity, grade 3 with progressing skeletal maturity, grade 4 with cessation of spinal growth, and grade 5 with cessation of increase in height.

The spinal curvature is measured using the Cobb method. To complete the measurement, one must first identify the end vertebrae. The end vertebrae are described as the most cephalad vertebra of a curve whose upper surface maximally tilts toward the curve's concavity and the most caudal vertebra with maximal tilt toward the concavity. Lines are drawn as extensions of the end vertebra from either end-plate or pedicle. The degree of curvature is measured as the angle formed by the intersection of lines perpendicular to these end vertebral lines (Dickson et al., 1984; Goldstein & Waugh, 1973). Minimal degree of curvature for diagnosis is 10° (Fig. 10-2). Computed tomography, conventional tomography, magnetic resonance imaging, myelography, and bone scans can provide additional information as necessary to aid in diagnosis and detection of spinal conditions.

Terminology

Spinal deformities are classified according to magnitude, location, direction, and etiology. Curvatures may be idiopathic, neuromuscular, or congenital and may further be classified by the area of the spine in which the apex of the curve is located: (1) cervical curve, between C1 and C6; (2) cervicothoracic curve, between C7 and T1; (3) thoracic curve, between T2 and T11; (4) thoracolumbar curve, between T12 and L1; (5) lumbar curve, between L2 and L4; and (6) lumbosacral curve, between L5 and S1. Direction of the curve is designated right or left by the side of the convexity of the deformity (Rothman & Simeone, 1982).

There are two major types of curvatures: structural and nonstructural. A nonstructural curve fully corrects clinically and radiographically on lateral bend toward the apex of the curve and lacks vertebral rotation. A nonstructural curve is usually nonpro-

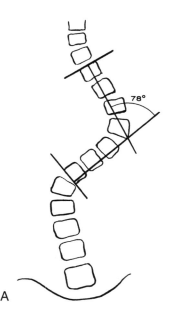
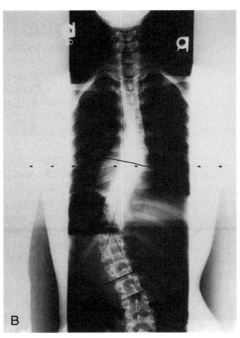

FIGURE 10–2. *A,* Cobb's method of measuring the angle of the curve in scoliosis (see text). *B,* The Cobb method of measuring the curve angle of scoliosis as seen on a radiograph. (*A,* From Tachdjian, MO. Pediatric Orthopedics, 2nd ed. Philadelphia: WB Saunders, 1990, p. 2285.)

78°

A

B

gressive and is most often caused by a shortened lower extremity on the side of the apex of the curve. It is essential, however, to watch nonstructural curves during growth because they may occasionally develop into structural deformities.

A structural curve cannot be voluntarily, passively, or forcibly fully corrected. Rotation of the vertebrae is toward the convexity of the curve. A fixed thoracic prominence or rib hump in a child with a thoracic deformity or a lumbar paraspinal prominence in a child with a lumbar curve is evidence of rotation when seen on clinical examination (Rothman & Simeone, 1982).

Idiopathic Scoliosis

Idiopathic scoliosis denotes a lateral curvature of the spine of unknown cause and is the most common form of scoliosis in children.

Etiology, Incidence, and Pathophysiology

Infantile idiopathic scoliosis develops in children younger than age 3, usually manifesting shortly after birth. The majority of the curves are left thoracic and occur more frequently in male infants. Eighty to ninety percent of these curves spontaneously resolve. Most of the remainder of cases progress throughout childhood, resulting in severe deformity. Because infantile idiopathic scoliosis is common in England and northern Europe, but rare in the United States, research suggests environmental factors in the development of the deformity (Rothman & Simeone, 1982).

Juvenile idiopathic scoliosis develops between age 3 years and before the onset of puberty. The most common curve is right thoracic, occurring in males and females with equal frequency and most often recognized around age 6 years. Juvenile idiopathic curves have a high rate of progression and result in severe deformity if untreated. A study by Wynne-Davies (1974) found the incidence of scoliosis in children younger than age 8 years to be 1.3%.

Adolescent idiopathic scoliosis categorizes curves manifesting at or around the onset of puberty. The prevalence of idiopathic scoliosis is 2 to 3% of children ages 7 to 16, with the majority of curves manifesting at the onset of puberty, and therefore classified as being adolescent idiopathic scoliosis (Bleck, 1991). Three to nine percent of these children have curves greater than 10° and require treatment (Dickson et al., 1984; Weinstein, 1989). The overall female-to-male ratio for prevalence of adolescent idiopathic scoliosis is 3.6:1. The female-to-male ratio is roughly equal (1.4:1) in curves of approximately 10°. With curve magnitude of 20° or greater, the female-to-male ratio increases to 6.4:1 (Weinstein, 1989). A greater percentage of curves will progress in the female patient, 19.3% compared with 1.2% of males. A large number of adolescent idiopathic scoliosis curvatures are structural at the time of detection, although flexibility and the progression of these curves vary. Structural curves have a greater tendency to progress throughout adolescence at an average rate of 1° per month if untreated, whereas the nonstructural curves may remain flexible enough to avoid becoming problematic (Rothman & Simeone, 1982).

An extensive amount of research has been devoted to discovering the cause of idiopathic scoliosis, but the mechanics and specific etiology are not clearly understood. A number of theories have been proposed that attempt to explain the mechanics of vertebral column failure and decompensation of the spine as seen in idiopathic scoliosis. These include insufficiency of the costovertebral ligaments, asymmetric weakness of the paraspinal musculature, unequal distribution of type I and type II muscle fibers, and collagen abnormalities. Clinical studies have focused on deviations in vibratory responses, proprioceptive deficits, and neurologic or vestibular dysfunction. No conclusive evidence has been found to indicate any of these factors as a cause of idiopathic scoliosis. In fact, it is now proposed that some of the clinical changes such as vibratory and proprioceptive deficits are actually secondary to, rather than a cause of, the existing spinal deformity (Dickson et al., 1984; McInnes et al., 1991). Byl and Gray (1993) report decreased performance of adolescents with idiopathic scoliosis, particularly those with severe curves, on complex balance activities especially when vision and proprioception were simultaneously challenged. The authors pose the question of whether balance changes are due to the structural impairment (scoliosis) or an underlying sensory impairment. They strongly suggest the need for longitudinal studies to determine if there is a predictive relationship between balance dysfunction and progressive scoliosis.

Although the specific etiology of idiopathic scoliosis is not known, data from studies by Wynne-Davies (1966, 1968) and Cowell and colleagues (1972) reflect the existence of a familial tendency. Familial prevalence of idiopathic scoliosis may reflect a growth pattern shared by families. The growth pattern and effects of biplanal spinal asymmetry during growth are discussed in a study by Dickson and associates (1984), which specifically examines the growth factors in the coronal and sagittal planes and their effect on progressive idiopathic scoliosis.

Structural changes vary with the degree of

scoliosis and affect the anatomy and physiology of the spine, with the greatest change at the apex of the curve (Tachdjian, 1990). Compression and distraction forces act on the growing spine to produce wedge-shaped vertebrae (larger on the convex side and smaller on the concave side). Associated changes are seen in the intraspinal canal and posterior arch, which may cause angulation and stretch on the spinal cord but rarely cause functional disturbances. Cord compression and functional changes occur most often secondary to an unusually tight dura mater, as seen in spines with marked dorsal kyphosis. Changes occurring on the concave side of the curvature include compression and degenerative changes of intravertebral disks and shortening of muscles and ligaments (Fig. 10–3). Changes in the thoracic spine directly affect the rib cage. The translatory shift of the spine causes an asymmetrically divided thorax, producing decreased pulmonary capacity on the convex side and increased pulmonary capacity on the concave side. Severe curves in the thoracic spine associated with increased angulation of the ribs posteriorly further reduce aeration of the lung on the convex side, potentially causing abnormal stresses on the heart and disturbed cardiac function (Dickson et al., 1984; Tachdjian, 1990). Structural changes cause cosmetic deformity that, in turn, affects appearance and may affect psychosocial well-being.

Natural History

A progressive curve is defined by a sustained increase of 5° or more on two consecutive examinations occurring at 4- to 6-month intervals. An untreated progressive curve has the potential to increase in magnitude in adult life. The following are the main factors that influence the probability of progression in the skeletally immature patient (Weinstein, 1989):

1. The younger the patient at diagnosis, the greater the risk of progression.
2. Double-curve patterns have a greater risk for progression than single-curve patterns.
3. The lower the Risser sign, the greater the risk of progression.
4. Curves with greater magnitude are at a greater risk to progress.
5. Risk of progression in females is approximately 10 times that of males with curves of comparable magnitude.
6. Greater risk of progression is present when curves develop before menarche.

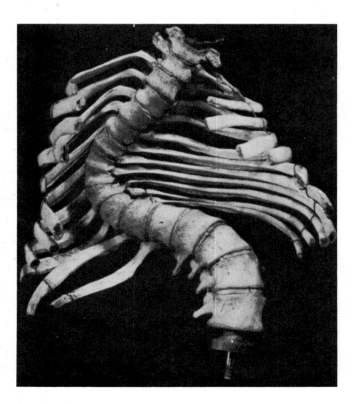

FIGURE 10–3. Anatomic specimen of the spine demonstrating structural changes of right thoracic scoliosis. Note vertebral wedging on the concave side and rotation of the vertebral bodies to the convexity of the curve. (From James, JIP. Scoliosis. Baltimore: Williams & Wilkins, 1967, p. 13. © 1967, Williams & Wilkins Co., Baltimore.)

Congenital Scoliosis

Etiology, Incidence, and Pathophysiology

Congenital scoliosis curves are caused by anomalous vertebral development. Congenital anomalies of the vertebrae can be attributed to failure of vertebral segmentation or failure of vertebral formation. Both pathologic processes are frequently seen in the same spine and may occur either at the same or at different levels. Location on the vertebrae (anterior, posterior, lateral, or a combination) determines the congenital deformity. Purely lateral deformity produces congenital scoliosis, and anterolateral and posterolateral deformities produce congenital kyphoscoliosis and lordoscoliosis, respectively (Winter, 1983, 1988).

A defect of segmentation is seen when adjacent vertebrae do not completely separate from one another, thereby producing an unsegmented bar, with no growth plate or disk between the adjacent vertebrae. A lateral, one-sided defect of segmentation produces severe progressive congenital scoliosis. Circumferential failure of segmentation produces en bloc vertebrae, an anomaly that results in loss of segmental motion and loss of longitudinal vertebral growth but no rotational or angular spinal deformity (Winter, 1983).

Defects of formation may be partial or complete. An anterior failure of formation of all or part of the vertebral body produces a kyphosis. A partial unilateral defect of formation of a vertebra produces a wedge-shaped hemivertebra (Fig. 10–4) with one pedicle and only one side with growth potential. A nonsegmented hemivertebra is completely fused to the adjacent proximal and distal vertebrae. A semisegmented hemivertebra is fused to only one adjacent vertebra and separated from the other by a normal end-plate and disk. A segmented hemivertebra is separated from both the proximal and distal vertebrae by a normal end-plate and disk. Hemivertebrae may be unbalanced, with the defect present on one side of the spine, or balanced, with different hemivertebrae present with defects on opposite sides of the spine compensating for any curves (Winter, 1983, 1988).

The etiology of congenital scoliosis involves fetal environmental factors that affect development at 45 to 60 days after fertilization (Winter, 1988). A study by Wynne-Davies (1975) is a comprehensive review of 337 patients with congenital spinal anomalies and their families. She found that an isolated anomaly, such as a hemivertebra, is a sporadic lesion with no increased risk of spinal deformities for subsequent births or for children of parents who have the deformity. Multiple spinal anomalies, with or without the presence of spina bifida, are believed to be related etiologically to spina bifida and therefore carry a 5 to 10% risk to subsequent siblings for any one of the anomalies. A review by Winter (1983) of 1250 patients with congenital spinal anomalies, however, found few familial relationships (only 13 of 1250). Conclusions were drawn that hemivertebrae carry an approximately 1% chance of occurring in a first-degree relative of a patient with a hemivertebra. A relationship between multiple congenital anomalies and spina bifida was not noted.

Other spinal anomalies or other organ system anomalies may be associated with congenital spinal malformations. One of these anomalies is diastematomyelia, a congenital malformation of the neural axis in which there is sagittal division of the spinal cord. Diastematomyelia is often associated with an osseous, fibrous, or fibrocartilaginous spur attached to one or more vertebral bodies and the dura mater. Clinical signs of a spinal dysraphism include a hair patch, unequal foot size, various foot

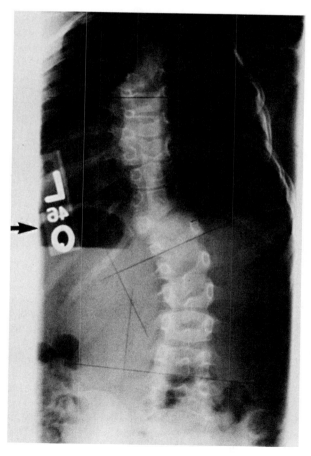

FIGURE 10–4. Radiograph of congenital scoliosis due to hemivertebrae of thoracic vertebrae. Compensatory scoliosis in the lumbar spine. (The arrow on the left indicates the hemivertebrae.)

deformities (e.g., cavus feet), and asymmetric lower extremity circumference and strength. Other associated defects include urinary tract anomalies, hearing deficits, facial asymmetries, and Sprengel's deformity, which is a partially undescended scapula that may cause apparent webbing or shortening of the neck and limited shoulder range of motion (ROM) (Winter, 1983).

The risk of progression can be analyzed by examining the growth potential of the congenital anomaly. Many congenital curves become stable and do not progress. The highest risk of progression is when there is asymmetric growth in which the convexity outgrows the concavity. This usually occurs when the anatomy of the convex side is relatively normal and the concave side is deficient. A shortened trunk may be the main deformity if both convex and concave growth deficiencies occur over multiple levels (Winter, 1988).

Treatment of Idiopathic and Congenital Scoliosis

Treatment decisions are based on skeletal maturity of the child, growth potential of the child, and curve magnitude. Options include nonsurgical methods, such as exercise, orthotic treatment, electrical stimulation, and surgical treatment.

Nonsurgical Methods

Idiopathic curves of less than 25°, curves of nonsurgical magnitude of any type in a skeletally mature patient, and nonprogressive congenital curves are evaluated by clinical examination every 4 to 6 months. Radiographs are obtained for congenital curves at each visit; however, unchanged results of a scoliometer examination may reduce the frequency of radiographs to every other visit depending on individual physician and institution practice.

A home exercise program designed to maintain or improve trunk and pelvic strength and flexibility is often prescribed for children with idiopathic or congenital scoliosis. Exercises include postural exercises (trunk extensor control, abdominal strengthening, gluteal strengthening), lateral flexion exercises, trunk shifts, stretching of pectorals and lower extremities, and respiratory exercises to increase chest capacity and maximize volume. In my clinical experience, compliance is often poor unless the child experienced back pain before diagnosis of scoliosis. Exercise as the sole treatment for prevention of progression of scoliotic curves has not been shown to be effective even if compliance is high (Lonstein & Renshaw, 1987).

ELECTRICAL STIMULATION

The use of electrical stimulation versus orthotic management is physician and rehabilitation center specific. Electrical stimulation is used on the convex side of the curve, in theory to produce sufficient stimulation to alter the direction of the deformity, decrease the pressure on the concave side of the curve, and allow for more normal vertebral growth. The stimulator is worn at night, and treatment continues until growth ceases, skin complications prevent further use, or curve progression continues. Indications for use are a skeletally immature child with an idiopathic curve of 10 to 40° (Eckerson & Axelgaard, 1984; Farady, 1983). Contraindications include inability of the patient to operate the unit, curves greater than 40°, heart disease, or thoracic hypokyphosis (Tachdjian, 1990).

Controversy surrounds the use of electrical stimulation as a viable treatment method for idiopathic scoliosis. Early studies indicated that curve stabilization occurred in 70 to 75% of patients (Brown et al., 1984) with good compliance and that potential for retention of curve correction was good (Eckerson & Axelgaard, 1984). More recent studies have found that electrical stimulation did not arrest progression or change the natural history of the curves when compared with control groups (Bertrand et al., 1992; Bylund et al., 1987). Electrical stimulation was found to be ineffective for double curves, and noncompliance rates were comparable to those of orthotic wear (Bertrand et al., 1992). Recent research, therefore, concluded that electrical stimulation had no effect on prevention of idiopathic curve progression, especially for patients with high-risk factors.

ORTHOTIC MANAGEMENT

Goals of orthotic management include halting curve progression, gaining some permanent correction, and allowing for continued spinal growth (Renshaw, 1985).

The principles of orthotic management are based on the biomechanical hypothesis that spinal stability is directly proportional to the end support of the spine and inversely proportional to spinal flexibility and the approximate square of its length. Therefore, the amount of load that may be placed on the spine before collapse can be increased by firm support at the upper and lower ends. An orthosis provides this support at the lower end of the spine anteriorly and laterally on the abdomen, posteriorly and laterally on the buttocks, and by contour over the iliac crests, effectively decreasing the lumbar lordosis. The upper end is supported by neck, shoulder, and spinal musculature; by central nervous system reflexes; and possibly by a throat mold. These end supports result in a functional shortening of the spinal column, decreased spinal flexibility, and increased resistance to buckling. Indirect forces are applied laterally by pads, flanges, or slings, thus providing lateral and rotational correction (Kehl & Morrissy, 1988; Renshaw, 1985).

The indication for orthotic use depends on curve type, magnitude, and location. Indications for orthotic management for children with idiopathic scoliosis are skeletal immaturity, a documented progressive curve of 20 to 29° or a curve at presentation of 30 to 40°, curve flexibility, and patient compliance (Green, 1986; Renshaw, 1985). A progressive curve is one that has increased at least 5° since detection. Rigid congenital curves do not respond well to orthotics, but an orthosis may be used to control compensatory, flexible curves resulting from a congenital anomaly in another part of the spine (Renshaw, 1985; Winter, 1988).

A Milwaukee brace or cervical-thoracic-lumbar-sacral orthosis (CTLSO) best treats a curve with an apex of T8 or above. A CTLSO consists of a pelvic girdle, a throat mold, and a metal suprastructure. Axillary slings, shoulder flange, and pads provide lateral or horizontal corrective forces giving three-point axially directed pressure. The Milwaukee brace was the only spinal orthosis available until the 1970s when the Boston bracing system was developed (Kehl & Morrissy, 1988; Renshaw, 1985).

The Boston system was designed to decrease costs, improve the acceptability of orthotic wear, and simplify construction (Farady, 1983). A series of 24 prefabricated polypropylene pelvic molds lined with polyethylene foam constitute the Boston system (Fig. 10–5). An orthotist molds the brace to the patient, adding lumbar pads and relief areas. The rigid shell provides a firm support, and the foam lining allows for comfort. A Boston brace is an example of a thoracolumbosacral orthosis (TLSO) and best treats a curve with an apex lower than T9 (Farady, 1983). A Boston brace may be modified by the addition of an extension on the concave side to achieve improved correction for curves with an apex at T7 to T9 (Kehl & Morrissy, 1988).

Other TLSO types include the Wilmington, Lyon, and Charleston models. A Wilmington TLSO (Fig. 10–6) is a total-contact, custom-molded orthosis that achieves maximal spinal correction by the tight contact and fit, not by pads and relief areas (Kehl & Morrissy, 1988). A Lyon orthosis is used to treat idiopathic scoliosis manifesting with thoracic hypokyphosis. A Charleston orthosis is used for idiopathic curves and worn only at night, because it is fabricated in the position of maximum side-bend

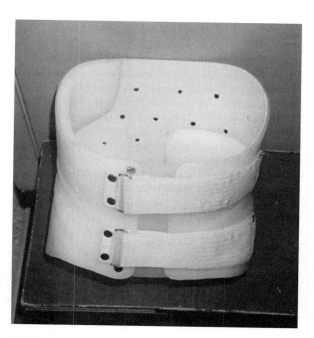

FIGURE 10–5. The Boston brace, underarm TLSO. Note pads for relief and pressure areas.

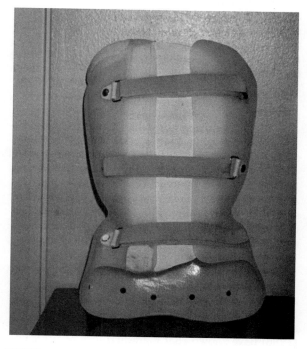

FIGURE 10–6. The Wilmington brace—a custom-molded, total-contact TLSO.

correction (Price et al., 1990). A long-term follow-up by Price and colleagues (1997) found that 65 of 98 patients showed improvement or less than 5° change in curvature and 17 patients progressed to the point of requiring surgery. These results indicate improvement of the natural history of adolescent idiopathic scoliosis and justify continued use of the Charleston brace (Price et al., 1997).

The active theory of orthotics is that curve progression is prevented by muscle contractions responding to the brace wear. A study by Wynarsky and Schultz (1989), however, showed no statistical difference between myoelectrical activity during braced and unbraced states of female patients being treated with the Boston brace for idiopathic scoliosis. The passive theory is that curve progression is prevented through the external forces of the brace on the spine.

Exercises to be performed while wearing the brace, such as pelvic tilts, thoracic flexion, and lateral shifts, are often taught to patients to improve the active forces. Studies have shown no statistical difference in curve stability between those patients who comply with orthotic wear and exercises and those who comply only with orthotic wear (Carman et al., 1985). A physical therapist's main role is to encourage physical activity of the patient (e.g., during physical education class, aerobics, dance) while wearing the orthosis to maintain balance, coordination, and strength and to develop good habits of achieving and maintaining cardiorespiratory fitness. Specific trunk exercises, such as those for unbraced scoliosis, may be taught to the patient to perform while out of the brace and are designed to maintain trunk strength and flexibility.

Orthotic treatment continues until the curve is no longer controlled (usually 40 to 45° or higher), curve progression persists, or skeletal maturity occurs, at which time weaning may begin. Twenty to twenty-six percent of orthotically treated curves will progress enough to require spinal fusion (Piazza & Basset, 1990). High-risk factors include younger age at curve detection, higher magnitude, and low Risser sign just as for untreated idiopathic scoliosis, although orthotic wear can positively influence the natural history of idiopathic scoliosis (Basset et al., 1986; Kehl & Morrissy, 1988).

The weaning process takes about 12 months from the time of skeletal maturity and consists of gradually decreasing the amount of time wearing the brace. Studies by Carr and associates (1980), Basset and colleagues (1986), and Emans and co-workers (1986) have shown that a gradual loss of curve correction occurs over 2 to 5 years following successful orthotic management. An orthotic treatment is considered successful if the curve magnitude at the end of treatment is within 5° of the magnitude at the start of treatment.

Surgical Methods

The major indication for spinal fusion is a documented progressive idiopathic curve that reaches 45° or greater. Curves greater than 40° are increasingly difficult to manage orthotically and also have significant risk of progression after skeletal maturity (Kostuik, 1990). The goals of spinal fusion are to halt the progression of the deformity to avoid the sequelae of pain and pulmonary dysfunction, achieve maximal correction in all three planes with minimal surgical risk, obtain a balanced trunk, and obtain a solid spinal arthrodesis (Drummond, 1991). The main objective of any scoliosis surgery is to obtain a solid arthrodesis because the fusion mass is ultimately what prevents further progression of the deformity (Drummond, 1991; Kostuik, 1990).

A posterior surgical approach is most often used for spinal fusion. Bone graft is packed into disk spaces and facet joints of the vertebrae after surgical exposure and preparation. The differences in posterior spinal fusions lie with the instrumentation used to obtain correction and protect the fusion. The Harrington rod system is the standard for comparison with newer instrumentation, although this system is rarely used today. The system consists of a distraction rod to the concave side and compression rod to the convex. The rods are attached to posterior spinal elements by hooks. This technique always requires postoperative immobilization of the trunk, does not allow for sagittal plane correction, and produces a flattened lumbar lordosis secondary to the distraction forces.

The Luque instrumentation consists of two L-shaped rods attached with sublaminar wiring. This system allows for load sharing because multiple segments are wired and is therefore best suited to patients with poor bone quality, anomalies of the posterior spinal elements, or poor muscle or skin quality (Drummond, 1991; Kostuik, 1990). The Luque system (Fig. 10–7) can prevent loss of lumbar lordosis and provide stabilization to the pelvis. The disadvantage is a risk of neurologic damage (Tachdjian, 1990). The Cotrel-Dubousset system (Fig. 10–8) uses two rods and compression or distraction hooks attached to either laminae or pedicles. The rods can be contoured to obtain sagittal plane correction, thus restoring lumbar lordosis and thoracic kyphosis (Drummond, 1991; Kostuik, 1990).

An anterior surgical approach includes opening of the thoracic cavity, resection of a rib, and excision through the diaphragm to expose the necessary vertebrae. To obtain correction and protect the spinal

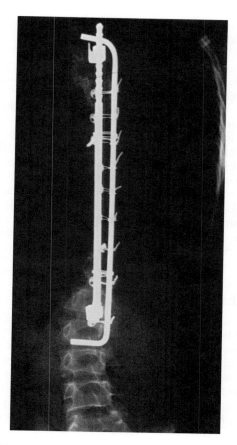

FIGURE 10–7. Radiograph of the Luque rod instrumentation system for corrective spinal surgery. Note the segmental wiring.

fusion, either Zielke or Dwyer screws are used on the vertebral bodies. Zielke screws are newer, provide control at each segment with a rod and screw, and allow for prevention of postinstrumentation kyphosis (Tachdjian, 1990). An anterior approach may be used to fuse a thoracolumbar or lumbar idiopathic scoliosis.

A two-stage procedure is used for higher-magnitude curves of severe kyphoscoliotic curves. An anterior approach is used for the release of anterior spinal ligaments, a discectomy, or a fusion with or without instrumentation. The procedure is completed by a posterior spinal fusion with instrumentation (Kostuik, 1990). Two procedures are necessary to gain range of the vertebral column for maximal correction of the curve and to provide fusion stability to prevent instrumentation failure or pseudarthrosis.

Anterior or posterior surgical approaches are used for fusion or congenital curves depending on the area of the spine where the anomaly occurs. Surgical

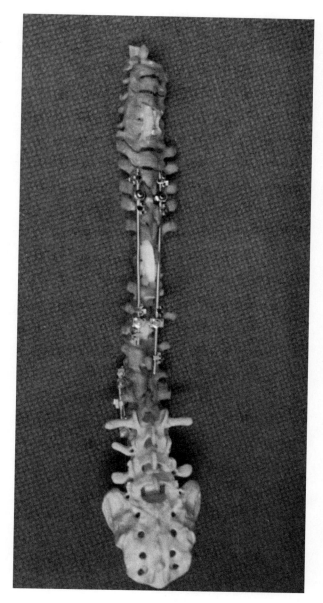

FIGURE 10–8. Cotrel-Dubousset instrumentation system implanted on a plastic spine.

methods for congenital scoliosis may include excision of the anomalous vertebrae, spinal fusion, or both. The fusion most often is performed in situ or without instrumentation on the convex side of the curve to prevent further curve progression because the goal of surgery is curve stabilization, not correction (Winter, 1983, 1988).

If a very young, skeletally immature patient has a significant curve that is not responsive to orthotic management, a procedure known as "rod without fusion" may be performed. A single, subcutaneous rod without compressive or distractive forces is placed along the scoliotic curve to control the direction of spinal growth. A fusion is not performed because this causes a cessation of growth at the fused segments of spine. An orthosis is prescribed for the patient for full-time wear to protect the instrumentation and control any decompensation of the trunk (Rothman & Simeone, 1982).

Postoperative Management

The postoperative use of an orthosis depends on the type of curve that was fused, the type of instrumentation used, and the postoperative alignment of the trunk. Nearly all congenital scoliosis curves require postoperative orthotic or plaster cast treatment to protect the in situ fusion, to promote healing or the fusion, and to help correct any compensatory curves. Idiopathic scoliotic curves managed with a two-stage procedure, Luque rods, or an anterior spinal fusion with instrumentation require orthotic use until the fusion mass is well formed as determined by radiographs. Currently, a child with idiopathic scoliosis who is treated with posterior spinal fusion and Cotrel-Dubousset instrumentation does not require postoperative bracing if the trunk is compensated and the correction is satisfactory.

The average length of a hospital stay for a posterior spinal fusion (or a one-stage procedure) is 5 to 9 days, with physical therapy initiated on the second postoperative day. A physical therapist's role following any spinal fusion procedure includes patient instruction in body mechanics for bed mobility, transfers, dressing, and ambulation. Trunk rotation is contraindicated; therefore the therapist must instruct the patient in log-rolling and in coming from a supine position to sitting without rotation. Shoes and socks are donned or removed with the legs in tailor position, with negligible forward flexion. The therapist may also instruct the patient in donning or removing of the orthosis while in bed, while from a side-lying to a supine position, or while standing with assistance (if not contraindicated by physician's orders). For the acute stage, donning or removing of the orthosis in bed is preferable. The patient is instructed in general ROM and strengthening exercises (without resistance) for the extremities such as isometric quadriceps sets, straight leg raises, supine abduction, and isometric gluteal sets. Because the patient's functional activities for the first 2 postoperative weeks are limited to showering and walking, the therapist's role is to encourage ambulation. Not only does this enable the patient to experience fewer side effects from bed rest, but it is also beneficial to the development of a strong, healthy fusion mass or arthrodesis.

On discharge from the hospital, the patient's postoperative activity remains restricted. In 1 month, the patient usually returns to school and can lift objects up to 5 pounds. At 3 months following surgery, bicycling, driving, swimming, and light jogging are allowed. The patient is able to lift objects weighing up to 10 pounds and also participate in noncontact sports (with physician approval) by 6 months postoperatively. By 1 year the patient may be involved in routine physical education classes, may lift more than 10 pounds, and may be active in other activities, such as skating, skiing, bowling, and amusement park rides. These guidelines are appropriate for the majority of patients with fusion of congenital and idiopathic curves regardless of which instrumentation is used.

Adults and Scoliosis

Two long-term longitudinal studies have been completed on scoliosis into adulthood. The first (Nachemson, 1968) reviewed 130 patients with untreated scoliosis of all types. Ninety percent (117 patients) were followed for 35 years. The results showed an overall mortality rate of twice the norm, with the group that had thoracic curves having a rate of four times the norm. There was an increase in death or disability at age 40, with 80% of the causes being cardiorespiratory conditions. The results also included the presence of back pain in 39 of 97 surviving patients.

In the second study, Nilsonne and Lundgren (1968) investigated 117 patients with idiopathic scoliosis with a maximal follow-up time of 50 years. The results showed a mortality rate 2.2 times higher than that of a control group. Pulmonary or cardiac failure was the cause of death in 60% of the scoliotic group, and 50% of the surviving scoliotic group were unable to work secondary to disabling symptoms. This study also reported that 70% of the female patients did not marry, perhaps because of cosmetic concerns.

The natural history of idiopathic scoliosis continues into adult life, because curves can progress after skeletal maturity. Risk of progression depends on curve magnitude and location (Lonstein & Winter, 1988). Curves of greater than 45° at the time of skeletal maturity have a higher risk of progressing and producing complications. Although thoracic and lumbar curves can both progress, progression in the thoracic region causes significant complications because of the effects on the heart and lungs. Complications of untreated scoliosis include severe cosmetic deformity and major disability, which may include pain, respiratory insufficiency, or right-sided heart failure (Rothman & Simeone, 1982). Considerations for adult treatment include back pain, compromised pulmonary function, psychosocial effects, and increased risk for premature death. The treatment plan is consistent with that for adolescent idiopathic scoliosis (Weinstein, 1989).

Neuromuscular Scoliosis

The terms *neuromuscular scoliosis* and *myopathic scoliosis* describe curves that are due to neurologic or muscular disorders (Raimondi et al., 1989). The curve presentation and risk of progression of neuromuscular scoliosis differ from idiopathic or congenital curves in some cases. Curves may be secondary to pelvic obliquity (Lonstein & Renshaw, 1987), unilateral or asymmetric spasticity of trunk musculature, athetosis, or asymmetric movement patterns (Tachdjian, 1990). Often a long "C-type" curve characterizes a neuromuscular curvature, but as compensatory curves become structural the pattern may change to an "S-type" curve (Fig. 10–9). A neuromuscular curve typically develops at a young age and tends to be progressive (Fisk & Bunch, 1979). The prevalence of spinal deformities varies with the type of neuromuscular disease.

The highest prevalence of spinal deformities (90–100%) occurs with a dystrophy diagnosis, such as spinal muscular atrophy or muscular dystrophy, and in spinal cord injuries that result in quadriplegia in infants or young children. There is a 60% prevalence of spinal deformity in patients with myelomeningocele and a 25% prevalence in patients with cerebral palsy (Lonstein & Renshaw, 1987).

Etiology and Risk Of Progression

The direct cause of neuromuscular scoliosis is unknown. One hypothesis is that spinal stability, which is directly proportional to the condition of the end support of the spine and inversely proportional to spinal flexibility and to the approximate square of spinal column length, is reduced in children with neuromuscular disease. Loss of muscle strength and loss of proprioception may also be factors in the development of scoliosis when it occurs in the relatively flexible and elongating spinal column of a child with a neuromuscular disease (Lonstein & Renshaw, 1987).

Treatment

Nonsurgical treatment of neuromuscular spinal curvatures includes clinical observation, radiograph examination, and orthotic management. Clinical ob-

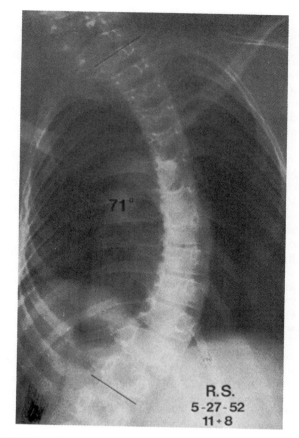

FIGURE 10–9. Severe neuromuscular scoliosis. (From Moe, JH, Winter, RB, Bradford, DS, Ogilvie, JW, & Lonstein, JE. Scoliosis and Other Spinal Deformities, 2nd ed. Philadelphia: WB Saunders, 1987, p. 277.)

servation allows thorough assessment of the child's present and potential function, level of comprehension, and ability to cooperate (Fisk & Bunch, 1979). Although no research studies have shown that custom seating is effective in reducing or preventing progression of curves, it is an important part of clinical treatment in which the physical therapist plays a vital role. A good postural support system allows the child to interact with the environment. These children often have multiple disabilities, which are best addressed by the team approach of a physical therapist, an occupational therapist, a physician, an equipment vendor, and an orthotist. Chapter 24 discusses seating options appropriate for this population.

The child with a neuromuscular curvature managed by orthotics has special needs that must be considered when ordering or fabricating seating systems. The orthosis eliminates the normal flexibility of the spine, which potentially reduces the child's ability to adjust the footrests, operate the brakes, and propel the chair. A child with a neuromuscular curve may demonstrate pelvic obliquity requiring specialized custom-molded seating to provide adequate support and pressure relief. Because these children may require lower extremity orthotics, adequate clearance in the seating device is necessary to accommodate orthoses.

Orthotic management might include the custom-molded, total-contact TLSO, underarm TLSO, or Milwaukee brace (Lonstein & Renshaw, 1987). The orthosis is worn during all upright (i.e., sitting or standing) activities and is usually not worn at night.

The use of an orthosis must provide curve stabilization without limiting the child's functional abilities. For example, attempting to control the lordosis in an ambulating child with muscular dystrophy would eliminate compensatory functional posture and result in earlier use of a wheelchair. An orthosis may be used before any measurable deformity is present to support the trunk. For example, a young child with spinal muscular atrophy may be fitted with a TLSO that has the anterior rib portion relieved and covered with elastic material to provide support for use during therapy, during feeding, and while standing in a standing frame. The use of a TLSO can improve head and upper extremity control. An orthosis should also be used to maintain alignment and provide trunk support for children with quadriplegic paralysis secondary to birth injuries or acquired spinal cord injuries. In these children, the use of an orthosis allows for upright orientation and may provide the support necessary for the child to operate a head switch or sip-and-puff mechanism to control an electric wheelchair.

An experimental method, just beginning to be researched, is the use of botulinum toxin type A in the treatment of neuromuscular curves in patients with other severe complicating diseases that have caused delays in surgery. Nuzzo and colleagues (1997) treated 12 children with botulinum type A, as a supplement other desirable treatment methods. Short-term results revealed no worsened scoliosis. All children had some degree of curve reduction, with some reduction as much as 50°.

If a neuromuscular scoliosis continues to progress, hygiene, nursing care, functional abilities, pulmonary function, and life expectancy may be affected. Once again, a team approach is preferred for optimal management of children with neuromuscular disease.

Surgical Options

Surgical methods for neuromuscular scoliosis are similar to those for idiopathic scoliosis. The curve may require both anterior and posterior fusion with instrumentation, posterior fusion with instrumentation, or fusion to the pelvis to correct obliquity and maintain symmetry. The goal of surgery is to achieve a stable and compensated spine.

An orthosis is always used postoperatively for support and immobilization of the fusion. Occasionally the patient may be placed in a body cast (Risser cast) in the operating room to protect against potential sheer stresses before the fabrication of a custom orthosis (Fisk & Bunch, 1979). The orthosis must be on the patient before initiation of out-of-bed mobility, unless otherwise specified by the physician.

The role of the physical therapist is similar to that for postoperative treatment of other curve types. The treatment may need to be modified to adjust to a patient's motor and cognitive abilities.

KYPHOSIS

A *kyphosis* is an abnormal posterior convexity of a segment of the spine. A spinal kyphosis may occur as a result of trauma, congenital conditions, or Scheuermann's disease or secondary to previous treatment of spinal tumors with laminectomy. Spinal kyphosis may also be found in children with osteochondrodystrophies, rickets, osteogenic imperfecta, idiopathic juvenile osteoporosis, neurofibromatosis, myelomeningocele, and spondyloepiphyseal dysplasia. Spinal kyphosis should be differentiated from postural roundback (Rothman & Simeone, 1982; Winter et al., 1973). The discussion in this section focuses on congenital kyphosis, Scheuermann's disease, and kyphosis in children with myelomeningocele.

Congenital Kyphosis

Congenital kyphosis results when the anterior part of the vertebra is aplastic or hypoplastic and posterior elements form normally. An anterior unsegmented failure of formation, or unsegmented bar, leads to progressive kyphosis. Congenital kyphoscoliosis or lordoscoliosis is the result when a combination of defective segmentation occurs at more than one location (Winter, 1983, 1988).

The natural history of congenital kyphosis includes progression, cosmetic deformity, back pain, and neurologic deficit. Congenital kyphosis is the most common cause of spinal cord compression caused by a spinal deformity (Winter et al., 1973). It is a potentially more debilitating deformity than congenital scoliosis without kyphosis. An anterior unsegmented bar at the thoracolumbar junction produces mild to moderate deformities but no reported paraplegia. Paraplegia is frequently noted with a progressive congenital kyphosis located in the upper thoracic spine when the posterior elements grow unaccompanied by anterior growth. The treatment of congenital kyphosis is surgery to prevent further progression (Winter, 1983).

Scheuermann's Disease

Scheuermann's disease is an often neglected deformity that develops during childhood and adolescence and is usually ascribed to poor posture. Diagnosis is made by these radiographic criteria: (1) irregular vertebral end-plates, (2) narrowing of the intervertebral disk space, (3) anterior wedging of 5° or greater of one or more vertebrae, and (4) kyphosis greater than 40° that is uncorrected on active hyperextension. Scheuermann's disease can be found in the thoracic spine, producing an increased kyphosis; in the thoracolumbar and lumbar spine, producing a neutral appearance in the sagittal plane; and, more rarely, in the cervical spine (Rothman & Simeone, 1982).

Little has been published on the pathophysiology of Scheuermann's disease. Cadaver dissections show that the anterior longitudinal ligament is thickened and taut as in other kyphoses and that the vertebral bodies are wedged and the disk spaces narrowed. The spongiosa and bone are irregular and can show disruption where Schmorl's nodules have fractured the bony tubercle. Growth plates are disorderly as a result of this disruption (Rothman & Simeone, 1982; Tachdjian, 1990).

Clinical findings include tight pectorals and hamstrings. An increased thoracic kyphosis with a compensatory increased lumbar lordosis and forward head posture are seen. Associated scoliosis is present in 30 to 40% of children with Scheuermann's disease. The disease has also been reported to be transmitted as an autosomal dominant trait with an incidence of 0.4 to 8.3%. Males and females are affected equally. Radiographic findings are often not seen until age 11 (Tachdjian, 1990). The chief complaint of patients is pain at the apex of the kyphosis.

Treatment

Treatment of Scheuermann's disease includes exercise, orthotic management, and surgical management. The prescribed exercises are specific for active trunk extensor strengthening, passive trunk stretching into extension, and general postural exercise (abdominals and gluteals). The child must be instructed to extend at the kyphotic section of the spine (usually thoracic) while maintaining a neutral or slightly flexed cervical and lumbar spine. Exercises addressing abdominal strengthening, especially of lower abdominals, are important to help maintain an upright posture and decrease lumbar lordosis. A patient may have hip flexion contractures from increased lumbar lordosis and increased anterior pelvic tilt, and limited hamstring length as measured by straight leg raising due to kyphotic and crouched posture in sitting and standing position. Stretching exercises are incorporated to improve overall alignment (Fig. 10–10). Exercise as the sole treatment has not been established as effective, although it has been shown to be beneficial in conjunction with other methods of treatment (Moe et al., 1987; Tachdjian, 1990).

Orthotic treatment is used when the kyphosis is greater than 50 to 60°. The use of a modified Milwaukee-type brace has a high reported success rate in the skeletally immature patient. The procedure is considered to be successful when the kyphosis decreases and vertebral bodies appear less wedge shaped on radiographs (Moe et al., 1987).

Surgical management is often a two-stage procedure, with anterior discectomy and intravertebral

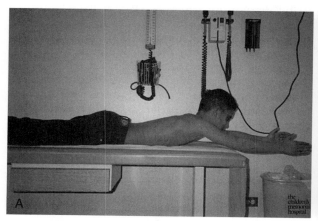 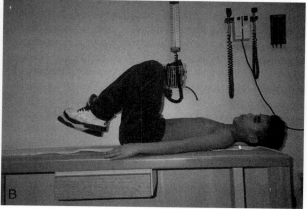

FIGURE 10–10. *A,* Active trunk extensor strengthening by prone lifts. *B,* Lower abdominal strengthening exercises.

grafting coupled with a posterior compression arthrodesis. Posterior fusion alone in a child with a fixed kyphosis greater than 60° may be subject to significant complications and loss of correction of kyphosis with instrumentation failure (Rothman & Simeone, 1982).

Postoperative treatment includes plaster casting, orthotic wear, or both. The orthotic of choice is usually a Milwaukee-type brace that may be modified to a TLSO after a 2- to 5-month postoperative period.

Postural Roundback

Postural roundback may often be confused with Scheuermann's disease; however, the kyphosis of postural roundback is not fixed and vertebrae show no end-plate irregularity. Exercise alone, as described for treatment of Scheuermann's disease, is the treatment of choice for this condition. If the kyphosis progresses to more than 60°, it may be treated with a Milwaukee brace to prevent permanent structural changes (Moe et al., 1987).

Kyphosis and Myelomeningocele

Spinal deformities are common in children with myelomeningocele. A congenital lumbar kyphosis, involving the portion of spine from the thoracolumbar junction to the sacrum, is unique to children with myelomeningocele.

Congenital kyphosis is easily recognized at birth because it is rigid and resistant to passive correction. Anatomically the pedicles are widely separated and protrude posterolaterally, accentuating the kyphotic appearance. The pedicles and laminae are splayed, pushing the deep back muscles to an anterior position. These deep back muscles may then serve as pathologic flexors of the lumbar spine. Often, owing to the level of deficit, the psoas muscle is the only innervated muscle. The force of the psoas, coupled with activity in the quadratus lumborum and anterior abdominals, may cause progressive deformity (Rothman & Simeone, 1982).

The congenital kyphosis may produce closure problems, caused by size and rigidity of the lesion. Orthopedic surgery, a kyphectomy or spinal osteotomy, may be done at the time of closure to help facilitate the procedure (Sharrad, 1968). Recurrent skin breakdown problems are common; therefore, special attention must be given to the use of adaptive equipment.

The kyphosis usually remains relatively stable until the child sits, using the hands for support. The child's sitting posture is marked by a forward trunk and sacral or lumbar sitting, instead of ischial weight bearing, and there may be a compensatory thoracic

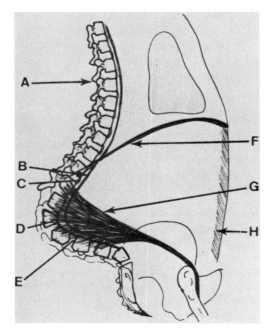

FIGURE 10–11. Drawing illustrating the deforming forces found in congenital lumbar kyphosis. *A,* Compensatory dorsal lordosis. *B,* Contracted anterior longitudinal ligament. *C,* Contracted anulus fibrosus. *D,* Wedge-shaped vertebral bodies. *E,* Intervertebral disks narrowed anteriorly with the nucleus pulposus shifted posteriorly. *F,* Diaphragm attached to the apex of the deformity. *G,* Psoas muscle is hypertrophied and bowstrings across the curve. *H,* Anterior abdominal musculature. (From Rothman, RH, & Simeone, FA. The Spine, 2nd ed. Philadelphia: WB Saunders, 1982, p. 252.)

lordosis. These children often develop respiratory complications when the anterior rib cage lies on the pelvic brim, causing the abdominal contents to be forced against the diaphragm, restricting excursion and respiratory function (Rothman & Simeone, 1982) (Figs. 10–11 and 10–12).

Treatment

Treatment of congenital kyphosis in children with myelomeningocele is limited. Bracing and stretching exercises are of no use because of the rigidity of the deformity and potential for skin breakdown. Exercises are useful in maintaining good range of motion at the hips and shoulders. The surgical procedure, a kyphectomy, is controversial and may produce only limited correction. The procedure requires further research.

Postoperative treatment may include plaster casting or orthotic treatment to protect the fusion.

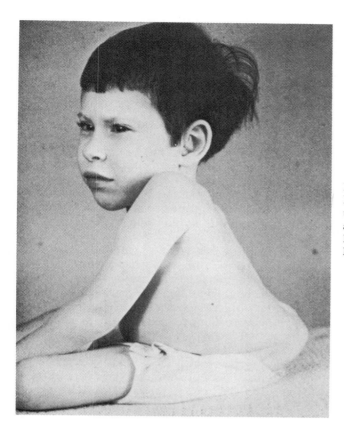

FIGURE 10–12. Nine-year-old with a congenital lumbar kyphosis. Typical sitting posture serves to accentuate the kyphosis. The child is sitting directly on the sacrum and the lower portion of the lumbar spine. (From Rothman, RH, & Simeone, FA. The Spine, 2nd ed. Philadelphia: WB Saunders, 1982, p. 252.)

Physical therapy is often involved to maximize endurance and mobility, as outlined in the section on surgery for idiopathic scoliosis.

LORDOSIS

An anterior convexity (or a posterior concavity) of a segment of spine is termed a *lordosis*. Congenital lordosis is the result of bilateral posterior failure of segmentation (Winter, 1983). Lordosis, both fixed and flexible, may be found in children with a variety of diagnoses. Lordosis in children with myelomeningocele usually occurs in the lumbar spine secondary to use of a tripod gait pattern. A lordosis may develop in the thoracic vertebrae to compensate for an increased lumbar kyphosis (Rothman & Simeone, 1982).

Children without motor deficits may have an increased lumbar lordosis. Assessment includes testing of lower extremity ROM, spinal flexibility, trunk and lower extremity strength, posture, and gait. Treatment includes abdominal strengthening (curls, crunches, and pelvic lifts), pelvic tilts in a supine position and standing, trunk extensor strengthening, and appropriate lower extremity stretching.

Spondylolisthesis

Spondylolisthesis is the forward translatory displacement of one vertebra on another, usually occurring at the fifth lumbar vertebra. Five types of spondylolysis and spondylolisthesis are classified by Wiltse and associates (1976):

1. *Dysplastic,* developing secondary to congenital malformations of the sacrum and posterior vertebral arch of L5. These malformations may include hypoplasia of the superior surface of the body of S1, hypoplasia-aplasia of the facets, elongation of the pars interarticularis, and spina bifida. The malformations decrease the efficiency of the posterior stabilizing system (Wiltse et al., 1976). The degree of slippage is usually severe and may produce neurologic deficits as the laminae of L5 are pulled against the dural sac (Tachdjian, 1990).

2. *Isthmic* describes slippage occurring secondary to an elongation of the pars interarticularis, a break

of the pars interarticularis, or a combination of both with the facets intact. A stress or fatigue fracture of the pars interarticularis is the basic pathologic occurrence. These pathogenic factors can cause elongation of the pars secondary to repeated microfractures that heal with the pars in an attenuated-elongated position. An isthmic spondylolisthesis may also be caused by an acute fracture of the pars (Tachdjian, 1990).

3. A *degenerative* type occurs in adults older than age 50 years and is caused by the structural destruction of the capsule and ligaments of the posterior joints producing hypermobility of the segment.

4. A *traumatic* type, more correctly defined as a fracture, is caused by a sudden fracture of the posterior arch of a vertebral segment. The fracture may occur at the pedicle, laminae, or facet, leaving the pars interarticularis intact.

5. *Pathologic* spondylolisthesis occurs most often secondary to an infectious disease that destroys the posterior arch of the vertebra (Wiltse et al., 1976).

Dysplastic and isthmic spondylolisthesis types are the most common in the pediatric population. Spondylolisthesis is further described by degree of severity as described by percentage of slippage, grades I to IV. Grade I is the mildest slippage at less than 25%. Grade II is 25 to 50% slippage. Grade III is 50 to 75%, and grade IV is greater than 75% slippage (Tachdjian, 1990; Wiltse et al., 1976).

Clinical Symptoms

A spondylolisthesis is often discovered on a radiograph taken for some other purpose. The clinical picture includes poor posture and increased lumbar lordosis in mild slippage. Higher-grade slippage may produce a flattened lumbar spine, a crease anteriorly at the umbilicus, and a prominent sacrum (Fig. 10–13). Symptoms may include low back pain relieved by rest, sciatic-type pain, local tenderness, hamstring spasm or tightness, and, in severe cases, torso shortening (Tachdjian, 1990).

Risk of Progression

The risk factors, clinically and radiographically, are similar to those for idiopathic scoliosis. Clinically, adolescents who are symptomatic are at a higher risk for increased slippage during their growth spurt. Females are at a greater risk than males, as are patients with increased ligament laxity, as in Down syndrome or Marfan syndrome. Radiographically, dysplastic types or patients with a 50% slippage, with a slip angle over 40 to 50°, or with bony instabilities or decreased anatomic stability of L5 and S1 are at greater risk for increased slippage (Moe et al., 1987; Tachdjian, 1990).

Nonsurgical Treatment

Observation is the treatment of choice, with asymptomatic spondylolisthesis causing less than 50% slippage. These children are routinely followed two times per year with clinical and radiographic examinations. Normal activities are allowed if the degree of slippage is less than 25%. Activities such as weight lifting and contact sports are restricted in patients with a slippage greater than 25%. Patients also learn lumbar stabilization exercises in which they are taught to maintain pain-free, neutral alignment of the pelvis and lumbar spine while they vary their positions. Exercises include bridging, wall squats, abdominal strengthening, prone gluteal strengthening, and supine exercises. A therapeutic exercise ball may be incorporated into the exercise session to allow patients to achieve and maintain neutral lumbar spine stabilization on a mobile surface.

A lumbosacral orthosis is used to manage the symptomatic patient with a slippage percentage of less than 25%. This treatment form is initially also used to conservatively treat patients with a slippage of 25 to 50%. If symptoms persist, surgery is indicated.

Surgical Treatment

The indications for surgery are persistent back pain despite conservative measures including physical therapy, greater than 50% slippage and associated gait deviations unresponsive to physical therapy, marked instability of the defect with slip progression, neurologic deficit, and persistent sciatic symptoms unresponsive to conservative measures (Tachdjian, 1990). The goals of surgery are to prevent further slippage, immobilize the unstable segment, prevent further neurologic deficit and relieve any nerve root irritation, and correct clinical symptoms of poor posture, gait, and decreased hamstring length (Tachdjian, 1990).

The surgical procedure most often performed is a posterolateral alar transverse process fusion. The fusion usually extends to L4 and is performed with an iliac bone graft. The patients are immobilized in a TLSO brace with a thigh extension for 6 weeks to 3 months and then in a TLSO until the fusion is solid (VanRens & VanHorn, 1982; Verbeist, 1979). Physical therapy is indicated for bed mobility, gait training, and activities of daily living and may be initiated to regain normal hamstring flexibility.

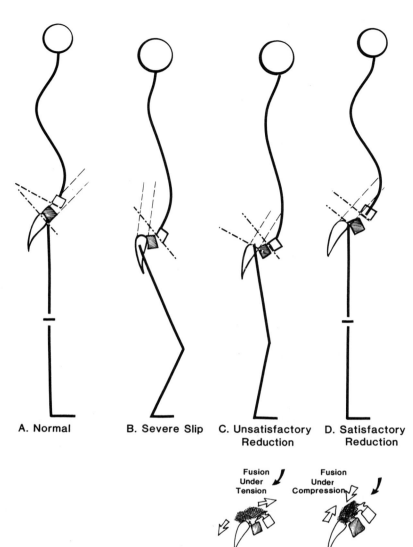

A. Normal   B. Severe Slip   C. Unsatisfactory Reduction   D. Satisfactory Reduction

Fusion Under Tension   Fusion Under Compression

E

FIGURE 10–13. *A,* Normal sagittal plane spinal alignment. *B,* Loss of alignment can be visualized following a severe L5 spondylolisthesis. The sacrum becomes vertical, and the resultant lumbosacral kyphosis "pushes" the lumbar spine forward. *C,* An unsatisfactory reduction occurs when L5 has little mobility and L4 lies anterior to the "anatomic zone" and is kyphotic in relationship to the sacrum. The fusion in this case will be under tension and less likely to hold. *D,* A satisfactory reduction occurs when L4 can be placed in the anatomic zone and oriented lordotic in relation to the sacrum. *E,* The more L4 can be positioned over the sacrum, the more posterior compressive forces will be directed across the fusion. In this position, sagittal plane alignment and hence deformity will be corrected. (From Moe, JH, Winter, RB, Bradford, DS, Ogilvie, JW, & Lonstein, JE. Scoliosis and Other Spinal Deformities, 2nd ed. Philadelphia: WB Saunders, 1987, p. 418.)

In severe cases associated with significant neurologic deficit, a decompression and posterior fusion procedure is indicated. A decompression consists of removal of the bony anatomy that is causing nerve root irritation. The segments are then fused posteriorly to prevent further slippage (VanRens & VanHorn, 1982; Verbeist, 1979). Anterior fusions have been performed with good results (Freebody, 1962); a posterior fusion is usually preferred, however, because it is less hazardous.

A reduction of the spondylolisthesis is indicated in cases in which the sacrum is in a vertical position causing a severe lumbosacral kyphosis that displaces the lumbar spine anteriorly (see Fig. 10–13). The result is a marked compensatory lumbar lordosis. A reduction of the slippage is followed by posterior fusion, anterior fusion, or a combination of surgical approaches.

SUMMARY

Scoliosis, kyphosis, and lordosis are common pediatric orthopedic conditions of the spine. We, as pediatric physical therapists, often concentrate our therapy for many types of patients on the trunk for midline activities, symmetry, and stability for movement, and therefore we can play a vital role in early detection of spinal deformities.

We encourage children to become active to allow for improved cardiorespiratory function, muscle strength, and endurance. We can provide a referral source for families, instruction in home exercises, input for selecting appropriate adaptive equipment and seating, and rehabilitative treatment following injury or surgery. We address issues concerning the spine on a daily basis and play an important role in achieving and maintaining good health through maximizing proper alignment and function.

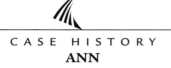

CASE HISTORY
ANN

Examination

Ann, a 15-year-old girl with a diagnosis of idiopathic scoliosis (curves measuring 45° right thoracic and 42° left lumbar), was referred to physical therapy for assessment and treatment. Ann wished to increase her participation in extracurricular activities and improve her overall physical endurance. Ann wore a Lyon-type TLSO full-time and knew that she would require a posterior spinal fusion in the future. The examination included testing of (1) lower extremity ROM; (2) lower extremity strength by manual muscle test; (3) trunk strength; (4) trunk flexibility; (5) trunk symmetry, including levels of bony prominences (i.e., iliac crest, inferior border of scapulae); (6) activity level; (7) posture; and (8) gait.

Evaluation

The evaluation of the test findings revealed decreased trunk flexibility in all planes (forward flexion by one half, lateral flexion by one third, and extension by one fourth) and limited hamstring length (145° popliteal angle bilaterally). Cosmetically, she was well compensated in her trunk with curves of essentially equal magnitude. No formal cardiopulmonary testing was performed; however, by patient history, Ann was unable to walk more than 15 to 20 minutes without fatigue.

Diagnosis

Ann had general deconditioning of the cardiopulmonary and musculoskeletal systems. Impairments included primary anatomic changes of the vertebrae and surrounding structures; decreased spinal, trunk, and lower extremity ROM secondary to full-time orthotic wear; decreased trunk strength secondary to inactivity; and decreased endurance secondary to limited activity caused by orthotic wear. Because physical therapy cannot change the underlying pathophysiology of the spine in scoliosis, the impairments of trunk strength, decreased flexibility, and decreased cardiopulmonary endurance were addressed.

Prognosis and plan of care

Physical therapy intervention was recommended for a short duration. Outcomes and goals were set to address improvement in trunk flexibility, increased cardiopulmonary fitness, and improved participation in extracurricular activities.

Intervention

The primary intervention in this case was patient-related instruction. Ann was instructed in proper body mechanics to adjust to limited trunk mobility and in trunk strengthening and flexibility exercises to be performed daily when not wearing the orthosis. The exercises (knees to chest, pelvic tilts, four-point trunk extensor strengthening, curl-ups, oblique curl-ups, lateral flexion, and trunk shift) were specifically designed to address trunk flexion, trunk rotation, abdominal strength, and trunk extensor–hip extensor strength while avoiding hyperextension of the spine. Her physical therapy also addressed her cardiorespiratory status. She was started on a daily walk-run program with a goal of 45 minutes three to five times per week. She also rode a stationary bicycle for 20 to 30 minutes during each treatment session.

In most instances, Ann was allowed to participate in noncontact, organized sports activities. The physical therapist encouraged wearing the orthosis when possible during these activities. The physical therapist also played an important role in helping Ann understand the importance of maintaining flexibility and strength in preparation for a faster recovery following her anticipated posterior spinal fusion.

A checklist system was used to follow Ann's compliance with home exercises and orthotic wear. After initial sessions for evaluation and teaching of a home program, Ann was followed in the clinic at regular intervals (6 to 8 weeks) to reevaluate strength, flexibility, and ROM as additional indicators of compliance.

Ann was very compliant with her flexibility and strengthening exercises. Her hamstring length improved to normal as measured by straight leg raise, her forward flexion was limited by one third, and she played on her school's basketball team. She was discharged from therapy after 3 months because she was continuing with a home program. She will undergo a posterior spinal fusion with Cotrel-Dubousset instrumentation in the future.

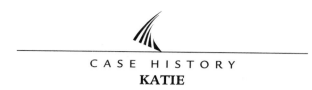

CASE HISTORY
KATIE

Examination

Katie, a 14-year-old girl with a diagnosis of athetoid cerebral palsy and a scoliosis measuring 54° (right thoracolumbar) out of brace and 42° in brace (custom-molded TLSO), was seen in a scoliosis clinic.

Katie received physical therapy twice weekly at her home. Her highest level of function was limited household ambulation. She is a potential surgical candidate.

The physical therapy examination included testing of (1) posture in prone, supine, sitting, and standing positions; (2) lower extremity ROM; (3) lower extremity manual muscle strength, including cortical control and in-pattern grades; (4) balance in sitting and standing positions; (5) tone; and (6) primitive reflexes.

Evaluation

Findings included bilateral hip flexion contracture of 15°; poor voluntary control of distal lower extremity musculature; ability to move from sitting to standing with minimal to moderate assistance by one person; athetoid/fluctuating tone; and present, but not obligatory, right asymmetric tonic neck reflex. Katie's disabilities and functional limitations included (1) inability to perform independent self-care owing to decreased balance; (2) inability to efficiently propel her manual wheelchair owing to orthotic wear; and (3) inability to independently obtain and maintain proper postural alignment of the trunk because of the influence of primitive reflexes, trunk weakness, abnormal tone, and decreased proprioception.

Diagnosis

Katie had limitations of her neuromuscular systems. Impairments included (1) primary anatomic changes in the vertebrae, supporting structures, and musculature of the trunk; (2) decreased midline orientation abilities due to spinal deformity and cerebral palsy; (3) decreased spinal mobility due to orthotic wear; and (4) decreased ability to use compensations of the trunk during household ambulation due to orthotic restrictions.

Prognosis and plan of care

It was determined that intensive physical therapy services for a short duration would be indicated to address functional outcomes. Physical therapy was used to address (1) assisted training in activities of daily living, (2) independent mobility with wheel-chair modifications or change to an electric device, (3) balance, (4) endurance for facilitated ambulation, and (5) postural alignment and midline orientation in all positions.

Intervention

Physical therapy was used to address impairment through services two to three times per week, emphasizing trunk strengthening (abdominals, gluteals, extensors), active-assistive ROM of bilateral lower extremities, and facilitated weight bearing and ambulation to improve endurance and function. Over 4 months, she progressed to require only minimal assistance for household ambulation.

The physical therapist plays a role in determining function, the effect of an orthosis on function, and the potential effect of surgical fusion on the child's function. To accomplish these objectives it is necessary to maintain verbal or written contact regarding the child's progress or regression with the child's orthopedic physician. In this particular case, surgery was postponed because the child was making improvements in independent household ambulation. Katie is expected to require surgery in the future, but her improved endurance and independence will give her an advantage for the procedure itself, as well as for recovery time.

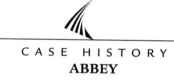

CASE HISTORY
ABBEY

Examination

Abbey, a 12-year-old girl with a diagnosis of grade III spondylolisthesis, was seen in a scoliosis clinic. A posture assessment, as well as ROM assessment, was completed.

Evaluation

Her clinical examination revealed (1) tight hamstrings with decreased ROM to 40° as measured by straight leg raising; (2) antalgic, crouch-type gait; (3) anterior abdominal crease at the level of the umbilicus; and (4) posterior pelvic tilt with prominent "heart-shaped" sacrum due to spasticity of the hamstrings because of nerve root irritation. Surgery was recommended for reduction of the spondylolisthesis coupled with a fusion. Postoperatively this child wore a TLSO for immobilization.

Diagnosis and prognosis

Her pathophysiologic features included (1) primary anatomic changes of the vertebrae and surrounding structures, (2) neurologic changes of the lower extremities secondary to nerve rootlet pressure caused by the primary slippage of the vertebrae, and (3) potential for permanent neurologic changes of lower extremities and bowel and bladder if no intervention occurred. The associated impairments and functional limitations expected if there was no surgical intervention include (1) low back pain; (2) potential for decreased lower extremity function due to neurologic changes; (3) altered gait; and (4) altered alignment of spine and pelvis causing difficulties with clothing, sitting for long periods of time, and endurance. After surgery, functional limitations included decreased trunk strength and limited participation in extracurricular activities.

Intervention

Physical therapy included hamstring stretching, body mechanics instruction, and gait reeducation. Physical therapy addressed the postsurgical issues through rehabilitation exercises once the fusion was stable. The child participated in pool activities, lumbar stabilization activities using the Swiss ball, and cardiovascular endurance activities after permission from her orthopedic surgeon. Proper surgical management and rehabilitation can allow the child to return to pain-free function.

References

Basset, GS, Burness, WP, & MacEwen, GD. Treatment of scoliosis with a Wilmington brace: Results in patients with 20-29 degree curves. Journal of Bone and Joint Surgery (American), 68:602-605, 1986.

Bertrand, SL, Drvaric, DM, Lange, N, Lucas, PR, Deutsch, SD, Herdon, JH, & Roberts, JM. Electrical stimulation for idiopathic scoliosis. Clinical Orthopedics and Related Research, 276:176-181, 1992.

Bleck, E. Annotation—Adolescent idiopathic scoliosis. Developmental Medicine and Child Neurology, 33:167-176, 1991.

Brown, JC, Axelgaard, J, & Howson, DC. Multicenter trial of a non-invasive stimulation method for idiopathic scoliosis: A summary of early treatment results. Spine, 9:382-387, 1984.

Byl, NN, & Gray, JM. Complex balance reactions in different sensory conditions: Adolescents with and without idiopathic scoliosis. Journal of Orthopaedic Research, 11:215-227, 1993.

Bylund, P, Aaro, S, Gottfries, B, & Jansson, E. Is lateral electric surface stimulation an effective treatment for scoliosis? Journal of Pediatric Orthopedics, 7:298-300, 1987.

Calvo, JJ. Observations on the growth of the female adolescent spine and its relationship to scoliosis. Clinical Orthopedics, 10:40, 1957.

Carman, D, Roach, JW, Speck, G, Wenger, DR, & Herring, JA. Role of exercises in the Milwaukee brace treatment of scoliosis. Journal of Pediatric Orthopedics, 11:65-68, 1985.

Carr, WA, Moe, JH, & Winter, RB. Treatment of idiopathic scoliosis in the Milwaukee brace, long term results. Journal of Bone and Joint Surgery (American), 62:8-15, 1980.

Cowell, HR, Hall, JN, & MacEwen, GD. Genetic aspects of idiopathic scoliosis. Clinical Orthopedics, 86:121-132, 1972.

Dickson, RA, Lawton, JD, Archer, JA, & Butt, WP. The pathogenesis of idiopathic scoliosis. Journal of Bone and Joint Surgery (British), 66:8-15, 1984.

Drummond, DS. A perspective on recent trends for scoliosis correction. Clinical Orthopedics and Related Research, 264:90-102, 1991.

Duval-Beaupere, G. The growth of scoliosis patients: Hypothesis and preliminary study. Acta Orthopaedica Belgica, 38:365-376, 1972.

Eckerson, LF, & Axelgaard, J. Lateral electrical surface stimulation as an alternative to bracing in the treatment of idiopathic scoliosis: Treatment protocol and patient acceptance. Physical Therapy, 64:483-490, 1984.

Emans, JB, Kaelin, A, Bancel, P, Hall, JE, & Miller, ME. The Boston bracing system for idiopathic scoliosis: Follow-up results in 295 patients. Spine, 11:792-801, 1986.

Farady, JA. Current principles in the non-operative management of structural adolescent idiopathic scoliosis. Physical Therapy, 63:512-523, 1983.

Fisk, JR, & Bunch, WH. Scoliosis in neuromuscular disease. Orthopedic Clinics of North America, 10(4):863-875, 1979.

Freebody, D. Lumbosacral fusion by the transperitoneal approach. Journal of Bone and Joint Surgery (British), 44:217, 1962.

Goldstein, LA, & Waugh, TR. Classification and terminology of scoliosis. Clinical Orthopedics, 93:10, 1973.

Green, N. Part-time bracing of adolescent idiopathic scoliosis. Journal of Bone and Joint Surgery (American), 68:738-742, 1986.

Kehl, DK, & Morrissy, RT. Brace treatment in adolescent idiopathic scoliosis: An update on concepts and technique. Clinical Orthopedics and Related Research, 229:34-43, 1988.

Kostuik, JP. Current concepts review operative treatment of idiopathic scoliosis. Journal of Bone and Joint Surgery (American), 72:1108-1113, 1990.

Lonstein, JE, & Renshaw, TS. Neuromuscular Spine Deformities. Instructional Course Lectures, Vol. 36. St. Louis: Mosby, 1987, pp. 285-304.

Lonstein, JE, & Winter, RB. Adolescent idiopathic scoliosis. Orthopedic Clinics of North America, 19:239-246, 1988.

McInnes, E, Hill, DL, Raso, VJ, Chetner, B, Greenhill, BJ, and Moreau, MJ. Vibratory response in adolescents who have idiopathic scoliosis. Journal of Bone and Joint Surgery (American), 73:1208-1212, 1991.

Moe, JH, Sundberg, AB, & Gustlio, R. A clinical study of spine fusion in the growing child. Journal of Bone and Joint Surgery (British), 46:784-785, 1964.

Moe, JH, Winter, RB, Bradford, DS, Ogilvie, JW, & Lonstein, JE. Scoliosis and Other Spinal Deformities, 2nd ed. Philadelphia: WB Saunders, 1987, pp. 162-228, 237-261, 347-368, 403-434.

Nachemson, A. A long term follow-up study of non-treated scoliosis. Acta Orthopaedica Scandinavica, 39:466-476, 1968.

Nilsonne, V, & Lundgren, KD. Long-term prognosis in idiopathic scoliosis. Acta Orthopaedica Scandinavica, 39:456-465, 1968.

Nuzzo, RM, Walsh, S, Boucherit, T, & Massood, S. Counterparalysis for treatment of paralytic scoliosis with botulism toxin type A. American Journal of Orthopedics, 26:201-207, 1997.

Piazza, MR, & Basset, GS. Curve progression after treatment with the Wilmington brace for idiopathic scoliosis. Journal of Pediatric Orthopedics, 10:39-43, 1990.

Price, CT, Scott, DS, Reed, FR, Jr, & Riddick, MF. Nighttime bracing for adolescent idiopathic scoliosis with the Charleston bending brace: Preliminary report. Spine, 15:1294-1299, 1990.

Price, CT, Scott, DS, Reed, FR, Jr, & Riddick, MF. Nighttime bracing for adolescent idiopathic scoliosis with the Charleston bending brace: Long-term follow-up. Journal of Pediatric Orthopedics, 17:703-707, 1997.

Raimondi, AJ, Choux, M, & Dirocco, C. The Pediatric Spine: II. Developmental Anomalies. New York: Springer-Verlag, 1989, pp. 189-220.

Renshaw, TS. Orthotic Treatment of Idiopathic Scoliosis and Kyphosis. Instructional Course Lectures, Vol. 34. St. Louis: Mosby, 1985, pp. 110-118.

Rothman, RH, & Simeone, FA. The Spine, 2nd ed. Philadelphia: WB Saunders, 1982, pp. 239–255, 263–282, 316–439.

Sharrad, WJW. Spinal osteotomy for congenital kyphosis in myelomeningocele. Journal of Bone and Joint Surgery (British), 50:466–471, 1968.

Tachdjian, MO. Pediatric Orthopedics, 2nd ed. Philadelphia: WB Saunders, 1990, pp. 1747, 2201–2320, 2380–2387.

Tanner, JM, & Whitehouse, RH. Clinical longitudinal standards for height, weight, height velocity and stages of puberty. Archives of Disease in Childhood, 51:170–179, 1976.

Tanner, JM, Whitehouse, RH, & Takaisni, M. Standards from birth to maturity for height, weight, height velocity and weight velocity: British children, 1965. Archives of Disease in Childhood, 47:454–471, 613–635, 1966.

VanRens, JG, & VanHorn, JR. Long-term results in lumbosacral interbody fusion for spondylolisthesis. Acta Orthopaedica Scandinavica, 53:383, 1982.

Verbeist, H. The treatment of lumbar spondyloptosis or impending lumbar spondyloptosis accompanied by neurologic deficit and/or neurogenic intermittent claudication. Spine, 4:68, 1979.

Weinstein, SL. Adolescent idiopathic scoliosis: Prevalence and natural history. Instructional Course Lectures, Vol. 38, Chap. 6. St. Louis: Mosby, 1989.

Wiltse, LL, Newman, PH, & MacNab, I. Classification of spondylolysis and spondylolisthesis. Clinical Orthopedics, 117:23, 1976.

Winter, RB. Congenital Deformities of the Spine. New York: Thieme-Stratton, 1983, pp. 6–10, 43–49.

Winter, RB. Congenital scoliosis. Orthopedic Clinics of North America, 19(2):395–408, 1988.

Winter, RB, Moe, JH, & Wang, JF. Congenital kyphosis: Its natural history and treatment as observed in a study of one hundred and thirty patients. Journal of Bone and Joint Surgery (American), 55:223–256, 1973.

Wynarsky, GT, & Schultz, AB. Trunk muscle activities in braced scoliosis patients. Spine, 14:1283–1286, 1989.

Wynne-Davies, R. Familial (idiopathic) scoliosis. Journal of Bone and Joint Surgery (British), 48:583, 1966.

Wynne-Davies, R. Genetic and environmental aspects. Journal of Bone and Joint Surgery (British), 50:24–30, 1968.

Wynne-Davies, R. The aetiology of infantile idiopathic scoliosis. Journal of Bone and Joint Surgery (British), 56:565, 1974.

Wynne-Davies, R. Congenital vertebral anomalies: Etiology and relationship to spina bifida cystica. Journal of Medical Genetics, 12:280–288, 1975.

Zaouss, AL, & James, JIP. The iliac apophysis and the evolution of curves in scoliosis. Journal of Bone and Joint Surgery (British), 40:442–453, 1958.

CHAPTER
11

Developmental Muscular Torticollis and Brachial Plexus Injury

ELLEN STAMOS NORTON, PT, PCS

Developmental muscular torticollis and brachial plexus injury are two of many conditions that must be considered diagnostically when a newborn has asymmetric posturing of the head. Although they are very different disorders and are discussed separately in this chapter, there are some common intervention strategies for these conditions. For example, range of motion (active and passive) must be maintained or increased in comfortable ways enlisting the participation of busy caretakers. Utilization of positioning during everyday activities is encouraged as a time-efficient way to address range-of-motion goals. In addition, strengthening activities during playtime that take advantage of normal reflexes and reactions are encouraged.

The etiology, examination, interventions, and expected outcomes of both developmental muscular torticollis and brachial plexus injury are discussed in this chapter.

DEVELOPMENTAL MUSCULAR TORTICOLLIS

Etiology

Developmental muscular torticollis (DMT), also referred to as congenital muscular torticollis or infantile torticollis, is characterized in an infant or child as persistent cervical lateral flexion to one side and generally rotation of the head to the opposite side. It is considered more a sign of an underlying disorder than an actual diagnosis. There are muscular and nonmuscular causes; the focus of this chapter is on the management of the muscular type of torticollis.

The etiology of DMT remains unclear. A palpable thickening, lump, pseudotumor, or hematoma may be present in the sternocleidomastoid muscle (SCMM). Figure 11–1 depicts the two origins and the insertion of the SCMM. Binder and colleagues (1987) and Cheng and Au (1994) report incidence of tumors in slightly more than one third of children with torticollis. Birth trauma to the SCMM, fetal malposition, uterine compression, and inflammatory conditions are other reported causes of DMT. Acquired torticollis after brachial plexus injury can be caused by prolonged positioning of an infant on one side. Davids and colleagues (1993) postulate that head position in utero can injure the SCMM, leading to a compartment syndrome. They propose that the mechanism of injury in these cases is therefore a kink or crush with subsequent ischemia, as opposed to stretch of the muscle. They confirm the existence of the compartment with injection studies in cadavers and during in vivo pressure studies in the presurgical and postsurgical release of the SCMM.

Nonmuscular causes of torticollis have been reported to account for approximately 18% of all cases of torticollis and include cervical skeletal malformation, subluxation of cervical vertebrae, herniated disk, posterior fossa tumor, extraocular muscle pare-sis, ocular strabismus or nystagmus, gastroesophageal reflux, and Sprengel's deformity or Klippel-Feil syndrome. A difficult, forceful delivery may also cause a clavicular fracture and brachial plexus injury leading to torticollis (Ballock & Song, 1996).

Pathophysiology

The palpable thickening or lump so frequently present in the SCMM is described by Porter and Blount (1995) as a pseudotumor, with an incidence of 4 per 1000 newborns. It is also referred to as an SCMM tumor of infancy or fibromatosis colli. They report that this painless, firm, fibrous mass commonly occurs in the sternal head and distal third of the SCMM. It occurs in infants at 2 to 4 weeks of age, gradually diminishing and disappearing clinically around 4 to 12 months of age. They suspect that 10 to 20% of these cases lead to residual fibrosis and torticollis.

The pathophysiology of the tumor involves ischemia, reperfusion, and neurologic injury to the SCMM similar to those that occur in a compartment syndrome (Davids et al., 1993). The nerve fiber damage then leads to muscle fiber degeneration and fibrosis of the muscle body. Microscopically there is replacement of the muscle fiber in various stages of degeneration with immature-appearing cellular fibrous tissue in younger children and mature-appearing noncellular collagen scarlike tissue in older children (Lin & Chou, 1997).

Ultrasonic examination of the tumor also shows fibrotic changes that are clearly differentiated from malignant soft tissue tumors. Lin and Chou (1997) performed 362 sonographic examinations on 197 children with DMT and found fibrous lesions in both the sternal and clavicular heads of the involved SCMMs in 76% of the children and in the sternal head in only 24% of the children. The extent of the fibrotic changes were represented by a ratio of the cross section of the lesion to muscle tissue. This ratio decreased with age as muscle fibers regenerated within the lesions. These fibrotic lesions persisted for as long as 15 years, even without clinical symptoms.

Plagiocephaly, cranial or facial deformation or asymmetry, is frequently present in DMT. This is probably the result of asymmetric forces on the growing cranium before or after birth.

Impairments

A shortened and fibrosed SCMM with a weakened contralateral SCMM will cause a child to laterally flex his head to the tight SCMM side and rotate it to the opposite side. Weakness of the contralateral SCMM has not been investigated, yet one may sus-

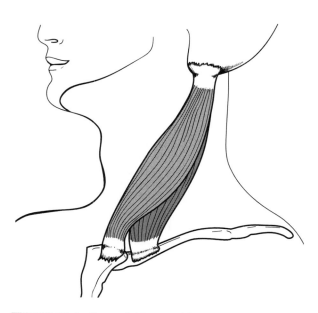

FIGURE 11–1. Sternocleidomastoideus muscle. The origin of the clavicular head is on the medial third of the clavicle, and the sternal head is on the anterior surface of the manubrium. The insertion is on the mastoid process and superior nuchal line of the occipital bone.

pect that the weakness may be due to the muscle's chronically overlengthened position or disuse in avoiding actions that cause pain. Some children will laterally flex and rotate to the same side, and in these cases a tight SCMM may not be the primary cause of asymmetry. If the torticollis does not resolve, facial asymmetry and plagiocephaly may develop and are unlikely to improve if already present.

A compensatory cervical and thoracic scoliosis can develop if a child is persistent in attempting to bring his eyes to a horizontal position when cervical motion is limited. Scoliosis was found in 5.8% of patients by Binder and colleagues (1987) in their long-term follow-up of 85 children with DMT.

Depending on the degree of range-of-motion limitation, these children may visually track in only one direction. They may strongly resist attempts to passively turn their heads in the restricted directions. Some parents report their children having aversive responses to their heads being touched if uncomfortable stretching exercises have been attempted.

Functional Limitations

No limitations in motor development other than in righting reactions should be expected in children with DMT. If motor delays are identified, further diagnostic examinations should be pursued. No studies have investigated the functional consequences of decreased cervical range of motion from torticollis or long-term outcomes with regard to neck pain. In their long-term follow-up of 2 to 23 years (mean = 4.7 years), Binder and colleagues (1987) reported that all sequelae were mild and did not pose serious cosmetic or functional problems. "Functional problems" were not described. No other long-term studies could be found that examined functional or quality-of-life outcomes in older children or adults.

Examination

A physician must rule out the many possible causes of torticollis discussed earlier. The physical therapist should be aware of the other causes of muscular and nonmuscular torticollis because the physician may misdiagnose a patient. Some physicians obtain cervical spine radiographs on all children with DMT. Ultrasound can provide diagnostic and prognostic information (Lin & Chou, 1997), and neurologic examinations may be necessary, possibly in conjunction with magnetic resonance imaging (MRI). In cases in which a child has a head tilt without limitations in range of motion, ocular dysfunction should be ruled out (Williams et al., 1996). Painful cervical conditions in the absence of typical DMT

findings may indicate inflammatory or central nervous system lesions. Ballock and Song (1996) suggest a pragmatic algorithm for evaluating children with DMT. It establishes indications for the many diagnostic examinations and tests available for differentially diagnosing a child with DMT.

Physical Therapy

History taking should include any other medical complications and pertinent medical information. Examples include hip dysplasia, type of delivery, birth weight and length, x-ray or other diagnostic imaging results, and previous interventions.

A range-of-motion examination includes documentation of the resting head position (described as lateral flexion or rotation left or right) with measurements of this resting position and active and passive cervical rotation and lateral flexion. Active cervical ranges can be measured as the child tracks and reaches or during head-righting reactions. Lateral head righting is examined by tilting the child to either side while held under the axilla. It is described as full if the eyes achieve a horizontal position. Frequently the weak side is slower to achieve its available range, even if the range is full. Neck flexor strength is examined using a pull-to-sit test. It is described as complete, incomplete, symmetric, or asymmetric.

A higher than normal incidence of hip dysplasia (10%) in children with torticollis has been reported (Porter & Blount, 1995). Therefore it is important to evaluate patients for any hip asymmetries. Asymmetries of even 5 to 10° in hip abduction may indicate hip dysplasia (see Chapter 16). Children with positive findings should be referred immediately back to their referring physician.

Facial asymmetry and plagiocephaly must be documented descriptively and subjectively. Photographs of the child's face from the front and head from the top are helpful in documenting facial asymmetry and plagiocephaly. The SCMM should be palpated for a lump or a tight feeling. The size, physical characteristics, and location of a lump should be documented.

Gross and fine motor development should be screened to help in ruling out any neurologic reasons for the torticollis. Again, the referring physician should be made aware of any abnormality.

Goals

The goals of no residual head tilt, full active and passive cervical range of motion, and normal cervical strength in all directions are reasonable goals to establish at an initial evaluation. Cheng and Au (1994) considered torticollis to be resolved when passive neck range was full or limited less than 5° with no palpable tumor. Any palpable tumors should resolve by 12 months.

Outcomes

There is a general consensus that outcomes are far better when treatment is initiated in the first year of life. The expected outcome is that the parent reports that any minor restrictions in range do not interfere with daily activities and that any minor residual craniofacial asymmetry is not noticeable. Head tilts that occur only when the child is fatigued should not be of great concern. In Taylor and Norton's (1997) study, 96% of the parents thought facial appearance was good to excellent and 100% thought head shape was good to excellent at an average of 14 months after the initial evaluation. No studies were found that reported long-term outcomes in relation to quality-of-life issues, psychologic effects of persistent craniofacial asymmetry, or possible pain related to unresolved range limitations.

Intervention

The management of DMT includes physical therapy, helmet therapy or craniotomy to reshape the skull, and surgery to release the tight SCMM or excise any pseudotumor. Prognosis is considered to be better if conservative treatment is begun before 1 year of age. The more invasive procedures are rare and reserved for children with persistent plagiocephaly and limited range of motion after 1 year of age.

Conservative treatment is a passive stretching program of the affected SCMM. Some therapists (Cheng & Au, 1994) use cervical manipulation or mobilization, yet no studies of its efficacy are available. Emery (1994) documents a passive stretching program that requires two people to implement. The program also includes positioning and handling instructions to parents. If the child has a head tilt of 6° or greater at 4.5 months, the use of a cervical orthosis is recommended. It is made of soft tubing, to be worn for active correction of torticollis. MacDonald (1996) advocates facilitation of active rotation activities to invoke the process of reciprocal inhibition, thereby reducing pain-related muscle spasms. Taylor and Norton (1997) describe a program that is mostly limited to home program instruction, using active range of motion and positioning to increase range of motion and strength of the affected soft tissues and muscles.

A comprehensive home program that includes the following key areas should be provided for parents of infants and children with DMT. Exercises should be simple, comfortable for the children, and incorporated into everyday child care routines to optimize compliance and effectiveness.

Range of Motion

Passive range of motion is an effective treatment tool if it is tolerated well by an infant. Under the age of 3 to 4 months, infants are not as resistant to passive stretching as older children may be. Passive stretching of the SCMM can be done by gently cradling the occiput on the involved side and the face on the opposite side and slowly moving into lateral flexion away from, and rotation toward, the tight SCMM. Straight rotation or lateral flexion away from the restricted directions can also be done if these are easier exercises for a parent to understand and perform. Clear written instructions to perform rotation to one side and lateral flexion to the opposite side will eliminate confusion about the unusual pull of this muscle.

If stretching is painful to a child, it will be poorly tolerated as evidenced by the child crying and strongly resisting the stretch. Parents will be hesitant to carry out exercises that cause discomfort to their child. A tight muscle can actually become stronger if a child resists against the stretch, furthering the muscle imbalance between the tight and weak side. Using active range of motion that is under the child's control will simultaneously strengthen the weakened muscles and elongate the shortened soft tissues.

Strengthening is achieved in the identified weak muscles using tracking and righting reactions. To increase rotation, visual tracking toward the affected SCMM can be used. These exercises should be done in a variety of positions such as supine, prone, reclining, and sitting (as developmentally appropriate). Gravity can be used as an assist when a muscle is weak. As the muscles gain strength, the activity should change to use gravity as resistance. One shoulder may need to be resisted to prevent the infant from using trunk rotation as a substitute for cervical rotation. To increase lateral neck flexion, lateral or optical righting (around 3–4 months) is used. Weight-shifting activities on a ball or on the lap are also effective. The use of a mobile surface enables the caretaker to elicit the correct combination of lateral cervical flexion and rotation to stretch the involved SCMM and obtain full participation of the weak SCMM. For example, while on a caregiver's lap, the child is encouraged to look and reach to the left while laterally flexing against gravity to the right, to stretch the left SCMM (Fig. 11–2). Another exercise is to hold the child around the upper trunk and tilt to the side. Doing this in front of a mirror elicits

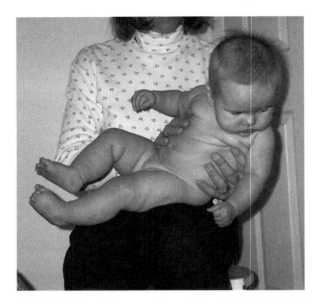

FIGURE 11–2. Active stretching of the tight (left) SCMM is achieved by eliciting head righting away from the tight SCMM and rotation toward the tight SCMM. Simultaneous strengthening of the weak contralateral side is occurring.

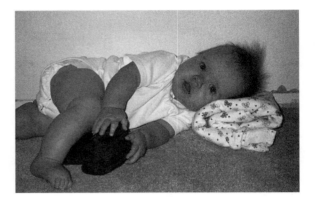

FIGURE 11–3. Passive, prolonged stretching is achieved by placing an infant in side-lying position with a folded receiving blanket under her head on the tight SCMM side. If the child rolls forward or back, she can be positioned against a supporting surface behind her with a small stuffed animal in front to prevent rolling forward.

a good response of head righting. When the eyes achieve a horizontal position, the child can be rotated in the correct direction for a full stretch of the SCMM as the child continues to focus on the reflection. The infant's attempt to achieve a horizontal position of the eyes may be slow and incomplete; therefore the infant must be given sufficient time to achieve maximal range.

Positioning

Positioning is another way to elongate shortened muscles in ways that do not elicit crying or resistance to stretch. The objectives are to create symmetry or prolonged stretches in a variety of positions and provide an opportunity and incentive for the child to perform active range of motion. During sleep, a child might tolerate a prolonged cervical stretch when placed in a side-lying position. A firm pillow made from a hand towel can be placed under the child's head to stretch the lateral flexion tightness (Fig. 11–3). This can also be done with very young infants when they are awake. The amount of stretch can be increased as the infant relaxes into the position. After a child falls asleep, positioning the head in a rotated position toward the tight SCMM is encouraged. Again, a towel folded like a wedge can be used to prevent the child's head from rotating back to the preferred position. The child's head may need to be repositioned several times during the nap. Bottle or breast feeding is also an efficient time to do

stretching. The infant can start in a relaxed position of comfort and can then be slowly moved into positions that the infant might normally resist. During free play, the child should be positioned supine, prone, or sitting in a manner that will encourage looking toward the affected SCMM and at general activity in a room.

Symmetry

Creating symmetry of the head, neck, and spine can be achieved in infant seats, high chairs, car seats, and other positioning devices. In addition to improving range of motion, these positions can aid in reshaping the infant's head by avoiding prolonged deforming forces on the same side of the head. The infant's positioning equipment is modified to achieve as much symmetry as possible by using a three-point system (Fig. 11–4). Toys can be suspended above many of these devices on the side the child must rotate toward. Parents can then make these adaptations to other positioning devices in their home or day care environment.

Parent Education

Parent education should be provided about the basic anatomy and kinesiology of the SCMM. The treatment philosophy of active range of motion and

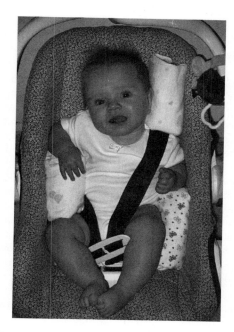

FIGURE 11–4. A three-point system is used in a car seat to achieve full spinal symmetry. Lateral cervical flexion is resisted by a small towel roll on the tight SCMM side. The towel roll at the contralateral trunk prevents the infant from merely being pushed to that side by the roll at the head. Toys are hung on the left to encourage cervical rotation to that side for a complete stretch of the SCMM.

positioning and avoidance of painful stretching should be explained. Caregivers should be encouraged to be creative in implementing the philosophy and therapeutic procedures in daily care and play routines, maximizing the time therapeutic intervention is occurring. A written home program should be provided once the therapist has identified the appropriate exercises and instructed the caregivers.

Follow-up sessions are used to reexamine the child, identify whether additional exercises are needed, or determine whether the parent can discontinue the program. As tracking, neck strength, and righting reactions emerge and improve with normal development, different exercises can be added to the program as needed. For example, a 2-month-old is not expected to perform lateral head righting. At 6 months, a full eyes-horizontal position should be present.

Surgery

Surgery is usually reserved for cases of persistent torticollis with significant deformity in children over 12 months of age. Davids and colleagues (1993) use the criterion of greater than 30° loss in range of motion (usually lateral flexion) or significant plagio-

cephaly before considering surgical intervention. Emery's (1994) findings demonstrate that torticollis tends to resolve when treatment is initiated before 2 years of age. Porter and Blount (1995) report that facial asymmetry will tend to resolve as long as growth potential exists, up to approximately 6 years of age. Therefore a truly comprehensive program that provides more than simple passive range of motion should be given a trial period to improve a child's torticollis before undergoing surgery. Porter and Blount (1995) report that surgical treatment usually consists of distal myomectomy or tenotomy of the SCMM. Severe fibrosis may require release of both SCMM heads. Other proposed techniques include open section of the SCMM, Z-plasty with lengthening, and complete excision of the muscle. Burstein and Cohen (1998) use an endoscopic surgical approach to release the SCMM fibers that leaves an inconspicuous scar in the scalp near the hairline. Postoperative splinting may be required, and postoperative physical therapy is typically recommended. The active exercises and positioning described in this chapter can be implemented when wound healing is sufficient.

Prognosis

The prognosis is considered good for children treated with a conservative program initiated in the first year of life. Full recovery (full range of motion) was achieved in all but 1 of 101 children treated for a mean duration of 4.7 months, even when treatment was not initiated until the second year of life (Emery, 1994). Emery (1994) found that children with masses, more severe restrictions in range of motion, and significant head tilts required longer treatment. Cheng & Au (1994) reported that 97% of all cases resolved with a conservative treatment program of passive and active range of motion and positioning. The duration of treatment ranged from 2 months for those with the least restricted range of motion initially to 5 months for those children with the most restricted range of motion.

Patients with fibrotic changes noted by ultrasound in the lower one third of the SCMM made up 14% of the group in Lin and Chou's (1997) study, and all of these patients recovered without surgery. Forty-eight percent had fibrotic changes in the middle and lower or middle third of the SCMM, and surgery was required in 6.3% of this group. The entire length of the muscle was involved in 38% of the children studied, with 26% of these undergoing surgery. Binder and colleagues (1987) reported torticollis resolving in 69.3% of 257 patients by 12 months of age with conservative treatment. In a long-term follow-up of 2 to 23 years (mean = 4.7 years), the most common sequela was persistent craniofacial asymmetry (45.9%). Intermittent head tilt associated with fatigue persisted in 24.7%, and scoliosis was present in 5.8% of the children. No dental problems were reported. In Taylor and Norton's (1997) study, good to excellent overall outcomes were documented in 96% of 23 children with an average of 3.8 treatments over an average time period of 2.9 months. Morrison and MacEwen (1982) reported 91 out of 113 children treated conservatively having good to excellent results based on a grading system incorporating range of motion and cranial facial asymmetry. No studies have reported incidence of neck pain on a long-term follow-up, a common problem in spastic torticollis in adults.

CASE HISTORY
MICHAEL

Michael was referred to physical therapy at the age of 4 months with a diagnosis of torticollis. His pediatrician initially recommended that the parents passively stretch his SCMM. No improvement was seen, despite resolution of an initial lump that the doctor had palpated in the SCMM. Cervical and hip x-rays had ruled out cervical pathology and hip dysplasia.

Clinical findings at 4 months included a resting position of Michael's head with rotation to the left of 35° and lateral flexion to the right of 45°. The right SCMM felt tight as compared with the suppleness of the left SCMM. When Michael's face was viewed from the front, the right eye was positioned lower than the left. When his head was viewed from the top, the right forehead and cheek and left posterior skull were flat as compared with a fullness of the opposite sides. All hip range-of-motion measurements were symmetric and within normal limits.

Cervical Range of Motion	Left	Right
Active rotation	80	35
Passive rotation	85	50
Active lateral flexion	−10	45
Passive lateral flexion	20	50

When pulled to sit, Michael demonstrated a slight lag that was asymmetric. When lateral head righting was tested, his eyes achieved a horizontal position quickly when tilted to the left. When tilted to the right, he lifted his head only partially through the range after holding the position for 5 to 10 seconds.

After the initial examination, Michael's parents were shown drawings of the SCMM, and its role in the cervical asymmetry was explained. The consequences of prolonged positioning of the head in one position

were discussed. Short- and long-term goals, functional outcomes, and prognosis were explained in detail. Exercises as described earlier in this chapter were taught to the mother. Michael did not like his head being passively ranged, yet he was a sound sleeper. His mother could incrementally move his head during naps into a position that stretched the SCMM. Because of the asymmetry noted when Michael was pulled to sit, she was instructed to work on neck flexor strengthening. She was to start with Michael supine, propped up slightly, and assist him at the shoulders in slowly flexing forward, waiting for active neck flexion. As the initial head lag resolved, he was to start the exercise from lying flat. These exercises were to be done in midline and partially to each side with the trunk rotated slightly. Using Michael's car seat, two receiving blankets, and a stuffed animal, a position of symmetry was created. Toys the mother had dangling from the carrying handle were moved to the right to encourage cervical rotation to that side.

The mother was instructed to spread the exercises out throughout the day during play and feeding times. She found that breast feeding him in the "football" hold (head at the breast, body under her arm and feet toward her back) allowed her free hand to easily cradle his head into the desired positions. A return appointment was scheduled for 1 month later. On return, the following examination results were determined. The resting tilt decreased to 20° of lateral flexion and 20° of rotation.

Cervical Range of Motion	Left	Right
Active rotation	80	65
Passive rotation	85	75
Active lateral flexion	Neutral	45
Passive lateral flexion	35	50

No facial asymmetry could be observed. There was still fullness of the left cheek and right posterior skull, but not as prominent as 1 month earlier. Pull-to-sit neck flexion was full, yet still slightly asymmetric. The parents were encouraged to continue the exercise program. The parents were instructed to resist the shoulder when practicing cervical rotation, begin cervical rotation against gravity (side lying), attempt holding positions longer for more prolonged stretches, and begin lateral head righting on moveable surfaces and in front of a mirror.

On the next visit 1 month later, the parents reported only rare times when they noticed head tilting and those were when Michael was tired. All cervical ranges were within normal limits and symmetric to within 5°. A screening of his motor development did not identify any developmental delays. Some minor plagiocephaly persisted, yet the mother reported not even noticing it, particularly because Michael's hair was getting thicker.

Michael was discharged at that time with instructions to return for follow-up if the head tilt or restrictions in range of motion reappeared.

A follow-up phone call to Michael's parents was made 6 months later. His father reported that the torticollis had resolved with no apparent residual impairment, functional limitations, or disability.

BRACHIAL PLEXUS INJURY

Etiology

Brachial plexus injuries (BPIs) can occur from a wide variety of traumas to the shoulder and spine. The focus of this chapter is on obstetric brachial plexus injuries, yet the concepts presented apply to resultant impairment, functional limitations, and disability caused by brachial plexus injury at any age.

Injury to the brachial plexus (Fig. 11–5) usually occurs during a difficult vaginal delivery. Traction on the newborn's shoulder during delivery of the head in a breech delivery can injure the cervical roots, fracture the clavicle or humerus, or sublux the shoulder. Forceful traction and rotation of the head during a vertex presentation to deliver the shoulder tends to injure the C5 and C6 roots. Complicating factors include maternal diabetes, high birth weight, prolonged maternal labor, a sedated hypotonic infant during delivery, shoulder dystocia (difficult delivery of the shoulder), a heavily sedated mother, breech delivery, and difficult cesarean extraction. Associated damage to the phrenic nerve at C4 is less common, yet will cause ipsilateral hemiparesis of the diaphragm. Other causes of damage to the plexus at any age include pressure from body casts or trauma to the shoulder of traction and abduction.

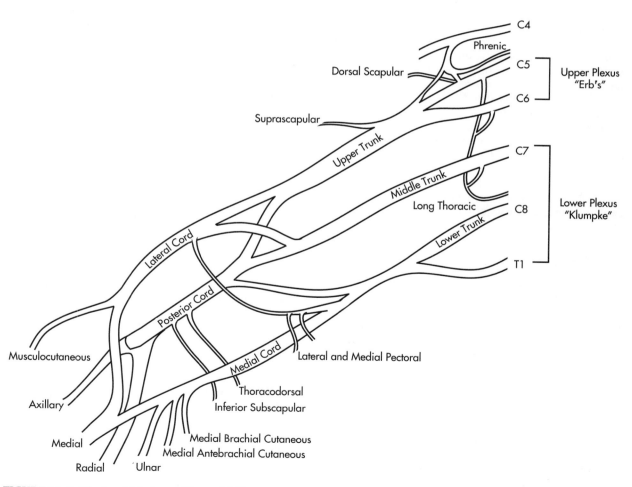

FIGURE 11–5. The brachial plexus. The variability in the impairments that a BPI can cause is easily understood, because the injury can occur at any point along the nerves as they branch off the spinal cord and weave into the brachial plexus.

Congenital anomalies such as cervical rib, abnormal thoracic vertebrae, or shortened scalenus anticus muscle can cause pressure on the lower plexus (Shepherd, 1991).

Pathophysiology

Damage can occur at the level of the nerve rootlet attached to the spinal cord, at the anterior or posterior rootlets, or distal to where the rootlets coalesce to form the mixed nerve root that exits the canal. Roots, trunks, divisions, cords, and peripheral nerves can all suffer neurotmesis (complete rupture), axonotmesis (neural sheath remains intact with disruption of the internal elements), or neurapraxia (temporary nerve conduction block). Partial or complete rupture may evolve into a neuroma and mass of fibrous tissue as disorganized neurons on the proximal end attempt to reach their distal end (Fig. 11-6). Hemorrhage into the subarachnoid space leads to presence of blood in the cerebrospinal fluid, which can be diagnostic of this more serious injury (Shepherd, 1991). Recovery is usually limited after ruptures. Prognosis after axonotmesis is better as the neurons reconnect more successfully through the intact neural sheath. Axon regrowth proceeds at approximately 1 mm per day, the majority of recovery usually taking 4 to 6 months in the upper arm and 7 to 9 months in the lower arm. Continued recovery can occur for up to 2 years in the upper arm and 4 years in the lower arm (Gilbert, 1995). Recovery after neurapraxia occurs as edema resolves and is usually quick and complete, sometimes within days. A combination of these lesions is common, which partially explains the irregularity of return of motor function in different muscles.

Impairments

There are several types of brachial plexus injuries. Erb's palsy is by far the most common (73%), involving the upper roots, C5 and C6. As a result of this injury, the child's shoulder is usually held in extension, internal rotation, and adduction; the elbow is extended; the forearm is pronated; and the wrist and fingers are flexed in the textbook "waiter's tip" position (Fig. 11-7) . Paralysis of the rhomboids, levator scapulae, serratus anterior, subscapularis, deltoid, supraspinatus, infraspinatus, teres minor, biceps, brachialis, brachioradialis, supinator, and long extensors of the wrist, fingers, and thumb can be expected. Grasp is left intact, but sensory loss is usually present. Elbow and finger extension is compromised if C7 is also involved. Klumpke's palsy is rare (2% of all cases) and involves the lower roots, C7, C8, and T1. The child's shoulder and elbow movements are

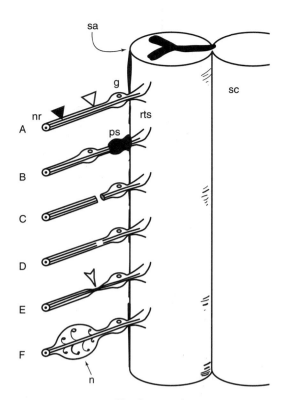

FIGURE 11-6. Types of birth injury lesions to the brachial plexus. *A*, Normal relationship of ganglion (g), subarachnoid space (sa), spinal cord (sc), rootlets (rts), neural elements (solid triangle), sheath elements (open triangle), and nerve root (nr). *B*, Avulsion with disconnection of the rootlets (anterior, posterior, or both) from the spinal cord, with formation of a pseudomeningocele (ps) at preganglionic location. *C*, Neurotmesis (rupture) with disconnection of both neural and sheath elements at postganglionic location. *D*, Axonotmesis with disconnection of neural elements and intact sheath elements at postganglionic location. *E*, Neuropraxic (arrowhead) conduction block without permanent structural lesion. *F*, Neuroma (n) with partial and complete disconnection of neural or sheath elements, with attempted aberrant regeneration. (From Laurent, JP, & Lee, RT. Birth-related upper brachial plexus injuries in infants: Operative and nonoperative approaches. Journal of Child Neurology, 9[2]:111–118, April 1994. Reprinted with permission from BC Decker, Inc.)

good with a resting position of forearm supination and paralysis of the wrist flexors and extensors and intrinsic muscles of the wrist and hand. Erb-Klumpke palsy is a combination of the injury to the upper and lower roots involving the C5 through T1 roots, resulting in total arm paralysis and loss of sensation. Involvement is usually unilateral yet is reported to be bilateral in 4% of cases (Laurent & Lee, 1994). The extent of the initial paralysis frequently

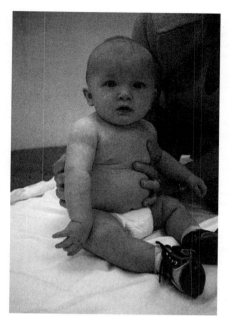

FIGURE 11–7. Infant with a Erb's palsy, a C5-C6 brachial plexus injury, resulting in the "waiter's tip" position of the upper extremity, which is typically observed with this type of injury.

recedes, with a total paralysis becoming limited to the upper roots. The pattern of motor loss does not always fit the classic definitions, indicating incomplete or mixed upper and lower types. Horner's syndrome, usually a result of avulsion of T1, can cause deficient sweating, recession of the eyeball, abnormal pupillary contraction, myosis, ptosis, and irises of different colors. Considered rare, Eng and colleagues (1978) reported 8 of 135 infants with BPI having Horner's syndrome.

During the period of neural regeneration, children use abnormal muscle substitutions that are the most advantageous given the innervated muscles available. For example, they may use wrist flexion with pronation for grasp. They may also neglect the extremity because of sensory loss or the comparative ease with which the opposite arm and hand accomplishes a task. These patterns of neglect or substitution are reinforced with repetition. The problems that arise from these repetitive patterns include soft tissue contracture and abnormal bone growth. The contractures most likely to develop are scapular protraction; shoulder extension, adduction, and internal rotation; elbow flexion or extension; forearm pronation; and wrist and finger flexion. These will obviously vary depending on the individual pattern of paralysis. Common orthopedic problems include flattening of the humeral head and hypoplasia of the

glenoid fossa with resultant glenohumeral subluxation or dislocation and posterior radial dislocation.

Torticollis can develop as a result of the child being positioned away from the involved arm or may be present from the same trauma that caused the BPI.

Functional Limitations

Functional limitations will vary greatly, depending on the extent of initial pathology, neurologic regeneration, and residual impairments. The primary functional limitations in children with BPI relate to an inability to reach, grasp, and perform tasks requiring bilateral manual abilities such as catching a large ball or lifting a large object. Activities of daily living that require bilateral upper extremity use will also be compromised. These would include donning and removing shirts and pants, tying shoes, and buttoning. Dressing aids may be necessary to achieve maximum independence. Studies have documented range-of-motion limitations of these children's affected arms, but no studies were found that reported functional limitations in dressing, eating, or participating in sports with or without aids or adaptations.

Normal developmental activities may be compromised as a result of BPI. Movement from prone or supine to sit may always be done from one side, thereby asymmetrically strengthening one side of the trunk or delaying balance reactions. The developmental milestone of creeping on all fours may not occur because the child may not be able to bear weight on the involved arm, and as a result the child may scoot around in sitting or progress straight to walking at the appropriate age.

Neglect of the involved limb or even self-abusive behavior such as biting can occur because of absent or abnormal sensation. Injuries such as burns, insect bites, and abrasions may go unnoticed if pain sensation is compromised.

Shoulder pain and neuritis in adults is a complication that can interfere not only with the function of the involved arm but also with other aspects of the individual's social or vocational activities.

Examination

Children may be referred to physical therapy in the days, weeks, months, or years after the initial injury. Physical therapy examination of these children's active and passive range of motion and sensory status is key in establishing a baseline of function and abilities. Screening the developmental status of the infant or child will ensure that other pathologic conditions are not missed. In the neonate, frequent reexamination serves to document motor recovery as neural regeneration occurs. These data aid in program planning whether it be therapeutic exercise, splinting, identification of surgical candidates, or discharge from intervention.

Grossman (1996) recommends physicians follow newborns at 2 weeks and at 1, 2, and 3 months of age. Infants not showing evidence of recovery may undergo an MRI to define the integrity of the nerve roots. Electromyography (EMG), although of little prognostic value, can determine the extent of involvement and is recommended as a preoperative baseline. Repeated EMG testing can alert the therapist to muscles that are undergoing reinnervation before obvious motor changes occur. Advances in MRI, EMG, computed tomography (CT), and CT with metrizamide (CT-myelogram) have aided in preoperative diagnosis and surgical planning, yet do not replace the careful physical examination of the clinical and functional consequences of neurologic damage and neural regeneration.

Range of Motion

Physical therapy examination of the neonate with BPI may be requested before discharge from the hospital. In any age child, range-of-motion measurements of the involved arm and cervical area are performed. All movements should be performed with great care because the child's joints can be unstable and the limbs may have sensory loss. Baseline range-of-motion data are essential for future identification of secondary contractures that could be avoided with appropriate intervention and to judge the effectiveness of interventions.

Motor Function

In the infant, the therapist can observe limb movement or muscle contractions when testing a variety of reactions and reflexes such as visual tracking, neck righting, Moro reflex, Galant reflex, parachute reaction, or the hand-placing reaction. Arm and head movement can be observed during wakeful play periods as a child tries to bring the hand to the mouth or reach for a toy, with care to document whether movements are with gravity eliminated or against gravity. Asymmetry of abdominal and thoracic movement may indicate phrenic nerve paralysis. Clarke and Curtis (1995) developed a muscle grading system called the "Active Movement Scale," which is an eight-grade scale designed to capture subtle but significant changes in movement of the arm (Table 11-1). They report that a study is underway to validate this assessment tool.

Older children can be examined using standard manual muscle tests, and dynamometers can provide

TABLE 11-1. Hospital for Sick Children Muscle Grading System—Active Movement Scale*

Observation	Muscle Grade
Gravity Eliminated	
No contraction	0
Contraction, no motion	1
Motion ≤½ range	2
Motion >½ range	3
Full motion	4
Against Gravity	
Motion ≤½ range	5
Motion >½ range	6
Full motion	7

*Full active range of motion with gravity eliminated (muscle grade 4) must be achieved before active range against gravity is scored (muscle grades 5 to 7).

From Clarke, HM, & Curtis, GC. An approach to obstetrical brachial plexus injuries. Hand Clinics, 11(4):567, November 1995.

objective measures of grasp strength. Patterns of movement, abnormal substitutions, and posturing of the arm as a result of muscle imbalance and sensory loss should also be documented.

Any spasticity would suggest an upper motor neuron lesion and therefore should not be present in a child with BPI. Further diagnostic evaluation by a neurologist is indicated if spasticity is found on examination.

Sensation

Examination of sensory loss in infants is not sensitive or reliable enough to document the clinical progression of neural regeneration. Attempts should be made, however, to identify areas on the involved extremity that may have compromised sensation. Narakas (1987) has developed the Sensory Grading System for children with BPI. A grade of S0 is no reaction to painful or other stimuli; S1 is reaction to painful stimuli, none to touch; S2 is reaction to touch, not to light touch; and S3 is apparently normal sensation. Sensory loss does not necessarily correspond to the extent of motor involvement (Eng et al., 1978); therefore care should be taken not to ignore this examination in children with milder involvement.

As neural regeneration proceeds, sensory loss may progress to hyperesthesia before achieving normal sensation (Narakas, 1987). Infants or older children may experience pain or discomfort in reaction to sensory stimulation and simple touch. This change should be documented and may indicate progression of regeneration.

More definitive sensory testing to a variety of stimuli such as heat, cold, light touch, and two-point

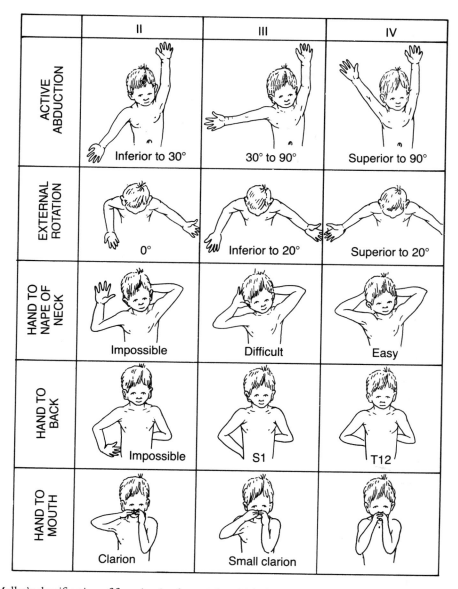

FIGURE 11–8. Mallet's classification of function in obstetric brachial plexus palsy. Grade 0 (not shown) is no movement in the desired plane, and grade V (not shown) is full movement. (From Gilbert, A. Obstetrical brachial plexus palsy. In Tubiana, R [Ed.], The Hand, Vol. 4. Philadelphia: WB Saunders, 1993, p. 579.)

discrimination is possible in older children, and specific areas of sensory loss can be mapped. Sensation may take as long as 2 years to recover.

Functional Status

Developmental tests of gross and fine motor performance can be used to establish and track any delays caused by the upper extremity impairment. Older children who can follow verbal commands or copy body positions can be assessed in their abilities to perform functional activities such as bringing hand to mouth for eating, bringing hand to head for brushing hair, and holding a variety of tools (e.g., toothbrush) sufficiently for their intended use. Videotaping of these activities is helpful. Gilbert (1993) described a classification of function in obstetric BPI that was developed earlier by Mallet. This scale (Fig. 11–8) is widely used when assessing children over age 3.

Electromyography

Findings from diagnostic EMG, although informative, are not accurate in predicting recovery or outcome and do not have consistent clinical correlation with the amount of strength in a muscle. Reinnervation after microsurgery can be identified by EMG immediately following surgery or in the following weeks and months, before clinical signs of motor return are present. This information may change a therapist's goals and intervention, and it may change a patient's prognosis significantly. Results would also assist in planning and implementing a program of functional electrical stimulation.

Outcomes and Goals

The ideal outcome for the neonate with BPI and a flaccid arm is complete return of sensation and motor control. The physical therapy goals during the first few months of recovery are preventive in nature. They include parent education, maintenance of range of motion and joint integrity, attainment of normal strength in all muscle groups, and normal development. As it becomes evident that complete return is not occurring, outcomes and goals must be revised. Depending on the extent of impairment, full range of motion and normal strength may remain a goal in the first 2 years of life, because continued neural regeneration or restored motor control through a variety of orthopedic and neurosurgical procedures may still be possible. As discussed earlier, the majority of spontaneous recoveries occur within 4 to 9 months, but continued recovery may occur up to 4 years after the injury (Gilbert, 1995).

At some point between 9 and 24 months of age, it may be apparent that significant neural regeneration is no longer occurring. Goals would need to be revised for children who lose range or plateau in their recovery over several months. Even with the most diligent home program implementation, full range of motion is difficult to maintain when muscle imbalance is present. Children with BPI continue to need monitoring of their range of motion and functional status. Every attempt should be made to continue encouraging functional bilateral activities. The desired outcomes at this time (2 years of age) would be that the child develop age-appropriate self-care skills such as dressing and grooming using either extremity and participate in age-appropriate movement activities and preschool programs. Goals would include maintaining or increasing range of motion and strength in movements critical to specific activities that the child is currently unable to perform. An example might be increasing elbow flexion from 40 to 90° and elbow strength from 2+ to 3+ in order to pick up objects from the ground with both hands and put them on a table. Decreased pain may also be a goal, with an outcome, for example, of being able to participate in a full game of soccer without shoulder pain.

Little information is available on long-term outcomes in adults with a history of BPI. An informal study of chat rooms on the Internet and conversations with some of these adults confirms that a number of adults are looking for treatment suggestions for persistent residual arm and shoulder pain. Gjorup (1965) published a long-term follow-up study of adults that included clinical examinations and a lengthy questionnaire of their functional and social status, their vocational and avocational activities, and their feelings about how BPI had affected their lives. Although this study is descriptive in nature, it is unique in its attempt to document how BPI affects people as adults. Out of 222 respondents, approximately one third thought they had a usable arm, one third thought they had a useless arm, and the remainder reported transitional stages between these extremes (Gjorup, 1965). Slightly more than one third thought they were disabled. Gjorup (1965) concluded that patients with BPI manage well socially, and no correlation was found between the severity of the arm defect and social status achieved by the patient. Further outcomes research using health-related quality-of-life measures as described by Jette (1993) would be helpful and possibly reassuring to parents in long-term planning for their children.

Intervention

The majority of infants (90–95%) with birth-related BPI require only physical therapy and no surgical intervention (Laurent & Lee, 1994). A consultation before discharge from the hospital may be performed; however, an initial rest period of 7 to 10 days is required to allow for reduction of hemorrhage and edema around the traumatized nerves. During this time, the involved limb is positioned gently across the abdomen. Lying on the involved limb is to be avoided.

After this initial period of immobilization, the physical therapist performs the baseline examinations described earlier in this chapter under Examination. A home program is developed for the parents that addresses all range of motion at risk for contractures, including precautions about any joints at risk for overstretching or dislocation. The physical therapist explains precautions regarding any areas of sensory loss and teaches the parents how to use positioning and therapeutic play during everyday activities to maintain range of motion and strengthen weak muscles.

Functional Training

The objective of the physical therapy program is to facilitate the highest functional outcome possible for the child, particularly in the areas of reach and grasp as they relate to meaningful, developmentally appropriate activities. As previously mentioned, children will use abnormal muscle substitutions that are the most advantageous given the innervated muscles available. The therapist intervenes in several ways, including facilitation of normal movement patterns while inhibiting substitutions during reach and weight-bearing activities. This intervention should be in the context of performing concrete versus abstract tasks. For example, strengthening of the shoulder flexors could be done by asking the child to lift 10 toy people up and into a doll house (a concrete task) instead of performing 10 repetitions of shoulder flexion (an abstract task). Van der Weel and colleagues (1991) describe the difference between concrete and abstract tasks in degrees to which the required act is directed toward controlling physical interaction with the environment or with the person's own body, as opposed to producing movement for its own sake. He found that active upper extremity range of motion was significantly greater in children with cerebral palsy when performing concrete as opposed to abstract tasks.

Careful attention to the scapula is critical during reaching activities, because paralysis of the rhomboids and contracture of the muscles that link the humerus to the scapula interfere with the normal 6:1 humeroscapular relation in the first 30° of movement. The scapula can be manually stabilized as the shoulder is assisted in flexion in reaching toward a toy. This activity achieves correct motor training and stretching at the same time.

A variety of opportunities should be provided for weak muscles to participate in normal movement patterns by eliminating gravity for very weak muscles, preventing substitutions, and manually guiding the extremity through movements to accomplish a task. Examples include hand to mouth; transferring objects; weight shifting on upper extremities in prone position, quadruped position, and sitting with hands in front or back; crawling; and reaching for toys placed at a variety of angles and heights from the child. Figure 11–9A illustrates a nonfunctional position that an infant with a classic C5, C6 injury may assume. Figure 11–9B demonstrates how manually guiding the shoulder into flexion and external rotation allows the infant to experience a normal, functional movement pattern and obtain sensory information through an open palm. The scapula is stabilized at the same time to allow for stretching of the soft tissues connecting the scapula to the humerus. Infants should be placed in a side-lying position on their uninvolved arm to avoid stresses on the involved arm and to free the weak arm to reach and play with toys placed in front of them. Gravity or toys held in the hand can be used as resistance as muscles gain strength. At times, the uninvolved arm may need to be gently restrained when encouraging the child to use the involved arm. Tactile stimulation or facilitation of the weak muscles with gentle joint compression in weight bearing is also helpful.

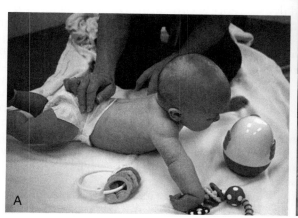 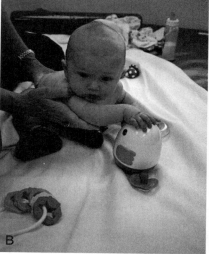

FIGURE 11–9. *A,* Infant with C5-C6 BPI trying to prop and reach. *B,* Infant assisted in reaching and grasping with manual guidance.

Normal developmental activities may be compromised as a result of BPI. Transitional movement into sitting may always be done from one side, and balance may be delayed. To address this reliance on one side, the activity can be practiced from the involved side using normal patterns. When sitting is achieved, shoulder abduction can be facilitated by challenging protective reactions to the involved side. Normal bilateral upper extremity use will also be delayed. Opportunities for the child to experience and practice two-handed activities such as holding balls or swinging can be provided.

In the older child who has not experienced return of motor function, adaptations and products to assist him in activities of daily living and sports should be made available for his consideration. Many products are available for performing a variety of daily tasks using only one hand, and families can be encouraged to design their own adaptations. Not every child or family wants to use these devices, and their opinions should be respected.

Range of Motion

Range of motion can be done in the context of normal developmental activities as described previously or positioning as described later in this chapter. Passive range of motion should never cause pain and should always be gentle. Overstretching can be harmful to joints and joint capsules that are already unstable. For example, forced supination of the elbow may compound the problem of radial head dislocation and ulnar bowing (Eng et al., 1978). Picking the child up under the axilla or by pulling on his arms is discouraged because these actions can overstretch the unprotected shoulder joint.

Prevention of scapulohumeral adhesions is one important goal. Parents should be educated about the anatomy and kinesiology of the glenohumeral joint. During reach, the scapula can be stabilized or restrained to allow for stretching of the muscles that link the scapula to the humerus, but not beyond 30° of abduction. Past that position, the scapula must rotate along with humeral external rotation to avoid harmful impingement on the acromion process.

Sensory Awareness

Sensory loss can lead to neglect or even self-mutilation. Parents must be precautioned about the risk of injuring body areas where sensation is compromised. They should watch for any signs of self-mutilation such as biting an insensate area. Enlisting the participation of the involved limb in activities previously mentioned or in holding a bottle gives the child the feeling of the extremity being a purposeful part of the body. Sensory perception can be enhanced by placing objects of different textures and temperatures in the hand, playing games such as finding toys under sudsy water or rice with the involved hand, or blindfolding the older child and having her name familiar objects placed in her hand. Range of motion can be accomplished by guiding the hand to different areas of the child's body to experience tactile stimulation. Parents themselves should be encouraged not to neglect the arm, but to caress and play with it as usual, while holding or guiding it through patterns that must be reinforced.

Positioning

Placing the child's arm in optimal positions is a time-efficient way to stretch limited ranges. As with the torticollis exercises, this can be done during feeding, carrying, or positioning in a car seat. When sleeping, the arm can be placed toward abduction, external rotation, elbow flexion, and forearm supination on a pillow to the child's side. As the child's arm relaxes during sleep, even more range can be attempted.

Splinting

Intermittent splinting of the wrist and fingers is sometimes indicated. Wrist splints may preserve the integrity of the tendons of the fingers and wrist until motor function returns. Resting night splints can help prevent wrist and finger flexion contractures. A wrist cock-up splint maintains a neutral alignment of the wrist yet frees the fingers for play. In an attempt to prevent adduction and internal rotation contractures, some have used a "statue of liberty" splint or an abduction splint. These are generally discouraged because there is evidence that they contribute to abduction contractures, hypermobility, and pathology of the glenohumeral and elbow joint (Price & Grossman, 1995; Shepherd, 1991).

Restraining splints such as air splints can be used on the uninvolved extremity to encourage use of the involved arm and hand. For example, elbow extension is limited on the uninvolved side, so the child would need to use his weaker arm to bring a toy to his mouth or self-feed. These should only be used for brief periods during the day with frustration levels monitored carefully. Some children will not tolerate them at all, particularly if it is unrealistic that the weaker arm could independently perform critical activities.

Neurosurgery

Microsurgical methods of reconstructing obstetric brachial plexus lesions in children are showing increasingly promising results as diagnostic and surgical techniques improve. Reports of improvement range from 75 to 95% (Sherburn et al., 1997); however, criteria for judging improvements are not standardized. Neurosurgery is reserved for the 5 to 10% of children not making spontaneous recoveries. Criteria for patient selection, timing of the intervention, and choice of surgical technique continue to be studied and debated.

In general, lack of improvement of at least one muscle grade in two of three muscle groups by 4 to 6 months of age would warrant serious consideration for surgery. Gilbert (1995) determined that operative repair of the brachial plexus was superior to spontaneous recovery in 436 children who underwent surgery. He operated at 3 months of age based on lack of biceps function at that time. Michelow and colleagues (1994) believe that many infants without biceps function at 3 months will show recovery by 9 months with outcome comparable to that of a child who has had surgery. They recommend surgery at 8 to 9 months of age in the absence of grade 4 biceps strength at that time. Laurent and Lee (1994) recommend that surgery be delayed to at least 4 to 6 months of age. They demonstrated improvement above preoperative status in 80% of infants with upper brachial plexus injury at 1 year after surgery. Antigravity function in the biceps and deltoid was achieved in 89% of their surgical patients. Based on historical controls, most of these children would not have been expected to gain this antigravity function. Sherburn and colleagues (1997) recommended surgical intervention in patients not having antigravity strength in the biceps, triceps, and deltoid by 6 months of age. Age at the time of surgery (mean =

10.5 months, range = 3 to 35 months) did not affect the results, which were 87.5% attaining antigravity strength in at least one muscle, 75% attaining antigravity strength in the biceps and triceps, and 50% attaining antigravity strength in the deltoid.

Neurosurgical techniques used in the treatment of BPI include nerve grafting, neuroma dissection and removal, neurolysis (decompression, removal of scar tissue), and direct end-to-end nerve anastomosis (Fig. 11–10).

Electrical Stimulation

Functional electrical stimulation (FES) is being used increasingly for children with BPI. Goals include improving sensory awareness and increasing strength and range of motion for functional purposes. Eng and colleagues (1978) promote its use in young infants with no voluntary motor unit activity and evidence of denervation in an effort to prevent atrophy while awaiting recovery. Stimulation is discontinued when recruitment patterns appear on EMG or no improvement is evidenced after several months of treatment. Eng and colleagues (1978) concluded that children gained better sensory awareness and decreased neglect from this intervention. In cases of denervation, a stimulator unit that delivers direct current is necessary. Cummings (1985) stated that stimulation of denervated muscle may have a trophic influence on axonal regeneration; however, this has not been studied in young children or in children with BPI. He describes in detail the use of electrical stimulation of denervated muscles, acknowledging the controversy in

PRE   POST

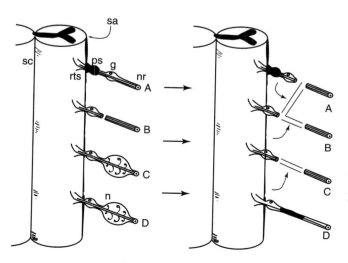

FIGURE 11–10. Neurosurgical procedures for BPI. *A,* Avulsion repair: graft (curved arrow) inserted between a rupture and the distal end of the avulsion. sa = subarachnoid space; sc = spinal cord; ps = pseudomeningocele; g = ganglion; rts = nerve rootlets; nr = nerve root. *B,* Rupture repair: graft (curved arrow) inserted to bypass disconnection. *C,* Neuroma excision: removal of neuroma (n) and grafting (curved arrow) the site. *D,* Neurolysis: removal of scar tissue (arrowhead). (From Laurent, JP, & Lee, RT. Birth-related upper brachial plexus injuries in infants: Operative and nonoperative approaches. Journal of Child Neurology, *9*[2]:111–118, April 1994. Reprinted with permission from BC Decker, Inc.)

the literature regarding its effectiveness. Others have suggested, however, that electrical stimulation may actually interfere with the process of neural regeneration.

The use of FES is also gaining popularity in postoperative programs. If a nerve that was previously denervated has gained innervation through microsurgery, FES can enhance the motor unit recruitment and provide a stronger contraction of the muscle. Electrically assisted strengthening, range of motion, and functional training can begin as the long process of reinnervation progresses.

There is a need for published research and guidelines on the use and efficacy of FES in children with BPI. Carmick (1993, 1997) has published guidelines for using FES with children with cerebral palsy. She emphasizes the importance of using FES as an adjunct to a dynamic systems or contemporary motor-learning physical therapy program utilizing task-specific activities during the sessions in which FES is administered. Until more research is available, it may be prudent to delay the implementation of an FES program until 18 months of age or older, when the majority of regeneration has occurred. Sensory loss should be carefully considered before implementing any program of FES.

Orthopedic Concerns and Surgery

Despite therapy and neurosurgery, contractures and secondary deformities are likely to occur in children who do not experience complete return. The severity and type of contracture will vary depending on the pattern of return and type of intervention the child has undergone. The most common injury, to C5 and C6, will likely result in absence or weakness of shoulder external rotation and abduction, elbow flexion, and forearm supination. Therefore the most common contractures are shoulder adduction and internal rotation, elbow flexion or extension (depending on the involvement of the triceps), and forearm pronation.

The main goal of orthopedic surgery is to provide the necessary active and passive range of motion that will enable the patient's hand to reach the head and mouth for meaningful activities of daily living. Price and Grossman (1995) provide a thorough discussion of historical and current orthopedic surgery for patients with BPI. Common surgeries include soft tissue releases (at muscle insertions or by Z-plasty), reductions of glenohumeral joint dislocations, transfers of muscles, and osteotomies. For example, Hoffer and Phipps (1998) achieved an increase in abduction of one grade and external rotation of two grades by releasing the pectoralis major, latissimus dorsi, and teres major and then transferring the latissimus dorsi and teres major to the rotator cuff. Functionally, the patients could then reach above their head for a variety of activities of daily living. Transferring a muscle can be expected to result in the loss of one muscle strength grade; therefore the muscle chosen for transfer should be as strong as possible before surgery. Grossman (1996) routinely performs releases of the subscapularis by 2 years of age on children with persistent internal rotation contractures. He recommends delaying hand and wrist reconstruction until 8 years of age when spontaneous recovery has reached a plateau and the child can fully participate in postoperative hand therapy. The literature reports a variety of surgeries that have been attempted with varying degrees of functional improvement (Hoffer & Phipps, 1998; Price & Grossman, 1995). Any parents pursuing orthopedic surgery for their child should become intimately knowledgeable of the most current research on the technique and outcome of any procedure being considered. Clearly identified functional goals should be established before any surgery.

Amputation of the involved arm has been suggested in the past and continues to be presented as a surgical option in a few centers. Most medical professionals, parents, and patients, however, do not think that this is a reasonable treatment option.

Parent Education

Providing parents with the resources at the end of this chapter is an important responsibility of the physical therapist. Parents can learn a great deal about the disorder and its treatment, follow current research, locate centers specializing in BPI, and network with other families. They should be educated before their search about the value of research from peer-reviewed journals versus anecdotal information.

Written parent educational materials translated into languages frequently spoken in the area serviced by the therapist are efficient tools to reinforce important information.

Parents should be made aware of orthopedic surgery and neurosurgery as options for their children. With the advent of managed care, physicians may be reluctant to recommend an evaluation for surgery if the client would need to go "off plan" for this specialized and expensive intervention. Parents may want to critically evaluate the success rate of any center they choose to provide these delicate surgeries. If they choose to travel to a center specializing in BPI surgery, there are sometimes resources to fund travel, lodging, and even treatment. These are best found through the agencies, support groups, and web sites listed at the end of this chapter.

Prognosis

Estimates of spontaneous recovery from BPI are difficult to establish because many children have neurapraxic lesions that resolve in several days, never entering into a study. Eng and colleagues (1978) classified 135 children with BPI into three groups based on residual deformities. The mildly affected group (70%) had minimal scapular winging, shoulder abduction of 90° or more, minimal limitation of shoulder rotation and forearm supination, normal hand function, and normal sweat and sensation. These patients were not considered to have functional problems, yet some of their involved limbs were shorter and smaller with some shoulder instability. The moderately affected group (22%) had moderate winging of the scapula, shoulder abduction less than 90° with substitution of the trapezius and serratus anterior in shoulder elevation, flexion contracture of the elbow, no forearm supination, weak wrist and finger extensors, good hand intrinsic muscles, and some loss of sweat and sensation. Eight percent were considered to have severe impairment with marked winging of the scapula, total loss of scapulohumeral rhythm, shoulder abduction less than 45°, severe elbow flexion contracture, no forearm supination, poor or no hand function, severe loss of sweat and sensation resulting in a small atrophic extremity, or agnosia in the arm.

Gilbert (1995) reported prognostic criteria established by Narakas on which many surgeons base their decisions for timing of surgery. Of 44 infants with BPI, all infants with complete recovery had contraction of the biceps and deltoid by the first month and normal contraction by the second month. A grade IV (good) outcome using Mallet's grading system (see Fig. 11-8) was not reached unless contraction of the biceps and deltoid began by the third month and was complete by the fifth month. Infants in whom neither the deltoid nor the biceps contracted by the third month could not be expected to have a good outcome. The biceps alone was chosen as a prognostic test given the difficulty in testing the deltoid.

Prevention

Risk factors for BPI can be identified before a birth. O'Leary (1992) identified maternal birth weight, prior shoulder dystocia, abnormal pelvis, maternal obesity, multiparity, and advanced maternal age as risk factors for delivering a child with shoulder dystocia. Cesarean section should be considered when a mother has multiple risk factors for a child being born with shoulder dystocia.

CASE HISTORY
BLAIR K.

Mrs. K. was at 36 weeks of gestation with her third child. She requested an ultrasound to determine the size of her baby because her second child had been born after 38 weeks of gestation at 9.7 pounds with the complication of shoulder dystocia. Her obstetrician reluctantly agreed. The fetus was estimated to be 7 pounds at 36 weeks of gestation. The physician declined Mrs. K.'s request to be induced or to have a cesarean section at 40 weeks. At 42 weeks of gestation, Mrs. K. was induced and delivered an 11-pound baby after a difficult delivery complicated by shoulder dystocia. Blair was in fetal distress with a limp left arm. Radiographs were inconclusive in establishing if there was a clavicular fracture. The intern told the family that Blair had Erb's palsy and that her hand would be in the waiter's tip position for life. On seeing the pediatric neurologist, the family was told that Blair had a "mild stretching" of the nerves, that the condition was not permanent, and that she would recover fully.

The physical therapist saw Blair on her second day of life, before discharge. The family was educated about the disorder, including precautions and prognosis. Instruction in range of motion and positioning was provided, with the parents given the opportunity to practice on a doll. They were told not to begin the exercises until the next week. They were given a packet of information on the diagnosis, exercises, terminology, support groups, and the National Brachial Plexus Association.

Initial examination at 2 days of age: Blair's left arm demonstrated no movement in the shoulder or arm except for palpable contractions in the pectoralis muscle. Her upper trapezius was active, which she used to splint the shoulder area, causing her left shoulder to be held close to her left ear. Range of motion was full in all joints. No reaction to pinching of the skin on the left arm was observed. A screening of her motor development was normal for a newborn.

Physical therapy was begun once a week at 3 weeks of age. Direct therapy was provided in the form of guided movements through developmentally appropriate gross and fine movement patterns as the weeks progressed. Tactile stimulation to individual muscles began to elicit muscle contractions in the triceps and pectoralis muscles after 4 weeks. About the same time, a weak grasp was developing when a finger was placed in Blair's hand. Range of motion in the cervical area and all upper extremity joints remained full.

The Internet and a local BPI support group provided a great deal of information to Blair's family in the ensuing weeks. The support group informed them about a hospital specializing in the management of BPI. Their local neurologist was not supportive of them pursuing surgical options for Blair because the neurologist thought the surgery was experimental. They decided to visit this hospital when Blair was 3 months of age.

3 months: Range of motion was full for all joints. Strength was returning to some muscle groups as follows: shoulder flexion (2), shoulder abduction (0), shoulder extension (2), elbow flexion (1), elbow extension (2), supination (0), wrist extension (1), and wrist flexion (3). Finger flexion and extension appeared normal. It was difficult to determine whether elbow flexion was being performed by the brachioradialis or biceps. Sensation was returning yet was not normal because responses to light touch did not elicit a response in the lower left arm.

Blair was taken to a hospital specializing in BPI at this time. She was evaluated and told to return at 6 to 7 months of age. Therapy continued once a week, and Blair continued to gain more strength in her shoulder, elbow, and hand. Her home program was modified weekly to add resistance in the form of gravity, hand-held toys, or bracelet weights to muscle groups gaining strength in the grade 3 to 4 range. Manual guidance techniques to emerging gross motor activities were taught. Careful attention was paid to identifying muscles regaining innervation and facilitating them appropriately. Other aspects of the treatment program were followed as described in the intervention section of this chapter.

6 months: Range of motion continued to be full. Blair no longer elevated her shoulder toward her ear. Strength was as follows: shoulder flexion (2+), shoulder abduction (0), shoulder extension (3), elbow flexion (1+), elbow extension (3), supination (0), wrist extension (1), and wrist flexion (3). Finger flexion and extension appeared normal. Wrist flexion was accompanied by a strong pull into ulnar deviation. A wrist cock-up splint to support weak wrist extension and prevent the ulnar deviation was provided for daytime use.

It was still unclear whether elbow flexion was being performed by the biceps, brachialis, or brachioradialis muscle. Developmentally, Blair progressed normally except for assuming quadruped and creeping, which she could not do. Sitting was asymmetric because she was afraid to shift her weight to the left (there were no functional protective reactions to that side). Weight-shifting activities on balls and the caregiver's lap while Blair was supported at the trunk were done while she was encouraged to reach for toys.

7 months: Blair returned to the hospital specializing in BPI. The family was instructed to come on a Monday and be prepared for possible exploratory surgery if indicated, on the following day. Exploratory surgery was recommended. Decisions on the surgery to be performed were determined at the time of exploration during which EMGs were performed. Nerve conduction to the deltoid was present, but not to the biceps. Surgery included removal of a neuroma and nerve grafting using the sural nerve as a donor. Blair was discharged on postoperative day 4, and her arm was placed in a sling for 10 days because of the nerve graft. Therapy resumed 10 days after surgery, twice a week. At this time, deltoid muscle activity could be palpated, but bicep strength remained at 1+. Two months after surgery, elbow flexion strength increased from 1+ to 2.

1 year: Range of motion continued to be full except for some mild scapulohumeral tightness. The left arm was slightly smaller in girth. Blair continued to prefer to use her right hand for activities of daily living, yet would use her left hand if encouraged to do so or if bilateral participation was required. Scapular winging was minimal, and based on Mallet's functional classification, Blair had grade III function. Active range was not full yet was functional for activities such as hand to mouth, using some shoulder abduction to substitute for decreased elbow flexion. She also used substitutions for the lack of wrist supination. Therapy continued once a week, and sensation and muscle strength continued to improve. Substitutions were being replaced with more normal movements, and new strategies for gaining and maintaining shoulder range were needed. Therapy activities included picking up objects from the floor and then placing them up on a table while a caregiver facilitated shoulder flexion with external rotation and forearm supination; use of a vibrator on the biceps during activities requiring elbow flexion, such as self-feeding; and utilization of fine motor skills, such as stacking rings, which requires elbow flexion and supination.

18 months: Electrical stimulation was prescribed at this time to stimulate the deltoid and biceps. Shoulder abduction was at 3−, elbow flexion 3−. Use of a stimulator that provided alternating current assisted these two active contractions to achieve close to full-range motions against gravity (3+). After 1 month of experimentation and parent instruction with the stimulator, therapy was reduced to once a week, and the parents used the stimulator 3 to 5 days a week for 30- to 60-minute sessions. At this age, Blair loved being prone on a platform swing doing push and pull activities that encouraged bilateral shoulder and elbow movements, and fast movements while prone over bolsters that elicited protective reactions and shoulder flexion.

2 years: Residual impairments at this time included mild sensory loss, decreased active shoulder and elbow range of motion (grade IV on Mallet's scale), and smaller limb girth. Passive range of motion was full, yet the family had learned that the shoulder would quickly become tight if exercises were neglected. Active ranges, as mentioned, were slightly limited yet functional for toothbrushing and hair brushing, with some substitution of shoulder abduction for lack of full elbow flexion. Some neglect of the involved arm was noticed in situations such as stair climbing because she would only use her uninvolved arm on a railing and in crayon-to-paper activities. No residual disability was apparent at this age; Blair performed all gross and fine motor activities at age-appropriate levels, with some abnormal substitutions. Electrical stimulation was discontinued because strength gains were occurring minimally. The frequency of physical therapy was decreased to once a month to monitor progress or regression and continue working on the acquisition of bilateral upper extremity skills without abnormal substitutions.

Recommended Resources

National Brachial Plexus/Erb's Palsy Association
nationalbpi@powernetonline.com
Note: This web site has many links to other BPI web sites.

"Outreach" Newsletter for consumers.
3116 E. Shea Blvd.
Box 250
Phoenix, AZ 85028-3294
E-mail: outreaching@compuserve.com

Carmick, J. Guidelines for the clinical application of neuromuscular electrical stimulation (NMES) for children with cerebral palsy. Pediatric Physical Therapy, 9:128–136, 1997.

Sheperd, RB. Brachial plexus injury. In Campbell, SK (Ed.), Pediatric Neurologic Physical therapy, 2nd ed. New York: Churchill Livingstone, 1991, pp. 101–130.

References

Ballock, RT, & Song, KM. The prevalence of nonmuscular causes of torticollis in children. Journal of Pediatric Orthopedics, 16:500–504, 1996.

Binder, H, Eng, GD, Gaiser, JF, & Koch, B. Congenital muscular torticollis: results of conservative management with long term follow-up in 85 cases. Archives of Physical Medicine and Rehabilitation, 68:222–225, 1987.

Burstein, FD, & Cohen, SR. Endoscopic surgical treatment for congenital muscular torticollis. Plastic and Reconstructive Surgery, 101: 20–24, 1998.

Carmick, J. Clinical use of neuromuscular electrical stimulation for children with cerebral palsy, part 1 and 2. Pediatric Physical Therapy, 9:128–136, 1993.

Carmick, J. Guidelines for the clinical application of neuromuscular electrical stimulation (NMES) for children with cerebral palsy. Pediatric Physical Therapy, 9:128–136, 1997.

Cheng, JCY, & Au, AWY. Infantile torticollis: a review of 624 cases. Journal of Pediatric Orthopedics, 14:802–808, 1994.

Clarke, HM, & Curtis, GC. An approach to obstetrical brachial plexus injuries. Hand Clinics, 11:563–580, 1995.

Cummings, JP. Conservative management of peripheral nerve injuries utilizing selective electrical stimulation of denervated muscle with exponentially progressive current forms. Journal of Orthopedic and Sports Physical Therapy, 7:11–15, 1985.

Davids, JR, Wenger DR, & Mubarak, S. Congenital muscular torticollis sequela of intrauterine or perinatal compartment syndrome. Journal of Pediatric Orthopedics, 13:141–147, 1993.

Emery, C. The determinants of treatment duration for congenital muscular torticollis. Physical Therapy, 74:29–36, 1994.

Eng, GD, Koch, B, & Smokvina, MD. Brachial plexus palsy in neonates and children. Archives of Physical Medicine and Rehabilitation, 59:458–464, 1978.

Gilbert, A. Obstetrical brachial plexus palsy. In Tubiana, R (Ed.), The Hand, Vol. 4. Philadelphia: WB Saunders, 1993, p. 579.

Gilbert, A. Long-term evaluation of brachial plexus surgery in obstetrical palsy. Hand Clinics, 11:583–593, 1995.

Gjorup, L. Obstetrical lesion of the brachial plexus. Acta Neurologica Scandinavica Supplementum, 18:31–58, 1965.

Grossman, JAI. Multidisciplinary treatment of patients with obstetrical brachial plexus palsy. Acta Neuropediatrica, 2:151–152, 1996.

Hoffer, MM, & Phipps, GJ. Closed reduction and tendon transfer for treatment of dislocation of the glenohumeral joint secondary to brachial plexus birth palsy. Journal of Bone and Joint Surgery (AM), 7:997–1001, 1998.

Jette, AM. Using health related quality of life measures in physical therapy outcomes research. Physical Therapy, 73:528–537, 1993.

Laurent, JP, & Lee, RT. Birth related upper brachial plexus injuries in infants: Operative and nonoperative approaches. Journal of Child Neurology, 9:111–117, 1994.

Lin, JN, & Chou, ML. Ultrasonographic study of the sternocleidomastoid muscle in the management of congenital muscular torticollis. Journal of Pediatric Surgery, 32:1648–1651, 1997.

MacDonald, J. Physiotherapy management of musculoskeletal anomalies—neonates and infants. In Burns, YR, & MacDonald, J (Eds.), Physiotherapy and the Growing Child. Philadelphia: WB Saunders, 1996, pp. 270–272.

Michelow, BJ, Clarke, HM, Curtis, CG, Zuker, RM, Seifu, Y, & Andrews, DF. The natural history of brachial plexus palsy. Plastic and Reconstructive Surgery, 93:675–680, 1994.

Morrison, D, & MacEwen, GD. Congenital muscular torticollis: observations regarding clinical findings, associated conditions, and results of treatment. Journal of Pediatric Orthopedics, 2:500–505, 1982.

Narakas, AO. Obstetrical brachial plexus injuries. In Lamb, DW (Ed.), The Hand and Upper Limb, Vol. 2: The Paralyzed Hand. Edinburgh: Churchill Livingstone, 1987, p. 116.

O'Leary, JA. Shoulder Dystocia and Birth Injury: Prevention and Treatment. New York: McGraw-Hill, 1992, pp. 11–24, 106–144.

Porter, SB, & Blount, BW. Pseudotumor of infancy and congenital muscular torticollis. American Family Physician, 52:1731–1736, 1995.

Price, AE, & Grossman, JAI. A management approach for secondary shoulder and forearm deformities following obstetrical brachial plexus surgery. Hand Clinics, 11:607–614, 1995.

Shepherd, RB. Brachial plexus injury. In Campbell, SK (Ed.), Pediatric Neurologic Physical Therapy, 2nd ed. New York: Churchill Livingstone, 1991, pp. 101–130.

Sherburn, EW, Kaplan, SS, Kaufman, BA, Noetzel, MJ, & Park, TS. Outcome of surgically treated birth-related brachial plexus injuries in twenty cases. Pediatric Neurosurgery, 27:19–27, 1997.

Taylor, JT, & Norton, ES. Developmental muscular torticollis: Outcomes in young children treated by physical therapy. Pediatric Physical Therapy, 9:173–178, 1997.

van der Weel, FRR, van der Meer, ALH, & Lee, DN. Effect of task on movement control in cerebral palsy: Implications for assessment and therapy. Developmental Medicine and Child Neurology, 33: 419–426, 1991.

Williams, CRP, O'Flynn, E, Clarke, NMP, & Morris, RJ. Torticollis secondary to ocular pathology. Journal of Bone and Joint Surgery (British), 78:620–624, 1996.

CHAPTER 12

Arthrogryposis Multiplex Congenita

MAUREEN DONOHOE, PT, PCS
DEBRA ANN BLEAKNEY, PT

Arthrogryposis multiplex congenita (AMC) is a nonprogressive neuromuscular syndrome that is present at birth. AMC is characterized by severe joint contractures, muscle weakness, and fibrosis. Although the child's condition does not deteriorate as a result of the primary diagnosis, the long-term sequelae of AMC can be very disabling. Functional limitations occur in mobility and activities of daily living (ADL) that can lead to varying degrees of disability.

Working with children with AMC presents the physical therapist with many challenges. Many children who have AMC are bright and motivated. Physical therapists must use their knowledge of biomechanics and normal development to maximize functional skills. Proper timing for therapeutic and medical interventions helps maximize the child's opportunities for independence. Creativity is needed to adapt equipment and the environment to allow the child with AMC to be as independent as possible.

In this chapter, we address the pathophysiology of AMC, its management from a medical and surgical perspective, physical therapy examination and evaluation, and specific physical therapy and team interventions used for children with AMC from infancy to adulthood.

INCIDENCE AND ETIOLOGY

Arthrogryposis is present in 1 of every 3000 to 4000 live births in the United States (Goodman & Gorlin, 1983). The etiology of AMC is unknown, but many different factors have been implicated. The insult, however, is believed to occur during the first trimester of pregnancy (Wynne-Davies et al., 1981). Insults occurring early in the first trimester have the potential for creating more involvement of the child than those that occur late in the first trimester. The basic pathophysiologic mechanism for the multiple joint contractures appears to be the lack of fetal movement (Tachdjian, 1990).

The various forms of arthrogryposis include a neuromuscular syndrome (7%); congenital anomalies (6%); chromosomal abnormalities (2%); contracture syndromes (35%); amyoplasia (43%), which is considered the "classic arthrogryposis"; and distal arthrogryposis (7%). Distal arthrogryposis, which affects primarily the hands and feet and is highly responsive to treatment, has a genetic basis and is inherited as an autosomal dominant trait (Hall et al., 1982). Gene mapping has been helpful in identifying those with arthrogryposis. Neuropathic arthrogryposis is found on chromosome 5 and can have survival motor neuron gene deletion (Burglen et al., 1996; Shohat et al., 1997). Distal arthrogryposis type I maps to chromosome 9 (Bamshad et al., 1994).

AMC is associated with neurogenic and myopathic disorders in which motor weakness immobilizes the fetal joints leading to joint contractures. It is not known whether all those with the neuropathic form of AMC have degeneration of the anterior horn cell, but of those studied postmortem, this is a consistent finding. A neurogenic disorder of the anterior horn cell is believed to cause muscle weakness with subsequent periarticular soft tissue fibrosis (Drummond et al., 1978; Goodman & Gorlin, 1983; Hall, 1989; Wynne-Davies et al., 1981). Because of the failure of the muscle to function, the joints in the developing fetus lack movement, which probably explains the stiffness and deformities of the newborn's joints. The fetus may have an imbalance in strength of oppositional muscle groups, creating the tendency toward a certain posture. For example, the fetus with good strength in the hamstrings and triceps brachii but weakness in the quadriceps and biceps brachii will have a flexed knee and extended elbow posture in utero. Decreased amniotic fluid throughout the pregnancy, but especially during the last trimester when the fetus is largest, may further inhibit freedom of movement in utero.

Although the etiology of AMC remains unknown, several factors have been implicated. Hyperthermia of the fetus is caused by a maternal fever greater than 37.8°C (100°F). Some mothers of children with AMC report having an illness with a fever for 1 to 2 days during the first trimester. Prenatal viral infection, vascular compromise between mother and fetus, or a septum in the uterus have all been suspected as causes of AMC (Wynne-Davies et al., 1981).

PROGRESS IN PRIMARY PREVENTION

Arthrogryposis appears to be a disorder of relatively recent origin because few middle-aged or elderly patients are reported (Wynne-Davies et al., 1981). Little progress has been made in the prevention of this rare disorder, given its nonspecific etiology. However, significant improvements have been made in the management of children with AMC.

DIAGNOSIS

No definitive laboratory studies exist that can diagnose AMC prenatally. The majority of AMC cases are not genetically based, and therefore prenatal amniocentesis or chorionic villous sampling may be inconsequential. If a parent or physician suspects that something is amiss, a detailed level II ultrasound evaluation can be helpful in identifying anomalies and decreased fetal movements. Ultrasound studies in subsequent pregnancies would help relieve parental anxiety.

During the first 6 months of life an immunoglobulin study may identify evidence of a viral infection. After that time, an ophthalmologist can examine the eye for pigment clumps on the retina, called chorioretinitis. This has no effect on vision but will establish whether the insult was a prenatal viral process.

Muscle biopsy in AMC varies with the muscle under study. Histologic analysis reveals that relatively strong muscles appear virtually normal, and very weak muscles reveal fibrofatty changes but may have normal muscle spindles. Embryologically, the muscles are formed normally but are replaced by fibrous and fatty tissue during fetal development (Hall, 1981, 1985). Neuropathic and myopathic changes can be seen in different muscles in the same patient with electromyographic testing (Sarwark et al., 1990). Muscle biopsies along with blood tests and clinical findings rule out progressive and fatal disorders while providing evidence to support the diagnosis of AMC.

CLINICAL MANIFESTATIONS

Clinical manifestations of AMC demonstrate great variability but generally include severe joint contractures and lack of muscle development or amyoplasia. The typical severely affected body parts in the AMC population include, in decreasing order of prevalence, the foot (67%), the hip (50%), the wrist (43%), the knee (41%), the elbow (30%), and the shoulder (4%) (Scott & Nicholson, 1992). One may see these percentages vary in the literature based on how the cases have been ascertained (i.e., care centers will see different mixes based on their specialty).

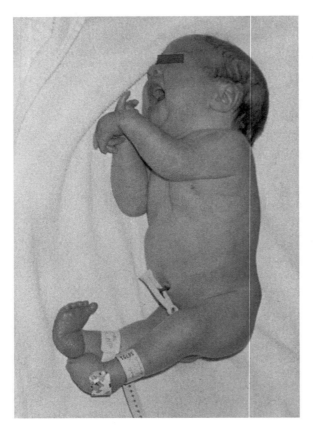

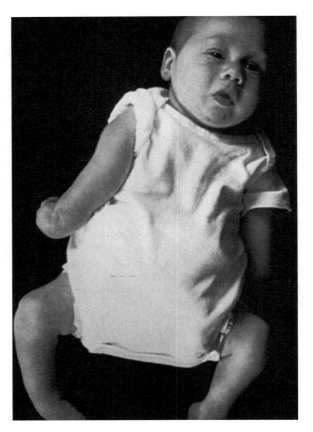

FIGURE 12–1. Infant with AMC with flexed and dislocated hips, extended knees, clubfeet (equinovarus), internally rotated shoulders, flexed elbows, and flexed and ulnarly deviated wrists.

FIGURE 12–2. Infant with AMC with abducted and externally rotated hips, flexed knees, clubfeet, internally rotated shoulders, extended elbows, and flexed and ulnarly deviated wrists.

There are two commonly seen variations of AMC. In one type, the child has flexed and dislocated hips, extended knees, clubfeet (equinovarus), internally rotated shoulders, flexed elbows, and flexed and ulnarly deviated wrists (Fig. 12–1). In another type, the child has abducted and externally rotated hips, flexed knees, clubfeet, internally rotated shoulders, extended elbows, and flexed and ulnarly deviated wrists (Fig. 12–2). Parents often describe the legs in the first type as jackknifed and in the second type as froglike. Because of the stiffness of the joints, extremity movements are described as wooden or marionette-like. The position of the upper extremities in the second type is described as the "waiter's tip" position owing to the internally rotated shoulder, extended elbow, pronated forearm, and flexed wrist. Common to both types are clubfeet, flexed and ulnarly deviated wrists, and internally rotated shoulders. Other associated characteristics may include scoliosis, dimpling of skin over joints, hemangiomas, absent or decreased finger creases, congenital heart disease, facial abnormalities, respiratory problems, and abdominal hernias. Intelligence and speech are usually normal.

MEDICAL MANAGEMENT

The main components of medical treatment include well-timed and surgical management (Hall, 1989; Palmer et al., 1985; St. Clair & Zimbler, 1985). Specific operations should be timed so that the child optimally benefits from the procedure. For example, clubfoot surgery, performed to allow plantigrade feet, is often deferred until the child is able to pull to stand and is interested in standing. The child can then easily self-stretch when standing and walking. One common clubfoot surgery is the posteromediolateral release. The entire hindfoot is opened during surgery so as to shorten the lateral column, lengthen the medial column, and lengthen the tendo

Achillis (Niki et al., 1997). Occasionally, this procedure includes using wires to realign the talus and the calcaneus. In severe cases of equinovarus and in cases in which this procedure fails, a talectomy is performed.

Children with AMC often have subluxed or dislocated hips. Dislocation is as frequently bilateral as unilateral. One dislocated hip is usually relocated to prevent secondary pelvic obliquity and scoliosis, unless the hip is extremely stiff (Sarwark et al., 1990; Staheli et al., 1987). Generally, if both hips are dislocated, they are not surgically reduced. However, there are those who advocate surgically reducing all dislocated hips. The most common approach to relocating the hips is through an anterolateral approach (MacEwen & Gale, 1983; Sarwark et al., 1990; Staheli et al., 1987; St. Clair & Zimbler, 1985; Szoke et al., 1996). It is more important to have mobile, painless, yet dislocated hips than to have very stiff but located ones. Prolonged immobilization following open or closed techniques can lead to the serious sequela of fused or stiff hips.

Moderate to severe contractures of the knee joint can be addressed surgically, but in the conservative approach one waits until the child is ambulating comfortably before surgical correction. Knee flexion contractures are most commonly associated with capsular changes within the joint. Medial and lateral hamstring lengthening or sectioning (if the muscle is fibrosed) along with a posterior capsulotomy of the knee joint may be performed (Tachdjian, 1990). These contractures inconsistently respond to hamstring lengthenings and posterior capsulotomy because there is a subsequent loss of muscle strength and risk of scar tissue leading to further joint stiffness and recurrence of the contracture. A distal femoral osteotomy is more frequently successful in realigning the joint and changes the arc of motion without risk of increased scar tissue and loss of strength (DelBello & Watts, 1996; Jayakumar, 1998) (Fig. 12–3). Knee extension contractures are frequently addressed by quadriceps lengthening if there is at least 25° of range of motion (ROM) in the knee. Intra-articular procedures such as a capsulotomy may be necessary if the knee is stiff. Some evidence suggests that knee extension contractures tend to have better results than knee flexion contractures when addressed surgically (Sodergard & Ryoppy, 1990). An important consideration before surgical intervention is determination of whether the limitation in ROM is creating functional problems with sitting or walking and if, indeed, the surgical intervention is likely to improve the child's function. For example, if the legs extend straight out when sitting, this position will interfere with sitting at school desks, in the car,

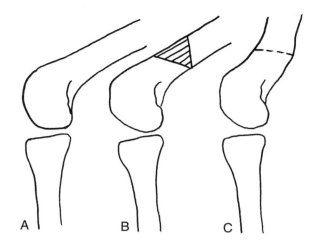

FIGURE 12–3. Diagram of a distal femoral wedge osteotomy performed to realign the contracted knee joint. A, Knee flexion contracture deformity before surgery. B, Distal femoral wedge osteotomy for reduction of the knee flexion deformity. C, Realignment after surgery.

and so on and may inhibit community involvement. The child participates in this decision-making process.

Restrictions in shoulder movement are rarely addressed through surgical interventions such as capsular or soft tissue releases because the musculature is usually inappropriate for transfer. If adequate muscle strength and control are present, surgery may be indicated to place wrists and elbows in positions of optimal function. One scenario involves a child with symmetric weakness or severe contractures of the upper extremities. In this case, a dominant arm can be identified for feeding (postured in flexion) and the other one for hygiene care (postured in extension) (Williams, 1973). If both arms are postured in extension, surgery would be necessary to position one arm in a functional flexion position. Such surgical considerations would include a pectoralis or triceps brachii transfer to give a child active elbow flexion with a posterior capsulotomy to allow for elbow flexion (Tachdjian, 1990). The muscle under consideration for transfer would need to be strong before transfer with adequate passive elbow flexion present. A consistent passive ROM and stretching program from birth is essential to maintain elbow motion for this type of surgery to be successful.

Wrists can be fused in positions for function if conservative splinting and stretching management have been unsuccessful. Wrists are fused in the dissimilar positions. Before a surgical wrist fusion, casting of the wrist for 1 week in the position of the potential fusion is suggested. During this time, the child's functional ADL skills are assessed while wearing the cast to ascertain the appropriateness of this potential surgery.

Scoliosis is frequently managed conservatively with bracing. In about one fifth of the children or adolescents with AMC, a long-C thoracolumbar scoliosis develops (Tachdjian, 1990). If the curve continues to progress, surgical fusion is considered. Most commonly, a posterior spinal fusion is performed. On large stiff curves, an anterior release of structures limiting spinal mobility may be necessary before the posterior spinal fusion to obtain satisfactory results. The type of fixation used is based on the orthopedist's preference (see Chapter 10).

IMPAIRMENT

Diagnosis and Problem Identification

The primary impairments in the child with AMC are joint limitations of movement and decreased muscle strength and bulk. Joint contractures are evident at birth, although a formal diagnosis of AMC may not be given at that time. In AMC, limitation of movement typically is seen in two or more joints in different body areas (Hall, 1989). No data are available to determine whether flexor or extensor musculature is most likely to be affected. From our experience, we have observed that approximately 65% of the children with AMC seen in our clinic have extended elbows; 35% have flexed elbows; 55% have extended knees; and 45% have flexed knees (Jayakumar, 1998).

Contractures can develop from an imbalance in muscle pull of agonist and antagonist muscles but also when symmetric weakness is present on all sides of the joint, thus hindering movement. Theoretically, this may be indicative of the point in fetal development at which the insult occurs. For example, because flexors develop before extensors in the upper extremity, a child may develop elbow flexion contractures but does not develop the usual strength in either the biceps or triceps brachii subsequent to the time of insult.

Decreased muscle bulk is evidence of muscle weakness secondary to decreased motor units in a muscle. Histologic analysis of muscles reveals nonspecific changes in the muscle such as fibrofatty scar tissue. Weakened muscles often have a fat layer around the muscle with dimpling of the skin. A muscle with a contracture but of normal strength through its available ROM may not have normal muscle bulk secondary to its inability to be active throughout the entire ROM.

Problem Identification by the Team

The team evaluation establishes a baseline from which to set realistic and functional goals. In addition to physical therapists, the primary intervention team consists of patients and their families and such medical professionals as orthopedists and geneticists, occupational therapists, and orthotists. Occasionally, speech pathologists, dentists or oral surgeons, and ophthalmologists are consulted as well. One of the goals of the primary team is to educate the family about AMC. Families are taught that arthrogryposis is a nonprogressive disorder but that without positioning, stretching, and strengthening, or possible surgery, the child's impairments could lead to further functional limitations and disability in daily life (Table 12–1).

During the initial examination by the team, photographs and videos are taken of the child depicting the child's position of comfort and detailing specific contractures such as clubfeet. This is an objective way to document changes that occur during growth and throughout splinting procedures and should be repeated every 4 months for the first 2 years.

In physical therapy, baseline goniometry is performed, documenting passive ROM and the resting position of each joint. ROM can be measured with a standard goniometer cut down to pediatric size. Active ROM is measured at the hips, knees, shoulders, elbows, and wrists. If possible, the same therapist consistently measures ROM for the child. Intratester and intertester reliability is determined for all therapists who evaluate children with AMC and should be checked annually. Functional ROM is also assessed to assist with visualizing the whole composite of motions and evaluating functional abilities. For example, functional active ranges include assessment of the hand to the mouth, ear, forehead, top of head, and back of neck.

A formal manual muscle test is performed when appropriate. Ascertaining muscle grades for infants and very young children is performed by using palpation, observation of the ability of extremities to move against gravity, and evaluation of gross motor function. The strength of the extensor muscles of the lower extremities is especially important to determine the appropriate level of bracing. Less than fair (grade 3/5) muscle strength in hip extensors will require bracing above the hip. Less than fair (grade 3/5) strength in knee extensors requires bracing above the knee. Corrected clubfeet require molded braces during growth to minimize problems of recurrent clubfeet. Children with poor upper extremity function and weak lower extremities may not be functional community ambulators as a result of

TABLE 12-1. **NCMRR Model of the Disabling Process for Children with AMC**

Pathophysiology	Impairments	Functional Limitations	Disability	Societal Limitations
Prenatal damage to the anterior horn cell resulting in neurogenic and myopathic disorder Decreased number of motor units within a muscle	Multiple joint contractures that can be progressive with growth Fibrotic joint capsule Strength limitation with imbalance of oppositional muscles Stronger muscles are often shortened	Limited functional mobility skills, including rolling, creeping, transitional movements, and higher-level mobility skills Limited ability to transfer Limited ambulation Posture and limited strength of upper extremity determine alternative mobility options Decreased endurance	Limited independence in self-care skills, including dressing and feeding Dependence in transfers for ADL, including toileting Inability to manage uneven terrain Limited endurance for ambulation Limited independence in wheelchair mobility without costly adaptations Limited participation in physical activities due to endurance and safety	Limited opportunity for play with young peers Inability to live independently Limited access to educational and work opportunities Limited access to a wide range of environments Health insurance may not pay for adaptations necessary for least restrictive mobility device Social isolation

NCMRR, National Center for Medical Rehabilitation Research.

decreased motor control and protective responses. Power mobility may be the most functional means of community locomotion.

Gross motor skills and functional levels of mobility and ADL are assessed. No current developmental tests have been designed for children with AMC, but these children usually score lower than average in formal gross motor tests secondary to inadequate strength and ROM in their extremities. Certain gross motor skills may never be attained owing to physical limitations. For example, some developmental milestones such as creeping may not be attained even though the child is able to stand and start to walk. Cognitively, children with AMC tend to score average to above average in formal developmental tests (Sarwark et al., 1990; Williams, 1978).

The therapist assesses the child for current and potential modes of functional mobility. This may include ambulation with assistive devices or the use of manual or power wheelchair or mobility devices. The therapist evaluates movement patterns and muscle substitutions used to accomplish each motor task or ADL skill.

Following assessment, a team treatment plan is established, incorporating the family early on as part of the team. The ultimate goal is to maximize the child's independence in ADL and mobility.

PHYSICAL THERAPY IN INFANCY

Physical limitations and deformities seen in infants with AMC include clubfeet, hip flexion con-

tractures, knee extension contractures, shoulder tightness (especially internal rotation), and elbow and wrist flexion contractures. At birth these children are commonly breech presentations. In another type, common posturing includes abducted and externally rotated hips, flexed knees, internally rotated shoulders, extended and pronated elbows, and flexed wrists. There may be asymmetric posturing of the extremities, which is especially problematic at the hip when dislocation of only one hip is present. The resulting asymmetry makes surgical correction the treatment of choice to relocate the hip and secondarily prevent pelvic obliquity and scoliosis.

Examination

Formal assessment of an infant with AMC begins as soon as possible after birth. The assessment consists of goniometry of passive ROM with reevaluation of ROM done on a monthly basis during this period. The therapist also documents the presence and strength of muscles based on observation of the child's movements and palpation of muscle contractions. Muscles of the trunk and upper and lower extremities are evaluated. Formal developmental assessment tools are occasionally used but reflect poorly on a child with AMC because strength and ROM limitations preclude the achievement of many motor milestones. These are the functional limitations and disabilities stemming from the initial impairments. Motor milestones in these children are often delayed or skipped. For example, because of development of good trunk control and balance and the ability to "hitch" on their buttocks, these children often bypass the creeping stage. Functional mobility and the mechanism used in attaining this mobility are more important to evaluate than is assignment of a developmental level or score. The therapist assesses rolling, prone tolerance, sitting control, scooting, creeping, crawling, transitional movements, and standing tolerance and upright mobility. Occupational therapy plays a key role in assessing feeding, ADL skills, and manipulation of objects. Physical therapists also assess the fit of any supportive or assistive devices that may have been issued.

Although it is not imperative to use formal scales in assessing these skills, some useful tests include the Alberta Infant Motor Scale, an observational tool for assessing motor milestones; the Pediatric Evaluation of Disability Inventory geared for tracking progress in children with disabilities and assessing functional limitations; the Bayley Scales of Infant Development; and the Peabody Developmental Motor Scales, in which gross motor change over time is assessed (see Chapters 1 and 2 on motor development and motor control).

Physical therapy goals for very young children include maximizing strength, improving ROM, and enhancing general sensorimotor development. Education of the family emphasizes instruction in proper positioning, stretching techniques, and the avoidance of potentially harmful activities.

Intervention Strategies

Intervention strategies focus on reducing the physical impairments through stretching, thermoplastic serial splinting, positioning, and strengthening activities. Intervention also addresses the functional limitations and disability through facilitation of developmental activities and teaching compensatory strategies, especially in ADL and alternative modes of mobility.

Development, Strength, and Mobility

Infants with the first type of AMC described earlier begin life with limited positioning options as a result of hip flexion contractures. Consequently, stretching hip flexors and prone positioning are encouraged within the first 3 months of life. Developmentally, these infants learn to roll or scoot on their bottoms as their primary means of floor mobility, because it is nearly impossible to comfortably assume the quadruped position without reinforcing a flexed posture of the upper extremities. Although

delayed in their ability to attain sitting independently, they are often able to do so by 15 months through trunk flexion and rotation. These children typically are able to stand when placed for over a year before pulling to stand is initiated by the child. Usually, the child attempts walking after clubfoot surgery is completed and the child has lower extremity orthotics.

In the past, clubfoot surgery was performed early but most often required revisions by the time the child was developmentally ready to walk. In our facility, we suggest postponement of surgery until after the first year of life so that the child has an opportunity to develop strength and a readiness to walk. Furthermore, the child is able to stand after clubfoot surgery and cast removal, which assists in stretching the feet into a plantigrade position and eliminates the need to perform multiple surgical revisions. Clubfoot surgery should be performed before 2 years of age when bony changes may occur that would necessitate more extensive osteotomy procedures rather than soft tissue releases. Also, most children begin some form of independent ambulation by the middle of their second year.

Infants with the second type of AMC posturing (hips externally rotated and flexed, knees flexed, elbows extended) have more positioning options. However, these children become frustrated with prone positioning secondary to their decreased ability to comfortably prop themselves up because of extended elbows. A towel roll or wedge under the infant's chest assists with increasing tolerance for this position. Positioning the hips in neutral rotation and neutral abduction is encouraged. Towel rolls can be placed along the lateral aspect of the thighs when the infant is sitting, and a wide Velcro band can be strapped around the thigh when the child is lying supine to keep the legs in more neutral alignment (Fig. 12-4). Developmentally, these children tend to be a little slower in attaining rolling but faster in attaining sitting and scooting than the children with the first type of posturing.

Although assuming the quadruped position and creeping are often feasible for this type of child, sitting and scooting are more energy efficient. Depending on muscle strength and the amount of bracing needed for standing, these children may never perform transitional movements from sitting to standing independently. They begin ambulating, as do their able-bodied counterparts, by the middle of their second year. Therapy focuses on addressing some key functional motor skills, such as rolling, sitting, hitching on the buttocks, standing, and strengthening those muscles that assist in maintain-

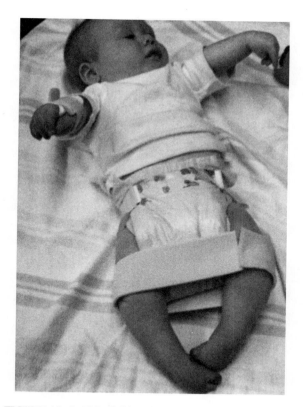

FIGURE 12–4. This child with AMC is wearing a wide Velcro band strapped around the thigh to keep the legs in more neutral alignment.

ing posture. The goal is reducing disability related to mobility.

Strengthening during the first 2 to 3 years is most frequently addressed through developmental facilitation and play. Dynamic strengthening of the trunk can be achieved by having the child reach for, swipe at, or roll toys in the positions of sitting and static standing or while straddling the therapist's leg so that the child must rotate the trunk. These maneuvers incorporate stretching and strengthening into the therapeutic play activity. One way to determine whether functional training is having a strengthening effect is to ascertain the child's improved ability to perform the task.

Self-care skills, feeding, and manipulation of objects are dependent on hand function and elbow flexibility. Those children with limited upper extremity strength may have significant functional limitations because of decreased ability to manipulate objects. Fortunately, these children tend to be resourceful in using other body parts, such as their feet or mouth, to manipulate objects when hands have inadequate strength and ROM. If the child has adequate ROM but inadequate strength, the child learns to support the arm on a leg or a table to assist in bringing the hand to the mouth. If the child is unable to get the hand to the mouth, adaptive equipment may make it possible to do some self-feeding. For example, if shoulder strength is absent, overhead arm slings are fashioned out of polyvinyl chloride piping and added to the high chair to permit finger feeding. If the upper extremities are postured in elbow extension, a typical and effective method of grasping an object is a hand cross-over maneuver, which affords some control and strength in holding or lifting an object. Toys can be adapted so that the child can operate them by use of a mercury switch attached to the head, whereby the position of the head activates the toy. These compensatory intervention strategies help decrease the child's disability by increasing independence in ADL.

Standing is an important component of therapy during the first and second years. Families are encouraged to begin standing the child at approximately 6 months of age, as is normally done with able-bodied children. During standing, lower extremities are held in as optimally corrected a position as possible before surgery through the use of splints. The sneakers can be wedged to accommodate the plantar flexion deformity and allow the child to bear weight throughout the plantar surface of the foot. Standing is initiated in a standing frame and progresses to independent static standing in the frame (Fig. 12–5). By 1 year of age, a child should be able to tolerate a total of 2 hours a day in the standing frame. This standing helps the child begin self-stretching of the feet and encourages the child to begin independent standing and walking. Dynamic standing is encouraged through games such as kicking a soccer or beach ball. Floor-to-stand activities usually do not begin to emerge until the child is ambulating securely, and sit-to-stand activities from a low chair usually begin to emerge when ambulation begins. Limitations in lower extremity strength and ROM can be addressed through splinting and bracing while the child is standing. Knee extension splints may be worn to compensate for muscle weakness and mediolateral instability of the knees.

Stretching and Splinting

Because stretching programs for joint contractures are imperative, parents and caregivers are taught a stretching regimen from the time of the initial evaluation. This intervention strategy addresses

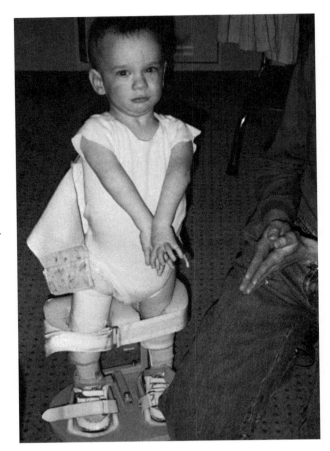

FIGURE 12–5. Child with AMC in a standing frame.

the primary impairment. A stretching program is divided into three to five sets a day with three to five repetitions during each set. Each repetition is held for 20 to 30 seconds. With the realization that this is a huge time commitment, families are taught to incorporate stretching into times when the child would normally have one-on-one time with the caregiver, such as lower extremity stretches during diaper changes and upper extremity stretches during feeding. Dressing and bath times are also opportunities for stretching, especially once the child is self-feeding and out of diapers. Stretching must be a daily lifelong commitment for a person with arthrogryposis, but consistent stretching is most critical during the growing years and especially within the first 2 years of life.

To maintain the prolonged effect of the stretch, the extremity is maintained in a comfortable position of stretch with thermoplastic splints. Attempting to maintain the maximum stretch, rather than a comfortable position, over prolonged periods will cause skin breakdown and intolerance to splints. Splints are adjusted for growth and improvements in ROM, usually every 4 to 6 weeks during infancy. When fabricating ankle-foot orthoses (AFOs) for clubfeet, the calcaneus must be aligned in a neutral position because this will affect the entire foot's position. If the calcaneus is allowed to move medially with respect to the talus, the forefoot will fall into an undesirable varus position. When the hindfoot and forefoot are in a neutral position between varus and valgus, splinting can address insufficient dorsiflexion of the hindfoot rather than forefoot. This will prevent the potential problem of a rocker-bottom foot. To be maximally effective, AFOs are worn 22 hours per day.

Knee contractures are addressed early using splinting and stretching. For the first 3 to 4 months, anterior thermoplastic knee flexion splints for extension contractures or posterior knee extension splints for knee flexion contractures are worn up to 20 hours per day. When the infant is older, we advise

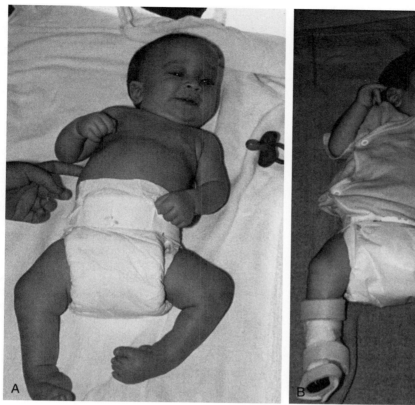
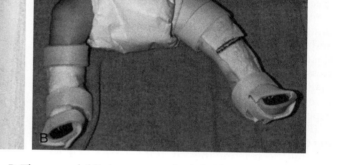

FIGURE 12–6. *A,* A child with AMC without leg splints. *B,* The same child's lower extremity is held out of the deforming positions through use of molded thermoplastic knee splints and AFOs.

that children not wear a knee flexion splint at greater than 50° of flexion for sleeping because this may encourage hip flexion contractures. Knee extension splints are worn for standing activities and sleeping, after 4 months, to encourage improved lower extremity positioning during independent floor mobility. Knee extension splints worn while sleeping also help stretch the hip flexors.

Newborns are provided with cock-up wrist splints, but splints for hands are generally provided only after 3 months of age. This allows the child to integrate the normal physiologic flexion before placing a stimulus across the palm. Two sets of hand splints are fabricated. For day use, the child wears dorsal cock-up splints with a palmar arch in a position of neutral deviation and a slight stretch into extension as tolerated. This allows the child to have fingers available to manipulate toys. For night wear, the splint is a dorsal cock-up splint with a pan to allow finger stretching when the child is sleeping.

When considering elbow splinting, note that function and independence in ADL are improved when one elbow is able to flex adequately to reach the mouth and one elbow is in adequate extension to reach the perineum. Other factors to consider include available muscle strength and ROM, response to stretching, and potential future surgical procedures. Elbow extension splints are best worn while sleeping, but elbow flexion splints and elbow flexion-assist splints tend to be most functional when worn during the day. This allows the child to experiment with the hand in a more functional position for most play activities.

In our experience, young children respond most readily to conservative treatment using serial splinting, frequent stretching, and proper positioning. In Figure 12–6A, the infant's posture is shown without leg splints. In Figure 12–6B, the infant's lower leg is held out of the deforming postures through molded thermoplastic knee and AFO splints. The key to this success is family training. Family training begins during the initial evaluation. The caretakers not only are given general information about arthrogryposis but they also receive information regarding their child's specific needs. Appropriate stretching exercises for involved joints are given with sketches or photographs to supplement the training. Subsequent visits to the physical therapist allow work on splint fabrication and modification and positioning. Developmental play ideas are incorporated into the exercises to help the child progress developmentally. Therapists also work with the family to adapt age-appropriate toys to stimulate the child physically and cognitively.

PHYSICAL THERAPY IN THE PRESCHOOL PERIOD

During the preschool period, the child's functional abilities and disabilities vary based on the degree of involvement. Poor upper extremity function from the contractures and lack of muscle strength limit the child's independence in feeding, dressing, and playing at a time when typical peers are relishing their independence. This may be particularly distressing for the parents, who are struck with the magnitude of the child's limitations when the child is no longer an infant in whom dependency is expected.

The impairments and functional limitations during this stage are similar to those found in the younger child. Restriction in joint ROM continues to be a problem secondary to rapid growth changes. Ambulation is often limited by decreased use of upper extremities and poor protective responses.

Examination

Passive and active ROM continue to be closely monitored by the therapist and caregivers. Proper fit of the splints is imperative in providing adequate stretch and positioning to impede the development of further deformities.

Functional muscle strength is an important component in the preschooler because it determines to a great degree the extent of bracing necessary and level of independence in self-care skills. Formal manual muscle testing, as defined by Kendall and colleagues (1993) or Daniels and Worthingham (1986), becomes more appropriate during this period because the child can comprehend verbal instructions. When testing strength, it is important to grade the resistance throughout the arc of motion because the child with AMC will frequently be strong in the midrange but unable to move the extremity to the shortened end range. This finding is significant because the end range is where the child needs to work the muscle to maintain stretch of the antagonist muscles.

Gait assessment should include distance, use of assistive devices, speed, symmetry of step length, gait deviations, and muscle activity. Some children ambulate as their primary means of locomotion; others rely on a stroller for community mobility. Mobility with wheelchairs is not usually addressed until school age when slow speed of ambulation, endurance, and safety concerns may preclude the child from interacting with peers.

Goals

Ability rather than disability must be stressed, with a strong emphasis on assisting the child through problem solving rather than through physical assistance. The ultimate goals for this age are to reduce the disability and enhance independent ambulation and mobility with minimum bracing and use of assistive devices. Physical and environmental structural barriers may limit achievement of some fine and gross motor skills, but social skill attainment is paramount. Another goal is for the team to work together to improve the child's function in basic ADL skills.

Intervention Strategies

The team will work together during the preschool period to solve basic ADL challenges, such as independent feeding and toileting. For example, the use of a lightweight reacher may assist with dressing skills. Preschoolers usually can self-feed with adaptive equipment. These children are often toilet trained but lack the ability to perform the task independently.

Stretching

The need for stretching at this age continues to be addressed despite the preschooler's decreased tolerance to passive stretching three to five times a day. Two times a day for the stretching program is more realistic and, in our experience, maintains ROM adequately in most cases. Families report that the best time for this is during dressing and bathing, which incorporates the program into an automatic part of the daily routine. Children can be taught how to assist with stretching through positioning. The child is also encouraged to verbally participate in the program, for example, by counting the number of repetitions. AFOs and positional splints continue to be worn to maintain the achieved positions.

Independent mobility in a safe and efficient manner is important for the preschooler to achieve and enhance social skills, as well as allow functional mobility. Independent ambulation with supportive bracing and with as few assistive devices as possible is stressed. Children with adequate strength and ROM who do not require bracing to walk generally need an AFO to prevent recurring clubfeet deformities. An articulating AFO, which provides forefoot control but allows for ankle dorsiflexion and stretch of the hindfoot during gait, is sometimes appropriate. Older preschoolers with AMC are generally in the level of bracing that will be continued throughout school age.

Bracing

Most braces now used are made of lightweight polypropylene and are more durable, less cumbersome, and more adjustable than the metal braces used previously. Children with knee extension contractures tend to require less bracing than those with knee flexion contractures. If there is any question about the child's ability to maintain an upright position without hip support, the child's first set of long leg braces, a hip-knee-ankle-foot orthosis, will include a pelvic band. This type of orthosis is used for several reasons. The family may perceive that the child is regressing if a pelvic band is found to be needed and then added after unsuccessful ambulation without the pelvic band. The pelvic band encourages neutral rotation and abduction of the lower extremities. The pelvic band can also facilitate full available hip extension, and the hips can be locked in that position for prolonged standing. Once the child is ambulating with both hips unlocked, without jackknifing at the hips during stance, the pelvic band can be removed.

Maintaining hip strength, especially when the pelvic band is removed, continues to be important. One activity is to have the child begin static and dynamic standing on the tilt board. The child also begins taking steps forward, backward, and sideways. Strengthening, as with progressive resistive exercises, may be appropriate at this time. Our clinical experience suggests that muscles may increase in strength by one-half muscle grade with exercise.

Ideally, the least amount of bracing is optimal, but if decreasing the bracing requires the child to use an assistive device that was previously unnecessary, the increased bracing may be more appropriate. A child with strong extensors such as the gluteus maximus and quadriceps is more functional than a child who requires bracing as a functional substitute for the extensors. The child with a good deal of bracing has difficulty donning and removing braces and is usually dependent for locking and unlocking hip and knee joints for standing and sitting.

Those children learning to walk may be limited in their independence if they do not have adequate strength and ROM to manipulate the assistive device, such as a walker, that is required to ambulate. Walkers are often heavy and cumbersome for the child, who may have inadequate protective responses in standing and upper extremity limitations. Thermoplastic material can be molded to the walker for forearm support when hand function is limited, affording the child added support and control (Fig. 12-7). Many children prefer to walk with someone rather than use a walker while they are gaining confidence in ambulatory skills. When learning to stand and walk, it is of utmost importance that the child learn how to use the head and trunk in order to stand and balance, and then weight shift for limb advancement. Those children who use ring- or trunk-supported walkers for ambulation often are delayed in learning these balance skills and are consequently limited in using upright control of balance for transfers and ADL.

Children with weak quadriceps and knee flexion contractures tend to ambulate with locked knee and ankle-foot orthoses. These braces can be fabricated

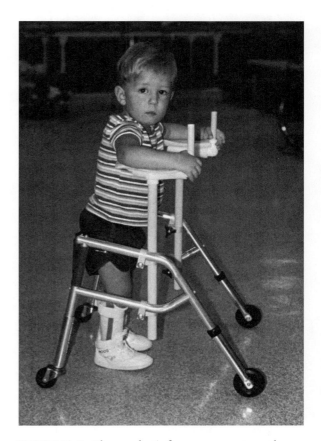

FIGURE 12–7. Thermoplastic forearm supports can be customized to the walker.

with dial knee locks so that the knee position can be adjusted to coincide with the changing state of the knee flexion contracture. This will afford the ongoing opportunity to stretch out the contracture. Shoes may need external wedges to compensate for hip and knee flexion contractures that interfere with static standing. The child should be able to comfortably balance with the feet plantigrade without upper extremity support. For walking, assistive devices can be customized with thermoplastic material to allow for less awkward hand grips. Very lightweight crutches can be custom-made of polyvinyl chloride pipe and thermoplastic material to give the child maximal independence (Fig. 12–8). Families may require assistance in identifying and removing environmental barriers that impede the child's independence.

Children in this age group are encouraged to participate in activities with children the same age in day care, swimming classes, and other peer group activities. They are encouraged to develop relationships with children who do not have disabilities, as well as with those who do. These relationships may influence the children to think and act not out of a response to disabilities but toward creative solutions. During the preschool period, many states mandate therapy services for children with special needs. Preschool services, as well as additional therapy services, are imperative for maximizing these children's skills for the demands they will encounter during school.

PHYSICAL THERAPY DURING THE SCHOOL-AGE AND ADOLESCENT PERIOD

The focus of physical therapy moves from the outpatient clinic into the classroom at this stage. The majority of children are mainstreamed, although they may have adaptive physical education, physical therapy, occupational therapy, and speech services to enhance the educational process.

Disabilities include limitations in mobility, now with the added constraints of needing to quickly traverse greater distances, which complicates the independent mobility issue. Efficient and independent dressing, feeding, and toileting abilities take on a more compelling nature. Joint contractures continue to be problematic especially through the last few growth spurts. This is a time when the adolescent is becoming more independent in self-care and adult monitoring of contractures tends to decrease. Appropriate intervention often is postponed or ignored because of time and social considerations.

Examination

The school therapist acts as a team member, addressing goals of the child and family in regard to enhancing the child's educational experience. The physical therapy examination determines what types of training and adaptive equipment are needed to achieve educational objectives. Functional ADL skills are assessed to ascertain how efficiency and independence can be improved.

Goals

During this period, the child with AMC must be responsible for self-care and for an exercise program to be performed to the best of the child's ability. The family must also become more responsible for expecting and allowing the child to be more independent. Addressing these goals reduces the overall disability. The goal of independence in mobility and

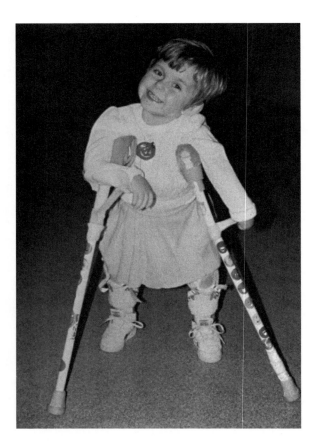

FIGURE 12–8. Child with AMC wearing polypropylene braces and using lightweight custom-made crutches constructed with polyvinyl chloride pipe.

keeping up with friends is important in the development of peer relationships. ROM continues to be a focus in management of impairment because a child with AMC will lose motion if he or she does not continue to stretch throughout the growing years. Teenagers who are going through their final growth spurt will often lose a significant amount of extension at the knees and the hips. If the teenager is not conscientious about night splint use and positioning for stretch, the ability to walk may be lost. Surgical intervention to regain ambulation skill during the second decade of life is not always an option.

Intervention Strategies

Dressing, toileting, and feeding may require adaptive equipment or setup for the child to be independent. Children with AMC require some selective pieces of adaptive equipment for achieving independence, but most are adaptable and innovative in using compensatory strategies rather than relying on assistive devices to achieve their goals. Frequently, classroom chairs and tables must be at custom-made heights to accommodate rising from a chair without manipulating brace knee locks. The desk top may need to be adjusted so that the child, by using a mouthstick or a wrist aid to hold crayons, can maneuver items on the desk or write (Fig. 12–9). Implementation of ideas such as these limits disability by providing the child with successful compensatory strategies.

Continued compliance with the customized splinting and stretching program is expected. Children at this age may lose a few degrees of motion during growth, but further regression may result in loss of function and independence. Surgical intervention is sometimes helpful to improve joint position. A self-stretching program, utilizing assistive straps, braces, and positioning, can be incorporated into the child's routine to promote independence in attaining goals. The adolescent must be permitted to help plan his or her schedule, or compliance can be expected to be poor. Adaptive physical education in school can be an adjunct to physical therapy for promoting strength, endurance, and mobility.

Speed and safety in independent mobility are important in the development of peer relationships. Families may be counseled during this time to look toward electrically powered mobility devices as an adjunct to previous mobility devices. Cumbersome bracing, inefficient gait, and poor upper extremity function can limit a child's ability to participate in playground or social activities. Alternative modes of mobility may allow the child to participate safely. Use of alternative modes need not preclude ambulation but rather provides supplemental mobility for safety and energy conservation. Most children can achieve functional household ambulation but require a wheelchair for efficient community mobility.

TRANSITION TO ADULTHOOD

We could find no published studies that address the transition to adulthood for children with AMC. Much of what we present in this section is derived from interviews with individuals with AMC. Disabilities in adulthood relate to continued problems achieving independence in ADL, ambulation, and mobility. Those who required assistance with ADL during their school-age years continued to require assistance throughout their lifetime but were able to achieve a degree of independence with feeding, dressing, and grooming using selected assistive ADL devices.

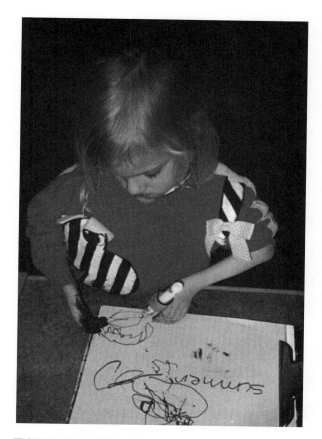

FIGURE 12–9. Child with AMC using a wrist aid to hold a crayon.

Problems

Some specific problems that occur in adults are arthritic changes in weight-bearing joints and overuse syndromes in muscles that are used for compensation or unique postures. Carpal tunnel problems and neuropathies may develop as a result of prolonged joint constrictions and deformities. Mobility problems emerging later in life may stem from secondary degenerative changes and muscle overuse syndrome (Hall, 1989). Manually or electrically powered wheelchairs, therefore, may be more commonly used than during the school-age years. Adults with AMC often use a wheelchair as their primary mode of mobility.

Advanced education is of utmost importance so that the adult with AMC becomes trained in a specialized skill or field. The type of work chosen will depend on the degree of functional limitations, education, and marketable skills. Desk work and computer work tend to be high employment options.

Many of the barriers that the adult with AMC will meet are physical barriers. Through the enactment of the Americans with Disabilities Act, attempts are being made to reduce the presence of these physical barriers. Through advancements in technology, patients with arthrogryposis have opportunities available to them to enhance their freedom of mobility and their career options. Assistive technology can be of value in helping the patient safely and efficiently achieve work and leisure goals. Adult rehabilitation facilities, although probably unfamiliar with AMC owing to the small number of adults who have AMC, can provide services regarding assistive technology and orthotics.

Technology for independent driving can provide customized equipment to accommodate the special needs of these drivers. Computerization and voice-activated equipment may provide new freedoms for this population.

Intervention Strategies

Once skeletal growth has stopped, stretching is not as imperative, but maintaining flexibility and proper positioning is encouraged to impede the further development of deformities. Those with AMC who used orthoses during the school-age years continue to do so throughout adulthood. Those who used only ankle-foot orthoses for clubfoot control tend not to need these orthoses once growth is complete. One intervention required is joint conservation, which addresses the secondary impairments resulting from degenerative changes.

Information about the long-term sequelae of AMC in relation to degenerative changes, mobility levels, and use of adaptive ADL devices is critical to providing the most effective therapy to persons with AMC. However, there is a lack of research regarding the extent of independence of these children, adolescents, and adults in the area of ADL, use of manual or power chairs, and ambulation ability. This lack of data may be because the children are followed early on within a medical model addressing their primary orthopedic concerns, but when they transfer to the educational setting and to less medical intervention they are lost to follow-up. To meet the objective of providing the most appropriate therapy to these children, a nationwide database on functional independent outcomes, mobility, and associated long-term problems must be established.

CONCLUSION

Arthrogryposis poses a variety of challenges for the health care team throughout the patient's lifetime. Although AMC is nonprogressive, its sequelae can be disabling. There is variability in clinical manifestations, but severe joint contractures and lack of muscle development are hallmarks of the disease. Each stage of development requires special attention for maximizing the child's function. An early goal of the team is to educate the family about AMC and to create the understanding that, without intervention, the child's impairments could lead to further functional limitations and disability. Early medical and therapeutic management includes vigorous stretching, splinting, positioning, and strengthening, which allow the child to develop optimal positions for functional ADL and enhance motor skill development. Timing of surgical procedures is critical to minimize intervention while maximizing benefits.

During infancy, motor milestones are often delayed or skipped, and determining functional mobility is more important than ascribing a developmental level. The intervention strategies focus on reducing physical impairments through serial splinting and strengthening and on facilitating developmental activities. Ambulation is a preliminary primary goal, but once the child reaches school age, the focus shifts toward more independent, functional, and safe mobility. During the school-age years, the child must become more responsible for stretching exercises because stretching is an integral part of the program throughout the growing years. The team emphasizes assisting the child with problem solving and working toward independent mobility. Adaptive equipment is often necessary to allow the child with AMC to be independent in mobility and self-care. A comprehensive and integrated team approach is critical in developing strategies to meet these challenges.

CASE HISTORY
WILL

Will was first seen by a physical therapist at 12 days of age. He was referred to physical therapy by our orthopedic department. During the initial evaluation, photographs were taken to document positions of his extremities. Will exhibited postures with extended elbows; flexed and pronated wrists; and hips in flexion, abduction, and external rotation (see Fig. 12-2). An x-ray examination determined that the right hip was dislocated. Formal goniometry was performed.

The family was instructed in passive ROM of the lower extremities during diaper changes and of the upper extremities during feeding. The following week, therapists fabricated customized low-temperature thermoplastic splints. These included AFOs, knee extension splints, and wrist splints. The infant was treated by physical therapists and occupational therapists every 3 to 4 weeks to adjust the splints and monitor the home program.

At 3 months of age, the therapists initiated the use of elbow flexion splints worn 23 hours per day. The family was taught to position the legs in a less abducted posture by wrapping a wide Velcro band around the thighs (see Fig. 12-4). Hip flexion contractures were reduced to 25° bilaterally, and hip adduction was to neutral (0°) bilaterally. Knee flexion contractures were 30° on the right and 25° on the left. Forefoot abduction was 0 to 5° on the right and 0 to 10° on the left.

Muscle testing determined by palpation and observation of active movement revealed active hip flexion, extension, and abduction. The hamstrings were active against gravity. The contractions of the quadriceps and plantar flexors were palpable. No biceps brachii contraction was palpable. There was, however, active shoulder flexion against gravity and at least fair strength of the pectoralis and triceps brachii. Ultrasound of the hips revealed that both hips were well seated.

At 6 months of age, Will began use of a standing frame using knee extension splints, AFOs, and wedged sneakers. At 7 months of age, Will began sitting independently once placed in that position. At 10 months, he was rolling for locomotion and was able to "commando crawl" occasionally. He was able to sit in a straddle position on the floor and tolerate dynamic challenges to his balance. He could move from supine to sitting while the lower extremities were stabilized.

Will was enrolled in a center-based early intervention program at 12 months of age. In this program, he received physical therapy three times a week with the goals of independent mobility, improving ROM through stretching and positioning, and work on pre-ambulation activities. Will was treated on a monthly outpatient basis through our clinic for program updates, and the family continued the stretching program two to three times per day. During this time, the potential use of adaptive equipment such as slings for play and feeding was explored. Splints were adjusted to accommodate the improving ROM.

At 14 months of age, Will independently maneuvered from prone to sitting by widely abducting his hips and using his arms to raise and lower his trunk. By 16 months of age, he could stand independently in leg splints and wedged sneakers, but his hips were very abducted and he required upper extremity support. A wide elastic strap was used in a figure-eight pattern around his thighs to reduce the abducted posture. Once this excessively abducted posturing was prevented, he was able to achieve a step but needed facilitation for weight shifting.

By 20 months of age, Will was excited about standing and wanted to stand all the time. When he was supported under the axillae, he would walk. At 22 months of age, Will underwent bilateral posterior mediolateral releases for his clubfeet, which were subsequently placed in casts for 8 weeks. During that time, he used a cart for mobility. After cast removal, custommade hip-knee-ankle-foot orthoses were fabricated and preambulation training began. He started standing with a posterior walker with the braces unlocked at the hips and rapidly progressed to taking two steps with the walker. During this period, Will received physical therapy three times per week, with concentration on independent standing and walking and adaptive aquatics two times per week. By 27 months of age, he was able to stand independently with both hips unlocked and could take two steps without upper extremity support.

At 30 months, Will was able to walk 600 feet with a walker and unlocked hip joints. He was also able to walk 6 feet without any assistive device. Gait training without the pelvic band on his braces was begun but required verbal cues to avoid abducting the lower extremities during gait.

At 7 years of age, Will is in second grade. He has had distal femoral osteotomies at the age of 6 for persistent knee flexion contractures. He had a triceps transfer and posterior elbow capsulotomy on the left upper extremity followed by a left wrist fusion into neutral at age 5 to allow for greater independence in ADL. He ambulates unlimited distances with knee-ankle-foot orthoses and is able to walk household distances without braces. He is able to toilet and feed himself independently.

At the current time, Will receives weekly educationally based physical therapy. Emphasis of therapy is independent mobility within the educational environment. Stair ambulation continues to be a challenge but is necessary for fire drills. He is working on managing his braces, including donning, removing, and locking. He is actively working on a self-stretching program with emphasis on stretching knees into extension. He continues working on managing books throughout the hallways and in the classroom. Power mobility has been discussed with Will and his family for middle school when his walking requirements will be more substantial.

CASE HISTORY
YURI

Yuri is a 14-year-old boy who lives in an urban environment. He attends ninth grade at his local high school. He is active with his friends, skateboarding throughout the neighborhood and playing the drums in a band. He lives with his parents, his 3-year-old brother, and his mobility dog Nancy in a small seventh floor apartment. Nancy helps Yuri in picking objects up off the floor, opening doors, and managing light switches. Yuri's primary means of mobility is ambulation with knee-ankle-foot orthoses and crutches with a swing-through gait pattern. He has a motorized scooter for long distances and school. A manual wheelchair is used for sports-related activities and is sometimes pulled by his dog. Yuri's daily routine involves lying on a wedge with weights on his hips and ankles for 30 minutes before independently donning his braces in the morning. He had been placed on consultative therapy services for the past year because of his physical limitations not interfering with his educational process. In the past year, the major change in his routine was that he no longer had someone closely tracking his joint contractures. In 1 year, his knee flexion contractures went from 45 to 85°. If his contractures progress further, he will no longer be able to lock his braces and therefore he will not be able to walk.

Yuri was referred to physical therapy at our clinic to improve his lower extremity alignment. He was deemed an inappropriate candidate for knee surgery because he had only a 20° arc of motion. If his knees were surgically extended, he would not have adequate knee flexion to sit in a chair.

Examination revealed that Yuri was sitting with his knees flexed more than 12 hours per day because of school and homework requirements. Much of that time he was actively swinging his feet because, he said, "It feels good to move." Yuri has 3/5 strength in his hamstrings and 1/5 strength in his quadriceps. Yuri sleeps with his hips and knees flexed. When walking, he is weight bearing on the end of the toe of his brace despite the fact that he has wedged sneakers.

Physical therapy involved negotiating what would be most effective for gaining ROM without limiting Yuri's independence. He was unwilling to have his braces extended further to give him a bigger stretch when locked because he would no longer be independent in lock management. He was molded for bivalved knee extension casts for night wear. He is having the posterior aspect of his knee ultrasounded while on stretch followed by extension activities in a standing position. Heel wedges were adjusted on his shoes to allow standing with the entire foot on the floor. Yuri is keeping his braces locked during the school day except for when he needs to maneuver into tight spaces with his scooter. He was willing to avoid swinging his feet when he realized that that motion was strengthening his contractures. Diligent work on Yuri's part resulted in a 30° decrease in knee flexion contractures in 3 months. He is now actively bearing weight on the full sole of his brace and has his braces extended to his end range at the knee.

Recommended Resources

Avenues: A National Support Group for Arthrogryposis Multiplex Congenita.
Web site: http://www.sonnet.com/avenues.
E-mail: avenues@sonnet.com.

Arthrogryposis Bulletin Board:
Web site: http://www.support-group.com/cgi-bin/sg/get_links?amc

National Arthrogryposis Foundation Video.
E-mail: GAF1016@aol.com.

Alfred I. duPont Hospital for Children:
Web site: http://www.kidshealthnetwork/ai/service/arthrogryposis.html.

References

Bamshad, M, Watkins, WS, Zenger, RK, Bohnsack, JF, Carey, JC, Otterud, B, Krakowiak, PA, Robertson, M, & Jorde, LB. A gene for distal arthrogryposis type I maps to the pericentromeric region of chromosome 9. American Journal of Genetics, 55:1153–1158, 1994.

Burglen, L, Amiel, J, Viollet, L, Lefebura, S, Burlet, P, Clermont, O, Raclin, V, Landriau, P, Verloes, A, Munnich, A, & Melki, J. Survival motor neuron gene deletion in arthrogryposis multiplex congenita–spinal muscular atrophy association. Journal of Clinical Investigation, 98(5):1130–1132, 1996.

Daniels, L, & Worthingham, C. In Venable, B (Ed.), Muscle Testing: Techniques of Manual Examination, 5th ed. Philadelphia: WB Saunders, 1986.

DelBello, DA,& Watts, HG. Distal femoral extension osteotomy for knee flexion contracture in patients with arthrogryposis. Journal of Pediatric Orthopedics, 16:122–126, 1996.

Drummond, DS, Siller, TN, & Cruess, RL. Management of arthrogryposis multiplex congenita. In AAOS Instructional Lectures, Montreal, Canada, 1978.

Goodman, RM, & Gorlin, RJ. Arthrogryposis. In Goodman, RM, & Gorlin, RJ (Eds.), The Malformed Infant and Child. New York: Oxford University Press, 1983, pp. 42–43.

Hall, JG. An approach to congenital contractures (arthrogryposis). Pediatric Annals, *10*:249–257, 1981.

Hall, JG. Genetic aspects of arthrogryposis. Clinical Orthopedics, *194*:44, 1985.

Hall, JG. Arthrogryposis. American Family Physician, *39*(1):113–119, 1989.

Hall, JG, Reed, SD, & Green, G. The distal arthrogryposis: Delineation of new entities—review and nosologic discussion. American Journal of Medical Genetics, *1*:185–239, 1982.

Jayakumar, S. Personal communication. Alfred I. duPont Institute, Department of Orthopedics, Wilmington, DE, July 1998.

Kendall, FP, McCreary, EK, & Provance, PG. Muscle and Function, 4th ed. Baltimore: Williams & Wilkins, 1993.

MacEwen, GD, & Gale, DI. Hip disorders in arthrogryposis multiplex congenita. In Katz, J, & Siffert, R (Eds.), Management of Hip Disorders in Children. Philadelphia: JB Lippincott, 1983, pp. 209–228.

Niki, H, Staheli, L, & Mosca, VS. Management of clubfoot deformity in amyoplasia. Journal of Pediatric Orthopaedics, *17*(6):803–807, 1997.

Palmer, PM, MacEwen, GD, Bowen, JR, & Matthews, PA. Passive motion therapy for infants with arthrogryposis. Clinical Orthopedics and Related Research, *194*:54–59, 1985.

Sarwark, JF, MacEwen, GD, & Scott, CI. Amyoplasia (a common form of arthrogryposis). Journal of Bone and Joint Surgery (American), *72*:465–469, 1990.

Scott, CI, & Nicholson, L. Personal communication. Alfred I. duPont Institute, Genetics Department, Wilmington, DE, 1992.

Shohat, M, Lotan, R, Magal, N, Shohat, T, Fishel-Ghodsian, N, Rotter, J, & Jaber, L. A gene for arthrogryposis multiplex congenita neuropathic type is linked to D5S394 on chromosome 5qter. American Journal of Human Genetics, *61*:1139–1143, 1997.

Sodergard, J, & Ryoppy, S. The knee in arthrogryposis multiplex congenita. Journal of Pediatric Orthopedics, *10*:177–182, 1990.

Staheli, LT, Chew, DE, Elliot, JS, & Mosca, VS. Management of hip dislocations in children with AMC. Journal of Pediatric Orthopedics, *7*:681–685, 1987.

St. Clair, HS, & Zimbler, S. A plan of management and treatment results in the arthrogrypotic hip. Clinical Orthopedics and Related Research, *194*:74–80, 1985.

Szoke, G, Staheli, LT, Jaffe, K, & Hall, J. Medial-approach open reduction of hip dislocation in amyoplasia-type arthrogryposis. Journal of Pediatric Orthopaedics, *16*:127–130, 1996.

Tachdjian, MO. Arthrogryposis multiplex congenita (multiple congenital contractures). In Tachdjian, M (Ed.), Pediatric Orthopedics. Philadelphia: WB Saunders, 1990, pp. 2086–2114.

Williams, PF. The elbow in arthrogryposis. Journal of Bone and Joint Surgery (British), *55*:834, 1973.

Williams, P. The management of arthrogryposis. Orthopedic Clinics of North America, *9*:67–88, 1978.

Wynne-Davies, R, Williams, PF, & O'Conner, JCB. The 1960s epidemic of arthrogryposis multiplex congenita. Journal of Bone and Joint Surgery (British), *63*:76–82, 1981.

Bibliography

Brown, LM, Robson, MJ, & Sharrard, WJW. The pathophysiology of arthrogryposis multiplex congenita neurologica. Journal of Bone and Joint Surgery (British), *62*:291–296, 1980.

Davidson, J, & Beighton, P. Whence the arthrogrypotic? Journal of Bone and Joint Surgery (British), *58*:492–495, 1976.

Fisher, RL, Johnstone, WT, Fisher, WH, & Goldkamp, OG. Arthrogryposis multiplex congenita: A clinical investigation. Journal of Pediatrics, *76*:255, 1970.

Hageman, G, Ippel, EP, Beemer, FA, DaPater, JM, Lindhout, D, & Willemse, J. The diagnostic management of newborns with congenital contractures and nosologic study of 75 cases. American Journal of Medical Genetics, *30*:883–904, 1988.

Hall, JG, Reed, SD, & Driscoll, EP. Amyoplasia: A common sporadic condition with congenital contractures. American Journal of Medical Genetics, *15*:579–590, 1983.

Hall, JG, Reed, SD, Scott, CI, Rogers, JG, Jones, KL, & Camarano, A. Three distinct types of X linked AMC seen in 6 families. Clinical Genetics, *21*:81–97, 1982.

Kamil, NI. A dynamic elbow flexion splint for an infant with arthrogryposis. American Journal of Occupational Therapy, *44*:460–461, 1990.

Lai, MM, Tettenborn, MA, Hall, JG, Smith, LJ, & Berry, AC. A new form of autosomal dominant arthrogryposis multiplex congenita. Journal of Medical Genetics, *28*:701–703, 1991.

Lloyd-Roberts, GC, & Lettin, AWF. Arthrogryposis multiplex congenita. Journal of Bone and Joint Surgery (British), *52*:494, 1970.

Mead, NG, Lithgaw, WC, & Sweeney, HJ. Arthrogryposis multiplex congenita. Journal of Bone and Joint Surgery (American), *40*:1285, 1958.

Robinson, RO. AMC: Feeding, language and other health problems. Neuropediatrics, *21*:177–178, 1990.

Sack, GH. A dominantly inherited form of AMC with unusual dermatoglyphics. Clinical Genetics, *14*:317–323, 1978.

Schiulli, C, Corradi-Scalise, D, & Donatelli-Schulthiss, ML. Powered mobility vehicles as aides in independent locomotion for very young children. Physical Therapy, *68*:997–999, 1988.

CHAPTER
13

Osteogenesis Imperfecta

DEBRA ANN BLEAKNEY, PT
MAUREEN DONOHOE, PT, PCS

Osteogenesis imperfecta (OI) is an inherited disorder of connective tissue. Other terms in the literature used to describe OI include fragilitas ossium and brittle bones. OI has an incidence of 1 in 20,000 live births, and its prevalence in the population is 16 per million (Wynne-Davies & Gormley, 1981). This disorder comprises a number of distinct syndromes and has great variability in its manifestations. The salient impairments of OI are lax joints, weak muscles, and diffuse osteoporosis, which results in multiple recurrent fractures. These recurring fractures, sustained from even minimal trauma, coupled with weak muscles and lax joints, result in major deformity. Additional impairments in OI with variable presentation include blue sclerae, dentinogenesis imperfecta, deafness, hernias, easy bruising, and excessive sweating. Without early and adequate intervention, these problems in children with OI may lead to irreversible deformities and disability. Physical therapy can have a positive impact on these children and their families. Therapists can accomplish this through strengthening exercises, adapting the environment, and educating the caregivers. Early physical therapy intervention helps prevent deformities and disability.

Too often children and adolescents with OI are overprotected as a result of the recurring fractures, leading to social isolation. This contributes to difficulty in interacting in peer play, adjusting to regular school, and achieving an independence level necessary to accomplish vocational goals. Because most children with OI have average or above-average intelligence, they may greatly benefit from a stimulating educational environment. These children usually become productive members of society. The management of their disabilities should therefore be directed toward obtaining optimal independence, social integration, and educational achievement. The overall prognosis of OI and its long-term sequelae depend on the severity of the disease, which ranges from severe to very mild. Likewise, the range of disability is from extremely severe, with death occurring at birth or shortly thereafter, to relatively mild, with no deformities.

In this chapter, we address the classification and pathophysiology of OI, medical and surgical interventions, physical therapy examination, and evaluation and interventions from infancy through adulthood. A case history of a child with OI is presented.

CLASSIFICATION

OI manifests as a group of impairments that vary in severity and that are marked by fragility of bone. It is not a single genetic disorder but is heterogeneous.

Because of the wide spectrum of this disease, there are many proposed classifications (Falvo et al., 1974; Sillence, 1981). Looser (1906) classified OI into two types: OI congenita and OI tarda. Seedorf (1949) further subclassified OI tarda into two types: tarda gravis and tarda levis. Historically, OI was classified based on clinical and descriptive characteristics (i.e., fracture healing and spinal deformities). The OI congenita and tarda classification system has clinical usefulness but does not reflect the scope of OI from a genetic or pathogenetic standpoint; however, the clinician will often see this classification system referenced in the literature and in patients' medical records.

Osteogenesis imperfecta congenita (OIC), the most severe and disabling form, is characterized by numerous fractures at birth, dwarfism, bowing or deformities of the long bones, blue sclerae (80% of cases), and dentinogenesis imperfecta (80% of cases). Infants with OIC have a poor prognosis, with a high mortality rate resulting from either intracranial hemorrhage at birth or recurring respiratory tract infections during infancy (Tachdjian, 1990).

Osteogenesis imperfecta tarda (OIT), considered the milder form of OI in which fractures occur after birth, has been subclassified based on either the degree of bowing of the extremities or the number of fractures. Bowing is a good measure of the severity of OI because it correlates with the number of fractures and the severity of subsequent deformity (Tachdjian, 1990). The degree of bowing also indicates the potential need for surgical intervention. The clinical characteristics of OIT type I include dentinogenesis imperfecta, short stature, and bowing of lower extremities, but the upper extremities are not bowed. Most children with OIT type I can ambulate but may need bracing. Surgery is often indicated for correction of the long bone deformity.

OIT type II is the least disabling form of OI in which fractures can occur in the first year of life or later. In contrast to OIT type I, there is no bowing of the long bones, and no deformities of the upper limbs are present. Most of these children approach average height. Prognosis for ambulation is excellent.

The classification system of OIC and OIT, although descriptive, has been deemed oversimplified by clinicians, geneticists, and biochemists. As a result of a comprehensive survey done by Sillence and Danks (1978), four distinct genetic types of OI have been delineated. This classification system includes clinical presentation, radiologic criteria, and mode of inheritance. The Sillence classification uses a numerical system rather than the more cumbersome descriptive classifications and correlates with morphologic and biochemical studies of OI (Sillence, 1981). A more recent theory suggests that the mode of inheritance in all forms of OI is dominant (Scott CI & Nicholson L, personal communication, 1993).

OI type I shows an autosomal dominant inheritance (Sillence, 1981; Sillence & Danks, 1978; Sillence et al., 1979). It is characterized by markedly blue sclerae throughout life, generalized osteoporosis with bone fragility, joint hyperlaxity, and presenile conductive hearing loss. These patients are generally short but are not as short as those with other forms of OI. At birth, weight and length are normal; short stature occurs postnatally. Dentinogenesis imperfecta is variably present. If dentinogenesis is not present, this type of OI is further subclassified as OI type IA; if dentinogenesis imperfecta is present, the subclassification is OI type IB. Fractures may be present at birth (10%) or may appear at any time during infancy and childhood (Sillence, 1981). The frequency and development of skeletal deformity are also variable. The birth and population incidence of OI type I is 1 in 30,000.

Based on the Sillence classification, OI type II is either a common autosomal dominant form or a rare autosomal recessive form. OI type II is lethal in the perinatal period. These infants may be stillborn. There is extreme bone fragility with minimal mineralization. Marked delay of ossification of the skull and facial bones is noted, and the long bones are crumbled (Tachdjian, 1990). The infants are small for their age and have characteristic short, curved, and deformed limbs. The incidence as reported by Sillence is 1 in 62,487 live births.

According to the Sillence classification, OI type III can be autosomal dominant or recessive but is heterozygous. This form is severe, and there is progressive deformity of the long bones, skull, and spine, resulting in very short stature. Usually, there is severe bone fragility, moderate bone deformity at birth, multiple fractures, and severe growth retardation. OI type III appears similar to the lethal perinatal OI type except that the lack of skull ossification is not as marked and birth weight and length are within normal range. Sclerae have a variable hue, tending to be bluish at birth but becoming less so with age. Dentinogenesis occurs in 45% of patients with OI type III. Hearing loss is common. As a result of the complications of severe kyphoscoliosis and resulting respiratory compromise, death occurs in childhood. OI type III is rare, and the exact incidence is not documented (Tachdjian, 1990).

OI type IV is rare and is inherited by autosomal dominant transmission. It is characterized by mild to moderate deformity and postnatal short stature. There is bone fragility and deformities of the long bones of variable severity. Sclerae tend to be normal, and dentinogenesis is common. Hearing loss is variable. The prognosis for ambulation is excellent (Byers, 1988). The exact incidence of OI type IV is unknown (Tachdjian, 1990).

Sillence (1981) has compared his proposed nomenclature with the congenita or tarda classification. He relates type I to the congenita and tarda form of OI, type II to the congenita form (always), and types III and IV to both congenita and tarda forms. Sillence acknowledges that difficulty exists in this comparison because any syndromes accompanied by the onset of fractures at birth may be classified as congenita, whereas children with types I, III, or IV could have their first fracture at any time (Table 13–1).

PATHOPHYSIOLOGY

In all forms of OI, a defect in collagen synthesis results from an abnormality in processing procollagen to type I collagen, apparently causing the bones to be brittle. This defect affects the formation of both enchondral and intramembranous bone. The collagen fibers fail to mature beyond the reticular fiber stage. Studies show that osteoblasts have normal or increased activity but fail to produce and organize the collagen (Ramser & Frost, 1966). Histologically, there is variability among the different types of OI. In the more severe congenita form, the proportion of primitive osseous tissue with a woven matrix is markedly greater than in the tarda form (Bullough et al., 1981; Falvo & Bullough, 1973). A relative abundance of osteocytes is present, but intracellular matrix is deficient. In Sillence classification OI type I, morphologic findings include an increased amount of glycogen in osteoblasts, mild hypercellularity of bone (Albright et al., 1975), and no abnormality in collagen fiber diameter (Doty & Matthews, 1971). In OI type II, morphologic findings include poorly ossified cortical bone (Follis, 1952), abnormally thin corneal and skin collagen fibers (Bluemcke et al., 1972), hypercellularity of secondary bone trabeculae and cortical bone (Sillence & Danks, 1978), and deficient osteoid with deposition of argyrophilic material or primary trabeculae (Follis, 1952). In types III and IV, morphologic findings include an increased amount of woven bone, increased cellularity, increased number of resorption surfaces, and wide osteoid seams (Falvo & Bullough, 1973).

Those persons who have inherited OI tend to have a similar, if not the same, collagen defect as their parent. First-generation OI tends to be caused by a novel mutation of the gene. This specific gene mutation can then be passed to offspring. Genetic counseling when OI is found gives parents an accurate estimate of the risk of recurrence and an understanding of clinical variabilities in their family. The degree of severity in families is also variable. A mildly affected patient could give birth to a severely affected child. Describing to the parents the lifestyle of a child with OI may have more meaning than quoting risk figures (Solomons & Millar, 1973).

MEDICAL MANAGEMENT

No consistently effective medications are available to strengthen skeletal structures and prevent fractures. Improvements in medical care for the treatment of respiratory tract infections and in orthopedic management contribute to the improved outlook for a child with OI. Life expectancy appears to be increasing, but limited gains have been made in improving functional abilities (Albright, 1981).

New areas of research in OI are in the field of gene therapy. Areas being investigated include cell replacement of the mutant gene, bone marrow transplants, and mutant allele suppression (Marini & Gerber, 1997).

Pharmacologic management for recurring fractures has included numerous medications and dietary supplements, all of dubious efficacy. Magnesium oxide, calcitonin, and fluoride have been administered in an attempt to decrease the frequency of fractures, but with inconsistent results. New research in postmenopausal women with osteoporosis has led to studies of children with OI using similar pharmacologic interventions. Positive results have been reported on the effects of such pharmacologic agents as bisphosphonates (Landsmeer-Beker, 1997). Sex hormones have been tried as a result of the clinical observation that fracture incidence diminishes after puberty. All of these regimens have been deemed ineffective as primary treatments in the prevention of fractures. Despite the fact that no dietary alterations have been shown to be effective, eating a well-balanced diet is highly recommended (Albright, 1981).

Once a fracture occurs, the bone is more susceptible to refracture. The already weakened structure predisposes the child to limb deformities from bowing of the long bones. Immobilization to assist in setting the bone in proper alignment can cause disuse osteoporosis, which, in turn, puts those fragile bones at greater risk of fracturing. Hence, a vicious cycle is created: osteoporosis leads to fractures, and immobilization secondary to fracture creates disuse osteoporosis, which leads to further fractures. The goal, then, is to limit immobilization of the extremi-

TABLE 13-1. **Classification of Osteogenesis Imperfecta**

Classification*	Inheritance	Fractures	Radiographic Features	Stature	Dentin	Sclerae	Hearing	Ambulation
Osteogenesis imperfecta congenita	Unknown	Extreme bone fragility at birth	Severe bowing of long bones	Dwarfism	Dentinogenesis imperfecta	Blue	Hearing loss	Nonambulatory
Osteogenesis imperfecta tarda type I	Unknown		Bowing of lower extremities	Short stature	Dentinogenesis imperfecta			Ambulation with braces
Osteogenesis imperfecta tarda type II	Unknown	Less disabling form	No bowing	Average height	Normal			Ambulatory
Osteogenesis imperfecta type IA	Autosomal dominant	Mild to severe bone fragility	Mildest form of OI	Short	Normal	Blue	Hearing loss	
Osteogenesis imperfecta type IB	Autosomal dominant	Mild to severe bone fragility	Mildest form of OI	Short	Dentinogenesis imperfecta	Blue	Hearing loss	
Osteogenesis imperfecta type IIA†	New autosomal mutation	Extreme bone fragility	Crumpled long bones, beaded ribs			Normal		
Osteogenesis imperfecta type IIB	New autosomal mutation	Extreme bone fragility	Crumpled long bones, normal ribs			Normal		
Osteogenesis imperfecta type IIC	New autosomal mutation	Extreme bone fragility	Long, thin fractured long bones, thin beaded ribs			Blue		
Osteogenesis imperfecta type III	Autosomal dominant (usual) Autosomal recessive (rare)	Variable bone fragility (often severe)	Progressive skeletal deformity (bowing)	Very short stature	Variable dentin abnormality	Variable; blue at birth	Hearing loss	
Osteogenesis imperfecta type IVA	Autosomal dominant	Bone fragility	Variable deformity	Short stature	Normal	Normal	Variable	Ambulatory
Osteogenesis imperfecta type IVB	Autosomal dominant	Bone fragility	Variable deformity	Short stature	Dentinogenesis imperfecta	Normal	Variable	Ambulatory

*Congenita and tarda are older forms of classification. OI types I through IV are based on the Sillence classification system.
†Osteogenesis imperfecta type II is lethal in the perinatal period.

ties as much as possible to prevent exacerbation of osteopenia and risk of more fractures.

Fractures in patients with OI generally heal within the normal healing time, although the resultant callus may be large but of poor quality. These fractures must be immobilized for pain relief and to promote healing in the correct alignment. Pseudarthrosis may occur when the fracture is not immobilized. Immobilization may be in the form of splinting with thermoplastic materials, orthoses, hip spica posterior shells, or casting. When there is malunion of fractures, angulation and bowing of the long bones occur, frequently accompanied by joint contractures. There may be disruption of the physis, resulting in asymmetric growth and deformity. When angulation occurs, mechanical forces tend to increase the deformity, thus aggravating the overall problem (Albright, 1981). The cartilaginous ends of the long bones are disproportionately large and have irregular articular surfaces. Fortunately, in nearly all patients with OI, the fracture rate diminishes near or after puberty.

The most successful means of fracture stabilization in long bones in OI is internal fixation with intermedullary rods (Jerosch et al., 1998). Although this method of stabilization is not without complications, the intramedullary rod can be helpful in preventing long bones from bowing after fractures and provides internal support to prevent further fractures. Indications for stabilization with rods include multiple recurring fractures and increasing long bone deformity that is interfering with orthotic fit and impairing function. The age of the patient and the size of the bone determine the type and timing of surgery. Intermedullary rod fixation of the femur is best done after 4 or 5 years of age when the thigh is not so short as to complicate surgery by compounding the technical difficulty. Surgical insertion of the rod in thin bones is also technically difficult.

The type of rod used depends on the type and severity of fracture. When a solid rod is used, bone growth may occur beyond the ends of the rods, necessitating reoperation later for placement of a longer rod. Because children with severe OI are at greater than normal anesthetic risk from potential respiratory compromise, the number of operative procedures is best kept to a minimum. Special instrumentation has been designed that "elongates" with the child's growth, eliminating the need for multiple reoperations as the bone grows (Fig. 13–1). These extensible intramedullary fixation devices were introduced by Bailey and Dubow (1965). They are used most frequently in the femur but may also be used in the humerus, tibia, and forearm. There is a high incidence of complications associated with using the intramedullary rods (Jerosch et al., 1998).

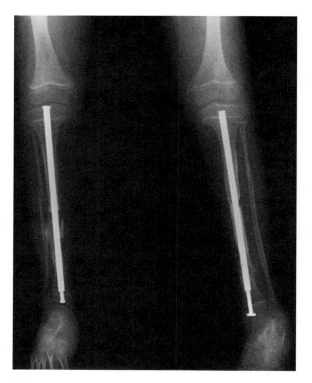

FIGURE 13–1. Extensible intramedullary fixation rods that elongate as the bone grows in a child with OI.

Problems exist with the control of rotation and migration when using extensible rods; thus postoperative casting may be necessary. Orthoses may be needed after insertion of the rod for further external support. Early weight bearing with orthotic support is initiated as soon as possible. With internal fixation, there is a risk of osteopenia around the rod, especially with the telescoping rods.

Spinal deformities, including scoliosis and kyphosis, occur in 50% of patients with OI, as a result of osteoporosis and vertebral compression fractures. Progressive spinal deformities such as scoliosis and pathologic kyphosis are more likely to occur in types III and IV than in type I (Engelbert et al., 1998). Kyphoscoliosis can be disabling and may be present in 20 to 40% of patients (Tachdjian, 1990). Unlike the typical population, kyphoscoliosis in the OI population can be progressive over a lifetime, which further compounds the patient's short stature. The most common curve is that of thoracic scoliosis. Scoliotic and kyphotic curves in patients with OI are not usually amenable to conservative bracing. The bones in children with OI usually cannot withstand the forces of the brace, and the result is rib deformities rather than the intended effect on the spine (Albright, 1981). In adolescents and adults with severe OI, the incidence of scoliosis is 80 to 90%. Surgical stabilization is often advocated for the management of these deformities, but there is little documentation of long-term outcome (Hanscom et al., 1992).

IMPAIRMENT

Diagnosis and Problem Identification

In the most severe forms of OI, the infant is born with multiple fractures sustained in utero or during the birth process. The prognosis of OI depends on its type. In the most severe forms these multiple fractures that have occurred in utero and during birth are associated with a high mortality rate. Prognostic indicators concerning survival and ambulation are the time of the initial fracture and the radiologic appearance of long bones and ribs at the time of the initial fracture. Spranger and associates (1982) devised a scoring system for providing an accurate prognosis for newborns with OI. This system coded the degree of skeletal changes based on clinical and radiographic findings in 47 cases. These investigators found that newborns who had marked bowing of their lower extremities but less severe changes in the skull, ribs, vertebrae, and arms and who had normal sclerae survived and had fewer fractures as they grew older. In the moderate and mild types, although the prognosis varies, there is a gradual tendency toward improvement when the incidence of fractures decreases after puberty.

If a family is known to be at risk of having a child with OI and the collagen defect has been identified in the parent, human chorionic villus biopsy can be done prenatally at 10 weeks of gestation to determine whether the child has the same defect. A prenatal ultrasound examination at 15 weeks of gestation can be helpful in identifying fractures, as well as possible mineralization problems (Byers, 1988).

The infant is usually of normal size at birth, but postnatal growth is impaired. Although no conclusive causative factors for this impaired growth are known, possible factors are the deformities themselves or abnormalities in the epiphyseal growth plates. The radiologic appearance of long bones associated with the most severe cases indicates bones with a thin radiolucent appearance. The malformed ribs affect respiratory function, which may lead to respiratory tract infections and reduced functional potential of the child.

Children with moderate OI are often identified after there have been several fractures from seemingly slight trauma. An example is a fractured humerus caused by the child holding onto a car seat while the caretaker is trying to get the child out of the car. Those children who begin having fractures of unknown origin at a young age can have collagen and biochemical studies done, usually from a skin biopsy. The tests can also be helpful in ruling out other disorders, such as idiopathic juvenile osteoporosis, leukemia, and congenital hypophosphatasia (which is fatal). No specific diagnostic abnormality indicating OI appears in laboratory tests; the diagnosis is made primarily from clinical and radiographic findings. In the infant, OI and achondroplasia are often confused because, in both conditions, children have large heads and short limbs. Radiographic reports, however, distinguish between the two.

Collagen and biochemical studies can assist in differentiating a battered infant from an infant with OI. Radiographic studies are helpful because fractures at the epiphysis are rare in OI but common in child abuse, in which there is also evidence of soft tissue trauma. Bruising is common to both the infant with OI and the battered infant, but the bruising will disappear when the battered infant is in a safe environment. Three of the most helpful radiographic views in diagnosing OI are those of the skull (Wormian bones), the lateral view of the spine (biconcave vertebrae or platyspondyly), and the pelvis (the beginnings of protrusio acetabuli) (Wynne-Davies & Gormley, 1981).

In the moderate to severe forms of OI, early childhood fractures lead to multiple recurring fractures because of the already weakened structure. The child develops limb deformities from bowing, which leads to impairment of mobility and of other functional skills. In the least severe forms of OI, because the first pathologic fractures occur later in childhood, there is less likelihood of recurring fractures with associated long bone deformities and therefore the best overall prognosis.

Engelbert and colleagues (1997), in a cross-sectional study of 54 children with OI, analyzed range of motion (ROM) and muscle strength for different types of OI. In OI type I, there was generalized hypermobility of the joints but without a decrease in ROM. In type III, extremities, especially the lower extremities, were severely malaligned. In type IV, upper and lower extremities were equally malaligned. Muscle strength in OI type I was normal except for periarticular muscles at the hip joint. In OI type III, however, muscle strength was severely decreased, especially around the hip joint. In OI type IV, the proximal muscles of both the upper and lower extremity were weak.

Team members other than physical therapists who have an important role in the management of OI are orthopedists, orthotists, occupational therapists, audiologists, dentists, and genetics professionals. Little progress has been made in the primary prevention of this disorder, nor has there been much improvement in the medical management. With technologic enhancements and advances in neonatal care, more of these infants are surviving and presenting a management challenge to health care professionals.

EXAMINATION, EVALUATION, AND INTERVENTION

Infancy

Typical disabilities seen in an infant with OI depend on the severity. In severe cases, the most serious impairments are those of rib and skull fractures, which could compromise pulmonary status and neural status, respectively. Because of possible cardiopulmonary compromise, time may be spent in the neonatal intensive care unit, which could lead to decreased parental interaction and bonding. If OI is moderate to severe, parents have increased anxiety about holding the infant for fear of fracturing the infant's bones. This may result in minimal contact and may decrease the mutually nurturing interaction vital to both parent and child. Children with severe OI who have reduced mobility from skeletal deformities may be unable to achieve age-appropriate activities of daily living (ADL) or play in the normal peer environment.

Infants with OI are at a very delicate stage of life. They are completely dependent on their caregivers and have special needs regarding handling, positioning, and playing. During this stage, minimizing fractures, the development of further muscle weakness, and joint laxity is paramount. This is accomplished primarily through a physical therapy home program and parental education for proper positioning and handling.

At birth the infant may be of normal size, but postnatal growth is almost always stunted. Typical disabilites of the infant include a relatively large head, with a soft and membranous skull, and deformed limbs, which are usually short in the more severe forms of OI. Other features include a broad forehead and faciocranial disproportions, which give the face a triangular shape. Radiographically, fractures present at birth may be in varying stages of healing. The bones of infants with severe OI are short and wide with thin cortices, and the diaphyses are as wide as the metaphyses. Crepitation can be palpated at fracture sites.

The physical therapist should be aware of the infant's medical history of past and present fractures and know the types of immobilizations employed before beginning the examination. The caregiver's handling and positioning techniques during dressing, diapering, and bathing are assessed. Assessing active, but not passive, ROM is essential. A standard goniometer can be used for measuring active ROM but may need to be cut down to a size suitable for the infant. Active ROM is measured at the hips, knees, ankles, shoulders, and elbows by lining up the goniometer at the axis of motion and, while observing the infant's movements, moving the goniometer through the observable range. Because passive ROM testing is contraindicated in these children, active ROM provides, at best, a close estimate and may vary during successive assessments. Functional ROM may prove more useful because it will assist in visualizing the whole composite of motions needed in functional abilities. For example, functional active ranges would include the extent to which the child can bring the hand to the mouth or reach to the top of the head. If possible, the same therapist measures ROM during reevaluations. Intrarater and interrater reliability is determined for therapists and is checked annually.

Assessing muscle strength is done through observation of the infant's movements and palpation of contracting muscles rather than by use of formal muscle tests. A gross motor developmental evaluation should also be performed because these children often have delayed development of gross motor skills secondary to fractures and muscular weakness. Delayed gross motor skills are functional limitations involving impaired achievement of motor milestones. Sitting by the age of 10 months is a good predictor of future walking ability (Daly et al., 1996) Some formal tests used include the Peabody Developmental Motor Scales (Folio & Fewell, 1983), which are normed and standardized; the Pediatric Evaluation of Disability Inventory (Haley et al., 1989), which is designed for tracking progress and assessing functional limitations; and the Bayley Scales of Infant Development (Bayley, 1993). Finally, it is important to assess the appropriateness of equipment used for seating, transporting, and encouraging independent mobility of the infant.

Physical therapy includes early parent education in proper handling and positioning techniques. Bathing, dressing, and carrying the infant are critical times when the infant is at risk for fractures (Binder et al., 1984). When handling the infant it is important that force not be put across the long bones; instead the head and trunk should be supported with the arms and legs gently draped across the supporting arm. Some parents feel most comfortable supporting the infant on a standard-size bed pillow for carrying at home. It is important, however, to change the carrying position of the infant periodically because he or she develops strength by accommodating to postural changes. Dressing and un-

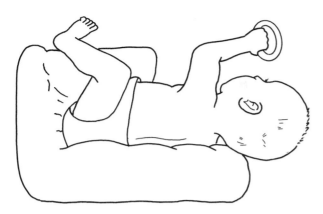

FIGURE 13–2. Infant positioned lying on side using rolls. Emphasis is on maintaining trunk alignment while allowing for active and spontaneous but safe movement.

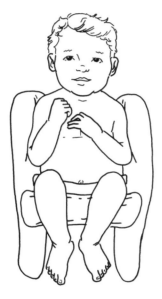

FIGURE 13–3. Infant positioned supine with hips in neutral rotation, with knees flexed, and supported through the trunk.

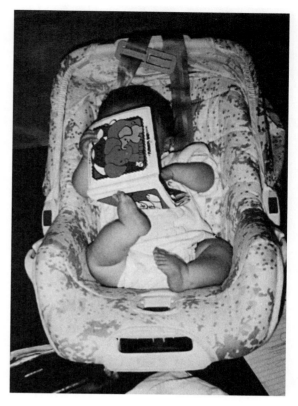

FIGURE 13–4. Child positioned poorly in an infant seat.

dressing can be facilitated by using loose clothing and front or side Velcro closures. Overdressing should be avoided to reduce excessive sweating. Proper diapering includes a technique of rolling the infant off the diaper and supporting the buttocks with one hand with the infant's legs supported on the caregiver's forearm while the other hand positions the diaper. The infant should never be lifted by the ankles. Bathing is done in a padded, preferably plastic, basin. Infant carriers that are designed to safely support the head, trunk, and extremities are frequently used for household transporting. The carrier can be customized, such as a one-piece molded thoracolumbosacral orthosis, which can incorporate the legs so that they will not dangle and sustain injury. The carrier minimizes stresses to the fragile bones while positioning and transporting the infant.

Proper positioning of the infant is a critical component of the home program and management of the infant with OI. One supported position is side lying with towel rolls along the spine and extremities so that they are aligned and protected while the child is allowed active movement (Fig. 13–2). A prone position over a towel roll or with a soft wedge under the chest (if prone position is tolerated) is an alternative. When supine, the infant needs support for the arms, and the hips should be in neutral rotation with the knees over a roll (Fig. 13–3). Positions should be changed frequently and should not restrict active spontaneous movement because this affords muscle strengthening and bone mineralization (Binder et al., 1984). Positioning is useful not only for the purpose of protection from fracturing but also for minimizing joint malalignment and deformities. Figure 13–4 is an example of an infant's legs being poorly positioned in a baby carrier. The same infant seat is

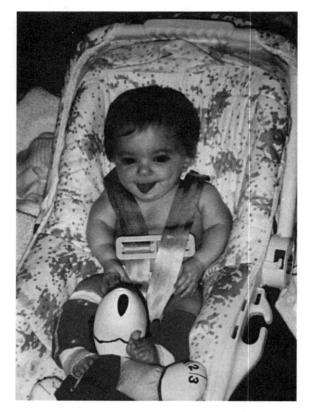

FIGURE 13–5. Child with improved positioning in infant seat.

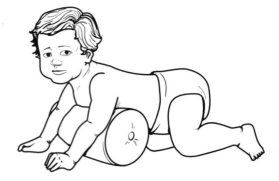

FIGURE 13–6. Infant positioned prone on a roll encourages weight bearing, extremity and trunk alignment, and strengthening of extensor musculature during developmental play.

modified with lateral leg pads to keep the infant's hips and legs in neutral alignment, along with lower leg molded plastic splints (Fig. 13–5). Varying the position of the infant promotes the development of age-appropriate development skills.

Promotion of sensorimotor developmental skills is an ongoing component in the management of the infant and child. Identification of appropriate and safe toys for a child, as well as comfortable play positions that promote development, is often addressed jointly by the occupational therapist and physical therapist. For example, lying prone on a soft roll or over a parent's leg allows for weight-bearing use of the arms with co-contraction of shoulder musculature and promotes active neck and back extensor muscle control (Fig. 13–6). Increasing muscle strength and support around the joint in activities such as this is especially important because the joint ligaments are lax. The prone-on-a-roll positioning also maintains good alignment of the extremities.

Developmental activities such as rolling and supported sitting should be encouraged as tolerated. In encouraging rolling, the infant's arm is placed along-

side his or her head, and then he or she attempts to roll over. Supported sitting is accomplished with seat inserts or corner chairs. Upright unsupported sitting can begin on the parent's lap with a pillow. When the child exhibits appropriate head control, short-sit and straddle activities can be done over the caregiver's leg or a roll but with avoidance of rotation across the lower extremity. These activities promote the development of protective and equilibrium responses and the beginning of protected weight bearing of the lower extremities. Many children with OI spend much time scooting on their buttocks before crawling is accomplished.

Awareness of proper handling while encouraging these developmental skills is of key importance. For instance, a pull-to-sit maneuver is contraindicated when using a distraction pull on the hands. Rather, this maneuver should be modified and facilitated by supporting the child around the shoulders while the child attempts to sit up. In working on trunk control over a ball, the therapist's hands are positioned on the pelvis and trunk rather than supporting or facilitating movement from the legs. Parents should be cautioned against using baby walkers and jumping seats because they do not foster proper positioning and weight bearing. Baby walkers tend to give parents a false sense that the infant is protected. The child may have difficulty controlling these devices, resulting in unnecessary fractures. A car seat can be adapted with foam behind the cover to ensure that the infant fits snugly in the seat with limited ability to fall sideways. The legs should be supported and not left to dangle. Padding can be rearranged in the seat to accommodate the various devices the child may be in for immobilization of fracture sites.

Active, spontaneous activity and exercise are encouraged in side-lying and supine positions, and in supported sitting, with the child reaching for, swiping at, rolling, and lifting lightweight toys of different textures. Pool exercises may begin as early as 6 months of age with the goals of promoting active exercise and weight bearing (Binder et al., 1984). Extremity movement may occur unobstructed as the child is supported in a neck or trunk flotation device accompanied by a parent or the therapist. Long-sleeved clothing may be used to distribute the absorbed water weight evenly over the length of the limb, thus introducing a resistive component to the exercise.

At this stage, goals include use of safe handling and positioning techniques by the caregivers and providing opportunities for development of age-appropriate skills. The intensity of treatment varies with the individual needs of the infant and family, but providing a home program and regular home visits by a physical therapist at least weekly is essential in ensuring that the environment is suitable for sensorimotor and cognitive development. The therapist can act as a resource and support for the caregivers as together they develop strategies to meet the challenges of safe caregiver handling, mobility, and developmental facilitation.

When fractures do occur, they may require splinting using a variety of materials such as perforated orthoplast or fiberglass. Ace wraps have been used to support and protect a limb in mild cases and in young infants. Fractures may heal within 2 weeks for the newborn and generally within the same time frame as other fractures in infancy (usually 6 weeks).

Preschool Period

The primary impairments of bone fragility, joint laxity, and reduced muscle strength continue to be present but are now accompanied by secondary impairments of disuse atrophy and osteoporosis from fracture immobilization (Fig. 13–7). Typical disabilities include the inability of the child to be as mobile as his or her peers, which will hamper play and socialization. This may affect the child's adjustment to regular school and hinder academic progress.

At this stage, muscles are usually weak as a result of immobilization and disuse. Developmental skills may continue to lag in the presence of frequent fractures and subsequent immobilizations, but cognitive skills should be appropriate for the child's age. When sustaining a fracture, these children complain of little pain and usually have minimal soft tissue trauma. There may be microfractures from repeated trauma at the epiphyseal plates, resulting in arrested growth and potential leg length discrepancy. In childhood, "popcorn calcifications" appear in the metaphyseal and epiphyseal areas of long bones

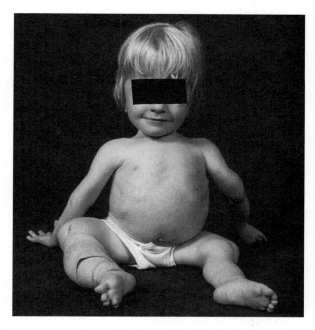

FIGURE 13–7. Child with OI showing joint laxity and bony deformities: femoral anterolateral bowing and tibial anterior bowing.

(Goldman et al., 1980). It is postulated that these are fragmentations of the cartilaginous growth plate.

If the child begins to walk without adequate support, there is further bending of the long bones as a result of abnormal stress on the weakened structure. Bowing occurs in the anterolateral direction in the femur and anteriorly in the tibia. In those children who do not walk, lack of the normal weight-bearing stress leads to a honeycomb pattern in the long bones.

Emphasis at this stage is on protected weight bearing and self-mobility for enhanced independence. Although proper positioning, handling, and transferring are still important, the emphasis shifts to the child's active participation in his or her care and safe independence. During this period, the child with OI should have adequate upright control and, at the very least, should be held in standing position, because early weight bearing appears to have some beneficial effect on the progression of the condition. When comparing radiographs of children with OI from the time of birth and later, the changing levels of bone density suggested that progressive osteoporosis had been superimposed on the basic bone defect (Bleck, 1981). Upper extremity bones were frequently more dense than those of the lower limbs and were less likely to fracture. This finding may be related to the use and stress put on upper extremity bones during ADL. A study by King and Bobechko in

1971 concluded that limb immobilization caused osteoporosis; thus, in the prevention of secondary impairment by osteoporosis in OI, stress on the bone through weight bearing is advocated. The management principle used to implement appropriate weight bearing is to stress the lower limb bones while supporting the weakened structures through compression of the musculature around the bone. Contour-molded orthoses can be used to provide this compression and support.

At this stage, an evaluation of modes of mobility and adapted equipment is essential. An assessment of modification needs to promote supported sitting and mobility is also important. Equipment requires constant updating because of the changing positional needs related to mobilization-immobilization status. Splinting needs and adaptive ADL equipment are assessed for fit and usefulness. Developmental assessment tools used may include the Peabody Developmental Motor Scales and the Pediatric Evaluation of Disability Inventory to assess gross motor function and functional limitations in children with disabilities, respectively.

Active exercise continues to be emphasized to increase muscle strength of the weakened muscles. Usually the hip extensor and abductor muscles are weak. Active exercise can be achieved primarily through developmental play. One developmental activity to increase weight bearing and maintain or increase strength in the quadriceps and hip extensor musculature involves having the child straddle a roll and come to stand with the therapist supporting the child's pelvis (Fig. 13–8). The therapist begins with the child sitting on a high roll that requires a small excursion of movement to go from sitting to standing and then gradually changes to using a lower roll. An active-resistive program graded for the patient's tolerance should be cautiously established. Use of light weights may be incrementally increased, but they should be attached close to large joints so as to avoid a long lever arm that increases the potential for fracture.

An aquatic exercise program is an excellent therapeutic program for the child with OI. It can be started at an early age and continue for a lifetime. There are many benefits to aquatic therapy, including the opportunity to socialize with peers in a safe environment, a safe method of strengthening muscles through resistance and assistance of the water, and the opportunity to improve cardiovascular fitness and to bear weight in a protected environment. The therapist can finely grade the progression of exercises in the pool by first using the buoyancy effect of the water to assist weak movements, then support the movements, and, finally, resist the movements. Exercises can be modified with floats by changing the length of the lever arm of the moving body part, through use of turbulence, and through altering the speed and direction of the movement. Pool exercises can also promote deep breathing to facilitate chest expansion and overall respiratory function, a goal that is especially important because chest deformities that may compromise breathing capacity are common. Certain precautions should be taken when considering pool therapy for the child with OI. The heat of the water creates a rise in body temperature and increases metabolism, which is frequently already elevated in these children. It is suggested, therefore, that the time, water temperature, and exercise activity level be closely monitored for each child. Pool sessions are generally limited to 20 to 30 minutes.

Pool exercise therapy may interrupt the cycle of further disuse and secondary complications from immobilization. Aquatic therapy is not only an ideal therapeutic modality for the child with OI but can also be a therapeutic, lifelong avocational activity that can ameliorate the effects of the disabling process.

One key goal to be emphasized for the preschool child is safe, independent mobility, which is certainly a challenge if the child has frequent fractures. The aim is to prevent a functional limitation of reduced mobility resulting from the initial impairment. Researchers such as Perrin and Gerrity (1984) theorize

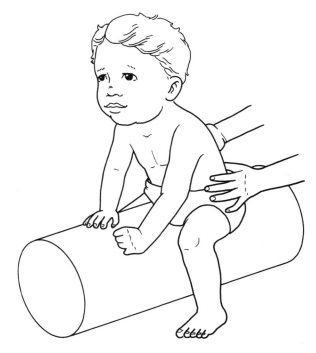

FIGURE 13–8. Straddle roll activity of supported sit-to-stand for lower extremity strengthening and weight bearing.

that disabilities in intellectual development may occur when children have limited mobility. Opportunities for multiple safe modes of mobility should be explored to expand the child's repertoire of environmental experiences. A scooter for sitting propelled with legs or hands may be useful (Fig. 13–9).

The degree of ambulation attainable varies for preschool children with OI. Those children with limited ambulatory skills may need formal gait training, as well as instruction of family members. Interest in standing often occurs in the child's second year of life. Factors affecting this ability include the degree of bowing in the extremities and the muscle strength of the limbs. Ambulation is often introduced in the pool, for protected weight bearing. Because the buoyancy of water provides support for the body, weight bearing on weakened extremities and unstable joints can be gradually introduced without fear of causing trauma. Weight relief depends on the proportion of the body below the water level. For maximum weight relief for ambulation, the child begins standing in the deeper end of the pool where the water level is at the child's neck. Over time, the child gradually progresses to bearing more weight in

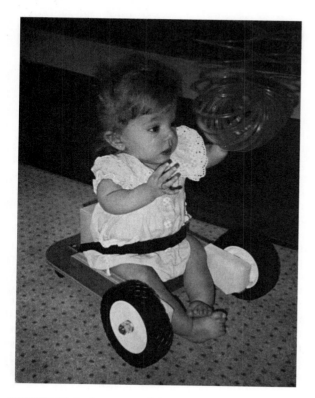

FIGURE 13–9. Scooter used for mobility that can be propelled by a child's legs or arms.

shallow water. If the child with OI is recovering from a fracture, it is recommended that thermoplastic splints be used to further protect the extremity while in the pool. General guidelines for walking reeducation in water according to Duffield (1983) suggest that a patient start in parallel bars or a walking frame with the therapist initially supporting the pelvis from the front. The patient practices weight shifts from side to side, forward, and backward and progresses to walking forward. The therapist cues the patient to lean slightly forward to counteract the upthrust of buoyancy, which tends to cause the child to overbalance backward. In this manner, protected walking for a child with OI can start much earlier than on a solid surface. Unsupported standing on solid ground is not recommended because it leads to rapid bowing of the long bones. When severe bowing of the extremities occurs, the child usually undergoes orthopedic surgery in the form of osteotomies. Age-appropriate lower extremity weight bearing is encouraged, although the child with moderate to severe OI needs external devices such as splints or braces to protect fragile long bones. Supported standing frames or orthoses such as hip-knee-ankle-foot orthoses (HKAFOs) are used.

In moderate to severe OI, braces and splints are usually required to begin standing activities on solid surfaces. Use of orthotics provides protected weight bearing needed to reduce the impact of stress on the osteoporotic bony deformities. Braces or splints are first used in conjunction with a standing frame. Prone standers with orthoses are used to grade the amount of weight born on the lower extremities with progression from an inclined position to an upright position. The child may be fitted with a containment-type brace fabricated of lightweight thermoplastic material. These plastic orthoses can be fabricated to conform to the contours of the limb to provide support for the weakened structures around the bone. Often the first braces used during the toddler stage are made without knee joints and may have a pelvic band for maximal support. The pelvic band and locked hips minimize femoral rotation (Gerber et al., 1990). Knee joints can be added to the orthosis when the limb grows and strength increases (Fig. 13–10). Some braces use a lightweight plastic clamshell design and are contoured for ischial weight bearing. The child usually progresses from maximally supportive bracing to less cumbersome bracing as bony alignment and strength factors permit. HKAFOs can be beneficial in reducing tibial bowing and progressing in gross motor skills (Gerber et al., 1990). In a study of the effects of withdrawal of bracing in children with OI, when children used HKAFOs, they were less sedentary, more upright, and likely to be more independent

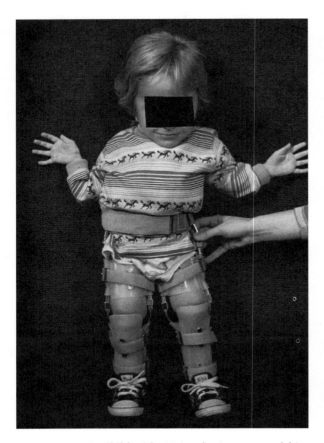

FIGURE 13–10. Child with OI in plastic contoured hip-knee-ankle brace.

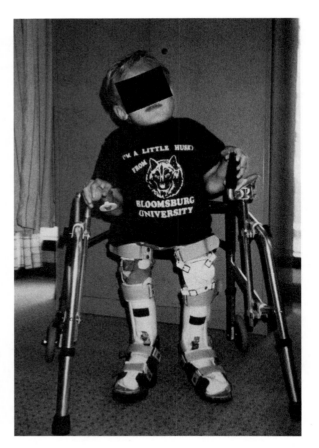

FIGURE 13–11. Child with OI with long leg braces and rear-wheeled walker.

than when not using the HKAFOs. A lower incidence of fracture was observed during periods of HKAFO use (Gerber et al., 1998).

Air splints have been used to prevent fractures and as a fracture management tool, either as a substitute for bracing or as a transition to bracing. Types of splinting include pneumatic trouser splints, which are used extensively in Europe. These air-filled trouser splints were introduced by Morel and Houghton (1982) for the support of the fragile long bones in OI. Morel has recommended that following the healing of the osteotomy for correction of long bone deformity these pneumatic splints be used for support. Letts and colleagues (1988) described pant orthoses called "vacuum pants" that were used in children with OI to enable weight bearing in a functional position during transition to knee-ankle-foot orthoses (KAFOs). Pneumatic trouser splints are not used in the United States, in part because of commercial unavailability and lack of familiarity with the splint. Therapy air splints such as the URIAS Pediatric C.P. Therapy Splints (J.A. Preston Corp., Jackson, MI) are

readily available, need not be custom-made, and afford some flexibility when inflated to allow ambulation. Scott (1990) used these splints for instituting graded weight bearing and gait training in a child with OI. Drawbacks of the air splints and pneumatic trousers are that they may be bulky and hot, so the child may not always tolerate them well.

The child graduates from using a standing frame with orthoses to ambulating in long leg braces with the knees locked in full extension. He or she then progresses from parallel bars to various walkers or crutches as limb strength and ability improve. A walker that supports the majority of body weight through the trunk and pelvis is often used to assist in weight bearing during initial overland ambulation. This walker supports weight by means of a trunk support cuff and a padded pommel that is positioned between the child's legs. Rear-wheeled and four-point walkers followed by canes or crutches (depending on the type and severity of OI) may be used (Fig. 13–11). Forearm attachments to walkers or crutches afford a degree of weight bearing distrib-

---

BOX 13–1. **Disabling Process in Children with Osteogenesis Imperfecta**

Pathophysiology	Impairments	Functional Impairments	Disability	Societal Limitations
Connective tissue disorder secondary to defect in collagen synthesis Brittle bones	Diffuse osteoporosis resulting in multiple recurrent fractures Weak muscles Joint laxity Bowing of long bones Scoliosis Kyphosis	Limited functional mobility skills, including rolling, creeping, transitional movements, and higher-level mobility skills Limited ability to transfer Limited ambulation Decreased endurance	Limited independence in self-care skills, including dressing and feeding Limited ability for ambulation on uneven terrain Limited independence in wheelchair mobility Limited participation in physical activites caused by endurance limitations and safety concerns	Limited peer play Infantilization Limited access to educational and work opportunities Limited access to wide range of environments Limited independent living Social isolation

---

uted throughout the forearm to reduce stress on the arm and wrist, as well as to relieve some weight bearing on the lower extremities. Some children ambulate without braces when their fracture rate decreases in later years.

Customized mobility caster carts may be fabricated to encourage independent mobility when the child is immobilized, enabling the child to explore his or her environment, gain some independence, and maintain strength in the upper extremities. When there is good head and trunk control and the child can cognitively and safely handle a mobility device, power mobility may be an adjunct to preventing disability by allowing the child to keep up and interact with peers. These alternative mobility modes do not preclude ambulation but are useful additional mobility options. Regardless of the mode of mobility used, it is imperative to provide the child with a degree of functional independence in the home and preschool environments.

School Age and Adolescence

Typical disabilities seen at this stage include inability to keep up with peers as a result of reduced mobility and limited independence in ADL (Box 13–1). Social skill development may also be hampered if the school-age child has been overprotected because of overwhelming fear and anxiety by caregivers regarding fracturing. This may have an impact on the school-age child's scholastic endeavors and future vocational achievements. Studies show that children with OI tend to be intelligent and

cheerful (Rezte, 1972). Parents and educators should encourage a positive attitude and excellence in school performance to prepare the child for a productive future.

At this age, the spine may show varying degrees of deformity. Usually there is scoliosis, kyphosis, or both, resulting from compression fractures of the vertebrae, osteoporosis, and ligamentous laxity. The child with moderate to severe OI shows marked bowing of the long bones from the multiple fractures and growth arrest at the epiphyseal plates. In the femur, the neck-shaft angle is decreased with a coxa vara deformity and acetabular protrusion. The tibia is anteriorly angulated, which, in combination with the angulation of the femur, results in an apparent knee flexion contracture. The patellofemoral joint frequently dislocates, predisposing the patient to falls and fractures. Pes valgus frequently occurs at the ankle. In the upper extremities, the humerus is angulated laterally or anterolaterally and the forearms are limited in rotation. The elbows often exhibit cubitus varus deformities, and elbow flexion contractures may be present.

Fractures tend to decrease markedly in frequency after puberty. Possible causes may be hormonal changes, increased awareness of how to prevent fractures, improvement in coordination, and increasing bone strength. Paradoxically, the adolescent who senses his or her increased stability and emerging independence may maximize involvement in activities, which increases the risk of more severe types of fractures. In an effort not to discourage these activities and independence, ongoing use of safe methods of mobility, caution, and responsible behavior should be stressed in patient instruction throughout childhood.

Physical therapy management at this stage involves other team members, including professionals in orthopedics, orthotics, occupational therapy, and rehabilitation engineering, to maximize the child's independence in ADL, mobility, endurance, problem solving, and adjustment to the school environment.

Children and adolescents should be encouraged to do their share of the chores at home within their functional capacity. This allows the child to feel valued and lessens sibling rivalry (Thompson, 1990).

In this period, physical therapy may be helpful in returning the child to premorbid mobility status after a series of immobilizations from prepubertal fractures. The child may also require changes in bracing to accommodate growth and body changes, such as increased or decreased mass. Lower extremity bracing continues to be of the lightweight plastic HKAFO or KAFO clamshell design, usually with joints.

Management of scoliosis and kyphosis is usually addressed by a spinal fusion, but the long-term results in maintaining alignment are questionable (Benson & Newman, 1981). Orthotic devices such as the Milwaukee brace and orthoplast jackets have been deemed ineffective in controlling scoliosis and kyphosis.

Along with occupational therapy, physical therapy can help maximize the child's independence by identifying safe, energy-efficient positions in which the child can work. Adaptive equipment is imperative for those with severe involvement. Occupational therapists, physical therapists, and rehabilitation engineers work together to adapt wheelchairs and seating and mobility devices to accommodate skeletal deformity, scoliosis, and kyphosis. A variety of lightweight and easily maneuverable manual wheelchairs can be adapted with seating inserts for trunk control and proper positioning. Plastic upholstery is usually unsatisfactory for the child with OI because of the propensity for excessive perspiration. Proper wheelchair positioning is critical for prevention of further disabling deformities and for protection of the exposed extremities from trauma.

Physical therapy continues throughout this stage to work on ambulation, endurance, and strength. Household ambulation is usually achieved with assistive devices if adequate upper extremity strength is present. Walkers with progression to canes or crutches are used. Toward adolescence, ambulation without braces is more conceivable than before because the fracture rate decreases. Many children with OI who have primarily used the wheelchair for mobility are now able to ambulate about the house

without any special change in their program. It is important to emphasize the maintenance of adequate skeletal alignment and maximal muscular strength throughout childhood to prepare for this improved function as an adolescent and adult. Community ambulation without braces, however, is not practical, given the patient's short stature, the energy expenditure required, and the reduced muscle power. Most school-age and older children with OI use wheelchairs for community ambulation (Bleck, 1981). Independence in mobility is paramount because it has been shown to correlate with the degree of adaptation to the community environment. In Bachman's (1972) study of the variables in children with disabilities that affected adaptation outside the school environment, it was reported that independence in travel away from home was the most significant factor.

Strengthening and endurance programs can be most successful when the child participates in developing a program that suits his or her interests and schedule. Programs can consist of progressive resistive exercises using incremental weights or adaptive sport activities. Enjoyable avocational activities that incorporate functional strengthening and mobility also must be stressed at this age. Although contact sports such as football, soccer, and baseball must be avoided, customized athletic and fitness programs are vital for youngsters with OI. These adaptive physical education activities can assist in improving physical health, finding a competitive outlet, helping to discover one's potential, and providing an opportunity to make friends (Patti, 1990). Activities may include swim team competition and wheelchair court sports such as tennis, badminton, and ping pong. The physical therapist's role is to set appropriate parameters for participation, to provide precautions, and to upgrade the level of activity progressively. Volunteer jobs and social opportunities, such as the Boy Scouts and Girl Scouts, encourage emotional growth and develop leadership skills. Volunteer jobs for the adolescent can be helpful when applying for future employment (Fehribach, 1990).

In an 8-year cumulative management program, Gerber and colleagues (1990) found that a comprehensive rehabilitation program, long leg bracing, and surgical procedures on the femur resulted in a high level of functional activity for children with OI along with an acceptable level of risk for fractures. The three-part program consisted of early intervention emphasizing positioning and handling, muscle strengthening and aerobic conditioning, and protected ambulation. Included in the program were strengthening exercises for the pelvic girdle and lower extremity musculature, pool exercises, molded seating, long leg bracing, and gait training. Of the 12 children studied, 10 became functional ambulators, whereas 2 were household ambulators. Five children walked or took steps without braces, and 6 ambulated without gait aids. No child primarily used a wheelchair. All children of school age were enrolled in regular neighborhood schools. The physical activity of these children was high in that they participated in peer activities and some sports. Fractures were not eliminated through bracing, but the fracture rate was deemed acceptable.

Transition to Adulthood

In the transition to adulthood, patients with OI are dealing with the secondary effects of disease because the fracture rate has declined or ceased by the late teen years. The onset of deafness in some children with OI will occur in adult life. Scoliotic curves are usually severe and continue to progress. The incidence of scoliosis approaches 80 to 90% in teenagers and adults (Albright, 1981). Patients with OI are especially susceptible to postmenopausal osteoporosis or the osteoporosis of immobilization (Sillence, 1981). No scientific data have been published on long-term sequelae for adults with OI. Adults with OI do, however, report problems with arthritic changes and back pain.

Emphasis of intervention during the transition to adulthood is on appropriate career placement, given the patient's intellectual capacity and consideration of the physical constraints. Because most patients with OI become productive members of society, optimal academic, social, and physical development will facilitate their opportunities to succeed in a competitive job market (Bleck, 1981). It is difficult to compete for jobs with physically healthy persons when life is complicated by repeated fractures, hospitalizations, and absences from work or school. Despite these problems, adults with OI tend to be ambitious and have low hostility levels. Half of adults with OI choose to marry and have children (Kiley et al., 1976). In a 1981 study by Bleck, 10 of 12 patients with OIC who had undergone early weight-bearing, orthotic, and mobility management programs attended regular educational facilities. Twelve patients with OIT who were managed by this program all attained complete independence in ADL, mobility, and ambulation (Bleck, 1981).

By the time these children reach adulthood, most use either manual or power wheelchairs for community mobility. Ambulation consists of household walking with an assistive device. Many of the children who previously relied on wheelchairs

for household ambulation no longer needed them because they improved in functional mobility as adults.

CASE HISTORY
RACHEL

Rachel is a 13-year-old girl with the diagnosis of osteogenesis imperfecta tarda I. She was born after a 38-week gestation with apparently normal fetal movements, and no abnormalities were perceived at birth. By the end of her second year, the diagnosis of OI was made based on clinical and radiographic findings. Before this her parents were questioned to rule out child abuse. Rachel's mother reports feeling high anxiety over the inherent accusations and her helplessness in explaining the fractures. Once the diagnosis was made, her anxiety was reduced, making education and training more effective.

Pathophysiologically, Rachel demonstrated general osteopenia and severe demineralization of the bilateral lower extremities with evidence of prior fractures of the shafts of long bones. This underlying pathophysiologic condition set the stage for her primary impairments—reduced mobility and strength as a result of the series of fractures.

Her early fractures, involving the clavicle and scapula, resulted from a fall she sustained at 18 months. At age 4, she fractured her right ulna, radius, and left tibia and fibula when she fell approximately 1.5 feet. At age 8, she sustained a fracture of the left tibia and growth plate. At age 9, she fractured her right tibia. Her fractures at age 10 involved the left distal femur and right distal tibia, both sustained while transferring from her wheelchair to a toilet. The patient again sustained a hairline fracture of her right distal tibia when her foot caught in a towel while showering.

The combination of these impairments, resulting in the cycle of immobilization and further disuse, rendered her condition disabling. Rachel was referred to our facility at age 10.

Femur fractures sustained at age 10 were managed with hip spica casts to allow continued weight bearing while the fractures were healing. Nevertheless, this series of fractures left Rachel virtually nonambulatory and with decreased ADL skills. In addition, she was afraid of attempting to walk again. At this point, Rachel's initial impairments had resulted in functional loss.

Rachel's disabilities included nonambulatory status, reduced endurance for community mobility using a wheelchair, and reduced independence at home in all of her self-care needs, such as toileting and bathing.

Specific impairments, functional limitations, and disabilities that physical therapy was intended to change included reduced ambulatory ability, reduced endurance and skill in wheelchair mobility, reduced strength in both the lower and upper extremities, and reduced ADL skills, particularly toileting and bathing. It was deemed necessary to provide Rachel with intensive rehabilitation with the goals of regaining lost ambulatory ability and functional ADL skills. In addition, weight management became a goal because she had gained weight secondary to her decreased activity level. Another complication to address was that of low back pain.

Physical therapy was used to prevent further secondary impairment with the goal of preserving and regaining as much function as possible. Specifically, for Rachel this was intended to retard the impairment and loss of function that had ensued from immobilization following the fractures.

The physical therapy program initially consisted of preambulation weight bearing and exercises (active and active-resistive exercises when possible). This was initiated in the pool, where protected weight bearing and graded resistive exercise could safely be monitored. Through the aquatics program, general conditioning, strengthening, and endurance could also be enhanced, thus addressing the weight and back pain concerns.

In conjunction with the aquatic program, Rachel gradually progressed to standing with a left HKAFO with drop-lock hinge for protected weight bearing and musculature support. During this time, graded manual and skateboard exercises (done in an antigravity horizontal plane) were accomplished primarily for lower extremity musculature strengthening and flexibility. Independence in a strengthening and flexibility (other than passive ROM) program was emphasized. Upper extremity exercises and activities were emphasized as well to improve strength needed for use in ambulation training with crutches and for wheelchair propulsion and transfer skills.

Ambulation training progressed from use of maximal support in which the HKAFO was locked at the knee and a walker was used as the assistive device with a contact guard. The goal was to progressively reduce the support of assistive devices and wean Rachel from use of the brace while she progressed in ambulatory endurance. During her 4-week admission, Rachel achieved household ambulation with the HKAFO on the left leg (knee unlocked) using Lofstrand crutches. She continued to use her wheelchair, which was once her major mode of mobility but was now

primarily for community mobility. Wheelchair adjustments were addressed, such as installing proper footrests to prevent a hyperextension injury, to prevent possible fracture to the ankles from otherwise dangling extremities, and to accommodate a leg length discrepancy. ADL were addressed in collaboration with the occupational therapist, and improvements were made in safer but independent transfer ability to the tub and toilet. An elevated toilet seat and nighttime commode helped Rachel achieve independence in toileting.

Also investigated was the use of hormonal therapy to either stimulate or arrest linear growth. A pediatric endocrinologist was consulted to consider the use of estrogen therapy to enhance her pubertal process and therefore reduce the likelihood of fractures. The conclusion from the endocrinologist was that he did not recommend use of estrogen therapy for Rachel because she had not yet completed 90% of her linear growth and estrogen therapy may decrease ultimate adult height.

In conclusion, Rachel benefited from the intensive and structured rehabilitation program in which she was an active participant both in the setting of her goals and in carrying them out now and in the future. Ultimately, she attained household ambulation status with braces and crutches, improved wheelchair propulsion skill and endurance for community mobility, and improved independence in ADL with the use of selected adaptive devices.

Although Rachel has endured setbacks, she has achieved greater independence in function and participated in community-based activities culminating in receipt of outstanding recognition and a medal in the state's annual wheelchair games. Academically and socially, Rachel interacts well with her peers and is attaining educational goals that will allow her to progress vocationally.

Recommended Resources

Osteogenesis Imperfecta Foundation, Inc.
804 W. Diamond Avenue, Suite 210
Gaithersburg, MD 20878
Phone: 301-947-0083

Osteogenesis Imperfecta National Capital Area, Inc.
Box 941
1311 Delaware Ave., SW
Washington, DC 20024
Phone: 202-265-1614

Children's Research Foundation for Osteogenesis Imperfecta
1027 Cambridge Street
Natrona Heights, PA 15065

Sillence, DO, & Barlow, KK. Osteogenesis Imperfecta: A Handbook for Medical Practitioners and Health Professionals. Sydney: IMS Publishing, 1992.

References

Albright, JA. Management overview of osteogenesis imperfecta. Clinical Orthopedics, *159*:80–87, 1981.

Albright, JP, Albright, JA, & Crelin, ES. Osteogenesis imperfecta tarda: The morphology of rib biopsies. Clinical Orthopedics, *108*:204–213, 1975.

Bachman, WH. Variables affecting post school economic adaptation of orthopedically handicapped and other health-impaired students. Rehabilitation Literature, *3*:98, 1972.

Bailey, RW, & Dubow, HI. Experimental and clinical studies of longitudinal bone growth utilizing a new method of internal fixation crossing the epiphyseal plate. Journal of Bone and Joint Surgery (American), *47*:1669, 1965.

Bayley, N. Bayley Scales of Infant Development, 2nd ed. San Antonio: Psychological Corporation, 1993.

Benson, DR, & Newman, DC. The spine and surgical treatment in osteogenesis imperfecta. Clinical Orthopedics, *159*:147–153, 1981.

Binder, H, Hawkes, L, Graybill, G, Gerber, NL, & Weintrob, JC. Osteogenesis imperfecta: Rehabilitation approach with infants and young children. Archives of Physical Medicine and Rehabilitation, *65*:537–541, 1984.

Bleck, EE. Nonoperative treatment of osteogenesis imperfecta: Orthotic and mobility management. Clinical Orthopedics, *159*:111–122, 1981.

Bluemcke, S, Niedorf, HR, Thiel, HJ, & Langness, U. Histochemical and fine structural studies on the cornea in osteogenesis imperfecta. Virchows Archiv. B, Cell Pathology, *11*:124–132, 1972.

Bullough, PG, Davidson, DD, & Lorenzo, JC. The morbid anatomy of the skeleton in osteogenesis imperfecta. Clinical Orthopedics, *159*: 42–57, 1981.

Byers, PH. Osteogenesis Imperfecta: An Update: Growth, Genetics and Hormones, Vol. 4, Part 2. New York: McGraw-Hill, 1988.

Daly, K, Wisbeach, A, Sampera, I, Jr, & Fixsen, JA. The prognosis for walking in osteogenesis imperfecta. Journal of Bone and Joint Surgery(British), *78*:477–480, 1996.

Doty, SB, & Matthews, RS. Electronmicroscopic and histochemical investigation of osteogenesis imperfecta tarda. Clinical Orthopedics, *80*:191–201, 1971.

Duffield, MH. Physiological and therapeutic effects of exercise in warm water. In Skinner, AT, & Thomson, AM (Eds.), Duffield's Exercise in Water, 3rd ed. London: Bailliere Tindall, 1983.

Engelbert, RHH, Gerver, WJM, Breslau-Siderius, LJ, van der Graaf, Y, Pruijs, HEH, van Doorne, JM, Beemer, FA, & Helders, PJM. Spinal complication in osteogenesis imperfecta: 47 patients 1–16 years of age. Acta Orthopaedica Scandinavica, *69*:283–286, 1998.

Engelbert, RHH, van der Graaf, Y, van Empelen, MA, Beemer, A, & Helders, PJM. Osteogenesis imperfecta in childhood: Impairment and disability. Pediatrics, *99*(2):E3, 1997.

Falvo, KA, & Bullough, PG. Osteogenesis imperfecta: A histometric analysis. Journal of Bone and Joint Surgery (American), *55*:275–286, 1973.

Falvo, KA, Root, L, & Bullough, PG. Osteogenesis imperfecta: A clinical evaluation and management. Journal of Bone and Joint Surgery (American), *56*:783–793, 1974.

Fehribach, G. Independent living. Presented before the Osteogenesis Imperfecta Foundation National Convention, Pittsburgh, 1990.

Folio, M, & Fewell, R. Peabody Developmental Motor Scales and Activity Cards. Allen, TX: DLM Teaching Resources, 1983.

Follis, RH, Jr. Osteogenesis imperfecta congenita: A connective tissue diathesis. Journal of Pediatrics, *41*:713–721, 1952.

Gerber, LH, Binder, H, Berry, R, Siegel, KL, Kim, HK, Weintrob, J, Lee,Y, Mizell, S, & Marini, J. Effects of withdrawal of bracing in matched pairs of children with osteogenesis imperfecta. Archives of Physical Medicine and Rehabilitation, *79*:46–51, 1998.

Gerber, LH, Binder, H, Weintrob, J, Grenge, DK, Shapiro, J, Fromherz, W, Berry, R, Conway, A, Nason, S, & Marini, J. Rehabilitation of children and infants with osteogenesis imperfecta: A program for ambulation. Clinical Orthopaedics and Related Research, *251*:254–262, 1990.

Goldman, AB, Davidson, D, Pavlov, H, & Bullough, PG. "Popcorn" calcifications: A prognostic sign in osteogenesis imperfecta. Radiology, *136*:351–358, 1980.

Haley, SM, Faas, RM, Coster, WJ, Webster, H, & Gans, BM. Pediatric Evaluation of Disability Inventory. Boston: New England Medical Center, 1989.

Hanscom, DA, Winter, RB, Lutter, L, Lonstein, JE, Bloom, B, & Bradford, DS. Osteogenesis imperfecta. Journal of Bone and Joint Surgery (American), *74*:598–616, 1992.

Jerosch, J, Mazzotti, I, & Tomasvic, M. Complications after treatment of patients with osteogenesis imperfecta with a Bailey-Dubow rod. Archives of Orthopaedic Trauma Surgery, *117*:240–245, 1998.

Kiley, L, Sterne, R, & Witkop, CJ. Psychosocial factors in low-incidence genetic disease: The case of osteogenesis imperfecta. Social Work in Health Care, *1*:409–420, 1976.

King, JD, & Bobechko, WP. Osteogenesis imperfecta: An orthopedic description and surgical review. Journal of Bone and Joint Surgery (British), *53*:72–86, 1971.

Landsmeer-Beker, EA. Treatment of osteogenesis imperfecta with the bisphosphonate olpadronate (dimethylaminohydroxypropylidene bisphosphonate). European Journal of Pediatrics, *156*:792–794, 1997.

Letts, M, Monson, R, & Weber, K. The prevention of recurrent fractures of the lower extremities in severe osteogenesis imperfecta using vacuum pants: A preliminary report in four patients. Journal of Pediatric Orthopedics, *8*:454–457, 1988.

Looser, E. Zur Kenntnis der Osteogenesis imperfecta congenita und tarda (sogenannte idiopathische Osteopsathyrosis). Mitteilungen Grenzgebieten Medizin und Chirurgie, *15*:161, 1906. (Translation: Toward an understanding of osteogenesis imperfecta and tarda [also known as idiopathic osteopsathyrosis]. Transactions of Fronteurs of Medicine and Surgery.)

Marini, JC, & Gerber, LH. Osteogenesis imperfecta: Rehabilitation and prospects for gene therapy. Journal of the American Medical Association, *277*:746–750, 1997.

Morel, G, & Houghton, GR. Pneumatic trouser splints in the treatment of severe osteogenesis imperfecta. Acta Orthopaedica Scandinavica, *53*:547–552, 1982.

Patti, G. Sports and OI. Presented before the Osteogenesis Imperfecta Foundation National Conference, Pittsburgh, 1990.

Perrin, EC, & Gerrity, PS. Development of children with a chronic illness. Pediatric Clinics of North America, *31*:19–31, 1984.

Ramser, JR, & Frost, HM. The study of a rib biopsy from a patient with osteogenesis imperfecta: A method using in vivo tetracycline labeling. Acta Orthopaedica Scandinavica, *37*:229–240, 1966.

Rezte, L. Osteogenesis imperfecta: Psychological function. American Journal of Psychiatry, *128*(12):1446–1540, 1972.

Scott, EF. The use of air splints for mobility training in osteogenesis imperfecta. Clinical Suggestions, *2*(1):52–53, 1990.

Seedorf, KS. Osteogenesis imperfecta: A study of clinical features and heredity based on 55 Danish families comprising 180 affected members. Opera ex Domo Biologiae Hereditariae Humanae Universitatis Hafniensis, Arhus: Universitetsforlaget, *20*:1–229, 1949.

Sillence, DO. Osteogenesis imperfecta: Expanding panorama of variants. Clinical Orthopaedics and Related Research, *159*:11–25, 1981.

Sillence, DO, & Danks, DM. The differentiation of genetically distinct varieties of osteogenesis imperfecta in the newborn period. Clinical Research, *26*:178A, 1978.

Sillence, DO, Senn, A, & Danks, DM. Genetic heterogeneity in osteogenesis imperfecta. Journal of Medical Genetics, *16*:101–116, 1979.

Solomons, CC, & Millar, EA. Osteogenesis imperfecta: New perspectives. Clinical Orthopaedics and Related Research, *96*:299–303, 1973.

Spranger, J, Cremin, B, & Beighton, P. Osteogenesis imperfecta congenita. Pediatric Radiology, *12*:21–27, 1982.

Tachdjian, MO (Ed.). Pediatric Orthopedics, Vol. 2, 2nd ed. Philadelphia: WB Saunders, 1990.

Thompson, CE. Raising a handicapped child. Presented before the Osteogenesis Imperfecta Foundation National Conference, Pittsburgh, 1990.

Wynne-Davies, R, & Gormley, J. Clinical and genetic patterns in osteogenesis imperfecta. Clinical Orthopaedics and Related Research, *159*:26–35, 1981.

C H A P T E R

14

Muscular Dystrophy and Spinal Muscular Atrophy

WAYNE A. STUBERG, PT, PhD, PCS

Neuromuscular diseases include disorders of the motor neuron (anterior horn cells and peripheral nerve), neuromuscular junction, and muscle. Muscular dystrophy (MD) and spinal muscular atrophy (SMA) are two prevalent, progressive neuromuscular diseases that require physical therapy. Progressive weakness, muscle atrophy, contracture, deformity, and progressive disability characterize both diseases. No cure is available for either disease. "Incurable," however, is not synonymous with "untreatable," and the physical therapist can be influential in prevention of complications, preservation of function, and issues concerning quality of life.

The objective of this chapter is to present an overview of the childhood forms of MD and SMA, including the role of the physical therapist as a member of the management team. The clinical presentation of the diseases is reviewed, and examination procedures are presented to assist the clinician in identifying impairments, functional limitations, and

disabilities associated with MD and SMA. Guidelines for physical therapy management are also outlined based on my clinical experience and review of related literature.

ROLE OF THE PHYSICAL THERAPIST

As a member of the management team in either the educational or medical setting, the physical therapist assists in the identification and amelioration of impairments, functional limitations, disabilities, or handicaps for persons with MD or SMA. The team often includes physician(s) (neurologist, orthopedist, or physiatrist), physical therapist, occupational therapist, speech therapist, educator, social worker, genetic counselor, psychologist, and orthotist. Because therapists typically maintain a higher frequency of contact with families, referral to and ongoing communication with other team members becomes an important issue in maintaining continuity of care.

The team approach should be family centered with a focus on collaborative goal setting among individuals with the disorder, family members, and professionals to ensure optimal care. By providing care using a family-centered philosophy, the pivotal role of the family is recognized and respected in the lives of persons with special health care needs.

Prevention is also an important role of the physical therapist. Stress on the child and family can be reduced and coping facilitated through accurate prognostic information and foreseeing signs that portend changing status that will result in increased disability. Examples of status change include the period before the loss of walking, before the need for architectural modifications to accommodate adaptive equipment for mobility, during transition from the educational environment, or during the terminal stages of the disease when the decision to use mechanical ventilation will be a major issue for the family.

Providing information to family members, persons with MD or SMA, and other members of the team regarding physical limitations and expected disabilities is an important role for the physical therapist. Resource materials for families (Ringel, 1987), teachers (Bleck & Nagel, 1982), or other members of the team can often eliminate misconceptions or false expectations. Many resource materials are available through the national Muscular Dystrophy Association (MDA) office (3300 East Sunrise Drive, Tucson, AZ 85718) or through state chapter MDA offices.

PHYSICAL THERAPY EXAMINATION AND EVALUATION

Although the progression of MD and SMA is relatively well known, the clinician must carefully observe the child for changes that require intervention modifications. As stated by Thomas McCrae (1870–1935), "More is missed by not looking than by not knowing" (Siegel, 1986). Ongoing dialogue with families is invaluable in identifying family-centered goals and the need for program modification.

The physical therapy examination is the initial step in management of the child with MD or SMA and should include those components identified in the "Guide to Physical Therapist Practice" (American Physical Therapy Association [APTA], 1997). Specifically, the following must be carefully examined:

1. History with family concerns
2. Aerobic capacity and endurance
3. Assistive and adaptive devices
4. Community and work (job/school/play) integration
5. Environmental, home, and job/school/play barriers
6. Gait, locomotion, and balance
7. Integumentary (when using orthoses, adaptive equipment, or wheelchair)
8. Muscle performance
9. Neuromotor development
10. Orthotic, protective, and supportive devices
11. Posture
12. Range of motion
13. Self-care and home management
14. Ventilation/respiration

Systematic documentation of disease progression is essential in timing of interventions during transitions from one functional status to another or during times of increased family need.

MUSCULAR DYSTROPHY

The etiology of MD is genetic inheritance. The pathophysiology underlying the disease is progressive loss of muscle contractility caused by the destruction of myofibrils. The specific cellular mechanism behind the destruction in Duchenne muscular dystrophy (DMD) and Becker muscular dystrophy (BMD) has been partially identified and is discussed later in the chapter. The rate of progression of myofibril destruction is variable among the various forms of MD, giving evidence for the possibility of more than one cellular mechanism in the destructive process.

The diagnosis of MD is confirmed by clinical examination and laboratory procedures, including electromyography, muscle biopsy, DNA analysis, and selected enzyme levels assayed from blood samples (Miller & Hoffman, 1994; Siegel, 1986). The criteria for classification of the various forms of MD include the mode of inheritance, age at onset, rate of progression, localization of involvement, muscle morphologic changes, and presence of a genetic marker if available. The MDA recognizes nine primary classifications of MD (Muscular Dystrophy Association, 1991). Table 14–1 lists the six most prevalent types that exhibit initial clinical signs in infancy, childhood, or adolescence. Emery-Dreifus MD (humeroperoneal) is very rare and is only discussed briefly. Limb-girdle MD may exhibit signs in the teenage years, but the onset of symptoms is more typically in early adulthood, and therefore, along with the adult-onset forms of MD, it is not discussed in this chapter. The reader should refer to texts on neuromuscular diseases by Brooke (1986), Siegel (1986), and Harper (1989) for further information on clinical presentation and general management of MD.

TABLE 14–1. **Classification of Muscular Dystrophy**

Type	Onset	Inheritance	Course
Duchenne	1–4 years	X-linked	Rapidly progressive; loss of walking by 9 to 10 years; death in late teens
Becker	5–10 years	X-linked	Slowly progressive; maintain walking past early teens; life span into third decade
Congenital	Birth	Recessive	Typically slow but variable; shortened life span
Congenital myotonic	Birth	Dominant	Typically slow with significant intellectual impairment
Childhood-onset facioscapulohumeral	First decade	Dominant/recessive	Slowly progressive loss of walking in later life; variable life expectancy
Emery-Dreifus	Childhood to early teens	X-linked	Slowly progressive with cardiac abnormality and normal life span

The primary impairment in MD is insidious weakness secondary to progressive loss of myofibrils. In the case of the congenital forms of MD the weakness is pronounced at birth and easily recognizable. In DMD, the weakness becomes evident by age 3 to 5 years. In congenital and congenital myotonic MD, contractures present at birth also cause primary impairment. The incidence of mental retardation is highest in congenital myotonic MD, but it is less frequently reported in DMD or the other childhood forms.

Secondary impairments in all forms of MD include the development of contractures and postural malalignment. Postural malalignment is seen in antigravity positions of sitting and standing and often includes development of scoliosis. Other secondary impairments include decreased respiratory capacity, easy fatigability, and occasionally obesity. Although significant intellectual impairment is not usual, IQ is commonly below average and reported in the range of 70 to 80 in DMD (Leibowitz & Dubowitz, 1981). This finding may be related to a loss of dystrophin in the brain, but the relationship has not been elucidated to date.

With the progression of muscle weakness, increasing caregiver assistance is required for persons with MD to carry out activities of daily living (ADL). Progressive disability is a hallmark of MD and requires multidisciplinary team management to minimize handicaps through the use of adaptive equipment and environmental adaptations.

Physical management in the treatment of MD is a key intervention because no drug or other therapy has been found to be curative (Brooke, 1986; DeSilva et al., 1987). Physical therapy has been used to prolong the child's independence, slow the progression of complications, and improve the quality of life.

Dystrophin-Associated Proteins and Muscular Dystrophy

Within the past 10 years significant advances have been made in the molecular genetics and biology of the muscular dystrophies. These advances have followed the identification of the genetic defect behind DMD and the missing protein dystrophin. Many other proteins that are associated with dystrophin have been found to be defective or missing in other forms of MD. The proteins are termed *dystrophin-associated proteins* (DAPs) (Brown, 1997). The DAPs form a complex of extracellular, transmembrane, and intracellular proteins that are represented in Figure 14–1.

Dystrophin acts as an anchor in the intracellular lattice to enhance tensile strength. The other proteins are thought to act as a physical pathway for transmembrane signaling, with the exception of sarcospan and the sarcoglycan complex, whose exact function is unknown. Absence of any transmembrane protein, however, would result in faulty mechanics of the cell membrane.

Duchenne Muscular Dystrophy

DMD is the most common X-linked disorder known, with an incidence of about 1 in 3500 live male births (MDA, 1991). The prevalence of DMD in the general population is reported at about 3 cases per 100,000 (Emery, 1993; Mostacciuolo et al., 1987). Longevity is variable from the late teens to early twenties up to the end of the third decade, depending on the rate of disease progression, presence of complications, and aggressiveness of respiratory care, including the use of assisted ventilation (Curran & Colbert, 1989).

Kunkel and associates (1985) identified the gene on the X chromosome (Xp21) that, when missing or

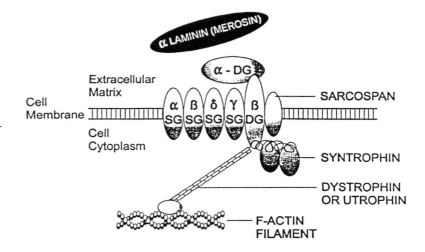

FIGURE 14–1. Dystrophin-associated protein complex. Cross-section through muscle membrane with intracellular, transcellular, and extracellular proteins.
SG = sarcogylcan, DG = dystroglycan.

defective, causes DMD and BMD, and Hoffman and associates (1987) then identified the protein (dystrophin) of the chromosome locus. Cloning of the dystrophin gene was the next major accomplishment, which provided a mechanism for prenatal or postnatal diagnosis and development of gene therapy (Koenig et al., 1987).

The etiology of muscle cell destruction in DMD and BMD is due to abnormal or missing dystrophin and its effect at the muscle cell membrane. Absent or abnormal dystrophin allows increased permeability of the cell (Arahata et al., 1988). Because several lytic enzymes within the muscle cell are activated by calcium, it is hypothesized that necrosis is due to an uncontrolled rise of calcium concentration in the cell, thereby activating proteolytic enzymes, leading to cell destruction (Mokri & Engel, 1975).

The focus of research for the treatment of DMD involves myoblast transfer therapy, gene replacement therapy, and attempts to increase production of other dystrophin-related sarcolemmal proteins (utropin). All therapies are in the experimental stage; myoblast transfer therapy is currently being evaluated in humans, the first human gene therapy trials for DMD using dystrophin are pending FDA approval, and no human trial work has begun on the use of utropin (Wahl, 1998).

In myoblast transfer therapy the embryologic precursor cells of skeletal muscle (i.e., myoblasts) are obtained from a histocompatible donor. The cells are then injected into the muscle of the individual with DMD with the hope that the normal myoblasts will grow, mutate with the surrounding cells that are lacking dystrophin, and result in development of dystrophin. The results of the research in animals have shown that donor myoblast cells fuse with the dystrophic cells to form a hybrid multinucleated cell that produces dystrophin (Partridge et al., 1978). Myoblast transfer therapy is currently controversial, with the research by Law and colleagues (1997) supporting its efficacy but earlier research reporting disappointing results (Karpati et al., 1992) and lack of substantiation by other laboratories for the findings of Law and associates.

Gene therapy research involves the introduction of the dystrophin gene that is packaged in a modified adenovirus called a vector. Lee and colleagues (1991) produced an entire dystrophin gene, and more recently Amalfitano and associates (1998) developed the vector for delivering the gene. The trial that is pending FDA approval will involve the injection of the vector into the bicep muscles of children age 5 to 7 years with a diagnosis of DMD.

Utropin is a muscle protein that has molecular similarity to dystrophin. Utropin levels in the muscle are high in the fetus and newborn but gradually diminish, until utropin is primarily found at the neuromuscular or musculotendinous junction in adults. It has been speculated that if utropin levels could be increased genetically through "upregulation," utropin might act as a substitute for abnormal or missing dystrophin. Work is also underway to stop the process of utropin decrease observed from childhood to adulthood. Utropin is found in the muscles of boys with DMD; therefore the use of utropin may be a more viable alternative to dystrophin because there may be an autoimmune response to dystrophin gene therapy in boys who genetically lack the protein (Tinsley & Davies, 1993).

Medical management of DMD has also included clinical trials of steroid therapy. DeSilva and

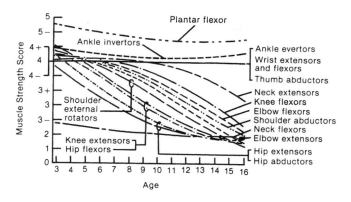

FIGURE 14–2. Muscle strength 50th percentile lines plotted against age of 150 children with DMD. (Redrawn from Brooke, MH. A Clinician's View of Neuromuscular Diseases, 2nd ed. Baltimore: Williams & Wilkins, 1986.)

colleagues (1987) have demonstrated evidence of significantly prolonged survival (up to 2 years) in a prednisone-treated versus control group study. A more recent study by Backman and Henriksson (1995) provided an excellent review of early steroid treatment studies and reported positive results in a 12-month, randomized, double-blind cross-over study using prednisolone in a group of 40 individuals with DMD or BMD. A significant increase in muscle strength was found in comparing the 6-month placebo versus 6-month prednisolone phases of the study.

Although it is commonly agreed that the prevention of contractures and deformity and the preservation of independent mobility are primary goals of a physical management program (Vignos, 1983), the prolongation of ambulation through surgery or orthotics has been controversial in DMD (Gardner-Medwin, 1979, 1980a). Some authors promote the use of surgery and lightweight bracing (Bach & McKeon, 1991; Heckmatt et al., 1985; Miller & Dunn, 1982; Siegel, 1975; Ziter & Allsop, 1979); others express skepticism about prolonging the inevitable in a progressive disease when the financial and emotional costs to the family may be very high (Gardner-Medwin, 1979).

Surgical management has focused on the control of lower extremity contractures, use of orthoses in conjunction with surgery to prolong ambulation, and spinal stabilization for control of scoliosis. Achilles tendon lengthenings and fasciotomies of the tensor fascia lata and iliotibial bands are two procedures commonly reported to be used in conjunction with orthotics and physical therapy to prolong ambulation (Bach & McKeon, 1991). Posterior tibialis transfer into the third cuneiform to reverse equinovarus deformity has also been reported (Roy & Gibson, 1970). Surgical management of scoliosis typically includes the use of spinal instrumentation with Luque rods (Marchesi et al., 1997).

Impairments, Functional Limitations, and Disability

Examination of the 4- to 5-year-old child demonstrates the onset of classical clinical features of DMD and the primary impairment of muscle weakness. The posterior calf is usually enlarged as a result of fatty and connective tissue infiltration, which corresponds to the term *pseudohypertrophic MD* that is used for the eponym DMD. The pseudohypertrophy can occasionally be seen to affect the deltoid, quadriceps, or forearm extensor muscle groups. Initial weakness of the neck flexor, abdominal, interscapular, and hip extensor musculature can be noted with a more generalized distribution with progression of the disease. Figure 14–2 demonstrates the trends of muscle strength decline up to age 16 years from a study by Brooke (1986). The data were obtained in a multiclinic study of 150 children with DMD over a follow-up period of 3 to 4 years. The data represent approximately 15 data points per boy as recorded during follow-up visits.

Muscle strength can be documented using manual muscle testing (MMT), which has been reported to have acceptable intrarater reliability (Florence et al., 1992), although it is not as accurate as using specialized devices such as a dynamometer. Instruments such as a handheld dynamometer (Stuberg & Metcalf, 1988) or strain gauge devices (Brussock et al., 1992) can be used to obtain objective strength recordings in the older child to assist in prediction

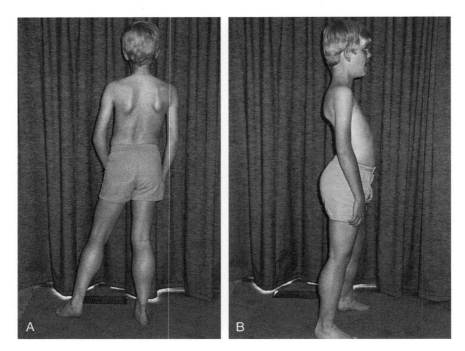

FIGURE 14-3. Typical standing posture of a 7-year-old boy with DMD. *A,* Posterior view; note the winging of the scapula, equinus contracture of the left ankle, and calf pseudohypertrophy. *B,* Lateral view; note increased lumbar lordosis.

of disability, such as the loss of independent ambulation.

No limitations in range of motion (ROM) are noted typically before 5 years of age in DMD. Mild tightness of the gastrocsoleus and tensor fascia lata muscles usually occurs first. The normal lordotic standing posture is increased, and mild winging of the scapulae is then seen as a compensation to keep the center of mass behind the hip joint to promote standing stability (Fig. 14-3). Scoliosis typically develops just before or during adolescence.

Infancy to Preschool-Age Period

No significant impairment, functional limitation, or disability is typically seen in the infant or toddler with DMD. Gardner-Medwin (1980b) reported that half of the children fail to walk until 18 months of age. Delay in walking, however, rarely leads to the diagnosis of DMD. Symptoms are seldom noted before age 3 to 5 years, unless there is a positive family history and caregivers are looking for early signs. The mean age at diagnosis is usually reported to be around 5 years (Miller & Dunn, 1982).

Although there is no significant disability in early childhood, many disability-related issues must be addressed. The family will have questions regarding peer interaction, routine activity level for the child, and the prognosis. The therapist must be aware of

each family's coping response, goals, and needed supports to provide family-centered care. This is the appropriate time to discuss with the family the social aspects of the disability and to answer questions without portraying a future without hope.

Early School-Age Period

The initial disability in DMD typically occurs by age 5 years and includes clumsiness, falling, and inability to keep up with peers while playing. The young child's gait pattern is only slightly atypical, with an increased lateral trunk sway (waddling). Attempts at running, however, accentuate the waddling progression, and neither running nor jumping is attained. The Gower sign (using the arms to push on the thighs to attain standing) is usually present after one or repeated trials of assuming standing position from sitting on the floor.

Stair climbing and arising to standing from the floor become progressively more difficult and signal the first significant functional limitation by age 6 to 8 years. Progressive changes in the gait pattern include the deviations of an increased base of support, pronounced lateral trunk sway (compensated Trendelenburg), toe-walking, and retraction of the shoulders with lack of reciprocal arm swing. Toe-walking initially may be a compensation for weakness of the abdominal and hip extensor muscles, resulting in lordosis and forward shift of the body's center of mass with later evidence of contracture of the posterior calf musculature.

Toe-walking caused by contracture of the posterior calf musculature, in-toeing with substitution of the tensor fascia lata to compensate for weakness of the iliopsoas muscles, falls resulting from progressive weakness, and complaints of fatigue while walking become increasingly frequent from age 8 to 10 years. A restrictive pattern of pulmonary impairment and progressive decline in maximal vital capacity also becomes increasingly evident (Galasko et al., 1995).

EXAMINATION CONSIDERATIONS

An examination to document functional impairment and disability progression is essential. Various formats have been reported (Brooke, 1986; Vignos et al., 1963) that are variations of the guidelines initially published by Swinyard and associates (1957). A classification system published by Vignos and colleagues (1963) is outlined in Box 14–1. A more detailed examination format for DMD has been published by Brooke and associates (1981), which includes pulmonary function and timed performance of activities (see Appendix I). Normative data for DMD has been published using the clinical protocol by Brooke and associates (1989). Other functional assessment tools, such as the Pediatric Evaluation of Disability Inventory (PEDI) (Haley et al., 1992) or School Function Assessment (SFA) (Coster et al., 1998), should also be considered for use to give more specific information on the child's functional skills. The PEDI, the SFA, or the Vignos (Brooke) functional testing format can be used for diagnosis of other types of MD or of SMA.

Muscle weakness is apparent in the school-age child by age 6 to 8 years and should be objectively documented using a handheld dynamometer (Stuberg & Metcalf, 1988), electrodynamometer (Saranti et al., 1980), isokinetic dynamometer (Molnar & Alexander, 1973; Scott et al., 1982), or other device. Use of a dynamometer in conjunction with manual muscle testing has been shown to provide reliable information on the progression of weakness in key muscle groups (Brussock et al., 1992; Fowler & Gardner, 1967; Stuberg & Metcalf, 1988). Contracture development should be documented using goniometry and a standardized protocol. Intrarater reliability of the measurements has been shown to be acceptable to provide objective information for program planning when a standardized measurement protocol is used (Pandya et al., 1985).

A clinical estimate of respiratory function can be obtained through measurement of respiratory rate and chest wall excursion (using a tape measure) and

---

> **BOX 14–1. Vignos Functional Rating Scale for Duchenne Muscular Dystrophy**
>
> 1. Walks and climbs stairs without assistance
> 2. Walks and climbs stairs with aid of railing
> 3. Walks and climbs stairs slowly with aid of railing (over 25 seconds for eight standard steps)
> 4. Walks, but cannot climb stairs
> 5. Walks assisted, but cannot climb stairs or get out of chair
> 6. Walks only with assistance or with braces
> 7. In wheelchair: sits erect and can roll chair and perform bed and wheelchair ADL
> 8. In wheelchair: sits erect and is unable to perform bed and wheelchair ADL without assistance
> 9. In wheelchair: sits erect only with support and is able to do only minimal ADL
> 10. In bed: can do no ADL without assistance
>
> Data from Vignos, PJ, Spencer, GE, & Archibald, KC. Management of progressive muscular dystrophy. Journal of the American Medical Association, *184*:103–112, 1963. Copyright © 1963, American Medical Association.

---

by noting the child's ability to cough and clear secretions. A portable spirometer is recommended to obtain a more direct and objective reading of expiratory capacity before the need for formal pulmonary function testing.

Physical therapy management typically begins when the child is initially diagnosed at age 3 to 5 years. Goals of the program are to provide family support and education, obtain baseline data on muscle strength and ROM, and monitor for the progression of muscle weakness that will lead to disability. Initial therapeutic input should not be burdensome to the child or family because the child is usually independent in all ADL before age 5 years. Information should be provided to the family pertaining to the therapist's role as a member of the management team. An appropriate activity level to avoid fatigue should be discussed with the family and school staff. Information on services through the local MDA office should be provided, including identification of support groups or contact families.

INTERVENTION CONSIDERATIONS

The role of exercise in the treatment of MD is controversial (Brooke, 1986; Fowler, 1982; Vignos, 1983). It is widely accepted that both overexertion (Johnson & Braddom, 1971; Vignos et al., 1963) and immobilization (Vignos et al., 1963) are detrimental. The use of graded resistive exercise has been reported to have a range of results from good (Vignos & Watkins, 1966) to limited (de Lateur & Giaconi, 1979) to adverse. Resistive exercise would theoretically be indicated with the disproportionate loss of type II (fast-twitch) muscle fibers in DMD (Edwards, 1980). However, the use of resistive exercise in the young school-age child should not be universally prescribed. Prescribing a submaximal exercise program early has been shown to have beneficial effects, but it should be offered only to families who have a specific desire to include it in the child's program. Consideration should be given to the fact that significant muscle weakness is not seen in the early stage of the disease and the use of an exercise program may be burdensome to the child and family.

If exercise is initiated early, the key muscle groups to be included are the abdominal, hip extensor and abductor, and knee extensor groups. Abdominal exercises should include trunk curls as opposed to sit-ups, which will primarily strengthen the hip flexors. Assistance may be required for neck flexor weakness, because the head typically cannot be flexed from a supine position. Cycling and swimming are excellent activities for overall conditioning and are often preferred over formal exercise programs (Gardner-Medwin, 1980b; Vignos, 1983). Standing or walking for a minimum of 2 to 3 hours daily is highly recommended (Siegel, 1978; Ziter & Allsop, 1976).

Breathing exercises have been shown to slow the loss of vital capacity and forced expiratory flow rate (Houser & Johnson, 1971; Rodillo et al., 1989). Game activities such as inflating balloons or using blow-bottles to maintain pulmonary function can easily be included in a home program and will decrease the severity of symptoms during episodes of colds or other pulmonary infections.

The use of electrical stimulation in DMD has also been suggested as a means of slowing the progression of weakness and improving function. Scott and co-workers (1986) studied the effect of low-frequency electrical stimulation on the tibialis anterior muscle of 16 children with DMD. A 47% increase in maximum voluntary contraction was observed in younger children following a stimulation protocol used for 8 weeks, with little change noted in older children. The authors concluded that the results were encouraging and that further study on muscle groups used for functional activities is needed.

One of the primary considerations in the early management program of the young school-age child is to retard the development of contractures. Contractures have not been shown to be preventable, but the progression can be slowed with positioning and an ROM program (Scott et al., 1981; Seeger et al., 1985; Wong & Wade, 1995; Ziter & Allsop, 1976).

The initial ROM program should include the gastrocsoleus and tensor fascia lata. Progressive contracture of the gastrocsoleus and tensor fascia lata corresponds to gait deviations of toe-walking and an increased base of support. Stretching for the gastrocsoleus can be done using a standing runner's stretch. The child stands at a supportive surface, places one leg back at a time with the knee straight, and leans forward. The position also assists with maintenance of hip flexor flexibility; however, specific stretching for the hip flexors should be included when any limitation is noted. Having the child lie supine with one thigh off the edge of a mat or bed and the other held to the chest (Thomas test position) can be used to stretch the hip flexors initially. An alternative method is discussed later for use as progression of hip extensor weakness evolves. A standing stretch for the tensor is accomplished by having the child stand with one side toward the supportive surface with the feet away from the wall and with the knee kept straight while leaning sideways toward the supportive surface.

A home ROM program should be emphasized for the young child and the family instructed in the stretching exercises. There is lack of agreement as to the frequency and duration of the stretching program. Suggested frequency of the program varies from once daily (Gardner-Medwin, 1980b; Miller & Dunn, 1982; Scott et al., 1981) to twice daily (Vignos et al., 1963; Ziter & Allsop, 1976), and duration from 1 repetition up to 10 (Vignos et al., 1963). Other authors have suggested a time frame of 10 (Ziter & Allsop, 1976) to 20 (Gardner-Medwin, 1980b) minutes to complete the stretching exercises. As a general recommendation, each movement should be repeated for 5 to 10 repetitions and with a 10-second hold in the stretched position. The stretch should be done slowly and should not be painful. Increased risk of injury with the loss of myofibrils and replacement by connective tissue is present because of decreased muscle elasticity, and caution in using excessive passive force is advised. Reassessment of the contracture progression should be used as the final guide to stretching frequency and duration.

The ROM program can often be supplemented as part of the physical education program at school. Special instruction should be provided to the physical education teacher to develop an adapted program, particularly if the teacher does not have an adapted physical education endorsement. General physical education activities will also require modification for the child's participation and should not be exhaustive. Physical fitness test activities such as push-ups, sit-ups, or timed running for long time periods should be modified or excluded to avoid fatigue or overwork weakness.

Night splints are helpful to slow the progression of ankle contractures. Scott and associates (1981) studied the efficacy of night splints and a home ROM program in a group of 59 boys diagnosed with

MD ranging in age from 4 to 12 years. The subjects were categorized into three groups based on compliance with splint wear and use of stretching. The group that followed through on the daily passive stretching program and use of the below-knee splints over the 2 years of the study demonstrated significantly less progression of Achilles tendon contractures and less deterioration in functional skills, leading to a longer period of independent walking. Boys in the group that did not follow through on the stretching or splint program lost independent walking at a younger age. Similar findings were reported in a study by Seeger and colleagues (1985) that compared the use of night splints, stretching, and surgery.

The use of prone positioning at night to slow progression of the hip and knee flexion contractures may be possible if tolerated by the child. The recommendation to have the child sleep prone with the ankles off the edge of the bed has not been shown to affect the progression of the contractures but theoretically is sound.

Scoliosis is not common when the child is ambulatory, but the spine should be checked routinely (Wilkins & Gibson, 1976; Ziter & Allsop, 1976). Alignment of the spine should be closely monitored as weakness progresses to the stage of making walking difficult. Postural analysis using the forward bend test is recommended to monitor spinal alignment for scoliosis. Presence of a rib hump with the forward bend test verifies a structural versus functional curve of the spine. Amendt and colleagues (1990) have demonstrated that a rib hump measuring at least 5° of inclination with a scoliometer is a reliable method and correlated to radiographic assessment. The study by Amendt and colleagues (1990) was, however, not inclusive of children with DMD but demonstrates an objective method of noninvasive screening for scoliosis. Orthopedic referral is indicated if a rib hump is documented.

Falls and complaints of fatigue while walking become increasingly more frequent as the child reaches age 8 to 10 years. Guarding during stair climbing or during general walking should be considered to ensure safety as balance becomes tenuous. A manual wheelchair with appropriate fit and accessories will allow for limited mobility as walking becomes more difficult. As progression of weakness in the trunk and hip girdle begins to make walking difficult, a similar amount of weakness of the shoulder girdle musculature is also present, making propulsion of a manual wheelchair difficult except on level and smooth surfaces such as linoleum. A motorized scooter should be considered to provide the child with independence, provided that access is available in the home and school (Fig. 14–4).

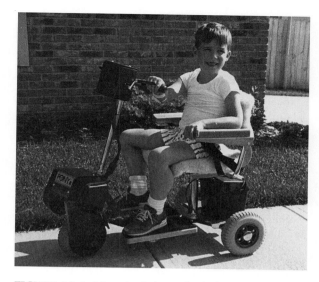

FIGURE 14–4. Motorized three-wheeled scooter for independence in distance mobility as an adjunct to walking. (OrthoKinetics, Inc., Waukesha, WI.)

Information should be made available to families concerning recreational activities provided through the local chapter of the MDA or other groups. Summer MDA camp is a wonderful experience for most children, and a support group is often developed for the child or family through participation in MDA or other group activities that provide not only physical but also emotional support.

Adolescent Period

Adolescence marks a time of significant disability progression as a result of the combined impact of muscle weakness and development of contractures. Walking is lost as a means of mobility, and increasing difficulty in general mobility with transfers is seen. Use of a manual wheelchair or powered mobility becomes necessary during adolescence. If powered mobility is used, assistance with finances for purchase of equipment or home modifications for access is typically needed, with coordination through a social worker or MDA patient services coordinator. Increasing difficulty with ADL, including dressing, transfers, bathing, grooming, and feeding, increases the involvement of the physical therapist and occupational therapist. Decisions regarding possible surgical intervention are also considered for the management of scoliosis or contractures or to prolong walking with the use of orthoses.

As muscle weakness becomes more pronounced in the trunk and hip musculature, and contractures of the hip flexors, tensor fascia lata, and gastrocsoleus progress, walking becomes increasingly difficult until cessation of independent walking occurs, usually by age 10 to 12 (Brooke, 1986). If orthoses are used to maintain a standing or walking program, they should be initiated before the child reaches the stage of being nonambulatory.

Various methods to predict the termination of walking have been reported. The inability to rise from the floor or climb stairs and reports of frequent falls often signal the impending termination of independent walking. If muscle strength has been routinely recorded using a dynamometer or other instrument, Vignos and Archibald (1960) and Scott and associates (1982) have reported cessation of walking when muscle strength in the lower extremities has decreased by 50%. An alternative method as shown in Figure 14–5 has been suggested by Siegel (1977). The knee extension lag while sitting and the hip extension lag while prone are assessed to predict the cessation of independent walking. If the combined lag is greater than 90°, the termination of independent ambulation is within a few months. Ziter and Allsop (1976) have reported using the point when the child is no longer able to ambulate for more than 1 hour during the day or requires external support as a signal to initiate bracing.

Monitoring and management of contractures becomes a key element in maintaining walking when the older child spends more time in sitting position. Because the hip extensor musculature is significantly weak in the early stage of the disease and weakness of the quadriceps muscles becomes pronounced by age 8 to 10 years, inability to maintain the center of gravity behind the hip joint or in front of the knee joint during stance will lead to loss of the ability to stand.

Manual stretching of the hip flexors, tensor fascia lata, and heel cords is necessary because the older child demonstrates difficulty in carrying out the exercises without assistance. Prone lying will help retard the development of hip and knee flexor contractures, but stretching of the hip flexors and tensor using the method shown in Figure 14–6 is recommended. The leg is initially positioned in abduction, then brought into the maximum allowable hip extension followed by hip adduction. A hamstring stretch can also be included in the exercise routine. However, a pattern of capsular tightness of the knee joint caused by prolonged sitting is more common than excessive hamstring contracture because use of the Gower maneuver to assume standing maintains flexibility of the hamstrings during the period of independent ambulation. If a hamstring stretch is used, the leg should be slightly abducted to minimize the subluxing force placed across the hip joint that is present when the leg is in the sagittal plane during the maneuver.

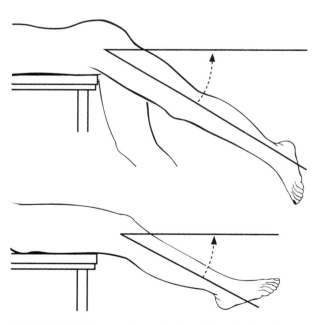

FIGURE 14–5. Prognostic method used by Siegel to determine cessation of independent walking caused by lack of antigravity hip and knee extensor torque. (Redrawn from Siegel, IM. Muscle and Its Diseases: An Outline Primer of Basic Science and Clinical Method. Chicago: Year Book Medical Publisher, 1986.)

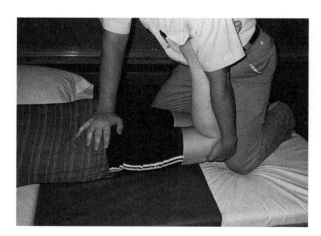

FIGURE 14–6. Prone stretching of the hip flexor, iliotibial band, and tensor fascia lata. The hip is first positioned in abduction and then moved into maximal hip extension and then hip adduction. The knee can be extended to provide greater stretch for the iliotibial band and tensor.

CONTINUATION OF STANDING OR WALKING

The use of orthoses for a standing program or continuation of supported walking is not appropriate for all individuals; in fact, it should be considered a personal rather than therapeutic decision. Although a standing program may be useful to slow the progression of contractures, a braced walking program has little long-term functional or practical application because the child will eventually use a wheelchair. Because surgery is often required in addition to orthotics for prolonged ambulation, both the parents and adolescent must agree in the management decision. Prolongation of ambulation through surgery and orthotics is not a common goal at our facility. Limited resources are more typically used for power mobility equipment, adaptive equipment, or environmental adaptations.

Prognostic factors for success that should be considered in making the decision to use orthoses include the residual muscle strength (approximately 50%) (Vignos, 1983); absence of severe contractures

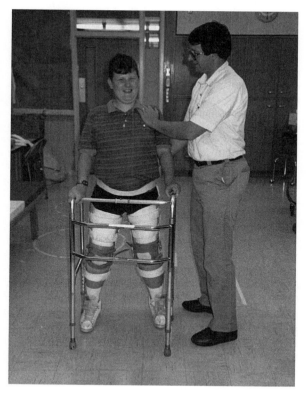

FIGURE 14–7. Polypropylene knee-ankle-foot orthosis and use of a reciprocating walker to promote walking for exercise in a 14-year-old boy with DMD. The reciprocating walker allows progression without picking up the device.

(Roy & Gibson, 1970; Spencer & Vignos, 1962); timely application of the braces (Bach & McKeon, 1991; Spencer & Vignos, 1962); residual walking ability (Vignos & Archibald, 1960); and motivation of the child and family (Bowker & Halpin, 1978). The degree of mental impairment, if present, and obesity should also be considered. The timely use of orthoses has been shown to prolong walking (Bach & McKeon, 1991; Bowker & Halpin, 1978; Heckmatt et al., 1985) and to increase the child's longevity (Bach & McKeon, 1991; Miller & Dunn, 1982; Vignos et al., 1963).

If the decision to use orthoses to prolong standing or walking is made, lightweight knee-ankle-foot orthoses (KAFOs) should be prescribed (Fig. 14–7) (Bowker & Halpin, 1978; Siegel, 1975). Ankle-foot orthoses are appropriate for positioning but often interfere with compensations required for balance during walking on nonlevel surfaces. A reciprocating or wheeled walker may be helpful when assistance for balance is needed. Assistive devices such as a standard walker, crutches, or canes are seldom functional because of the degree of proximal shoulder girdle and upper extremity muscle weakness. Standby assistance should be provided when KAFOs are used, owing to the risk of injury with falls. Closer guarding and increased assistance will be needed as the weakness progresses. Transfers to and from standing are dependent because the knee of the KAFO must be locked to provide stability. The KAFOs can then be used for continuation of a standing program even after walking is no longer possible.

Surgical intervention is commonly needed in conjunction with the use of braced walking as contractures progress. Documented indications for surgery include ankle plantar flexion contractures of greater than 10°, iliotibial band contractures greater than 20°, or knee-hip flexion contractures greater than 20° but less than 45° (Bowker & Halpin, 1978). Subcutaneous tenotomy of the Achilles tendon and fasciotomy of the iliotibial bands are the most commonly reported surgical procedures (Bach & McKeon, 1991; Bowker & Halpin, 1978; Siegel et al., 1972; Vignos, 1983). Transfer of the posterior tibialis tendon is occasionally used for correction of the equinovarus foot posture.

An intensive postoperative management program is essential to retard the effects of immobilization (Siegel et al., 1986). Standing in the plaster casts can be done on the first or second postoperative day. Gait training is begun as tolerated, and general conditioning exercises for the hips, trunk, and upper extremities are recommended. Breathing exercises should also be stressed. A smooth transition from the casts to bracing is ensured by having the child fitted for the KAFOs before hospitalization.

Standing pivot transfers must eventually be replaced by one- or two-person lifts or use of equipment as a result of the development of knee and hip flexion contractures and pronounced weakness of the lower extremities. Transfers to and from the wheelchair, toilet, tub, car, and furniture usually become dependent by age 12 to 14. A sliding board, manual lift, or Hoyer lift can be used during transfers. Proper instruction for transfers is needed because the degree of trunk muscle weakness makes sitting balance tenuous by this stage. If the caregiver is using manual lifting for transfers, he or she should be observed for and instructed in proper body mechanics and safety. A Hoyer lift can be used for transfers to and from the wheelchair particularly when the adolescent is large or obese. A hammock-style sling should be used with the lift to provide adequate head and trunk support during transfers. A tub lift or bath bench for bathing will be needed and a wheeled commode-shower chair considered depending on bathroom accessibility.

MOBILITY AND SPINAL ALIGNMENT

A power scooter as shown in Figure 14–4 should be considered as an initial power wheelchair prescription for the child who is hesitant to use a power wheelchair when walking is no longer possible. The scooter is often more easily accepted by the child and may be used for transition to a standard power wheelchair. If a power scooter is initially used, transition to a power wheelchair will be necessary when the adolescent is seen propping on the arm rests for trunk control. Asymmetric sitting postures must be aggressively managed owing to the correlation of increased sitting time and poor sitting posture with the onset of scoliosis. When limited resources are an issue, which is typically the case for children in managed care, a power wheelchair should be acquired without consideration for a scooter.

A manual wheelchair will be needed if nonaccessible areas for a powered wheelchair are encountered in the usual environment. Architectural barriers in the home or inability to transport a power wheelchair may also necessitate the use of a manual wheelchair.

Fit of the wheelchair must be closely monitored to provide adequate support. The reader should refer to Chapter 24 for information on wheelchairs and postural support systems. Special attention should be given to alignment of the spine and pelvis and to the need for customized accessories or modifications. Accessories to be considered for the manual or power wheelchair prescription should include a solid back and seat, lateral trunk support, lumbar support, adductor pads, seat belt, and chest strap. The footrests should be modified to support the ankle in a neutral position. Additional items that may be appropriate include a tray; head support, if needed; or coated push rims, if the child has the strength to propel the wheelchair. A reclining back will allow a position change while sitting in the wheelchair and will help deter flexion contracture formation at the hip, or a tilt-in-space reclining option can be considered to allow for pressure relief. Midline placement of the control stick on a power wheelchair may be considered to assist in symmetric trunk alignment. If a cushion is required, it should maintain the pelvis in a level position.

Maintaining the spine in a neutral or slightly extended position is essential to retard the formation of a scoliosis. The spine should be in slight extension to increase weight bearing through the facet joints, minimize truncal rotation and lateral flexion, and slow the progression of scoliosis formation (Gibson et al., 1978; Wilkins & Gibson, 1976). Scoliosis is seen in approximately 25% of individuals before the cessation of walking (Miller et al., 1992). Poor sitting posture, in addition to muscle weakness, has been shown to accelerate scoliosis formation and progression (Gibson & Wilkins, 1975). The onset of scoliosis is typically seen by age 10 to 14 years (Ziter & Allsop, 1976). Spinal orthoses may also retard the progression of scoliosis, although they have not been shown to prevent development of a significant scoliotic curve (Cambridge & Drennan, 1987; Colbert & Craig, 1987). Custom-molded seating inserts, corsets, and modular seating inserts are options to provide trunk support in an attempt to slow the progression of the scoliosis. A study comparing the three methods of spinal control in a cohort of 24 boys with DMD concluded that the progression of the curvature was not significantly changed by either method, nor was one found to be superior in controlling the progression (Colbert & Craig, 1987; Seeger et al., 1984).

Early surgical intervention is recommended for the control of scoliosis through the use of segmental spinal instrumentation with Luque rods (Marchesi et al., 1997; Miller et al., 1992). Miller and associates (1992) report improved quality of life, attainment of a balanced sitting posture, and more normal alignment following surgical intervention for scoliosis. Pulmonary complications are reported as minimal if forced vital capacity is at least 35% of normal age-predicted values.

EXERCISE AND CUSTOM EQUIPMENT

With the cessation of walking in late childhood or early adolescence, the emphasis of an exercise program should shift from the lower extremities to active-assistive and active exercises of the upper extremities. More important, however, active exercise should be encouraged by having the adolescent assist as much as possible in ADL such as grooming, upper body dressing, and feeding through consultation with an occupational therapist. Key muscle groups for maintenance of strength for transfers include the shoulder depressors and triceps. The shoulder flexor and abductor and elbow flexor muscle groups are key areas for exercises to maintain routine ADL such as self-feeding and hygiene. Weakness of the upper arm musculature by 16 years of age makes ADL such as dressing, feeding, or hygiene extremely difficult.

The ROM program will require further modification as the adolescent becomes nonambulatory. Stretching of the aforementioned lower extremity joints should be continued with stretching of the shoulder and elbow included. Limitation in shoulder flexion and abduction, elbow extension, forearm supination, and wrist extension are most common.

The family will need to consider additional equipment or home modifications as their child reaches adolescence. A van with a lift or ramp will be needed to transport a power wheelchair. Modification of the bathroom can significantly assist the family by using a wheeled commode chair for toileting and a bath chair and handheld shower for bathing. A tub lift is a second option for bathing. A urinal should be available at home or school to decrease the frequency of transfers to the toilet. Modifications of the bed are also frequently required because the adolescent is unable to change position. An airflow mattress, eggcrate foam cushion, or hospital bed are all possibilities to be considered. A positioning program to include position changes at night is necessary for adolescents who are thin to provide comfort and ensure against skin breakdown. Customized foam wedges fabricated by the therapist may also be helpful in positioning at night.

Transition to Adulthood

The transition to adulthood marks a time of continued progression of disability with greater reliance on assistive technology for environmental access and increased need for assistance to carry out routine ADL. Mobility using a power wheelchair is necessary because upper extremity and truncal weakness will typically not allow use of a motorized scooter. Assistance for ADL, including dressing, transfers, and bathing, is now required. Hygiene about the face and feeding become increasingly difficult but usually remain manageable. Many social issues also arise with the completion of educational programming and transition to a prevocational, vocational, or home environment on a more full-time basis. Another major issue that requires thoughtful consideration by the family, individual, and management team is the utilization of assisted ventilation with progressive respiratory involvement at the terminal stage of the disease.

All transfers require assistance during late adolescence and by adulthood typically require use of a Hoyer or other mechanical lift. A high-backed sling seat is indicated because head and trunk control is minimal with the progressive weakness.

Depending on the availability of funding, accessibility, and family choice, a power recline feature on the wheelchair may be available. If not, a regular schedule for pressure relief through lateral weight shifting with assistance is needed. A properly fitting and well-tolerated cushion to avoid skin breakdown becomes an important area of intervention with loss of the ability to weight shift in the wheelchair. Skin breakdown is not a typical problem in DMD, but a cushion should be considered. A Jay Medical cushion (Jay Medical, Boulder, CO) is often well tolerated and provides a firm base of support to control pelvic obliquity, yet the gel inserts can be adjusted to allow for adequate pressure distribution. A customized insert will be needed if deformity becomes severe (e.g., severe scoliosis without surgical stabilization).

A ball-bearing feeder may be required to assist arm movement when progression of upper extremity weakness makes independent feeding difficult (Chyatte et al., 1965). The device can also be used to assist with general use of the arms in conjunction with activities at a table, such as when using a computer. Coordination of planning with an occupational therapist to address feeding and dressing issues is needed to identify solutions to increased dependence in feeding, dressing, and hygiene.

To maintain independence in environmental access, consideration for using environmental control devices should be given. An environmental control unit included on the power wheelchair can be used to independently access the lights, telephone, television, motors on doors, or a computer, to name just a few applications. Computer access for vocational applications such as word processing or avocational activities such as games is available.

Breathing exercises, postural drainage, or intermittent pressure breathing treatments should be included in the management program based on results of pulmonary evaluation (Rodillo et al., 1989). Specific tests of pulmonary function that document respiratory status include forced vital capacity (amount of air expired following a maximal inspiration) and peak expiratory flow rate (highest flow rate sustained for 10 ms during maximal expiration). In addition to the breathing exercises and assisted coughing, the family and caregivers should be instructed in the technique of postural drainage.

Close monitoring of respiratory function should become routine with increasing age because respiratory failure or pulmonary infection is the major contributing factor to death in 75% of children with DMD (Gilroy & Holliday, 1982). Longevity in DMD can be significantly prolonged by assisted ventilation (Alexander et al., 1979; Bach et al., 1987; Curran & Colbert, 1989). However, a survey of MDA-sponsored clinics reports that only 26% of clinic directors offered ventilatory aid for acute respiratory failure (Bach, 1992). Bach (1992) stresses the need for health care professionals to explore attitudes toward mechanical ventilation because our perceived impression of patient desires may often be incorrect. The use of intermittent positive-pressure breathing, negative pressure ventilators, and suctioning may be considered for the chronic hypoventilation related to weakness of respiratory musculature (Hill et al., 1992).

A power-controlled bed to allow elevation of the head for respiratory management should be considered. Use of a bed with elevating capability also allows for greater ease in transfers, and height adjustment promotes use of proper body mechanics by family members for activities that require assistance such as dressing. Mattress selection should also be reviewed with the family because an airflow mattress may be needed when increasing dependence for bed mobility is encountered. Use of an airflow mattress may decrease the frequency of need for turning and repositioning at night. If sitting in a wheelchair is no longer tolerated in the later stages of the disease, elevation of the head of the bed becomes beneficial for reading or watching television. An easel will be required for reading.

Although it may be assumed by care providers that the quality of life and therefore satisfaction are significantly reduced for severely disabled individuals with DMD, this notion may be incorrect. In a survey of 82 ventilator-assisted individuals with DMD, Bach and colleagues (1991) concluded that the vast majority of individuals had a positive affect and were satisfied with life despite the physical dependence. Furthermore, it was found in a survey of 273 physically intact health care professionals that they significantly underestimated patient life satisfaction scores, and therefore they may make patient management recommendations based on their attitudes rather than the patient's wishes. The article by Bach and colleagues (1991) points out that we need to constantly inquire and objectively assess family and individual needs when interacting to provide therapeutic programs. Curran and Colbert (1989) have reported an average increase in longevity from 19 years 9 months to 25 years 9 months in individuals who use ventilatory assistance.

Respiratory insufficiency is a hallmark sign of the preterminal stage of DMD (Newsom-Davis, 1980). Progressive muscular weakness results in decreased ventilatory volumes caused by restriction of chest wall excursion. Coordination of care with the respiratory therapist is essential when clinical findings of respiratory muscle weakness, inability to cough, or chest wall restrictions are observed (Burke et al., 1971). Severe oxygen desaturation leading to a comatose state is evidence of the terminal stage of the disease.

Members of the team often become involved in answering questions regarding death. The physical therapist should be aware of the stages of disease progression and especially the preterminal signs to avoid making inappropriate comments concerning prognosis. Often little needs to be said, but rather a good listening ear is needed to help the family work through the crisis that is ever pending. It is often a comfort to individuals with DMD or family members that the end may come as a sleep without wakening. The person with DMD and his family members may indicate the need for additional support, but if issues are not being resolved adequately by the support that is available, consideration for involvement by a psychologist, counselor, clergy member, MDA support group, or other trained professional is indicated. Literature is available through the MDA to comfort family members, and texts are available if the family is interested (Kushner, 1981; Tatelbaum, 1980).

Becker Muscular Dystrophy

BMD, a more slowly progressive variant of DMD, has an incidence of about 1 in 20,000 births and a prevalence of 2 to 3 cases per 100,000 population (Emery, 1993; Mostacciuolo, 1987). The impairments and disabilities of BMD closely resemble those of DMD; however, the progression is significantly slower, with a longevity into the forties (Emery & Skinner, 1976; Gilroy & Holliday, 1982). The genetic defect for BMD is located on the same gene as that for DMD only in a different area; therefore dystrophin is present in reduced amounts rather than completely absent as in DMD, which may explain the slower progression of clinical symptoms (Kingston et al., 1983).

Initial clinical symptoms are typically not identified in boys with BMD before late childhood or early adolescence. Emery and Skinner (1976) found the mean age at onset of symptoms to be 11 years, inability to walk at 27 years, and death at 42 years. The authors point out, however, that the range of walking cessation is very wide. Perhaps one of the best functional discriminators between BMD and DMD is that 97% of adolescents with DMD are using a wheelchair for mobility by age 11 years, whereas 97% of adolescents with BMD are still walking (Emery & Skinner, 1976). Another discriminator is the frequent complaint of muscle cramping in individuals with BMD that is rarely reported in DMD (Dubowitz, 1992).

The impairments of BMD are the same as in DMD, although less severe, and the initial disability includes frequent falls and clumsiness in the mid to late teens. The pattern of weakness is the same as in DMD, and pseudohypertrophy of the calves may be present. The incidence of contracture, scoliosis, and other skeletal deformities is lower in BMD. Although not as severe as in DMD, hip, knee, and ankle plantar flexor muscle contractures can be present when walking is no longer possible. The use of night splints to maintain ankle dorsiflexion ROM is often indicated, along with a home program of heel cord stretching. Significant disability will develop by the midtwenties, requiring the use of power mobility and consideration for use of orthoses to maintain walking. KAFOs can also be used to prolong walking; however, braced ambulation will not be functional for community access but rather as a means of exercise. The general goals and management procedures outlined in the section on DMD are the same for BMD, including the progression from walking to use of power mobility.

Because the person with BMD lives much longer than someone with DMD, transition planning following school and assistance with living arrangements into adulthood become major issues. Vocational or avocational choices should be made with the disease progression and disability level in mind. Vocational rehabilitation services should be initiated before completion of high school to allow adequate time for evaluation. Governmental support through Medicaid, Social Security benefits, or other sources may be needed to offset expenses to allow for independent living because adaptive equipment and an attendant will be needed. Ongoing medical services are available through the MDA. No data are available regarding the number of individuals who go to college or become employed following high school, but with the assistive technology available to promote independence, either option can be explored.

Congenital Muscular Dystrophy

Congenital myopathies as a diagnostic category consist of many diseases, including congenital MD. Congenital MD is not a single clinical entity, and up to four different forms have been reported. The four types reported by Brooke (1986) are (1) congenital MD with central nervous system (CNS) disease

(Fukuyama type), (2) congenital MD without CNS damage, (3) atonic sclerotic type, and (4) stick man type. The last two types are extremely rare, and the reader should refer to the text by Brooke (1986) for additional information because only the first two types are discussed here. The mode of inheritance in congenital MD is reported as autosomal recessive (Muscular Dystrophy Association, 1991). Although all forms are rare, the range of severity and disability varies significantly among types.

Currently, no definitive information is available regarding longevity in the various forms of congenital MD other than case reports. McMenamin and associates (1982) reported on a cohort of 24 patients with congenital MD, of whom 4 had died between the ages of 5 and 8 years, and 4 between the ages of 18 and 24 years. The oldest patient in the study was 23 years of age.

In congenital MD with associated CNS disease (Fukuyama type), mental retardation and seizures are common along with moderate to severe hypotonia at birth and the presence of contractures (Fukuyama et al., 1981). Magnetic resonance imaging reveals nonspecific cerebral malformations and occasionally lissencephaly as pathologic features of the CNS disease. Contractures typically involve the lower extremities (hips and knees) and elbows. Other commonly reported dysmorphic features include congenital dislocation of the hips, pectus excavatum, pes cavus, kyphoscoliosis, and an unusually long face. Weakness of the extraocular muscles, optic atrophy, and nystgmus have been reported (Brooke, 1986). Children with this type of MD rarely attain the ability to walk.

The early management program in children with congenital MD with nervous system disease should focus on family instruction, developmental activities to address delays in gross motor skill development, and aggressive management of contractures. Attention to positioning is necessary to guard against secondary deformity resulting from gravitational effects on the trunk with presence of moderate to severe hypotonia. Early intervention by an occupational therapist to address feeding and oral motor control issues is commonly coordinated with physical therapy. Impaired respiratory function and pulmonary complications are hallmark features of congenital MD. The family should be instructed in chest physical therapy, such as postural drainage, and consultation with a respiratory therapist may be needed on an ongoing basis.

Because many children with congenital MD and associated nervous system disease do not attain walking, maximizing functional skills in sitting becomes a primary goal of the physical therapy management program as the child ages. Therapeutic exercise to improve head and trunk control should be aggressively addressed with use of adaptive equipment to slow the progression of spinal deformity and contractures and to maximize access to the environment. Because mental retardation is common, power mobility may not be an option. Additional management issues for children with significant hypotonia are discussed later in the chapter in the section on acute SMA.

Congenital Muscular Dystrophy without Central Nervous System Disease

In congenital MD without CNS disease, the typical clinical presentation includes hypotonia and weakness, frequently with contractures, and a delay in acquisition of motor milestones. Infants with this form of congenital MD may demonstrate a rapid progression of muscle weakness with loss of skills (Donner et al., 1975), slow progression, static neuromotor status (McMenamin et al., 1982), or slow improvement (Jones et al., 1979). Two subcategories of this form of MD have been identified based on the presence or absence of the muscle protein merosin (alpha-laminin). In the case of merosin-deficient congenital MD the gene locus is 6q2; the locus of the merosin-positive form is yet to be determined.

Jones and associates (1979) reported on a cohort of 27 children with congenital MD, all younger than age 18 years. The authors subdivided the group into severe (those who never walked and demonstrated severe weakness, $n = 19$) and mild (those who walked independently before age 2 years, $n = 8$). Sixteen of the children were reported to demonstrate a general improvement in strength with increasing age, 8 remained static, and 2 demonstrated progressive weakness. One child was only 2 months of age and progress was not reported. The follow-up period was 5 years.

Muscle weakness and contractures are the primary impairment; however, intellectual impairment may also limit attainment of functional skills. Muscles innervated by the cranial nerves may be involved, requiring a feeding program that is coordinated with occupational therapy. Contractures must be managed aggressively with a home ROM program including manual stretching, positioning, and splinting. Because many of the children have a potential to develop walking, the ankle plantar flexion contractures may require orthopedic intervention if the contractures cannot be managed conservatively. McMenamin and co-workers (1982) reported significant developmental delay in all cases of congenital MD. The average age for attainment of independent

sitting was 11.5 months and 2.6 years for walking. Only 15 of the 26 infants attained independent walking.

Functional limitations, such as delayed acquisition of gross motor skills, should not be managed by extensive direct service therapy programs because a slower rate of skill progression is expected. Because many children begin to walk within the first 2 to 3 years, information can be provided to the family concerning probable rates of motor skill acquisition, and unrealistic therapeutic expectations should be avoided. Because there is a wide range of functional deficits in children with congenital MD, care must be taken in predicting functional gross motor outcomes.

Childhood-Onset Facioscapulohumeral Muscular Dystrophy

Facioscapulohumeral MD is rare, with an incidence of 3 to 10 cases per million births (Stevenson et al., 1990). The disorder is inherited as autosomal dominant or recessive with the genetic defect on chromosome 4q35. The disorder affects males and females equally. Childhood-onset facioscapulohumeral MD typically demonstrates the onset of clinical signs within the first 2 years but without significant impairment or disability until later in the first decade. Contractures are seldom a problem.

Infancy and Preschool-Age Period

The impairment of muscle weakness about the face and shoulder girdle is typically the only prominent feature of the disease during the infant and preschool-age period. Parents report that the child may sleep with the eyes partially open, and on physical examination weakness of the facial musculature is predominant. Children are frequently unable to whistle, and drinking with a straw may be difficult. When asked to purse the lips together and puff the cheeks out, the child is unable to maintain the cheeks out when even the slightest pressure is applied. The child's smile is also masked because of the weakness, thereby hindering communication as a result of inconsistency between what is spoken and the affect displayed.

Children with childhood-onset facioscapulohumeral MD typically develop independence in walking without significant delay. An excessive lordotic posture during walking is a classic clinical feature with progression of weakness. The scapulae are widely abducted and outwardly rotated, giving evidence of the degree of interscapular muscle weakness.

School-Age Period

Progressive disability occurs during the school-age period, with weakness becoming more generalized throughout the trunk, shoulder, and pelvic girdle musculature. Progression of childhood-onset facioscapulohumeral MD is more insidious than the adult form, and independent walking may be lost by the end of the first decade (Gardner-Medwin, 1980b).

The severe winging of the scapula, a hallmark feature of the adult form of the disease, becomes more prominent with age in activities such as reaching overhead. Management should focus on instruction to the child and family on activities to avoid that promote fatigue and on guarding against heavily resisted upper extremity activity. Studies of adults with facioscapulohumeral MD comparing dominant with nondominant arm strength have shown that mechanical factors play a significant role in progression of muscle weakness (Brouwer et al., 1992; Johnson & Braddom, 1971).

As weakness of the hip and knee extensors progresses, the use of KAFOs should be considered for assisted walking and transfers. When walking becomes increasingly difficult, power mobility using a scooter or power wheelchair should be considered because the degree of upper extremity weakness will not allow independence in propulsion of a manual wheelchair.

Transition to Adulthood

No specific prognostic information on the longevity of individuals with childhood-onset facioscapulohumeral MD is available, and therefore transition planning from the educational environment should be a goal of the therapy program. If severe weakness is present and significant assistance from the family is needed, individuals may not desire to plan for living outside the family home. If independent living is desired, coordination of planning with an attendant will be necessary and evaluation for accessibility issues will need to be completed. Assistance through vocational rehabilitation services should be coordinated with transition planning if vocational goals are identified.

Congenital Myotonic Muscular Dystrophy

Myotonic MD has the highest incidence of the dystrophies at 3 to 5 cases per 100,000 population (Gardner-Medwin, 1980a). Congenital myotonic MD is rare and demonstrates severe clinical features of the adult-onset diagnosis. Inheritance is reported as autosomal dominant with genetic defect of chromosome 19 affecting males and females equally (Harley et al., 1991).

Children with congenital myotonic MD are almost exclusively born to mothers with myotonic MD, and a "maternal factor" has been hypothesized by Harper (1989). Two variations within the congenital form are reported. Most children demonstrate severe hypotonia and weakness at birth; however, a few children first have only signs of mental retardation by age 5 years and no significant motor impairment as infants. Because the children who initially have only mental impairment follow a progression of motor impairment similar to that of adult-onset myotonic MD, the infancy-onset form is discussed in this section of the chapter.

Mental retardation in congenital myotonic MD is common. A mean IQ of 66 was reported by Harper (1975a). There is no evidence of progressive deterioration of mental function. A study by Rutherford and co-workers (1989) including 14 children provides prognostic information regarding survival and the relationship to mechanical ventilation. No infant in the study survived who required mechanical ventilation for longer than 4 weeks.

Infancy

If the child survives the early weeks of life, the prognosis is one of steady improvement in motor function over the first decade, with most children developing independent walking (Harper, 1975a, 1989). A follow-up study by O'Brien and Harper (1984) of 46 children reported only 4 children who died outside the neonatal period at ages 4, 18, 19, and 22 years. Four additional children demonstrated a more significant disability associated with a poor prognosis, and none was older than age 30 years. Information is lacking on the longevity of individuals who survive to adulthood with congenital myotonic MD.

Severe weakness and partial paralysis of the diaphragm at birth are clinical features that often suggest the diagnosis of congenital myotonic MD. Myotonia (delay in relaxation after muscular contraction), a hallmark feature of adult myotonic MD, is typically not evident at birth in the congenital form but rather develops by 3 to 5 years of age (Brooke, 1986). Myotonia in congenital myotonic MD is typically not considered to be a significant impairment or a cause of functional limitations in comparison with the degree of weakness that is present. The symptoms of myotonia, however, are increased with fatigue, cold, or stress (Siegel, 1986). Typical facial features include a short median part of the upper lip, which gives the mouth an inverted-V shape. Facial movements are limited, with muscles innervated by the cranial nerves involved in the severe weakness pattern. Severe respiratory impairment is prominent in the newborn period, requiring resuscitation and assisted ventilation in most cases. Talipes equinovarus contractures are reported in over 50% of children, and a general pattern of arthrogryposis occurs in less than 5% (Harper, 1989).

Progressive improvement in gross motor skills can be expected if the child survives the newborn period. The presence and degree of intellectual impairment becomes a major factor in the progression of milestone acquisition. The development of hip abduction and external rotation contractures should be closely monitored if leg movement and habitual positioning favor the development of secondary impairment.

Harper (1989), in a cohort of 70 children with congenital myotonic dystrophy, reported that hypotonia is rarely prominent beyond age 3 to 4 years. Children typically develop walking, but further motor impairment follows the clinical progression of adult-onset disease without definitive data being available into adulthood to document disease progression.

Consultation with a respiratory therapist on pulmonary care will be needed until the infant is weaned from assisted ventilation. Feeding may require the use of a nasogastric tube during the newborn period or early infancy, and initiation of a feeding program should be coordinated with an occupational therapist. A swallowing study may be indicated to evaluate potential for aspiration when the feeding program is initiated. If the newborn survives early respiratory difficulties, progressive improvement in pulmonary function is usually seen without need for ongoing intervention.

Talipes equinovarus contractures should be aggressively managed in infancy with casting, taping, and exercises but may ultimately require orthopedic intervention. Ankle-foot orthoses or night splints may be indicated based on individual needs. In addition to home instruction for ROM activities to manage contractures, the family should be provided with a general program of activities to promote gross motor skill development. Because the natural progression of the disease is improvement of motor function, consultation rather than a direct service program is indicated, unless surgical intervention for contracture management is required.

School-Age Period

Consultation for development of adaptive physical education activities will be needed during the school-age period. Other physical therapy–related activities will depend on the use of orthoses and progression of gross motor skill development. Spe-

cific therapeutic exercise programs for strengthening have not been reported but may be indicated in addition to ROM activities.

Transition to Adulthood

The natural progression of myotonic MD is insidious weakness of the distal upper and lower extremity musculature and progressive increase in myotonia, leading to increasing disability. Children with congenital myotonic MD will demonstrate progression in the disease as described for adults, but typically at an earlier stage, usually by the middle of the second decade. The reader should refer to references on adult myotonic MD for further information on clinical course and management (Brooke, 1986; Harper, 1989; Siegel, 1986).

Emery-Dreifus Muscular Dystrophy

Emery-Dreifus MD is inherited as an X-linked recessive disorder characterized by weakness predominantly in a humeroperoneal distribution and with variable facial involvement (Pinelli et al., 1987). Limited information is available in the literature, but the disorder resembles facioscapulohumeral MD in certain persons. The gene locus is at Xq28, and the missing protein has been identified as emerin. Onset of muscle weakness is typically in the first decade, and progression is very slow (Brooke, 1986).

Ankle equinus and elbow flexion contractures are common. Contracture of muscles of the neck and spine, resulting in limited flexion ROM, is reported (Brooke, 1986). Weakness of the elbow flexor and extensor musculature is the initial pattern of muscle involvement. Cardiac abnormalities are common, with sudden death (in persons ranging in age from 25 to 56 years) reported by Pinelli and colleagues (1987) in a large family cohort with bradyarrhythmias.

Physical therapy management is limited during the childhood period because disability is not common. Independent walking is typically maintained into adulthood without significant disability. An ROM program for contracture prevention is advised, but orthopedic intervention is common to correct the Achilles tendon contractures (Shapiro & Specht, 1991). Holter monitoring is advised when cardiac abnormalities are identified, and pacemakers are used to control rhythm.

SPINAL MUSCULAR ATROPHY

Classification of SMA into four groups is based on clinical presentation and progression (Table 14–2). Types I and II are commonly referred to

TABLE 14–2. **Classification of Spinal Muscle Atrophy**

Type	Onset	Inheritance	Course
Childhood-onset, type I, Werdnig-Hoffmann (acute)	0–3 mo	Recessive	Rapidly progressive; severe hypotonia; death within first year
Childhood-onset, type II, Werdnig-Hoffmann (chronic)	3 mo–4 yr	Recessive	Rapid progression that stabilizes; moderate to severe hypotonia; shortened life span
Juvenile-onset, type III, Kugelberg-Welander	5–10 yr	Recessive	Slowly progressive; mild impairment

as acute and chronic Werdnig-Hoffmann disease, respectively, type III as Kugelberg-Welander disease, and type IV as adult-onset SMA.

Diagnosis and Pathophysiology

SMA comprises the second most common group of fatal recessive diseases after cystic fibrosis (Pearn, 1980). The pathologic feature of SMA is abnormality of the large anterior horn cells in the spinal cord. The number of cells is reduced, and progressive degeneration of the remaining cells is correlated with loss in function.

The diagnosis of SMA is confirmed by clinical examination and laboratory procedures, including electromyography, muscle biopsy, and genetic testing (Brooke, 1986; MacKenzie et al., 1994). Electromyographic findings include fibrillation and fasciculation potentials, repetitive discharge, excessive polyphasic potentials, and increased amplitude and duration of the motor unit potentials consistent with chronic denervation and reinnervation of muscle. Nerve conduction velocities are normal. The muscle biopsy demonstrates changes that are typical of a disease involving denervation (i.e., large groups of atrophic fibers are dispersed among groups of normal or hypertrophic fibers). The absence of fibrosis around the atrophic groups on the muscle biopsy helps delineate SMA from DMD.

SMA is typically inherited as autosomal recessive with the genetic defect on chromosome 5 (Gilliam et al., 1990). An autosomal dominant inheritance has been reported that tends to manifest with clinical signs later in the first decade and demonstrates a slower progression (Emery et al., 1976; Pearn, 1978; Zellweger et al., 1972). The sex-linked recessive form demonstrates clinical findings similar to those of BMD with onset later in the first decade, a slow progression, and calf muscle hypertrophy (Bundey & Lovelace, 1975; Gamstrop, 1967; Pearn, 1978). The greatest variation in the clinical course of SMA is seen with the autosomal recessive mode of inheritance.

The gene for SMA, termed *survival motor neuron* (SMN), was discovered in 1994 by MacKenzie and colleagues (1994) on chromosome 5q13 and is responsible for the production of a protein bearing the same name. The SMN protein is involved in maintenance of the anterior horn cell and when missing results in a lack of survival of the cell, leading to apoptosis (programmed cell death). In addition to the SMN gene another defect of the gene in a near locus results in the lack of formation of neuronal apoptosis inhibitory protein (NAIP), which has also been shown to play a role in SMA. The lack of the NAIP protein may be the explanation for the premature cell death seen in SMA and in association with the SMN gene defect (Robinson, 1995).

The incidence of Werdnig-Hoffmann disease is 1 in 15,000 to 25,000 live births (Pearn, 1973; Pearn et al., 1973), and the incidence of Kugelberg-Welander disease is reported as 6 cases per 100,000 live births (Winsor et al., 1971). Specific information on the incidence of the other forms is variable because of inconsistency of classification criteria and is based on the clinical heterogeneity of the disease.

One criterion for classification of SMA is the level of functional ability (Dubowitz, 1989). The more typical classification criteria are multifactorial and involve age at onset of the first clinical signs, pattern of muscle involvement, age at death, and genetic evidence (Pearn, 1980).

SMA is a heterogeneous disorder containing several different clinical presentations and rates of progression. Progressive SMA of early childhood (type I) was first reported by Werdnig and Hoffmann in the late 1800s (Hoffmann, 1893; Werdnig, 1894). A more slowly progressive form of SMA (type III) with onset usually between the ages of 2 and 9 years was reported by Kugelberg and Welander (1956) and also by Wohlfart and colleagues (1955). Werdnig-Hoffmann disease and Kugelberg-Welander disease have therefore become the eponyms for early-onset and juvenile-onset SMA, with many authors preferring to use the numeric classification system as outlined above in Table 14–2.

Pearn (1980), in a large multicenter study in England, reported SMA type II and III to be the most frequent, accounting for approximately 47% of the population. The next most prevalent forms were

SMA type I at about 27% and adult-onset type IV at 8%; the other 18% had mixed classifications, including distal involvement, neurogenic SMA, SMA of adolescence with hypertrophied calf muscles, and childhood-onset SMA with cerebellar and optic atrophy.

No cure or treatment is available for SMA, but physical therapy is commonly advocated (Brooke, 1986; Hausmanowa-Petrusewicz, 1978; Marshall, 1984; Watt & Greenhill, 1984). The prognosis is variable, but grave indicators for long-term survival include early age at onset (before 4 months of age) that is often noted as weak fetal movement; fasciculations of the tongue in infancy; and severe, generalized weakness, particularly of the trunk and proximal musculature (Gamstrop, 1967).

Acute Childhood Spinal Muscular Atrophy (Type I)

Impairments, Functional Limitations, and Disability

The primary impairment in all forms of SMA is muscle weakness secondary to progressive loss of anterior horn cells in the spinal cord. Weakness is particularly pronounced in the acute and chronic childhood forms (types I and II) within the first 4 months. The cranial nerves are inconsistently involved in childhood-onset SMA, with rare involvement with juvenile onset. Contractures may be a primary impairment in acute-onset SMA, with reports of talipes equinovarus or other intrauterine deformities secondary to limited fetal movement. Muscle fasciculations, including fasciculations of the tongue, are most commonly reported in children with acute-onset SMA (Namba et al., 1970). Unlike the faces of children with myotonic or facioscapulohumeral MD, children with acute childhood SMA appear alert and responsive. Respiratory distress is present early, and significant effort to augment breathing by use of the abdominal musculature is typical.

Secondary impairments in acute-onset SMA include the development of scoliosis and often contractures. It is widely reported in the literature that all children with SMA develop scoliosis, usually requiring surgical intervention (Granata et al., 1989c; Lonstein, 1989). Other secondary impairments include decreased respiratory capacity and easy fatigability. Because only the passage of time will allow differentiation of children with acute versus chronic childhood SMA, treatment should begin early with a focus on feeding, ROM, positioning, respiratory care, and selected developmental activities.

Infancy

In acute childhood SMA, weak or absent fetal movement during the last months of pregnancy is commonly reported by the mother. Significant weakness is present at birth or develops within the first 4 months, which manifests as inability to perform antigravity movements with the pelvic or shoulder girdle musculature and typical posturing in a gravity-dependent position (Fig. 14–8). The proximal musculature of the neck, trunk, and pelvic and shoulder girdles demonstrates the greatest weakness. Limited antigravity movement of distal upper and lower extremity musculature is present, and a positioning program in the newborn period or at the onset of symptoms is necessary. Use of wedges should be considered to avoid supine positioning in the presence of respiratory distress. If the supine position is used, rolled towels or bolsters are needed to keep the upper extremities positioned in midline and to prevent lower extremity abduction and external rotation. The side-lying position allows midline head and hand use for play without having to work against gravity. Prone positioning on wedges should be limited or not used, owing to the effort required for head righting to interact with the environment.

Respiratory care is a central focus of the habilitation program in acute childhood SMA. Children frequently require intubation for respiratory distress and tracheostomy. Coordination with nurses and respiratory therapists on a program that includes suctioning, assisted coughing, and postural drainage is necessary. The use of supported sitting should be closely monitored for spinal alignment and respiratory response. Use of an elastic binder around the abdomen in sitting may be useful for children who demonstrate a marked reduction in oxygen saturation when seated.

ROM exercises should be carried out to ensure maintenance of flexibility and comfort. Flexion contractures of the hips, knees and elbows, hip abductors, ankle plantar flexors, and positional torticollis are deformities that can be avoided with a comprehensive ROM and positioning program (Binder, 1989). The exercise program should also include limited activities for strengthening, such as lightweight toys or rattles with Velcro straps around the wrists or mobiles positioned close to the hands for easy access. The use of hammocks has also been advocated to provide the child with the opportunity for movement with only slight movements of the body (Eng, 1989a, 1989b). Developmental activities such as the use of supported sitting for the development of head control should be of short duration to avoid fatigue.

Head control fails to develop or is significantly impaired in acute childhood SMA. The child is unable to lift the head from a prone position to clear

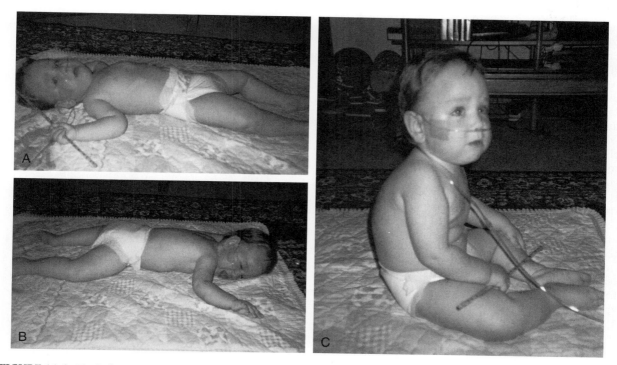

FIGURE 14–8. Typical postures seen in a young child with SMA in supine *(A)*, prone *(B)*, and sitting *(C)* positions. Note the limited antigravity control and dependent posturing.

the airway. Early developmental postures such as prone on elbows are not attained. The use of developmental exercise in acute childhood SMA is controversial but should be considered if the child tolerates the activities, because a few children with chronic childhood SMA exibit clinical signs of weakness in the first year of life and as a result may be misdiagnosed as having acute SMA.

In conjunction with an occupational therapist, a feeding program that is safe and not excessively exhausting should be implemented. Small, frequent feedings may be necessary, and breast feeding may be difficult (Eng, 1989b). Special care with feeding is necessary to avoid aspiration and secondary respiratory problems.

Although death secondary to pneumonia or other respiratory complications is typical within a few months to a few years in acute childhood SMA, the child's death is usually not a struggle, owing to the degree of weakness and apnea (Eng, 1989b; Gamstrop, 1967). The mean age of death is reported to be 6 months, with a range from 1 to 21 months reported by Merlini and associates (1989). Counseling and support for the parents and family is an extremely important component in the management of these children.

Chronic Childhood Spinal Muscular Atrophy (Type II)

Impairments, Functional Limitations, and Disability

The onset of significant weakness in chronic childhood SMA usually appears within the first year. The course of the disease may be widely variable. Pearn and colleagues (1978) reported on the clinical progression in a cohort of 141 children. The authors reported that 95% of the children demonstrated clinical signs before age 3 years. Forty-six percent never walked (even with orthotics), 38% were able to walk unaided at some stage, and the median age at death exceeded 10 years.

Eng (1989b) has reported three separate subgroupings within type II based on the pattern of presentation and progression. In the most severely involved group, the children never developed the ability to sit alone and respiratory capacity was significantly reduced. In the intermediate group, the children sat alone but never developed the ability to walk and demonstrated a regression of forced vital capacity to 45% by age 10 years. In the final group, independent walking was attained but half of the children lost this ability toward the end of the first decade. Interestingly, in the group of patients who remained ambulatory in the study by Eng (1989b), forced vital capacity was maintained at 90% as compared with 65% for those who lost independent walking during the first decade. The results of the study led Eng to conclude that forced vital capacity may be a physiologic predictor of walking duration.

Contractures are infrequently an impairment in chronic SMA. The distribution of weakness is similar to acute childhood SMA with primary proximal involvement, but of much less severe degree. Weakness is usually greatest in the hip and knee extensors and trunk musculature. Involvement of the distal musculature appears later in the course of the disease and is less severe than the proximal involvement (Namba et al., 1970). Involvement of the cranial nerves is reported but not considered to be a typical feature of SMA other than in the acute childhood form. Fasciculations of the tongue are reported in approximately one half of the children (Pearn et al., 1973). A tremor may also be noted and is considered by several authors as substantiating the diagnosis (Brooke, 1986; Moosa & Dubowitz, 1973).

Infancy

Because the clinical presentation and progression of chronic childhood SMA are highly variable, the management program must address the major disability at each point in time. Approximately 15% of children have impairments within the first 3 months, and the remaining children have impairments by 18 months (Merlini et al., 1989). The program for the newborn with chronic SMA should be similar to that for children with acute SMA. Some children may develop the ability to stand, but few are able to use walking as a primary means of mobility.

Sitting posture is an area of primary concern in the management program with children who demonstrate significant weakness, requiring head and trunk control in antigravity positions. A molded sitting support orthosis as shown in Figure 14–9 provides optimal contouring of the torso for support in sitting, or a thoracolumbosacral orthosis (TLSO, or "body jacket") can also be used. Developmental activities provided on an ongoing basis are indicated to develop gross motor skills. Therapy sessions should be kept short to avoid fatigue and should emphasize selected developmental areas during each session because tolerance to handling in multiple positions is usually limited. Instruction with the family for carryover and the use of adaptive equipment for proper positioning are crucial in slowing the deforming effects of gravity on the spine when the child is sitting or standing.

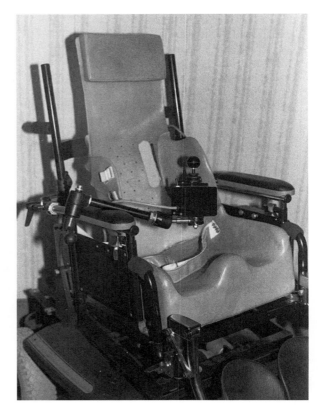

FIGURE 14–9. Custom-molded sitting-support orthosis to provide trunk support in sitting.

If the child is not standing by the age of 16 to 18 months, adaptive equipment for standing should be considered. The rate of fracture in SMA has been reported to range from 12 to 15%, and weight bearing has been shown to decrease the frequency of lower extremity fractures (Ballestrazzi et al., 1989). A supine stander is recommended for children without adequate head control. Orthopedic consultation for a corset or TLSO should be considered for use in standing to maintain trunk alignment if the adaptive equipment does not provide adequate control.

Preschool-Age and School-Age Period

In the toddler, orthotics for standing might be considered (lightweight KAFOs); however, the progression of weakness may make walking an unrealistic goal. In a report of promotion of walking in 12 children with intermediate SMA (ages 13 months to 3 years), Granata and associates (1989a) described success in attaining assisted ambulation, with 58% of the children using orthoses. Although the findings are preliminary, these investigators also report less severity of scoliotic curves in the children who used the orthoses in comparison with a control group of children with SMA.

If a walking program is initiated, training in the parallel bars followed by use of a walker or other device to allow greater independence is desired. Close monitoring of safety with supported walking is necessary owing to the degree of weakness present and the potential for serious injury with a fall. The incidence of hip dislocation and contractures has also been reported as less when a supported walking program is used (Granata et al., 1989b).

Independence with mobility other than walking is a primary goal for the child who will not develop independence in walking or when walking is no longer possible. Because most power scooters do not provide adequate trunk control, use of a power wheelchair is indicated. If an orthopedic appliance is not used, close attention to fit is needed with use of lateral trunk supports and a trunk harness. Consideration should also be given to changing the side of the joystick every 6 months to avoid a pattern of leaning to one side. Prognosis for children with chronic childhood SMA is dependent on frequency and severity of pulmonary complications. Severe contractures as a result of prolonged sitting and progression of scoliosis are common, necessitating implementation of a consistent ROM program. Surgical intervention for spinal stabilization is an option if pulmonary function testing indicates a good prognosis for survival of the surgical intervention.

Transition to Adulthood

Survival into adulthood is extremely variable in chronic childhood SMA and depends on the progression of muscle weakness and secondary deformities. Because of the significant degree of muscle weakness, assistance is typically required for transfers and many ADL. An attendant or family member is needed to provide assistance for general ADL. Intelligence is rarely affected, and therefore vocational goals in areas of interest should be explored through vocational rehabilitation services.

An aggressive program of pulmonary care is required, including breathing exercises and postural drainage. The ROM program should also be continued to control progression of the contractures unless a pattern of stability is recorded.

Juvenile-Onset Spinal Muscular Atrophy (Type III)

Juvenile-onset SMA may demonstrate symptoms of weakness within the first year of life in the proximal hip and shoulder girdle musculature, but more typically the onset is later in the first decade. Rarely

are bulbar signs seen with the disease. Calf pseudohypertrophy is reported in approximately 10% of the cases. Fasciculations are noted in about half of the patients, and minimyoclonus may be a primary impairment noted on examination but rarely interferes with function (Brooke, 1986; Dorscher et al., 1991).

Impairments, Functional Limitations, and Disability

In a study by Dorscher and colleagues (1991) reviewing the status of 31 patients with Kugelberg-Welander disease, proximal lower extremity weakness was the most common impairment reported. Secondary impairments included postural compensations resulting from the muscle weakness, contractures, and occasionally scoliosis. An increased lumbar lordosis and compensated Trendelenburg gait pattern are common postural compensations for proximal muscle weakness of the lower extremities. Ankle plantar flexion contractures are occasionally reported but not with the frequency seen in DMD, which aids differentiation of the two diseases. Scoliosis was reported in about 20% of patients by Dorscher and colleagues (1991) but was reported in all patients by other researchers (Granata et al., 1989b). In adolescents with type III SMA the incidence of scoliosis and its severity are related to the degree of weakness and functional status. Individuals who maintain independent walking have a lower incidence of scoliosis and less severe curves if scoliosis develops.

School-Age Period

A similar clinical presentation to DMD is seen in juvenile-onset SMA. The initial disability usually becomes apparent within the first decade and includes difficulty in arising from the floor, climbing stairs, and keeping up with peers during play, and a waddling gait, which becomes more pronounced with attempts at running. Unlike DMD, no significant disability of upper extremity function is usually noted and proximal upper extremity strength is well preserved. Walking can usually be maintained lifelong as the primary means of ambulation. In those cases when weakness is noted before 2 years of age, however, a wheelchair or scooter may ultimately be required for mobility over long distances.

Management for the adolescent with juvenile-onset SMA is consistent with the concepts previously presented in this chapter. ROM exercises should be prescribed where appropriate, and selected strengthening exercises may be indicated to maintain functional skills. Adaptive equipment for mobility is not usually indicated, but a power scooter for long-distance mobility may be needed in certain cases. If performance of ADL becomes a problem, collaboration with an occupational therapist to address concerns may also be needed.

Transition to Adulthood

Difficulty in ADL that requires lifting of moderately heavy objects overhead can be expected, and vocational activities that involve manual labor are not recommended. Because the life span is not significantly shortened, vocational planning is needed. No significant disability requiring adaptive equipment or environmental access is usually required until later in adulthood.

CASE HISTORY
DONALD

Each of the two cases that are presented began before development of the "Guide to Physical Therapist Practice" (APTH, 1997). However, the reports are presented with reference to the guide to assist the practitioner in application of the guide to clinical practice.

Donald is 26 years old and from a family with six siblings (three brothers and three sisters). Three of the four boys were diagnosed with DMD. No family history of neuromuscular disease had been reported previously, and diagnosis followed medical examination of Donald's older brother at age 5 years for clumsiness and frequent falls. Donald was 3 years of age at the time of diagnosis.

At the time of diagnosis Donald's management program would be included in Musculoskeletal Practice Pattern C: Impaired Muscle Performance of the "Guide to Physical Therapist Practice" (APTH, 1997). He exibited no significant gait deviations but had mild shoulder girdle and trunk flexor muscle weakness, evidence of a Gower sign after the third attempt to rise to standing from the floor, and pseudohypertrophy of the posterior calf musculature.

A physical therapy examination at age 8 years revealed a gait pattern typical for DMD as previously described. No significant disability was noted, and impairments were only minimal. Donald was independent on stairs using a handrail but demonstrated a two-foot-per-step progression. Functional status corresponded to grade 2 on the scale published by Vignos and associates (1963) (see Box 14-1). ROM was within normal limits, with the exception of mild limitation of ankle dorsiflexion with the knee in extension. Muscle strength was quantified with manual muscle

testing and recorded as fair plus in the shoulder and hip girdle musculature, poor in the abdominals, and good minus in the intermediate and distal upper and lower extremities. A home program was provided that included daily ROM of the posterior calf musculature and instruction on general activities to avoid excessive fatigue. Services were coordinated by the local MDA clinic with a follow-up visit every 6 months.

Donald's initial disability was related to independent mobility with progressive loss of walking, which by age 12 involved inability to climb stairs and increased frequency of falls with attempts to walk on uneven surfaces. Furniture and walls were commonly used for balance. He was independent in scooting on the floor and used crawling for additional mobility at home. Although he was not able to stand from the middle of the floor, he was able to pull up to standing at a supportive surface. Night splints were initiated to augment the ROM program for the ankle plantar flexion contractures, and a manual wheelchair was provided for assistance with long-distance mobility. Muscle strength demonstrated progressive decline, with manual muscle testing measuring poor grades for the proximal hip and shoulder girdle musculature, fair plus grades for knee extension, and a Vignos scale rating of 5. Mild tightness of the iliotibial band was present, and limitation of full hip and knee extension was noted. The ROM program was expanded to include the additional areas of tightness. With the progression of impairments beyond muscle function, a shift in Musculoskeletal Practice Pattern C to D: Impaired Joint Mobility, Muscle Function, Muscle Performance, and Range of Motion Associated with Capsular Restriction would be indicated.

By age 15, Donald was walking only short distances, and primarily for mobility within the home. A three-wheeled motorized scooter was provided for distance mobility, and Donald was independent in all transfers from the scooter. A raised toilet seat and tub bench were provided for the bathroom. He received adapted physical education and consultative physical therapy as a related service in the educational setting. He was followed through the MDA clinic, and Donald's home program was augmented by a school program including standing using a prone stander, ROM exercises three times per week, and adaptive physical education activities for general mobility and upper and lower extremity strengthening.

Progressive weakness and flexion contractures at the hip and knee resulted in the loss of walking when Donald was 17. It should be noted that this is exceptionally late for the loss of walking because 10 to 11 years is more typically reported (Brooke, 1986). Because Donald's older brother had died following complications from a fracture resulting from a fall while wearing KAFOs, Donald and the family decided

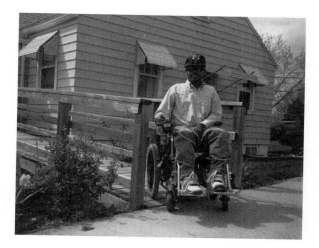

FIGURE 14–10. Donald using power mobility.

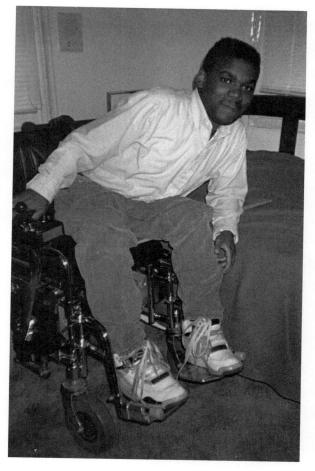

FIGURE 14–11. Donald demonstrating sliding board transfer technique used for chair-to-bed transfers.

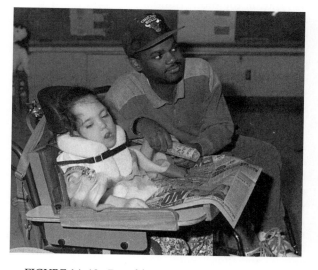

FIGURE 14–12. Donald assisting student in art class.

against continuation of a walking program using orthoses. A daily standing program at school was maintained until progression of the contractures resulted in a need to discontinue the program because orthopedic intervention was not desired by the family.

Currently at age 26, Donald is at stage 8 on Box 14–1. He is living in an apartment with a full-time home health aide. The scoliosis that was documented 6 years ago has not progressed, nor has it required any intervention. Donald uses a power wheelchair with joystick control as shown in Figure 14–10 owing to progression of upper extremity weakness and a need to provide greater trunk support in sitting. Assistance is required for all transfers, for bathing, and for dressing. A tub bench is used. Donald is independent with eating and personal hygiene such as brushing his teeth. Donald requires assistance for bed mobility. The sliding board transfer demonstrated in Figure 14–11 became too difficult 3 years ago, requiring use of a manual lift or Hoyer for all transfers.

Donald, or, as he prefers, "The Duckman," graduated from high school in 1980 and is currently not working. He assisted as an aide for an art teacher at a school for children with multiple disabilities (Fig. 14–12) until 3 years ago, when his upper extremity weakness progressed to the point where he decided to stop. He has worked with vocational rehabilitation services that resulted in two different jobs during the past 3 years, but after two recent hospitalizations for pneumonia he has decided to pursue avocational goals.

Although Donald is currently not having any symptoms of respiratory distress, consideration of using Cardiopulmonary Practice Pattern H: Impaired Ventilation and Respiration with Potential for Respiratory Failure would be appropriate for many individuals at this stage of the disease.

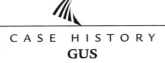

CASE HISTORY
GUS

Gus is a bright and inquisitive 7-year-old boy with a diagnosis of type I SMA. He is shown as a 25-month-old child in Figure 14–8. He was born at 32 weeks of gestation without significant neonatal complications and was discharged after 4 days. The only concerns during the early neonatal period were problems tolerating formula and frequent episodes of choking. Gus is an only child.

Gus's mother reported that he had a spontaneous and interactive smile with cooing at 2 months of age, midline play with shaking and banging of toys by 5 months, but delayed head control, no rolling, and limited movement at 5 months. At this time, the pediatrician stated concern about Gus's developmental delays in head control and rolling, but because of family history of later motor milestone development, further evaluation was not completed until the next well-baby checkup at 8 months of age. His management program with the guide would begin with Neuromuscular Practice Pattern A: Impaired Motor Function and Sensory Integrity Associated with Congenital or Acquired Disorders of the Central Nervous System in Infancy, Childhood, and Adolescence or Cardiopulmonary Practice Pattern H: Impaired Ventilation and Respiration with Potential for Respiratory Failure.

At 9 months, Gus was referred to an MDA clinic for further examination. He was noted to lie quietly supine with limited spontaneous movement. He would play with a toy while supine and roll to side lying but was unable to roll to prone. Verbalizations were frequent. In the prone position, limited head righting into extension was noted, and the mother reported limited use of this position because Gus often fussed when placed prone. Head-righting reactions in supported sitting were developed, and he was able to maintain propped sitting momentarily. Fasciculations of the tongue were noted. Following electromyographic testing and a muscle biopsy, the diagnosis of SMA was confirmed.

Home-based physical therapy services were authorized following the diagnosis, and services were coordinated through hospital visits for medical follow-up. Equipment included a customized seating insert and mobility base for transportation. A therapy program was carried out at home with Gus's mother as the primary caregiver. The program included instruction on positioning and handling for ADL, therapeutic exercise to facilitate head and trunk control, reaching games, and ROM. Pulmonary care instructions were given by a respiratory therapist. Routine pulmonary care included use of a percussor and nebulizer every 4 hours during the day.

At almost 2 years of age, Gus was able to prop sit when placed and roll independently from supine to side lying and vice versa. Other developmental skills required assistance. Higher developmental gross motor skills were not attained, and today at age 7 assistance is given for all transfers and positioning. He is, however, independent with mobility using his power wheelchair (Fig. 14–13).

A standing frame was used from age 2 to 3, but it was discontinued because of progression of his hip and knee flexion and ankle plantar flexion contractures. Other equipment includes a bath chair and extra pillows that are used for positioning at night.

Medical intervention has been required for feeding impairments. Choking with feeding continued to be a concern, and a fundoplication and placement of a gastric button were performed when Gus was 11 months of age. At 3 years of age a jejunostomy was performed because of problems with reflux and has worked well since that time.

Medical intervention has also been required for respiratory impairments. At 20 months of age concern was expressed by Gus's mother about his breathing at night, and after further evaluation oxygen by means of

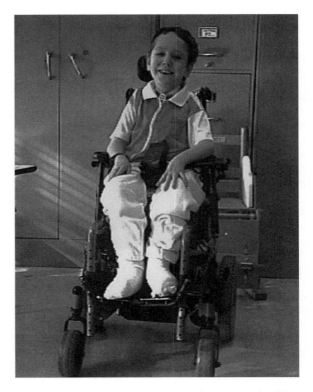

FIGURE 14–13. Gus at age 7 years in his power wheelchair and seating system.

a nasal cannula was initiated. After recurrent pneumonias a tracheostomy was placed at 6 years of age, with only two episodes of pneumonia after that time. He was able to be weaned from the oxygen following the tracheostomy. Gus does use an assisted breathing device at night along with an apnea monitor and a pulse oximeter. He receives pulmonary treatments by the family or nurse every 6 hours using a nebulizer and percussor. He is suctioned as required.

Even though Gus's prognosis is not hopeful, he is a warm and intelligent child who is busy exploring his world. He takes delight in new adventures and brings great happiness to all those who care for him, especially his mother.

SUMMARY

Muscle weakness and contracture are hallmark features of the childhood forms of muscular dystrophy and spinal muscle atrophy. A background knowledge of therapeutic exercise, functional use of orthoses and adaptive equipment, and strategies to minimize disabilities secondary to these impairments allow the physical therapist to bring unique information and skills to the management team.

Many of the disorders significantly reduce longevity. Therefore the patient's quality of life and attention to how the family copes with the stress should be included in the team's intervention program. Providing the children and families with support and realistic expectations is an ongoing challenge. Support groups or contact with another family that has had a similar experience can often help the family work through crisis periods, particularly when extended family support is not available.

Through the combined perspectives and innovative solutions of team members, a comprehensive program can be provided that takes into consideration the multifaceted demands of each individual and family. A philosophy of using a family-centered approach to care will help ensure that needs are met to the best of the team's ability.

ACKNOWLEDGMENTS

My personal thanks goes to the children and their families who contributed to my knowledge of MD and SMA that made the writing of this chapter possible. Many challenges, accomplishments, disappointments, joys, and tears have paved the way. Special thanks to Donald and Gus and their families for sharing their stories, and to Becky, who first inspired me to take this path of clinical work.

Recommended Resources

Muscular Dystrophy Association
http://www.mdausa.org/home.html.

Recommended Texts

Brooke, MH. A Clinician's View of Neuromuscular Diseases, 2nd ed. Baltimore: Williams & Wilkins, 1986.
Siegel, IM. Muscle and Its Diseases: An Outline Primer of Basic Science and Clinical Method. Chicago: Year Book Medical Publishers, 1986.

References

Alexander, MA, Johnson, EW, Petty, J, & Stauch, D. Mechanical ventilation of patients with late stage Duchenne muscular dystrophy: Management in the home. Archives of Physical Medicine and Rehabilitation, 60:289–292, 1979.

Amalfitano, A, Hauser, MA, Hu, H, Serra, D, Begy, CR, & Chamberlain, JS. Production and characterization of improved adenovirus vectors with the E1, E2b, and E3 genes deleted. Journal of Virology, 72(2):926–933, 1998.

Amendt, LE, Ause-Ellias, KL, Eybers, JL, Wadsworth, CT, Nielsen, DH, & Weinstein, SL. Validity and reliability testing of the scoliometer. Physical Therapy, 70:108–117, 1990.

American Physical Therapy Association (APTA). Guide to physical therapist practice. Physical Therapy, 77(11):1155–1674, 1997.

Arahata, K, Ishiura, S, & Ishiguro, T. Immunostaining of skeletal and cardiac muscle surface membrane with antibody against Duchenne muscular dystrophy peptide. Nature, 333:861–863, 1988.

Bach, JR. Ventilator use by Muscular Dystrophy Association patients. Archives of Physical Medicine and Rehabilitation, 73:179–183, 1992.

Bach, JR, Campagnolo, DI, & Hoeman, S. Life satisfaction of individuals with Duchenne muscular dystrophy using long-term mechanical ventilatory support. American Journal of Physical Medicine and Rehabilitation, 70:129–135, 1991.

Bach, JR, & McKeon, J. Orthopaedic surgery and rehabilitation for the prolongation of brace-free ambulation of patients with Duchenne muscular dystrophy. American Journal of Physical Medicine and Rehabilitation, 70:323–331, 1991.

Bach, JR, O'Brien, J, Krotenberg, R, & Alba, AS. Management of end stage respiratory failure in Duchenne muscular dystrophy. Muscle and Nerve, 10:177–182, 1987.

Backman, E, & Henriksson, KG. Low-dose prednisolone treatment in Duchenne and Becker muscular dystrophy. Neuromuscular Disorders, 5(3):233–241, 1995.

Ballestrazzi, A, Gnudi, A, Magni, E, & Granata, C. Osteopenia in spinal muscular atrophy. In Merlini, L, Granata, C, & Dubowitz, V (Eds.), Current Concepts in Childhood Spinal Muscular Atrophy. New York: Springer-Verlag, 1989, pp. 215–219.

Binder, H. New ideas in the rehabilitation of children with spinal muscular atrophy. In Merlini, L, Granata, C, & Dubowitz, V (Eds.), Current Concepts in Childhood Spinal Muscular Atrophy. New York: Springer-Verlag, 1989, pp. 117–128.

Bleck, EE, & Nagel, DA. Physically Handicapped Children: A Medical Atlas for Teachers. New York: Grune & Stratton, 1982, pp. 385–394.

Bowker, JH, & Halpin, PJ. Factors determining success in reambulation of the child with progressive muscular dystrophy. Orthopedic Clinics of North America, 9:431–436, 1978.

Brooke, MH. A Clinician's View of Neuromuscular Diseases, 2nd ed. Baltimore: Williams & Wilkins, 1986.

Brooke, MH, Fenichel, GM, Griggs, RC, Mendell, JR, Moxley, R, Florence, J, King, WM, Pandya, S, Robinson, J, Schierbecker, J, Singnor, L, Miller, JP, Gilder, BF, Kaiser, KK, Mandel, S, & Arfken, C. Duchenne muscular dystrophy: Patterns of clinical progression and effects of supportive therapy. Neurology, 39:475–481, 1989.

Brooke, MH, Griggs, RC, Mendell, JR, Fenichel, GM, Shumate, JB, & Pellegrino, RJ. Clinical trial in Duchenne dystrophy: I. The design of the protocol. Muscle and Nerve, 4:186–197, 1981.

Brouwer, OF, Paderg, GW, Van Der Ploeg, RJO, Ruys, CJM, & Brand, R. The influence of handedness on the distribution of muscular weakness of the arm in facioscapulohumeral muscular dystrophy. Brain, 115:1587–1598, 1992.

Brown, RH. Dystrophin-associated proteins and the muscular dystrophies. Annual Review of Medicine, 48:457–66, 1997.

Brussock, CM, Haley, SM, Munsat, TL, & Bernhardt, DB. Measurement of isometric force in children with and without Duchenne's muscular dystrophy. Physical Therapy, 72:105–114, 1992.

Bundey, S, & Lovelace, RE. A clinical study of chronic proximal spinal muscular atrophy. Brain, 98:455–472, 1975.

Burke, SS, Grove, NM, & Houser, CR. Respiratory aspects of pseudohypertrophic muscular dystrophy. American Journal of Diseases of Children, 121:230–234, 1971.

Cambridge, W, & Drennan, JC. Scoliosis associated with Duchenne muscular dystrophy. Journal of Pediatric Orthopedics, 7:436–440, 1987.

Chyatte, SB, Long, C, & Vignos, PJ. Balanced forearm orthosis in muscular dystrophy. Archives of Physical Medicine and Rehabilitation, 46:633–636, 1965.

Colbert, AP, & Craig, C. Scoliosis management in Duchenne muscular dystrophy: Prospective study of modified Jewett hyperextension brace. Archives of Physical Medicine and Rehabilitation, 68:302–304, 1987.

Coster, W, Deeney, T, Haltiwanger, J, & Haley, S. School Function Assessment. San Antonio, TX: Therapy Skill Builders, 1998.

Curran, FJ, & Colbert, AP. Ventilator management in Duchenne muscular dystrophy and postpoliomyelitis syndrome: Twelve years' experience. Archives of Physical Medicine and Rehabilitation, 70:180–185, 1989.

deLateur, BJ, & Giaconi, RM. Effect on maximal strength of submaximal exercise in Duchenne muscular dystrophy. American Journal of Physical Medicine, 58:26–36, 1979.

DeSilva, S, Drachman, DB, Mellitis, D, & Kuncl, RW. Prednisone treatment in Duchenne muscular dystrophy. Archives of Neurology, 44:818–822, 1987.

Donner, M, Rapola, J, & Somer, H. Congenital muscular dystrophy: A clinico-pathological and follow-up study of 15 patients. Neuropediatrics, 6:239–258, 1975.

Dorscher, PT, Mehrsheed, S, Mulder, DW, Litchy, WJ, & Ilstrup, DM. Wohlfart-Kugelberg-Welander syndrome: Serum creatine kinase and functional outcome. Archives of Physical Medicine and Rehabilitation, 72:587–591, 1991.

Dubowitz, V. The clinical picture of spinal muscular atrophy. In Merlini, L, Granata, C, & Dubowitz, V (Eds.), Current Concepts in Childhood Spinal Muscular Atrophy. New York: Springer-Verlag, 1989, pp. 13–19.

Dubowitz, V. The muscular dystrophies. Postgraduate Medical Journal, 68:500–506, 1992.

Edwards, RHT. Studies of muscular performance in normal and dystrophic subjects. British Medical Bulletin, 36:159–164, 1980.

Emery, AEH. Duchenne muscular dystrophy. Oxford: Oxford University Press, 1993.

Emery, AEH, Hausmanowa-Petrusewicz, I, Davie, AM, Holloway, S, Skinner, R, & Borkowska, J. International collaborative study of spinal muscular atrophies: I. Analysis of clinical and laboratory data. Journal of Neurologic Science, 29:83–94, 1976.

Emery, AEH, & Skinner, R. Clinical studies in benign (Becker-type) X-linked muscular dystrophy. Clinical Genetics, 10:189–201, 1976.

Eng, GD. Therapy and rehabilitation of the floppy infant. Rhode Island Medical Journal, 72:367–370, 1989a.

Eng, GD. Rehabilitation of the child with a severe form of spinal muscular atrophy (type I, infantile or Werdnig-Hoffman disease). In Merlini, L, Granata, C, & Dubowitz, V (Eds.), Current Concepts in Childhood Spinal Muscular Atrophy. New York: Springer-Verlag, 1989b, pp. 113–115.

Florence, JM, Pandya, S, King, WM, Robinson, JD, Baty, J, Miller, JP, Schierbecker, J, Signore, LC. Intrarater reliability of manual muscle test (Medical Research Council Scale) grades in Duchenne's muscular dystrophy. Physical Therapy, 72(2):115–122, 1992.

Fowler, WM. Rehabilitation management of muscular dystrophy and related disorders: I. The role of exercise. Archives of Physical Medicine and Rehabilitation, 63:208–210, 1982.

Fowler, WM, & Gardner, GW. Quantitative strength measurements in muscular dystrophy. Archives of Physical Medicine and Rehabilitation, 48:629–644, 1967.

Fukuyama, Y, Osaw, M, & Suzuki, H. Congenital muscular dystrophy of the Fukuyama type: Clinical, genetic and pathological considerations. Brain and Development, 3:1–29, 1981.

Galasko, CSB, Williamson, JB, & Delany, CM. Lung function in Duchenne muscular dystrophy. European Spine, 4:263–267, 1995.

Gamstrop, I. Progressive spinal muscular atrophy with onset in infancy or early childhood. Acta Paediatrica Scandinavica, 56:408–423, 1967.

Gardner-Medwin, D. Controversies about Duchenne muscular dystrophy: II. Bracing for ambulation. Developmental Medicine and Child Neurology, 21:659–662, 1979.

Gardner-Medwin, D. Rehabilitation in muscular dystrophy. International Rehabilitative Medicine, 2:104–110, 1980a.

Gardner-Medwin, D. Clinical features and classification of the muscular dystrophies. British Medical Bulletin, 36:109–115, 1980b.

Gibson, DA, Koreska, J, & Robertson, D. The management of spinal deformity in Duchenne's muscular dystrophy. Clinical Orthopedics, 9:437–450, 1978.

Gibson, DA, & Wilkins, KE. The management of spinal deformities in Duchenne's muscular dystrophy. Clinical Orthopedics, 108:41–51, 1975.

Gilliam, TC, Brzustowicz, LM, & Castilla, LH. Genetic homogeneity between acute and chronic forms of spinal muscle atrophy. Nature, 345:823–825, 1990.

Gilroy, J, & Holliday, P. Basic Neurology. New York: Macmillan, 1982.

Granata, C, Magni, E, Sabattini, L, Colombo, C, & Merlini, L. Promotion of ambulation in intermediate spinal muscle atrophy. In Merlini, L, Granata, C, & Dubowitz, V (Eds.), Current Concepts in Childhood Spinal Muscular Atrophy. New York: Springer-Verlag, 1989a, pp. 127–132.

Granata, C, Marini, ML, Capelli, T, & Merlini, L. Natural history of scoliosis in spinal muscular atrophy and results of orthopaedic treatment. In Merlini, L, Granata, C, & Dubowitz, V (Eds.), Current Concepts in Childhood Spinal Muscular Atrophy. New York: Springer-Verlag, 1989b, pp. 153–164.

Granata, C, Merlini, L, Magni, E, Marini, ML, & Stagni, SB. Spinal muscular atrophy: Natural history and orthopaedic treatment of scoliosis. Spine, 14:760–762, 1989c.

Haley, SM, Coster, WJ, Ludlow, LH, & Haltiwanger, JT. Pediatric Evaluation of Disability Inventory (PEDI): Development, Standardization and Administration Manual. Boston: New England Medical Center Hospital, 1992.

Harley, HG, Walsh, KV, Rundle, S, Brook, JD, Sarfarazi, M, Koch, JL, Harper, PS, & Shaw, DJ. Localization of the myotonic dystrophy locus to 19q13.2-19q13.3 and its relationship to twelve polymorphic loci on 19q. Human Genetics, 87:73–80, 1991.

Harper, PS. Congenital myotonic muscular dystrophy in Britain: I. Clinical aspects. Archives of Disease in Childhood, 50:505–513, 1975a.

Harper, PS. Myotonic Dystrophy, 2nd ed. Major Problems in Neurology, Vol. 21. Philadelphia: WB Saunders, 1989.

Hausmanowa-Petrusewicz, I. Spinal Muscular Atrophy: Infantile and Juvenile Type. Springfield, VA: US Department of Commerce, National Technical Information Service, 1978.

Heckmatt, JZ, Dubowitz, V, & Hyde, SA. Prolongation of walking in Duchenne muscular dystrophy with lightweight orthoses: Review of 57 cases. Developmental Medicine and Child Neurology, 27:149–154, 1985.

Hill, NS, Redline, S, Carskadon, MA, Curran, FJ, & Millman, RP. Sleep-disordered breathing in patients with Duchenne muscular dystrophy using negative pressure ventilators. Chest, *102*:1656–1662, 1992.

Hoffman, EP, Brown, RH, & Kunkel, LM. Dystrophin: The protein product of the Duchenne muscular dystrophy locus. Cell, *51*:919–928, 1987.

Hoffmann, J. Ueber chronische spinale Muskelatrophie im Kindesalter, auf familiar Basis. Deutsche Zeitschrift fur Nervenheilkunde, *3*:427, 1893.

Houser, CR, & Johnson, DM. Breathing exercise for children with pseudohypertrophic muscular dystrophy. Physical Therapy, *51*: 751–759, 1971.

Johnson, EW, & Braddom, R. Over-work weakness in facioscapulohumeral muscular dystrophy. Archives of Physical Medicine and Rehabilitation, *52*:333–336, 1971.

Jones, R, Khan, R, Hughes, S, & Dubowitz, V. Congenital muscular dystrophy: The importance of early diagnosis and orthopaedic management in the long-term prognosis. Journal of Bone and Joint Surgery (American), *61b*:13–17, 1979.

Karpati, G, Holland, P, & Worton, RG. Myoblast transfer in DMD: Problems in the interpretation of efficiency (Letter). Muscle and Nerve, *15*:1209–1210, 1992.

Kingston, HM, Harper, PS, Pearson, PL, Davies, KE, Williamson, R, & Page, D. Localization of the gene for Becker muscular dystrophy. Lancet, *2*:1200, 1983.

Koenig, M, Hoffmann, EP, & Pertelson, CK. Complete cloning of the Duchenne muscular dystrophy (DMD) cDNA and preliminary genomic organization of the DMD gene in mouse and affected individuals. Cell, *50*:509–517, 1987.

Kugelberg, E, & Welander, L. Heredofamilial juvenile muscular atrophy simulating muscular dystrophy. Archives of Neurology and Psychiatry, *75*:500, 1956.

Kunkel, LM, Monaco, AP, Middlesworth, W, Ochs, SD, & Latt, SA. Specific cloning of DNA fragments absent from the DNA of a male patient with an X chromosome deletion. Proceedings of the National Academy of Science, USA, *82*:4778–4782, 1985.

Kushner, HS. When Bad Things Happen to Good People. London: Pan Books, 1981, pp. 54–79.

Law, PK, Goodwin, TG, Fang, Q, Quinley, T, Vastagh, G, Hall, T, Jackson, T, Deering, MB, Duggirala, V, Larkin, C, Florendo, JA, Li, LM, Yoo, TJ, Chase, N, Neel, M, Krahn, T, & Holcomb, RL. Human gene therapy with myoblast transfer. Transplantation Proceedings, *29*:2234–2237, 1997.

Lee, CC, Pearlman, JA, Chamberlain, JS, & Caskey, CT. Expression of recombinant dystrophin and its localization to the cell membrane. Nature, *349*:334–336, 1991.

Leibowitz, D, & Dubowitz, V. Intellect and behavior in Duchenne muscular dystrophy. Developmental Medicine and Child Neurology, *23*:557–590, 1981.

Lonstein, JE. Management of spinal deformity in spinal muscular atrophy. In Merlini, L, Granata, C, & Dubowitz, V (Eds.), Current Concepts in Childhood Spinal Muscular Atrophy. New York: Springer-Verlag, 1989, pp. 165–173.

MacKenzie, AE, Jacob, P, Surh, L, & Besner, A. Genetic heterogeneity in spinal muscle atrophy: A linkage analysis-based assessment. Neurology, *44*(5):919–924, 1994.

Marchesi, D, Arlet, V, Stricker, U, & Aeibi, M. Modification of the original luque technique in the treatment of Duchenne's neuromuscular scoliosis. Journal of Pediatric Orthopaedics, *17*:743–749, 1997.

Marshall, CR. Medical treatment of spinal muscular atrophy. In Gamstorp, I, & Sarnat, HB (Eds.), Progressive Spinal Muscular Atrophies. International Review of Child Neurology Series. New York: Raven Press, 1984, pp. 163–171.

McMenamin, JB, Becker, LE, & Murphy, EG. Congenital muscular dystrophy: A clinical/pathological report of 24 cases. Journal of Pediatrics, *100*:692–697, 1982.

Merlini, L, Granata, C, Capelli, T, Mattutini, P, & Colombo, C. Natural history of infantile and childhood spinal muscular atrophy. In Merlini, L, Granata, C, & Dubowitz, V (Eds.), Current Concepts in Childhood Spinal Muscular Atrophy. New York: Springer-Verlag, 1989, pp. 95–100.

Miller, F, Moseley, CF, & Koreska, J. Spinal fusion in Duchenne muscular dystrophy. Developmental Medicine and Child Neurology, *34*:775–786, 1992.

Miller, G, & Dunn, N. An outline of the management and prognosis of Duchenne muscular dystrophy in Western Australia. Australian Pediatric Journal, *82*:277–282, 1982.

Miller, RG, & Hoffman, EP. Molecular diagnosis and modern management of Duchenne muscular dystrophy. Neurology Clinics, *12*(4): 699–725, 1994.

Mokri, B, & Engel, AW. Duchenne dystrophy: Electron microscopic findings pointing to a basic or early abnormality in the plasma membrane of the muscle fiber. Neurology, *25*:1111–1120, 1975.

Molnar, GE, & Alexander, J. Objective, quantitative muscle testing in children: A pilot study. Archives of Physical Medicine and Rehabilitation, *54*:224–228, 1973.

Moosa, A, & Dubowitz, V. Spinal muscular atrophy in childhood: Two clues to clinical diagnosis. Archives of Disease in Childhood, *48*: 386–388, 1973.

Mostacciuolo, ML, Lombardi, A, Cambissa, V, Danieli, GA, & Angelini, C. Population data on benign and severe forms for X-linked muscular dystrophy. Human Genetics, *75*:217–220, 1987.

Muscular Dystrophy Association. Facts About Muscular Dystrophy. Tucson, AZ: Muscular Dystrophy Association, 1991.

Namba, T, Aberfeld, DC, & Grob, D. Chronic proximal spinal muscular atrophy. Journal of Neurologic Science, *11*:401–423, 1970.

Newsom-Davis, J. The respiratory system in muscular dystrophy. British Medical Bulletin, *36*:135–138, 1980.

O'Brien, T, & Harper, PS. Course, prognosis and complications of childhood-onset myotonic dystrophy. Developmental Medicine and Child Neurology, *26*:62–67, 1984.

Pandya, A, Florence, JM, King, WM, Robinson, JD, Oxman, M, & Province, MA. Reliability of goniometric measurements in patients with Duchenne muscular dystrophy. Physical Therapy, *65*:1339–1342, 1985.

Partridge, TA, Grounds, M, & Sloper, JC. Evidence of fusion between host and donor myoblasts in skeletal muscle grafts. Nature, *273*: 306–308, 1978.

Pearn, JH. The gene frequency of acute Werdnig-Hoffman's disease (SMA type 1): A total population survey in northeast England. Journal of Medical Genetics, *10*:260–265, 1973.

Pearn, JH. Autosomal dominant spinal muscular atrophy: A clinical and genetic study. Journal of Neurologic Science, *38*:263–275, 1978.

Pearn, JH. Classification of spinal muscular atrophies. Lancet, *1*:919–922, 1980.

Pearn, JH, Carter, CO, & Wilson, J. The genetic identity of acute spinal muscular atrophy. Brain, *96*:463–470, 1973.

Pinelli, G, Dominici, P, Merlini, L, DiPasquale, G, Granata, C, & Bonfiglioli, S. Cardiologic evaluation in a family with Emery-Dreifus muscular dystrophy. Giornale Italiano di Cardiologia, *17*:589–593, 1987.

Ringel, SP. Neuromuscular Disorders: A Guide for Patient and Family. New York: Raven Press, 1987.

Robinson, A. Programmed cell death and the gene behind spinal muscle atrophy. Canadian Medical Association Journal, *153*(10): 1459–1462, 1995.

Rodillo, E, Noble-Jamieson, CM, Aber, V, Heckmatt, JZ, et al. Respiratory muscle training in Duchenne muscular dystrophy. Archives of Disease in Childhood, *64*:736–738, 1989.

Roy, L, & Gibson, DA: Pseudohypertrophic muscular dystrophy and its surgical management: Review of 30 patients. Canadian Journal of Surgery, *13*:13–20, 1970.

Rutherford, MA, Heckmatt, JZ, & Dubowitz, V. Congenital myotonic dystrophy: Respiratory function at birth determines survival. Archives of Disease in Childhood, *64*:191–195, 1989.

Saranti, AJ, Gleim, GW, & Melvin, M. The relationship between subjective and objective measurements of strength. Journal of Orthopedic Sports and Physical Therapy, 2:15–19, 1980.

Scott, OM, Hyde, SA, Goddard, C, & Dubowitz, V. Prevention of deformity in Duchenne muscular dystrophy: A prospective study of passive stretching and splintage. Physiotherapy, 67:177–180, 1981.

Scott, OM, Hyde, SA, & Goddard, E. Quantification of muscle function in children: A prospective study in Duchenne muscular dystrophy. Muscle and Nerve, 5:291–301, 1982.

Scott, OM, Vrbova, G, Hyde, SA, & Dubowitz, V. Responses of muscles of patients with Duchenne muscular dystrophy to chronic electrical stimulation. Journal of Neurology, Neurosurgery and Psychiatry, 49:1427–1434, 1986.

Seeger, BR, Caudrey, DJ, & Little JD. Progression of equinus deformity in Duchenne muscular dystrophy. Archives of Physical Medicine and Rehabilitation, 66:286–288, 1985.

Seeger, BR, Sutherland, AD, & Clark, MS. Orthotic management of scoliosis in Duchenne muscular dystrophy. Archives of Physical Medicine and Rehabilitation, 65:83–86, 1984.

Shapiro, F, & Specht, L. Orthopaedic deformities in Emery-Dreifus muscular dystrophy. Journal of Pediatric Orthopedics, 11:336–340, 1991.

Siegel, IM. Plastic-molded knee-ankle-foot orthosis in the management of Duchenne muscular dystrophy. Archives of Physical Medicine and Rehabilitation, 56:322, 1975.

Siegel, IM. The Clinical Management of Muscle Disease: A Practical Manual of Diagnosis and Treatment. Philadelphia: JB Lippincott, 1977.

Siegel, IM. The management of muscular dystrophy: A clinical review. Muscle and Nerve, 1:453–460, 1978.

Siegel, IM. Muscle and Its Diseases: An Outline Primer of Basic Science and Clinical Method. Chicago: Year Book Medical Publishers, 1986.

Siegel, IM, Miller, JE, & Ray, RD. Subcutaneous lower limb tenotomy in the treatment of pseudohypertrophic muscular dystrophy. Archives of Physical Medicine and Rehabilitation, 53:404–406, 1972.

Spencer, GE, & Vignos, PJ. Bracing for ambulation in childhood progressive muscular dystrophy. Journal of Bone and Joint Surgery (American), 44:234–242, 1962.

Stevenson, WG, Perloff, JK, Weiss, JN, & Anderson, TL. Facioscapulohumeral muscular dystrophy: Evidence for selective, genetic electrophysiologic cardiac involvement. Journal of the American College of Cardiology, 15:292–299, 1990.

Stuberg, WA, & Metcalf, WM. Reliability of quantitative muscle testing in healthy children and in children with Duchenne muscular dystrophy using a hand-held dynamometer. Physical Therapy, 68:977–982, 1988.

Swinyard, CA, Deaver, GG, & Greenspan, L. Gradients of functional ability of importance in rehabilitation of patients with progressive muscular and neuromuscular diseases. Archives of Physical Medicine, 38:574, 1957.

Tatelbaum, J. The Courage to Grieve. London: Heinemann, 1980.

Tinsley, JM, & Davies, KE. Utropin: A potential replacement for dystrophin. Neuromuscular Disorders, 3(5/6):537–539, 1993.

Vignos, PJ. Physical models of rehabilitation in neuromuscular disease. Muscle and Nerve, 6:323–338, 1983.

Vignos, PJ, & Archibald, KC. Maintenance of ambulation in childhood muscular dystrophy. Journal of Chronic Diseases, 12:273–290, 1960.

Vignos, PJ, Spencer, GE, & Archibald, KC. Management of progressive muscular dystrophy. Journal of the American Medical Association, 184:103–112, 1963.

Vignos, PJ, & Watkins, MP. The effect of exercise in muscular dystrophy. Journal of the American Medical Association, 197:121–126, 1966.

Wahl, M. Gene therapy trials. Quest, 5(1):9–10, 1998.

Watt, JM, & Greenhill, B. Commentary: Rehabilitation and orthopaedic management of spinal muscle atrophy. In Gamstorp, I, & Sarnat, HB (Eds.), Progressive Spinal Muscular Atrophies. International Review of Child Neurology Series. New York: Raven Press, 1984.

Werdnig, G. Eie fruhinfantile progressive spinale Amyotrophie. Archives fur Psychiatrie Nervenkrankheiten, 26:706–744, 1894.

Wilkins, KE, & Gibson, DA. Patterns of spinal deformity in Duchenne muscular dystrophy. Journal of Bone and Joint Surgery (Am), 58:24–32, 1976.

Winsor, EJ, Murphy, EG, Thompson, MW, & Reed, TE. Genetics of childhood spinal muscular atrophy. Journal of Medical Genetics, 8:143–148, 1971.

Wohlfart, G, Fex, J, & Eliasson, S. Hereditary proximal spinal muscular atrophy: A clinical entity simulating progressive muscular dystrophy. Acta Psychiatrica Neurologica Scandinavica, 30:395–406, 1955.

Wong, CK, & Wade, CK. Reducing iliotibial band contractures in patients with muscular dystrophy using custom dry floatation cushions. Archives of Physical Medicine and Rehabilitation, 76:695–700, 1995.

Zellweger, H, Simpson, J, McCormick, WF, & Ionaseslu, V. Spinal muscular atrophy with autosomal dominant inheritance. Neurology, 22:957–963, 1972.

Ziter, FA, & Allsop, KG. The diagnosis and management of childhood muscular dystrophy. Clinical Pediatrics, 15:540–548, 1976.

Ziter, FA, & Allsop, KG. The value of orthoses for patients with Duchenne muscular dystrophy. Physical Therapy, 59:1361–1365, 1979.

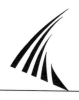

Clinical Protocol for Functional Testing in Duchenne Muscular Dystrophy*

A. Pulmonary.
  1. Forced vital capacity.
  2. Maximum voluntary ventilation.
B. Functional grade (arms and shoulders). Select one.
  1. Starting with arms at the sides, the patient can abduct the arms in a full circle until they touch above the head.
  2. Can raise arms above head only by flexing the elbow (i.e., shortening the circumference of the movement) or using accessory muscles.

If 1 or 2 is entered above, how many kilograms of weight can be placed on a shelf above eye level, using one hand?

  3. Cannot raise hands above head but can raise an 8 oz glass of water to mouth (using both hands if necessary).
  4. Can raise hands to mouth but cannot raise an 8 oz glass of water to mouth.
  5. Cannot raise hands to mouth but can use hands to hold pen or pick up pennies from the table.
  6. Cannot raise hands to mouth and has no useful function of hands.
C. Pulmonary.
  1. Maximum expiratory pressure.
D. Time to perform functions. Enter time in seconds. T = tried but failed to complete by time limit of 120 seconds.
  1. Standing from lying supine.
  2. Climbing four standard stairs (beginning and ending standing with arms at sides).
  3. Running or walking 30 feet (as fast as is compatible with safety).
  4. Standing from sitting on chair (chair height should allow feet to touch floor).
  5. Propelling a wheelchair 30 feet.
  6. Putting on a T-shirt (sitting in chair—see instructions).
  7. Cutting a 3 × 3-inch premarked square from a piece of paper with safety scissors (lines do not need to be followed precisely).
E. Functional grade (hips and legs). Select one.
  1. Walks and climbs stairs without assistance.
  2. Walks and climbs stairs with aid of railing.
  3. Walks and climbs stairs slowly with aid of railing (over 12 seconds for four standard stairs).
  4. Walks unassisted and raises from chair but cannot climb stairs.
  5. Walks unassisted but cannot rise from chair or climb stairs.
  6. Walks only with assistance or walks independently with long leg braces.
  7. Walks in long leg braces but requires assistance for balance.
  8. Stands in long leg braces but is unable to walk even with assistance.
  9. Is in wheelchair.
  10. Is confined to bed.

*From Brooke, MH, Griggs, RC, Mendell, JR, Fenichel, GM, Shumate, JB, & Pellegrino, RJ. Clinical trial in Duchenne dystrophy: I. The design of the protocol. Muscle and Nerve, 4:186–197, 1981.

CHAPTER
15

Limb Deficiencies and Amputations

MEG STANGER, PT, PCS, MS

The child with an amputation is defined as a person with an amputation who is skeletally immature because the epiphyses of the long bones are still open (Aitken, 1963). Amputations can be classified as congenital or acquired. Annual surveys of child amputee clinics in the United States indicate that 60% of childhood amputations are congenital and 40% are acquired (Tooms, 1992). Krebs and Fishman's (1984) study of 4105 children with limb deficiencies supports these findings. Krebs and colleagues (1991) further extrapolated from the data to estimate that the United States would be likely to experience 5525 new cases of childhood amputations per year, with 3315 of these amputations being congenital.

Many different factors must be considered in the management of children with a limb deficiency or amputation. These factors differ from those involved in the management of adults with a limb deficiency or amputation because as children grow their musculoskeletal systems continue to develop. Children also are emotionally immature and variably dependent on adults for care and decision making regarding surgical and prosthetic issues (Tooms, 1985).

In this chapter the etiology of limb deficiencies and amputations in children, surgical management, physical therapy intervention relative to a child's age and developmental function, and pediatric prosthetic options are discussed. Emphasis is on the aspects of management that differ from those encountered by adults with amputations. The role of the physical therapist includes education to parents of infants and children with limb deficiencies, development and progression of postoperative exercise programs, training in mobility and self-care skills, and providing input to both parents and the child or adolescent regarding prosthetic options. Studies have shown that children with limb deficiencies who participated in extensive rehabilitation programs have vocational skills with high employment potential (Tebbi, 1993).

CONGENITAL LIMB DEFICIENCIES

Classification

Various classification systems of congenital limb deficiencies have been developed. Greek terminology has been used to describe various deficiencies but is often inaccurate and ambiguous (Day, 1991). Frantz and O'Rahilly (1961) developed a classification system based on embryologic considerations and the absent skeletal portions. Swanson and colleagues (1968) modified that system with a classification system of seven categories based on embryologic failure: (1) failure of formation of parts (arrest of development), (2) failure of differentiation (separation of parts), (3) duplication, (4) overgrowth, (5) undergrowth (hypoplasia), (6) congenital constriction band syndrome, and (7) generalized skeletal deformities. Further modifications were made by the International Society for Prosthetics and Orthotics (ISPO) in 1973 and 1989. The classification developed by the ISPO has now been accepted and published as an international standard, International Standards Organization (ISO) 8548-1:1989, "Method of Describing Limb Deficiencies Present at Birth" (Day, 1991).

The ISO/ISPO classification of congenital limb deficiency is restricted to skeletal deficiencies described on anatomic and radiologic bases only; Greek terminology, such as hemimelia and phocomelia, is avoided because of its lack of precision and difficulty of translation into languages that are not related to Greek (Day, 1991). Deficiencies are described as either transverse or longitudinal. In transverse deficiencies the limb has developed normally to a particular level beyond which no skeletal elements exist, although digital buds may be present. A transverse deficiency is described by naming the segment in which the limb terminates and then describing the level within the segment beyond which no skeletal elements exist (Day, 1991) (Fig. 15–1).

In longitudinal deficiencies there is as a reduction or absence of an element or elements within the long axis of a limb. Normal skeletal elements may be present distal to the affected bones. A longitudinal deficiency is described by naming the bones affected in a proximal-to-distal sequence and stating whether each affected bone is totally or partially absent (Day, 1991) (Fig. 15–2).

Etiology

To fully understand the etiology of congenital limb deficiencies, a basic knowledge of embryonic skeletal development is necessary. Limb buds first appear at the end of the fourth week of embryonic development, arising from mesenchymal tissue. During the next 3 weeks the limb buds grow and differentiate into identifiable limb segments (Moore, 1982). Development of limb buds occurs in a proximodistal sequence, with the upper limb developing ahead of the lower limb by several days. The mesenchymal tissue undergoes chondrification to become cartilaginous models of individual bones (Tooms, 1985). By the end of the seventh week a recognizable embryonic skeleton is present. Teratogenic factors must therefore be present at some time between the third and seventh weeks of embryonic development to produce a limb deficiency.

Brent (1985) reviewed human malformations and found that in 60 to 70% of cases the cause is unknown. Several teratogenic factors have been identified (e.g., thalidomide, contraceptives, irradiation) as possible causative factors for congenital limb deficiencies. Genetic factors have also been linked with some congenital limb deficiencies, such as Holt-Oram, Fanconi, Nager, and thrombocytopenia-absent radius syndromes (Lenz, 1980). The limb deficiency may be the result of sporadic genetic mutation (Lenz, 1980). For most children born with a limb deficiency, however, the cause is unknown.

Levels of Limb Deficiency

The clinical presentation of a child with a congenital limb deficiency depends on the type, level, and number of deficiencies. Almost any combination or variety of limb deficiency is possible, but some are more common, and these are discussed here in detail. Between 20 and 30% of children have limb deficiencies affecting more than one limb (Krebs & Fishman, 1984; Tooms, 1985) (Fig. 15–3).

Most transverse deficiencies are unilateral, with the transverse below-elbow limb deficiency being the most common (Wright & Jobe, 1991) (Fig. 15–4). Rudimentary finger vestiges called nubbins may be present. This type of deficiency occurs more frequently in females, with a left-sided predominance of almost 2:1 (Shurr & Cook, 1990).

A complex lower extremity congenital limb deficiency has been termed *proximal femoral focal deficiency* (PFFD). Aitken (1969) first described this deficiency, which includes absence or hypoplasia of the proximal femur with varying degrees of involvement of the acetabulum, femoral head, patella, tibia, and fibula. The deficiency may be unilateral or bilateral. Aitken describes four classes of severity, A

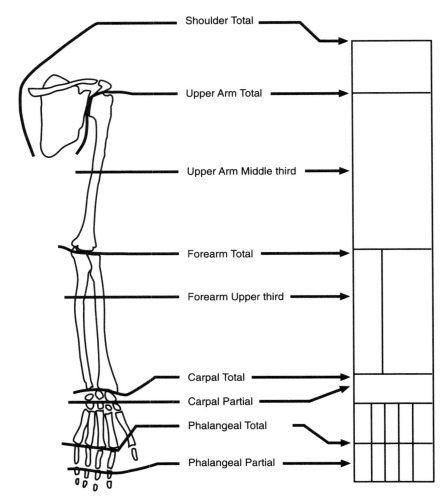

FIGURE 15-1. Examples of transverse deficiencies at various levels of the upper extremity. (From Day, HJ. The ISO/ISPO classification of congenital limb deficiency. In Bowker, JH, & Michael, JW [Eds.], Atlas of Limb Prosthetics: Surgical, Prosthetic, and Rehabilitation Principles, 2nd ed. St. Louis: Mosby, 1992, p. 747.)

through D, with class A exhibiting the least involvement (Fig. 15-5).

The clinical manifestations of a child with PFFD are relatively typical. They include a shortened thigh that is held in flexion, abduction, and external rotation; hip and knee flexion contracture; and severe leg length discrepancy, with the foot often at the level of the opposite knee. These children also have instability of the knee joint secondary to absent or deficient cruciate ligaments and a 70 to 80% incidence of total longitudinal deficiency of the fibula. Fifteen percent of children with PFFD have bilateral involvement (Epps, 1983). The incidence of PFFD is reported to be 1 per 50,000 live births, and it is usually of unknown etiology (Herzenberg, 1991).

ACQUIRED AMPUTATIONS

Acquired amputations account for approximately 40% of childhood amputations. Of these, 70 to 85% can be attributed to trauma (Challenor, 1992). The remainder of acquired amputations in children are the result of disease (most frequently tumors but also infection and vascular malformations). Ninety percent of acquired amputations involve only one limb, and the lower extremity is involved in 60% of cases (Tooms, 1985) (Figs. 15-6 and 15-7).

Traumatic Amputations

Accidents involving farm machinery and power tools are the leading causes of acquired amputations

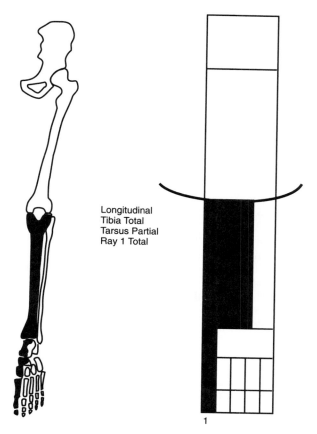

Longitudinal
Tibia Total
Tarsus Partial
Ray 1 Total

1

FIGURE 15–2. Example of a longitudinal deficiency of the lower extremity. (From Day, HJ. The ISO/ISPO classification of congenital limb deficiency. In Bowker, JH, & Michael, JW [Eds.], Atlas of Limb Prosthetics: Surgical, Prosthetic, and Rehabilitation Principles, 2nd ed. St. Louis: Mosby, 1992, p. 748.)

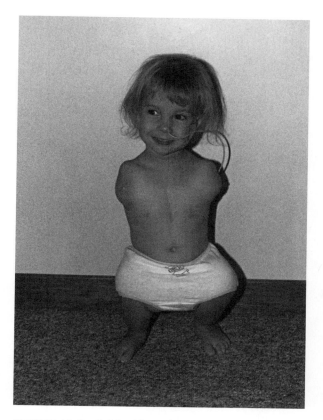

FIGURE 15–3. Child with multiple congenital limb deficiencies including bilateral transverse upper arm deficiency and bilateral proximal femoral focal deficiency.

in the pediatric population, followed closely by vehicular accidents, gunshot wounds, and railroad accidents (Tooms, 1992). Incidences vary according to age and geographic location. Lawn mowers and household accidents account for most amputations in the 1- to 4-year-old population. Vehicular accidents, power tools and machinery, and gunshot wounds are common causes of traumatic amputations in the older child (Tooms, 1992).

Disease-Related Amputations

Sarcoma of Bone

Primary bone tumors are rare in children, accounting for 5% of cancers in children younger than 15 years of age (Miller, 1995). Annual incidence rates for childhood bone cancers in the United States are 5.5 per million for whites and 4.3 per million for African-Americans. This represents approximately a 1 in 12,000 chance of developing a bone malignancy before 15 years of age (Robison et al., 1991). Osteosarcoma and Ewing's sarcoma are the most common of the primary bone tumors and account for 89% of malignant bone tumors in children (Robison et al., 1991). Childhood cancer statistics are based on children younger than 15 years of age; however, both osteosarcoma and Ewing's sarcoma continue to be seen in the late teenage years and beginning of the third decade of life with incidence rates comparable to the 10- to 14-year-old population.

OSTEOSARCOMA

Osteosarcoma is a primary malignant tumor of bone derived from bone-forming mesenchyme in which the malignant proliferating spindle cell stroma produces osteoid tissue or immature bone. The cause of osteosarcoma is unknown; however,

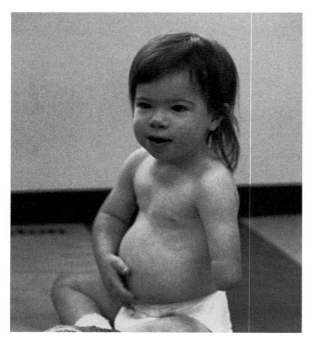

FIGURE 15–4. Child with congenital transverse below-elbow limb deficiency.

osteosarcoma has been linked with exposure to ionizing radiation (Link et al., 1991b; Meyers, 1987a). A viral cause has also been suggested based on evidence that bone sarcomas can be induced through viruses in animals, but this has not been replicated in humans (Link & Eilber, 1988; Link et al., 1991b).

Osteosarcoma represents 50% of bone cancers in children in the United States. The overall annual incidence rate is 3.3 cases per million children under age 15 years. There is a slightly higher incidence among females and among African-Americans compared with whites. The peak incidence rate is 13 years of age for females and 14 years for males (Gurney, 1995). Approximately 80% of childhood cases are diagnosed between 10 and 14 years of age (Robison et al., 1991).

The peak incidence of osteosarcoma coincides with the pubertal growth spurt, and it occurs most frequently at the metaphyseal portion of the most rapidly growing bones in adolescence. As a result, the distal femur, proximal tibia, and proximal humerus are the most common sites for osteosarcoma. This finding supports the theory that these rapidly growing cells are susceptible to oncogenic agents or mitotic errors and that osteosarcoma is the result of an aberration of the normal process of bone growth and remodeling (Link & Eilber, 1988; Link et al., 1991b; Meyers, 1987a).

EWING'S SARCOMA

Ewing's sarcoma is an undifferentiated round cell tumor. The tumor infiltrates bone marrow and subsequently adjacent soft tissue. Primary sites for Ewing's sarcoma are the weight-bearing bones of the lower extremity or pelvis. Ewing's sarcoma tends to occur in the diaphysis of long bones. The cause is unknown; however, radiation does not increase the risk (Link et al., 1991b).

Ewing's sarcoma is less common than osteosarcoma and represents 39% of bone tumors in children (Robison et al., 1991). The overall incidence rate in the United States is 2.8 cases per million children under 15 years of age with an extremely low rate in African-Americans of 0.3 cases per million children. Eighty percent of patients are younger than 20 years of age; the peak incidence is 8.3 years for males and 13 years for females. Slightly more males than females are diagnosed with Ewing's sarcoma (Link et al., 1991b; Gurney, 1995).

DIAGNOSIS

The initial complaint for both osteosarcoma and Ewing's sarcoma is pain at the site of the tumor with or without a palpable mass. Localized swelling is present in 63% of children with Ewing's sarcoma. Systemic symptoms are rare in osteosarcoma unless widespread metastatic disease is present. On the other hand, systemic symptoms, most commonly fever and weight loss, are present in 25% of children with Ewing's sarcoma at the time of diagnosis (Link et al., 1991b). If fever is present, Ewing's sarcoma may be mistakenly suspected to be chronic osteomyelitis (Miser et al., 1988b). The most common site for tumors in children with osteosarcoma is the knee. Fifty percent of tumors arise from the distal femur and proximal tibia (Link et al., 1991b; Meyers, 1987a). Common sites for Ewing's sarcoma include the diaphyses of the weight-bearing bones of the lower extremity, the pelvis, and the humerus (Link et al., 1991b; Meyers, 1987b).

Because the initial complaint for both osteosarcoma and Ewing's sarcoma is pain at the site of the tumor, diagnosis is often delayed. Duration of symptoms before diagnosis averages 3 months for osteosarcoma and up to 6 months for Ewing's sarcoma (Link et al., 1991b). Children presenting to a physical therapist with a complaint of pain, which is often chronic, a negative history of injury, and no evidence of musculoskeletal abnormalies should be referred for further medical workup to rule out a malignant bone tumor.

The key to diagnosis of a bone tumor is a radiologic evaluation (Link et al., 1991b). Plain-view x-ray films, computed tomography, or magnetic resonance imaging will reveal evidence of a mass and

TYPE		FEMORAL HEAD	ACETABULUM	FEMORAL SEGMENT	RELATIONSHIP AMONG COMPONENTS OF FEMUR AND ACETABULUM AT SKELETAL MATURITY
A	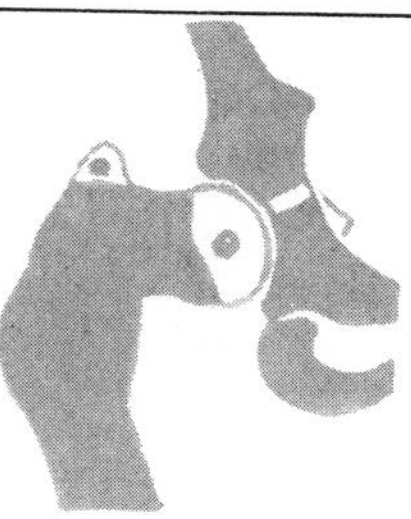	Present	Normal	Short	Bony connection between components of femur Femoral head in acetabulum Subtrochanteric varus angulation, often with pseudarthrosis
B	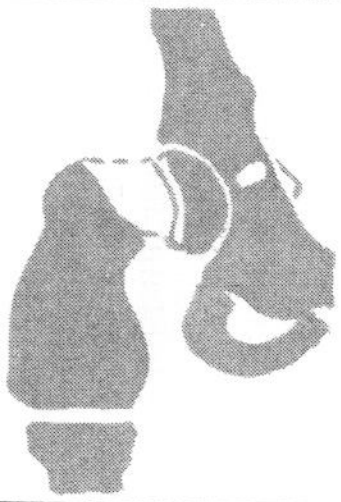	Present	Adequate or moderately dysplastic	Short, usually proximal bony tuft	No osseous connection between head and shaft Femoral head in acetabulum
C	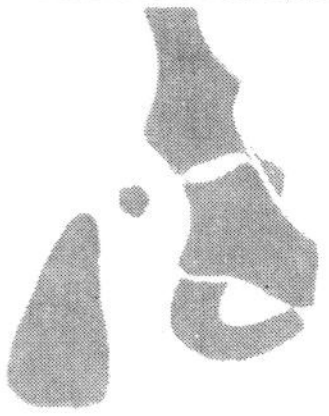	Absent or represented by ossicle	Severely dysplastic	Short, usually proximally tapered	May be osseous connection between shaft and proximal ossicle No articular relation between femur and acetabulum
D	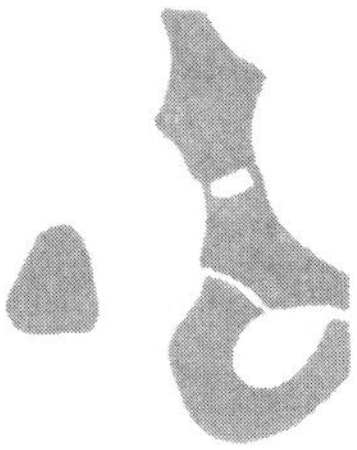	Absent	Absent Obturator foramen enlarged Pelvis squared in bilateral cases	Short, deformed	(none)

FIGURE 15–5. Aitken classification of proximal femoral focal deficiency. (From Tachdjian, MO [Ed.]. Pediatric Orthopedics, 2nd ed. Philadelphia: WB Saunders, 1990, p. 556.)

bony destruction. A definitive diagnosis is made through biopsy and histologic examination (Meyers, 1987a, 1987b). To complete the workup, a bone scan and chest computed tomography are performed to determine the extent of metastases.

Medical Management of Malignancies

Medical management of bony tumors and neoplasms includes several goals: (1) complete and permanent control of the primary tumor, (2) control and prevention of microstatic and metastatic dis-ease, and (3) preservation of as much function as possible. Local control of the primary tumor is most often achieved through surgery and radiation therapy. Surgical options include amputation and numerous limb-sparing procedures. Which surgical procedure is selected varies depending on location and size of tumor, extramedullary extent, presence or absence of metastatic disease, and the child's age, skeletal development, and lifestyle. Control of microstatic and metastatic disease is achieved through radiation therapy and adjuvant chemotherapy (multidrug chemotherapy).

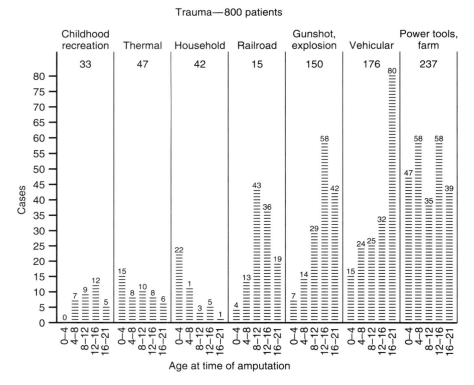

FIGURE 15–6. Etiology of acquired amputations resulting from trauma. (From Juvenile Amputee Course Manual. Evanston, IL: Northwestern University Medical School Prosthetic-Orthotic Progam, 1983.)

Radiation Therapy

Radiation therapy directs high-energy emissions at the tumor. The energy from the radiation disrupts the structure of atoms and damages essential molecules, including the chromosomes. Cell reproductive capacity is therefore compromised, leading to tumor cell death (Link, 1982). Damage can occur to surrounding normal tissue as well.

Osteosarcoma is generally unresponsive to radiation therapy. Osteosarcoma cells seem to repair themselves after radiation injury, whereas Ewing's sarcoma is highly responsive to radiation therapy (Link & Eilber, 1988; Link et al., 1991b; Miser et al., 1988b). Local control of Ewing's sarcoma may be achieved with moderately high doses of radiation to the entire bone and a boost of radiation to the primary tumor.

The side effects of radiation therapy are related to the primary site of the tumor, volume, dose rate, age of the patient, and use of chemotherapy. Acute side effects are seen in rapidly dividing tissues such as the skin, bone marrow, and gut. Common side effects are red and tender skin, mouth sores from irradiation to mucous membranes, and nausea and vomiting from irradiation to the abdomen. Irradiation of extremities produces few acute side effects (Link et al., 1991b). Children receiving radiation therapy may exhibit a decreased activity level secondary to nausea and vomiting, poor appetite secondary to mouth sores, and generalized malaise. Their physical therapy sessions may need to be altered on a daily basis to accommodate their changing energy levels. Children wearing a prosthesis must be monitored closely for skin irritation and breakdown.

Late side effects of radiation include fibrosis of soft tissues, bony changes ranging from osteoporosis to fractures, and growth disturbances, including damage to the epiphyseal plate and bowing of the metaphysis. Greater growth disturbances are found in younger children (Goldwein, 1991). Butler and colleagues (1990) reported that 77% of patients with Ewing's sarcoma who received radiation therapy developed a leg length discrepancy; in 58% of these patients the leg length discrepancy was significant enough to require treatment. If possible, attempts are made to shield the epiphyseal plate at the opposite end of the involved bone to minimize the radiation-linked growth retardation and still allow for some growth of the extremity. For some young children, an amputation may produce a more func-

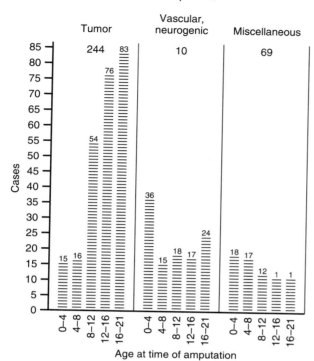

FIGURE 15–7. Etiology of acquired amputations resulting from disease. (From Juvenile Amputee Course Manual. Evanston, IL: Northwestern University Medical School Prosthetic-Orthotic Program, 1983.)

tional extremity than an extremity that is significantly shortened as a result of radiation therapy.

Secondary malignant neoplasms resulting from radiation therapy of the primary tumor are well documented. Meadows and colleagues (1985) cite data indicating that 3 to 12% of survivors of childhood cancer develop secondary neoplasms. Tucker and colleagues (1987) also report an increased risk of developing secondary bone tumors after receiving radiation therapy for childhood cancers.

Chemotherapy

The use of adjuvant chemotherapy has increased the survival rates for both osteosarcoma and Ewing's sarcoma. Children treated with surgery or radiation therapy alone have a poor prognosis, with 9 to 25% achieving 5-year survival (Link & Eilber, 1988; Miser et al., 1988a). Chemotherapy is used to control micrometastatic disease that is present but undetectable at diagnosis. It may also be used to control the size of the primary tumor. Preoperative chemotherapy may shrink the local tumor, making limb-sparing surgery a more feasible option or reducing the level of the amputation.

Five-year disease-free survival rates for children with Ewing's sarcoma treated with a combination of radiation therapy, chemotherapy, and in some cases surgery vary from 60 to 80% (Meyers, 1987b; Miser et al., 1988a). Survival rates are better for children whose tumors are more distal, rather than located on the axial skeleton, and for patients with no metastases at the time of diagnosis. Overall survival rates for children with osteosarcoma treated with a combination of surgery and chemotherapy have also drastically improved from 20% in the 1970s to 60 to 65% more recently (Link et al., 1991a; Meyers & Gorlick, 1997).

Chemotherapy agents are circulated in the bloodstream and so are delivered to all tissues of the body. They enter the cells and disrupt metabolic processes, especially cell division (Link, 1982). The result is death of the invaded cells. Malignant cells are killed, but normal cells may also be damaged or killed. Typical side effects of chemotherapy include nausea and vomiting, hair loss, anemia, neutropenia, and thrombocytopenia. Most of these side effects are reversible (Link, 1982). Some chemotherapeutic agents produce more specific and dose-related side effects. Therapists treating children receiving chemotherapy should be aware of how these side effects and possible complications will affect therapy (Table 15-1). The linear growth of children is slowed during the time period of intensive chemotherapy. After cessa-

TABLE 15–1. **Chemotherapy Agents**

Agent	Side Effects and Adverse Reactions	Therapy Concerns
Doxorubicin (Adriamycin)	Alopecia (hair loss), myelosuppression, orogastrointestinal reactions (oral reddening, ulcers, nausea, vomiting; more serious adverse reactions include diarrhea, dysphagia, gastrointestinal bleeding), myocardial toxicity (can lead to cardiac failure).	Extravasation can occur with intravenous administration. Reactions include stinging and burning sensation, possible cellulitis, blistering, and tissue necrosis. Life-threatening arrhythmias may occur during or within a few hours of administration. Cardiac failure is not often favorably affected by medical or physical support and must be detected early for successful treatment.
Bleomycin (Blenoxane)	Toxic to skin and lung tissues. Skin reactions include erythema, tenderness, hyperpigmentation. Pulmonary toxicities occur in 10% of patients. Pneumonitis may progress to pulmonary fibrosis and death.	Dyspnea is earliest symptom of pulmonary toxicity. Fine rales on auscultation. Pulmonary function test changes include decrease in total lung volume and decrease in vital capacity, but they are not predictive of development of pulmonary fibrosis. Pulmonary toxicity monitored through x-ray changes.
Dactinomycin (actinomycin D) (Cosmegen)	Orogastrointestinal reactions, alopecia, myelosuppression, liver toxicity.	Can impair wound healing. Corrosive to soft tissue. If extravasation occurs, severe damage to soft tissues will occur and can lead to contractures. Severe skin reactions occur where there has been previous irradiation.
Cyclophosphamide (Cytoxan) Dacarbazine (DTIC)	Alopecia, nausea and vomiting, myelosuppression, hemorrhagic cystitis. Myelosuppression, anorexia, nausea and vomiting, myalgias, malaise, alopecia.	Can impair wound healing. Must force liquids to control cystitis. Extravasation after intravenous administration produces severe local pain and stinging; can result in tissue damage.
Methotrexate	Potential for serious toxicity. Toxicity is function of dose and duration of treatment. Orogastrointestinal reactions, myelosuppression, hepatic or renal damage occur with prolonged use. Leukoencephalopathy reported in patients with osteosarcoma. Neurologic effects include behavioral changes, abnormal reflexes, and focal sensorimotor signs. Pulmonary symptoms include dry nonproductive cough, fever, dyspnea, hypoxemia, and chest x-ray infiltrate.	After discontinuation of methotrexate, complete recovery not always noted with leukoencephalopathy. Blurred vision, headaches, aphasia, and hemiparesis are other neurologic adverse reactions seen with methotrexate. Seizures have led to coma in children. May be administered with anticonvulsants if on large doses.
Vincristine (Oncovin)	Alopecia, constipation, nausea and vomiting, hypertension and hypotension, neuromuscular side effects, cranial nerve manifestations, seizures.	Monitor cardiovascular status. Neuromuscular side effects include pain distally, loss of deep tendon reflexes, footdrop, with progression to contractures, gait abnormalities, ataxia. Splinting may be helpful to avoid contractures. Extravasation during administration can lead to cellulitis. Paralysis of cranial nerves may be seen; most comonly affected muscles are extraocular and laryngeal.
Cisplatin (Platinol)	Nausea and vomiting, myelosuppression, cumulative renal toxicity, ototoxicity, peripheral neuropathies. Ototoxic effects can be more severe in children than in adults.	Ototoxicity may include tinnitus or hearing loss in high-frequency range. Occasionally may affect ability to hear normal conversation. Peripheral neuropathies may be irreversible and can include loss of motor function.

Data from Physicians' Desk Reference. Oradell, NJ: Medical Economics, 1993.

tion of chemotherapy, linear growth continues with no marked height differences noted in adulthood (Glasser et al., 1991).

SURGICAL OPTIONS IN THE MANAGEMENT OF ACQUIRED AND CONGENITAL LIMB DEFICIENCIES

Amputation in the Management of Traumatic Injuries and Malignant Tumors

Although most of the basic premises related to management of adults with amputations apply to children, there are important differences. First, skeletal immaturity and future growth are important factors when considering surgical alternatives. Physes should be preserved whenever possible to ensure continued growth of the limb. For the upper extremity the majority of growth occurs in physes around the shoulder and wrist, whereas in the lower extremity the physes around the knee account for most of the growth (Herzenberg, 1991).

Second, the fact that amputation through long bones may result in terminal overgrowth is an important point that should not be overlooked. Terminal overgrowth is a painful, spikelike prominence of new bone on the transected end of the residual limb. Significant pain can interfere with weight bearing and wearing of the prosthesis. The spikelike growth is not the result of growth from the proximal epiphysis but rather represents osteogenic activity of the periosteum (Gillespie, 1990). Terminal overgrowth occurs most frequently in the humerus, followed in order of incidence by the fibula, tibia, and femur (Herzenberg, 1991; Kruger, 1980). Surgical options include revisions and bone capping. The possibility of terminal overgrowth should not be a reason to elect higher-level amputation, such as a knee disarticulation rather than a below-knee amputation. As in adults, length of the lever arm, function of the extremity, and prosthetic fit remain important considerations when deciding on the level of amputation. Saving the child's life is, of course, the most important consideration, whether the amputation is the result of a malignancy or trauma.

Finally, wound healing in children is rarely a concern as it may be in adults with peripheral vascular disease. Skin grafts therefore may be used to close the amputation site in preference to performing a higher-level amputation for a child with a traumatic injury.

Acquired amputations secondary to trauma may result in a short residual limb. This is especially true of an above-knee amputation in which the distal physes have been resected. It may be possible to increase the length of a residual limb in older children by using one of the limb-lengthening techniques (see Chapter 16 for a discussion of limb-lengthening techniques). Lengthening of a short residual limb may increase the efficiency of gait and promote a better prosthetic fit (Eldridge et al., 1990).

The traditional approach for malignant bone tumors has been amputation of the limb in which the tumor is found. The surgical margin for an amputation is usually 6 to 7 cm above the most proximal medullary extent of tumor as defined on computed tomography or magnetic resonance imaging. This level of surgical margin allows for removal of microscopic tumor and skip lesions while allowing for the greatest amount of residual limb length for the individual. Studies have shown only a 5% local recurrence rate using this level of surgical margin (Link & Eilber, 1988; Link et al., 1991b).

For those tumor sites that are in the proximal humerus or femur, amputation results in severe loss of function. For example, a tumor of the proximal humerus treated by amputation would leave the patient with severely diminished function as a result of loss of the hand. Therefore most surgeons elect not to perform an amputation, if possible, for tumors of the upper extremity. Amputation for tumors of the pelvis or proximal femur also result in complete loss of the limb or a very short residual limb, which makes functional ambulation with a prosthesis difficult. Some limb-sparing procedures may result in a more functional extremity than an amputation without decreasing the expected rate of survival for the child. The decision regarding an amputation is based on expectations regarding control of the primary tumor and survival of the child and the functional use of the extremity.

Amputation to Revise Congenital Limb Deficiencies to Improve Function

Rarely is an amputation necessary with upper extremity limb deficiencies, but it may be indicated for some children with lower extremity limb deficiencies. A child with bilateral PFFD, however, may be more functional without any surgery. They will be of short stature but will walk quite well (Herzenberg, 1991). For cosmesis, extension prostheses may be an option.

The surgical treatment of a child with unilateral PFFD is case specific. If the child has a stable hip and foot and a significant portion of normal femur is present, one of the limb-lengthening procedures may be appropriate. Most surgeons agree that 60% of predicted femoral length must be present for a lengthening procedure to be a viable alternative (Gillespie, 1990; Herzenberg, 1991). If limb lengthening is not an option, the typical surgical intervention for

PFFD is a knee arthrodesis and foot amputation. Usually the Syme or Boyd amputation is recommended. A Syme amputation involves complete removal of the foot, including the calcaneus, followed by sectioning of the distal tibia perpendicular to the weight-bearing line (Tachdjian, 1990a). A Boyd amputation preserves the calcaneus, providing a more bulbous surface for weight bearing, as well as preserving leg length (Herzenberg, 1991). The knee is usually fused to form one long bone for fitting of an above-knee prosthesis (Herzenberg, 1991; Koman et al., 1982) (Fig. 15–8).

Amputation may also be an option for a child with a longitudinal tibial or fibular total deficiency in which a significant limb length difference exists along with deformity of the foot. Frequently the foot is positioned in equinovalgus with absent lateral rays. If the leg length difference is too significant for limb-lengthening techniques or epiphysiodesis of the uninvolved leg, or if the ankle is significantly unstable, a Syme or Boyd amputation may lead to a more functional lower extremity with the addition of a prosthesis. When considering an amputation for a child, it is important that alternatives are discussed with the family and child and that the ultimate lifestyle goals are known.

Rotationplasty

Rotationplasty, or a turnabout procedure, is a typical option for children with congenital limb deficiencies, specifically PFFD, as well as for those with bony tumors of the proximal tibia or distal femur. This procedure involves excision of the distal femur and proximal tibia; 180° rotation of the residual lower limb, including the distal femur and proximal tibia, ankle joint, foot, and neurovascular supply; and reattachment to the proximal femur (Fig. 15–9). The ankle then functions as a knee joint, with ankle plantar flexion used to extend the "knee" and ankle dorsiflexion to flex the "knee" (Herzenberg, 1991; Kotz & Salzer, 1982). Rotationplasty requires a functioning hip joint and ankle joint. In the case of malignant tumors, the tumor cannot have invaded the surrounding soft tissue, especially the neurovascular supply.

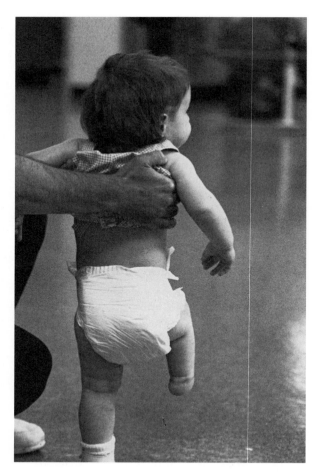

FIGURE 15–8. Child with unilateral proximal femoral focal deficiency following a Boyd amputation of his foot. Note popliteal crease near the diaper line indicating where his knee is located.

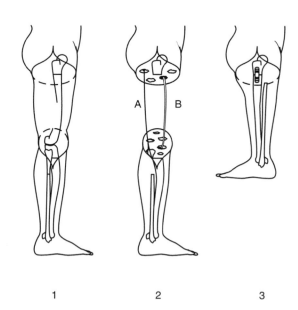

FIGURE 15–9. A schematic illustration of a rotationplasty procedure. Neurovascular structures (*A* and *B*) are left intact and wrapped into the existing space when the tibia is reattached to the femur.

The advantages of a rotationplasty are the increased limb length, improved prosthetic function with the ankle serving as a knee joint, improved weight-bearing capacity, and elimination of the problems of terminal overgrowth and pain from neuromas or phantom limb sensations (Kotz & Salzer, 1982). Weight is borne through the heel, which is more suitable for weight bearing than the end of a residual limb. Rotationplasty also allows for some growth of the leg. With an appropriate prosthesis, children who have had a rotationplasty procedure can run, jump, and play with their peers.

Disadvantages are cosmesis and derotation of the foot. Critics of rotationplasty cite poor cosmesis and psychologic issues as a deterrent to the procedure. In my experience with children who underwent a rotationplasty for either a tumor or congenital PFFD, cosmesis was not a complaint from the child or the child's parents. Krajbich and Bochmann (1992) cite their experience of 27 children with osteosarcoma who underwent a rotationplasty. Twenty-two of these children are alive with no evidence of metastatic disease. No long-term complications related to cosmesis and psychologic decompensation were reported; in fact, virtually all of the children with a rotationplasty now actively participate in sports and other activities with their peers. Before a rotationplasty it may be helpful for parents and the child to meet another child who has had the rotationplasty performed. Certainly, the cosmetic disadvantages must be discussed.

When the procedure is performed on young children, derotation of the foot may occur requiring rerotation of the limb. The limb may derotate secondary to the spiral pull of the muscles proximal and distal to the osteotomy (Tachdjian, 1990a). Both Krajbich and Bochmann (1992) and Gillespie (1990) discuss surgical options to limit derotation of the limb after a rotationplasty. Derotation is more common in children younger than 10 years of age and is most frequently seen in children when a rotationplasty is performed at 3 or 4 years of age (Gillespie, 1990).

Limb-Sparing Procedures

With the use of chemotherapy, improvements in diagnostic imaging to determine tumor margins, and new techniques of reconstruction, amputation is not always the treatment of choice for children with bony malignancies. Limb-sparing or limb-salvage procedures may be an alternative to amputation for some children with malignant bone tumors. Limb-sparing procedures involve resection of the tumor and reconstruction of the limb to preserve function without amputation of the limb. Reconstruc-

tion of the limb may include excision of bone without replacement of the excised area or replacement with an allograft or endoprosthetic implant.

The selection of appropriate children for limb-sparing surgery is critical. The goal of saving the limb should never compromise the goal of removing all gross and microscopic tumor (Link et al., 1991b). Limb-sparing surgery is contraindicated if the tumor has invaded the surrounding soft tissue to a large extent, if it involves the neurovascular supply, or if a wide surgical margin cannot be achieved (Finn & Simon, 1991). In addition, limb-sparing surgery for the lower extremity of a young child may not be beneficial when the child is skeletally immature and may be left with a severe leg length discrepancy and nonfunctional lower extremity. In these cases amputation may be a better choice than limb-sparing surgery.

Autologous grafts are rarely appropriate because long segments of bone usually must be excised. Replacement of the excised bone with a near-equal length of noninvolved bone from another portion of the body is often not possible. Cadaver allografts are another option. If a short segment of bone is replaced with an allograft, the graft provides a latticework into which the child's bone grows so that eventually the allograft is incorporated into the host bone. For this reason, successful allografts provide a durable implant that does not loosen over time.

Allografts have been most successful in children when used to replace a portion of the shaft of a bone. Growth centers are left undisturbed, allowing full growth of the limb. Allografts have also been used to replace the epiphysis as well as the metaphysis of a bone. When allografts are used as a joint arthrodesis, the results are less favorable, especially surrounding the knee joint. Often there is insufficient soft tissue remaining to allow significant coverage of the new graft. In addition, a portion of the physes surrounding the knee joint is removed, limiting the potential growth of the limb.

Allografts remain a viable surgical alternative for children nearing skeletal maturity or those children requiring only excision of a portion of the shaft of the bone. Bone grafting is contraindicated with the use of postoperative radiation therapy because of the possible development of pseudoarthrosis.

At times a tumor may be excised without replacing the excised bone. The proximal fibula may be resected if the soft tissue involvement is minimal and the peroneal nerve is not included in the soft tissue involvement. The biceps femoris tendon and fibular collateral ligament are reattached to the lateral condyle of the tibia (Tachdjian, 1990b). After healing, full knee motion and a normal gait pattern can be expected. The Tikhoff-Linberg procedure has been successfully used for osteosarcomas involving the proximal humerus when the brachial plexus is not included in the soft tissue involvement. With this procedure the proximal humerus is excised and not replaced. The remaining muscles of the upper arm are reattached to the trapezius and pectoralis muscles to suspend the remaining portion of the humerus (Springfield, 1991). The shoulder is unstable, but the elbow and hand are functional. With the increased use of endoprosthetics, a humeral device could be implanted to provide added stability and function to the shoulder area (Link & Eilber, 1988). In either case the functional outcome is superior to that following amputation of the entire upper extremity.

Endoprosthetic devices are ultimately an extension of joint arthroplasty procedures. These manufactured devices are implanted in the area of the excised bone and can be custom-designed for the proximal humerus, elbow, proximal and distal femur, and proximal tibia. They have the advantage of being able to provide a functional joint as well as providing structural integrity to replace that of excised bone (Link et al., 1991b). Problems include loosening of the prosthesis, infection, and mechanical failure of the device (Kenan & Lewis, 1991; Unwin & Walker, 1995). Children and adolescents may be very active and create vigorous stresses on prosthetic implants that lead to failures and the need for replacement of the devices over time. They may also not be appropriate for the young, skeletally immature child because these devices may not allow for growth.

Some endoprosthetic designs incorporate a telescoping unit that can be expanded to accommodate growth. Expansion of the prosthesis involves a minor surgical procedure at periodic intervals. The expandable prosthesis may function as the permanent prosthesis after skeletal maturity has been achieved or may need to be replaced by a conventional endoprosthesis if the device provides for poor function of the limb (Kenan & Lewis, 1991; Schindler et al., 1997; Unwin & Walker, 1996).

Clinical experience has shown that complications will occur with all telescoping endoprosthetic implants over time (Schindler et al., 1997). Loosening of the prosthesis occurs after a mean of 5 years with improvement noted with biologic fixation of the device versus use of cement. Infections occur most frequently 2 to 3 years after the implant when a lengthening procedure is performed. Newer models of implants have improved on mechanical failures and have minimized the invasiveness of the lengthening procedure. Several reports demonstrate effective growth of the child's limb with the use of an endoprosthetic device with gains of up to 7 or 8 cm in length (Kenan & Lewis, 1991; Schindler et al., 1997).

Several studies have reported comparable long-term survival rates between groups undergoing amputation versus a limb-sparing procedure (Eckhardt et al., 1985; Sim et al., 1985). The data are thought to indicate that limb-sparing surgery is as effective in controlling the tumor as amputation when adjuvant chemotherapy is used and when particular attention is given to patient selection, surgical margins, and surgical techniques. Limb-sparing procedures for the upper extremity clearly result in improved function for the patient when compared with amputation and the use of a prosthesis. More debate centers around limb-sparing techniques of the lower extremity and their functional results for the young child (Finn & Simon, 1991; Simon, 1991). Limb-sparing surgery is often not appropriate for the child with a congenital limb deficiency. First, most children with limb deficiencies have associated problems of the involved extremity. Second, they may have an unstable ankle joint for weight bearing, or their residual limb may be too short. Third, limb-sparing procedures, especially those involving the use of endoprosthetic devices, do not allow for the growth that these young children will experience in their uninvolved limb.

Limb Replantation

For children with traumatic amputations, limb replantation may be a surgical option. As with other surgical options, the goal of replantation is directed not only at preserving the amputated limb but also at restoring pain-free function to the extremity that is superior to the function obtained with a prosthesis. For an upper extremity, replantation entails elbow and hand function, as well as distal sensation. Replantation of a lower extremity must provide a painless, sensate extremity capable of bearing weight during normal daily activities (Gayle et al., 1991).

Contraindications for replantation include warm ischemic time of more than 10 hours; severe joint destruction or crush injury resulting in an immobile extremity; peripheral nerve injury that would limit return of sensation; and substantial soft tissue damage (Gayle et al., 1991). Replantation may be a surgical option for children who are skeletally immature. If epiphyseal plates are preserved and revascularized, normal bone growth can be expected (Gayle et al., 1991).

Physical therapy is indicated for these children for wound care, control of edema, joint range of motion (ROM), strengthening, ambulation, and self-care activities. Rehabilitation will include close communication with the physician and family instruction both while the child is in the hospital and as an outpatient.

Phantom Limb Sensations

Phantom limb sensations are an occurrence in many adults with amputations, but few reports are available concerning children with phantom limb sensations. Some persons may believe that if young children do not complain of phantom limb pain, they therefore must not have any pain. Phantom limb sensations are rarely reported before age 6 years (Jenson & Rasmussen, 1989; Setoguchi & Rosenfelder, 1982). Simmel (1962) reported that the incidence of phantom limb sensations increases with the age of the child so that all children older than 8 years of age reported some degree of phantom limb sensations. Mount (1989) expounds on accepted theories of pain in children and suggests that young children are more disturbed by visually painful experiences such as a cut finger or a venipuncture than by internal pain and have not yet learned the potential negative responses of internal sensations. Young children may also not be able to appropriately verbalize the sensations they may be experiencing.

The phantom limb sensations and pain of adolescents can become intense. If left untreated, phantom limb sensations can become debilitating and interfere with prosthetic wear and daily activities. Some teenagers are able to control the sensations through rubbing or massaging the uninvolved limb at similar points to those in which they are experiencing the phantom limb sensations of the amputated limb. Others feel more in control by keeping a daily log of their sensations and reporting the pain intensities on one of a variety of pain scales. For some adolescents the use of analgesics may be beneficial. If available, a referral to a pain management team should be instituted for children undergoing amputations.

PHYSICAL THERAPY INTERVENTION FOR THE CHILD WITH A LIMB DEFICIENCY OR AN ACQUIRED AMPUTATION

The parents are an integral part of the rehabilitation team for a child with an amputation or a limb deficiency. The rehabilitation team should also include an orthopedist, a prosthetist, and a physical therapist who are experienced in the management of children with amputations. This may often mean traveling to a major medical center for periodic assessments and prosthetic adjustments. Physical therapy can be delivered in the local community if available, but the therapist must be in communication with the managing rehabilitation team.

The overall goals of physical therapy are to facilitate as normal a sequence of development as possible for the child, prevent or minimize the development of impairments or functional limitations, and prevent disability. Impairments can include joint contractures and weakness with resultant functional limitations of limited mobility and a lack of independence in self-care skills. Physical therapy goals are directed toward preventing joint contractures, minimizing muscle strength imbalances, preventing skin breakdown, and developing independence with mobility and self-care skills. Ideally these goals are accomplished through physical therapy intervention for the child, child or parent instruction, and follow-up of a child's progress and functional outcomes. The child's age, type of limb deficiency or level of amputation, and other medical factors will all influence the intensity of physical therapy needed.

Functional outcomes can be assessed using current assessment tools. However, these assessment tools may not be able to determine the functional effectiveness of various prosthetic options. Currently, insurance companies and state-funded programs will opt for the prosthetic options that are less costly if outcomes are not present to justify the more expensive options. An outcome measure, the Child Amputee Prosthetics Project–Functional Status Inventory (CAPP-FSI), is currently being revised and validated. The CAPP-FSI is an outcome measure that includes a behavioral inventory to assess the functional status of children with upper or lower limb deficiencies (Pruitt et al., 1996).

Infancy and Toddler Period

An infant with a limb deficiency should be referred for an initial examination by a pediatric orthopedist and a physical therapist shortly after birth. Monitoring by the physical therapist with suggestions to parents regarding positioning and stretching may be all that is needed initially. The motor development of children with multiple limb deficiencies or upper extremity deficiencies may become delayed or impaired owing to their inability to use their arms for such activities as pushing up to sit, crawling, and pulling to stand. Physical therapy is necessary to monitor the infant's developmental progress, ROM, and strength needed for later prosthetic use and for the parents' comfort with their child's progress. This can be accomplished through periodic physical therapy examinations and evaluations, optimally at 1-month intervals, with updated parent instruction provided.

Generally, infants with limb deficiencies do not develop contractures after birth, but ROM should be carefully monitored according to individual needs.

The parents of a child with a PFFD may benefit from instruction to decrease the hip flexion and abduction contractures that are typically noted at birth and will later interfere with prosthetic fit. Most children with upper extremity limb deficiencies will maintain ROM and strength through their developmental activities.

Careful monitoring of the developing infant is necessary to evaluate ROM, functional strength, weight-bearing capabilities, and posture while prone, sitting, and standing. Often a child with a limb deficiency will tend to bear weight asymmetrically in prone and sitting activities. Some children will take increased weight on their limb-deficient side to free their noninvolved side for reaching and movement. Other children may take more weight through their noninvolved side because of weight-shifting and balance difficulties. Suggestions may be given to the parents and therapy provided to encourage weight-shifting activities to improve symmetry. For the child with an upper limb deficiency this will encourage the co-contraction of shoulder musculature needed later for prosthetic use. For the child with a lower limb deficiency this encourages assumption of an erect trunk with normal balance reactions. Shifting weight to the limb-deficient side is also important for preprosthetic training needed for standing and ambulation activities.

If an infant is not progressing developmentally, direct physical therapy intervention may be warranted to provide alternative methods of achieving the normal developmental sequence. For example, a child with bilateral upper extremity limb deficiencies may need assistance to learn to stand from sitting or to safely learn to balance in standing.

A child is usually fitted with a prosthesis at a developmentally appropriate age. A child with a lower extremity deficiency will therefore be fitted for a prosthesis when weight bearing is appropriate and the child is beginning to pull to stand (between 8 and 10 months of age depending on the child's developmental progress). A child with a unilateral PFFD may have a Syme or Boyd amputation and be fitted with a prosthesis after surgery (Herzenberg, 1991; Koman et al., 1982). A child with an upper extremity limb deficiency may be fitted with a prosthesis to assist with early playing skills in sitting or even earlier to assist with weight-bearing skills while prone. A child is best fitted with an upper extremity prosthesis between 6 and 8 months of age or when sitting can be done independently (Krebs et al., 1991; Setoguchi & Rosenfelder, 1982).

When a child first receives a prosthesis, the fit and alignment as well as the overall function of the prosthesis are assessed. The initial session is spent on instructing the parents in proper donning of the prosthesis, in checking the skin, and in developing a wearing schedule. The initial goal is to have the infant or toddler wear the prosthesis comfortably for as many hours a day as possible and for the parents to be comfortable in donning and removing the prosthesis. The prosthesis may be removed for naps and should be removed when the child sleeps at night.

A child with an upper extremity prosthesis may initially ignore it. The focus of therapy should be on having the child wear the prosthesis while playing and to begin to use it for bimanual play such as manipulating and holding large toys and during gross motor activities such as pushing up to sitting, protective reactions, and propping in sitting.

The child's first upper extremity prosthesis may have one of several terminal device options (Fig. 15-10). A young infant may have a passive hand that is cosmetically appealing but nonfunctional. As the child begins to engage in bimanual play, either a simple split hook (Hosmer Dorrance, Campbell, CA) or a Child Amputee Prosthetics Project (CAPP) (Hosmer Dorrance, Campbell, CA) terminal device is more functional. The split hook is similar to that used with adult prosthetics except smaller. The CAPP was designed specifically for children, is cosmetically more appealing than a hook terminal device, is safer than a hook for a young child, and provides an efficient grip without requiring great operating force (Gover & McIvor, 1992). The goal for the young child at this time is to adjust to the weight of a prosthesis, to begin to use it to manipulate larger toys, and to shake or remove toys placed in the terminal device by an adult (Setoguchi & Rosenfelder, 1982) (Fig. 15-11).

A child is not expected to begin to operate the terminal device until 18 months of age or later (Gover & McIvor, 1992; Patton, 1989; Setoguchi & Rosenfelder, 1982). An active terminal device and cable as needed should be added to the child's prosthesis by 18 months of age. Training to operate the terminal device is dependent on the child's developmental level. Children can be taught to release objects placed in their terminal device at 15 months of age (Patton, 1989). Generally, children are taught to open the terminal device, place objects in it, and then release them, in that order (Gover & McIvor, 1992; Setoguchi & Rosenfelder, 1982). This corresponds with the normal developmental sequence of learning to grasp before learning to release objects. The therapist must be familiar with the mechanism that controls the terminal device because it can differ from child to child, depending on the design of the device. The CAPP and Hosmer Dorrance hook are

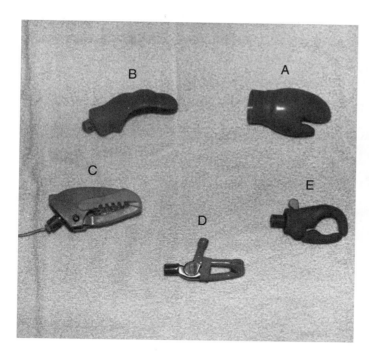

FIGURE 15–10. Terminal device options: *A*, Baby Mitt (Hosmer Dorrance, Campbell, CA). *B*, Sport Mitt (Therapeutic Recreation Systems, Boulder, CO). An infant size is suitable for crawling infants. *C*, Child Amputee Prosthetics Project (CAPP) (Hosmer Dorrance) voluntary-opening device. *D*, Hosmer Dorance 12P infant voluntary-opening hook. *E*, Anatomically Designed-Engineered Polymer Technology (ADEPT) (Therapeutic Recreation Systems) infant voluntary-closing hook.

voluntary-opening terminal devices; forward reaching of the arm pulls the cable tight and activates opening of the terminal device. Children with a transverse deficiency of the upper arm will need to use scapular abduction to activate opening of the terminal device with the elbow locked; control of the prosthetic elbow comes at a later age. The ADEPT (Therapeutic Recreation Systems, Boulder, CO) hook is a voluntary-closing terminal device designed to mimic forward reaching to grasp or close on an object (Fig. 15–12). Enhanced motor development has been reported with the early fitting of a voluntary-closing terminal device (DiCowden et al., 1987).

Children younger than 2 years of age with a lower limb deficiency or above-knee amputation are often fitted with a prosthesis without a knee (Fig. 15–13). The goal is to begin weight-bearing and ambulation activities and to progress to learning control of a prosthetic knee when they are closer to 3 years of age.

When fitting a toddler with a lower extremity prosthesis, normal stance and gait patterns for their developmental age should be kept in mind. Children 1 year of age stand and walk with a wide base of support and exhibit increased hip external rotation during swing phase (Sutherland, 1984). For this reason, a toddler's prosthesis may need to be aligned

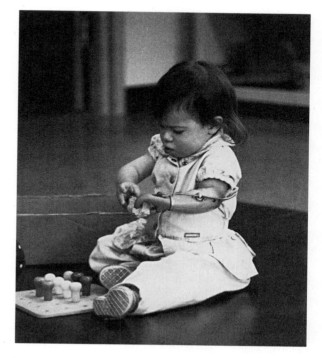

FIGURE 15–11. Child engaging in bimanual play wearing below-elbow prosthesis with an ADEPT voluntary-closing hook.

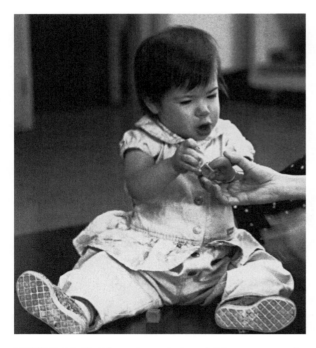

FIGURE 15–12. Therapist assisting child to operate the terminal device.

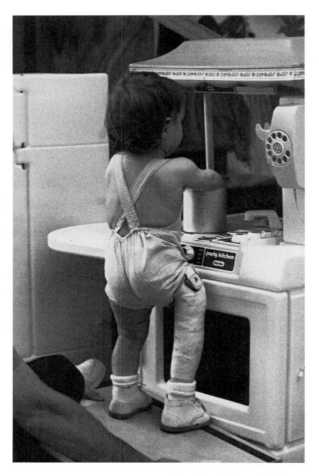

FIGURE 15–13. Fourteen-month-old child with lower extremity prosthesis without a knee component.

with more hip abduction than that provided to an older child.

Because a goal of physical therapy is symmetry of posture and movements during developmental activities, proper alignment and controlled weight-shifting and balance activities are emphasized for children with a lower limb prosthesis. Many children with lower limb prostheses do not require an assistive device for ambulation; however, initial gait training with an assistive device promotes a reciprocal gait pattern and an erect trunk. As the child develops balance and is able to control weight shifting, he or she will naturally discard the assistive device when he or she is comfortable with independent ambulation.

Preschool- and School-Age Period

When a child attends a preschool or kindergarten class for the first time, many anxieties may resurface for the parents of a child with a limb deficiency. Parents will worry that their child may not fit in or will look different from his or her peers. This is also an age by which typical children have achieved independence with activities of daily living skills such as eating and dressing and their social relationships with peers increase. The preschool years should emphasize development of independence in self-care skills, mobility, and acquisition of school skills such as coloring, cutting, and writing. If these skills are achieved during the preschool years, the child will enter school with minimal or no functional limitations or disabilities.

The child with an upper limb deficiency should be able to activate the terminal device of the prosthesis by this age. Children using an above-elbow prosthesis can begin learning to control the elbow by 3 or 4 years of age. Most above-elbow prostheses have a dual cable system that allows the child to control both elbow flexion and extension and forearm pronation and supination. With control of the elbow and forearm the terminal device of the prosthesis becomes more functional in a variety of positions.

Emphasis should always be on assisting the child to learn skills that are appropriate for his or her age. Play skills involving manipulation of smaller objects, using the prosthesis to hold and turn paper for coloring and cutting activities, holding the handlebars of a tricycle, and self-dressing and feeding skills are important. A child with a unilateral upper limb prosthesis will always use it as a helper hand and not as the dominant hand.

For those children with bilateral upper limb deficiencies the use of a prosthesis should be carefully monitored. These children should always be allowed to use their feet or mouth for play and self-care activities. A prosthesis may aid these children for only some periods of the day and may actually limit their function during some activities.

Myoelectric prostheses are an option that should be discussed with the parents of a preschool-age child with an upper limb deficiency. These prostheses are not body-powered but are controlled by surface electrodes in the prosthetic socket that receive electrical signals from residual limb muscles to activate a motor-driven hand (Singer & Lombardo, 1992). The use of a myoelectric prosthesis is most successful when fitting occurs between 3 and 5 or 6 years of age (Gover & McIvor, 1992). Advantages of a myoelectric prosthesis are improved cosmesis and functional use of the hand with minimal physical effort. Disadvantages include weight of the prosthesis, cost, electric components that require repair, and lack of durability (Gover & McIvor, 1992). If a child is fitted with a myoelectric prosthesis, therapy is necessary to learn to control the hand and use the prosthesis functionally.

Children with a lower limb deficiency, including those children with ulilateral PFFD, should be functional ambulators at this age. A child with a below-knee limb deficiency should be wearing a prosthesis for most of the day and engaging in normal activities with peers. The child with an above-knee limb deficiency should be ready to begin ambulation with a prosthesis with a knee joint by around age 3 years. Initially, children are usually given a constant-friction knee joint. They may need a short period of physical therapy to learn control of the knee joint and weight-shifting activities without falling.

During the preschool years some surgery is usually necessary for the child with a unilateral PFFD. Arthrodesis of the knee joint, usually performed between 2.5 and 4 years of age, increases the lever arm of the thigh and decreases the hip and knee flexion contractures (Gillespie, 1990; Koman et al., 1982). Femoral or tibial epiphysiodesis may be performed at the time of knee arthrodesis. The ultimate goal is for limb length on the prosthetic side to be 5 cm shorter than that of the contralateral femur. This enables the prosthetic knee joint to be at approximately the same level as the contralateral knee joint at maturity (Epps, 1983). Placement of the prosthetic knee joint at the same level as the contralateral knee joint allows for improved cosmesis and improved gait.

For the child with an acquired lower extremity amputation an immediate-fit prosthesis is usually used. This may not be the case if significant trauma was present to the surrounding tissue or if skin grafting was necessary after the injury. The physical therapy examination and evaluation focuses on sensitivity of the residual limb, active movement, strength, bed mobility, transfers for toileting and getting out of bed, and ambulation. The goals of postoperative physical therapy are similar to those developed for an adult with an amputation.

Children are more likely to move about after an amputation than an adult, so contractures are less likely to occur. However, some children undergoing chemotherapy are extremely ill and weak and may tend to lie in bed with their residual limb propped on pillows. They must be monitored for developing contractures, and parents and nursing staff must be instructed in ROM exercises and positioning of the residual limb.

Gait training should begin as soon as cleared by the physician. Young children can safely learn to ambulate with an immediate-fit prosthesis using a walker or crutches. If a child has been hospitalized for a period of time, strengthening exercises of the uninvolved leg and the residual limb may be necessary.

After the removal of the immediate-fit prosthesis the child is fitted with a permanent prosthesis. The exception to this would be a child who is undergoing chemotherapy. These children tend to have weight fluctuations secondary to side effects of the medications. They are better fitted with a socket that allows for weight fluctuations, such as one with Velcro closures. Children with above-knee amputations should be fitted with a prosthesis with a knee joint. Most children with an above-knee amputation will initially require a pelvic strap to help hold the prosthesis in place. Some children may do well with a suction socket and no straps. Instruction must be given to both the parents and the child in donning and removing the prosthesis, care of the prosthesis, skin checks, and wear schedule.

The child who undergoes a rotationplasty is usually casted to allow for healing of the bone. The cast may incorporate a pylon to permit the shortened leg to contact the ground for safe ambulation using a walker or crutches. After the cast is removed and the bone is healed the child with a rotationplasty must work on increasing ROM at the ankle joint, which functions as the child's knee. For ambulation and sitting, 0 to 20° of ankle dorsiflexion is more than adequate. Some children will be able to achieve 30° of ankle dorsiflexion, which will allow for some squatting activities and facilitate bike riding. Maximal plantar flexion will allow for greater extension of the leg in stance. Optimal plantar flexion ROM is at least 45 to 50°; the prosthetist can align the prosthesis to achieve an additional few degrees of plantar flexion for stance. Exercises should begin gently and progress to active and resistive exercises.

The child who undergoes a rotationplasty is fitted with a custom-made prosthesis that incorporates the foot in a position of maximum plantar flexion and allows it to act as a knee joint. An external knee hinge joint must be used with an attached thigh cuff. The prosthesis is usually held in place with a pelvic strap.

A child who has had a limb-sparing procedure will also require physical therapy after surgery. Lower extremity procedures usually require a period of non–weight bearing. Rehabilitation for children with a limb-sparing procedure to either the upper or lower extremity includes exercise through active movement with a progression to strengthening exercises. The progression of the intervention is dictated by the procedure that was performed, the surgeon's protocols, and the amount of bone replaced. Children who have had a limb-sparing procedure involving the femur will also frequently require physical therapy after a lengthening procedure of the endoprosthetic implant. Range of motion of the knee often becomes restricted, similar to that seen with children who undergo limb-lengthening techniques (see Chapter 16).

Gait training for all children at this age will focus on symmetry and the normal characteristics of gait, such as stride length, step length, and velocity, and all skills that the child needs to participate in play and games with other children. When initially learning to ambulate or after a surgical procedure, most children will use an assistive device. As balance and ambulation speed improve and postsurgical limitations are lifted, many children will begin to discard the assistive device. The assistive device should only be discarded, however, if the child's ambulation is safe and speed is functional to keep pace with the child's peers.

During the school-age years the physical therapist should instruct the child in running techniques so that the child may participate in play and games with her or his peers. This is the age range at which the child may also show an interest in participating in various amputee sports or recreational programs.

When attending school for the first time, the child will be questioned about the prosthesis and assistive devices. This is especially true of a child with an upper limb deficiency. A meeting before the beginning of school with the child and his or her parents, the child's teacher, and perhaps the child's physical therapist may be helpful to allay any concerns and to answer or develop a way to answer the questions of the child's peers. The child with a unilateral limb deficiency or amputation should succeed in school with minimal adaptations.

The child with bilateral upper limb deficiencies may need to use a tape recorder or computer to assist with writing skills. In school, a child with bilateral upper limb deficiencies may be able to carry papers or books in the classroom between the chin and shoulder. The child also may use the mouth for manipulation and holding objects such as pencils. Whether the child uses his or her feet in school for manipulation or grasping is something that should be clearly discussed with the child, parents, and teacher before school entrance. Many children opt not to use their feet for grasping objects in public as they get older; however, this can limit their independence, especially with toileting and feeding. If a child is adept with the use of his or her feet and is independent and chooses to use the feet, this should not be discouraged. If the teacher displays a supportive attitude toward the child's use of the feet, the child's classroom peers will soon view this as usual procedure in their classroom. The ultimate outcome is for the child to be functional in our society as an adult; this may mean use of the feet or a combination of use of the feet and prostheses.

Adolescence and Transition to Adulthood

Adolescence, with its hallmark concerns of appearance and acceptance by peers, relationships with the opposite sex, career decisions, and the struggle for independence, can be a trying time for anyone. Disability and societal limitations may become apparent during adolescence. The majority of teenagers with a congenital limb deficiency have been adjusting both functionally and emotionally from birth. At this point in their lives they are part of a social network of friends, realize the support of their families, and have attempted and succeeded at various activities in school and the community. They will be dealing with these adolescent issues right alongside their peers, although increased fears concerning dating and social acceptance can be typical at this time and participation in school athletic activities may be limited. A higher percentage of children and adolescents with congenital limb deficiencies exhibit greater behavioral and emotional problems and lower social competence than their peers without a disability (Varni & Setoguchi, 1992).

An amputation of a limb during the adolescent years adds quite an emotional burden to a teenager, who must deal with the loss of a body part and the grieving process and may be facing the possibility of death. Added to the physical appearance difficulties are the possible side effects such as hair loss from chemotherapy. A teenager who is facing a possible amputation as the result of cancer should be included, if he or she desires, in discussions of treatment options, including surgical options. Obviously, this is not possible if the amputation is the result of sudden trauma.

Health care professionals have reasoned that limb-sparing procedures offer cosmetic advantages and an increased quality of life compared with an amputation. Prevailing thought also assumed that limb-sparing surgery offers a more functional outcome than an amputation. However, studies have shown that no significant difference exists in quality of life between adolescents and young adults with amputations compared with those who underwent a limb-sparing procedure (Postma et al., 1992; Weddington et al., 1985). The studies do report that adolescents with an amputation exhibit a lower self-esteem and those who underwent a limb-sparing procedure exhibit more physical complaints.

The immediate postoperative concerns and physical therapy intervention for adolescents undergoing an amputation or a limb-sparing procedure are similar to those described for school-age children. If an immediate-fit prosthesis is not used, teenagers are more likely to develop edema of their residual limb following surgery. In that case, wrapping of the residual limb or fitting with a shrinker sock should be instituted.

Teenagers who sustain a lower extremity amputation are fitted with a prosthesis when the residual limb has stabilized. They should be involved in the fitting of the prosthesis and in deciding on the design of the socket and type of knee joint and foot to be used. For most teenagers a large variety of prosthetic options are available. These should be fully discussed with the teenager and parents, and the choice should complement the lifestyle of the user. Both the teenager and his or her family should be cautioned that the prosthesis will not function or look exactly like the contralateral limb.

Many teenagers with a high above-knee amputation will attempt to ambulate with a prosthesis but will ultimately opt for no prosthesis and crutches. A gait with crutches is faster and more energy efficient. The decision to use or not to use a prosthesis should be the child's and not be based on society's idea of the most appropriate physical appearance. Some teenagers use a prosthesis for certain activities and not for others. The ultimate outcome is for them to be comfortable with their peers and interact with their peers in school and socially.

The use of prosthetics varies for teenagers with upper limb deficiencies. For those who have become adept with a prosthesis since early childhood, they probably will continue to use their prosthesis. The teenager who has an upper limb amputation may learn to operate a body-powered above- or below-elbow prosthesis. To become functional with the prosthesis requires much practice, and the teenager may opt not to use one.

One major milestone for teenagers is the acquisition of a driver's license. Nearly all teenagers with a limb deficiency or amputation can learn to drive. Hand controls can be used for the teenager with bilateral PFFD or with bilateral lower extremity amputation as the result of trauma. For the teenager with a unilateral upper limb deficiency or amputation, minimal adjustments will be necessary. Driving can be done by using the sound hand, or a driving ring can be attached to the steering wheel. The prosthetic terminal device, preferably a hook, slips into the ring to assist wth controlling the steering wheel and easily slips out of the ring in emergencies. Driving becomes more difficult for the teenager with bilateral upper limb deficiencies or amputations. A driving ring may be used by the dominant limb. Controls such as light switches or turn signals may need to be moved to the dominant side and within reach of the limb or can be operated by the driver's knee. Unless specifically trained in the area of driver education, physical therapists should assist the teenager and his or her parents to seek information and driver training from a local rehabilitation center.

Career and college decisions are also made during adolescence. Some teenagers may work at a part-time job during high school. All teenagers with limb deficiencies or amputations eventually seek employment. At times, adjustments must be made to a prosthesis, such as a specific terminal device, to assist the young adult in his or her particular career area. Going to college is a true test of independence with self-care skills. Some individuals with bilateral upper limb deficiencies or multiple limb deficiencies will always require some degree of assistance with self-care activities. Toileting, especially wiping after defecation, and dressing, specifically managing underpants and bras, are self-care activities for which it is difficult for anyone with bilateral upper limb deficiencies or short above-elbow amputations to achieve total independence. This does not preclude attending college or independent living, but an aide or other arrangements may be needed. Creativity, experimentation, and talking with other teenagers or adults with limb deficiencies can often produce strategies for accomplishing difficult tasks. High employment rates, active lifestyles, and marriage are reported for adults who underwent an amputation as a child or adolescent (Tebbi, 1993).

OVERVIEW OF PROSTHETICS

Upper Extremity Prosthetics

Upper extremity prosthetic components include a terminal device, a wrist unit, possibly an elbow unit, a socket, and possibly a harness and cable system. Terminal devices range from the passive baby mitten to a myoelectric hand. Terminal devices often used in pediatrics include the baby mitt, cosmetic hand, CAPP, and various hooks, including the Dorrance and ADEPT models (see Fig. 15–10). The child's age and size, as well as the parents' and child's desires and functional goals, determine the appropriate terminal device. The wrist unit allows forearm pronation and supination and accommodates the terminal device.

As a child's activities change, different terminal devices may be needed. Various recreational terminal devices are available to allow participation in a variety of sports activities (Krebs et al., 1991; Michael et al., 1990). Teenagers may desire a cosmetic hand for social activities and a functional terminal device for daily activities.

Most upper limb prostheses are suspended with a harness system. Two basic systems are used: the chest strap and the figure-eight. The chest strap or harness fits over the shoulder of the involved limb and around the chest to secure the prosthesis without limiting movement of the shoulders. The figure-eight harness securely anchors the prosthesis so that the child may activate the cable system of an above-elbow prosthesis (Setoguchi & Rosenfelder, 1982). Suction sockets are available for young children. A simple suction socket may be all that is necessary to suspend a below-elbow prosthesis of an infant or toddler. When the cable for the terminal device is added to the prosthesis, an above-elbow pad or cuff to secure the cable can be incorporated. A shoulder disarticulation prosthesis is secured with a chest strap and often with a thigh strap for the young child. A thigh strap can provide added power to operate the control system of a shoulder disarticulation prosthesis and may provide more excursion than the chest strap (Setoguchi & Rosenfelder, 1982).

Lower Extremity Prosthetics

Until recently few options for the foot were available in pediatric lower extremity prosthetics. The SACH (Otto Bock Orthopedic, Plymouth, MN) foot has long been the mainstay for pediatric prosthetic

feet and continues to be used for young toddlers. The new designs in adult energy-storing prosthetic feet are now making their way into pediatric prosthetics. Pediatric sizes are available in the Seattle Lightfoot (Model and Instrument Development, Seattle, WA), SpringLite (SpringLite, Salt Lake City, UT), and Flex-Foot (Flex-Foot Inc., Laguna Hills, CA). Many school-age children and adolescents may also be fitted with a STored ENergy (STEN) (Kinsley Manufacturing, Costa Mesa, CA) prosthetic foot or a College Park Foot/Ankle System (College Park, Fraser, MI) (Fig. 15–14).

The shank of a lower extremity prosthesis is either an exoskeletal or an endoskeletal design. Exoskeletal shanks are fabricated of wood covered with hard plastic, and endoskeletal shanks consist of a pylon made of ultralight material, such as graphite or titanium, and covered with foam. Teenagers prefer en-

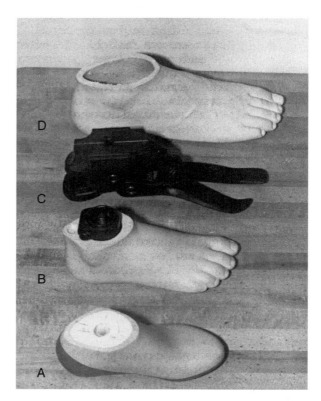

FIGURE 15–14. Prosthetic feet options. *A,* Solid-ankle cushion heel (SACH) assembly (Kinsley Manufacturing Co., Costa Mesa, CA; Otto Bock Orthopedic Industries, Inc., Minneapolis, MN). *B,* Seattle LightFoot Child's Play (Model and Instrument Development, Seattle, WA). *C,* College Park Foot/Ankle System (College Park Industries, Fraser, MI), which allows increased inversion/eversion mobility through graded ankle bushings. *D,* Cosmetic cover for College Park Foot/Ankle System.

doskeletal shanks because of their cosmesis and decreased weight. The durability of exoskeletal shanks is often more appropriate for the younger child.

Knee unit availability is often limited by the child's size. Most prostheses for children utilize a constant-friction knee. A constant-friction knee is set to function at a certain walking speed. If the speed of walking increases, the prosthesis lags behind because the shank cannot swing through as quickly as the uninvolved limb. Another type of knee joint available for the pediatric population is a polycentric knee with a four-bar linkage mechanism (Fig. 15–15). A polycentric knee mimics the anatomic knee joint to increase stability. The axis of motion is posterior during stance to provide added stability and anterior during swing to shorten the shank and assist with clearance. This added stability in addition to the light weight of both the constant-friction knee and the four-bar linkage mechanism make them favored knee joints for the preschool- and school-age child with an amputation.

A larger variety of knee units are available for teenagers, including hydraulic and pneumatic knees.

Hydraulic and pneumatic knee units are variable-friction units that allow variable walking and running speeds. Variable-friction units are equipped with a swing control mechanism that sets the drag of the shank through swing phase and a stance control unit that permits knee flexion during stance without collapse of the leg. Swing and stance control mechanisms are excellent options for active teenagers, especially those engaged in physical activities. Drawbacks of hydraulic and pneumatic knees are the added weight to the prosthesis, cost, and intricacy of adjustments.

Like adult sockets, pediatric socket design has changed in recent years. Movement is away from the bony weight bearing of patellar tendon–bearing below-knee sockets and quadrilateral above-knee sockets toward more evenly distributed pressures (Michael et al., 1990). Children of all ages can be fitted with a narrowed medial-lateral ischial containment socket (Fig. 15–16). For children with an above-knee amputation, the narrowed medial-lateral socket with ischial containment more evenly distributes weight-bearing pressures and allows less lateral movement of the distal femur, thereby providing more stability during stance. Some children, however, prefer a quadrilateral socket, and some teenagers with a large fatty residual limb are more comfortable in a quadrilateral socket (Fig. 15–17).

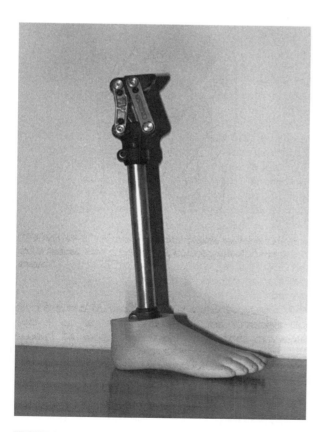

FIGURE 15–15. Prosthetic knee component with four-bar linkage mechanism.

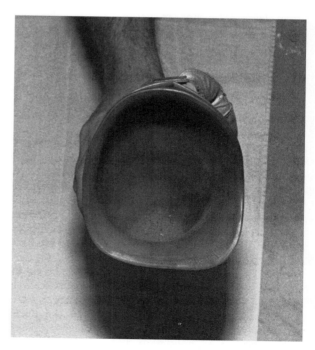

FIGURE 15–16. Narrowed medial-lateral ischial containment socket.

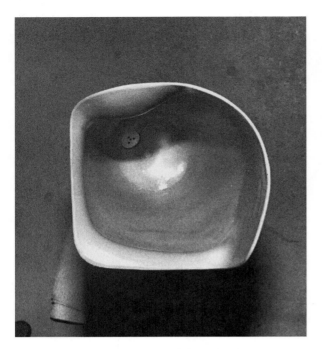

FIGURE 15–17. Quadrilateral socket.

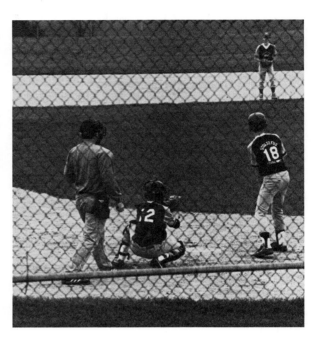

FIGURE 15–18. Catcher is an adolescent with a left below-knee amputation.

Because teenagers and children are generally very active, a well-fitting above-knee or below-knee socket is essential. During prosthetic fitting and socket design a clear plastic check socket may be used to easily identify areas of pressure and allow modification before the final socket is fabricated. Colloidal suspensions such as dental alginate can be added to a socket to fill any empty spaces during weight bearing to further distribute pressures within the prosthesis (Michael et al., 1990).

Infants and toddlers will require some type of suspension in addition to a suction socket. A Silesian belt works well for younger children with an above-knee amputation or PFFD; preschoolers can become independent in its use. By school age most children will not require this additional suspension. For active children and those participating in athletics, neoprene sleeves or the newer roll-on silicone sheaths provide excellent suspension of the prosthesis for children and adolescents with a below-knee or an above-knee amputation.

Children with a rotationplasty use a prosthesis that incorporates the plantar-flexed foot in the socket. The socket is essentially a below-knee socket with a thigh cuff attachment and external hinges for the knee joint. A Silesian belt may be needed for suspension.

Children of all ages with a limb deficiency or amputation should be encouraged to participate in activities with their peers. Many children may want to participate in sports at either a recreational or a competitive level (Fig. 15–18). There are many prosthetic options available that promote participation in various sports. Recreational prosthetics options are too numerous to mention for this discussion, and the reader is referred to other resources. Kegel (1986, 1992) discusses sports options in detail. Information is also available on various upper extremity terminal devices for recreational and sports activities (Michael et al., 1990; Radocy, 1992). Kegel (1992) includes a comprehensive resource list outlining sporting associations, camps for persons with amputations, and suppliers of specialized equipment and devices.

Ultimately, any prosthesis for a child must have some cosmetic appeal and be more functional than the limb without a prosthesis (Fig. 15–19). Decision making for infants' and toddlers' prosthetic needs should include the parents, orthopedist, prosthetist, and physical therapist. The older child should be included in the decision-making process.

Appropriate prosthetic components are costly, and a full prosthesis must be replaced at least every 12 to 18 months for growing children and adolescents. If an adolescent chooses to participate in sports or swimming activities, an additional prosthesis or components may be required. Third-party payers are reluctant to pay for multiple prostheses or myoelectric devices. Currently, some health maintenance organizations will pay for only one prosthesis in a lifetime.

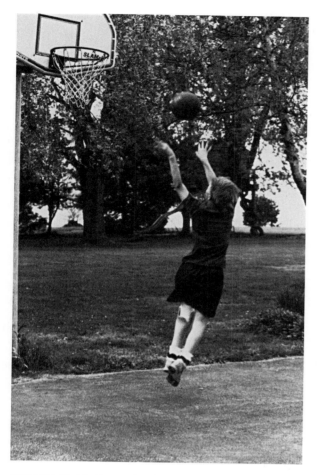

FIGURE 15–19. Recreational and social activities should not be limitations or obstacles for children with limb deficiencies or amputations.

Studies are beginning to examine the cost-effectiveness of surgical procedures and various prosthetic options. Grimer (1997) compared long-term costs of limb-sparing procedures to amputation with a prosthesis. Limb-sparing procedures are more costly initially, but amputations for children or adolescents are very costly over time because of the need for multiple and sophisticated prostheses. The development of a functional outcome measure, the CAPP-FSI, may assist the rehabilitation team and families in justifying specific prosthetic components or the more expensive myoelectric prostheses.

SUMMARY

The etiology and classification of congenital limb deficiencies and the causes of acquired amputations were reviewed in this chapter. An overview of the medical and surgical management of congenital limb deficiencies and amputations was presented. Treatment of a child with a congenital limb deficiency or amputation is complex and must involve a team of professionals who recognize the impact of various treatment options on the child's function in both the home and school environment and ultimately as an independent adult. Treatment options that involve careful planning and discussion with the family include surgical options, the use of chemotherapy and radiation therapy for children with malignant tumors, and prosthetic options. Each child must be assessed as an individual, with consideration given to the child's age and musculoskeletal development, immediate and long-term functional abilities, family and child's activity level and lifestyle choices, and prosthetic and physical therapy intervention needed to meet the child's goals.

The recent proliferation of prosthetic designs and materials available to the pediatric population has opened up many options for recreation and sports, vocation, and self-care, as well as early fitting of infants and toddlers with prostheses. Research is needed in the pediatric population to determine which surgical options, prosthetic designs, terminal devices, and materials best improve function, increase comfort, or decrease energy consumption. Physical therapists can easily contribute their expertise to the literature, as well as initiate clinical research to investigate the effectiveness of various treatment options and prosthetic designs.

CASE HISTORY
SCOTT

Scott is a 7-year-old boy with a congenital right PFFD, Aitken type B. Aitken type B classification signifies presence of an acetabulum and femoral head, although the acetabulum may be dysplastic; ossification of the capital femoral epiphysis is delayed; the proximal portion of the femur is displaced laterally and upward; the femoral neck contains defective cartilage that fails to ossify; and the shaft of the femur is short and deformed (Tachdjian, 1990a). A radiologic assessment shortly after birth revealed an absence of the right distal femoral epiphysis, absence of right proximal tibial and fibular epiphyses, and a fibrous connection between the femoral head and proximal femur. A Boyd amputation of the right foot was performed at 8 months to allow for fitting of a lower extremity prosthesis and weight bearing. By 18 months Scott was walking independently with a prosthesis without a knee joint. He was followed every 3 to 4 months in an amputee clinic and seen by an orthopedist, a prosthetist, and a physical therapist, but he did not receive intensive physical therapy except for a short period after receiving his first prosthesis.

A knee fusion was performed at 3 years of age to improve the lever arm length needed for an efficient gait. A metaphyseal-epiphyseal synostosis with bone grafting was also performed at that time to achieve stability in the region of the proximal femur. After cast removal, Scott was fitted with a new prosthesis with a knee joint, and regular physical therapy sessions for 6 weeks were begun. Both Scott and his parents expressed the goal of a return to independent ambulation with his new prosthesis. Scott also wanted to learn to run fast. Therapy focused on strengthening of right lower extremity musculature, especially hip abduction motions, and decreasing the hip flexion contracture, along with gait training with a prosthetic knee.

At the end of 6 weeks of therapy, Scott was ambulating independently without an assistive device, was able to kick a ball with his noninvolved leg, and was able to run. Scott's running was equal to the speed of his 4-year-old sibling, but asymmetric step lengths necessitated a hop-run pattern. He was pleased with his running speed, and his mother was happy that he was not falling.

Scott presently attends the first grade in his local school. He wears his prosthesis throughout the day. He continues to ambulate independently, runs and climbs with his peers at recess, and is learning to ride a bicycle. He has been independent with donning and removing the prosthesis for several years. Before the start of his first year in school, Scott, his mother, and his physical therapist met with his teacher to discuss Scott's PFFD, use of a prosthesis, and his ability levels. Scott readily answers any questions his peers may ask about his prosthesis. At this time Scott requires no extra help in class or at school.

Scott will probably need to undergo a left distal femoral epiphysiodesis and right proximal tibial epiphysiodesis at age 9 or 10 years to ensure equal knee joint lengths at maturity. He continues to be followed at 6-month intervals in an amputee clinic by an orthopedist, a prosthetist, and a physical therapist.

CASE HISTORY
ANDREW

Andrew is a 6-year-old boy who was diagnosed with Ewing's sarcoma of the right distal femur at 3 years of age. He had no metastases at the time of diagnosis. Andrew underwent a course of preoperative chemotherapy to destroy any micrometastatic disease. Surgical options were discussed with the family, including amputation and rotationplasty. At his young age an amputation would result in a very short above-knee residual limb. Limb-sparing procedures were not possible because of his young age and significant skeletal immaturity. For these reasons, radiation therapy was not used for local tumor control. A rotationplasty was chosen because it afforded a longer residual limb with more function than an above-knee amputation.

Postoperatively, Andrew was placed in a hip spica cast with his right ankle incorporated in approximately 45° of plantar flexion. A pylon was attached to the cast on the right. He received twice-daily physical therapy while an inpatient with the goals of ambulation with a walker and maintenance of upper body strength. He continued on chemotherapy postoperatively. Andrew was discharged home able to walk with a walker in the hip spica cast; the pylon attachment allowed for earlier and safer postoperative ambulation.

After cast removal Andrew received twice-weekly physical therapy to improve ROM and strength of his right ankle joint. His mother was instructed in a home program of ROM and strengthening exercises. A right ankle plantar flexion contracture was present after cast removal, but dorsiflexion to the neutral position was achieved within 1 week. Two weeks after cast removal right ankle motion was as follows: dorsiflexion 0 to 30° and plantar flexion 0 to 50°. Andrew could actively move his foot through available ranges, and resistive exercises were added. Cosmetically, Andrew exhibited no problems looking at or manipulating his foot. Both of his parents had met and spoken with a child who had had a rotationplasty before Andrew's surgery. His mother often expressed the feeling that dealing with the appearance of a "backward foot" was nothing compared with dealing with Andrew's cancer and unknown fate.

Following cast removal Andrew had been fitted with a prosthesis with external knee hinges, a thigh cuff, and a Silesian belt. Family goals related to physical therapy were for Andrew to walk independently and engage in play activities with his older siblings. Andrew's parents were instructed in donning the prosthesis, increasing wearing time, skin checks, and gait training for Andrew using a walker. The parents were able to incorporate wearing of the prosthesis into Andrew's daily routine and readily encouraged ambulation for functional activities within their home. Andrew discarded the walker on his own for independent ambulation.

Presently, Andrew attends fourth grade in his neighborhood school. He runs, climbs on playground equipment, and rides a skateboard. Andrew is monitored for recurrence of his cancer and is followed in an amputee clinic at 6-month intervals. During the summer he goes to the community pool with his family and swims without the prosthesis. He has also participated in Little League within his community. He performs well academically in school and is becoming skilled on the computer. So far Andrew's mother states that he has not expressed any anger at the cosmesis of his leg. She has noticed stares from persons at the pool, but they quickly accept Andrew once they are aware of his medical history.

CASE HISTORY
JENNIFER

Jennifer is a 17-year-old girl who underwent a left above-knee amputation at age 14 secondary to osteosarcoma of the left distal femur. Limb-sparing procedures could not be done because the tumor encompassed both vascular and nerve supplies. Her residual limb after the amputation is very short. Before the amputation, Jennifer was a ninth-grade student who actively participated on community and school sports teams. She is described by her parents as very outgoing with lots of friends. From the onset, Jennifer's goal was to play varsity-level high school sports.

Jennifer was fitted with an immediate-fit prosthesis in the operating room, but this had to be removed after several days when she developed open sores on her residual limb secondary to an allergic reaction. She was instructed in gait training with crutches, residual limb ROM, and wrapping to control edema and was discharged. She returned weekly to the hospital for chemotherapy and was monitored by a physical therapist at these visits. She was fitted with a temporary prosthesis with an expandable socket with Velcro closures after her wounds healed. Jennifer was very excited about receiving a prosthesis so she could run and play sports again.

Physical therapy sessions were begun three times a week when Jennifer received her prosthesis. Wearing time, skin checks, donning and removing the prosthesis, and gait training were reviewed with her and her parents. Jennifer gradually increased her prosthesis wearing time, wore it to school, and carried out her exercises. She quickly became very disenchanted with the prosthesis because she could not run and play sports as she could previously. (Note: The physical therapist should have assisted Jennifer early on with modifications of her goals. Jennifer could participate in competitive sports but not in the immediate time frame that she was seeking nor most likely against her able-bodied peers. Information about amputee sports programs should have been introduced to Jennifer early in her rehabilitation.)

She continued to go out socially with her friends. Gradually, Jennifer became less and less active, gained weight, and wore her prosthesis less and less. She eventually chose not to wear her prosthesis and opted for ambulation with forearm crutches. She continues to attend high school, occasionally watches her friends participate in sports, and is now working at a part-time job. Her parents sought counseling to assist Jennifer emotionally. They also enrolled her in a summer sports camp and a ski weekend for adolescents with amputations. She enjoyed those opportunities but did not use her prosthesis to participate in the activities.

In the past year, Jennifer has begun looking into getting her driver's license and has applied to work at a camp for children with amputations as a counselor. In conversations, she states that she might like to get a new prosthesis, but at this time she appears content and functional without a prosthesis. Whether Jennifer goes on to further schooling, her career choice, and her use of a prosthesis are all decisions she has to make. She has a supportive family and network of friends to help her with these decisions.

Recommended Resources

Amputee Coalition of America
6300 River Road, Suite 27
Rosemont, IL 60018-4226
Phone: 708-698-1633

Association of Children's Prosthetic-Orthotic Clinics (ACPOC)
P.O. Box 94020
Department 851-0950W
Palatine, IL 60094-4020

United Amputee Services Association, Inc.
P.O. Box 4277
Winter Park, FL 32793-4277
Phone: 407-678-2920

Recommended Reading

Bowker, JH, & Michael, JW (Eds.). Atlas of Limb Prosthetics: Surgical, Prosthetic, and Rehabilitation Principles. Part V: The child amputee, 2nd ed. St. Louis: Mosby, 1992, pp. 729–907.

Challenor, Y. Limb deficiencies in children. In Molnar, GE (Ed.), Pediatric Rehabilitation, 2nd ed. Baltimore: Williams & Wilkins, 1992, pp. 400–424.

Gover, AM, & McIvor, J. Upper limb deficiencies in infants and young children. Infants and Young Children, 5:58–72, 1992.

Jain, S. Rehabilitation in limb deficiency. 2. The pediatric amputee. Archives of Physical Medicine and Rehabilitation, 77(3 suppl): S9–S13, Review.

Krebs, DE, Edelstein, JE, & Thornby, MA. Prosthetic management of children with limb deficiencies. Physical Therapy, 71:920–934, 1991.

Setoguchi, Y, & Rosenfelder, R (Eds.). The Limb Deficient Child. Springfield, IL: Charles C. Thomas, 1982.

References

Aitken, GT. Surgical amputation in children. Journal of Bone and Joint Surgery (American), 45:1735–1741, 1963.

Aitken, GT. Proximal femoral focal deficiency: Definition, classification, and management. In Proximal Femoral Focal Deficiency: A Congenital Anomaly. Washington, DC: National Academy of Sciences, 1969.

Brent, RL. Prevention of physical and mental congenital defects: The scope of the problem. In Marios, M (Ed.), Progress in Clinical and Biological Research, Vol. 163A. New York: Alan R Liss, 1985, pp. 55–68.

Butler, MS, Robertson, WW, Rate, W, D'Angio, GJ, & Drummond, DS. Skeletal sequelae of radiation therapy for malignant tumors. Clinical Orthopedics and Related Research, 251:235–239, 1990.

Challenor, Y. Limb deficiencies in children. In Molnar, GE (Ed.), Pediatric Rehabilitation, 2nd ed. Baltimore: Williams & Wilkins, 1992, pp. 400–424.

Day, HJB. The ISO/ISPO classification of congenital limb deficiency. Prosthetics and Orthotics International, 15:67–69, 1991.

DiCowden, M, Ballard, A, Robinette, H, & Ortiz, O. Benefit of early fitting and behavior modification training with a voluntary closing terminal device. Journal of the Association of Children's Prosthetic Orthotic Clinics, 22:47–50, 1987.

Eckhardt, JJ, Eilber, FR, Grant, TT, Mirra, JM, Weisenberger, TH, & Dorey, FJ. Management of stage IIB osteogenic sarcoma: Experience at the University of California, Los Angeles. Cancer Treatment Symposia, 3:117–129, 1985.

Eldridge, JC, Armstrong, PF, & Krajbich, JI. Amputation stump lengthening with the Ilizarov technique. Clinical Orthopedics and Related Research, 256:76–79, 1990.

Epps, CH. Proximal femoral focal deficiency. Journal of Bone and Joint Surgery (American), 65:867–870, 1983.

Finn, HA, & Simon, MA. Limb-salvage surgery in the treatment of osteosarcoma in skeletally immature individuals. Clinical Orthopedics and Related Research, 262:108–118, 1991.

Frantz, CH, & O'Rahilly, R. Congenital skeletal limb deficiencies. Journal of Bone and Joint Surgery (American), 43:1202–1204, 1961.

Gayle, LB, Lineaweaver, WC, Buncke, GM, Oliva, A, Alpert, BS, Billys, JB, & Buncke, HJ. Lower extremity replantation. Clinics in Plastic Surgery, 18:437–447, 1991.

Gillespie, R. Principles of amputation surgery in children with longitudinal deficiencies of the femur. Clinical Orthopedics and Related Research, 256:29–38, 1990.

Glasser, DB, Duane, K, Lane, JM, Healey, JH, & Caparros-Simon, B. The effect of chemotherapy on growth in the skeletally immature individual. Clinical Orthopedics and Related Research, 262:93–100, 1991.

Goldwein, JW. Effects of radiation therapy on skeletal growth in childhood. Clinical Orthopedics and Related Research, 262:101–107, 1991.

Gover, AM, & McIvor, J. Upper limb deficiencies in infants and young children. Infants and Young Children, 5:58–72, 1992.

Grimer, RJ, Carter, SR, & Pynsent, PB. Cost-effectiveness of limb salvage for bone tumors. Journal of Bone and Joint Surgery (British), 79:558–561, 1997.

Gurney, J, Severson, RK, Davis, S, & Robison, LL. Incidence of cancer in children in the United States. Cancer 75(8):2186–2195, 1995.

Herzenberg, JE. Congenital limb deficiency and limb length discrepancy. In Canale, ST, & Beatty, JH (Eds.), Operative Pediatric Orthopedics. St. Louis: Mosby, 1991, pp. 187–251.

Jenson, TS, & Rasmussen, P. Phantom pain and related phenomena after amputation. In Melzack, W, & Wall, PD (Eds.), Textbook of Pain, 2nd ed. New York: Churchill Livingstone, 1989, pp. 508–519.

Kegel, B. Sports for the Leg Amputee. Redmond, WA: Medic Publishing, 1986, pp. 5–72.

Kegel, B. Adaptations for sports and recreation. In Bowker, JH, & Michael, JW (Eds.), Atlas of Limb Prosthetics: Surgical, Prosthetic, and Rehabilitation Principles, 2nd ed. St. Louis: Mosby, 1992, pp. 623–654.

Kenan, S, & Lewis, MM. Limb salvage in pediatric surgery: The use of the expandable prosthesis. Orthopedic Clinics of North America, 22(1):121–131, 1991.

Koman, LA, Meyer, LC, & Warren, FH. Proximal femoral focal deficiency: Natural history and treatment. Clinical Orthopedics and Related Research, 162:135–143, 1982.

Kotz, R, & Salzer, M. Rotation-plasty for childhood osteosarcoma of the distal part of the femur. Journal of Bone and Joint Surgery (American), 64:959–969, 1982.

Krajbich, JI, & Bochmann, D. Van Nes rotation-plasty in tumor surgery. In Bowker, JH, & Michael, JW (Eds.), Atlas of Limb Prosthetics: Surgical, Prosthetic, and Rehabilitation Principles, 2nd ed. St. Louis: Mosby, 1992, pp. 885–899.

Krebs, DE, Edelstein, JE, & Thornby, MA. Prosthetic management of children with limb deficiencies. Physical Therapy, 71:920–934, 1991.

Krebs, DE, & Fishman, S. Characteristics of the child amputee population. Journal of Pediatric Orthopedics, 4:89–95, 1984.

Kruger, LM. Recent advances in surgery of lower limb deficiencies. Clinical Orthopedics and Related Research, 148:97–105, 1980.

Lenz, W. Genetics and limb deficiencies. Clinical Orthopedics and Related Research, 148:9–17, 1980.

Link, MP. Cancer in Childhood: Physically Handicapped Children. New York: Grune & Stratton, 1982, pp. 43–58.

Link, MP, & Eilber, F. Osteosarcoma. In Pizzo, PA, & Poplack, DG (Eds.), Principles and Practice of Pediatric Oncology. Philadelphia: JB Lippincott, 1988, pp. 689–711.

Link, MP, Goorin, AM, Horowitz, M, Meyer, WH, Belasco, J, Baker, A, Ayala, A, & Shuster, J. Adjuvant chemotherapy of high-grade osteosarcoma of the extremity. Clinical Orthopedics and Related Research, 270:8–14, 1991a.

Link, MP, Grier, HE, & Donaldson, SS. Sarcomas of bone. In Fernbach, DJ, & Vietti, TJ (Eds.), Clinical Pediatric Oncology, 4th ed. St. Louis: Mosby, 1991b, pp. 545–575.

Meadows, AT, Baum, E, Fossati-Bellani, F, Green, D, Jenkin, RD, Marsden, B, Nesbit, M, Newton, W, Oberlin, O, & Sallan, SG. Second malignant neoplasms in children: An update from the late effects study group. Journal of Clinical Oncology, 3:532, 1985.

Meyers, PA. Malignant bone tumors in children: Osteosarcoma. Hematology/Oncology Clinics of North America, 1:655–666, 1987a.

Meyers, PA. Malignant bone tumors in children: Ewing's sarcoma. Hematology/Oncology Clinics of North America, 1:667–673, 1987b.

Meyers, PA, & Gorlick, R. Osteosarcoma. Pediatric Clinics of North America, 44(4):973–989, 1997.

Michael, JW, Gailey, RS, & Bowker, JH. New developments in recreational prostheses and adaptive devices for the amputee. Clinical Orthopedics and Related Research, 256:64–75, 1990.

Miller, RW, Young, JL, & Novakovic, B. Childhood cancer. Cancer, 75(S):395–405, 1995.

Miser, JS, Kinsella, TJ, Triche, TJ, Tsokos, M, Forquer, R, Wesley, R, Horvath, K, Belasco, J, Longo, DL, Steis, R, Glatstein, E, & Pizzo, PA. Preliminary results of treatment of Ewing's sarcoma of bone in children and young adults: Six months of intensive combined modality therapy without maintenance. Journal of Clinical Oncology, 6:484–490, 1988a.

Miser, JS, Triche, TJ, Pritchard, DJ, & Kinsella, T. Ewing's sarcoma and the nonrhabdomyosarcoma soft tissue sarcomas of childhood. In Pizzo, PA, & Poplack, DG (Eds.), Principles and Practice of Pediatric Oncology. Philadelphia: JB Lippincott, 1988b, pp. 659–688.

Moore, KL. The Developing Human, 3rd ed. Philadelphia: WB Saunders, 1982, pp. 366–368.

Mount, BM. Psychological and social aspects of cancer pain. In Melzack, W, & Wall, PD (Eds.), Textbook of Pain, 2nd ed. New York: Churchill Livingstone, 1989, pp. 610–623.

Patton, JG. Developmental approach to pediatric prosthetic evaluation and training. In Atkins, DJ, & Meier, RH (Eds.), Comprehensive Management of the Upper-Limb Amputee. New York: Springer-Verlag, 1989, pp. 137–149.

Postma, A, Kingma, A, De Ruiter, JH, Koops, HS, Veth, RPH, Goeken, LNH, & Kamps, WA. Quality of life in bone tumor patients comparing limb salvage and amputation of the lower extremity. Journal of Surgical Oncology, 51:47–51, 1992.

Pruitt, SD, Varni, JW, & Setoguchi, Y. Functional status in children with limb deficiency: Development and initial validation of an outcome measure. Archives of Physical Medicine and Rehabilitation, 77:1233–1238, 1996.

Radocy, B. Upper-limb prosthetic adaptations for sports and recreation. In Bowker, JH, & Michael, JW (Eds.), Atlas of Limb Prosthetics: Surgical, Prosthetic, and Rehabilitation Principles, 2nd ed. St. Louis: Mosby, 1992, pp. 325–344.

Robison, LL, Mertens, A, & Neglia, JP. Epidemiology and etiology of childhood cancer. In Fernbach, DJ, & Vietti, TJ (Eds.), Clinical Pediatric Oncology, 4th ed. St. Louis: Mosby, 1991, pp. 11–28.

Schindler, OS, Cannon, SR, Briggs, TWR, & Blunn, GW. Stanmore custom-made extendible distal femoral replacements. Journal of Bone and Joint Surgery (British), 79(6):927–937, 1997.

Setoguchi, Y, & Rosenfelder, R (Eds.). The Limb Deficient Child. Springfield, IL: Charles C. Thomas, 1982.

Shurr, DG, & Cook, TM. Prosthetics and Orthotics. East Norwalk, CT: Appleton & Lange, 1990, pp. 183–193.

Sim, FH, Ivins, JC, Taylor, WF, & Chao, EYS. Limb-sparing surgery for osteosarcoma: Mayo Clinic experience. Cancer Treatment Symposia, 3:139–153, 1985.

Simmel, ML. Phantom experiences following amputation in childhood. Journal of Neurology, Neurosurgery, and Psychiatry, 25:69–78, 1962.

Simon, MA. Limb salvage for osteosarcoma in the 1980's. Clinical Orthopedics and Related Research, 270:264–270, 1991.

Singer, MB, & Lombardo, JR. Training can be fun at Shriner's myoelectric camp. Occupational Therapy Week, April 1992, pp. 24–25.

Springfield, DS. Musculoskeletal tumors. In Canale, ST, & Beatty, JH (Eds.), Operative Pediatric Orthopedics. St. Louis: Mosby, 1991, pp. 1073–1113.

Sutherland, DH. Gait Disorders in Childhood and Adolescence. Baltimore: Williams & Wilkins, 1984, pp. 14–27.

Swanson, AB, Barsky, AJ, & Entin, MA. Classification of limb malformations on the basis of embryological failures. Surgical Clinics of North America, 48:1169–1179, 1968.

Tachdjian, MO. Congenital deformities. In Tachdjian, MO (Ed.), Pediatric Orthopedics, Vol. 1, 2nd ed. Philadelphia: WB Saunders, 1990a, pp. 104–687.

Tachdjian, MO. Tumors and tumerous conditions of bone. In Tachdjian, MO (Ed.), Pediatric Orthopedics, Vol. 2, 2nd ed. Philadelphia: WB Saunders, 1990b, pp. 1186–1189.

Tebbi, CK. Psychological effects of amputation in sarcoma. In Humphrey, GB, Koops, HS, Molenaar, WM, & Postma, A (Eds.), Osteosarcoma in Adolescents and Young Adults. Boston: Kluwer Academic, 1993, pp. 39–44.

Tooms, RE. The amputee. In Lovell, WW, & Winter, RB (Eds.), Pediatric Orthopedics, 2nd ed. Philadelphia: JB Lippincott, 1985, pp. 999–1053.

Tooms, RE. Acquired amputations in children. In Bowker, JH, & Michael, JW (Eds.), Atlas of Limb Prosthetics: Surgical, Prosthetic, and Rehabilitation principles, 2nd ed. St. Louis: Mosby, 1992, pp. 735–741.

Tucker, MA, D'Angio, GJ, Boyce, JD, Strong, LC, Li, FP, Stovall, M, Stone, BJ, Green, DM, Lombardi, F, Newton, W, Hoover, RN, & Fraumeni, JF. Bone sarcomas linked to radiotherapy and chemotherapy in children. New England Journal of Medicine, 317:588, 1987.

Unwin, PS, & Walker, PS. Extendible endoprosthesis for the skeletally immature. Clinical Orthopedics and Related Research, 322:179–193, 1996.

Varni, JW, & Setoguchi, Y. Screening for behavioral and emotional problems in children and adolescents with congenital or acquired limb deficiencies. American Journal of Diseases in Childhood, 146:103–107, 1992.

Weddington, WW, Segraves, KB, & Simon, MA. Psychological outcome of extremity sarcoma survivors undergoing amputation or limb salvage. Journal of Clinical Oncology, 3:1393–1399, 1985.

Wright, PE, & Jobe, MT. Congenital anomalies of the hand. In Canale, ST, & Beatty, JH (Eds.), Operative Pediatric Orthopedics. St. Louis: Mosby, 1991, pp. 253–330.

Orthopedic Conditions

JUDY LEACH, PT

In the course of their careers, physical therapists may meet patients with a wide variety of diagnoses or they may tend to specialize in one particular area. Almost without exception, however, a strong grounding in orthopedics is a necessary part of a therapist's academic and clinical experience. For therapists specializing in the assessment and treatment of children, this orthopedic knowledge is especially necessary and the acquisition of it particularly challenging because of one immutable fact—children grow. The human skeleton undergoes an incredible amount of growth and change in the years between birth and skeletal maturity. What may be considered "normal" at one age can be decidedly abnormal at another. For example, most infants have bowlegs (genu varum), but significant genu varum in an 8-year-old child would be cause for concern.

The rotational alignment of the lower extremity provides another example of the need for physical therapists to be familiar with the growth and development of the musculoskeletal system. Internal tib-

ial torsion in the infant is commonly seen and considered normal for age. However, a high degree of internal tibial torsion in a 5-year-old child is an impairment that may produce a significant functional deficit, such as difficulty running and frequent falls, and require surgical correction.

In addition, as physical therapy practice becomes more autonomous, the burden and the challenge of timely identification of problems outside our scope of practice that require referral to other specialists are responsibilities we should all welcome and view as a necessary service to our patients.

In this chapter I do not attempt an exhaustive review of all the orthopedic conditions that affect children. A number of excellent texts already accomplish that (Scoles, 1988; Tachdjian, 1990; Wenger & Rang, 1993). Instead, specific areas of concern to the physical therapist and commonly seen conditions will be highlighted in the hope that this will provide a basic framework for further independent study. Torsional conditions, angular conditions, developmental dysplasia of the hip, causes of limp in children, back pain, and leg length inequality are discussed.

TORSIONAL CONDITIONS

A chief complaint of either in-toeing or out-toeing is probably the most common reason for elective referral of a child to an orthopedist. Even though these rotational conditions in the lower extremities usually do not require any treatment, they are often a source of significant concern to parents and other family members. This concern is often enhanced by the comments of neighbors, teachers, and strangers on the street—"Why does your child walk funny?" This group has been described by Dr. Mercer Rang as "the worried well," an apt phrase that indicates the strong concern of the family and others involved with the child over alignment conditions that are often part of the spectrum of normal musculoskeletal development.

Numerous differences of opinion exist on how to define torsional conditions, how to measure them, and especially on how to treat them, or if they should be treated at all. Most treatment with special shoes, casts, or braces has no proven efficacy, and many orthopedists believe that persistent deformity beyond skeletal maturity is unusual and significant functional disability rare (Bruce, 1996). Unfortunately the term torsional *deformities* is used in the literature, at national meetings, and in verbal discussions. Patients and parents hear the term *deformity*, and their worst fears are validated. The terms *condition* or *variation* produce less anxiety and are usually more anatomically correct. The Subcommittee on Torsional Deformity of the Pediatric Orthopaedic Society of North America has recommended a classification system in which normal limb alignment and joint range of motion (ROM) are defined as those occurring within two standard deviations of the mean. These are termed *rotational variations*. Those falling outside the two standard deviations are termed *torsional deformities* (Scoles, 1988).

Obtaining a History

A specific history provides a wealth of information regarding possible causative factors and indications for possible treatment. Specific information obtained may also direct the examiner to expand the examination to rule out other, more severe, conditions that may initially cause a chief complaint of in-toeing or out-toeing. Relevant information to be elicited from the parents includes the following:

1. *Birth history.* Was the infant full term or premature? Was it a vaginal or cesarean delivery? Was oligo-

hydramnios (deficiency of amniotic fluid) present? How many times has the mother been pregnant? What is the birth order of the patient? Many of the torsional problems seen in infants are "packaging" defects (i.e., caused by a restricted intrauterine environment). It is easy to imagine that an infant's lower limbs may "grow" into a particular position if one visualizes a full-term 9-pound fetus in the womb of a gravida 1, para 1 mother.

2. *Age when in-toeing or out-toeing was noted.* Has it improved or worsened since first noted? Has there been any prior treatment? For the walking child, at what age did the child start to walk independently? In the differential diagnosis, there should be an increased index of suspicion when a child has a history of prematurity, difficult birth, or delayed motor milestones or has significant in-toeing or out-toeing that is worsening with time or is very asymmetric. Children with mild spastic diplegia may have in-toeing, and children with Duchenne muscular dystrophy may have out-toeing and flat feet. Conditions such as these must be ruled out.

3. *Family history.* In many cases there is a positive family history for in-toeing or out-toeing, and this should be noted, especially if treatment was undertaken.

4. *Sleeping and sitting positions.* Sleeping prone with the legs internally rotated encourages persistent internal tibial torsion and metatarsus adductus (Staheli, 1977). Sitting in a W-sit position encourages the persistence of femoral anteversion.

Clinical Examination: In-Toeing and Out-Toeing

Clinical examination of the child should include documentation of the foot progression angle in standing or walking, hip rotation ROM, thigh-foot axis, and alignment of the foot. These four components form the torsional profile described by Staheli (1977). In a later study, Staheli and colleagues (1985) described means and ranges for these parameters in 1000 normal children and adults.

Foot Progression Angle

Foot progression angle (FPA), or "the angle of gait," is defined as the angle between the longitudinal axis of the foot and a straight line of progression of the body in walking (Staheli, 1977). The child is observed while walking, and a value is assigned to the angle of both the right and the left foot. This is a subjective determination and represents an average of the angles noted on multiple steps. There are various footprint techniques to measure FPA, but these are time consuming and usually not practical in a clinical situation. In-toeing is expressed as a negative value (e.g., −30°), and out-toeing is expressed as a positive value (e.g., +20°). This angle gives an overall view of the degree of in-toeing or out-toeing in the walking child. The FPA can also be assessed in supported stance for the child who is not yet walking independently. FPA is variable during infancy. During childhood and adult life, it shows little change, with a mean of +10° and a normal range of −3 to +20° (Staheli et al., 1985).

Hip Rotation, Femoral Anteversion, and Retroversion: Examination

Hip rotation ROM is measured most accurately in the prone position, with the hip in a position of neutral flexion/extension. (An extremely frightened, crying child can be examined more easily by having the parent stand up and hold the child against the chest, facing the parent. This allows the child's hips to hang into neutral flexion/extension, and the examiner can then bend the child's knees and evaluate the hip rotation range.) This hip rotation measurement will be a reflection of the flexibility of the soft tissues and the version of the femur.

Version is the normal angular difference between the transverse axis of each end of a long bone. The terms *femoral anteversion* (FA) and *retroversion* refer to this relationship between the neck of the femur and the femoral shaft, ending in the femoral condyles, that dictates the position of the femoral head when the knee is pointing straight ahead (Fig. 16–1). If the femoral head is directed anteriorly, the hip is in anteversion (or "anteverted") and the patient will usually have more hip internal rotation (IR) than external rotation (ER) ROM, assuming no soft tissue tightness. If hip IR is measured at 70° and ER at 25°, for example, the child is said to have FA and may in-toe when walking. In retroversion, the femoral head is directed posteriorly when the knee is aligned straight ahead and the patient will have greater ER range.

Femoral and tibial torsion, or version, can be measured by computed tomography (CT). However, clinical measurements of hip IR and ER have been found accurate for diagnosing rotational abnormalities. Cahuzac and co-workers (1992) found that relationships between FA and hip IR were significant, as were relationships between the clinical and CT values of femoral and tibial torsion. Stuberg and associates (1989) found a discrepancy of 10 to 15° between clinical goniometric assessment and CT analysis of femoral torsion, with goniometric measurements less than the femoral anteversion measured by CT. Clinical measurements are sufficient for documentation in the majority of patients with benign rotational problems.

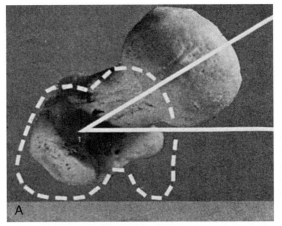

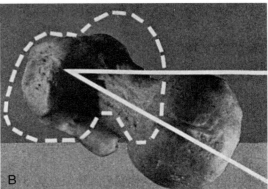

FIGURE 16–1. *A*, Femoral anteversion. *B*, Femoral retroversion. In the femur, version is the angular difference between the transcondylar axis of the knee and the axis of the femoral neck (a line drawn between the center of the femoral head and the center of the base of the femoral neck). (From Salter, RB. Textbook of Disorders and Injuries of the Musculoskeletal System. Baltimore: Williams & Wilkins, 1970, p. 48. © 1970, The Williams & Wilkins Co.)

The sum of hip IR and ER is usually 120° up to age 2 years; over age 2 it is 95 to 110° (Engel & Staheli, 1974). Most infants have FA and also have contractures of the hip external rotator muscles at birth (from the intrauterine position) that mask the anteversion; they tend to hold their legs in an abducted/externally rotated position. True femoral retroversion in an infant is rare; it is usually tightness in the hip lateral rotator muscles and capsular ligaments that is producing the externally rotated position, masking the femoral anteversion (Pitkow, 1975). Gradually the tightness of the hip soft tissues stretches out, and the true anteversion of the femur becomes more apparent. This process is often described incorrectly as "femoral anteversion increases"—the amount of femoral version is in fact decreasing, but it is more easily visualized because

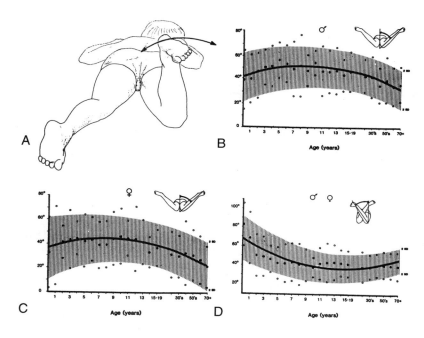

FIGURE 16–2. *A*, Hip rotation is measured with the patient prone, knee flexed to 90°. Means for hip rotation in midchildhood and in older subjects. *B*, Medial rotation in males: 50 (range 25–65°). *C*, Medial rotation in females: 40 (range 15–60°). *D*, Lateral rotation: 45 (range 25–65°), with no gender difference. (From Staheli LT, Corbett, M, Wyss, C, & King, H. Lower extremity rotational problems in children. Journal of Bone and Joint Surgery [American], *67*:39–47, 1985.)

the muscle tightness of the lateral rotators is decreasing. The FA becomes increasingly more apparent as the child approaches 5 to 6 years of age, as the soft tissue tightness resolves. It has been measured by radiographs and CT in typically developing children, and the average shows a gradual decrease with age: 35° at age 1 year, to 21° at age 9 years, to 15.5° in adults (Crane, 1959; De Alba, 1998; Fabry et al., 1973; Shands & Steele, 1958). By midchildhood, the femoral head and neck have usually assumed a relatively more neutral position in relationship to the femoral shaft and children typically have approximately equal amounts of hip IR and ER (Fig. 16–2).

Femoral Anteversion: Treatment

Many types of treatment have been tried to correct FA, including braces, twister cables, and special shoes. None of these has been proven effective in clinical trials. Anecdotal evidence of their efficacy abounds, with a tendency to ignore the natural history of the condition (i.e., that spontaneous improvement will occur). One reasonable recommendation is to have the child avoid W-sitting (reverse tailor sitting) and to encourage tailor sitting in maximum external rotation. If significant FA is still present at age 10 to 14 years and resulting in cosmetically unappealing in-toeing, surgical correction in the form of femoral derotation osteotomies may be considered, although the possible operative risks may outweigh the benefits of realignment. Surgical intervention may be warranted and has proven suc-

cessful in children with severe symptomatic torsional malalignment with excessive FA or external tibial torsion (ETT) associated with patellofemoral pathology, where conservative treatment has failed (Cameron and Saha, 1996; Delgado et al., 1996; Meister & James, 1995; Turner, 1994).

Thigh-Foot Axis, Tibial Torsion: Examination

The alignment of the lower leg can be measured by documenting the thigh-foot axis, which is a reflection of the version of the tibia. Tibial torsion is assessed using the thigh-foot angle, the angular difference between the longitudinal axes of the thigh and foot, as measured in the prone position with the knee flexed. Some examiners measure tibial torsion with the child sitting and the knee flexed to 90°. Tibial torsion can also be described as the angle formed by a straight-line axis through the knee and the axis through the medial and lateral malleoli. By convention, internal tibial torsion (ITT) is expressed as a negative value, such as "tibial torsion of −30." External tibial torsion is expressed as a positive value.

The tibia is usually medially rotated in infants (ITT) as a result of intrauterine positioning (Hensinger & Jones, 1981). Spontaneous derotation on the long axis takes place during growth. The tibia gradually rotates out into ETT, especially during the first 6 months of independent walking, or by approximately 18 months of age. The normal range of thigh-foot angle is between 0 and 30° of ETT, with a mean of approximately 10° during most of childhood (Staheli & Engel, 1972). Scoles (1988) described the following approximate thigh-foot normative angles:

Birth: −15° (normal range −30 to +20°)
Age 3: +5° (normal range −10 to +20°)
Midchildhood to skeletal maturity: +10°
    (normal range −5 to +30°)

ITT in infancy is often not apparent to the parents or the casual examiner because the hips have external rotation muscle contractures and the infant's legs tend to assume an abducted and externally rotated position. The ITT may become noticeable only as the hip contractures stretch out resulting in a more neutral position of the hip, and especially when the child begins to walk independently.

Internal Tibial Torsion: Treatment

Controversy exists regarding appropriate treatment of ITT, as it does in FA. Many orthopedists believe that it should not be treated at all because the natural history of the condition is gradual improvement. The very small percentage of children who do not improve and who have a significant functional deficit as a result of ITT can be treated surgically at a later date with external rotational osteotomy of the tibia and fibula. A different school of thought relies on natural improvement up to about 18 months of age, and at that age advocates treating persistent ITT with a Friedman counter splint (a flexible leather strap) or a Denis Browne bar (a metal bar) for night wear, usually for about 6 months. These devices attach to shoes and hold the feet in an externally rotated position.

There may be an association of increased incidence of knee osteoarthritis in adults with decreased ETT or true ITT (Turner, 1994; Yagi, 1994). Turner (1994) observed that patients with patellofemoral instability had greater than normal ETT and patients with panarticular osteoarthritis had decreased ETT, and he noted that abnormal torsion causes gait adaptations that affect external loading on the knee joint.

Metatarsus Adductus

Alterations in alignment of the foot can be divided into two categories: positional or "packaging" problems caused by a restricted intrauterine environment and "manufacturing" defects or true congenital abnormalities such as talipes equinovarus. Metatarsus varus, also called metatarsus adductus (MTA), is one of the most commonly seen positional conditions in infants; Moreuende and Ponseti (1996) note the possibility of a developmental abnormality of the

medial cuneiform as a pathogenic factor. In MTA the forefoot is curved medially, the hindfoot is in the normal slight valgus position, and there is full dorsiflexion ROM. The degree of MTA can be graded as I—mild, II—moderate, and III—severe. Having the child stand on the glass plate of a photocopying machine and xeroxing the feet is an easy, quick way to document the amount of metarsus adductus. Some clinicians use grade ½ to describe dynamic MTA: the foot looks straight at rest, but when the child walks there is a dynamic forefoot varus due to muscle action, with medial motion of the great toe, described as a "searching great toe" (Staheli, 1977). Treatment is rarely required for mild cases (grade I), which usually resolve on their own, generally by about age 4 to 6 months. Moderate cases (grade II) may be treated with stretching exercises and corrective shoes (straight-last or reverse-last shoes or both). Severe cases may be treated with manipulation and serial casting, followed by corrective shoes. Another school of thought advocates no conservative treatment, recommending surgical correction at a later age for those feet that do not improve with time. Thirty-one patients (45 feet) followed an average of 32 years, 6 months, by Farsetti and colleagues (1994) demonstrated good results in all feet with passively correctable MTA that had no treatment. Twenty-six (90%) of the 29 feet with moderate or severe MTA treated with serial manipulation and casting had good results.

Clubfoot

A condition often confused with MTA is the congenital deformity of clubfoot, or talipes equinovarus (TEV). First described by Hippocrates, the forefoot in this condition is curved in medially (adducted), the calcaneus is small, the hindfoot is in varus, and there is equinus of the ankle. The calf and the foot are generally smaller on the involved side. In some children, TEV is just one manifestation of more serious malformations such as myelomeningocele or arthrogryposis. Typical congenital clubfoot is probably the result of abnormal intrauterine restriction in a genetically predisposed individual. It occurs in 1 per 1000 live births, with a 2:1 male-to-female ratio (Scoles, 1988; Wynne-Davies, 1964).

Treatment consists of manipulation and serial casting, which is most effective if started immediately after birth, often followed by surgical correction from 3 months to 1 year of age, depending on the surgeon's preference. Occasionally a positional clubfoot is seen in which the deformity is similar to that described earlier but can be treated successfully with manipulation and casting, with no surgery needed.

Calcaneovalgus

Calcaneovalgus is a common positional foot problem in newborns. In this condition, the result of a large infant in a small space, the forefoot is curved out laterally, the hindfoot is in valgus, and there is full or excessive dorsiflexion. The dorsum of the foot may actually be touching the anterior surface of the leg at birth. The positional calcaneovalgus foot corrects spontaneously and does not require treatment. It must be distinguished from more severe conditions, such as a calcaneovalgus foot caused by a vertical talus. In this condition, the talus is vertically oriented and the navicular is displaced onto the dorsal surface of the talus. The forefoot is dorsiflexed, but the hindfoot is plantar flexed, and the foot bends at the instep. This characteristic position is described as a rocker-bottom deformity of the foot, and the foot is much more rigid than the typical calcaneovalgus foot.

Foot Alignment Problems: Summary

Table 16–1 is a decision matrix that provides a quick and easy way to categorize foot conditions (Wenger & Leach, 1986).

Torsional Profile

The components that may contribute to in-toeing are femoral anteversion, internal tibial torsion, and metatarsus adductus. Those that may contribute to out-toeing are ER contractures of the hip (and, rarely, femoral retroversion), external tibial torsion, and calcaneovalgus. The foot progression angle can be viewed as the "summation" of the rotational alignment of the three segments of the lower limb: the hip and femur, the lower leg, and the foot. For example, significant FA at the hip may be balanced by ETT, with a straight foot (no MTA or calcaneovalgus). The foot progression angle would be 0/0 (right/left) with the feet pointing straight ahead. When a child toes in or toes out, the condition is usually bilateral, but occasionally one sees "windswept" lower extremities, with one limb toeing in and the other limb toeing out.

An example of a torsional profile of a typically developing 8-month-old infant might be as follows:

	Right	Left
Foot progression angle	—	—(not yet standing)
Internal rotation of hip	20°	20°
External rotation of hip	90°	90°
Thigh-foot angle	0°	0°
Foot	Neutral	Neutral

When supported in upright, the legs would be positioned in external rotation, the usual position for the lower extremities in infancy. The torsional profile of a 5-year-old child with in-toeing might look like this:

	Right	Left
Foot progression angle	−40°	−30°
Internal rotation of hip	70°	70°
External rotation of hip	20°	20°
Thigh-foot angle	−10°	+ 15°
Foot	Grade I MTA	Neutral

From this discussion, it is clear that one must determine which component(s) of the lower extremity is causing the torsional impairment and then treat that level, if treatment is indicated. For example, using heavy, high-topped orthopedic shoes will not correct femoral anteversion. In fact, the child will probably be more clumsy and stumble more frequently. The concept of a natural history of improvement with time is also pivotal. It is important not to extoll the virtues of various treatments too vigorously, because it is difficult to differentiate benefits obtained from the treatment versus benefits that occurred simply with the passage of time as a result of skeletal maturation.

In children with neuromuscular diseases such as cerebral palsy, the basic examination format described previously is useful in helping to delineate the child's problems with gait. In addition to this assessment, which mainly addresses bony alignment, one must, of course, document muscle tone, muscle

---

TABLE 16–1. **Decision Matrix for Foot Deformity**

	Metatarsus Varus	Clubfoot	Calcaneovalgus
Side view (Can foot dorsiflex?)	Yes	No	Yes
Foot shape (viewed from bottom)	Kidney shaped (deviated medially)	Kidney shaped	Banana shaped (deviated laterally)
Heel position	Valgus	Varus	Valgus

strength, and motor control. Abnormalities in any of these areas can cause in-toeing or out-toeing, either alone or in conjunction with skeletal malalignment. An example would be a child with cerebral palsy who ambulates with a foot progression angle of −40°/−30°. This may be due to a combination of FA, ITT, MTA, and spasticity in the hip adductors, medial hamstrings, and posterior tibialis muscles. By contrast, a child with Duchenne muscular dystrophy may ambulate with an in-toeing gait at age 6 because of FA and then gradually develop an out-toeing gait by age 10, resulting from resolution of the FA and increasing weakness of the gluteus maximus and quadriceps muscles, plus tightness in the iliotibial band and plantar flexors.

Another area of assessment and treatment in which this multilevel concept is useful is in measurement of other gross motor activities, such as sitting. Many children with increased tone, as well as children with hypotonia, will W-sit. This postural preference is frequently ascribed to problems with spasticity, or it is thought of as a compensatory mechanism to achieve better sitting balance. However, a more detailed examination might reveal that the child has, in addition to spasticity or poor balance, significant FA that simply does not allow comfortable sitting with the hips in external rotation.

ANGULAR CONDITIONS

Genu varum (bowlegs) and genu valgum (knock-knees) are similar to torsional conditions in that they are commonly seen in typically developing children and a specific natural history has been described that results in normal skeletal alignment at maturity.

Moderate genu varum, often referred to as physiologic bowing (apex laterally), is normal for newborns and for infants before they are walking. This physiologic genu varum generally resolves, and the child gradually develops genu valgum between 2 and 4 years of age. By age 3 years, 80% of children have mild knock-knees. This valgus angulation generally corrects by 5 to 7 years of age, and the child is left with a "normally" straight leg. The normal tibiofemoral angulation in adults is 7 to 9° of valgus in females and 4 to 6° in males (Scoles, 1988). Cahuzac and colleagues (1995) measured the tibiofemoral angle clinically in 427 children ages 10 to 16 years and found that girls had a constant valgus (5.5°), whereas the boys showed a varus evolution (4.4°) during the last 2 years of growth. Bowlegs and knock-knees tend to run in families, however, and some children will inherit this genetic predisposition to one or the other in adulthood.

Genu Varum

Examination

Genu varum can be documented by having the child lie supine and approximating the medial malleoli, and then measuring the distance between the femoral condyles or at the knee joint line. The child must be undressed, with diaper removed, for this measurement to be accurate. A plastic triangle with centimeters marked on both sides is useful, allowing the examiner to easily obtain accurate measurements, especially of a wiggling child.

Infants usually have ITT and genu varum, and this combination tends to make the child look "bowlegged and pigeon-toed," causing many parents and others great concern. Even when the genu varum has resolved and the child may actually have developed genu valgum, the presence of ITT may make the child look bowlegged.

Treatment

"Physiologic" (normal) genu varum does not usually require treatment unless it persists after age 2 years and either shows no tendency to correct or is actually worsening. This latter condition may require bracing in hip-knee-ankle-foot orthoses (HKAFOs) or knee-ankle-foot orthoses (KAFOs) with no knee joint or a hinged knee joint that can be locked. Surgical correction is sometimes required, although this is rare.

Differential Diagnosis

When a child develops severe genu varum, especially after 4 years of age or with worsening over time, systemic disorders such as vitamin D–resistant rickets must be ruled out, along with a variety of skeletal dysplasias and other conditions that cause genu varum. Radiographs are used to rule out idiopathic tibia vara, also known as Blount's disease. The first case of infantile tibia vara was reported in 1922, and Blount presented a complete description of the condition in 1937. In Blount's disease, increased compressive forces across the medial aspect of the knee cause growth suppression of the proximal tibia physis, resulting in a bowleg deformity (Thompson & Carter, 1990).

In Blount's disease, a characteristic breaking of the medial metaphysis is noted on radiographs, especially in younger children. In 1952 Langenskiold described six stages of infantile tibia vara based on their radiographic appearance (Langenskiold, 1989). Tibia vara is usually seen in children under 3 years of age, although it may be found in older children. Children with Blount's disease may clinically resemble those with physiologic genu varum except that they are often obese and also have a lateral thrust of the knee during stance phase of gait. Blount's disease requires aggressive treatment, with bracing in full HKAFOs worn 23 hours per day recommended for patients under 3 years of age (Johnson, 1990). Surgical correction by proximal tibial osteotomy is sometimes performed. To ensure a better outcome, it should be done before permanent physeal damage has occurred, as shown by Hofmann and colleagues (1982) in their series of 19 knees (12 patients) evaluated at a mean of 12 years after osteotomy. Twelve knees were symptomatic, and 8 of those had early degenerative changes. Poor results were directly correlated to the amount of physeal damage.

Physiologic genu varum must also be distinguished from anterolateral bow of the tibia, usually noted at birth (Hensinger & Jones, 1981). In this extremely serious condition, radiographs demonstrate a tibia with a narrowed, sclerotic intramedullary canal; the majority fracture in the first year of life. Both tibia and fibula fail to unite; hence the name "pseudoarthrosis of the tibia." Protective bracing and surgical treatment may be helpful, but many eventually require amputation because of persistent pseudoarthrosis.

Genu Valgum

Examination and Treatment

Like genu varum, genu valgum can occasionally persist beyond the age range when one expects the legs to become generally straight; many of these children are overweight and have an out-toeing foot progression angle, an awkward gait, and flat feet. Genu valgum can be measured by documenting the intermalleolar distance in supine or standing, with the medial aspect of the knees lightly touching each other.

Children with significant femoral anteversion may often appear knock-kneed. Once again, a clear understanding of the three-level concept of torsional conditions and the angular conditions of genu varum and genu valgum is necessary to define the specific problem(s). Krivickas (1997) noted that athletes are predisposed to developing overuse injuries by both extrinsic factors (e.g., training errors) and intrinsic or anatomic factors, such as malalignment of the lower extremities. Genu varum or valgum, along with torsional malalignment, may predispose athletes to knee extensor mechanism injuries, iliotibial band syndrome, stress fractures, and plantar fasciitis.

If severe, physiologic genu valgum can be safely and effectively corrected by stapling of the medial femoral growth plate, and genu varum by stapling of the lateral growth plate, in the teenage years (Mielke & Stevens, 1996). This allows the other side of the femoral growth plate to continue growing, and the leg gradually grows into better alignment. A second option for surgical treatment is femoral osteotomy.

FLAT FOOT

The subject of flexible flat feet is a controversial one, with a variety of players: unconcerned children, usually with no foot pain and no disability; concerned parents who frequently were treated in childhood for flat feet and now demand treatment for their child; physical therapists concerned about the abnormal appearance of the foot and ankle and the possible secondary effects on the more proximal joints; and various other medical practitioners, some well intended, who provide arch supports that need frequent replacement in a growing child.

Examination

Children with flexible flat feet have a normal-appearing arch in sitting and when asked to walk "on their toes" in maximum plantar flexion. In standing, however, the longitudinal arch decreases or disappears. This is usually due to normal ligamentous laxity, and the child will typically demonstrate laxity throughout the upper and lower extremities, as evidenced by hyperextension at the elbows and knees and ability to approximate the thumb to the forearm. The fat pad noted in the medial part of the foot in many infants and toddlers contributes to the flat-footed appearance. A wide variation of rate and onset of arch development was noted in the 160 children studied by Engel and Staheli (1974). Volpon (1994) documented static footprints on 672 children, and found rapid spontaneous plantar arch development between 2 and 6 years of age. An interesting study by Sachithanandam and Joseph (1995) of 1846 skeletally mature individuals in India found a significantly higher prevalence of flatfoot in those who began to wear shoes before age 6 years. They also noted a higher prevalence of flat foot in obese individuals and those with ligament laxity.

Treatment

A great deal of anecdotal evidence but little scientific proof exists to support the use of special shoes or arch supports for the treatment of flexible flat feet in children. In a prospective study Wenger and colleagues (1989) concluded that wearing corrective shoes or inserts for 3 years does not alter the natural history. They studied 129 children randomly assigned to three groups treated with (1) corrective orthopedic shoes, (2) Helfet heel-cups (Apex Foot Health, South Hackensack, NJ), or (3) custom-molded plastic inserts, with a fourth group as controls. The minimum 3 years of treatment was completed by 98 patients with documented compliance. All groups showed significant improvement, including the control group, and there was no significant difference between the control group and the treated patients.

It has been widely documented that a low arch is usually less of a problem in adulthood than high-arched (cavus) feet. Most pediatric orthopedists now counsel parents regarding the natural history of improvement in flat feet through childhood and advise the use of a lightweight running shoe as the only recommendation. Using shoes with a good arch support and a strong counter will not correct the flat foot but can help decrease wear on the medial border of shoes, thereby decreasing the expense of frequent shoe purchases.

Differential Diagnosis and Treatment

A tendo Achillis contracture can produce a secondary flat foot. Examples of conditions in which this may occur are cerebral palsy, congenital or familial tight heel cords, and muscular dystrophy. A fixed valgus of the hindfoot causing symptoms such as pain, callus, ulceration, poor brace tolerance, and excessive shoe wear can be relieved by tendo Achillis lengthenings and other soft tissue and osseus procedures (Mosca, 1995).

Children occasionally have an extra ossicle located at the medial border of the navicular, called an accessory navicular, frequently associated with flat feet. This condition may become symptomatic in late childhood or early adolescence, resulting in pain over the ossicle and along the medial arch, and can be corrected surgically.

A small subgroup of children with flat foot have a rigid, painful foot with limited subtalar motion. Some of these children carry the diagnosis of peroneal spastic flat foot, because of clonus in the peroneal muscles, and may be referred for physical therapy (Kelo & Riddle, 1998). These children deserve further diagnostic scrutiny and a workup for tarsal coalition. (See section on causes of limping later in this chapter for more information on this condition.)

DEVELOPMENTAL DYSPLASIA OF THE HIP

The term *developmental dysplasia of the hip* (DDH) is replacing the term *congenital dysplasia of the hip*. The term *DDH* is also used as an abbreviation for developmental dislocation of the hip. The term *developmental dysplasia* includes hips that may have been normal, or believed to be normal, at birth but subsequently are documented to have dysplasia. Ilfeld and co-workers (1986) noted that delayed diagnosis of dislocation is not evidence that these hips were "missed" by inadequate examinations. They describe a separate entity of the delayed subluxed or dislocated hip, possibly the result of a dynamic process due to an increased acetabular index.

The term *dysplasia* describes abnormal development or growth. Normal muscle balance and a femoral head that is concentric, congruent with, and seated deep within the acetabulum are necessary prerequisites for normal hip development. The concave acetabulum develops in response to a spherical femoral head, and the depth normally increases with growth.

The incidence of hip dysplasia in the United States is 1 per 100 persons for dysplasia or subluxation and 1 per 1000 persons for dislocation (Mubarak et al., 1987). Prompt recognition and treatment of DDH, preferably in the newborn period, provides the best chance for subsequent optimal hip development and a normal hip at skeletal maturity.

The etiology of DDH is thought to be multifactorial. In the early fetal period, measurements of femoral head coverage and acetabular anteversion do not show significant variation through the embryonic and early fetal stages (6 to 20 weeks), and the hip stays well covered (Lee et al., 1992). Dislocated fetal hips tend to appear only in the last trimester.

Factors that predispose an infant to DDH include mechanical, physiologic, and environmental factors. Mechanical factors are a small intrauterine space and tight abdominal wall of a primipara mother, breech presentation, and positioning of the fetal hip against the mother's sacrum in utero (Hensinger & Jones, 1981). Physiologic factors include maternal hormonal influence of estrogen and relaxin and the resulting ligamentous laxity of the female infant (Wynne-Davies, 1970). This is thought to account for the 6:1 female-to-male incidence of DDH. Environmental or cultural factors include strapping the child's lower extremities in extension, such as on a cradle board, noted in the Eskimo and some other Native American cultures. Cultures in which infants are routinely carried with their hips in flexion and wide abduction in cloth slings on the mother's back or astride her hip have a decreased incidence of DDH.

Mechanical factors can act to restrict the position of the head, neck, and feet of the developing fetus, as well as the hips. Problems associated with DDH include a 20% incidence of congenital muscular torticollis (Hummer & MacEwen, 1972), although Walsh and Morrissy (1998) report that the rate of hip disease in those with torticollis is approximately 8%. A 10% incidence of metatarsus adductus or calcaneovalgus is reported in patients with DDH (Dunn, 1976).

Examination

Based on a careful clinical examination, newborn hips can be classified as follows (Mubarak et al., 1987):

1. Normal—no instability noted.
2. Subluxatable (9.8/1000) (Tredwell & Bell, 1981)—the femoral head is in the socket but can be partially displaced out to the acetabular rim.
3. Dislocatable (1.3/1000)—the femoral head is reduced but can be dislocated with a Barlow maneuver.
4. Dislocated but reducible (1.2/1000)—the femoral head is out of the acetabulum at rest but can be reduced with an Ortolani maneuver.
5. Dislocated but not reducible—seldom encountered in the newborn to 2-month-old age group. When seen, this type of dislocation is usually teratologic, occurring before birth, usually from a neurologic or muscular abnormality such as myelomeningocele or arthrogryposis.

Clinical examination includes documentation of the ROM of hip abduction in flexion. Most infants have 75 to 90° of abduction. Significant limitation or an asymmetry of even 5 to 10° may indicate hip dysplasia and warrants further workup. Other clinical findings may include asymmetric thigh folds, pistoning, apparent (not true) femoral shortening with uneven knee heights (positive Galeazzi sign), and positive Barlow or Ortolani signs (Fig. 16-3).

The infant must be completely relaxed for the Barlow and Ortolani maneuvers to have reliable diagnostic value. Even slight muscular contraction around the hip can obscure the instability and negate the examination. These two signs of hip instability usually will disappear by 2 to 3 months of age, because the hip either improves in stability and stays in the socket or becomes fixed in a dislocated position. Often limited hip abduction may be the only clinical sign of hip dysplasia in the infant older than 1 month. It continues to be the most reliable clinical

finding in older infants and toddlers with dysplasia. Further diagnostic studies are warranted if there are positive findings on clinical examination and even with a normal clinical examination but a high index of suspicion because of multiple risk factors, such as a female first-born child with breech presentation and a family history of DDH.

The use of ultrasonography to examine infant hips is routine in Europe (Graf, 1992) and becoming standard in the United States. It is recognized as more accurate and helpful than radiographs in infants. It is useful in the newborn and up to 3 to 6 months of age, before the femoral head starts to ossify and obscure the structures deep to it, although it may be effective in children up to 1 year of age (Harcke, 1992). The secondary ossification center is present in 80% of children at age 6 months (Scoles et al., 1987). Ultrasonography allows assessment of the cartilaginous structures not visualized on plain radiographs and allows stress testing (to document instability), with the additional advantage of no radiation exposure. It is a useful tool in both the diagnosis and management of DDH, documenting reduction of the dislocated hip in the Pavlik harness (Taylor & Clarke, 1997) and providing information on the status of the hip to aid decisions on altering or stopping treatment. Provision of ultrasound in pediatric orthopedic offices is becoming more common and has been shown to be efficient, cost effective, and convenient for parents and the treating physician (Davids et al., 1995).

The use of ultrasound screening for DDH in newborns has been studied, especially in Europe. Rosendahl and colleagues (1994) did a randomized, controlled trial of 11,925 newborns and found no significant reduction in prevalence of late DDH in the screened group compared with the unscreened group. Donaldson and Feinstein (1997) support targeting high-risk infants for supplemental ultrasound screening as being effective and less expensive than generalized screening.

Radiographs, rather than ultrasound, are used for older infants. Because of the need for a radiograph of the uninvolved side for comparison, and because of the frequency of bilateral involvement, the standard radiograph is an anterior-posterior view of the pelvis. Many parameters of hip development can be measured on hip radiographs (Hensinger & Jones, 1981). Scoles and colleagues (1987) studied 50 boys and 50 girls at each of six age levels: 3, 6, 9, 12, 18, and 24 months. They documented a decrease in acetabular index with age and concluded that this was a helpful parameter in following hip development (Fig. 16-4). Smith JT and colleagues (1997) propose that appearance of the teardrop is the earliest radiographic sign

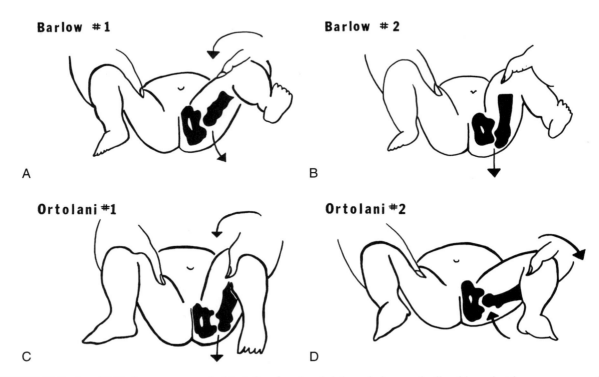

FIGURE 16–3. *A* and *B*, Barlow maneuver: the hip is first flexed and abducted, then gradually adducted with pressure exerted in a posterior direction. Dislocation of the femoral head over the posterior acetabular rim indicates an unstable hip. The head may slide to the edge of the socket (subluxatable) or may dislocate out of the acetabulum (dislocatable). *C* and *D*, Ortolani test: In the Ortolani positive hip, the hip is dislocated in a position of flexion and adduction. Gentle flexion, abduction, and slight traction (the Ortolani maneuver) reduce the hip. A positive Ortolani sign indicates a more unstable hip than a positive Barlow sign. (From Mubarak, SJ, Leach, J, & Wenger, DR. Management of congenital dislocation of the hip in the infant. Contemporary Orthopaedics, *15*:29–44, 1987.)

FIGURE 16–4. Radiographic parameters of hip development involve use of the Hilgenreiner line (H) and Perkin's line (P) to document proximal and lateral migration of the femoral head, with disruption of Shenton's line (crosshatched line). The acetabular index (AI) is the most helpful documentation of acetabular development. In the drawing above, the AI of the left hip is increased, documenting acetabular dysplasia, and Shenton's line is broken, indicating subluxation of the left hip. (From Mubarak, SJ, Leach, J, & Wenger, DR. Management of congenital dislocation of the hip in the infant. Contemporary Orthopaedics, *15*: 29–44, 1987.)

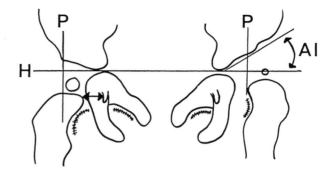

that a stable, concentric reduction of the hip has been achieved. Hips can be classified radiographically as acetabular dysplasia (without subluxation or dislocation); subluxated, with associated acetabular dysplasia; and dislocated.

Between 18 and 24 months of age children with hip dislocation usually have an abnormal gait. With unilateral dislocation the child will limp, demonstrating a positive Trendelenburg sign on the involved side in the stance phase of gait. With bilateral dislocation the child will have a waddling gait.

Treatment

BIRTH TO 9 MONTHS

The Pavlik harness was first described by Dr. Arnold Pavlik, who originally called his treatment device "stirrups." Modifications have been made in the design of the device, but the principles of treatment and the requirements of the harness remain essentially the same as described by him over 40 years ago (Pavlik, 1950). He stressed that one of the main advantages of the harness over casts was that it allowed active motion, thereby decreasing the incidence of avascular necrosis (AVN) (Pavlik, 1957).

The Pavlik harness restricts hip extension and adduction and allows the hips to be maintained in flexion and abduction, the "protective position" (Fig. 16–5). Studies with newborn pigs show hip dislocation precipitated by maintaining the hips in extension (Salter, 1968). The position of flexion and abduction enhances normal acetabular development, and the kicking motion allowed in this "human" position (not as radical as the "frog" position) stretches the contracted hip adductors and promotes spontaneous reduction of the dislocated hip. Because of the biologic plasticity of growing bone, positioning the hip in flexion/abduction can promote acetabular development.

Complications of use of the Pavlik harness include AVN of the femoral head, femoral nerve palsy, inferior dislocation, and erosion of the posterior rim of the acetabulum. Essentially all of these complications can be avoided by using a Pavlik harness of proper design, educating the caregiver to apply it correctly, and monitoring the status of the hip carefully over the entire treatment period (Mubarak et al., 1981). The prognosis with Pavlik harness treatment is excellent: 90 to 95% success in cases of subluxation and dysplasia and approximately 85% success in cases of dislocation (Fig. 16–6).

If a brief trial (up to 3 weeks) with the Pavlik harness is not successful in reducing a dislocated hip, surgical treatment is indicated. This may include a period of 2 to 3 weeks of traction to reduce the incidence of AVN of the femoral head. Home

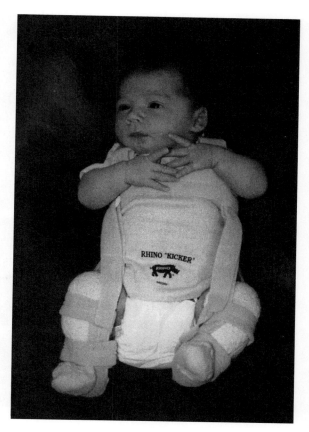

FIGURE 16–5. The Pavlik harness can be used to reduce a dislocated hip, to stabilize a lax hip, and to treat acetabular dysplasia.

traction is a safe, effective, and much less expensive alternative to the 2- to 3-week admission required for hospital traction (Mubarak et al., 1986). Surgery includes an arthrogram to define the anatomic landmarks of the femoral head and acetabulum and to detect the presence of soft tissue (pulvinar) interposition between the head and acetabulum; adductor tenotomy; closed or (if necessary) open reduction of the hip; and application of a spica cast.

AGE 9 MONTHS AND OLDER

In infants more than 9 months of age who are beginning to walk independently, an abduction orthosis should be considered as an alternative to the Pavlik harness for treatment of acetabular dysplasia with or without subluxation. This orthosis should be designed so the child can walk in it. For dislocatable or dislocated hips diagnosed in the 6- to 18-month age group, surgical treatment is usually required. Treatment falls into a gray zone in the 18- to 24-month age group, when either open or closed reduc-

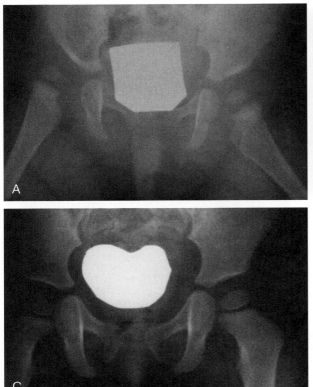

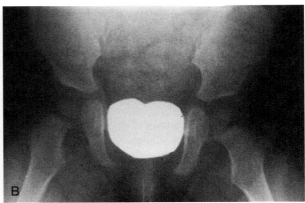

FIGURE 16–6. *A*, Age 4 months: right hip dislocated, severe acetabular dysplasia. *B*, Age 7 months: treated with a Pavlik harness for 3 months full time. Right hip is reduced; continued acetabular dysplasia. Patient continued Pavlik harness treatment for 3 more months, part time (night and naps only). *C*, Age 15 months: both hips centered in the acetabulae with good acetabular development bilaterally.

tion may be used. Olney and colleagues (1998) used a one-stage procedure combining open reduction and pelvic and femoral osteotomies with success, in patients ranging in age from 15 to 117 months.

The diagnosis of hip dislocation in the child age 2 years or older is generally considered to mandate open reduction, because the results of closed reduction are not predictable in these older children. Instead of prior traction, femoral shortening (where a segment of the femoral shaft is removed) is often used (Galpin et al., 1989) to reduce the compressive forces on the femoral head once it is reduced back into the acetabulum. (In 1995 Wenger and colleagues described special circumstances in which femoral shortening may also be used in the child younger than 2 years.) Older children with continuing acetabular dysplasia will benefit from a pelvic osteotomy, as the remodeling potential of the acetabulum decreases with age. Three-dimensional computed tomographic analysis (3DCT) helps define the nature and degree of acetabular and femoral deformity and can be used to evaluate the results of the surgery (Kim & Wenger, 1997a; Smith et al., 1997).

A number of children with acetabular dysplasia are never diagnosed as infants or toddlers. With mild dysplasia, they will walk without a limp, have essentially normal hip ROM, and can actively participate in all childhood activities, including sports. However, the hip is like a tire that is out of round—you can drive on it for quite a few miles, but uneven wear will occur. The dysplastic hip, especially the one with subluxation, also develops uneven wear with subsequent articular cartilage damage. The person may develop degenerative arthritis, hip pain, and limp as early as the late teens. Very mild dysplasia may go undetected for many decades and be diagnosed later in life when the patient develops degenerative hip joint disease. The age at symptom onset in untreated patients with subluxation is variable, with the mean in the midthirties for women and the midfifties for men (Weinstein, 1992). Many middle-aged adults requiring total hip replacement had DDH that was never diagnosed and treated or was treated in childhood without full resolution. A number of studies have documented the association of osteoarthritis (OA) in adults who have residual hip dysplasia (Michaeli et al., 1997) and the increased technical difficulties of total hip arthroplasty with high acetabular component failure rates (Jasty et al., 1995).

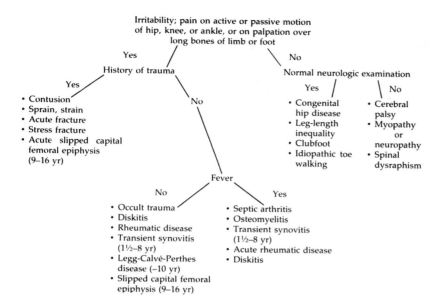

FIGURE 16–7. A clinical decision tree for children with a limp. (From Scoles, PV. Pediatric Orthopedics in Clinical Practice, 2nd ed. St. Louis: Mosby, 1988, p. 21.)

However, the results of Lane and colleagues (1997) did not support the hypothesis that mild acetabular dysplasia accounts for a substantial proportion of hip OA in adult women.

CAUSES OF LIMPING IN CHILDREN

The acute onset of limp in a child can present a diagnostic dilemma. In this section chronic causes of limp, such as those due to muscle weakness, are not discussed. A review of conditions that cause acute limping will provide an overview of a wide range of orthopedic conditions affecting children. Some are transitory and benign, whereas others can result in lifelong disability, especially if not treated promptly and effectively. A clinical decision tree, as shown in Figure 16–7, is useful in identifying those problems that need immediate medical or surgical attention.

Examination

A careful workup is required when a child has a limp. A detailed history must be taken, including a description of any recent illness or injury that may be related. The examiner should be aware, however, that children do fall frequently and that parents may relate the onset of the limp to a fall or other injury that often turns out to be unrelated. Physical examination includes observational gait analysis, which usually will indicate which leg is involved and perhaps even the location within the leg. An example of an antalgic gait deviation is the Trendelenburg sign, a lean toward the involved side in the stance phase, usually caused by a hip problem. A "sore foot gait"

describes a decreased stance time on the involved side and decreased roll-off. This usually results from a problem in the foot, ankle, or lower leg, for example, a toddler's fracture of the tibia.

The physical examination should include a complete assessment of the spine, hips, thighs, knees, lower legs, ankles, and feet, including the uninvolved side for comparison. ROM, strength, presence of muscle atrophy, swelling, redness, increased warmth, and pain to palpation must all be assessed. The way in which a child performs functional activities, such as moving from the floor to standing, crawling, and achieving a comfortable sitting position, can provide important information. For example, a child may refuse to walk because of pain but may crawl easily, indicating that the problem is probably in the lower part of the leg rather than the hip or knee. A child may be able to walk short distances with no significant gait deviations but be reluctant to walk because of pain and may move into the seated position with difficulty and sit with a rigidly fixed spine, indicating a problem in the back, such as diskitis.

Other Diagnostic Tests

In addition to a careful clinical examination, additional tests are often indicated. Radiographs can document fractures or other bony abnormalities, although some occult fractures are not identifiable on radiography until 10 to 14 days after onset, when a repeat radiograph may document callus formation. Laboratory examination of blood samples provides information regarding the presence of infection or other acute processes. The erythrocyte sedimentation rate (ESR) and C-reactive protein (CRP) can indicate the presence of acute inflammation, as well as response to treatment. More complex diagnostic studies may also be needed to define the problem or evaluate the treatment efficacy. These include bone scans, magnetic resonance imaging (MRI) (for soft tissue), and CT (for bony structures).

Many causes of limp in children are easily treated on a routine basis, and some require no treatment beyond observation. Many are age dependent in part, and certain common diagnoses are seen most frequently within one of three age groups: birth to 5 years, 5 to 10 years, and 10 to 15 years. Two common causes of limp can occur in any age group: soft tissue injuries (e.g., contusions, ligament and tendon injuries) and fractures. Spine injury or disease may also cause a limp, at any age, with diskitis being the most common pediatric spinal infection (Glazer & Hu, 1996).

Common Diagnoses by Age Group

Birth to Age 5 Years

OSTEOMYELITIS

Osteomyelitis is an infection of a bone by bacterial organisms. In children, this infection is usually seen in the metaphyseal area. In some cases of osteomyelitis, the infection starts in the bony metaphysis and spreads to the adjacent joint, creating a septic arthritis. Osteomyelitis can be extremely and rapidly destructive, causing permanent damage that can have lifelong consequences for the child. The most common sites of infection are the distal femur and proximal tibia. The origin of the infection is usually hematogenous (blood-borne) and the portal of entry is usually through the skin, secondary to infected scratches, boils, or sore throat (Salter, 1970). It may occasionally result from an open fracture or a penetrating injury. For example, lawn mower injuries, estimated to be 85% preventable by the Research Committee of the Pediatric Orthopedic Society of North America, can result in multiple complications, including osteomyelitis (Loder et al., 1997).

The child with osteomyelitis can present with a high fever, chills, severe pain, swelling, and tenderness over the metaphysis of the involved bone. In this age group, the child may refuse to walk. Newborns and children with osteomyelitis of the smaller bones tend to be less sick, with fewer symptoms. The leukocyte count and ESR are usually elevated but occasionally normal. The bone scan is positive early. Needle aspiration may be diagnostic in only about 60% of children (Hughes & Aronson, 1994). Sonography can be useful in early diagnosis with early findings of intra-articular fluid collection or subperiosteal

abcess formation, preceding radiographic changes (Riebel et al., 1996). Radiographs are usually normal initially, with early bone destruction not demonstrated until 7 to 14 days after onset. Subperiosteal new bone formation indicates periosteal stripping with formation of subperiosteal pus; at this stage, the cortex is already dead.

Acute hematogenous osteomyelitis can be fatal as a result of overwhelming septicemia, and treatment must be instituted on an emergency basis. It consists of aspiration, antibiotics, and immobilization of the affected part, and possibly surgical decompression if gross purulence is identified. Surgical drainage is usually required when the diagnosis is delayed. Delayed treatment may be lifesaving by controlling the septicemia but may be ineffective in controlling progression of the pathologic process within the bone.

SEPTIC ARTHRITIS

Septic arthritis (pyogenic arthritis) is defined as an infection of a joint caused by bacterial organisms. This is an extremely threatening condition, because a joint may be destroyed within 48 hours of onset of symptoms. Septic arthritis causes destruction of articular cartilage and long-term growth arrest (Fig. 16–8). The resulting deformities may be permanent and have a wide-ranging, lifelong impact affecting the person's gait, participation in sports, and choice of occupation and leisure activities.

Staphylococcus aureus is the most common organism (Bennett & Namnyak, 1992), and *Haemophilus influenzae* may also be seen in children younger than 3 years of age. The organism enters the joint by hematogenous spread (e.g., from an ear infection), direct spread (from adjacent osteomyelitis), or direct inoculation (from a foreign body, needle, or surgical penetration of a joint). An increased incidence of septic arthritis in children with human immunodeficiency virus infection has been noted (Hughes & Aronson, 1994). The hip joint is the most commonly involved in this age group, followed by the knee. Septic arthritis of the hip is particularly devastating in the newborn, because the cartilaginous femoral head can be completely destroyed. Even milder cases have potentially lifelong effects because the increased intra-articular pressure can occlude the blood supply to the femoral head, causing AVN.

The child usually has acute onset of irritability, fever to 104°F (40°C), refusal to move the affected limb, and a warm, swollen joint held in flexion. Laboratory data show an elevated leukocyte count and ESR. Radiographs and ultrasound examination may show a distended joint capsule. In older children and adolescents there tends to be a more subtle clinical presentation. These patients often do walk and will allow motion. Subjective discomfort and febrile epi-

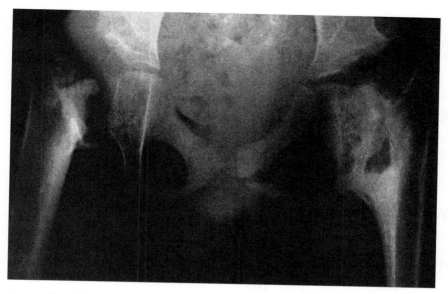

FIGURE 16–8. Septic arthritis of both hip joints in a 5-year, 9-month-old boy treated 17 days after onset of symptoms. Both capital epiphyses are destroyed, and the triradiate cartilage of both hips is sclerosed and irregular, with dysplastic acetabulae. The left hip is ankylosed. (From Bennett, OM, & Namnyak, SS. Acute septic arthritis of the hip joint in infancy and childhood. *Clinical Orthopaedics and Related Research, 281:*123–132, 1992.)

sodes can be prolonged. The incidence of AVN is higher in the older age group (Dales & Hoffinger, 1993). Interestingly, newborns may also have few clinical symptoms, and severe systemic symptoms are rarely seen. Local signs of warmth, swelling, and tenderness may be present. Usually the newborn is unwilling to use an extremity, described as "pseudoparalysis of infancy" (Hensinger & Jones, 1981). Treatment of septic arthritis consists of immediate aspiration and drainage and intravenous administration of antibiotics. A recent study of 200 children treated for septic arthritis in two large tertiary care children's hospitals demonstrated that early conversion from intravenous to oral antibiotics was safe and effective (Newton PO, personal communication, 1998).

TRANSIENT SYNOVITIS

Transient synovitis (also known as toxic synovitis) is probably the most common cause of a painful hip in children younger than 10 years of age. This condition affects males more than females, in a 4:1 ratio. The child has gradual or acute onset of limp. There may be occasional periods when the child refuses to walk. The child usually complains of mild to moderate hip pain but may complain of knee pain, because hip pain is often referred to the knee. Mild fever may be present, with normal leukocyte count and ESR. The cause is unclear, but often a history can be elicited of a recent upper respiratory tract infection or other illness. The treatment is symptomatic, con-

sisting of limitation of activity, bed rest, and use of crutches if the child is old enough to manage them. Symptoms usually resolve in about 7 days. Occasionally a child will have recurrent hip synovitis, and a small percentage of these patients later develop Legg-Perthes disease.

OCCULT FRACTURES

A usually benign condition causing a limp in children is an occult fracture. A commonly seen example is a hairline fracture of the tibia called a toddler's fracture. The child usually refuses to walk or walks with a limp, has no history of significant trauma, and has no fever or signs of infection. Laboratory data are normal, and radiographs of the painful area are usually normal initially. The child can be treated with a splint or cast for comfort and observed closely for signs of incipient infection. If an occult fracture is present, radiographs in 10 to 14 days often show evidence of callus (new bone formation) and the diagnosis can be confirmed in retrospect.

KOHLER SYNDROME

Kohler syndrome is an osteochondrosis affecting the navicular bone, usually occurring in children between ages 2 and 9 years. It was first described by Alban Kohler, a German radiologist (Wenger & Rang, 1993). The child usually has localized pain in the area of the navicular bone and a limp. Radiographic changes are characteristic, with the navicular being sclerotic and small compared with the opposite side. All of these cases resolve with time. Children with limited ambulation as a result of severe pain may be best managed with a brief period of casting.

Other orthopedic conditions that can cause an acute limp in children from birth to age 5 years include juvenile rheumatoid arthritis (see Chapter 8), nonaccidental trauma (fractures or soft tissue injuries), hemophilia (see Chapter 9), diskitis, discoid meniscus, popliteal cysts, foreign bodies, and bone tumors.

Ages 5 to 10 Years

Various types of osteochondroses are common causes of limp in the 5- to 10-year-old age group and in the 10- to 15-year-old age group. These are idiopathic conditions (of unknown cause) characterized by a disorder of endochondral ossification. Many may be microtrauma fractures or growth plate injuries not appreciated on plain radiographs. They may be due to repetitive trauma with weight bearing (Lovell & Winter, 1978).

PERTHES DISEASE

Legg-Calvé-Perthes disease is a condition in children who may be referred to physical therapy for treatment of the resulting muscle weakness, ROM limitations, and gait deviations. It was initially described in the early 1900s by three separate authors, Arthur T. Legg in the United States, Georg Perthes in Germany, and Jacques Calvé in France, and is defined as AVN of the ossific nucleus of the femoral head caused by loss of blood supply. The medial femoral circumflex artery is the principal vessel in the complex vascular distribution in the neck and head of the femur.

Legg-Calvé-Perthes disease usually occurs in children between ages 3 and 12 and most commonly in boys ages 5 to 7 years (Wenger et al., 1991). The male-to-female ratio is 4:1 (Catteral, 1971). These children are frequently small for their age, with retarded bone age (Loder et al., 1995), and very active. There is a high frequency of learning disabilities (Lahdes-Vasama et al., 1997). The disease is bilateral in 20% of cases. The cause is not yet defined, but it occasionally follows repeated episodes of transient synovitis of the hip. There may be a number of pathologic processes that cause an interruption of the blood flow in vessels ascending the femoral neck, including increased joint pressure secondary to synovitis. There is a relationship of Legg-Calvé-Perthes disease to parental cigarette smoking during pregnancy, secondhand smoke, hypofibrinolysis, and thrombophilia (Glueck et al., 1997, 1998). The disease is self-limiting and always heals spontaneously in 1 to 3 years' time, as the femoral head revascularizes (Catterall, 1971). Many but not all patients have good clinical outcomes, with good hip ROM and no pain with activity. Prognostic factors include age at onset (younger children tend to do better), extent of the disease, the amount of femoral head deformity, and the amount of incongruity between the femoral head and acetabulum, because hip joint growth and development depends on a well-located, centered, spherical femoral head (Weinstein, 1997).

Patients tend to have a limp and frequently have a positive Trendelenburg sign resulting from pain or hip abduction weakness. Limited hip ROM is noted, especially in hip abduction and internal rotation. The child complains of pain in the groin, hip, or knee (referred pain). Children who have knee pain may have multiple radiographs of both knees and may be referred to physical therapy for treatment of their "knee pain" (Tippett, 1994). A careful clinical examination and observational gait analysis usually provide the information needed to avoid this situation, with clear indication that the problem is in the hip, not the knee. The radiographic findings reflect the temporary interruption of blood flow, with necrosis, possible subchondral fracture, collapse of the femoral head, and then regeneration of bone in the secondary ossification center. The radiographic "sagging rope" sign results from a portion of the femoral head (false head) protruding anterolaterally and inferiorly (Kim et al., 1995). Two commonly used methods of grading the femoral head changes radiographically are the Catterall grouping (Catterall, 1971) and more recently the Herring lateral pillar classification (Herring et al., 1992), which has been noted to be a better predictor of final outcome (Farsetti et al., 1995; Ismail & Macnicol, 1998).

Controversy exists regarding the appropriate treatment for Legg-Calvé-Perthes disease, or whether treatment is even necessary. The goal of treatment is to maintain the spherical shape of the femoral head (because it may tend to flatten if left untreated) and to prevent extrusion of the enlarged femoral head (coxa magna) from the joint. Treatment is based on the principle of "containment," preserving the contour of the femoral head and keeping it centered in the acetabulum during the active phase of the disease to prevent premature degenerative arthritis. If the entire femoral head cannot be contained, it is still important to obtain and maintain hip motion, especially hip abduction, and to relieve the commonly seen hinge abduction (Reinker, 1996).

Treatment methods include observation only, ROM exercises, bracing, Petrie casts (two long leg casts with a bar between, holding the hips abducted and internally rotated), and surgery (Wang et al.,

1995). Proximal femoral varus derotation osteotomy (VDRO) decompresses the femoral head, centers it more deeply in the acetabulum when the limb is in the weight-bearing position, and allows long-term remodeling (Eckerwall et al., 1997; Wenger et al., 1991). A pelvic osteotomy may be used alone or combined with VDRO for certain patients (e.g., with a femoral head so large or subluxated that femoral osteotomy alone will not contain the head). A prophylactic trochanteric arrest is often performed to prevent trochanteric overgrowth and the resulting hip abductor muscle weakness (Matan et al., 1996). Kim and Wenger (1997b, 1997c) described the concept of "functional retroversion" and "functional coxa vara" of the deformed femoral head in severe Legg-Calvé-Perthes disease and discussed the use of valgus-flexion-internal rotation femoral osteotomy and acetabuloplasty for correction.

DISCOID LATERAL MENISCUS

The lateral meniscus can develop an abnormal discoid shape, possibly caused by hypermobility, because the more firmly attached medial meniscus rarely develops this discoid shape. A discoid lateral meniscus may become symptomatic, usually between ages 4 and 12 years (Scoles, 1988). It can cause pain, locking, or clicking of the knee, "giving way," and limp. Twenty-five percent of patients have unilateral symptoms but bilateral discoid menisci, and many symptomatic knees also have a meniscal tear (Connolly et al., 1996). In severe cases, meniscectomy provides generally good results (Washington et al., 1995).

SEVER DISEASE

Sever disease, or calcaneal apophysitis, is an osteochondrosis caused by trauma (e.g., traction of the tendo Achillis). This results in the fragmentation or avulsion of cartilage at the point of attachment, disruption of chondrogenesis, reparative callus, fibrosis, and ossification (Siffert, 1981). The child usually has pain in the heel area, exacerbated by sports and especially by running. The condition is usually self-limiting. It may be treated symptomatically with rest, ice, heel cups, heel lifts, reduced activity, and tendo Achillis stretching exercises. A short leg walking cast may be used to relieve severe pain.

GROWING PAINS

"Growing pains" is a diagnosis frequently made by parents and probably is an entity, observable in children when increased stresses occur in the musculoskeletal system, often during periods of rapid growth. Growing pains is a diagnosis of exclusion; that is, all other more serious conditions must be ruled out. The child usually has aching in the legs (typically bilateral and generalized), usually at night and after high levels of activity during the day. Reassurance, symptomatic treatment such as massage and acetaminophen, and time usually resolve the symptoms. The child should be evaluated further if the pain increases or becomes localized or if other symptoms such as chronic fatigue appear.

Transient hip synovitis, described in the birth to age 5 years section, can also be seen in this older age group.

Ages 10 to 15 Years

SLIPPED CAPITAL FEMORAL EPIPHYSIS

Ambroise Pare first described slipped capital femoral epiphysis (SCFE) in 1572. SCFE (also called epiphysiolysis) occurs when the growth plate of the proximal femoral physis is weak and becomes displaced ("slips") from its normal position. This disorder is classified into three subtypes:

1. Acute: occurs with significant trauma and causes immediate, severe pain and restricted hip abduction and internal rotation.
2. Acute-on-chronic: the patient has already experienced some aching in the hip, thigh, or knee for weeks or even months as a result of a chronic slip. Then, with a significant trauma, the epiphysis suddenly slips farther and acute symptoms are noted.
3. Chronic: in this most common form the child has a history of limp and pain, often for weeks or months, and loss of hip motion, especially internal rotation and abduction.

The cause of SCFE is unclear, although many consider it to be part of a generalized metabolic disorder of puberty. It is thought to involve a mechanical failure of the growth plate to resist displacement (Weiner, 1996). It is probably due to alterations in hormonal balance, with or without the stress imposed by acute trauma or the chronic shearing stresses of weight bearing. The incidence of SCFE is 0.71 to 3.41 per 100,000 (Scoles, 1988). African-Americans are more frequently affected than the Caucasian population. Loder reported (1996a, 1996b) on an international multicenter study of 1630 children with 1993 slips. Frequency of slips in various populations worldwide is reviewed, and Loder even notes seasonal variations—in children living north of 40°N latitude, slips occur more often in the summer months. Males are more affected than females, with a 2:1 to 3:1 male-to-female ratio (Scoles, 1988). SCFE occurs about 2 years earlier in males than females and is closely related to the onset of puberty. Slips are bilateral in one quarter to one third of cases (Hurley et al., 1996) and may be more common in younger (11 years, 7 months or less) than older boys (Stasikelis et al., 1996). Obesity is reported in as many as 75% of patients. There is also an association of SCFE in patients with endocrine disorders (Loder et al., 1995) and renal failure and secondary hyperparathyroidism; these slips are usually stable and bilateral (Loder & Hensinger, 1997).

The patient usually has an antalgic limp and pain in the groin, often referred to the anteromedial aspect of the thigh and knee. As with other hip disorders, patients may have only thigh or knee pain and may be referred to a physical therapist for treatment. Knowledge of SCFE and a high index of suspicion will facilitate prompt referral by the physical therapist to an orthopedic surgeon (Pellecchia et al., 1996). The leg is usually held in ER, both when supine and when standing. Decreased hip motion is noted in flexion, abduction, and IR. With attempts to flex the hip, the leg moves into ER.

Radiographs demonstrate that the initial displacement is usually posteriorly and inferiorly and therefore may be missed on an anterior-posterior view. A "frog" view of both hips is needed for diagnosis. Slips are classified as grade I (displacement of the femoral head up to one third of the width of the femoral neck), grade II (more than one third but less than one half), and grade III (more than one half) (Fig. 16–9). MRI has been found to delineate physeal changes preslip, as well as SCFE, sometimes earlier than radiographs and CT (Umans et al., 1998).

The goals of treatment are to keep the displacement to a minimum, maintain motion, and delay or prevent premature degenerative arthritis. Treatment is by surgical fixation, using one or two pins or screws, usually in situ (Crawford, 1996) (Fig. 16–10). Percutaneous pin fixation of chronic slips is safe and effective (Rostoucher et al., 1996; Samuelson & Olney, 1996). With higher degrees of slip, the procedure becomes more technically difficult and the incidence of pin penetration into the joint increases, leading to an increased incidence of chondrolysis (Aronson et al., 1992). Chondrolysis (acute cartilage necrosis of the femoral capital epiphysis) is a severe complication of treated and untreated SCFE with no completely successful treatment (Lubicky, 1996; Warner et al., 1996). There is also a significant danger of AVN with severe and acute slips (Rattey et al., 1996), especially if a forceful reduction is attempted and especially if reduction is attempted with chronic slips. However, Peterson and colleagues (1997) found no increased risk of AVN with manipulative reduction in acute slips, with a 7% incidence in hips reduced less than 24 hours after presentation to a care provider. In unilateral injuries, the contralateral hip may be stabilized prophylactically (Hagglund, 1996; Kumm et al., 1996).

Even though surgically stabilized, most hips with SCFE develop some degenerative changes in later life, especially those with higher-grade slips, along with the complications of chondrolysis and AVN. These can affect the person's choice of occupation and recreational activities as an adult and cause secondary impairments, including hip pain. Goodman and colleagues (1997) examined hip joints in 2665 adult human skeletons and found an 8% prevalence of postslip morphology. They determined that it was

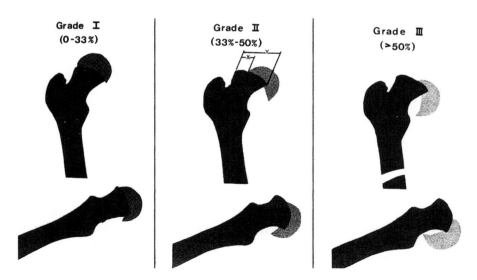

FIGURE 16–9. Classification of the three grades of slipped capital femoral epiphysis. (From Lovell, WW, & Winter, RB [Eds.]. Pediatric Orthopaedics. Philadelphia: JB Lippincott, 1978, p. 767.)

a major risk factor for development of OA, unrelated to age. This provides a good example (along with DDH and Legg-Calvé-Perthes disease) of how a developmental condition in childhood can cause disability later in life. The most severely involved patients may require hip arthrodesis as a salvage procedure (Schoenecker et al., 1997).

OSGOOD-SCHLATTER SYNDROME

Osgood-Schlatter disease, or syndrome, is characterized by activity-related pain and swelling at the insertion of the patellar tendon on the tibial tubercle caused by minor degrees of separation of the tibial tubercle (Salter & Harris, 1963). An association with patella alta has been demonstrated. This increase in patellar height requires an increase in force needed from the quadriceps for full extension and could be responsible for this apophyseal lesion (Aparicio et al., 1997). Unlike SCFE, it is not felt to be an abnormality of physeal development or structure (Yashar, 1995). It may manifest as acute, severe pain, causing a child to limp, or be noted by the child over a period of months as low-grade discomfort, usually brought on by running or playing sports. Treatment consists

of application of ice and rest, decreasing activity, and avoidance of all squatting and jumping activities. Use of a neoprene knee brace may prove helpful. Severe cases may require cast immobilization initially. The condition is usually self-limiting and resolves when the tubercle fuses to the main body of the tibia, usually around age 15 years.

OSTEOCHONDRITIS DISSECANS

Osteochondritis dissecans (OD) is a lesion affecting subchondral bone and the articular surface of a joint. The mechanism producing this disorder is believed to be ischemic necrosis, but the cause is unclear (probably trauma). It is frequently asymptomatic. OD is most commonly noted in the distal femur, usually on the lateral surface of the medial femoral condyle, although it may occur in other areas such as the femoral capital epiphysis (Wood et al., 1995) or the talus (Higuera et al., 1998). The child with OD of the distal femur presents with pain, swelling around the knee, and an antalgic gait. If the fragment separates, the loose body may cause locking of the joint. The lesion is identified as a radiolucent area, usually on the posteromedial aspect of the

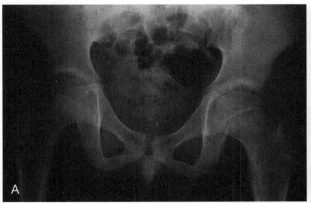

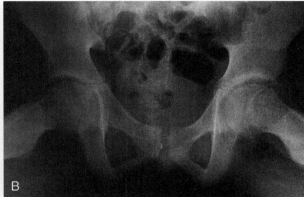

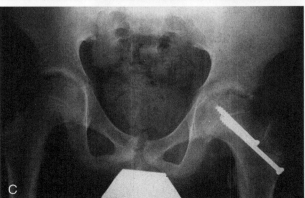

FIGURE 16–10. *A,* Twelve-year-old boy with a 4-month history of hip pain, exacerbated by jumping off a picnic table 2 days previously. The slipped capital femoral epiphysis is not clearly identified on the anterior-posterior view. *B,* Frog view demonstrates a slipped capital femoral epiphysis on the left, thought to be an acute-on-chronic slip by history. *C,* Treatment with percutaneous pin fixation was successful.

distal femur, and thus often cannot be visualized on a straight anterior-posterior radiograph; a notch, or tunnel, view is needed (Fig. 16–11). In mild to moderate cases the treatment may consist of cast immobilization and then graduated activity with quadriceps strengthening exercises. Most cases of OD of the distal femur are self-limiting and heal without surgical intervention. If the defect has separated and an intra-articular loose fragment is present and causing symptoms, surgical treatment is effective in skeletally immature patients. Surgery can include removal or fixation of the loose body, bone grafting, and drilling through the cartilage into the bone in the base of the defect to stimulate healing by growth of new bone (Anderson & Pagnani, 1997; Anderson et al., 1997).

TARSAL COALITION

Tarsal coalition is a failure of segmentation of the hindfoot bones. The connecting tissue may be fibrous, cartilaginous, or bony. Calcaneonavicular and talocalcaneal coalitions are the most common (Fig. 16–12). There may be multiple coalitions in the same foot (Clarke, 1997). Tarsal coalition usually produces symptoms between ages 8 and 12 years when the abnormal cartilaginous bar begins to ossify. The child usually has foot pain, limp, and a rigid flat foot with decreased subtalar motion and peroneal spasm; there may be a history of frequent sprains. The coalition may be defined on plain radiographs of the foot (oblique views). Often CT or MRI provides the most definitive information about the site of the bridging, especially in talocalcaneal coalition. Surgical excision of the coalition is frequently necessary and is usually successful in relieving symptoms (Comfort & Johnson, 1998).

ADDITIONAL CAUSES OF LIMP

Patellofemoral pain and recurrent patellar subluxation or dislocation are two common causes of limp in this age group (see Chapter 17 for a detailed discussion). Monoarticular inflammatory arthritis and gonococcal arthritis also can cause acute onset of limp in a child.

Many types of neoplasms and related bone lesions can cause a child to limp. Commonly seen conditions include osteoid osteoma, unicameral bone cyst, osteochondroma (single or multiple), enchondroma, aneurysmal bone cyst, eosinophilic granuloma, and nonossifying fibroma. Symptoms may include limp, pain, and pathologic fracture through the lesion.

MISCELLANEOUS CONDITIONS

Back Pain

Back pain in adults is frequently mechanical, but back pain in children (especially preadolescents) is often the result of organic causes (Thompson, 1993). Examples of etiology include spondylolysis and spondylolisthesis, infection (e.g., discitis or osteomyelitis), and either benign or malignant tumors. Complaints of back pain in children persisting for more than 1 to 2 weeks should be taken seriously. The

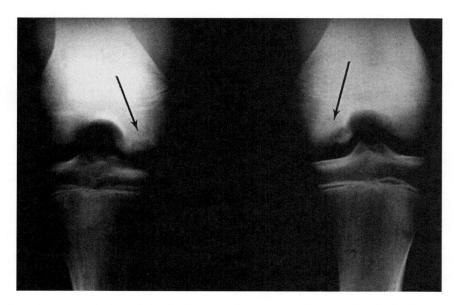

FIGURE 16–11. A notch, or tunnel, view of the distal femurs demonstrates the osteochondritis dissecans lesions, noted by arrows.

child should be referred to a physician for an appropriate workup, especially if the pain is accompanied by fever, neurologic signs, or night pain.

Idiopathic Toe-Walking

A number of children tend to toe-walk some of the time when first walking independently. A smaller subset persist in toe-walking, yet have no history of prematurity or difficult delivery and no evidence of hypertonicity or abnormal developmental reflexes that might lead to a diagnosis of cerebral palsy. This "idiopathic toe-walking" (ITW) usually responds well to a conservative treatment program of therapeutic exercise to stretch the gastrocnemius and soleus muscles and strengthen the ankle dorsiflexors. With significant tendo Achillis contractures, pa-

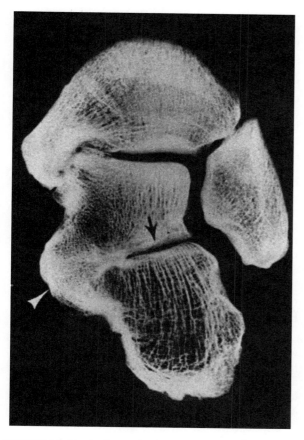

FIGURE 16–12. Radiograph of a coronal section of the foot in a cadaver, demonstrating a talocalcaneal coalition affecting the middle facets of the talus and calcaneus *(arrowhead)* and a normal posterior subtalar joint *(arrow)*. (From Pineda, C, Resnick, D, & Greenway, G. Diagnosis of tarsal coalition with computed tomography. Clinical Orthopaedics and Related Research, *208*:282–288, 1986.)

tients may require serial casting, perhaps with short leg cutout casts to encourage active dorsiflexion. Operative treatment is rarely required and carries the risk of overlengthening, which can cause a serious functional deficit. Stricker and Angulo (1998) compared outcomes in 85 children with ITW and found that patients in the observation only group and the cast or brace group showed little change in passive dorsiflexion and poor parental satisfaction. They surgically treated 15 of 85 children with more severe equinus contractures, resulting in improved dorsiflexion and parental satisfaction.

Differences in knee and ankle kinematics between patients with ITW and spastic diplegia can be documented on gait analysis (Kelly et al., 1997). These children may have "soft" neurologic signs, such as a mild residual asymmetric tonic neck reflex in the quadruped position. Shulman and colleagues (1997) prospectively studied 13 children with persistant toe-walking and found that 10 of 13 had speech or language deficits, with fine motor (4 patients) and gross motor (3 patients) delays as well. There is also a group of idiopathic toe-walkers in which a family history of toe-walking can be documented. This is an autosomal dominant pattern described by Katz and Mubarak (1984).

Achondroplasia

Achondroplasia (dwarfism) is the most common of a large group of conditions known as the osteochondrodysplasias. The incidence is approximately 1 per 10,000 births. It is an autosomal dominant condition with about 90% of cases representing a new mutation (Smith & Jones, 1982). Orthopedic manifestations of this condition include frontal bossing, cuboid-shaped vertebral bodies that may cause narrowing of the spinal canal and cord compression, with short pedicles, lumbar lordosis, short tubular bones, and short trident-shaped hands. The incidence of neurologic complications secondary to spinal abnormalities ranges from 20 to 47%; frequently the symptoms are subtle (Ruiz-Garcia et al., 1997). Persons with achondroplastic dwarfism have abnormal length ratios of limbs to trunk, with more shortening of the proximal segments, in contrast to persons classified as midgets, who have proportionate limb and trunk ratios. Some centers advocate surgical lengthening of the lower extremities for children with dwarfism (Yasui et al., 1997).

Many infants demonstrate hypotonia with transient kyphotic deformity. In 10 to 15% of children this may result in fixed angular kyphosis with serious neurologic sequelae later in life. Discouraging early unsupported sitting is effective, and bracing can also be used (Pauli et al., 1997).

LEG LENGTH INEQUALITY

Leg length inequality (LLI) is also called leg length discrepancy (LLD) and is often defined as 2.5 cm or greater difference in length. Differences smaller than this tend not to cause clinical problems. The difference in leg lengths may be due to relative overgrowth or shortening.

Etiology

The etiology of leg length inequality is divided into a number of categories: trauma, congenital, neuromuscular, acquired diseases, infections causing physeal growth arrest, tumors, and vascular disorders. Types of trauma include epiphyseal and diaphyseal injuries. Epiphyseal injuries with growth plate closure may be asymmetric, such as a fracture involving the medial epiphysis of the distal femur. This type of injury can result in an angular deformity (varus) as well as shortening of the femur.

Congenital disorders include hemihypertrophy, in which one half of the body (the arm and leg) is larger than the other, or hemiatrophy, in which one half of the body is smaller than the other. These can sometimes be difficult to distinguish, necessitating a decision on which arm and leg best "match" the rest of the body. Proximal focal femoral deficiency, congenital coxa vara, fibular and tibial hemimelia, and other focal dysplasias are additional causes of leg length inequality (see Chapter 15). DDH can also cause a leg length discrepancy, due either to an apparent femoral shortening noted when the hip is dislocated or actual shortening caused by femoral head AVN. Surgical treatment of DDH can change the leg length, including VDRO (shortens the femur) and pelvic osteotomies that may add up to 1 inch to the height of the pelvis.

Neuromuscular disorders can cause asymmetric growth of lower extremity bones. Decreased growth in the affected leg may be due to decreased muscle forces in weak or paralyzed muscles. Examples of this include myelodysplasia, poliomyelitis, and hemiplegia caused by congenital or acquired cerebral palsy. However, not all cases of LLI should be corrected. A child with hemiplegia will have a short lower limb on the affected side. Because of weakness and spasticity in that leg, foot clearance may be difficult as a result of decreased hip and knee flexion and equinus positioning of the foot and ankle. The shortness of the leg makes foot clearance in swing easier. A similar situation may be encountered in patients with polio who may advance a weakened leg more easily if it is short.

Acquired conditions such as Legg-Calvé-Perthes disease and SCFE can result in a shortened lower extremity, usually as a result of AVN of the femoral head or occasionally as the result of surgical treatment. Fibrous dysplasia and tumors, including benign bone cysts and malignant neoplasms, can change leg length. This can occur either through interference with growth centers by the disease process or secondarily as a result of fracture or surgical treatment.

Impairments

The effects of LLI vary widely among patients because of the patient's perception of the problem, the actual amount of difference and how well the patient physically compensates for it, the possibility of progression of the inequality and the overall picture of muscle strength, motor control, and ROM. If the discrepancy is marked or compensation is limited, poor cosmesis may be evident, and a significant increase in energy expenditure may be required to walk. Musculoskeletal adaptations and compensations may result. These secondary impairments include pelvic obliquity with changes in spinal alignment that can cause a functional scoliosis or low back pain (9 of 16 patients in a study by Bhave and colleagues, 1996). Other musculoskeletal adaptations may be required at the hip, knee, and ankle, including ipsilateral equinus, pelvic tilt, and contralateral knee flexion. These problems may be significant but easily accommodated because of the inherent energy and motivation usually present in children. However, in adulthood the factors of increased size and weight, increased energy expenditure to walk, increased sensitivity regarding the poor cosmesis of a lurching gait, or long-term effects of asymmetric lumbosacral spinal alignment may combine to significantly reduce the person's ability to walk and even render him or her nonambulatory.

Examination

The physical therapy examination for patients with LLI starts with obtaining a complete history, including any previous treatment. The physical examination incorporates the following elements: clinical analysis of gait, including observation of spine and lower extremity alignment and substitution patterns; observation of the patient with and without assistive devices and shoe lift in gait on level ground, ramps, stairs, and in functional activities, such as rising from a chair to standing and getting down to the floor and back up to standing; measurement of ROM and muscle strength of the trunk, hips, knees, ankles, and feet; body measurements, including both sitting and standing height, weight, and arm span; and leg length measurements.

Two options are available for clinical measurement of leg lengths. One is to level the pelvis in standing, using blocks under the short leg and then measuring the height of the blocks. The other is to measure the legs using various landmarks: anterior-superior iliac spine to medial malleolus, anterior-superior iliac spine to lateral malleolus, anterior-superior iliac spine to heel pad, and umbilicus to heel pad. In a patient without significant lower extremity contractures, leveling the pelvis in standing with blocks may be the most accurate (reproducible). Radiographic measurement of leg lengths is usually done with scanograms. The patient is positioned on the x-ray table with a ruler alongside the legs, and three radiographs are taken on the same cassette, at the level of the hips, knees, and ankles, with the patient held motionless. These three views with the ruler markings next to them allow the examiner to measure the length of the femur and the tibia and combine them for the total leg length. Landmarks commonly used are the top of the femoral head, the bottom of the medial femoral condyle, and the tibial plafond. A film of the left wrist and hand should be performed in conjunction with the scanogram. This allows determination of the skeletal age of the patient, using a reference such as Greulich and Pyle (1950).

A range of measurement error is present in the use of any of these techniques. Validity of the measurement is affected by hip and knee flexion contractures that "shorten" the leg. Determination of bone age is somewhat subjective. These and other factors make both clinical and radiographic leg length determinations an inexact science. The percentage of growth inhibition must also be determined because this assists in estimating the eventual discrepancy at maturity. For example, a 10% inhibition of growth in the short leg may result in a minor discrepancy when the child is quite young. When the leg is 20 cm long, a 10% shortening is 2 cm. However, when the leg is 70 cm long a 10% inhibition of growth will result in a shortening of 7 cm, which is significant.

The most helpful information is gained if the patient can be followed with serial measurements over time, both clinically and by scanogram. Scanogram measurements of total length of both the long and the short leg and the skeletal age at the time of each scanogram can be plotted on the Moseley graph, which depicts past growth and predicts future growth (Moseley, 1977) (Fig. 16–13). Observing the child longitudinally allows more accurate planning for treatment, avoiding errors that are possible when making decisions based on a single measurement.

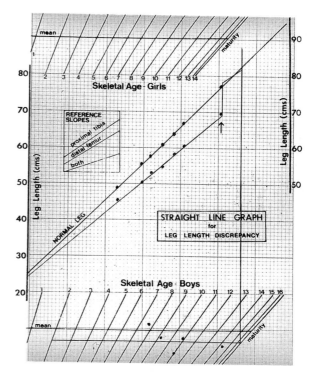

FIGURE 16–13. An example of the use of the Moseley graph to plot a patient's serial scanogram measurements and bone ages to determine the discrepancy at maturity and the possibilities for surgical intervention. Growth of the short leg is depicted by the line below the normal leg line. The increase in the length of the short leg (*arrow*) shows the effects of a leg-lengthening procedure. The two legs are approximately equal at skeletal maturity.

The LLD at the time of skeletal maturity can be predicted to assist in timing of surgery. The effects of surgery can also be plotted on the graph to predict the alteration in leg lengths and the eventual impact on discrepancy at skeletal maturity.

Treatment

Treatment of LLI can be conservative or surgical. Conservative treatment consists of observation only or use of a shoe lift. Surgical treatment is directed at either shortening the long leg or lengthening the short leg. Some patients need both to achieve equality at maturity. Shortening the long leg in the growing child is achieved by epiphysiodesis, the surgical physeal arrest of one or more growth centers in the long leg. This can be an open procedure or can be done percutaneously (Horton & Olney, 1996; Metaizeau et al., 1998). This allows the short leg to "catch up" in length. The fastest growing growth plate in the leg is the distal femur, followed by that of the proximal tibia. The percentages of growth of the leg that occur at each center have been defined as proximal femur 30% and distal femur 70% of the total length of the femur and proximal tibia 60% and distal tibia 40% of the total length of the tibia (Moseley, 1977). The percentages of growth for the entire leg are proximal femur, 15%; distal femur, 35%; proximal tibia, 30%; and distal tibia, 20%. Timing of the epiphysiodesis is obviously crucial. Future growth of each leg must be predicted and the surgery performed at a time when the amount of growth denied the long leg will match the amount of growth still available in the short leg, allowing them to be approximately equal in length at skeletal maturity. If epiphysiodesis is performed too early, the long leg may actually become the short leg, with an obviously less than optimal surgical result. One other option for shortening the long leg is a shortening osteotomy, usually considered in a skeletally mature patient who is not a candidate for epiphysiodesis.

Epiphysiodesis can also be performed on only the medial or lateral part of the growth plate to correct angular deformities. For example, a fracture of the distal femur may cause damage to the medial aspect of the distal femoral growth plate. The lateral part of the growth plate continues to function normally and the leg grows into varus, which also produces a functional shortening. If the medial portion of the growth plate is still open, stapling of the lateral portion can allow the femur to gradually grow out of varus. This type of surgery may also include resection of a bony bar on the involved side of the growth plate.

Limb Lengthening

Surgical lengthening of the short leg has appeal as a treatment alternative because the surgery is performed on the affected leg, not the "normal" leg, and the opportunity exists for correction of discrepancies of much greater magnitude. Criteria for leg lengthening include a discrepancy of greater than 4 to 6 cm, adequate soft tissue mobility available to allow correction, and a stable joint above and below, although unstable joints can be protected with an external frame. A decision must be made whether to lengthen the femur or the tibia or both. Ideally the final result will be fairly equal leg lengths and equal knee heights in standing. If the discrepancy is too large to be amenable to these procedures, as in some cases of proximal focal femoral deficiency, amputation of the distal segment to allow the use of a prosthesis would be considered to be the most practical alternative (see Chapter 15). Another option is a rotationplasty of the affected limb (Torode & Gillespie, 1983).

Limb lengthening was first reported in the literature by Codivilla in Italy in 1905 (Coleman & Scott, 1991), and the field has expanded significantly since that time. Two biologic approaches to lengthening exist: 1) lengthening through bone and 2) lengthening by physeal distraction. Physeal distraction includes the option of subacute epiphysiolysis, initially described by Monticelli and Spinelli and called chondrodiatasis (Coleman & Scott, 1991). It consists of gradual distraction of the growth plate using a circular fixator, leading to a sudden rupture of the growth plate 3 to 4 days after the procedure begins. This is rarely used except for adolescent limb lengthening near the end of the patient's growth, because it may lead to premature closure of the growth plate.

A number of devices have been developed for lengthening bone, including diaphyseal lengthening devices (Wagner, unilateral frame) and metaphyseal lengthening devices, such as the Ilizarov (circular frame), Monticelli-Spinelli (circular frame and half ring), and DeBastiani (Orthofix unilateral frame) devices (Coleman & Scott, 1991). The Wagner technique for lengthening through bone, used extensively in the United States from 1970 to 1990, involves an osteotomy of the bone followed by rapid distraction, with cancellous bone grafting and plating of the distraction gap (Wagner, 1978).

Dr. Gavriil Abramovich Ilizarov first developed his technique and device in Russia to treat World War II veterans and later widened the applications (Ilizarov & Ledyaev, 1969). The Ilizarov method of slow distraction does not use bone grafting of the distraction gap. The circular design and the custom fitting of the external fixator allows simultaneous correction of rotational and angular deformities, as well as achieving the lengthening (Stanitski et al., 1996). The standard rate of distraction is usually about 1 mm per day. The frequency of distraction is usually four times per day (0.25 mm each time). After the desired correction has been achieved, the fixator is left in place to allow consolidation of new bone. Aaron and Eilert (1996) noted few complications with the multiaxial Ilizarov external fixator compared with the Wagner method. Many applications of the Ilizarov technique are currently in use for both adult and pediatric disorders, including limb length discrepancy, angular deformities such as adolescent Blount's disease, congenital tibial pseudarthrosis, resistant or recurrent clubfeet, correction of forearm or humeral shortening and deformity due to trauma or infection, and others (Rajacich et al., 1992). Another, more controversial, indication for leg lengthening is its bilateral use in patients with achondroplasia to achieve a more normal height (Paley, 1988).

Paley and colleagues (1997) have described femoral lengthening over an intramedullary (IM) nail. The IM nail is inserted concomitantly with the external fixator. Once the distraction phase is completed the nail is locked with two screws and the external fixator is removed. The IM nail then protects the bone from fracture during the consolidation phase, and the decreased time with external fixation allows earlier rehabilitation. Monolateral external fixation can be used to lengthen bones in patients with LLI or short stature if angular correction is not needed (Noonan et al., 1998).

Complications of lengthening procedures can be divided into five categories: bone, joint, nerve, muscle, and vascular complications. Bone complications include angulation, delayed union or nonunion, fractures, pin tract infections, and osteomyelitis. Joint complications include cartilage degeneration, stiffness, subluxation, or dislocation. Nerves can suffer stretch paralysis that may be transient or permanent. Complications of muscle include weakness, contracture, and ischemia. There may also be vascular complications, such as a transient hypertension, probably due to stretching of the sciatic nerve, although this has not been well documented. A higher rate of complications has been noted in patients whose LLI is secondary to an underlying bone disorder (Naudie et al., 1998). As defined by Paley (1990), "problems" following lengthening procedures represent difficulties that do not require operative intervention, "obstacles" require operative intervention, and true "complications" include all problems that do not resolve by the end of treatment.

Children undergoing leg lengthening must adjust to the pain of the procedure, which can be significant and extended (Young et al., 1994). The child may experience frustration, anger, and fear because of the temporary loss of independence inherent in the procedure. Difficult behavior may require intervention by a psychologist to assist the child and family in developing appropriate coping strategies. Candidates for surgical lengthening must be extremely motivated, with a supportive and committed family. Successful limb lengthening also mandates a comprehensive medical care system, with knowledgeable, experienced physicians, nurses, and therapists to guide the patient and family through the process.

Role of Physical Therapy in Limb Lengthening

Physical therapy involvement with the child undergoing limb lengthening may vary with the patient and the institution in which the procedure is performed. An excellent description of the physical therapy goals and program for these patients is provided by Simard and colleagues (1992). They describe the preoperative and postoperative phases of intervention in patients undergoing leg lengthening by the Ilizarov technique. Before the surgery, the physical therapy examination includes the following components: muscle strength, passive ROM, sensation, girth of thighs and calves, leg length discrepancy, and joint stability. Bony deformities, if present, are described. Posture, gait, and functional mobility skills are documented. The patient is fitted with crutches and instructed in their use, maintaining restricted weight bearing on the involved leg. In conjunction with the patient, parents, and any other caregivers involved, a program of home exercise and postoperative positioning and splinting is developed, as well as stretching and strengthening exercises to use in preparation for surgery.

The greatest challenges for the physical therapist treating children in the postoperative phase include promoting weight bearing in the presence of significant pain, maintaining the child's ROM, and motivating the patient to continue with the program both in the hospital and at home over the long period of treatment. There can also be significant difficulty in obtaining funding for physical therapy because insurance carriers usually want documentation of improved function during the treatment period. For the patient undergoing leg lengthening by the Ilizarov technique, the goal is to maintain ambulation, joint ROM, and strength while undergoing the lengthening, with a long-term goal of improved function after the device is removed.

The postoperative phase includes instruction in functional activities, active assistive and isometric exercise, proper positioning of the extremity, gait training with progressive weight bearing as tolerated, and pin care. Modalities such as ice or transcutaneous electrical nerve stimulation may be useful for pain management. Dynamic splinting may be used in the limb-lengthening stage to provide low-intensity, prolonged stretch to joints with significantly limited ROM. Exercise techniques useful throughout the Ilizarov lengthening include both closed- and open-chain exercise for strengthening and active-assistive or passive exercise for ROM. A stationary bicycle and treadmill may be used. After removal of the fixator, the patient may require additional gait training, monitoring and adjusting of the exercise program, and possibly refitting and retraining with orthotic or prosthetic devices worn preoperatively. Throughout the course of treatment, children are encouraged to participate in their usual school and leisure activities to the fullest extent possible.

CASE HISTORY
AMY

Amy was referred for orthopedic consultation at 1 day of age. The following clinical findings were documented: positive Galeazzi sign on the left with the femur approximately 2 cm short, hip abduction right/left 70°/40°, 2 cm shortening of the left tibia measured clinically, a band in the area of the left fibula, and calcaneovalgus of the left foot. Radiographs showed both hips located, with coxa vara and decreased femoral neck length, a slight bow of the left femur, shortening of the left femur by 2 cm and the left tibia 1 cm compared with the right, and complete absence of the left fibula. The diagnosis was made of left proximal focal femoral deficiency and absent left fibula.

The following summary documents the progression of Amy's limb length discrepancy as she grew older and her treatment:

1 month:	Physical therapy—home exercise program
10 months:	Excision of fibular anlage, peroneus longus muscle lengthening; scanogram showed 5.6 cm of shortening
13 months:	Fitted with a step-in prosthesis, follow-up physical therapy. Options for treatment: (1) knee fusion and Syme amputation, followed by fitting with a below-knee prosthesis; (2) maintain use of her step-in prosthesis; (3) modified rotationplasty. Her parents opted for a prosthesis.
2 years:	Using step-in prosthesis, able to run and jump; left leg 7.3 cm short by scanogram
3 years:	Left leg 9.2 cm short, continuing with the 20% inhibition of growth noted earlier
8 years:	Left leg 12.7 cm short; able to ski with step-in prosthesis
9 years, 9 months:	Left Salter pelvic osteotomy to correct mild acetabular dysplasia

At age 10 years, through use of the Canadian Occupational Performance Measure, it was clarified that the most important concerns of Amy and her parents included her awkward gait and poor cosmesis. The poor cosmesis had only recently become a concern for Amy, due to her increasing awareness of how she was viewed by her peers. In addition, Amy felt that she was limited in her athletic abilities because of her leg length discrepancy and she wanted very much to participate more actively in competitive sports.

Examination of Amy's left leg showed significant impairments, including shortening of the femur and tibia, external rotational deformity of the femur, genu valgum secondary to a hypoplastic lateral femoral condyle, an apex medial bow in the tibia, and equinus of the ankle. Her projected leg length inequality at skeletal maturity was 18 cm.

Working in concert, Amy's physical therapist and orthopedic surgeon recommended a limb-lengthening procedure. This was agreed to by the child and family, who were very much against the only other alternative of amputation. Long-term goals of the surgery included independent ambulation without bracing or assistive devices, a smoother gait with decreased energy expenditure, increased agility in sports, improved cosmesis, and possibly decreased potential for future disability resulting from greatly disparate leg lengths.

Surgery consisted of application of Ilizarov frames to the left femur, tibia, and foot to accomplish femoral lengthening, rotational and angular correction, and tibial lengthening and angular correction. A tendo Achillis lengthening was also performed. Amy's initial lengthening was 0.25 mm four times a day, in both the femur and tibia. This rate provided 1 mm of lengthening in each bone every 24 hours.

The following summary documents her progress during the course of postoperative treatment:

3 weeks:	Attending school part time. Knee extension—15°; physical therapy program of active and active-assistive ROM and strengthening exercises
4 weeks:	Left tibia subluxating posteriorly on femur; rate of lengthening decreased temporarily
3 months:	Foot frame removed; weight bearing as tolerated; ongoing exercise program of ROM exercises of left knee and ankle, strengthening exercises for quadriceps, hip abductor, and hip extensor muscles; able to exercise in pool
7 months:	Tibial frame removed with 3 cm of tibial lengthening achieved; knee passively taken through ROM at the time of surgery, to aid in ROM exercises postoperatively
8 months:	Resumed an aggressive knee ROM exercise program; care was taken to support the tibia just distal to the knee during exercise, avoiding a long lever arm across the regenerate bone site
9 months:	Losing knee ROM; continuous passive motion machine instituted 4 hours per day; dynamic splint also used

10 months:	Femoral frame removed with 13 cm of femoral lengthening achieved
10.5 months:	5-day history of deformity of the proximal femur and increased pain; diagnosis of femoral fracture through one of the half-pin sites; closed reduction, insertion of distal femoral traction pin, and application of Neufeld traction
11 months:	Further closed reduction, removal of traction pin, and application of a spica cast
12 months:	Total contact HKAFO, with free hip, knee, and ankle joints; worn full time, with time out for bathing; ROM exercise (active only)
13 months:	Radiographs showed evidence of an additional, healing pathologic stress fracture of the femur
14.5 months:	Able to walk well with HKAFO and one crutch, no pain; extensive stretching and strengthening program through physical therapy, physical education at school, and home exercise program

Even with the added complication of femoral fractures, Amy achieved good results from her surgery. Of the original projected discrepancy of 18 cm, a total of 16 cm was gained through the femoral and tibial lengthenings, and her knees were essentially level. This abbreviated documentation of the process can only hint at the incredible amount of work, time, and commitment required by this type of treatment on the part of everyone involved.

ACKNOWLEDGMENTS

I would like to thank C. Douglas Wallace, MD, for his review and helpful comments for this chapter.

References

Aaron, AD, & Eilert, RE. Results of the Wagner and Ilizarov methods of limb-lengthening. Journal of Bone and Joint Surgery (American), 78:20–29, 1996.

Anderson, AF, & Pagnani, MJ. Osteochondritis dissecans of the femoral condyles. Long-term results of excision of the fragment. American Journal of Sports Medicine, 25:830–834, 1997.

Anderson, AF, Richards, DB, Pagnani, MJ, & Hovis, WD. Antegrade drilling for osteochondritis dissecans of the knee. Arthroscopy, 13:319–324, 1997.

Aparicio, G, Abril, JC, Calvo, E, & Alvarez, L. Radiologic study of patellar height in Osgood-Schlatter disease. Journal of Pediatric Orthopaedics, 17:63–66, 1997.

Aronson, DD, Peterson, DA, & Miller, DV. Slipped capital femoral epiphysis: The case for internal fixation in situ. Clinical Orthopaedics and Related Research, 281:115–122, 1992.

Bennett, OM, & Namnyak, SS. Acute septic arthritis of the hip joint in infancy and childhood. Clinical Orthopaedics and Related Research, 281:123–132, 1992.

Bhave, A, Herzenberg, JE, & Paley, D. Gait asymmetries with leg length discrepancy (LLD): Symmetry after leg lengthening. Pediatric Orthopaedic Society of North America Annual Meeting, scientific poster, 1996.

Bruce, RW, Jr. Torsional and angular deformities. Pediatric Clinics of North America, 43: 867–881, 1996.

Cahuzac, JP, Hobatho, MC, Baunin, C, Boulot, J, Darmana, R, & Autefage, A. Classification of 125 children with rotational abnormalities. Journal of Pediatric Orthopaedics, Part B, 1:59–66, 1992.

Cahuzac, JP, Vardon, D, & Sales de Gauzy, J. Development of the clinical tibiofemoral angle in normal adolescents. A study of 427 normal subjects from 10 to 16 years of age. Journal of Bone and Joint Surgery (British), 77:729–732, 1995.

Cameron, JC, & Saha, S. External tibial torsion: An underrecognized cause of recurrent patellar dislocation. Clinical Orthopaedics and Related Research, 328:177–184, 1996.

Catterall, A. The natural history of Perthes' disease. Journal of Bone and Joint Surgery (British), 53:37–53, 1971.

Clarke, DM. Multiple tarsal coalitions in the same foot. Journal of Pediatric Orthopaedics, 17:777–780, 1997.

Coleman, SS, & Scott, SM. The present attitude toward the biology and technology of limb lengthening. Clinical Orthopaedics and Related Research, 264:76–83, 1991.

Comfort, TK, & Johnson, LO. Resection for symptomatic talocalcaneal coalition. Journal of Pediatric Orthopaedics, 18:283–288, 1998.

Connolly, B, Babyn, PS, Wright, JG, & Thorner, PS. Discoid meniscus in children: Magnetic resonance imaging characteristics. Canadian Association of Radiology Journal, 47:347–354, 1996.

Crane, L. Femoral torsion and its relation to toeing-in and toeing-out. Journal of Bone and Joint Surgery (American), 41:421–428, 1959.

Crawford, AH. Role of osteotomy in the treatment of slipped capital femoral epiphysis. Journal of Pediatric Orthopaedics (British), 5:102–109, 1996.

Dales, MC, & Hoffinger, SA. Septic hip in older children and adolescents (Abstract). Proceedings of the American Academy of Orthopaedic Surgeons Annual Meeting, San Francisco. American Academy of Orthopaedic Surgeons, 1993.

Davids, JR, Benson, LJ, Mubarak, SJ, & McNeil, N. Ultrasonography and developmental dysplasia of the hip: A cost-benefit analysis of three delivery systems. Journal of Pediatric Orthopaedics, 15:325–329, 1995.

De Alba, CC, Guille, JT, Bowen, JR, & Harcke, HT. Computed tomography for femoral and tibial torsion in children with clubfoot. Clinical Orthopaedics and Related Research, 353:203–209, 1998.

Delgado, ED, Schoenecker, PL, Rich, MM, & Capelli, AM. Treatment of severe torsional malalignment syndrome. Journal of Pediatric Orthopaedics, 16:484–488, 1996.

Donaldson, JS, & Feinstein, KA. Imaging of developmental dysplasia of the hip. Pediatric Clinics of North America, 44:591–614, 1997.

Dunn, PM. Perinatal observations of the etiology of congenital dislocation of the hip. Clinical Orthopaedics and Related Research, 119:11–22, 1976.

Eckerwall, G, Hochbergs, P, Wingstrand, H, & Egund, N. Magnetic resonance imaging and early remodeling of the femoral head after femoral varus osteotomy in Legg-Calvé-Perthes disease. Journal of Pediatric Orthopaedics (British), 6:239–244, 1997.

Engel, GM, & Staheli, LT. The natural history of torsion and other factors influencing gait in childhood. Clinical Orthopaedics and Related Research, 99:12–17, 1974.

Fabry, G, MacEwen, D, & Shands, AR. Torsion of the femur: A follow-up study in normal and abnormal conditions. Journal of Bone and Joint Surgery (American), 55:1726–1738, 1973.

Farsetti, P, Tudisco, C, Caterini, R, Potenza, V, & Ippolito, E. The Herring lateral pillar classification for prognosis in Perthes disease. Late results in 49 patients treated conservatively. Journal of Bone and Joint Surgery (British), 77:739–742, 1995.

Farsetti, P, Weinstein, SL, & Ponseti, IV. The long-term functional and radiographic outcomes of untreated and non-operatively treated metatarsus adductus. Journal of Bone and Joint Surgery (American), 76:257–265, 1994.

Galpin, RD, Roach, JW, Wenger, DR, Herring, JA, & Birch, JG. One-stage treatment of congenital dislocation of the hip in older children, including femoral shortening. Journal of Bone and Joint Surgery (American), 71:734–741, 1989.

Glazer, PA, & Hu, SS. Pediatric spinal infections. Orthopaedic Clinics of North America, 27:111–123, 1996.

Glueck, CJ, Brandt, G, Gruppo, R, Crawford, A, Roy, D, Tracy, T, Stroop, D, Wang, P, & Becker, A. Resistance to activated protein C and Legg-Perthes disease. Clinical Orthopaedics and Related Research, 338:139–152, 1997.

Glueck, CJ, Freiberg, RA, Crawford, A, Gruppo, R, Roy, D, Tracy, T, Sieve-Smith, L, & Wang, P. Secondhand smoke, hypofibrinolysis, and Legg-Perthes disease. Clinical Orthopaedics and Related Research, 352:159–167, 1998.

Goodman, DA, Feighan, JE, Smith, AD, Latimer, B, Buly, RL, & Cooperman, DR. Subclinical slipped capital femoral epiphysis. Relationship to osteoarthrosis of the hip. Journal of Bone and Joint Surgery (American), 79:1489–1497, 1997.

Graf, R. Hip sonography—how reliable? Sector scanning versus linear scanning? Dynamic versus static examination? Clinical Orthopaedics and Related Research, 281:18–21, 1992.

Greulich, WW, & Pyle, SI. Radiographic Atlas of Skeletal Development of the Hand and Wrist. Stanford, CA: Stanford University Press, 1950.

Hagglund, G. The contralateral hip in slipped capital femoral epiphysis. Journal of Pediatric Orthopaedics (British), 5:158–161, 1996.

Harcke, HT. Imaging in congenital dislocation and dysplasia of the hip. Clinical Orthopaedics and Related Research, 281:22–28, 1992.

Hensinger, RH, & Jones, ET. Neonatal orthopaedics. In Oliver, TK (Ed.), Monographs in Neonatalogy. New York: Grune & Stratton, 1981.

Herring, JA, Neustadt, JB, Williams, JJ, Early, JS, & Browne, RH. The lateral pillar classification of Legg-Calvé-Perthes disease. Journal of Pediatric Orthopaedics, 12:143–150, 1992.

Higuera, J, Laguna, R, Peral, M, Aranda, E, & Soleto, J. Osteochondritis dissecans of the talus during childhood and adolescence. Journal of Pediatric Orthopaedics, 18:328–332, 1998.

Hofmann, A, Jones, RE, & Herring, JA. Blount's disease after skeletal maturity. Journal of Bone and Joint Surgery (American), 64:1004–1009, 1982.

Horton, GA, & Olney, BW. Epiphysiodesis of the lower extremity: Results of the percutaneous technique. Journal of Pediatric Orthopaedics, 16:180–182, 1996.

Hughes, LO, & Aronson, J. Skeletal infections in children. Current Opinions in Pediatrics, 6:90–93, 1994.

Hummer, CD, & MacEwen, GD. The coexistence of torticollis and congenital dysplasia of the hip. Journal of Bone and Joint Surgery (American), 54:1255–1256, 1972.

Hurley, JM, Betz, RR, Loder, RT, Davidson, RS, Alburger, PD, & Steel, HH. Slipped capital femoral epiphysis. The prevalence of late contralateral slip. Journal of Bone and Joint Surgery (American), 78:226–230, 1996.

Ilfeld, FW, Westin, GW, & Makin, M. Missed or developmental dislocation of the hip. Clinical Orthopaedics and Related Research, 203:276–281, 1986.

Ilizarov, GA, & Ledyaev, VI. The replacement of long tubular bone defects by lengthening distraction osteotomy of one of the fragments. Vestnik. Khururgii, 6:78, 1969. (Translated by Schwartzman, V. Clinical Orthopaedics and Related Research, 280:7–10, 1992.)

Ismail, AM, & Macnicol, MF. Prognosis in Perthes' disease: A comparison of radiological predictors. Journal of Bone and Joint Surgery (British), 80:310–314, 1998.

Jasty, M, Anderson, MJ, & Harris, WH. Total hip replacement for developmental dysplasia of the hip. Clinical Orthopaedics and Related Research, 311:40–45, 1995.

Johnson, CE. Infantile tibia vara. Clinical Orthopaedics and Related Research, 255:13–23, 1990.

Katz, MM, & Mubarak, SJ. Hereditary tendo Achillis contractures. Journal of Pediatric Orthopaedics, 4:711–714, 1984.

Kelly, IP, Jenkinson, A, Stephens, M, & O'Brien, T. The kinematic patterns of toe-walkers. Journal of Pediatric Orthopaedics, 17:478–480, 1997.

Kelo, MJ, & Riddle, DL. Examination and management of a patient with tarsal coalition. Physical Therapy, 78:518–525, 1998.

Kim, HT, Eisenhauer, E, & Wenger, DR. The "sagging rope sign" in avascular necrosis in children's hip diseases—confirmation by 3D CT studies. Iowa Orthopaedic Journal, 15:101–111, 1995.

Kim, HT, & Wenger, DR. "Functional retroversion" of the femoral head in Legg-Calvé-Perthes disease and epiphyseal dysplasia: Analysis of head-neck deformity and its effect on limb position using three-dimensional computed tomography. Journal of Pediatric Orthopaedics, 17:240–246, 1997a.

Kim, HT, & Wenger, DR. Surgical correction of "functional retroversion" and "functional coxa vara" in late Legg-Calvé-Perthes disease and epiphyseal dysplasia: Correction of deformity defined by new imaging modalities. Journal of Pediatric Orthopaedics, 17:247–254, 1997b.

Kim, HT, & Wenger, DR. The morphology of residual acetabular deficiency in childhood hip dysplasia: Three dimensional computed tomographic analysis. Journal of Pediatric Orthopaedics, 17:637–647, 1997c.

Krivickas, LS. Anatomical factors associated with overuse sports injuries. Sports Medicine, 24:132–146, 1997.

Kumm, DA, Schmidt, J, Eisenburger, SH, Rutt, J, & Hackenbroch, MH. Prophylactic dynamic screw fixation of the asymptomatic hip in slipped capital femoral epiphysis. Journal of Pediatric Orthopaedics, 16:249–253, 1996.

Lahdes-Vasama, TT, Sipila, IS, Lamminranta, S, Pihko, SH, Merikanto, EO, & Marttinen, EJ. Psychosocial development and premorbid skeletal growth in Legg-Calvé-Perthes disease: A study of nineteen patients. Journal of Pediatric Orthopaedics (British), 6:133–137, 1997.

Lane, NE, Nevitt, MC, Cooper, C, Pressman, A, Gore, R, & Hochberg, M. Acetabular dysplasia and osteoarthritis of the hip in elderly white women. Annals of Rheumatic Disorders, 56:627–630, 1997.

Langenskiold, A. Tibia vara: A critical review. Clinical Orthopaedics and Related Research, 246:195–206, 1989.

Lee, J, Jarvis, J, Uhthoff, HK, & Avruch, L. The fetal acetabulum. Clinical Orthopaedics and Related Research, 281:48–55, 1992.

Loder, RT. The demographics of slipped capital femoral epiphysis. An international multicenter study. Clinical Orthopaedics and Related Research, 322:8–27, 1996a.

Loder, RT. A worldwide study on the seasonal variation of slipped capital femoral epiphysis. Clinical Orthopaedics and Related Research, 322:28–36, 1996b.

Loder, RT, Brown, KL, Zaleske, DJ, & Jones, ET. Extremity lawn-mower injuries in children: Report by the Research Committee of the Pediatric Orthopaedic Society of North America. Journal of Pediatric Orthopaedics, 17:360–369, 1997.

Loder, RT, Farley, FA, Herring, JA, Schork, MA, & Shyr, Y. Bone age determination in children with Legg-Calvé-Perthes disease: A comparison of two methods. Journal of Pediatric Orthopaedics, 15:90–94, 1995.

Loder, RT, & Hensinger, RN. Slipped capital femoral epiphysis associated with renal failure osteodystrophy. Journal of Pediatric Orthopaedics, 17:205–211, 1997.

Loder, RT, Wittenberg, B, & DeSilva, G. Slipped capital femoral epiphysis associated with endocrine disorders. Journal of Pediatric Orthopaedics, 15:349–356, 1995.

Lovell, WW, & Winter, RB. Pediatric Orthopaedics, Vols. I and II. Philadelphia: JB Lippincott, 1978.

Lubicky, JP. Chondrolysis and avascular necrosis: Complications of slipped capital femoral epiphysis. Journal of Pediatric Orthopaedics (British), 5:162–167, 1996.

Matan, AJ, Stevens, PM, Smith, JT, & Santora, SD. Combination trochanteric arrest and intertrochanteric osteotomy for Perthes' disease. Journal of Pediatric Orthopaedics, 16:10–14, 1996.

Meister, K, & James, SL. Proximal tibial derotation osteotomy for anterior knee pain in the miserably malaligned extremity. American Journal of Orthopaedics, 24:149–155, 1995.

Metaizeau, JP, Wong-Chung, J, Bertrand, H, & Pasquier, P. Percutaneous epiphysiodesis using transphyseal screws (PETS). Journal of Pediatric Orthopaedics, 18:363–369, 1998.

Michaeli, DA, Murphy, SB, & Hipp, JA. Comparison of predicted and measured contact pressures in normal and dysplastic hips. Medical Engineering & Physics, 19:180–186, 1997.

Mielke, CH, & Stevens, PM. Hemiepiphyseal stapling for knee deformities in children younger than 10 years: A preliminary report. Journal of Pediatric Orthopaedics, 16:423–429, 1996.

Moreuende, JA, & Ponseti, IV. Congenital metatarsus adductus in early human fetal development: A histologic study. Clinical Orthopaedics and Related Research, 333:261–266, 1996.

Mosca, VS. Calcaneal lengthening for valgus deformity of the hindfoot. Results in children who had severe, symptomatic flatfoot and skewfoot. Journal of Bone and Joint Surgery (American), 77:500–512, 1995.

Moseley, CF. A straight-line graph for leg-length discrepancies. Journal of Bone and Joint Surgery (American), 59:174–179, 1977.

Mubarak, SJ, Beck, L, & Sutherland, D. Home traction in the management of congenital dislocation of the hips. Journal of Pediatric Orthopaedics, 6:721–723, 1986.

Mubarak, SJ, Garfin, SR, Vance, R, McKinnon, B, & Sutherland, D. Pitfalls in the use of the Pavlik harness for treatment of congenital dysplasia, subluxation, and dislocation of the hip. Journal of Bone and Joint Surgery (American), 63:1239–1248, 1981.

Mubarak, SJ, Leach, JL, & Wenger, DR. Management of congenital dislocation of the hip in the infant. Contemporary Orthopaedics, 15:29–44, 1987.

Naudie, D, Hamdy, RC, Fassier, F, & Duhaime, M. Complications of limb-lengthening in children who have an underlying bone disorder. Journal of Bone and Joint Surgery (American), 80:18–24, 1998.

Noonan, KJ, Leyes, M, Forriol, F, & Canadell, J. Distraction osteogenesis of the lower extremity with use of monolateral external fixation. Journal of Bone and Joint Surgery (American), 80:793–806, 1998.

Olney, B, Latz, K, & Asher, M. Treatment of hip dysplasia in older children with a combined one-stage procedure. Clinical Orthopaedics and Related Research, 347:215–223, 1998.

Paley, D. Current techniques of limb lengthening. Journal of Pediatric Orthopaedics, 8:73–92, 1988.

Paley, D. Problems, obstacles, and complications of limb lengthening by the Ilizarov technique. Clinical Orthopaedics and Related Research, 250:81–104, 1990.

Paley, D, Herzenberg, JE, Paremain, G, & Bhave, A. Femoral lengthening over an intramedullary nail. Journal of Bone and Joint Surgery (American), 79:1464–1480, 1997.

Pauli, RM, Breed, A, Horton, VK, Glinski, LP, & Reiser, CA. Prevention of fixed, angular kyphosis in achondroplasia. Journal of Pediatric Orthopaedics, 17:726–733, 1997.

Pavlik, A. Stirrups as an aid in the treatment of congenital dysplasias of the hip in children. LeKarskeListy 5(3-4):81–85, 1950. (Translated by Bialik, V, & Reis, ND. Journal of Pediatric Orthopaedics, 9:157–159, 1989.)

Pavlik, A. The functional method of treatment using a harness with stirrups as the primary method of conservative therapy for infants with congenital dislocation of the hip. Zeitschrift fur Orthopadie und Ihre Grenzgebeit 89:341, 1957. (Translated by Peltier, LF. Clinical Orthopaedics and Related Research, 281:4–10, 1992.)

Pellecchia, GL, Lugo-Larcheveque, N, & Deluca, PA. Differential diagnosis in physical therapy evaluation of thigh pain in an adolescent boy. Journal of Orthopedic and Sports Physical Therapy, 23:51–55, 1996.

Peterson, MD, Weiner, DS, Green, NE, & Terry, CL. Acute slipped capital femoral epiphysis: The value and safety of urgent manipulative reduction. Journal of Pediatric Orthopaedics, 17:648–654, 1997.

Pineda, C, Resnick, D, & Greenway, G. Diagnosis of tarsal coalition with computed tomography. Clinical Orthopaedics and Related Research, 208:282–288, 1986.

Pitkow, RB. External rotation contracture of the extended hip. Clinical Orthopaedics and Related Research, 110:139–144, 1975.

Rajacich, N, Bell, DF, & Armstrong, PF. Pediatric applications of the Ilizarov method. Clinical Orthopaedics and Related Research, 280: 72–80, 1992.

Rattey, T, Piehl, F, & Wright, JG. Acute slipped capital femoral epiphysis. Review of outcomes and rates of avascular necrosis. Journal of Bone and Joint Surgery (American), 78:398–402, 1996.

Reinker, KA. Early diagnosis and treatment of hinge abduction in Legg-Perthes disease. Journal of Pediatric Orthopaedics, 16:3–9, 1996.

Riebel, TW, Nasir, R, & Nazarenko, O. The value of sonography in the detection of osteomyelitis. Pediatric Radiology, 26:291–297, 1996.

Rosendahl, K, Markestad, T, & Lie, RT. Ultrasound screening for developmental dysplasia of the hip in the neonate: The effect on treatment rate and prevalence of late cases. Pediatrics, 94:47–52, 1994.

Rostoucher, P, Bensahel, H, Pennecot, GF, Kaewpornsawan, K, & Mazda, K. Slipped capital femoral epiphysis: Evaluation of different modes of treatment. Journal of Pediatric Orthopaedics (British), 5:96–101, 1996.

Ruiz-Garcia, M, Tovar-Baudin, A, Del Castillo-Ruiz, V, Rodriguez, HP, Collado, MA, Mora, TM, Rueda-Franco, F, & Gonzalez-Astiazaran, A. Early detection of neurological manifestations in achondroplasia. Child's Nervous System, 13:208–213, 1997.

Sachithanandam, V, & Joseph, B. The influence of footwear on the prevalence of flat foot. A survey of 1846 skeletally mature persons. Journal of Bone and Joint Surgery (British), 77:254–257, 1995.

Salter, RB. Etiology, pathogenesis and possible prevention of congenital dislocation of the hip. Canadian Medical Association Journal, 98:933–945, 1968.

Salter, RB. Textbook of Disorders and Injuries of the Musculoskeletal System. Baltimore: Williams & Wilkins, 1970.

Salter, RB, & Harris, WR. Injuries involving the epiphyseal plate. Journal of Bone and Joint Surgery (American), 45:587–622, 1963.

Samuelson, T, & Olney, B. Percutaneous pin fixation of chronic slipped capital femoral epiphysis. Clinical Orthopaedics and Related Research, 326:225–228, 1996.

Schoenecker, PL, Johnson, LO, Martin, RA, Doyle, P, & Capelli, AM. Intra-articular hip arthrodesis without subtrochanteric osteotomy in adolescents: Technique and short-term follow-up. American Journal of Orthopaedics, 26:257–264, 1997.

Scoles, PV. Pediatric Orthopaedics in Clinical Practice, 2nd ed. Chicago: Year Book, 1988.

Scoles, PV, Boyd, A, & Jones, PK. Roentgenographic parameters of the normal infant hip. Journal of Pediatric Orthopaedics, 7:656–663, 1987.

Shands, AR, & Steele, MK. Torsion of the femur: A follow-up report on the use of the Dunlap method for its determination. Journal of Bone and Joint Surgery (American), 40:803–816, 1958.

Shulman, LH, Sala, DA, Chu, ML, McCaul, PR, & Sandler, BJ. Developmental implications of idiopathic toe walking. Journal of Pediatrics, 130:541–546, 1997.

Siffert, RS. Classification of the osteochondroses. Clinical Orthopaedics and Related Research, 158:10–18, 1981.

Simard, S, Marchant, M, & Mencio, G. The Ilizarov procedure: Limb lengthening and its implications. Physical Therapy, 72:25–34, 1992.

Smith, BG, Millis, MB, Hey, LA, Jaramillo, D, & Kasser, JR. Postreduction computed tomography in developmental dislocation of the hip. Part II: Predictive value for outcome. Journal of Pediatric Orthopaedics, 17:631–636, 1997.

Smith, DW, & Jones, KL. Recognizable Patterns of Human Malformation, Vol. VII. Major Problems in Clinical Pediatrics. Philadelphia: WB Saunders, 1982.

Smith, JT, Matan, A, Coleman, SS, Stevens, PM, & Scott, SM. The predictive value of the development of the acetabular teardrop figure in developmental dysplasia of the hip. Journal of Pediatric Orthopaedics, 17:165–169, 1997.

Staheli, LT. Torsional deformity. Pediatric Clinics of North America, 24:799–811, 1977.

Staheli, LT, Corbett, M, Wyss, C, & King, H. Lower extremity rotational problems in children. Journal of Bone and Joint Surgery (American), 67:39–47, 1985.

Staheli, LT, & Engel, GM. Tibial torsion: A method of assessment and a study of normal children. Clinical Orthopaedics and Related Research, 86:183–186, 1972.

Stanitski, DF, Shaheheraghi, H, Nicker, DA, & Armstrong, PF. Results of tibial lengthening with the Ilizarov technique. Journal of Pediatric Orthopaedics, 16:168–172, 1996.

Stasikelis, PJ, Sullivan, CM, Phillips, WA, & Polard, JA. Slipped capital femoral epiphysis. Prediction of contralateral involvement. Journal of Bone and Joint Surgery (American), 78:1149–1155, 1996.

Stricker, SJ, & Angulo, JC. Idiopathic toe walking: A comparison of treatment methods. Journal of Pediatric Orthopaedics, 18:289–293, 1998.

Stuberg, WA, Koehler, A, Wichita, M, Temme, J, & Kaplan, P. A comparison of femoral torsion assessment using goniometry and computerized tomography. Pediatric Physical Therapy, 1:115–118, 1989.

Tachdjian, MO. Pediatric Orthopaedics, Vols. 1–4, 2nd ed. Philadelphia: WB Saunders, 1990.

Taylor, GR, & Clarke, NM. Monitoring the treatment of developmental dysplasia of the hip with the Pavlik harness. The role of ultrasound. Journal of Bone and Joint Surgery (British), 79:719–723, 1997.

Thompson, GH. Back pain in children: An instructional course lecture. Journal of Bone and Joint Surgery (American), 75:928–938, 1993.

Thompson, GH, & Carter, JR. Late onset tibia vara (Blount's disease). Clinical Orthopaedics and Related Research, 255:24–35, 1990.

Tippett, SR. Referred knee pain in a young athlete: A case study. Journal of Orthopedic and Sports Physical Therapy, 19:117–120, 1994.

Torode, IP, & Gillespie, R. Rotationplasty of the lower limb for congenital defects of the femur. Journal of Bone and Joint Surgery (British), 65:569–573, 1983.

Tredwell, SJ, & Bell, HM. Efficacy of neonatal hip examination. Journal of Pediatric Orthopaedics, 1:61–65, 1981.

Turner, MS. The association between tibial torsion and knee joint pathology. Clinical Orthopaedics and Related Research, 302:47–51, 1994.

Umans, H, Liebling, MS, Moy, L, Haramati, N, Macy, NJ, & Pritzker, HA. Slipped capital femoral epiphysis: A physeal lesion diagnosed by MRI, with radiographic and CT correlation. Skeletal Radiology, 27:139–144, 1998.

Volpon, JB. Footprint analysis during the growth period. Journal of Pediatric Orthopaedics, 14:83–85, 1994.

Wagner, H. Operative lengthening of the femur. Clinical Orthopaedics and Related Research, 136:125–142, 1978.

Walsh, JJ, & Morrissy, RT. Torticollis and hip dislocation. Journal of Pediatric Orthopaedics, 18:219–221, 1998.

Wang, L, Bowen, JR, Puniak, MA, Guille, JT, & Glutting J. An evaluation of various methods of treatment for Legg-Calvé-Perthes disease. Clinical Orthopaedics and Related Research, 314:225–233, 1995.

Warner, WC, Jr, Beaty, JH, & Canale, ST. Chondrolysis after slipped capital femoral epiphysis. Journal of Pediatric Orthopaedics (British), 5:168–172, 1996.

Washington, ER, III, Root, L, & Liener, UC. Discoid lateral meniscus in children. Long-term follow-up after excision. Journal of Bone and Joint Surgery (American), 77:1357–1361, 1995.

Weiner, D. Pathogenesis of slipped capital femoral epiphysis: Current concepts. Journal of Pediatric Orthopaedics (British), 5:67–73, 1996.

Weinstein, SL. Congenital hip dislocation: Long range problems, residual signs and symptoms after successful treatment. Clinical Orthopaedics and Related Research, 281:69–74, 1992.

Weinstein, SL. Natural history and treatment outcomes of childhood hip disorders. Clinical Orthopaedics and Related Research, 344:227–242, 1997.

Wenger, DR, & Leach, J. Foot deformities in infants and children. Pediatric Clinics of North America, 33:1411–1427, 1986.

Wenger, DR, Lee, CS, & Kolman, B. Derotational femoral shortening for developmental dislocation of the hip: Special indications and results in the child younger than 2 years. Journal of Pediatric Orthopaedics, 15:768–779, 1995.

Wenger, DR, Mauldin, D, Speck, G, Morgan, D, & Lieber, RL. Corrective shoes and inserts as treatment for flexible flatfoot in infants and children. Journal of Bone and Joint Surgery (American), 71:800–810, 1989.

Wenger, DR, & Rang, M. The Art of Pediatric Orthopaedics. New York: Raven Press, 1993.

Wenger, DR, Ward, WT, & Herring, JA. Current concepts review: Legg-Calvé-Perthes disease. Journal of Bone and Joint Surgery (American), 73:778–788, 1991.

Wood, JB, Klassen, RA, & Peterson, HA. Osteochondritis dissecans of the femoral head in children and adolescents: A report of 17 cases. Journal of Pediatric Orthopaedics, 15:313–316, 1995.

Wynne-Davies, R. Family studies and the cause of congenital clubfoot: Talipes equinovarus, talipes calcaneovalgus and metatarsus varus. Journal of Bone and Joint Surgery (British), 46:445–463, 1964.

Wynne-Davies, R. Acetabular dysplasia and familial joint laxity: Two etiological factors in congenital dislocation of the hip. Journal of Bone and Joint Surgery (British), 52:704–716, 1970.

Yagi, T. Tibial torsion in patients with medial-type osteoarthrotic knees. Clinical Orthopaedics and Related Research, 302:52–56, 1994.

Yashar, A, Loder, RT, & Hensinger, RN. Determination of skeletal age in children with Osgood-Schlatter disease by using radiographs of the knee. Journal of Pediatric Orthopaedics, 15:298–301, 1995.

Yasui, N, Kawabata, H, Kojimoto, H, Ohno, H, Matsuda, S, Araki, N, Shimomura, Y, & Ochi, T. Lengthening of the lower limbs in patients with achondroplasia and hypochondroplasia. Clinical Orthopaedics and Related Research, 344:298–306, 1997.

Young, N, Bell, DF, & Anthony, A. Pediatric pain patterns during Ilizarov treatment of limb length discrepancy and angular deformity. Journal of Pediatric Orthopaedics, 14:352–357, 1994.

C H A P T E R
17

Sports Injuries in Children

DONNA BERNHARDT-BAINBRIDGE, PT, ATC, EdD

On playgrounds, fields, and courts, and in gyms and pools, more children than ever before are playing or competing in sports. No fewer than 50 million children and adolescents take part in school-sponsored or extracurricular athletics. Seventy-five percent of American middle and junior high schools had significant competitive sports programs by 1981 (Stanitski, 1989). More than 1.85 million girls and 3.5 million boys participated in varsity athletics in the 1980–1981 school year, a gain of 5.9% in girls' participation and a decline of 0.4% in boys' participation over previous years. Thirty million youngsters age 6 to 21 years were involved in out-of-school programs (Mueller & Blythe, 1982). By 1987 6.5 million teenagers regularly participated in com-petitive high school team sports (Birrer & Brecher, 1987). In 1989 half of all males and one fourth of all females age 8 to 16 years (approximately 7 million) were engaged in competitive, organized school sports (Stanitski, 1989).

The issue of sports injury in children can no longer be ignored. The child, however, is not just a small adult. Children have different structural and physiologic components that must be specifically addressed (Stanitski, 1997). This chapter will provide an extensive overview of sports medicine in the youth population for the pediatric therapist. The purpose of the chapter is to review the elements of prevention and to discuss the factors that increase risk of sports-related injury in able and disabled children. The types and sites of sports injuries and those injuries unique to the child will be addressed, as well as guidelines for rehabilitation.

INCIDENCE OF INJURY

The incidence of injury has escalated as participation has increased. Although broad epidemiologic information is lacking because of varying methodologies and definitions of injury, many studies have documented risk in sports participation (Davis et al., 1993; DiScala et al., 1997). One of the earliest studies, completed over a 2-year period (1973–1975) in four Seattle high schools, demonstrated 1181 injuries in 3049 students who participated in 19 different sports (Garrick, 1982). Sprains and strains accounted for 60.5% of all injuries. The sports that placed boys most at risk were football, which accounted for 50% of total injuries, followed by wrestling (17.5%) and track (10%). Injuries in girls occurred largely in tennis (38%), gymnastics (20%), and basketball (15%). The highest proportion of fractures, contusions, and strains occurred in boys, whereas a greater percentage of overuse injuries was noted in girls. Sprains were documented equally in both groups.

When Garrick (1982) related the total number of injuries to total participants, he noted boys to have an 85% injury rate whereas girls had only a 22% injury rate. If, however, injuries received in football and wrestling were not included, the injury rate for the genders was similar (27% for boys, 22% for girls). Snively and co-workers (1981) compared boys and girls who participated in eight similar sports and reported no difference in overall injury rate. Other researchers concurred with these findings (Backx et al., 1989; Kvist et al., 1989; Lodge et al., 1990; McLain & Reynolds, 1989).

A Dutch study further suggested that sports characterized by contact, repetitive jumping, and indoor activities create the most risk (Backx et al., 1991). Athletic trainers in four high schools (Whieldon & Cerny, 1990) reported that collision sports such as football and wrestling generated the highest injury rates, followed by contact sports such as baseball and basketball. Boys had higher injury rates than girls only in contact sports.

Many studies have documented injury rates in specific sports. Youth football (played by children age 8 to 15 years) was shown to cause an overall injury rate of 5%, with 61% classified as moderate and 39% as major injuries, although permanent disability was rare. Fractures of the upper extremity were the most common injury. Both the injury rate and the site of injury change with age (Goldberg et al., 1988; Halpern et al., 1987). Injuries in high school athletes

occurred primarily in the lower extremity and especially affected the knee. Forty percent of injuries were sprains and strains, 25% were contusions, and only 10% were fractures (Halpern et al., 1987).

Injuries related to soccer occur with an incidence of 10.6 injuries per 1000 hours of play in girls and of 7.3 injuries per 1000 hours of play in boys (Backous et al., 1988). The incidence of injury in both groups increased at 14 years of age and continued at a higher rate as the participants became older. The authors noted that 70% of the injuries were to the lower extremities, with a total of 84.2% represented by contusions, sprains, and strains (Backous et al., 1988). Keller and colleagues (1987) postulated that ball and body momentum increased with age and affected injury rates. They suggested that the greater incidence of head and upper extremity injuries in young soccer players could be related to lack of technical expertise, weakness of dental tissues, and increased ball-to-head weight ratios. Overall injury rates were higher in outdoor than in indoor soccer (Hoff & Martin, 1986; Keller et al., 1987). Players of outdoor soccer experienced more strains, fractures, cuts, and infections; dental and upper extremity injuries and tendinitis occurred more frequently in players of indoor soccer. The cleanliness, traction, and shock absorption of the playing surface, the weather, the perimeter boards, and the pace of play were all postulated to influence injury characteristics.

A study that evaluated track and field athletes from 17 teams found one injury for every 5.8 males and every 7.5 females. The majority of injuries (83%) involved the lower extremities, with sprinting responsible for 46% of all injuries (Watson & DiMartino, 1987). Another research group evaluated the members of 12 high school ice hockey teams (Gerberich et al., 1987). Seventy-five injuries in 100 players were documented, with 22% of these injuries to the head and neck. Ski injury patterns of children under 18 years of age were assessed by Shorter and colleages (1996). In a 5-year period, 38 patients were seen with head injuries (27), extremity fractures (13), and trunk or spinal injuries (13). Fifty-eight percent of injuries were the result of collisions.

Several studies have assessed injuries in recreational sports. Retsky and associates (1991) assessed the U.S. Consumer Product Safety Commission injury frequency estimates for skateboarding. A marked increase in injuries was noted: 19,182 injuries were reported in 1984, and 37,180 injuries were reported in 1985. Injuries occurred with greater frequency in children age 10 to 14 years. More frequent head and neck trauma occurred in children younger than 5 years of age, and more severe head and neck injuries were reported in older children. Older children experienced more injuries to the extremities than younger children. Powell and colleagues (1997) studied bicycle injuries in preschoolers. They noted 4041 injuries in a 10-year period with 5% of those injured under 5 years of age. An escalation of injuries has been noted in in-line and roller skating (Powell & Tanz, 1996). The 1993 rate for injury in in-line skating was 31 per 100,000, and the rate was 95 per 100,000 for roller skating.

The trampoline is another emerging source of injury. Smith and Shields (1998) documented 214 injuries in 1995 through 1997. The children were supervised in 55.6% of the injury occasions. Many other recreational activities such as dancing, dirt biking, and tag football cause injury, but no data on the types or incidence of injury have been collected in children.

The incidence of catastrophic injuries and fatalities in high school and college athletes has been documented for the years 1982 through 1988 (Mueller & Cantu, 1990). A total of 218 injuries, including 44 fatalities, 74 nonfatal but permanent injuries resulting in severe functional neurologic disability, and 100 serious injuries with no permanent functional neurologic disability, were reported in high school athletes. During the same period 76 indirect deaths caused by heart failure, heat stroke, sickle cell crisis, or asthma occurred in the following sports, which are listed in decreasing order of number of deaths: football, wrestling, basketball, track, and baseball. Even lower in incidence of injury or death were cross-country, soccer, gymnastics, ice hockey, and swimming. Attention to the causes of severe injuries or deaths, such as overaggression in hockey, grading of risk in gymnastics, improper padding of landing pits, insufficient clearance at field events, and takeoff dives into shallow water, will assist in their elimination.

Lack of fitness has been associated with injury in both children and adults (Birrer & Levine, 1987; Macera et al., 1989). Fitness levels have declined for boys older than age 14 and for girls older than age 12. One third of American children younger than age 8 are overweight. Fifty percent of children in grades 5 through 12 do not get the vigorous activity necessary to maintain or improve cardiovascular status. Forty percent of children between 5 and 8 years of age show at least one risk factor for heart disease (Schlicker et al., 1994).

PREVENTION OF INJURIES

The key to management of sports injuries in children is prevention. As discussed in Chapter 5, children need proper physiologic conditioning, strength, and flexibility to participate safely in an organized or recreational athletic endeavor. Al-
though lack of fitness, strength, and flexibility does not preclude participation, remediation must be built into conditioning and training programs to decrease the risk of injury. The major elements in the process of injury risk management are preparticipation examination, conditioning and training, proper supervision, protection of the body, and environmental control.

Preparticipation Examination

The preparticipation examination is the initial step in the process of injury prevention. The American Medical Association Committee on Medical Aspects of Sports constructed a Bill of Rights for the Athlete, one part of which is a thorough preseason history and medical examination. The purposes are fivefold: (1) to determine the general health of the athlete and detect conditions that place the participant at additional risk; (2) to identify relative or absolute medical contraindications to participation; (3) to identify sports that may be played safely; (4) to assess maturity and overall fitness; and (5) to educate the athlete. These examinations are also necessary to meet legal and insurance requirements in many states (Bar-Or et al., 1988).

The usefulness of these assessments in identifying children at risk has been demonstrated. In one study, 15% of participants had conditions requiring further evaluation, although only 9 of 701 were excluded. One third of the musculoskeletal problems identified were previously unknown to the primary care physician (Goldberg et al., 1980). In another study it was noted that in the 1977–1978 and 1978–1979 school years, respectively, 3.2% and 6.5% of athletes had abnormalities severe enough to require further evaluation. Only 0.3% were excluded from participation (Linder et al., 1981). In a study to assess utilization of preseason assessment, questionnaires were mailed to 300 secondary schools. Seventy-one percent of schools used a health history form, and 94.2% administered preseason physical examinations to all interscholastic athletes. It was noted, however, that the health forms were not specific to sports, were evaluated by individuals who were not competent for the task, were not available during the season, and were not followed by appropriate student counseling (Harvey, 1982).

Most states require either an individual examination or a multistation screening. The merits and disadvantages of these methods have been evaluated. The primary physician performing an individual examination knows or has access to the athlete's health records, can discuss sensitive health or personal issues, and may be most qualified to oversee any necessary follow-up care. The time and cost are a disadvantage of the individual examination. Additionally, disparate knowledge and interest among physicians regarding sports and the requirements to participate may hinder effective evaluation for all participants. The multistation examination is more cost efficient and time efficient and provides a thorough and appropriate screening for all potential participants. Professional experts assess each athlete in the area of her or his specialization (Table 17–1), increasing the probability of detection of abnormalities (Bar-Or et al., 1988; Harvey, 1982).

The frequency of the preparticipation examination is being debated. Although annual evaluations are most traditional (McKeag, 1985; Powell, 1987), many clinicians advocate evaluation before each season (Micheli & Stone, 1984). The American Academy of Pediatrics (1989) recommends a biannual complete evaluation followed by an interim history before each season. The schedule that meets the primary objectives of the academy, however, is a complete entry-level evaluation followed by a limited annual reevaluation that includes a brief physical examination (to evaluate height, weight, blood pressure, and pulse; perform auscultation; examine the skin; and test visual acuity), a physical maturity assessment if previous level was less than Tanner stage IV, and an evaluation of all new problems (Powell, 1997).

The components of the preparticipation examination are the medical history; the physical examination, including cardiovascular and eye examinations; musculoskeletal assessment; body composition and height and weight determination; specific field testing; and readiness, both physical and psychologic. The examination should be completed 6 weeks before the practice season to allow adequate time for further evaluation or for correction of any problems (Bar-Or et al., 1988; Lehman, 1988; Linder et al., 1981; Lombardo, 1991; McKeag, 1985; Rooks & Micheli, 1988). The components of the examination should be tailored to the specific demands of the sport.

History

The medical history is the cornerstone of the medical evaluation (Bar-Or et al., 1988; Lombardo, 1991; McKeag, 1985) and will identify 63 to 74% of problems affecting athletes (Goldberg et al., 1980). Forms that are short, easy to complete, and written in lay terms are preferable (Fig. 17–1). Forms should be completed by the athlete and parent or legal guardian and then signed by the parent or legal guardian. Content areas that should be particularly noted include exercise-induced syncope or asthma; family history of heart disease or sudden death; history of loss of consciousness, concussion, or neurologic conditions; history of heat stroke; medications; allergies; history of musculoskeletal dysfunction; dates of hospitalizations or surgery; absence or loss of a paired organ; and immunizations.

Physical Examination

The physical examination is used to evaluate areas of concern identified by the history. The minimally sufficient examination includes cardiovascular and eye examinations, a maturity assessment, and a review of all body systems. Blood pressure should be measured using appropriately sized sphygmomanometer cuffs for accuracy (Lombardo, 1991; McKeag, 1985). The 95th percentile upper limit values for normal blood pressure are 110/75 mm Hg below age 6, 120/80 mm Hg for 6- to 10-year-olds, 125/85 mm Hg for 11- to 14-year-olds, and 135/90 mm Hg for 15- to 18-year-olds (Cooper, 1991). A diagnosis of hypertension requires three abnormal readings. If blood pressure is elevated, repeat measures should be taken later in the examination or the next day (Feld et al., 1998). High blood pressure requires further evaluation by the personal physician for clearance to participate in sports (Lombardo, 1991). The remainder of the cardiovascular screening evaluation assesses peripheral pulses and heartbeat for symmetry and rate. Auscultation of the heart should be performed with the young person both seated and supine (Lombardo, 1991). As many as 85% of youths have benign heart murmurs. Various maneuvers such as squat to stand, Valsalva, and

TABLE 17–1. Multistation Preparticipation Assessment

Station	Personnel
Sign-in/instructions	Ancillary personnel/coach
Height/weight/vital signs	Nurse, exercise physiologist, athletic trainer, or physical therapist
Visual examination	Nurse or coach
Medical examination	Internist or family practitioner
Orthopedic evaluation	Physician or physical therapist
Flexibility assessment	Physical therapist or athletic trainer
Strength evaluation	Physical therapist, athletic trainer, or exercise physiologist
Body composition	Exercise physiologist, physical therapist, or athletic trainer
Speed, agility, power, balance, endurance	Exercise physiologist, coach, or athletic trainer
Assessment/clearance	Physician

deep inspiration can differentiate functional from pathologic murmurs (Bar-Or et al., 1988). Arrhythmias are not abnormal in children, but increases in premature ventricular contractions with exercise require further assessment. Paroxysmal supraventricu-

lar tachycardia, once evaluated, is not a reason for disqualification (Bar-Or et al., 1988; Powell, 1987).

Visual acuity is tested using a Snelling chart and should be correctable to 20/200. Any inequality of pupil diameter or reactivity should be noted so

Name _____   Date of Birth _____
Address _____   Class _____
Parents _____   Phone # _____
Physician _____
Sports _____   _____

Fill in details of "YES" answers in space below:

	Yes	No
1. Have you ever been hospitalized?		
Have you ever had surgery?	___	___
2. Are you currently taking medication?	___	___
3. Do you have any allergies (medicines, bees)?	___	___
4. Have you ever passed out during exercise?	___	___
Have you ever been dizzy during exercise?	___	___
Have you ever had chest pain?	___	___
Do you tire more quickly than your friends during exercise?	___	___
Have you ever had high blood pressure?	___	___
Have you ever been told you have a heart murmur?	___	___
Have you ever had racing of your heart or skipped beats?	___	___
Has anyone in your family died of heart problems or a sudden death before age 40?	___	___
5. Do you have any skin problems? (itching, moles, breaking out)	___	___
6. Have you ever had a head injury?	___	___
Have you ever been knocked out?	___	___
Have you ever had a seizure?	___	___
Have you ever had a stinger or burner?	___	___

7. Have you ever injured (sprained, dislocated, fractured, etc.):

___ Hand	___ Shoulder	___ Thigh
___ Wrist	___ Neck	___ Knee
___ Forearm	___ Chest	___ Shin/Calf
___ Elbow	___ Back	___ Ankle
___ Arm	___ Hip	___ Foot

	Yes	No
8. Have you ever had heat cramps?		
Have you ever been dizzy or passed out in the heat?	___	___

9. Have you ever had:

___ Mononucleosis	___ Diabetes
___ Hepatitis	___ Headaches (frequent)
___ Asthma	___ Eye injuries
___ Tuberculosis	___ Stomach ulcer

	Yes	No
10. Do you use special pads or braces?	___	___
11. When was your last tetanus shot?	___	
12. When was your first period?	___	
When was your last period?	___	

Explain YES answers here:

_____
_____
_____
_____
_____
_____
_____

Parent's signature: _____

FIGURE 17–1. Medical questionnaire. (From Lombardo, J. Preparticipation examination. In Cantu, R, & Micheli, L [Eds.], ACSM's Guidelines for the Team Physician. Philadelphia: Lea & Febiger, 1991.)

responses after potential injury can be compared with this baseline value. Uncorrectable legal blindness (acuity less than 20/200 or absence of an eye) requires counseling regarding participation in collision or contact sports. The importance of protective eyewear for athletes who wear glasses or have unilateral vision should be stressed (Bar-Or et al., 1988; Lombardo, 1991).

Pulmonary status is determined by symmetry of diaphragmatic excursion and breath sounds. Children with asthma, including exercise-induced asthma, should be allowed to participate in activities if the condition is properly controlled with medication (Lombardo, 1991; Wiens et al., 1992). Abdominal assessment determines rigidity, tenderness, organomegaly, or the presence of masses. Participation by any athlete with organomegaly is restricted until further tests determine the cause of the enlarged organ (Bar-Or et al., 1988; McKeag, 1985; Powell, 1987).

Careful examination of the skin is vital in examination of all persons, but it is particularly important for those who will participate in contact sports. Participation in these sports should be deferred for children with evidence of any communicable skin disease, such as impetigo, carbuncles, herpes, scabies, and louse or fungal infections (Bar-Or et al., 1988; Lombardo, 1991; McKeag, 1985).

Genitourinary examination of males is used to assess the child for testicular presence, descended testicles, and possible inguinal hernia. The genital examination is deferred in girls unless a history of amenorrhea or menstrual irregularity warrants referral. A maturational index should be determined for all athletes so that appropriate matching of age and sport can occur (McKeag, 1985). Guidelines for staging of secondary sexual characteristics are reliable, proven, and practical (Table 17–2).

The musculoskeletal screening examination should include assessment of posture with particular attention to atrophy, spinal asymmetry, pelvic level, discrepancy of leg lengths, and lower extremity deformities such as genu valgus or varus, patellar deformities, and pes planus. Gait should be examined with the child walking and running, as well as walking on toes and heels. Passive range of motion and two-joint musculotendinous flexibility should be screened, using the Thomas, Ober, and Ely tests. Muscle strength can be assessed using a manual muscle test, handheld dynamometer, or isokinetic device. Special stability testing of the shoulders, knees, and ankles should be conducted if the child has had a previous injury or if the current assessment indicates that instability may be present (Powell, 1987) (see Appendix I).

Body Composition

Height and weight should be assessed and results compared with standard growth charts. Weight, however, gives no specific assessment of the percentage of lean mass and fat tissue. Assessment of subcutaneous body fat provides a more specific evaluation of body composition, although fat thickness varies from birth to adolescence (see Chapter 5). The most practical method for screening is skinfold measurement. This method has demonstrated correlations of .70 to .85 with hydrostatic weighing if performed by

TABLE 17–2. **Maturity Staging Guidelines**

Male		
Pubic Hair	**Penis**	**Testis**
None	Preadolescent	
Slight, long, slight pigmentation	Slight enlargement	Enlarged scrotum, pink slight ruga
Darker, starts to curl, small amount	Longer	Larger
Coarse, curly, adult type, but less quantity	Increase in glans size and breadth of penis	Larger, scrotum darker
Adult—spread to inner thighs	Adult	Adult

Female	
Pubic Hair	**Breasts**
Preadolescent (none)	Preadolescent (no germinal button)
Sparse, lightly pigmented, straight medial border of labia	Breast and papilla elevated as small mound; areolar diameter increased
Darker, beginning to curl, increased	Breast and areola enlarged; no contour separation
Coarse, curly, abundant, but less than adult	Areola and papilla form secondary mound
Adult female triangle and spread to medial surface	Mature, nipple projects, areola part of general breast contour

From McKeag, D. Preseason physical examination for the prevention of sports injuries. Sports Medicine, 2:425, 1985.

an experienced examiner (Going, 1988). Although the criterion ranges for body fatness related to optimal health are 15 to 25% for girls and 10 to 25% for boys (Lohman, 1992), 20% for girls and 12% for boys are ideal for most activities (Bar-Or et al., 1988). Elevated body fat levels may indicate the need for weight reduction. Low weight or low body fat warrants a thorough evaluation of eating habits, weight loss, and body image to rule out the possibility of an eating disorder. High weight and very low body fat could signal use of anabolic steroids, growth hormone, or other performance-enhancing drugs (Lombardo, 1991; McKeag, 1985). Because of unorthodox weight loss methods, nutritional content and patterns should also be evaluated, especially in those athletes who must "make weight" (Perriello et al., 1995).

The physical examination would be incomplete without a thorough evaluation for possible use of pharmacologic ergogenic aids. Observation for physical symptoms and signs, as well as careful examination, can reveal potential abuse. The most frequently used drugs, particularly in sports requiring muscle power, are anabolic steroids. Although reliably reported data are difficult to obtain, probably more than 1 million individuals in the United States use steroids (Yesalis et al., 1989). The most compelling reasons for taking steroids are to increase body weight and muscle mass, decrease fatigue, and increase aggressive behavior. The adverse effects, including hypertension, hepatitis, testicular atrophy, loss of libido, hepatic carcinoma, and premature epiphyseal closure, far outweigh the benefits of these drugs (Birrer & Brecher, 1987; Haupt, 1989; Hickson et al., 1989; Laseter & Russell, 1991; Sachtelben et al, 1993). Warning signs of steroid abuse include irritability; sudden mood swings; puffiness in face, upper arms, and chest; sudden increases in blood pressure and weight; yellowish coloration around the fingernails and eyes; hirsutism; and deepening of voice and acne in girls (Haupt, 1989; Hickson et al., 1989; Nevole & Prentice, 1987; Perry, 1985; Yesalis et al., 1989).

Diuretics are frequently used to "make weight" for an event or to mask drug usage (Grana & Kalenak, 1991). Performance may, however, be decreased as a result of dehydration or electrolyte losses (Birrer & Brecher, 1987; Grana & Kalenak, 1991). Likewise, stimulants, such as caffeine and amphetamines, are commonly abused in an effort to increase performance in sports. They serve only to mask normal fatigue and to increase aggression, hostility, and uncooperativeness and can lead to addiction and death (Wagner, 1991).

The use of barbiturates, antidepressants, and beta blockers has been noted in sports in which fine control is required, such as shooting and archery.

Although they do calm the nervous system and lower heart rate, even therapeutic doses may cause bronchospasm, hypotension, and bradycardia (Millar, 1990).

Natural elements such as human growth hormone, vitamins, and amino acids have been touted in popular literature as aids for growth, performance, immunity, and healing and are widely used by both high school and college, as well as professional, athletes (Sobal & Marquart, 1994; Williams, 1994). Some of these substances are widely publicized by popular athletes (e.g., Andro used by Mark McGwire during the 1998 baseball season). Although normal dosage may provide some benefits, minimal data exist to support their use (Clarkson, 1996; Haupt, 1993; Williams, 1994). Overdosage of both fat- and water-soluble vitamins can cause damage to liver and kidney (Millar, 1990).

The use of recreational drugs, including nicotine, smokeless tobacco, alcohol, marijuana, cocaine, and even heroin, is increasing among youth (Creath et al., 1988; Sobal & Marquart, 1994). Symptoms including agitation, restlessness, insomnia, difficulty with short-term memory or concentration, or decline in performance might signal behavior indicative of substance abuse (Clarkson, 1996; Green, 1990).

Specific Field Tests

Field testing is done to assess specific athletic potential in a specific sport. The components assessed are muscle strength, muscle power, endurance, speed, agility and flexibility, and cardiovascular performance (Bar-Or et al., 1988).

General muscle strength can be assessed with a maximal activity pertinent to the sport, such as bench presses, pull-ups, or push-ups for the upper extremities and leg presses or sit-ups for the lower extremities. Endurance can be assessed by performing as many repetitions of the task as possible. Muscle power can be evaluated with vertical jumping, performing a standing long jump, or throwing a medicine ball, as appropriate.

Speed is evaluated using a 40- or 50-yard dash, and agility can be assessed with the Vodak agility test (Gaillard et al., 1978) or a similar battery of tests. The most common, standardized methods of assessing flexibility are the sit and reach test, which has norms for children, and active knee extension performed in a supine position with the hips flexed to 90° (Hunter et al., 1985). Cardiovascular performance is most easily assessed using a submaximal test on an appropriate device, such as a cycle ergometer, treadmill, or upper-body ergometer. A field test for cardiovascular performance is the 12-minute run or the timed 1.5-mile run (Bar-Or et al., 1988).

TABLE 17–3. **Sports Classification System**

| | | Noncontact | | |
| | | Strenuous | Moderately Strenuous | Nonstrenuous |
Contact Collision	**Limited Contact Impact**			
Boxing	Baseball	Aerobic dancing	Badminton	Archery
Field hockey	Basketball	Crew	Curling	Golf
Football	Bicycling	Fencing	Table tennis	Riflery
Ice hockey	Diving	Field		
Lacrosse	Field	Discus		
Martial arts	High jump	Javelin		
Rodeo	Pole vault	Shot put		
Soccer	Gymnastics	Running		
Wrestling	Horseback riding	Swimming		
	Ice skating	Track		
	Roller skating	Weight lifting		
	Skiing			
	Cross-country			
	Downhill			
	Water			
	Softball			
	Squash, handball			
	Volleyball			

From American Academy of Pediatrics Committee on Sports Medicine. Recommendations for participation in competitive sports. Pediatrics 81:737, 1988.

From Lombardo, J. Preparticipation examination. In Cantu, R, & Micheli, L (Eds.), ACSM's Guidelines for the Team Physician. Philadelphia: Lea & Febiger, 1991, p. 74.

The outcome of the preparticipation examination is a definition of clearance to participate in sports. Clearance can be unrestricted for any sport or restricted to specific types of sports in the following manner: (1) no collision (violent, direct impact) or contact (physical touching); (2) limited contact or impact; or (3) noncontact only. The American Academy of Pediatrics has developed a classification system for sports activities (Table 17–3) and recommendations for restriction of participation (Table 17–4) that are excellent guides in making decisions for individual athletes. All decisions or recommendations for further evaluation should be thoroughly discussed with the athletes and their parents (Bar-Or et al., 1988; Powell, 1987).

Training Program

The preseason examination provides a clear definition of the individual athlete's areas of strength and limitations (Fig. 17–2). The next appropriate step in prevention is the development of an individualized training plan designed to address the particular problems of the athlete as they relate to the requirements of the sport(s). This program could be developed by a sports physical therapist, athletic trainer, or exercise physiologist involved in the preseason screening. Once developed, it should be taught to the athlete, the parent, and the coach.

The training program should be a systematic, progressive plan to address the athlete's weaknesses and to maximally condition the athlete for participation. Training consists of off-season, preseason, in-season, and postseason programs for year-round conditioning and for development of appropriate peak performance. Components should include energy training (aerobic foundation and anaerobic training), muscle training (strength, endurance, flexibility, and power), speed, and proper nutrition. A well-developed, variable, and well-paced program will avoid boredom and potential overuse injury. The psychologic effects of year-round training, or exercise in general, are controversial and not well documented. The risk-benefit ratio, however, tends to favor exercise for improvement of mood, self-concept, and work behavior when competition is sensibly controlled (Brown, 1982).

Energy Training

The basis of energy training, a strong aerobic base, should be developed during the off-season. Good training consists of low-intensity, long-duration activity with natural intervals of low- and moderate-intensity work that is sport specific. Swimming would be a good choice for the field athlete, and cycling or running is appropriate for those in track, soccer, and football. Training on hills or perfor-

TABLE 17–4. **Recommendations for Participation**

	Contact/ Collision	Limited Contact/Impact	Noncontact		
			Strenuous	Moderately Strenuous	Nonstrenuous
Atlantoaxial instability *Swimming: no butterfly, breast stroke, or diving starts	No	No	Yes*	Yes	Yes
Acute illnesses *Needs individual assessment, e.g., contagiousness to others, risk of worsening illness	*	*	*	*	*
Cardiovascular					
Carditis*	No	No	No	No	No
Hypertension					
Mild	Yes	Yes	Yes	Yes	Yes
Moderate	*	*	*	*	*
Severe	*	*	*	*	*
Congenital heart disease	†	†	†	†	†
*Needs individual assessment †Patients with mild forms can be allowed a full range of physical activities; patients with moderate or severe forms, or who are postoperative, should be evaluated by a cardiologist before athletic participation.					
Eyes					
Absence or loss of function of one eye	*	*	*	*	*
Detached retina	†	†	†	†	†
*Availability of American Society for Testing and Materials (ASTM)— approved eye guards may allow competitor to participate in most sports, but this must be judged on an individual basis. †Consult ophthalmologist					
Inguinal hernia	Yes	Yes	Yes	Yes	Yes
Kidney: absence of one	No	Yes	Yes	Yes	Yes
Liver: enlarged	No	No	Yes	Yes	Yes
Musculoskeletal disorders	*	*	*	*	*
*Needs individual assessment					

From Lombardo, J. Preparticipation examination. In Cantu, R, & Micheli, L (Eds.), ACSM's Guidelines for the Team Physician. Philadelphia: Lea & Febiger, 1991, p. 74.

mance of similar resistance efforts should be done once weekly. Children exhibit less efficient movement patterns and a lower maximal acidosis level. They are less able to withstand high temperatures secondary to a greater rate of heat exchange and less sweat production (Bar-Or, 1995; Stanitski, 1997). Consequently, intense training in the extreme heat and hard training involving long durations should be minimized until puberty. This avoidance of excessive exercise also helps avert early burnout (Sharkey, 1991).

Anaerobic training programs consist of exertion at 85 to 90% of maximal heart rate for short periods. Anaerobic drills develop a person's ability to tolerate the production of excess lactic acid. Twice-weekly anaerobic training should be performed for maximal benefit. Methods including interval training, fartlek (speed play, or alternate fast and slow running in natural terrain), and pace training are variations of the anaerobic method. Sport-specific anaerobic skills should be developed during preseason and early-season activities (Sharkey, 1991). Young children are

TABLE 17–4. Recommendations for Participation—cont'd

	Contact/ Collision	Limited Contact/Impact	Noncontact		
			Strenuous	Moderately Strenuous	Nonstrenuous
Neurologic					
History of serious head or spine trauma, repeated concussions, or craniotomy	*	*	Yes	Yes	Yes
Convulsive disorder					
Well controlled	Yes	Yes	Yes	Yes	Yes
Poorly controlled	No	No	Yes†	Yes	Yes‡
*Needs individual assessment					
†No swimming or weight lifting					
‡No archery or riflery					
Ovary: absence of one	Yes	Yes	Yes	Yes	Yes
Respiratory					
Pulmonary insufficiency	*	*	*	*	Yes
Asthma	Yes	Yes	Yes	Yes	Yes
*May be allowed to compete if oxygenation remains satisfactory during a graded stress test					
Sickle cell trait	Yes	Yes	Yes	Yes	Yes
Skin: boils, herpes, impetigo, scabies	*	*	Yes	Yes	Yes
*No gymnastics with mats, martial arts, wrestling, or contact sports until not contagious					
Spleen: enlarged	No	No	No	Yes	Yes
Testicle: absent or undescended	Yes*	Yes*	Yes	Yes	Yes
*Certain sports may require protective cup					

From Lombardo, J. Preparticipation examination. In Cantu, R., & Micheli, L (Eds.), ACSM's Guidelines for the Team Physician. Philadelphia: Lea & Febiger, 1991, p. 74.

less able to use muscle glycogen and produce lactic acid, so this training is difficult for young athletes and has only minor fitness benefits until they mature. Some training should be used, however, to achieve relaxation and mechanical efficiency at these levels.

Strength Training

Weight training in children has been controversial because of concerns regarding injury to growing bones and the questionable efficacy of this type of training to increase strength. Several research studies have demonstrated that strength can be improved by systematic overload of muscle in postpubescent athletes with similar results as in adults (Pfeiffer & Francis, 1986; Sailors & Berg, 1987; Sewall & Micheli, 1986).

The area of greatest debate in strength training is how it affects the prepubescent athlete. Because the levels of circulating androgens are low, questions of efficacy have been raised. Several studies have demonstrated that, although little increase in muscle bulk occurs, definite changes in strength can be achieved through controlled weight training in this group (Ramsey et al., 1990; Servedio et al., 1985; Sharkey, 1991; Weltman et al., 1986). The trends documenting increased twitch torque and motor unit activation suggest neuromuscular changes, including motor learning and reduction of inhibition (Ramsey et al., 1990; Sharkey, 1991). All authors firmly state, however, that weight lifting in the prepubescent athlete should follow a thorough preparticipation screening for constitutional or anatomic abnormalities (Sewall & Micheli, 1986; Sharkey, 1991). The program should be closely monitored by an adult with emphasis on form and technique and with careful spotting. Movements should be nonballistic with avoidance of extremely heavy weights. The training apparatus should be scaled to fit the athlete (Kraemer & Fleck, 1993).

Athletic fitness scorecard for boys

Test	0 Below average	1 Above average	2 Good	3 Very good	4 Excellent
Strength Pull-ups (no)	Fewer than 7	7 to 9	10 to 12	13 to 14	15 or more
Power Long jump (in)	Fewer than 85	85 to 88	89 to 91	92 to 94	95 or more
Speed 50-yd dash (sec)	Slower than 6.7	6.7 to 6.4	6.3 to 6.0	5.9 to 5.6	5.5 or less
Agility 6-c agility (c)	Fewer than 5-5	5-5 to 6-3	6-4 to 7-2	7-3 to 8-1	8-2 or more
Flexibility Forward flexion (in)	Not reach ruler	1 to 2	3 to 5	6 to 8	9 or more
Muscular endurance Sit-ups (no)	Fewer than 38	38 to 45	46 to 52	53 to 59	60 or more
Cardiorespiratory endurance 12-min run (mi)	Fewer than 1½	1½	1¾	2	2¼ or more

YOUR SCORE

	Strength	Power	Speed	Agility	Flexibility	Muscular endurance	Cardiorespiratory endurance
Your Score							
Rating (0–4)							

Athletic fitness scorecard for girls

Test	0 Below average	1 Above average	2 Good	3 Very good	4 Excellent
Strength Pull-ups (no)	Fewer than 2	2 to 3	4 to 5	6 to 7	8 or more
Power Long jump (in)	Fewer than 63	63 to 65	66 to 68	69 to 71	72 or more
Speed 50-yd dash (sec)	Slower than 8.2	8.2 to 7.9	7.8 to 7.1	6.9 to 6.0	5.9 or less
Agility 6-c agility (c)	Fewer than 3-5	3-5 to 4-3	4-4 to 5-2	5-3 to 6-2	6-3 or more
Flexibility Forward flexion (in)	Fewer than 3	3 to 5	6 to 8	9 to 11	12 or more
Muscular endurance Sit-ups (no)	Fewer than 26	26 to 31	32 to 38	39 to 45	46 or more
Cardiorespiratory endurance 12-min run (mi)	Fewer than 1¼	1¼	1½	1¾	2 or more

YOUR SCORE

	Strength	Power	Speed	Agility	Flexibility	Muscular endurance	Cardiorespiratory endurance
Your Score							
Rating (0–4)							

FIGURE 17–2. Athletic fitness scorecards. (Reproduced with permission from *Patient Care,* October 30, 1988, Copyright © Medical Economics Publishing, Montvale, NJ 07645. All rights reserved.)

Guidelines for strength training are provided in Table 17–5. Athletes will increase strength at a rate of 1 to 3% per week with strength training routines (Sharkey, 1991). Most strength training occurs during the late off-season and preseason periods. Programs should be sport specific both for the muscles used and the rests between sets. For example, a wrestler, gymnast, or sprinter may take 60- to 90-second rests between exercise bursts whereas a distance runner may move slowly and continuously through all exercises with little rest (Rooks & Micheli, 1988). When athletes have achieved the adequate level for their sport, they should work on the appropriate type of muscle endurance (Table 17–6) with one set of higher-resistance training per week to maintain strength. Endurance work begins in late preseason and continues during the early in-season period.

Power is the ability to do work over a given period of time. As such, it involves both strength and speed in a sport-specific movement. Power is usually developed by performing 15 to 25 repetitions of three sets at 30 to 60% of maximal effort as fast as possible. Although power develops slowly in children, some training can help a child develop the neuromuscular skill of quick movement against low resistance (Sharkey, 1991). Because of the requirements of power training, variable-resistance devices that allow control of speed or resistance are the best approach. Plyometrics, or muscle stretch followed by a burst of contraction, is another available form of power training. Because body weight is approximately 33% of maximal leg strength, these exercises fit the power prescription. An example of a plyometric exercise is step jumping (Voight & Draovitch, 1991).

Power training can cause muscle soreness and potential injury if conducted improperly. Proper technique includes adequate warm-up; slowly increased intensity; performance of jumping activities on dirt, grass, or soft surfaces; and thorough stretching after each session.

Achieving joint and musculotendinous flexibility is an essential part of any training program. Although the effects of flexibility on injury prevention are unclear, enhanced joint mobility, improved comfort of the muscle crossing the joint, and increased blood supply have been documented (Rooks & Micheli, 1988). Stretching is most effective if non-ballistic. Effective methods include static or proprioceptive neuromuscular stretching. The young athlete should be placed on a daily program that stretches all areas of the extremities and trunk with emphasis on the body parts to be used in the sport. Stretches should be easy and simple and demand appropriate levels of neuromuscular control for the age of the child (Rooks & Micheli, 1988).

TABLE 17–5. **Guidelines for Pediatric Weight Training**

Ages	9–11	12–14	15–16	17+
Exercises per body part	1	1	2	>2
Sets	2	3	3–4	4–6
Repetitions	12–15	10–12	7–11	6–10
Maximum weight (resistance)	Very light	Light	Moderate	Heavy

From Rooks, D, & Micheli, L. Musculoskeletal assessment and training: The young athlete. Clinics in Sports Medicine, 7(3):663, 1988.

TABLE 17–6. **The Strength-Endurance Continuum**

Strength	Short-Term Endurance	Intermediate Endurance
Maximum force 6–10 RM	Persistence with heavy load 15–25 RM	Persistence with intermediate load 30–50 RM
3 sets	3 sets	2 sets
3 times/week	3 times/week	3 times/week
Contractile protein (actin and myosin)	Some strength and anaerobic metabolism (glycolysis)	Some endurance and anaerobic metabolism
Connective tissue		Slight strength improvement
Oxygen intake	Oxygen intake	Endurance

From Sharkey, B. Training for sport. In Cantu, R, & Micheli, L (Eds.), ACSM's Guidelines for the Team Physician, Philadelphia: Lea & Febiger, 1991.

Speed

Because the proportion of fast twitch fibers in muscle is inherited, speed is "born" in the child (Sharkey, 1991; Smith MJ, 1983). All athletes, however, can train the intermediate fibers and improve the components of reaction and movement time. Faster reactions are taught in sport-specific practice drills such as starts, acceleration drills, or play drills that gradually narrow choice. Movement time is enhanced from a base of flexibility and strength with ballistic motions, sprint loading (explosive jump or throw), overspeed, or resisted sprinting (Sharkey, 1991).

Nutrition

Many general articles have been written on nutritional requirements for athletes (Bauman, 1986; Clark, 1991) with recent revisions for pediatric and adolescent athletes (Cooper, 1991; Peterson & Peterson, 1988; Sanders, 1990). The preparticipation screening includes components of a nutritional assessment: skinfold measurements, height, and weight. Skinfold standards for the triceps and calf in children allow one to determine whether the child is overfat (Cooper, 1991). The ideal range for adolescent males is 10 to 18% total body fat, and in females the range is 15 to 25% total body fat (Bar-Or et al., 1988; Cooper, 1991). The body fat percentage can be matched to the approximated body fat values developed for various sports, although percentages are not well standarized for younger athletes (Klish, 1995).

Caloric requirements for children are age dependent and vary directly with body weight and surface area. Generally, a young child requires more calories than an adolescent or adult—36 to 40 calories per pound per day (Cooper, 1991; Peterson & Peterson, 1988). An additional caloric load is necessary depending on the level of energy output. An approximation for energy expenditure, based on a child weighing 100 lb, is 4 kcal/min for low-intensity activities, 4 to 7 kcal/min for moderate-intensity activities, and greater than 7 kcal/min for high-intensity activities (Peterson & Peterson, 1988). A more complex, but also more accurate, method is to multiply ideal weight in pounds times 10 for basal calories. Basal activity calories are then calculated by multiplying weight in pounds times 3 for sedentary activity, times 5 for moderate activity, and times 10 for vigorous activity. The additional requirements of the sports activity are determined by adding 10 to 14 calories per minute for boys and 9 to 12 calories per minute for girls. For example, an active female gymnast who weighs 92 pounds requires 920 basal calories plus 920 basal activity calories. Her daily 2-hour workout requires another 1200 calories (10 calories times 120 minutes). Her total caloric need is 3040 calories (Birrer & Brecher, 1987).

Protein requirements of the preadolescent and adolescent athlete approximate those of the adult, but younger athletes have increased protein needs for growth. Small children have special iron needs, as do females after menarche (Peterson & Peterson, 1988; Sanders, 1990). Recommended dietary allowances for children are presented in Table 17–7.

The child needs more fluid per proportional weight than the adult. A useful formula for daily water requirements of children is 100 ml/kg/day for the first 10 kg of weight, 50 ml/kg additional for the next 10 kg of weight, and 25 ml/kg additional for the next 10 kg of weight. Above 30 kg of weight the requirements should approximate adult values (64 oz of liquid daily) (Ziegler, 1982).

The training diet of the young athlete should routinely consist of 50 to 55% carbohydrate, 15% protein, and 30 to 35% fat, of which only 10% is saturated. Smaller, growing muscles cannot store glycogen as efficiently as larger, strong muscles, so more complex carbohydrates may be necessary if the child complains of fatigue (Peterson & Peterson, 1988). The basic food groups should be included in these plans with attention to total caloric intake (Food Guide Pyramid, 1992). Additional supplements are not necessary if the diet is adequate and may even be dangerous in the growing child (Clarkson, 1996). Glycogen loading, or increased amounts of glycogen to increase muscle stores to two to three times their normal levels, is not recommended in young children or in early adolescence because of the side effects of muscle stiffness and water retention. Glycogen loading can be used with caution by teenagers (Birrer & Brecher, 1987).

Dietary recommendations differ during the four phases of training and competition. In the postseason and off-season periods, the athlete should receive all nutritional and caloric needs for optimal weight; during the preseason and in-season periods, optimal weight and performance should guide the nutritional balance and caloric load. The pregame meal should be eaten 2 to 3 hours before competition to guarantee digestion in the stomach and upper intestine. The meal should be easy to digest; be low in fat, protein, salt, and bulk; and have abundant liquid content and complex carbohydrates for adequate energy and hydration. Examples are waffles, pasta, sandwiches, or liquid meals. The goal during competition is maintenance of adequate hydration (and glycogen for endurance events). Postcompetition meals should immediately replenish glycogen stores and restore fluid balance. Two cups of water should be consumed for each pound lost

(Clark, 1991; Grana & Kalenak, 1991; Peterson & Peterson, 1988).

Alterations in weight can and should be made carefully. Weight gain diets should have a similar composition to the training diet but include additional calories. An added 1000 calories a day will result in a gain of 2 lb weekly. This gain will occur in lean body tissue if the child is moderately active. Determination of whether an athlete is overfat or overweight must be made before recommendation of a diet for weight loss. If the athlete is excessively fat or has too great a percentage of body fat in relation to total body composition, careful structure of a training plan can convert fat to lean muscle mass. If an athlete is also overweight, a weight loss diet of composition similar to that of the normal athlete but with 1000 fewer calories per day should be constructed. This will result in a safe loss of 2 lb weekly. Additional exercise will hasten weight loss and maintain firmness of body tissue (Peterson & Peterson, 1988).

Proper Supervision

The first in the series of supervisors is the coach, the key to a successful sports program. Approximately 20 million children, however, are coached by 2.5 million adult volunteers with varying levels of expertise. The American Academy of Pediatrics has stated that coaches should encourage preparticipation screenings every 1 to 2 years, enforce use of warm-up procedures, require suitable protective equipment, and enforce rules concerning safety. In addition, it recommends completion of a certification program that covers teaching techniques, basic sports skills, fitness, first aid, sportsmanship, enhancement of self-image, and motivational skills (American Academy of Pediatrics, 1989).

Qualified officials and professional medical personnel at games and practices are the second level of supervision. These individuals provide game control and immediate injury containment on site. Medical personnel could include physicians, physical therapists, or athletic trainers who have certification in basic first aid and cardiopulmonary resuscitation techniques in addition to their medical skills (American Academy of Pediatrics, 1989; Puffer, 1991).

Protection

Outfitting the child athlete with proper equipment should be mandated and enforced for the protection of the participants. Equipment must be appropriate for the sport. High quality and proper fit

TABLE 17–7. **Recommended Daily Dietary Allowances for the Growing Child**

		Males				Females			
Age (yr):	4–6	7–10	11–14	15–18	4–6	7–10	11–14	15–18
Calories	1800	2100	2800	3000	1800	2100	2100	2100
Protein (g)	30	36	44	54	30	36	44	48
Fat-soluble vitamins								
A (IU)	2000	2500	3300	5000	2000	2500	4000	4000
D (IU)	100	100	100	100	100	100	100	100
E (IU)	9	10	12	15	9	10	12	12
Water-soluble vitamins								
Ascorbic acid (mg)	40	40	45	45	40	40	45	45
Folacin (μg)	200	300	400	400	200	300	400	400
Niacin (mg)	12	16	18	20	12	16	16	14
Riboflavin (mg)	1.1	1.2	1.5	1.8	1.1	1.2	1.3	1.4
Thiamin (mg)	0.9	1.2	1.4	1.5	0.9	1.2	1.2	1.1
B_6 (mg)	0.9	1.2	1.5	2.0	0.9	1.2	1.6	2.0
B_{12} (μg)	1.5	2.0	3.0	3.0	1.5	2.0	3.0	3.0
Minerals								
Calcium (mg)	800	800	1200	1200	800	800	1200	1200
Phosphorus (mg)	800	800	1200	1200	800	800	1200	1200
Iron (mg)	10	10	18	18	10	10	18	18
Magnesium (mg)	200	250	350	400	200	250	300	300
Trace elements								
Iodine (μg)	30	110	130	150	80	110	115	115
Zinc (mg)	10	10	15	15	10	10	15	15

From Ziegler, M. Nutritional card of the pediatric athlete. Clinics in Sports Medicine, *1*(3):375, 1982. Adapted from Food and Nutrition Board, National Academy of Sciences–National Research Council, 1974.

are essential to correct function (Stanitski, 1989). Proper footwear with adequate cushioning, rearfoot control, and sole flexibility for the sport should be required (Segesser & Pforringer, 1989; Trepman & Micheli, 1988). Protective padding in contact or kicking sports, such as shoulder and shin pads, should be recommended.

Protective headgear for contact and collision in football, baseball, and hockey is necessary to limit the number of head and neck injuries. Schuller and colleagues (1989) have demonstrated a lower risk of auricular damage in wrestlers wearing headgear (26% incidence) versus those with no headgear (52% incidence). Helmets should be approved by the National Operating Committee on Standards for Athletic Equipment and the American National Safety Institute (Grana & Kalenak, 1991; Objective testing group certifies head protection, 1988).

Eye injuries have been on the increase in recent years, particularly in racquet sports, baseball, and basketball (Napier, 1996; Stock & Cornell, 1991; Strahlman et al., 1990). An estimated 100,000 sports-related eye injuries occur yearly and are the most common cause of eye trauma in children younger than age 15 years (Stock & Cornell, 1991) (Box 17-1). Eye protectors that dissipate injury to a wider area without reducing visual field should be required in racquet sports, ice hockey, baseball, basketball, and football and during use of air-powered weapons. They should be cosmetically and functionally acceptable and made of impact-resistant material. Polycarbonate is the most impact- and scratch-resistant material. A list of high-risk sports and recommended protection is given in Table 17-8. All eye protectors should be approved by either the Canadian Standards Association or the American Society for Testing and Materials.

Studies have highlighted the incidence of oral and facial injuries in many sports, particularly football, hockey, baseball, basketball, wrestling, and boxing (Maestrello-deMoya & Primosch, 1989). Youth baseball generated the greatest number of head and face injuries in 1980 (Castaldi, 1986). Before mandatory use of mouthguards, oral trauma constituted 50% of all football injuries (McNutt et al., 1989). The mandatory use of mouthguards has cut the injury rate of oral trauma in football to less than 1% of all injuries (Kerr, 1986). The mouth protector serves to prevent injury to the teeth and lacerations of the mouth.

BOX 17-1. **Sports Associated with Eye Injury at Various Ages**

Children (5 to 12 years of age)
  Baseball
  Basketball
  Soccer
  BB gun injuries
Adolescents (13 to 21 years of age)
  Basketball
  Football
  Ice hockey
  Soccer
Adults (21 years of age and older)
  Racquetball
  Squash
  Tennis
  Badminton

From Stock, J, & Cornell, M. Prevention of sports-related eye injury. American Family Practice, 44:516, 1991; published by the American Academy of Family Physicians.

TABLE 17-8. **Risk Level for Eye Injury with Recommendations for Protective Eyewear**

Risk	Sport	Protective Wear
Unacceptable	Boxing	Not applicable
Very high	Ice hockey	Helmet with full visor
	Squash	Polycarbonate sports protector
	Badminton	Polycarbonate sports protector
	Basketball	Polycarbonate sports protector
	Men's lacrosse	Helmet with full visor
High	Racquetball	Polycarbonate sports protector
	Baseball	Polycarbonate sports protector
	Cricket	Helmet with full visor
	Field hockey	Helmet with full visor
	Rugby football	Debatable
	Soccer	Debatable
	Water polo	Polycarbonate goggles
	Shooting	Polycarbonate sports protector
	Women's lacrosse	Helmet with full visor
Moderate	Tennis	Plastic lens spectacles
	American football	Helmet with polycarbonate visor
Low	Golf	Sports protector if one-eyed
	Volleyball	Sports protector if one-eyed
	Skiing	UV filter goggles ± helmet
	Cycling	Sports protector ± helmet
	Fishing	Polycarbonate protector if one-eyed
	Swimming	Goggles if in water for long periods
	High diving	Not feasible
	Track & field	None required

From Jones, N. Eye injury in sport. Sports Medicine, 7:178, 1989.

Because it absorbs blows to the oral and facial structures, it also prevents fractures, dislocations, and concussions. It should position the bite so the condyles of the mandible do not contact the fossae of the joints. These mouthguards should be inexpensive, strong, and easy to clean and should not interfere with speech or breathing. They should be used alone in field hockey, rugby, wrestling, basketball, and other field events and used in conjunction with face protectors in football, ice hockey, baseball, and lacrosse (Grana & Kalenak, 1991; Kerr, 1986).

Environmental Control

Assessment and control of the environment is also vital to the safety of the child athlete. The playing area should be well lighted and maintained for safety. Surfaces should be free from obstacles and smooth and even, with good shock-absorbing qualities (wood as opposed to concrete). Modifications of equipment that have been shown to decrease injury (e.g., breakaway bases) should be installed. Sports equipment and playing environments should be scaled down to the size of the athlete (Stanitski, 1989).

Ambient temperature and humidity should be carefully monitored. Children have a greater surface area per body weight, so their rate of heat exchange is greater with lower ability to endure exercise in climatic extremes. They also have a distinctly deficient ability to perspire, so they carry a larger heat load. They acclimatize less efficiently and require more "exposures" for acclimatization to occur (Bar-Or, 1995; Squire, 1990). Exercise should be modified if the temperature is above 80°F or if relative humidity is above 95% (Peterson & Peterson, 1988). The recommendations for exercise and hydration in relation to the environment are noted in Tables 17–9 and 17–10.

Dehydration can be avoided by drinking plenty of liquid before, during, and after play. Thirst is not a valid indicator of the amount of water needed, so every pound lost should be replaced with 2 cups of water (Peterson & Peterson, 1988). The American College of Sports Medicine recommends that 400 to 500 ml of water be ingested before distance running. They further recommend water intake every 35 to 45 minutes of football practice and nude weighing before and after practice. If residual weight loss from day to day exceeds 2 to 3 pounds, practice is restricted until water is replenished (Ziegler, 1982). Table 17–10 outlines the recommended amount and time of fluid breaks for degree of weight loss.

The American Academy of Pediatrics has established guidelines on dangerous sports. It does not recommend boxing or trampoline jumping for any growing child (Mellion, 1988). One pediatric sports

TABLE 17–9. Wet-Bulb Temperature and Field Precautions

Temperature	Precaution
Under 68°F	No precautions necessary except close observation of those squad members most susceptible to heat illness (those who lose over 3% of their body weight as determined from weight chart).
69–79°F	Insist that unlimited amounts of drinking water be given on the field. Ice water is preferable.
Over 80°F	Lighten the practice routine or practice in shorts. Withhold susceptible players from participation. Whenever the humidity is over 95%, alter practice as described for "Over 80."

From Murphy, R. Heat illness in the athlete. In Athletic Training, Schering Symposium, Nashville, 1984, p. 2.

TABLE 17–10. Recommended Fluid Intake and Availability for a 90-Minute Practice

Weight Loss		Minutes between Water Break	Fluid per Break	
lb	kg		oz	ml
8	3.6	*		
7.5	3.4	*		
7	3.2	10	8–10	266
6.5	3.0	10	8–9	251
6	2.7	10	8–9	251
5.5	2.5	15	10–12	325
5	2.3	15	10–11	311
4.5	2.1	15	9–10	281
4	1.8	15	8–9	251
3.5	1.6	20	10–11	311
3	1.4	20	9–10	281
2.5	1.1	20	7–8	222
2	0.9	30	8	237
1.5	0.7	30	6	177
1	0.5	45	6	177
0.5	0.2	60	6	177

From Peterson, M, & Peterson, K. Eat to Compete: A Guide to Sports Nutrition. Chicago: Year Book Medical, 1988, p. 182.
*No practice recommended.

orthopedist recommends that children younger than age 14 not be allowed to run distances greater than 10 km because of the effects of repetitive trauma on growing bone (Physician urges caution for child marathoners, 1982).

RISK FACTORS FOR INJURY

Injury can be the result of a single macrotrauma or of repetitive microtrauma (Micheli, 1991). Seven risk factors for repetitive trauma, or "overuse," have been identified: (1) training errors; (2) musculotendinous imbalances of strength, flexibility, or bulk; (3) anatomic malalignment of the lower extremity; (4) improper footwear; (5) faulty playing surface; (6) associated disease states of the lower extremity such as old injury or arthritis; and (7) growth factors (Maffulli, 1990; Micheli, 1983; Taimela et al., 1990).

Training Error

Training error is frequently the cause of overuse injuries in children, as it is in adults. The evolution of sport-specific camps from the generalized summer camp experience has dramatically increased the daily level of participation. The sudden transition from casual play to 6 or 8 hours of intense participation has contributed to the incidence of overuse injury in children.

Muscle-Tendon Imbalance

Muscle-tendon imbalance can occur in strength, flexibility, or bulk. Until recently, little attention was paid to conditioning in children. This attitude may have been appropriate for free play activities but not for organized sport. The repetitive, often predictable, demands of a sport may result in imbalances of muscle and tendon unless the child is on a well-designed training plan. For example, a baseball pitcher or swimmer who does the breast stroke might develop a loose anterior capsule and a tight posterior capsule, a situation that could lead to impingement or anterior shoulder subluxation. Repetitive running creates strength and tightness in the quadriceps femoris and triceps surae muscles with relatively weaker hamstrings. This could be problematic if pace and hence stride length are increased.

Anatomic Malalignment

Anatomic malalignment can be a factor in the occurrence of injury because the body may not be able to compensate for the malalignment under the demands of a sport. Femoral anteversion in a young dancer can cause excessive tibial external rotation and ankle pronation as substitutes for natural hip external rotation. Hyperlordosis of the spine or hyperextension of the knee creates abnormal loading on portions of the joint, leading to pain. Pes planus can increase the valgus moment at the knee, as well as allowing the weight of the body to land on a flexible foot. This malalignment can cause pain and abnormal wear on the medial knee joint and foot.

Footwear and Playing Surface

Well-fitting shoes with a firm heel counter, slight heel lift, and flexible toe box are essential for the young athlete. Inadequate footwear that does not support the structures of the foot while playing can lead to a number of foot and lower extremity problems. The shoe should compensate for changes in alignment and shock absorption. Likewise, improper playing surfaces can predispose the child to knee pain, shin splints, or stress fractures. These symptoms have been associated with playing on hard, banked surfaces or synthetic courts, as opposed to clay and hardwood surfaces (O'Neill & Micheli, 1988).

Associated Disease States

Associated disease is occasionally an issue, as in the child with previous Legg-Calvé-Perthes disease who has limited hip rotation. Likewise, a child with juvenile rheumatoid arthritis or hemophilia may have exacerbations of joint pain or synovitis with participation in sports.

Growth

The first aspect of growth that is a factor in overuse injuries is the articular cartilage (Fig. 17–3). Clinical and biomechanical evidence suggests that growing cartilage has low resistance to repetitive loading, resulting in microtrauma to either the cartilage or the underlying growth plate. Damage may result in osteoarthritis or growth asymmetry (Micheli, 1983).

The growing articular cartilage is also less resistant to shear, particularly at the elbow, knee, and ankle. Repetitive shear has been implicated in osteochondritis dissecans of the capitellum in Little League pitchers and of the proximal and distal femur and talus in runners. Studies postulate that a segment of subchondral bone becomes avascular and separates with its articular cartilage from the surrounding bone to become a loose body (Maffulli, 1990). Shear stress has further been implicated in epiphyseal displacement (Micheli, 1983).

The final site of growth cartilage weakness is the apophysis. Increasing evidence suggests that traction apophysitis, such as Osgood-Schlatter disease, Sever disease, and irritation of the rectus femoris or sartorius muscle origins, is the result of degeneration of the growth center with tiny avulsion fractures and associated healing (Maffulli, 1990; Micheli, 1983; O'Neill & Micheli, 1988).

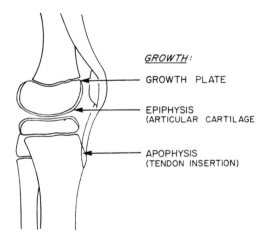

GROWTH:

GROWTH PLATE

EPIPHYSIS
(ARTICULAR CARTILAGE)

APOPHYSIS
(TENDON INSERTION)

FIGURE 17–3. Sites of susceptibility of the growth cartilage. (From Micheli, L. Overuse injuries in children's sports: The growth factor. Orthopedic Clinics of North America, *14*:341, 1983.)

The second element of growth involved in overuse injury is the process itself. Longitudinal growth occurs in the bones, with secondary elongation of the soft tissues. During periods of rapid bone growth ("growth spurts") the musculotendinous structures tighten and cause loss of flexibility. A coincidence of overuse injury and growth spurt has been noted (Micheli, 1983).

TYPES OF INJURIES

Although injuries in children have some similarity to those in adults, several are peculiar to the growing child. These specific injuries fall into three categories: (1) fractures, (2) joint injuries, and (3) muscle-tendon unit injuries (Micheli, 1983; O'Neill & Micheli, 1988).

Fractures

A relatively new injury in children is the stress fracture, which usually results from repetitive microtrauma or poor training. Repetition causes cancellous bone fractures as opposed to cortical bone fatigue in adults (Coady & Micheli, 1997; Maffulli, 1990). These cancellous bone fractures are often imperceptible on radiographs until 6 to 8 weeks after the onset of pain. Stress fractures cause persistent, activity-related pain that can be reproduced by indirect force to the bone. Suspicion based on clinical signs and symptoms can be reinforced by bone scans if diagnostic uncertainty exists.

Growth plate or epiphyseal fractures are peculiar to the child. The cartilaginous growth plate is less resistant to shear or tensile-deforming force than either the ligament or bony cortex, so mechanical disruption frequently occurs through the plate itself, usually in the zone of hypertrophy (Maffulli, 1990). This disruption can be caused by a single macrotrauma, such as jumping, or by repetitive microtrauma as in distance running. The potential for problems from epiphyseal fracture depends on the specific plate involved and on the extent of the injury. Decreased limb length, angular deformity, joint incongruity, and premature closure are frequent sequelae (Maffulli, 1990; Micheli, 1984). Shaft fractures are usually noted in the older child who is approaching adult status.

Joint Injuries

Joint injuries in the young athlete include ligamentous sprains, internal derangement, and musculotendinous insertional injuries. These can result from a single discrete injury or from repetitive trauma. The diagnosis of sprain must be made carefully in the child. During a growth spurt, ligaments may be stronger than the growth plate, so excessive bending or twisting forces cause the plate rather than the ligament to yield. Severe ligamentous injuries can occur, however, so careful examination is necessary to differentiate among these injuries (Micheli, 1983; Trepman & Micheli, 1988).

Repetitive microtrauma of the joint articular cartilage often results in softening, followed by frank shredding and thinning of the surface. Compression to the joint causes exacerbation of the symptoms, such as pain, edema, and decreased functional use of the joint (Trepman & Micheli, 1988).

Muscle-Tendon Unit Injuries

Another area at particular risk of injury in the growing child is the insertion of the musculotendinous unit into the bone through the epiphyseal cartilage. Growth occurs at the apophyseal growth plate, where tendons and ligaments are attached. During growth spurts the increased tension on the attachments often leads to detachment of the structure at the apophysis (avulsion fracture). Tendonitis occurs much less frequently in the child than in the adult because the insertion becomes symptomatic before the tendon (Micheli, 1983, 1984; Trepman & Micheli, 1988).

Irritation of the insertional area of the musculotendinous unit, the enthesis, can cause pain and inflammation. This area is highly vascular and metabolically active. During exercise, when blood is diverted to the active muscle, these areas may suffer periods of ischemia (Maffulli, 1990). The symptoms cause inhibition of muscle activity with resultant weakness and loss of flexibility. The weakness and tightness then lead to greater irritation and pain (O'Neill & Micheli, 1988).

Children can overuse muscles, resulting in strain, just like adults. The increase in muscle volume during exercise may cause exertional compartment syndromes. Muscle hernias, however, occur in children secondary to tight fascial or musculotendinous structures (Trepman & Micheli, 1988).

SITES OF INJURY

The anatomy and the factor of growth combine to make certain injuries more likely and more serious in the various segments of the child's body.

Brain and Cervical Injuries

The incidence of central nervous system injury in children is low, varying from 1 to 5% of sports-related injuries, but these cases constitute 50 to 100% of the deaths from injury. Cervical spine injuries result in 30 to 50% of cases of childhood quadriplegia (Bruce et al., 1982). The rate of spinal cord injuries in children younger than age 11 years is low, but it escalates dramatically in the 15- to 18-year-old age bracket. Because the brain and spinal cord are largely incapable of regeneration, these injuries take on a singular importance (Cantu, 1988).

Participation in several sports carries a particularly high risk for head and neck injuries. Football accounts for 40% of all concussion injuries in school sports. The incidence of serious head injuries has decreased by 60% over the past 20 years, probably because of use of better equipment. Fatalities in children younger than age 12 have not been reported, but the mortality rate is 0.44 per 100,000 participants in tackle football. The incidence of serious head injury is still 0.75 to 1.5 per 100,000 participants per season, with a mortality rate of 0.5 to 1.09 per season (Bruce et al., 1982). Severe injuries, however, often result in quadriplegia and total disability. Rugby, a popular collision sport outside the United States, has head and neck injury rates similar to those of American football. Wrestling has the second highest injury rate of all high school sports, although the central nervous system injury rate is low. The rate of concussion is 1.7% of all wrestling injuries as a result of direct blows or falls (Bruce et al., 1982). Baseball accounts for a large number of concussions secondary to collision with the bat, other players, or the ball, although exact incidence figures have not been reported. Diving accounts for 3 to 18% of all cervical spine injuries in young people (Bruce et al., 1982).

TABLE 17–11. Grading of Severity of Concussion

Grade	Severity
1 (mild)	No loss of consciousness; posttraumatic amnesia 30 minutes
2 (moderate)	Loss of consciousness <5 minutes or posttraumatic amnesia >30 minutes
3 (severe)	Loss of consciousness 5 minutes or post-traumatic amnesia 24 hours

Adapted from Cantu, R. Guidelines to return to contact sports after a cerebral concussion. Physician and Sportsmedicine, 14:76, 1986. Reproduced with permission of McGraw-Hill, Inc.

Concussion, or temporary disturbance of brain function, results from a traumatic blow to the head. Symptoms are caused by biomechanical or physiologic aberrations, but no permanent pathologic process occurs (Birrer & Brecher, 1987). Concussions are graded according to duration of unconsciousness (Table 17–11). Because of the occurrence of second impact syndrome, in which a series of insults can lead to cerebral damage when one impact would not, decisions regarding return to play are critical. No universally accepted criteria for return to play exist, but Table 17–12 contains recommendations based on the severity and incidence of prior concussion (Birrer & Brecher, 1987; Bruce et al., 1982; Cantu, 1988). Postconcussion syndrome, which is characterized by headache, irritability, labyrinthine disturbance, and impaired memory and concentration, is rare but suggests altered neurotransmitter function. Further evaluation is warranted before clearance to play is granted (Cantu, 1988).

The leading cause of death from head injury is intracranial hemorrhage. The most rapidly progressing and universally fatal disorder if missed is the epidural hematoma. Symptoms include initial preservation of consciousness with increasingly severe headache, lethargy, and focal neurologic signs. It is frequently associated with temporal bone fracture. An acute subdural hematoma is the most common fatal head injury and should always be considered as a possible diagnosis in the athlete who loses and does not regain consciousness. A chronic subdural hematoma should be suspected in the athlete who is not quite the same for days or weeks after a head injury. Signs may include headache or mild mental, motor, or sensory signs and symptoms (Cantu, 1988).

The intracerebral hemorrhage is also rapidly progressive because the bleeding is into the brain itself. No lucid interval is noted, and death often occurs before arrival at a hospital. The subarachnoid hemorrhage is a brain contusion that causes headache and associated neurologic deficits that are

TABLE 17–12. Guidelines for Return to Play after Concussion

Grade	First Concussion	Second Concussion	Third Concussion
1 (mild)	May return to play if asymptomatic* for 1 week	Return to play in 2 weeks if asymptomatic at that time for 1 week	Terminate season; may return to play next season if asymptomatic
2 (moderate)	Return to play after asymptomatic for 1 week	Minimum of 1 month; may return to play then if asymptomatic for 1 week; consider terminating season	Terminate season; may return to play next season if asymptomatic
3 (severe)	Minimum of 1 month; may then return to play if asymptomatic for 1 week	Terminate season; may return to play next season if asymptomatic	

Adapted from Cantu, R. Guidelines to return to contact sports after a cerebral concussion. Physician and Sportsmedicine, 14:79, 1986. Reproduced with permission of McGraw-Hill, Inc.

*No headache, dizziness, or impaired orientation, concentration, or memory during rest.

dependent on the area of the brain involved. All injured athletes with potential intracranial hemorrhages should be transported to a hospital for further evaluation and medical or surgical management (Bruce et al., 1982).

Most neck injuries are caused by hyperflexion or hyperextension. Hyperflexion injuries, the most common, result from spearing or butt blocking (Fig. 17–4). Because of the poorly developed musculature in youngsters and the commonly associated fracture, hyperflexion injury can be serious. Hyperextension injuries often occur even in the absence of severe force because the anterior neck musculature is weaker than the posterior musculature. Common causes are face or head tackling (Fig. 17–5). Hyperextension injury with a rotatory component is the most common cause of nerve root damage (Birrer & Brecher, 1987). Evaluation of these injuries should always include radiographs of the cervical spine. In the adolescent the second cervical vertebra is normally displaced posteriorly over the third secondary to hypermobility. This pseudosubluxation is normal and not the result of injury (Cantu, 1988) but should be referred for assessment.

Another common injury is a "burner," which is a traction injury to the brachial plexus. It is caused by a forceful blow to the head from the side or from depression of the shoulder while the head and neck are fixed. Repeated injuries may cause weakness of the deltoid, biceps, and teres major muscles, which should be resolved with strengthening exercises. If the use of a collar or a change in technique or neck strength does not solve the problem, cessation of participation is warranted (Cantu, 1988).

Thoracic and Lumbar Spinal Injuries

Spinal injuries can occur in both the thoracic and the lumbar areas, although thoracic injuries are rare.

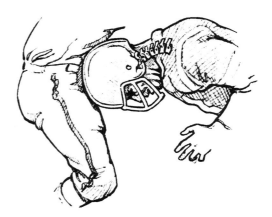

FIGURE 17–4. Hyperflexion damage from head butting. (From Birrer, R, & Brecher, D. Common Sports Injuries in Youngsters. Oradell, NJ: Medical Economics, 1987, p. 36.)

Costovertebral injury secondary to compression of the rib cage in a pileup in football or from a forceful takedown in wrestling can injure the costovertebral articulations. Complaints include pain and muscle spasm along the associated rib. Axial compression forces on a preflexed spine, as in sledding or tobogganing, can fracture the vertebrae, particularly at the vulnerable T12–L1 level. These injuries can cause pain but are frequently asymptomatic (Birrer & Brecher, 1987).

The most common injuries in the lumbar spine are spondylolysis and spondylolisthesis. One study of 3132 competitive athletes ages 15 to 27 years noted an incidence of spondylolysis of 12.5% (Rossi & Dragoni, 1990). Repeated hyperflexion and hyperextension in football blocking, clean and jerk lift, diving, pole vaulting, wrestling, high jump, or gymnastic maneuvers can place excessive forces on the pars interarticularis and cause a stress fracture.

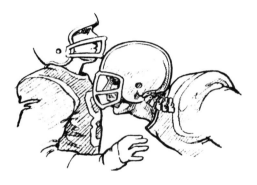

FIGURE 17–5. Hyperextension injury from face blocking. (From Birrer, R, & Brecher, D. Common Sports Injuries in Youngsters. Oradell, NJ: Medical Economics, 1987, p. 38.)

Spondylolisthesis, or fracture and slippage of one vertebra on another, usually L5 over S1, is most common at ages 9 to 14 years. Loading of a bilateral spondylolysis, in which there is a defect in the bony connection of the posterior arch with the vertebral body, can cause a spondylolisthesis, as can traumatic or repetitive bilateral loading of a normal spine. The slippage is graded from 1 to 4, depending on the degree of slippage. Athletes with grade 2 or greater slippage should be counseled against participation in weight lifting, baseball, diving, gymnastics, or wrestling. Participation in basketball or football is permissible with use of a brace (Birrer & Brecher, 1987). The growth spurt in the spine causes lumbar lordosis secondary to the enhanced anterior growth with posterior tethering by the heavy lumbodorsal fascia. This biomechanical situation increases the tendency of posterior element failure at the pars and perhaps at the disc (Micheli, 1983). Athletes with spondylolysis are managed in a brace until healing occurs. Physical therapy is indicated to maintain flexibility in the lumbosacral spine and the spinal and hip musculature and to improve trunk and abdominal muscle strength while braced. Surgery is indicated only in cases of unstable lesions or nerve root compression (Birrer & Brecher, 1987).

The true incidence of disc lesions in young athletes is unclear, but several studies have demonstrated disturbing data. Although acute trauma has a role in this condition, degenerative changes of the vertebral bodies and intervertebral joints may be the leading factor, with trauma as only the precipitating incident (Maffulli, 1990).

Shoulder Injuries

Specific shoulder injuries can be predicted based on the biomechanics of the sport and the age of the athlete. Football, wrestling, and ice hockey cause upper extremity fractures and dislocations, and sports with repeated overhead activities contribute to overuse injuries. The hyperelasticity of juvenile joints, particularly the shoulder, makes them vulnerable to passive and dynamic instability patterns that can predispose the shoulder to injury (Ireland & Andrews, 1988).

Acromioclavicular sprains may occur in the immature athlete without clavicular fracture. The most common mechanism is direct force from a fall or blow to the lateral aspect of the shoulder or a fall on an outstretched arm (Birrer & Brecher, 1987; Micheli, 1984; Nevaiser, 1986). Grade I and II sprains are more common in the athlete whose skeleton is immature. Grade III sprains commonly rupture the dorsal clavicular periosteum, but the acromioclavicular and coracoclavicular ligaments remain intact (Ireland & Andrews, 1988). These lesions are treated symptomatically with rest, ice, compression, and elevation (RICE) in a sling. Exercises are often necessary to increase scapulothoracic and glenohumeral mobility and strength (see rehabilitation source material in Appendix II).

Fractures are most common in the middle third of the clavicle from a direct blow. These can be actual fractures in the older child or greenstick fractures in the youngster. They are managed with a figure-of-eight strap until healed.

Because the proximal humerus is an area of bone growth, fractures are more common in children than in adults, who are more prone to dislocation. Epiphyseal displacements occur in the younger child, and metaphyseal fractures are more common in the older child or adolescent (Micheli, 1984). After healing, therapeutic intervention to normalize mobility and strength of the scapular, shoulder, and elbow muscles is frequently indicated.

Little League shoulder, a relatively common injury in young pitchers and catchers, involves a fracture of the proximal humeral growth plate secondary to rotatory torque. Any athlete who complains of proximal shoulder pain in the absence of trauma should be suspected of having an epiphyseal fracture until proven otherwise. The athlete should not do any throwing until the pain subsides (Ireland & Andrews, 1988).

Frank anterior subluxation and dislocation of the glenohumeral joint is rare in children but common in adolescents. Because of the laxity of juvenile joints, a blow or forceful maneuver in abduction, external rotation, or extension can dislodge the head of the humerus (Birrer & Brecher, 1987; Ireland & Andrews, 1988; Nevaiser, 1986). This condition is common in throwing or racquet sports, gymnastics, and swimming. Patients with posterior glenohumeral instability respond better to conservative strengthening of appropriate musculature than those with anterior instability, although a program of scapular and shoulder muscle strengthening in a biomechanically correct range of motion should be attempted. Motion should be limited to ranges that prevent chronic subluxation. Surgery is more often an option with anterior or multidirectional instability than in posterior instability (Ireland & Andrews, 1988).

Rotator cuff tears are not as common in the skeletally immature athlete as in the older athlete. They occur in throwing and racquet sports, as well as from direct contact blows in collision sports. These tears can be treated successfully with arthroscopic surgery and rehabilitation that includes strength and endurance training for all scapular and shoulder muscles, as well as training with correct biomechanical movements of the shoulder complex (Ireland & Andrews, 1988; Nevaiser, 1986).

Rotator cuff impingement syndrome (Fig. 17-6) is a frequent injury in athletes younger than 25 years of age. More than 50% of swimmers age 12 to 18 years complain of shoulder pain (Birrer & Brecher, 1987). One hypothesis is that these athletes develop a characteristic contracture around the shoulder with loss of internal rotation at 90° of abduction and with increased external rotation in all positions of abduction. This might reflect a tightened posterior and a loosened anterior capsule, suggesting a tendency to subluxate anteriorly. Conservative physical therapy with normalization of mobility and strength has been successful in resolving the primary instability (Micheli, 1983). All positions of impingement (anterior, lateral, or overhead) should be avoided until the child is free of pain.

Elbow Injuries

Supracondylar fracture of the humerus is the second most common fracture in the skeletally immature client. Most of these fractures occur in the age group of 5 to 10 years. They are the result of significant forces into extension. Avulsion fractures of the medial epicondyle are not uncommon and are associated with elbow dislocations or throwing injuries. Anatomic reduction usually requires internal fixation with early protected range of motion to avoid loss of extension (Ireland & Andrews, 1988). Subsequent to healing, normalization of mobility and strength of the elbow and forearm are necessary for full function.

Repetitive microtrauma from pitching may result in epiphyseal fracture of the radial head. Loss of extension and supination with a history of repetitive loading of the radiocapitellar joint indicates fracture. A radial head fracture is treated with rest

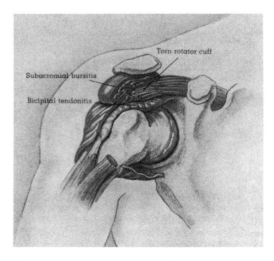

FIGURE 17-6. Common causes of impingement. (From Birrer, R, & Brecher, D. Common Sports Injuries in Youngsters. Oradell, NJ: Medical Economics, 1987, p. 61.)

(DaSilva et al., 1998; Ireland & Andrews, 1988). Jerking of the elbow in the child younger than 7 years old can subluxate the radial head because of the poor development of the annular ligament. The child positions the injured arm in flexion and pronation, dangling it at the side of the body (Birrer & Brecher, 1987; Micheli et al., 1980).

Elbow dislocation is seen in contact sports secondary to a fall on an abducted, extended arm. Early reduction will avoid neurovascular damage, and further evaluation and radiographs are necessary to assess the presence of associated fracture. Early protected mobility is necessary to preserve normal elbow motion (Birrer & Brecher, 1987; Ireland & Andrews, 1988). Physical therapy to normalize elbow and forearm mobility and to improve strength at the elbow, forearm, and hand is appropriate.

Little League elbow commonly results from the extreme valgus stress placed on the epicondyles during the acceleration phase of pitching (Fig. 17-7). If this is not recognized and regular throwing continues, mild separation of the medial epicondyle with hypertrophy, irregularity, fragmentation, and avulsion can occur. The most serious damage is the jamming of the radial head against the capitellum on the lateral side, a finding that occurs in 8 to 10% of young pitchers. The results of this jamming can be osteochondritis of the capitellum, avascular necrosis of the radial head, and loose bodies within the joint. Treatment is RICE and rest from throwing (Birrer & Brecher, 1987). Eventual alteration of throwing technique may be necessary.

Tennis elbow is seen in a variety of racquet sports as a result of repeated injury to the lateral epicon-

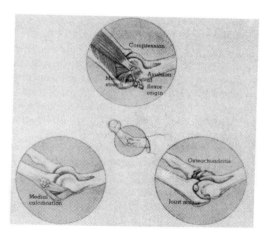

FIGURE 17–7. Little League elbow. (From Birrer, R, & Brecher, D. Common Sports Injuries in Youngsters. Oradell, NJ: Medical Economics, 1987, p. 74.)

dyle. A faulty stroke initiates the process. The resulting friction between the extensor muscles, the lateral epicondyle, and the radial head causes irritation, microtears in the extensor muscle origin, and adhesions between the annular ligament and the joint capsule. Using tightly strung racquets, racquets with small handles, and old tennis balls will aggravate the situation. Rehabilitation to decrease irritation, reduce adhesions, and strengthen the forearm and hand musculature is required. Alteration of technique and equipment, such as enlargement of the racquet grip area or reduction of string tension, is helpful (Birrer & Brecher, 1987; Knowles et al., 1987).

Wrist and Hand Injuries

Because of the inherent complexity of the anatomy of the wrist joint, potentially serious injuries may be missed or underdiagnosed. Careful diagnosis using knowledge of biomechanics of the wrist and hand is crucial (Birrer & Brecher, 1987; Micheli, 1984).

Fractures about the wrist follow an age-related pattern. In the young child a torus, or buckle fracture, of the distal radial epiphysis is common after a fall. Clinical signs are minimal pain and tenderness, so careful radiologic examination is necessary. Simple splinting is adequate for healing (Birrer & Brecher, 1987; Micheli, 1984). Metaphyseal fractures of the distal radius and ulna are more common in the child. Often displaced, they require reduction with the use of anesthesia. In the younger adolescent, fractures through the growth plate are common, again from falls, and require operative reduction to minimize trauma to the growth plate (Micheli,

1984). Rehabilitation to regain normal forearm and wrist mobility as well as wrist and grip strength is desirable. Stress injuries to the distal radial epiphysis have been noted in athletes such as gymnasts who bear weight on their hands. Complaints of pain with wrist dorsiflexion and of wrist stiffness are common. Radiographs demonstrate a widened epiphysis, cystic changes, and breaking of the distal metaphysis. Management consists of cessation of gymnastics with or without casting (Simmons & Lovallo, 1988).

Although fracture of most carpal bones is rare, fracture of the navicular or scaphoid bone is common in children from 12 to 15 years of age. This fracture results from a fall on the dorsiflexed hand of an outstretched arm. Although the fracture is not readily visible on a radiograph, early diagnosis is important because of the high incidence of avascular necrosis and nonunion. If tenderness in the anatomical snuffbox occurs with a high degree of suspicion of fracture, use of a short-arm spica cast will be adequate management (Birrer & Brecher, 1987; Micheli, 1984; Simmons & Lovallo, 1988).

Because the hand and fingers are so essential in most sports, the small structures absorb tremendous forces of initial contact (Birrer & Brecher, 1987). Injuries are therefore common. Dislocations are uncommon in the child's hand because the forces necessary to produce these injuries are usually dissipated by producing a fracture. If dislocations do occur, it is usually in the adolescent and in patterns similar to those in an adult. Thus the most common dislocation occurs at the carpometacarpal joint of the thumb, usually secondary to axial compression forces on the thumb tip in contact sports. Although reduction is easy, maintenance is not, and chronic instability can result. The thumb is put in a short-arm thumb spica, and participation in sports should be avoided for 6 weeks. A short opponens splint is advisable for the initial 6 weeks of reentry to play (Simmons & Lovallo, 1988).

Dorsal dislocation of the thumb metacarpophalangeal joint is the most common dislocation in the hand of a child. A fall or forceful contact hyperextends the metacarpophalangeal joint. If the proximal phalanx is parallel to the metacarpal, the volar plate has been avulsed and surgical reduction is necessary. Cast immobilization for 3 weeks with sports participation permitted is adequate for healing. Physical therapy may be indicated to normalize thumb mobility and strength following casting. Metacarpophalangeal dislocations in the fingers are rare except for those that affect the index finger. After this injury is reduced, splinting in flexion for 3 weeks with immediate mobilization after splint removal is the treatment of choice (Birrer & Brecher, 1987; Simmons & Lovallo, 1988).

Joint injuries are common in ball sports and skiing. The metacarpophalangeal joint of the thumb is the most commonly injured joint in skiers. The majority of these injuries in youth are bony gamekeeper's thumb in which the ulnar collateral ligament avulses a segment of bone, as compared with the purely ligamentous injury in adults. If the bony fragment lies close to its origin, good results are obtained with use of a short-arm thumb spica for 6 weeks, followed by exercises to normalize mobility and strength. Athletic participation, even molding the cast to fit the ski pole, can be allowed. If the radiograph is negative, integrity of the ulnar collateral ligament must be established by assessing radial deviation in extension and 30° of flexion. Deviation of greater than 30° indicates at least a partial tear. No firm end point in full extension or greater than 45° of deviation in flexion indicates full ligamentous tear with volar plate injury, which will require surgical repair (Birrer & Brecher, 1987; Simmons & Lovallo, 1988). Hand therapy is necessary to regain normal mobility, strength, and pinch.

Jammed fingers are common injuries in all age groups. Axial compression force to the fingertips causes distal interphalangeal flexion with proximal interphalangeal hyperextension. Reduction is easily accomplished by distal traction. Buddy taping will allow the athlete to return to play (Birrer & Brecher, 1987; Simmons & Lovallo, 1988). Caution should be exhibited, however, because fractures through the growth plate of the phalanx are common. These intra-articular, or neck, fractures have a great tendency to displace and then require open reduction with internal fixation (Micheli, 1984). In the absence of a fracture or dislocation, damage to the collateral ligaments can occur and is managed in similar fashion. Jamming at the distal interphalangeal joint can result in "mallet finger," or tearing of the terminal extensor tendon with or without a bony fragment. This injury is easily managed with use of a dorsal extension splint for 6 to 8 weeks. If active and passive extension ranges are equal at 6 weeks, active flexion can be initiated. If not, splinting is continued for another month. Participation is allowed with the splint in place (Birrer & Brecher, 1987; Simmons & Lovallo, 1988).

Pelvis and Hip Injuries

Because the hip and pelvis have complex ossification patterns and fuse late in childhood, the possibility for injury is high. The acetabulum has three sections joined by triradiate cartilage. Likewise, three ossification centers exist on the femoral head: the capital femoral epiphysis, the greater trochanter, and the lesser trochanter. The circular vascularity of the femoral head and neck also creates risk for injury in the growing child (Waters & Millis, 1988).

Fractures are uncommon but can occur in the epiphyseal plate, the femoral neck, or the subtrochanteric area. Slipped capital femoral epiphysis is not caused by sports but must be suspected in any athlete with persistent hip or knee pain and a limp. It occurs during the rapid growth in adolescence in either obese or very thin males. Surgical reduction with internal fixation is necessary (see Chapter 16).

Fractures of the neck or subtrochanteric area are rare but can be the result of severe trauma, usually incurred during contact sports such as football and rugby. Surgical reduction is necessary to maintain position (Waters & Millis, 1988). More common are avulsion fractures from a sudden violent muscular contraction or excessive muscle stretch. The most common sites are the anterior-superior iliac spine (origin of the sartorius), the ischium (hamstring origin) (Fig. 17–8), the lesser trochanter (insertion of the iliopsoas), the anterior-inferior iliac spine (rectus femoris origin), and iliac crest (abdominal insertion). These injuries are classic in sprinting, jumping, soccer, football, and weight lifting. Rest with gradual increase of excursion to full mobility followed by progressive resistance exercise and reintegration to play is the treatment sequence (Birrer & Brecher, 1987; Micheli & Smith, 1982; Waters & Millis, 1988). One less traumatic overuse parallel of avulsion is iliac apophysitis, which usually affects adolescent track, field, or cross-country athletes or dancers. Repeated contraction of the tensor fascia lata, rectus femoris, sartorius, gluteus medius, and oblique abdominal muscles causes nonspecific pain and tenderness over the iliac crest. Rest helps this problem

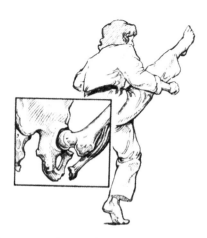

FIGURE 17–8. Avulsion of the ischial tuberosity. (From Birrer, R, & Brecher, D. Common Sports Injuries in Youngsters. Oradell, NJ: Medical Economics, 1987, p. 101.)

(Birrer & Brecher, 1987), but often exercises to increase strength and normalize two-joint muscle flexibility are required.

Stress fractures and osteitis pubis are being diagnosed more frequently as a result of repetitive microtrauma in runners or athletes who have suddenly increased their involvement in jumping or kicking activities. Persistent pain and tenderness in the groin with limited mobility and activity-related increases in pain could signal either of these conditions. Radiographs showing inflammation, demineralization, and sclerosis confirm the diagnosis of osteitis pubis, but a bone scan is necessary to diagnose a stress fracture. Stress fractures have been seen in the pelvis at the junction of the ischium and pubic ramus and in the femoral neck and shaft (Birrer & Brecher, 1987; Waters & Millis, 1988). Relative rest, use of crutches, and restriction from percussive activities (running and jumping) are required for resolution of these disorders.

Snapping hip syndrome is an overuse problem noted in gymnasts, dancers, and sprinters. The term *snapping hip syndrome* can refer either to irritation of the iliotibial band over the greater trochanter with hip motion or to tenosynovitis of the iliopsoas tendon near its femoral insertion. Usually, relative rest, use of appropriate modalities, stretching, and improved muscle strength overcome these symptoms (Micheli, 1983; Waters & Millis, 1988).

A serious condition seen in the young athlete age 5 to 12 years is avascular necrosis of the femoral head. Activity can irritate the synovium, leading to joint effusion and reduction of the blood supply to the femoral head. The initial complaint is nonspecific hip pain, but radiographs demonstrate periosteal rarefaction followed by sclerosis and irregular collapse of the humeral head. Bracing or surgery may be required, depending on the degree of progression of the problem (Birrer & Brecher, 1987; Micheli, 1983) (see Chapter 16).

Contusions are common, but the most frequent is the hip pointer. This iliac crest contusion is caused by a driving blow by a helmet, occurring typically in football or hockey. The overlying muscle is damaged with a resultant subperiosteal hematoma. RICE and padding will resolve this problem with time (Birrer & Brecher, 1987). Occasionally, use of ultrasound evaluation and soft tissue mobilization along with stretching may be necessary.

Knee Injuries

As the largest joint in the body and one with minimal anatomic protection, the knee is the focal point of stress forces applied along the tibia and femur. Consequently, it is not only the site of macrotrauma but also the most frequent site of overuse injury (Birrer & Brecher, 1987; Stanitski, 1997).

Fractures about the knee, although not frequent, are significant for their possible influences on growth. Distal femoral epiphyseal fractures occur in the young athlete as a consequence of twisting injuries. Careful open anatomic reduction with internal fixation is necessary to avoid subsequent growth disturbances (Steiner & Grana, 1988). Physical therapy is usually necessary for children who sustain distal femoral or proximal tibial epiphyseal fractures. Either open reduction with internal fixation or casting causes loss of knee and ankle mobility and decreased thigh and calf muscle strength. Rehabilitation to reverse these effects and retrain the youngster in balance and agility skills is necessary.

Fractures of the proximal tibial epiphysis are rare but treacherous because of associated popliteal artery damage and compartment syndrome. More common is fracture of the tibial tuberosity alone or in association with the proximal tibia. These are most common at the end of adolescence in jumping sports such as basketball and track. These fractures can be managed with extension casting if minimal displacement has occurred or with internal fixation if displaced. Growth disturbances are rare because of the late occurrence of the fracture (Mirby et al., 1988; Steiner & Grana, 1988). Stress fractures were rare but are being reported more commonly in the tibias of runners and swimmers. Reduction of the loading stress of running or of turns in swimming is suggested until healing occurs (Steiner & Grana, 1988). Ligament injuries are becoming more common in the young athlete, with one study reporting medial collateral ligament injury in children as young as 4 years of age (Steiner & Grana, 1988). All ligament injuries should be assessed for coincident physis fractures (Steiner & Grana, 1988). Medial collateral ligament tears in youth can include both the superficial and the capsular components of the ligament. Nonoperative treatment with splinting and avoidance of valgus stress has been successful in adolescents, so it may be possible to obtain equally good results in younger children (Steiner & Grana, 1988). Physical therapy to retain or improve lower extremity strength and coordination, especially in the thigh and calf, is often needed.

Most anterior cruciate ligament tears in the preteen group are in fact avulsion fractures at the tibial insertion. The fracture of the tibial spine usually occurs through the cancellous bone, demonstrating avulsion of the tibial spine on a radiograph. The mechanism of injury is typically a bicycle accident or a fall in preteens and a contact sport in adolescents. Casting in 30° of knee flexion is accepted practice for minimally displaced fractures, but internal fixation is needed for full displacement of the fragment. Midsubstance tears of the anterior cruciate ligament are most common in the adolescent. An increase in injury rates has been noted in female basketball players. Traditional reconstructive procedures are avoided because of fear of injury to the growth plate with the proximal tibial drill hole. Classic management is functional bracing and development of muscular strength and balance for knee stability (Steiner & Grana, 1988; Zarins, 1982).

Internal derangement of the knee joint can be either juvenile osteochondritis dissecans or meniscal injury. The etiology of juvenile osteochondritis dissecans is still an enigma. Compression of the tibial spine against the medial femoral condyle, interruption of the vascularity, anatomic variations in the knee, and abnormal subchondral bone are all possible causes. Athletic children do not seem to be at greater risk for this injury than more sedentary children. The most common sites of involvement are the lateral side of the medial femoral condyle and the lateral femoral condyle in the weight-bearing region or posteriorly. The condition usually causes pain, recurrent swelling, or catching in the knee. Pain is usually evident as the tibia rotates internally and the knee extends from a flexed position (Birrer & Brecher, 1987). Because these lesions have a poor prognosis after skeletal maturity, every attempt should be made to gain healing before growth plate closure. In the child younger than 15 years of age, diminished activity to the point of not bearing weight is suggested. Drilling of the condyles with removal of fragments is recommended in children older than 15 years of age. This procedure usually necessitates restriction of running and jumping for at least 6 weeks with concomitant intensive rehabilitation to regain strength, balance, and agility in the lower extremity (Grana & Kalenak, 1991; Steiner & Grana, 1988).

The challenge of meniscal injuries in the young athlete is accurate diagnosis. Often the initial incident is forgotten and clinical testing is less diagnostic than in the adult. Arthroscopic excision or repair is the treatment of choice if conservative management fails. Excision necessitates physical therapy to regain mobility and strength deficits. Meniscal repair further requires limitations of knee mobility and weight bearing while healing occurs. Discoid lateral meniscus, which is particularly common in the Japanese, can create joint line tenderness, decreased joint mobility, effusion, and, most notably, a prominent snap in the lateral compartment as the knee is extended (Steiner & Grana, 1988). Normal menisci do not go through a discoid stage during development. The complete type of discoid meniscus, producing symptoms in late adolescence, is distinguished by

intact peripheral attachments. Good results are obtained with saucerization of the meniscus. The Wrisberg type of discoid meniscus, which is more common in the pediatric group, has an attachment only through the ligament of Wrisberg and can be resolved by cutting the ligament and removing the portions with no peripheral attachments (Steiner & Grana, 1988).

The majority of problems at the knee in children are disorders of the patellar mechanism (Birrer & Brecher, 1987; Micheli, 1983; Steiner & Grana, 1988). Macrotrauma, repetitive microtrauma, and growth all can contribute to the disorders of the patellofemoral joint. Patellofemoral pain is the most frequent problem in the young athlete. Malalignment of the patellofemoral joint is the major cause of this pain. Several factors can cause or contribute to this malalignment. Anatomic factors such as patella alta, large Q angle, hip anteversion, flattened lateral femoral condyle, shallow femoral groove, or pes planus and hyperpronation can cause abnormal tracking of the patella during knee motion. Acquired factors such as weakness of the medial quadriceps, tension in the lateral retinaculum and lateral soft tissues, or ligamentous laxity can affect patellar alignment and tracking (Fig. 17–9). The malalignment can assume one of three different patterns: (1) lateral subluxation and tilting, (2) lateral subluxation alone, or (3) isolated tilting. The source of pain has been postulated to be the increased stress on the subchondral bone from abnormal patellar stresses, increased tension in the lateral retinaculum, or formation of

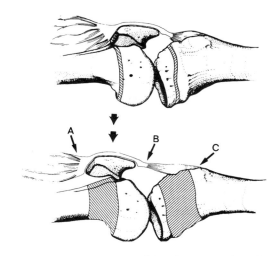

FIGURE 17–9. Tension resulting from growth. Pain may occur at the patella *(A)*, lower pole of the patella *(B)*, or patellar tendon insertion on the tibia *(C)*. (From Micheli, L. Overuse injuries in children's sports: The growth factor. Orthopedic Clinics of North America, *14*:353, 1983.)

synovitis from articular cartilage degeneration (Steiner & Grana, 1988). Management of patellofemoral pain can be conservative or surgical. Conservative management consists of relative rest, balancing of muscle strength and length, and correction of abnormal biomechanics with patellar taping or orthotics. Surgical options include arthroscopic shaving, lateral retinacular release, or patellar realignment (Micheli, 1983; Steiner & Grana, 1988).

Apophysitis, or degeneration of the ossification centers where tendons attach with chronic inflammation and microavulsion, is common in the knee in girls between ages 8 and 13 years and in boys between 10 and 15 years. These can result from longitudinal traction with bone growth or from repetitive activity of sports participation. The most common apophysitides are Osgood-Schlatter disease of the tibial tubercle and Sinding-Larsen-Johansson disease at the inferior pole of the patella. Careful differential diagnosis is necessary to correctly identify these disorders (see Chapter 16). Relative rest, maintenance of quadriceps muscle strength with pain-free exercise, and possible extension splinting are treatment options (Birrer & Brecher, 1987; Maffulli, 1990; Micheli, 1983; Steiner & Grana, 1988).

Infrapatellar tendinitis or traction irritation at the inferior pole, otherwise known as jumper's knee, is noted most frequently in the older adolescent. The etiology includes involvement in sports that require running, jumping, climbing, or kicking. RICE with subsequent strengthening of the knee musculature is important in treatment. Assessment of two-joint muscle length is vital because tightness of the hamstrings muscles or iliotibial band may increase the flexion moment at the knee (Birrer & Brecher, 1987; Micheli, 1983; Steiner & Grana, 1988).

Patellar subluxation or dislocation can be seen in young athletes secondary to the stresses of sports requiring cutting and twisting such as soccer, dancing, cheerleading, gymnastics, and track jumping events or as a result of a direct blow to the knee. Imbalance of the length or strength of the extensor muscles, the hamstrings, the retinaculum, or the iliotibial band, as well as anatomic malalignments such as genu valgus, patella alta, or shallow condylar cup, can be etiologic factors. Management of patellar instability may include bracing in conjunction with physical therapy to normalize length-strength relationships. Failure of conservative management, although the exception, may necessitate surgical intervention to realign the patella by release of the tight structures or by alteration of the line of pull of the infrapatellar tendon (Grana & Kalenak, 1991; Micheli, 1983).

Ankle and Foot Injuries

Because of the peculiarities of their growing skeleton and their penchant for ingenious physical activity, children suffer from foot and ankle problems that may not have counterparts in the adult (McManama, 1988; Santopietro, 1988). Injuries to the distal tibial and fibular growth plates are common in the young athlete. Gregg and Das (1982) have classified growth plate injuries into a clinically useful system (Fig. 17–10). The most common fractures to the ankle in the skeletally immature athlete are the Salter-Harris type 1 and 2 injuries to the

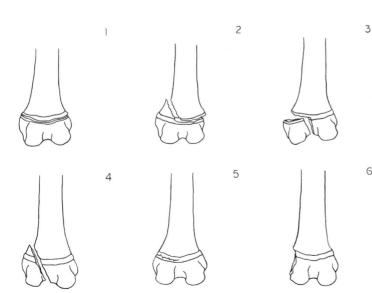

FIGURE 17–10. Modified Salter-Harris classification of growth plate injuries: 1. Disruption entirely confined to the growth plate; distraction or slip injury. 2. Fracture line runs partially through the growth plate, then extends through the metaphysis. 3. Fracture line runs partially through the growth plate, then extends through the epiphysis. 4. Combined disruption of metaphysis, growth plate, and epiphysis. 5. Crush or compression injury of growth plate. 6. Abrasion, avulsion, or burn of the perichondrial ring of the growth plate. (From Gregg, J, & Das, M. Foot and ankle problems in the preadolescent and adolescent athlete. Clinics in Sports Medicine, 1:133, 1982.)

distal fibula. Although these fractures can occur with adduction and abduction injury to the distal tibia, they frequently occur alone as a result of inversion injury. Treatment with immobilization in a short leg cast for 4 to 6 weeks is suggested, although the fracture will usually heal even if untreated (McManama, 1988). Physical therapy after casting to increase ankle and foot mobility and strength and to improve balance may be indicated.

Type 2 injury of the distal tibia is a result of ankle pronation and eversion. Common in football and soccer players, this injury is frequently associated with greenstick fracture of the distal fibula. Care must be taken to reduce these fractures and immobilize them in a long leg cast with knee flexion to prevent impaction of the tibial metaphysis into the growth plate. The results of this type of fracture are unpredictable; occasionally angulation or premature closure of the plate occurs (McManama, 1988; Santopietro, 1988). The most common mechanism of injury in type 3 and 4 fractures of the medial malleolus is ankle supination or inversion. Adduction injuries appear in approximately 15% of these injuries and are characterized by medial displacement of part or all of the distal tibial epiphysis. The affected children are usually young, so the incidence of growth disturbance is higher. Internal fixation with restoration of ankle joint congruity is critical (McManama, 1988).

Because of the porosity of the bones of the foot in a child, stress fractures are common in the metatarsals in all jumping and distance running activities. If suspected by local tenderness that is aggravated with activity, these injuries should be casted for 3 weeks. After casting, one can progressively and slowly increase activities to former levels over 3 more weeks (McManama, 1988; Santopietro, 1988).

Several types of ischemia can occur in the bones of the child's foot. Freiberg infarction, or avascular necrosis of the metatarsal epiphysis, occurs in those who walk or perform on their toes. Initial synovitis is followed by sclerosis, resorption, plate fracture and collapse, and bone re-formation. It does not affect children younger than age 12 years. Most commonly affected is the second metatarsal head. Treatment consists of cessation of toe-walking, use of high-heeled shoes, and jumping. A negative-heel shoe is fitted. Kohler disease is seen in active boys age 3 to 7 years who have a tendency to cavus feet. Focal tenderness and swelling around the navicular bone are noted clinically. The radiograph reveals sclerosis and irregular rarefaction indicative of ischemia. Conservative treatment calls for use of a walking cast for 6 to 8 weeks followed by use of an arch support and limitation of activity for another 6 weeks (McManama, 1988).

Although ankle sprains can occur in the young athlete, epiphyseal fractures are more common. Sprains occur in the older adolescent near the end of growth. The common cause of injury is landing on the lateral border of a plantar-flexed foot (Fig. 17–11). Management is similar to that in adults. Surgery is indicated only in multiple sprains with gross instability.

Apophysitis of the calcaneus is an Osgood-Schlatter syndrome of the foot (Fig. 17–12). It is seen

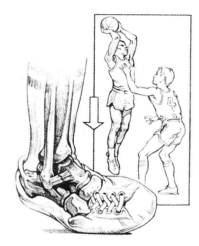

FIGURE 17–11. Plantar flexion–inversion injury. (From Birrer, R, & Brecher, D. Common Sports Injuries in Youngsters. Oradell, NJ: Medical Economics, 1987, p. 120.)

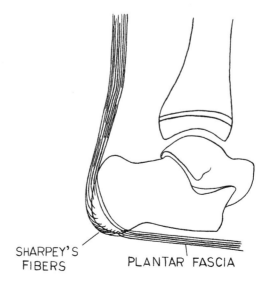

SHARPEY'S FIBERS   PLANTAR FASCIA

FIGURE 17–12. Insertion of Sharpey's fibers from the Achilles tendon into the calcaneal apophysis. (From Gregg, J, & Das, M. Foot and ankle problems in the preadolescent and adolescent athlete. Clinics in Sports Medicine, 1:140, 1982.)

most frequently in basketball and soccer players with complaint of heel pain on running. The usual age of occurrence is 8 to 13 years. Frequently, tight heel cords, a tendency toward in-toeing, and forefoot varus are noted. Treatment consists of heel cord stretching and initial use of a heel lift in well-constructed shoes (Doxey, 1987).

REHABILITATION AND RETURN TO PLAY

Contrary to some opinions, the young athlete will not return to normal function spontaneously. Children and adolescents require supervised rehabilitation programs that begin with first aid on the field of play (Davis, 1986; Stanitski, 1989). The goal of first aid is to contain the extent of injury and reduce any possibility of further harm. The long-term goal of rehabilitation is return to play in a safe manner. Short-term goals should include the accomplishment of the component skills needed to reach the long-term goal. The general process of rehabilitation should emphasize maintenance of cardiovascular skills while normalizing mobility and flexibility. Emphasis then shifts to normalization of muscular endurance and strength, of both the injured area and the entire extremity. Eventually attention is directed toward resumption of purposeful, controlled movements at the appropriate speed (Davis, 1986). Utilization of the "10% rule"—no weekly increase greater than 10% of the previous level—is a safe progression for training (Trepman & Micheli, 1988).

Complete rehabilitation is synonymous with return to play. Premature return to activity courts reinjury and the development of chronic problems (Stanitski, 1989). The criteria for return include no edema; full, pain-free, biomechanically normal mobility; normal strength by objective testing; and normal completion of appropriate functional tests such as vertical leap, hopping, running, or cutting activities (Davis, 1986). Supportive or protective devices such as orthoses or braces may be used to supplement rehabilitation and to provide stability and anatomic alignment (Trepman & Micheli, 1988).

THE YOUNG ATHLETE WITH A PHYSICAL DISABILITY

Children with a disability have the same basic needs as their able-bodied peers. With the approval in the United States of Public Law 94-142, the Rehabilitation Act of 1973, and the Americans with Disabilities Act in 1991, a variety of physical activity and sports programs are now available to those with impairments (Bernhardt, 1985b; Birrer & Brecher, 1987; McCormick, 1985). Several studies have demonstrated that those with physical disabilities do indeed participate in sports. In a survey of 100 persons with lower extremity amputations, 60% were active in sports. Younger persons of both genders were most active (Kegel et al., 1980). Of a group of 67 individuals with spinal cord injury, 72% participated in sports at least once weekly. These sports included basketball, swimming, weight lifting, road racing, and boating. The group included 19 athletes currently involved in competition (Curtis et al., 1986).

Both psychologic and physiologic benefits of sports participation have been demonstrated in individuals with disabilities. Self-concept and self-acceptance were shown to be equal or greater in athletes of various ages with disabilities when compared with control subjects who were able-bodied (Jackson & Davis, 1983; Patrick, 1984; Sherrill et al., 1990). Wheelchair basketball players had significantly better mental profiles than players who were able-bodied and nonathletes (Paulsen et al., 1991). When novice and veteran wheelchair athletes were compared, the novice group had lower perceived social adequacy and lower self-perception, suggesting that sports participation might change these perceptions in a positive way (Patrick, 1984). Among children with limb deficiencies, athletic competence was one predictor of higher perceived physical appearance and, in turn, lower levels of depression and higher self-esteem (Varni & Setoguchi, 1991).

Disability often causes some reduction of fitness relative to the general population (Jackson & Davis, 1983). Several research studies have demonstrated, however, that fitness training in those with disabilities can reverse this reduction of physiologic status. In classic studies by Zwiren and Bar-Or (1975) and others, the physiologic capabilities of athletes who participated in wheelchair sports were shown to be only 9% lower than those of athletes without disabilities and fully 50% greater than those of sedentary individuals who used wheelchairs. Other studies have confirmed these findings (Bernhardt, 1985a; Jackson & Davis, 1983). Decreases in body fat and increases in muscle strength and endurance, often beyond that of individuals without disabilities, have also been documented (Jackson & Davis, 1983). In a comparison of the health and functional status of athletes and nonathletes with spinal cord injuries, the athletes had only 2.4 physician visits per year compared with 6.7 physician visits for the nonathletes. Although they were involved in sports significantly more hours per week (10.2 ± 9.6 hours for athletes; 4.9 ± 4.1 hours for nonathletes), the athletes on average had fewer hospitalizations, decubitus ulcers, medical complications, and hours of required attendant care. The researchers concluded that the medical risks associated with intense sports activity for those with spinal cord injuries are minimal (Curtis et al., 1986).

Preparticipation Examination

Preparticipation assessment of a young person with a disability is similar to that of someone who is able-bodied, and it can be conducted in a multistation fashion. Several areas, however, must be more thoroughly addressed. The personnel performing the assessment must understand not only the physical, physiologic, and psychologic requirements of the sport but also the potential medical risks of participation. The physically challenged athlete may be prone to additional injury or illness secondary to the disability. In addition, the physician may be involved in classification of the athlete depending on the type and severity of the disability and must be aware of international and national classification systems (Bernhardt, 1991; Jackson & Davis, 1983).

The history should include the date of the onset of disability. Description and dates of all medical problems, hospitalizations, and operations before and after the onset of disability should be included. Releases for participation from all attending physicians are required. Thorough documentation of medications for comparison with lists of permissible drugs is necessary (Bernhardt, 1991).

Physical examination must include documentation of level of understanding, vocalization, communication abilities, and hearing. Flexibility should be evaluated because greater than normal muscle length may be required for certain activities (e.g., flexible hips for positioning in sports wheelchair). Special consideration should be given to instability in specific disability groups, such as the propensity for cervical instability and subluxation in Down syndrome (Cantu, 1988). Complete assessment of all sensory systems is required for classification and safety. Documentation of the presence of abnormal muscle tone and primitive, protective, or pathologic reflexes is critical for participation in sports such as archery, horseback riding, and swimming. Assessment of integrity and toughness of the skin and documentation of any history of skin problems are vital in any athlete with sensory impairment (Bernhardt, 1991).

The level of sitting and standing posture and balance as it pertains to the sport is critical for effective and safe participation. The athlete who skis while seated or rides horseback must have adequate balance to perform. The athlete can be placed in a mock-up situation for assessment if necessary. Assessment of gait is mandatory in all clients who are ambulatory. The pattern and efficacy, as well as assistive devices needed, must be reviewed. Estimation of locomotor endurance is helpful.

The assessment of gross and fine motor skills should be performed in tasks similar to those required by the sport. Bilateral comparisons and timing and quality should be noted (Bernhardt, 1991). Muscle strength and endurance should be assessed, if possible, with either manual or mechanical methods. Although this area has received little attention, dominant hand grip force can be used as a partial predictor of upper body strength (Jackson et al., 1981; Jackson & Davis, 1983). Davis (1981) has also shown that a good relationship exists between upper body isokinetic strength and habitual activity.

Physiologic assessment should include nutritional analysis, body composition measurement, and exercise testing. Exercise testing may be advisable for assessment of cardiopulmonary functional capacity or the efficacy of medications. Testing must often be adjusted for the disability, such as armcrank, wheelchair, or single leg ergometry (Bernhardt, 1985a, 1991; Jackson & Davis, 1983). Field testing can be completed as long as standard testing principles are followed (Crews, 1982; Kofsky et al., 1983). Although maximal oxygen consumption is the best single indicator of cardiovascular fitness, submaximal testing can be performed as an estimation of maximal capacity.

For many athletes with a disability, equipment is part of their participation. Specially designed wheelchairs, skiing outriggers, ergonomic racquet handles, rotation platforms for field events, and custom prostheses are but a few of the technologic advances that have made sports more assessible. The assessor should check the equipment for function, fit, safety, and conformity to rules of competition or participation (Bernhardt, 1991).

Training Programs

Persons with disabilities should be placed on training programs in a manner similar to those who are able-bodied (Bernhardt, 1985a, 1985b; Curtis, 1981a, 1981b) (Fig. 17–13). Several studies have evaluated the efficacy of these training programs in various disability groups. Research on wheelchair training demonstrated increases in maximal oxygen uptake, decreases in exercise and resting heart rate, and increases in maximal work capacity. Documented increases in muscle force and endurance and peak force have been noted after strength training (Hutzler et al., 1998; Lintunen et al., 1995; Veeger et al., 1991).

Injury Data

Little information has been gathered on the incidence and type of sports injuries that occur in persons who are disabled. Although several studies have

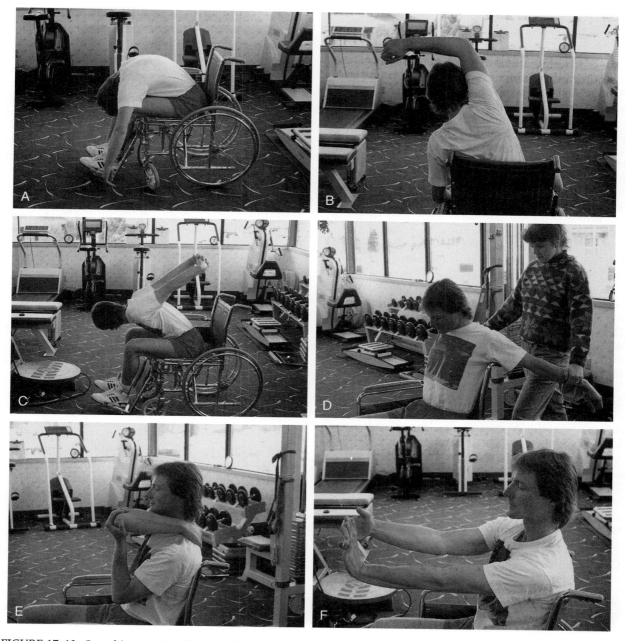

FIGURE 17–13. Stretching exercises for the athlete in a wheelchair. *A*, Exhale; lean forward to touch ground. *B*, Lift one arm over head and lean to side. Repeat with opposite side. *C*, Exhale, clasp hands, lean forward, and lift arms high in back. *D*, Pull arms to side with palms facing forward. Pull back with elbows straight. *E*, Bend arm across chest. Reach for opposite blade. Push on elbow. Repeat. *F*, Straighten elbow. Push wrist and fingers back. Repeat with opposite side.

appeared in the literature, they have had small sample sizes and select groups of individuals with specific disabilities. An exception was a survey distributed to 1200 athletes in regional wheelchair competition during 1981. One hundred two male and 27 female athletes responded. Thirty-two differ-

ent sports were represented by the group. Seventy-two percent of all athletes had sustained at least 1 injury, with some reporting as many as 14 injuries. The most prevalent injuries were soft tissue trauma (33%), blisters (18%), and lacerations or abrasions (17%). The majority of the injuries occurred in the upper extremity. Most of the injuries were associated with track (26%), basketball (24%), and road racing (22%) (Curtis, 1982). A survey of the 1990 Junior National Wheelchair Games demonstrated injury rates of 97% in track, 22% in field events, and 91% in swimming among 83 athletes (Wilson & Washington, 1993).

A study of the injuries at the Special Olympic games demonstrated that 3.5% of the athletes required care for an injury or illness. Track and field events consumed the least time but had the greatest injury rate (McCormick et al., 1990). Data from the International Flower Marathon showed that 19 athletes experienced 20 medical problems, many caused by climate and spills. Problems were more frequent in groups with disabilities caused by paraplegia and polio. Thirteen medical problems were classified as injuries: five were ulcers and abrasions and eight were soft tissue injuries (Hoeberigs et al., 1990).

The largest study, a retrospective survey of 426 athletes participating in the 1989 competitions of the National Wheelchair Athletic Association (NWAA), the United States Association for Blind Athletes (USABA), and the United States Cerebral Palsy Association (USCPA), demonstrated that 32% of the respondents had at least one time-loss injury. Twenty-six percent of all injuries were from the NWAA, with 57% of this total at the shoulder and elbow. Fifty-three percent of all USABA athletes' injuries were in the lower extremity. The injuries in the USCPA athletes were noted in all areas. Injury rates were the same for athletes with or without disabilities (Ferrara et al., 1992). Thus very limited data are available that document the occurrence or management of injuries in the athlete with a disability. Research is needed to address these issues before further conclusions can be drawn.

CONCLUSION

Young athletes, whether able-bodied or disabled, are not just small adults. They have unique issues in sports participation that must be specifically addressed. Recognition of these unusual qualities is necessary for effective prevention and management of sports-related injuries.

Physical therapists should play a significant role in the total management of the child athlete. The broad-based and eclectic medical background of physical therapists makes them ideal professionals for the assessment and rehabilitation of sports injuries in athletes with full or altered physical capabilities. Depending on advanced experience or certification in sports physical therapy, athletic training, or exercise physiology, they may be the primary medical professional to administer total management from prevention to return to participation after injury.

If lacking in expertise or time, a physical therapist may alternatively work with a certified athletic trainer and an exercise physiologist to provide comprehensive sports safety management. The certified trainer is appropriately skilled to assist with preparticipation screenings and to provide on-site coverage of practices and games with immediate triage and injury management. The exercise physiologist plays an integral part in the preseason screening and in conditioning and training programs. The physical therapist can provide assessment and total rehabilitation of sports injuries and aid in phasing the athlete back to play with appropriate progression, supportive devices, or medical limitations. The certified trainer or the exercise physiologist often works with the physical therapist in the return-to-play planning and follow-up.

The goal of these programs is to promote the health and safety of the young athlete. All those involved should work in a manner appropriate to their education, skills, and practice statutes as members of a team, including coaches and parents, toward the goal of safe, rewarding, and successful participation in sport and recreation.

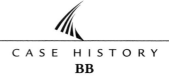

CASE HISTORY
BB

BB is a 14-year-old boy who decided to go out for eighth-grade football as a lineman. Two weeks into fall practice he noted left knee pain, especially when in a crouching position, running or cutting, or on stairs. He further experienced left upper back pain. He reported a history of a back injury when loading hay several months ago, but stated that it had improved until football. When questioned, he reported no off-season preparation for football.

His examination revealed tenderness at the inferior patellar pole and over the length of the patellar tendon. He had no tenderness at the tendon insertion on the tibial tuberosity. Knee flexion was limited by 20° when compared with the right, although knee extension was full. Girth measurements of his midthigh and calf were 1 inch smaller on the left. He had a slight antalgic gait with decreased flexion in swing and increased stance time. Active knee extension (popliteal angle) was −50°, indicating hamstring inflexibility.

Examination of his upper back area demonstrated tenderness (6/10) with palpation and use of the rhomboid and lower trapezius muscles on the left. He had a 30° decrease in shoulder flexion and abduction. Strength in the rhomboids was 4/5, lower trapezius 3+/5. His posture was guarded on the left with rounding and depression of his shoulder complex.

A diagnosis of left patellar tendinitis, inferior pole irritation, and strain of the left rhomboid and lower trapezius was made. He received two treatments in the clinic consisting of warmth and inferential stimulation followed by myofascial stretching. He was instructed in stretching for the muscles that elevate the shoulder and adduct the scapula. He was shown shoulder and scapular isolation exercises and correct postural alignment. Additionally, he was given a short home program to increase hamstring flexibility and quadriceps strength. His program consisted of squats, lunges with weights, and 4-inch lateral step-ups to be done on nongame days.

By his second visit, his knee pain was minimal and occasional. Hamstring flexibility had increased 5°. Scapular soreness was decreased (4/10) but still present with play. Postural alignment was now good. He had been compliant with his home program.

His program was advanced to include shoulder and scapular endurance and strength exercises with green Theraband. He was advanced to 6-inch step-ups and single-leg squats and toe raises. He was instructed to continue his home program and report in 2 weeks.

When he called, his knee pain had resolved, and he could perform functional tests equally well on both legs. His scapular pain was only slight, and he could play without soreness. He was instructed to increase to blue theraband and continue his lower extremity exercises. He will come in after football for an off-season program.

CASE HISTORY
NE

NE was a star basketball player in her senior year. She landed off balance during a midseason game and fell, twisting her right knee. Immediate field examination revealed tenderness over the medial joint line. She demonstrated +2 laxity on a Lachman test and could not bear weight on her leg.

Follow-up 2 days later by her orthopedist confirmed the probability of anterior cruciate ligament (ACL) injury. An MRI demonstrated both an ACL tear and medial meniscal damage. She was referred for preoperative rehabilitation and scheduled for surgery in 2 weeks.

Initial examination revealed an edematous knee with some bruising. Her gait was antalgic with decreased heel strike and push-off, limited knee motion, and minimal comfortable weight bearing. Although her thigh and calf girth measurements were unchanged, the tone of her right quadriceps was decreased. She performed only a 3+/5 quadriceps isometrically. Knee mobility was −12° extension, 80° flexion. Her pain level was 5 on a scale of 1 through 10, and she had difficulty sleeping.

Before surgery, she began a program to reduce edema, increase knee mobility, normalize gait, and maintain leg strength. Her treatment included cooling, inferential stimulation, and gait training. She was instructed in wall slides and heel slides, as well as straight-leg raising (SLR) and short arc knee extension. The final goals for this 2-week period were full knee mobility, normal gait without device, no edema, and strength 80% of normal knee.

Her final preoperative visit consisted of reevaluation and teaching. The surgical procedure, use of crutches, and postsurgical rehabilitation were explained. She was fit for and instructed in the use of a continuous passive motion (CPM) machine and a cooling unit.

Postsurgical rehabilitation after her patellar tendon graft began on postoperative day 1. She was placed in a CPM machine and gradually increased in flexion to 60°. She was instructed in quadriceps setting and assisted SLR. Her CPM mobility was reinforced by supine knee flexion against a wall. Her postoperative brace was unlocked, and she was instructed in correct gait pattern with weight bearing to tolerance with crutches.

Her program progressed from edema and pain reduction, knee mobility, and gait training to endurance and then strength exercises. The CPM was discontinued when she could actively achieve 110° of knee flexion. The majority of her strength exercises were closed-chain exercises with emphasis on correct technique through full available range of motion. She progressed to one crutch, then to no device when her gait was normal without assistance. She was seen three times weekly in the clinic with a full home program.

She was compliant and progressed steadily. Three months after surgery, she was fitted with a functional brace and instructed in a home training program. At this time, mobility and gait were normal. Knee stability was excellent. Thigh and calf strength were still only 50%.

She was monitored every 2 weeks until 5 months, then monthly for 1 year. She was tested on an isokinetic dynamometer at 6 months and 12 months. At the end of 1 year, her strength was 95% of her uninjured leg, so her brace was discontinued and she was released to full function.

References

American Academy of Pediatrics. Organized athletics for preadolescent children. Pediatrics, 84:583–584, 1989.

Backous, DD, Triedl, KE, Smith, NJ, Parr, TJ, & Carpine, WD. Soccer injuries and their relation to physical maturity. American Journal of Diseases in Children, 148:839–842, 1988.

Backx, FJ, Beijer, HJ, Bol, E, & Erich, WB. Injuries in high-risk persons and high-risk sports: A longitudinal study of 1818 school children. American Journal of Sports Medicine, 19:124–130, 1991.

Backx, FJ, Erich, WB, Kemper, AB, & Verbeek, AL. Sports injuries in school-aged children: An epidemiological study. American Journal of Sports Medicine, 17:234–240, 1989.

Bar-Or, O. The young athlete: Some physiological considerations. Journal of Sports Sciences, 13:S31–S33, 1995.

Bar-Or, O, Lombardo, JA, & Rowland, TW. The preparticipation sports exam. Patient Care, October 1988, pp. 75–102.

Bauman, M. Nutritional requirements for athletes. In Bernhardt, DB (Ed.), Sports Physical Therapy. New York: Churchill Livingstone, 1986, pp. 89–105.

Bernhardt, DB. Exercise testing and training for disabled populations: The state of the art. In Bernhardt, DB (Ed.), Recreation for the Disabled Child. New York: Haworth Press, 1985a, pp. 3–25.

Bernhardt, DB. The competitive spirit. In Bernhardt, DB (Ed.), Recreation for the Disabled Child. New York: Haworth Press, 1985b, pp. 77–86.

Bernhardt, DB. The physically challenged athlete. In Cantu, RC, & Micheli, LJ (Eds.), ACSM's Guidelines for the Team Physician. Philadelphia: Lea & Febiger, 1991, pp. 242–251.

Birrer, RB, & Brecher, DB. Common Sports Injuries in Youngsters. Oradell, NJ: Medical Economics, 1987.

Birrer, RB, & Levine, R. Performance parameters in children and adolescent athletes. Sports Medicine, 4:221–237, 1987.

Brown, RS. Exercise and mental health in the pediatric population. Clinics in Sports Medicine, 1:515–527, 1982.

Bruce, DA, Schut, L, & Sutton, LN. Brain and cervical spine injuries occurring during organized sports activities in children and adolescents. Clinics in Sports Medicine, 1:495–514, 1982.

Cantu, R. Head and spine injuries in the young athlete. Clinics in Sports Medicine, 7:459–472, 1988.

Castaldi, CR. Sports related oral and facial injuries in the young athlete: A new challenge for the pediatric dentist. Pediatric Dentistry, 8:311–316, 1986.

Clark, N. Nutrition: Pre-, intra-, and postcompetition. In Cantu, RC, & Micheli, LJ (Eds.), ACSM's Guidelines for the Team Physician. Philadelphia: Lea & Febiger, 1991, pp. 58–65.

Clarkson, PM. Nutrition for improved sports performance. Current issues on ergogenic aids. Sports Medicine, 21:393–401, 1996.

Coady, CM, & Micheli, LJ. Stress fractures in the pediatric athlete. Clinics in Sports Medicine, 16:225–238, 1997.

Cooper, K. Kid Fitness. New York: Bantam Books, 1991.

Creath, CJ, Shelton, WO, Wright, JT, Bradley, DH, Feinstein, RA, & Wisniewski, JF. The prevalence of smokeless tobacco use among adolescent male athletes. Journal of American Dental Association, 116:43–48, 1988.

Crews, D. Field testing the wheelchair athlete. Sports n' Spokes, March/April 1982, p. 37.

Curtis, KA. Wheelchair sportsmedicine: II. Training. Sports n' Spokes, July/August 1981a, pp. 16–19.

Curtis, KA. Wheelchair sportsmedicine: III. Stretching. Sports n' Spokes, September/October 1981b, pp. 16–18.

Curtis, KA. Wheelchair sportsmedicine: IV. Athletic injuries. Sports n' Spokes, January/February 1982, pp. 20–24.

Curtis, KA, McClanahan, S, Hail, KM, Dillon, D, & Brown, KF. Health, vocational and functional status in spinal cord injured athletes and nonathletes. Archives of Physical Medicine and Rehabilitation, 67:862–865, 1986.

DaSilva, MF, Williams, JS, Fadale, PD, Hulstyn, MJ, & Erhlich, MG. Pediatric throwing injuries about the elbow. American Journal of Orthopedics, 27:90–96, 1998.

Davis, GM. Cardiorespiratory fitness and muscle strength in lower-limb disability. Canadian Journal of Applied Sports Sciences, 6:159–165, 1981.

Davis, JM. Rehabilitation of sports injuries: A practical approach. In Bernhardt, DB (Ed.), Sports Physical Therapy. New York: Churchill Livingstone, 1986, pp. 155–171.

Davis, JM, Kuppermann, N, & Fleisher, G. Serious sports injuries requiring hospitalization seen in a pediatric emergency department. American Journal of Diseases of Children, 147:1001–1004, 1993.

DiScala, C, Gallagher, SS, & Schneps, SE. Causes and outcomes of pediatric injuries occurring at school. Journal of School Health, 67:384–389, 1997.

Doxey, GE. Calcaneal pain: A review of various disorders. Journal of Orthopedic and Sport Physical Therapy, 9:25–32, 1987.

Feld, LG, Springate, JE, & Waz, WR. Special topics in pediatric hypertension. Seminars in Nephrology, 18:295–303, 1998.

Ferrara, MS, Buckley, WE, McCann, BC, Limbird, TJ, Powell, JW, & Robl, R. The injury experience of a competitive athlete with a disability: Prevention implications. Medicine and Science in Sports and Exercise, 24:184–188, 1992.

Food Guide Pyramid. Washington, DC: U.S. Department of Agriculture, 1992.

Gaillard, B, Haskell, W, Smith, N, & Ogilvie, B. Handbook for the Young Athlete. Palo Alto, CA: Bull Publishing, 1978, pp. 32–33.

Garrick, JG. Epidemiological perspective. Clinics in Sports Medicine, 1:13–18, 1982.

Gerberich, SG, Finke, R, Madden, M, Priest, JD, Aamoth, G, & Murray, K. An epidemiological study of high school ice hockey injuries. Childs Nervous System, 3:59–64, 1987.

Going, S. Physical best: Body composition in the assessment of youth fitness. Journal of Physical Education, Recreation and Dance, 59(9):32–36, 1988.

Goldberg, B, Rosenthal, PP, Robertson, LS, & Nicholas, JA. Injuries in youth football. Pediatrics, 81:255–261, 1988.

Goldberg, B, Saranti, A, Witman, P, Gavin, M, & Nicholas, J. Preparticipation sports assessment: An objective evaluation. Pediatrics 66:736–745, 1980.

Grana, WA, & Kalenak, A. Clinical Sports Medicine. Philadelphia: WB Saunders, 1991.

Green, GA. Drugs, athletes, and drug testing. In Sanders, B (Ed.), Sports Physical Therapy. Norwalk, CT: Appleton & Lange, 1990, pp. 95–111.

Gregg, JR, & Das, M. Foot and ankle problems in the preadolescent and adolescent athlete. Clinics in Sports Medicine, 1:131–147, 1982.

Halpern, B, Thompson, N, Curl, WW, Andrews, J, Hunter, SC, & Boring, JR. High school football injuries: Identifying the risk factors. American Journal of Sports Medicine, 15:316–320, 1987.

Harvey, J. The preparticipation examination of the child athlete. Clinics in Sports Medicine, 1:353–369, 1982.

Haupt, HA. Drugs in athletics. Clinics in Sports Medicine, 8:561–582, 1989.

Haupt, HA. Anabolic steroids and growth hormone. American Journal of Sports Medicine, 21:468–474, 1993.

Hickson, RC, Ball, KL, & Falduto, MT. Adverse effects of anabolic steroids. Medical Toxicology and Adverse Drug Exposure, 4:254–271, 1989.

Hoeberigs, JH, Deberts-Eggen, HB, & Debets, PM. Sports medical experience from the International Flower Marathon for disabled wheelers. American Journal of Sports Medicine, 18:418–421, 1990.

Hoff, GL, & Martin, TA. Outdoor and indoor soccer: Injuries among youth players. American Journal of Sports Medicine, 14:231–233, 1986.

Hunter, SC, Etchison, WC, & Halpern, B. Standards and norms of fitness and flexibility in the high school athlete. Athletic Training, Fall 1985, pp. 210–212.

Hutzler, Y, Ochana, S, Bolotin, R, & Kalina, E. Aerobic and non-aerobic arm-cranking outputs of males with lower limb impairments: relationship with sport participation intensity, age, impairment with functional classification. Spinal Cord, 36:205–212, 1998.

Ireland, ML, & Andrews, JR. Shoulder and elbow injuries in the young athlete. Clinics in Sports Medicine, 7:473–494, 1988.

Jackson, RW, & Davis, GM. The value of sports and recreation for the physically disabled. Orthopedic Clinics of North America, 14:301–315, 1983.

Jackson, RW, Davis, GM, Kofsky, PR, Shepard, RJ, & Keene, GCR. Fitness levels in the lower-limb disabled. In Transactions of the 27th Annual Meeting of the Orthopedic Research Society, Vol. 6. Rosemont, IL: Orthopedic Research Society, 1981.

Kegel, B, Webster, JC, & Burgess, EM. Recreational activities of lower extremity amputees. Archives of Physical Medicine and Rehabilitation, 61:258–264, 1980.

Keller, CS, Noyes, FR, & Buncher, CR. The medical aspects of soccer injury epidemiology. American Journal of Sports Medicine, 15: 230–236, 1987.

Kerr, IL. Mouth guards for the prevention of injuries in contact sports. Sports Medicine, 5:415–427, 1986.

Klish, WJ. Childhood Obesity: Pathophysiology and treatment. Acta Pediatrica Japan, 37:1–6, 1995.

Knowles, KG, Yakavonis, VJ, & George, F. Overuse syndromes about the elbow. Postgraduate Advances in Sports Medicine, II(VIII): 3–17, 1987.

Kofsky, PR, Davis, GM, Shepard, RJ, Jackson, RW, & Keene, GC. Field testing: Assessment of physical fitness of disabled youth. Journal of Applied Physiology, 51:109–120, 1983.

Kraemer, WJ, & Fleck, S. Strength Training for Young Athletes. Champaign, IL: Human Kinetics, 1993.

Kvist, M, Kujala, UM, Heinonen, OJ, Vuori, IV, Aho, AJ, Pajulo, O, Huintsa, A, & Parvinen, T. Sports-related injuries in children. International Journal of Sports Medicine, April 1989, pp. 81–86.

Laseter, JT, & Russell, JA. Anabolic steroid-induced tendon pathology: A review of the literature. Medicine and Science in Sports and Exercise, 23:1–3, 1991.

Lehman, L. The preseason athletic screening examination. Medical Times, 116(8):29–31, 1988.

Linder, CW, DuRant, RH, Seklecki, RM, & Strong, WB. Preparticipation health screening of young athletes. American Journal of Sports Medicine, 9:187–193, 1981.

Lintunen, T, Heikinaro-Johansson, P, & Sherrill, C. Use of Perceptual Physical Competence Scale with adolescents with disabilities. Perceptual Motor Skills, 80:571–577, 1995.

Lodge, JF, Langley, JD, & Begg, DJ. Injuries in the 14th and 15th years of life. Journal of Paediatric and Child Health, 26:316–322, 1990.

Lohman, TG. Advances in Body Composition Assessment. Champaign, IL: Human Kinetics Publishers, 1992.

Lombardo, JA. Preparticipation examination. In Cantu, RC, & Micheli, LJ (Eds.), ACSM's Guidelines for the Team Physician. Philadelphia: Lea & Febiger, 1991, pp. 71–94.

Macera, CA, Jackson, KL, Hagenmaier, GW, & Kronenfeld, JJ. Age, physical activity, physical fitness, body composition, and incidence of orthopedic problems. Research Quarterly for Exercise and Sport, 60:225–233, 1989.

Maestrello-deMoya, MG, & Primosch, RE. Orofacial trauma and mouth-protector wear among high school varsity basketball players. ASDC Journal of Dentistry in Children, 56:36–39, 1989.

Maffulli, N. Intensive training in young athletes. Sports Medicine, 9:229–243, 1990.

McCormick, D. Handicapped skiing. In Bernhardt, DB (Ed.), Recreation for the Disabled Child. New York: Haworth Press, 1985, pp. 27–44.

McCormick, DP, Niebiehr, VN, & Risser, WL. Injury and illness surveillance at local Special Olympic Games. British Journal of Sports Medicine, 24:221–224, 1990.

McKeag, D. Preseason physical examination for prevention of sports injuries. Sports Medicine, 2:413–431, 1985.

McLain, LG, & Reynolds, S. Sports injuries in a high school. Pediatrics, 84:446–450, 1989.

McManama, GB. Ankle injuries in the young athlete. Clinics in Sports Medicine, 7:547–562, 1988.

McNutt, T, Shannon, SW, Wright, JT, & Feinstein, RA. Oral trauma in adolescent athletes: A study of mouth protectors. Pediatric Dentistry, 11:209–213, 1989.

Mellion, MB (Ed.). Office Management of Sports Injuries and Athletic Problems. Philadelphia: Hanley & Belfus, 1988.

Micheli, LJ. Overuse injuries in children's sports: The growth factor. Orthopedic Clinics of North America, 14:337–360, 1983.

Micheli, LJ. Musculoskeletal trauma in children. In Green, M, & Haggerty, RJ (Eds.), Ambulatory Pediatrics III. Philadelphia: WB Saunders, 1984, pp. 95–208.

Micheli, LJ. The child athlete. In Cantu, RC, & Micheli, LJ (Eds.), ACSM's Guidelines for the Team Physician. Philadelphia: Lea & Febiger, 1991, pp. 228–241.

Micheli, LJ, Santore, R, & Stanitski, CL. Epiphyseal fractures of the elbow in children. American Family Physician, November 1980, pp. 107–116.

Micheli, LJ, & Smith, AD. Sports injuries in children. Current Problems in Pediatrics, 12:1–54, 1982.

Micheli, LJ, & Stone, KR. The pre-sports physical: Only the first step. Journal of Musculoskeletal Medicine, May 1984, pp. 56–60.

Millar, AL. Ergogenic Aids. In Sanders, B. (Ed.), Sports Physical Therapy. Norwalk, CT: Appleton & Lange, 1990, pp. 79–93.

Mirby, J, Besancenot, J, Chambers, RT, Durey, A, & Vichard, P. Avulsion fractures of the tibial tuberosity in the adolescent athlete. American Journal of Sports Medicine, 16:336–340, 1988.

Mueller, F, & Blythe, C. Epidemiology of sports injuries in children. Clinics in Sports Medicine, 1(3):343–352, 1982.

Mueller, FD, & Cantu, RC. Catastrophic injuries and fatalities in high school and college sports, Fall 1982–Spring 1988. Medicine and Science in Sports and Exercise, 22:737–741, 1990.

Napier, SM, Baker, RS, Sanford, DG, & Easterbrook, M. Eye injuries in athletics and recreation. Surv Ophthalmologia, 41:229–244, 1996.

Nevaiser, RJ: Injuries to and developmental deformities of the shoulder. In Bora, FW (Ed.), The Pediatric Upper Extremity. Philadelphia: WB Saunders, 1986, pp. 235–246.

Nevole, GJ, & Prentice, WJ. The effect of anabolic steroids on female athletes. Athletic Training, 22:297–299, 1987.

Objective testing group certifies head protection. Occupational Health and Safety, March 1988, pp. 18–20.

O'Neill, DB, & Micheli, LJ. Overuse injuries in the young athlete. Clinics in Sports Medicine, 7:591–610, 1988.

Patrick, GD. Comparison of novice and veteran wheelchair athletes' self-concept and acceptance of disability. Rehabilitation Counseling Bulletin, 27:186–188, 1984.

Paulsen, P, French, R, & Sherrill, C. Comparison of mood states of college able-bodied and wheelchair basketball players. Perceptual Motor Skills, 73:396–398, 1991.

Perriello, VA, Jr, Almquist, J, Conkwright, D, Jr, Cutter, D, Gregory, D, Pitrezzi, MJ, Roemmich, J, & Snyders, G. Health and weight control management among wrestlers. A proposed program for high school athletes. Virginia Medical Quarterly, 122:179–183, 1995.

Perry, A. Distinction between drug use and abuse. Athletic Training, Summer 1985, pp. 114–116.

Peterson, M, & Peterson, K. Eat to Compete: A Guide to Sports Nutrition. Chicago: Year Book Medical, 1988.

Pfeiffer, RD, & Francis, RS. Effects of strength training on muscle development in prepubescent, pubescent and postpubescent males. Physician and Sports Medicine, 14:134–143, 1986.

Physician urges caution for child marathoners. Physician and Sports Medicine, 10:26, 1982.

Powell, EC, & Tanz, RR. In-line skate and rollerskate injuries in children. Pediatric Emergency Care, 12:259–262, 1996.

Powell, EC, Tanz, RR, & DiScala, C. Bicycle-related injuries among preschool children. Annals of Emergency Medicine, 30:260–265, 1997.

Powell, J. 636,000 injuries annually in high school football. Athletic Training, 22:19–22, 1987.

Puffer, JC. Organizational aspects. In Cantu, RC, & Micheli, LJ (Eds.), ACSM's Guidelines for the Team Physician. Philadelphia: Lea & Febiger, 1991, pp. 95–100.

Ramsey, JA, Blunkie, C, Smith, K, Garner, S, MacDougall, JD, & Digby, GS. Strength training effects in prepubescent boys. Medicine and Science in Sports and Exercise, 22:605–614, 1990.

Retsky, J, Jaffe, D, & Christoffel, K. Skateboarding injuries in children: A second wave. American Journal of Disease in Children, 145:188–192, 1991.

Rooks, DS, & Micheli, LJ. Musculoskeletal assessment and training: The young athlete. Clinics in Sports Medicine, 7:641–677, 1988.

Rossi, F, & Dragoni, S. Lumbar spondylolisthesis: Occurrence in competitive athletes. Journal of Sports Medicine and Physical Fitness, 30:450–452, 1990.

Sachtelben, TR, Berg, KE, Elias, BA, Cheatham, JP, Felix, FL, & Hofschire, PJ. The effects of anabolic steroids on myocardial structure and cardiovascular fitness. Medicine and Science in Sports and Exercise, 25:1240–1245, 1993.

Sailors, M, & Berg, K. Comparison of responses to weight training in pubescent boys and men. Journal of Sports Medicine, 27:30–37, 1987.

Sanders, B (Ed.). Sports Physical Therapy. Norwalk, CT: Appleton & Lange, 1990.

Santopietro, FJ. Foot and foot-related injuries in the young athlete. Clinics in Sports Medicine, 7:563–589, 1988.

Schlicker, SA, Borra, ST, & Regan, C. The weight and fitness status of United States children. Nutritional Review, 52:11–17, 1994.

Schuller, DE, Dankle, SK, Martin, M, & Strauss, RH. Auricular injury and the use of headgear in wrestlers. Archives of Otolaryngology—Head and Neck Surgery, 115:714–717, 1989.

Segesser, B, & Pforringer, W (Eds.). The Shoe in Sport. Chicago: Year Book Medical, 1989.

Servedio, FJ, Bartels, RL, Hamlin, D, Teske, T, Schaffer, T, & Servedio, A. The effect of weight training using Olympic style lifts on various physiological variables in prepubescent boys. Medicine and Science in Sports and Exercise, 17:228, 1985.

Sewall, L, & Micheli, LJ. Strength training for children. Journal of Pediatric Orthopedics, 6:143–146, 1986.

Sharkey, B. Training for sports. In Cantu, RC, & Micheli, LJ (Eds.), ACSM's Guidelines for the Team Physician. Philadelphia: Lea & Febiger, 1991, pp. 34–47.

Sherrill, C, Hinson, M, Gench, B, Kennedy, SO, & Low, L. Self-concepts of disabled youth athletes. Perceptual Motor Skills, 70:1093–1098, 1990.

Shorter, NA, Jensen, PE, Harmon, BJ, & Mooney, DP. Skiing injuries in children and adolescents. Journal of Trauma, 40:997–1001, 1996.

Simmons, BP, & Lovallo, JL. Hand and wrist injuries in children. Clinics in Sports Medicine, 7:493–512, 1988.

Smith, GA, & Shields, BJ. Trampoline-related injuries to children. Archives of Pediatric and Adolescent Medicine, 152:694–699, 1998.

Smith, MJ. Muscle fiber types. Orthopedic Clinics of North America, 14:403–412, 1983.

Snively, RA, Grove, WA, & Ellis, D. High school sports injuries. Physician and Sports Medicine, 9(8):46–55, 1981.

Sobal, J, & Marquart, LF. Vitamin/mineral supplement use among high school athletes. Adolescence, 29:835–843, 1994.

Squire, DL. Heat illness. Fluid and electrolyte issues for pediatric and adolescent athletes. Pediatric Clinics of North America, 37:1085–1109, 1990.

Stanitski, C. Common injuries in preadolescent athletes. Sports Medicine, 7:32–41, 1989.

Stanitski, CL. Pediatric and adolescent sports injuries. Clinics in Sports Medicine, 16:613–633, 1997.

Steiner, ME, & Grana, WA. The young athlete's knee: Recent advances. Clinics in Sports Medicine, 7:527–546, 1988.

Stock, JG, & Cornell, FM. Prevention of sports-related eye injury. American Family Practice, 44:515–520, 1991.

Strahlman, E, Elman, M, Daub, E, & Baker, S. Causes of pediatric eye injuries. A population-based study. Archives of Ophthalmology, 108:603–606, 1990.

Taimela, S, Kujala, UM, & Osterman, K. Intrinsic risk factors and athletic injuries. Sports Medicine, 9:205–215, 1990.

Trepman, E, & Micheli, LJ. Overuse injuries in sports. Seminars in Orthopedics, 3:217–222, 1988.

Varni, JW, & Setoguchi, Y. Correlates of perceived physical appearance in children with congenital/acquired limb deficiencies. Journal of Development and Behavior in Pediatrics, 12:171–176, 1991.

Veeger, HE, Hadj Yahmed, M, van der Woude, LH, & Charpentier, P. Peak oxygen uptake and maximal power output of Olympic wheelchair-dependent athletes. Medicine and Science in Sports and Exercise, 23:1201–1209, 1991.

Voight, M, & Draovitch, P. Plyometrics. In Albert, M (Ed.), Eccentric Muscle Training in Sports and Orthopaedics. New York: Churchill Livingstone, 1991, pp. 45–73.

Wagner, JC. Enhancement of athletic performance with drugs. An overview. Sports Medicine, 12:250–265, 1991.

Waters, PM, & Millis, MB. Hip and pelvic injuries in the young athlete. Clinics in Sports Medicine, 7:513–526, 1988.

Watson, MD, & DiMartino, PP. Incidence of injuries in high school track and field athletes and its relation to performance ability. American Journal of Sports Medicine, 15:251–254, 1987.

Weltman, AC, Janney, CB, Rains, CB, Strand, K, Berg, B, Tippitt, S, Wise, J, Cahill, BR, & Katch, FI. The effects of hydraulic resistance strength training in pre-pubescent males. Medicine and Science in Sports and Exercise, 18:629–638, 1986.

Whieldon, TJ, & Cerny, FJ. Incidence and severity of high school athletic injuries. Athletic Training, 25:344–350, 1990.

Wiens, L, Sabath, R, Ewing, L, Gowdamarajan, R, Portnoy, J, & Scagliotti, D. Chest pain in otherwise healthy children and adolescents is frequently caused by exercise-induced asthma. Pediatrics, 90:350–353, 1992.

Williams, MH. The use of ergogenic aids in sports: Is it an ethical issue? International Journal of Sports Nutrition, 4:120–131, 1994.

Wilson, PE, & Washington, RL. Pediatric wheelchair athletics: Sports injuries and prevention. Paraplegia, 31:330–337, 1993.

Yesalis, CE, Wright, JE, & Bahrke, MS. Epidemiological and policy issues in the measurement of long term health effects and anabolic-androgenic steroids. Sports Medicine, 8:129–138, 1989.

Zarins, B. Knee injuries in sports. New England Journal of Medicine, 318:950–961, 1982.

Ziegler, MM. Nutritional care of the pediatric athlete. Clinics in Sports Medicine, 1:371–381, 1982.

Zwiren, L, & Bar-Or, O. Response to exercise of paraplegics who differ in conditioning level. Medicine and Science in Sports, 7:94–98, 1975.

Selected Special Musculoskeletal Tests

Differential Diagnosis	Test Performed
Acromioclaviclar separation	Horizontal adduction in flexion and internal rotation
	Step deformity
	Stress test with hand weight
Shoulder impingement	Neer impingement test
	Painful arc
Shoulder instability	Anterior-posterior translation
	Inferior glide in abduction
	Apprehension test
	Sulcus test
Rotator cuff injury	Clunk test
	Drop arm test
	Impingement tests
	Instability tests
Patellar instability	Apprehension test
	Glide test
	Static/dynamic medial-lateral position
	Patellar motion in knee flexion-extension
Patellar dysfunction	Crepitus
	Patellar compression test
	Patellar grind test
	Anterior-posterior tilt
	Patellar rotation
	Ballotable patella
	Q angle
Ligamentous laxity (knee)	Lachman test
	Losee test
	Posterior drawer/drop
	Valgus/varus stress tests
Ankle instability	Talar tilt (medial-lateral)
	Anterior drawer
	Single-limb balance

A P P E N D I X

II

Resource List

ORGANIZATIONS

Accessibility Information Center
National Center for a Barrier Free Environment
1140 Connecticut Avenue, NW
Washington, DC 20036

American Academy of Orthopaedic Surgeons
222 South Prospect Avenue
Park Ridge, IL 60068

American Academy of Pediatrics
141 Northwest Point Blvd.
Elk Grove, IL 60009-0927

American Wheelchair Pilots Association
1621 East 2nd Avenue
Mesa, AZ 85204

Breckenridge Outdoor Recreation Center
P.O. Box 697
Breckenridge, CO 80424

Bureau of Outdoor Recreation
Department of the Interior
Washington, DC 20240

Courage Center
3915 Golden Valley Road
Golden Valley, MN 55422

Drug Hotline
800-223-0393

U.S.O.C. Sports Medicine and Science Division

Handicapped Scuba Association
1104 El Prado
San Clemente, CA 92672

National Archery Association
1750 East Boulder Street
Colorado Springs, CO 80909

National Foundation for Horsemanship for the Handicapped
Box 462
Malvern, PA 19355

National Handicapped Sports and Recreation Association
P.O. Box 18664, Capitol Hill Station
Denver, CO 80218

National Information Center for Handicapped Children and Youth
P.O. Box 492
Washington, DC 20013

National Wheelchair Athletic Association
2107 Templeton Gap Road
Colorado Springs, CO 80907

National Wheelchair Basketball Association
110 Seaton Bldg.
University of Kentucky
Lexington, KY 40506

National Wheelchair Marathon
15 Marlborough Street
Belmont, MA 02178

National Wheelchair Racquetball Association
c/o American Amateur Racquetball Association
815 North Weber
Colorado Springs, CO 80903

National Youth Sports Foundation
10 Meredith Circle
Needham, MA 02192

North American Riding for the Handicapped Association
Box 100
Ashburn, VA 22011

Recreation and Athletic Rehabilitation-Education Center
University of Illinois
1207 South Oak Street
Champaign, IL 61820

Skating Association for the Blind and Handicapped
3236 Main Street
Buffalo, NY 14214

Vinland National Center
3675 Ihduhapi Road
Loretto, MN 55347

Voyageur Outward Bound
Box 250
Long Lake, MN 55356

Wilderness Inquiry II
1313 Fifth Street, SE
Minneapolis, MN 55414

BIBLIOGRAPHY

Rehabilitation

Albert, M. Eccentric Muscle Training in Sports and Orthopaedics. New York: Churchill Livingstone, 1991.

Andrews, J, & Harrelson, GL. Physical Rehabilitation of the Injured Athlete. Philadelphia: WB Saunders, 1992.

Arnheim, D. Modern Principles of Athletic Training, 7th ed. St. Louis: Mosby, 1989.

Booher, J, & Thibodeau, G. Athletic Injury Assessment. St. Louis: Mosby, 1985.

Chu, D. Jumping into Plyometrics. Champaign, IL: Human Kinetics, 1992.

Coaches' and Trainer's Guide to Nonprescription Medications
Upjohn
Box 307
Coventry, CT 06238

DeValentine, SJ (Ed.). Foot and Ankle Disorders in Children. New York: Churchill Livingstone, 1992.

Donatelli, R, & Wooden, MJ (Eds.). Orthopaedic Physical Therapy. New York: Churchill Livingstone, 1989.

Garrick, JG, & Webb, DR. Sports Injuries: Diagnosis and Management. Philadelphia: WB Saunders, 1990.

Gould, J, & Davis, G (Eds.). Orthopaedic and Sports Physical Therapy. St. Louis: Mosby, 1985.

Hoppenfeld, S. Physical Examination of the Spine and Extremities. New York: Appleton-Century-Crofts, 1976.

Kessler, R, & Hertling, D. Management of Common Musculoskeletal Disorders. Philadelphia: Harper & Row, 1983.

Kibler, WB. The Sport Preparticipation Fitness Examination. Champaign, IL: Human Kinetics, 1990.

Kraemer, W, & Fleck, S. Strength Training for Young Athletes. Champaign, IL: Human Kinetics, 1993.

Kuprian, W (Ed.). Physical Therapy for Sports. Philadelphia: WB Saunders, 1982.

Magee, DJ. Orthopedic Physical Assessment, 2nd ed. Philadelphia: WB Saunders, 1992.

McLaren, DS, Burman, D, Belton, NR, & Williams, AF (Eds.). Textbook of Paediatric Nutrition, 3rd ed. New York: Churchill Livingstone, 1992.

McLatchie, GR (Ed.). Essentials of Sports Medicine. New York: Churchill Livingstone, 1986.

Nickel, VL, & Botte, MJ (Eds.). Orthopaedic Rehabilitation, 2nd ed. New York: Churchill Livingstone, 1992.

O'Donoghue, DH (Ed.). Treatment of Injuries to Athletes, 4th ed. Philadelphia: WB Saunders, 1984.

Orthopedic Clinics of North America. Philadelphia: WB Saunders, 1992.

Perrin, D (Ed.). Journal of Sports Rehabilitation. Champaign, IL: Human Kinetics, 1992.

Reid, DC. Sports Injury Assessment and Rehabilitation. New York: Churchill Livingstone, 1992.

Reider, B (Ed.). Sports Medicine: The School Age Athlete. Philadelphia: WB Saunders, 1991.

Rowland, TW (Ed.). Exercise and Children's Health. Champaign, IL: Human Kinetics, 1990.

Rowland, TW (Ed.). Pediatric Exercise Science. Champaign, IL: Human Kinetics, 1992.

Rowland, TW (Ed.). Pediatric Laboratory Exercise Testing. Champaign, IL: Human Kinetics, 1993.

Roy, W, & Irwin, R. Sports Medicine: Prevention, Evaluation, Management, and Rehabilitation. Englewood Cliffs, NJ: Prentice-Hall, 1983.

Sportsmediscope. U.S.O.C. Sports Medicine and Science Division Newsletter.

Strauss, RH (Ed.). Sports Medicine, 2nd ed. Philadelphia: WB Saunders, 1991.

Stretching Charts
P.O. Box 44646
Tacoma, WA 98444

Strickland, JW. Hand Injuries in Athletes. Philadelphia: WB Saunders, 1992.

Subotnick, SI (Ed.). Sports Medicine of the Lower Extremity. New York: Churchill Livingstone, 1989.

Parental and Coaching Information

Access National Park: A Guide for Handicapped Visitors
U.S. Government Printing Office
Washington, DC 20402

Cooper, KH. Kid Fitness. New York: Bantam Books, 1991.
Exceptional Parent
605 Commonwealth Avenue
Boston, MA 02215

Facile Fashions, Irwin/Taylor
80 Superior Road
Rochester, NY 14625

Human Kinetics Publishers
Box 5076
Champaign, IL 61825-5076

Sports and Physical Education Videos and Books
The Athletic Institute
200 Castlewood Drive
North Palm Beach, FL 33408-5697

Sports n' Spokes
Paralyzed Veterans of America
5201 North 19th Avenue
Phoenix, AZ 85015

U.S. Department of Health and Human Services, Alcohol, Drug Abuse and Mental Health Administration, Washington, DC.

MANAGEMENT OF NEUROLOGIC IMPAIRMENT

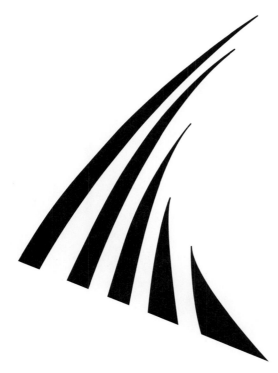

DARL W. VANDER LINDEN, PT, PhD

Section Editor

CHAPTER
18

Developmental Coordination Disorders

KATHRYN STEYER DAVID, PT, PCS, MS

Why are some children considered to be born athletes or graceful dancers? Why do other children always seem to be falling over their feet or bumping into walls? When is clumsiness considered a normal part of growing up, and when is it abnormal? What can physical therapists do to help children with a developmental coordination disorder (DCD)?

Physical therapists have a unique service to offer individuals with DCD. Their background in normal and abnormal motor control, motor learning, and motor development can be used to individually assess, plan programs for, treat, and educate children with DCD, as well as consult with their families. As members of a collaborative team, physical therapists can influence functional outcomes for a group of individuals with very real problems that are often overlooked by members of the medical and educational community.

This chapter describes the process of differential examination that allows a physical therapist to make evaluation and diagnostic decisions regarding goals, outcomes, and interventions for a child with DCD. Evidence is presented to support the need for a multidisciplinary, environmentally referenced, age-appropriate examination followed by an emphasis on selective intervention for collaborative family and school consultation and training at key points during a child's developmental years. A case study illustrates the decision-making stages for a child with DCD from age 19 months through high school. A list of important resources for physical therapists and parents of children with DCD completes the chapter.

DEFINITIONS

Many professionals have attempted to identify and define variables related to incoordination. Different terms have been used in different professions, and the resulting confusion has often inhibited dialogue and limited the generalization of research. The disorder currently identified in the fourth revised edition of the *Diagnostic and Statistical Manual of Mental Disorders* (DSM-IV) (American Psychiatric Association, 1994) is *developmental coordination disorder*. DCD is diagnosed when motor coordination is markedly below expected levels for the child's chronologic age and intelligence, significantly interferes with academic achievement or activities of daily living, is not due to a general medical condition, does not meet criteria for a pervasive developmental disorder, and, if mental retardation is present, the motor difficulties are in excess of those usually associated with mental retardation. DCD would be included under the "Guide to Physical Therapist Practice" (American Physical Therapy Association, 1997) diagnostic group 5A, Impaired Motor Function and Sensory Integrity Associated with Congenital or Acquired Disorders of the Central Nervous System in Infancy, Childhood, and Adolescence (pp. 1371–1382). I have chosen to use the term *developmental coordination disorder* because it highlights movement as the primary focus of the nonprogressive motor abnormalities identified initially in childhood, but often observed throughout an individual's life span. This term is meant to be closely synonymous with the terms *developmental clumsiness, clumsy child,* and *developmental apraxia* (Gubbay, 1975). *Incoordination* has also been associated with a variety of other terms such as *visuomotor problems, dyspraxia,* and *somatodyspraxia* (Missiuna & Polatajko, 1994). The last two terms are used most frequently by occupational therapists when they discuss sensory integration theory and practice.

By definition, motor incoordination caused by or closely associated with mental retardation, genetic disorders (e.g., Down syndrome), neurologic disorders (e.g., cerebral palsy, traumatic brain damage, Friedreich's ataxia), brain tumors, or loss of sensory function (e.g., visual, auditory) is not discussed in this chapter. One should always consider the possibility, however, that DCD can occur along with any of these other diagnoses. It has long been recognized that children with cerebral palsy often exhibit agnosic and apraxic defects that compound the problem of integration of movement (Gubbay, 1975). Deciding when motor incoordination is caused by or closely associated with another disorder such as cerebral palsy rather than occurring along with, but not caused by, that disorder is an important program planning decision. The specific combination of DCD, learning disability, prematurity, and spastic diplegia is further explored in this chapter because it is a combination of which physical therapists need to be especially aware.

INCIDENCE

Just as the term *DCD* and associated terms are difficult to define, the incidence of each is equally unclear. Gubbay (1975) believed that at least 5% of the school-age population displayed clumsiness or DCD. The DSM-IV estimates that as many as 6% of children between 5 and 11 years of age have DCD. Other estimates project that 5 to 10% of the school-age population display minimal brain dysfunction (MBD) with soft neurologic signs (Gaddes, 1985; Gillberg et al., 1982) and that 98% of children with MBD have motor problems, as evidenced by poor, slow, labored handwriting (Clements et al., 1971). Reports indicate that children with educationally identified learning disability are 5 to 6% of the school-age population (U.S. Department of Education, 1997), and it is estimated that 90% of children with learning disability have motor coordination or visuomotor problems (Tarnopol & Tarnopol, 1977). Obviously the problem of motor incoordination exists whether or not it can be consistently categorized and quantified.

Gubbay (1975) believed so strongly that clumsiness should be studied by the medical community as an entity separate from MBD or learning disability that he created a standardized battery of eight tests for physicians to use. A survey was conducted on 992 children and normative data were collected on 919 children ages 8 to 12 years. Children were identified as clumsy based on the number of failures for their age. For example, an 8-year-old was identified as clumsy when there were six or more failures, whereas a 12-year-old was identified when there were two or more failures. On this basis, Gubbay identified 32 children as clumsy and 14 children as borderline clumsy, resulting in a sample of 56 children who were matched to a control group of children of the same sex, age, and classroom. Most of Gubbay's conclusions regarding clumsiness are based on this descriptive study.

PATHOPHYSIOLOGY

No specific pathologic process or single neuroanatomic site has been associated with DCD (Box 18-1). Gaddes (1985) believed that motor clumsiness may find its origin in dysfunction of the cerebellum, of one of the two cerebral motor strips, or of the efferent motor pathways or in some imbalance in one or more of the sensory neural mechanisms. From a systems perspective, smooth motor functioning depends not only on an intact central nervous system but also on use of appropriate, environmentally referenced inputs. Roy and Square (1985) argue that control of praxis involves both top-down and bottom-up influences that operate in

BOX 18–1. **The Disabling Process in Children with Developmental Coordination Disorders**

Pathophysiology	Impairments	Functional Limitations	Disability	Societal Limitation
Heterogeneous central nervous system sites Prenatal, perinatal, and neonatal insults	Soft signs: Poor strength Poor coordination Jerky movements Poor visual perception Joint laxity Poor spatial organization Inadequate information processing Poor sequencing Poor feedback Poor short- and long-term memory	Awkward gait Delayed and poor quality of fine and gross motor skills, such as hopping, jumping, ball skills, and threading beads Delayed oral-motor skills Low self-esteem Distractibility	Dependent self-help skills Limited participation in physical education Poor written communication Poor language skills and social interaction Depression Low academic achievement	Limited indoor and outdoor play with peers Strained child-parent relationships Social isolation Limited vocational success Design of objects such as tamper-proof packaging

parallel. According to Gubbay (1975), clumsiness could be regarded as an all-inclusive end-product of differing etiologies, implying a heterogeneous pathophysiology.

By definition, DCD is not related to muscle pathology, peripheral sensory abnormality, or central nervous system damage that causes spasticity, athetosis, or ataxia. Hypotonia, however, is sometimes associated with motor clumsiness as a neurologic soft sign (Schoemaker et al., 1994). Among infants with low birth weight but no major congenital problems, infants with truncal or lower extremity hypotonia had the worst developmental outcome (Georgieff et al., 1986). Gubbay (1975) found, however, that hypotonia was not more prevalent in children with clumsiness than in a control group. The exact cause of excessive hypotonia and its specific relationship to DCD is not clear and warrants further study.

Studies have been inconclusive in correlating abnormal electroencephalographic findings (Gubbay, 1975) or abnormal results of computed tomographic scans (Knuckey et al., 1983) with clumsiness in children. Either the abnormal findings were not of sufficient magnitude to account for the clumsiness or were not directly related to one anatomic site or pathologic process.

The extent to which research with adults can be applied to children is unclear. The similarities between children with developmental dyspraxia and adults with apraxia have not been thoroughly researched (Cermak, 1985). Some studies with adults have searched for an anatomic site to explain apraxia (Geschwind, 1975; Volpe et al., 1982; Watson et al.,

1986); other theories support a concept of apraxia as an integration problem involving the entire brain (Faglioni & Basso, 1985; Luria, 1966; Roy & Square, 1985). Current theories suggest that multiple mechanisms are involved with praxis and that lesions at any of the multiple pathways can result in one of the many forms of apraxia (Kertesz, 1985) (Fig. 18–1). Kertesz believes that the anterior half of the periventricular white matter and the frontal lobe are the most frequent location of lesions resulting in apraxia. Interestingly, spastic diplegia is the most common form of cerebral palsy likely to result from damage to the periventricular white matter in premature infants (Soltesz & Brockway, 1989). This may be the link between the observed simultaneous occurrence of prematurity, spastic diplegia, and DCD in some children.

Although no certain way of preventing DCD is known, some hypotheses can be made about the causes of DCD. DCD has been associated with perinatal abnormalities of anoxia at birth (Gubbay, 1975). In a later study (Gubbay, 1978) it was found that 50% of children identified as clumsy had prenatal, perinatal, or neonatal risk factors. Infants with low birth weight, especially those with increasing grades of intracranial hemorrhage, score lower on motor development when tested at various ages from infancy through early elementary school years (Hertzig, 1981; Jongmans et al., 1993). Als (1986) has suggested that better prenatal care, perinatal monitoring, and newborn care may decrease the occurrence of developmental motor incoordination problems.

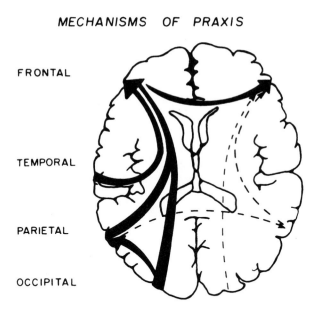

MECHANISMS OF PRAXIS

FRONTAL

TEMPORAL

PARIETAL

OCCIPITAL

FIGURE 18-1. Diagrammatic representation of the neural mechanisms of praxis. Interruption of this network at any point may result in apraxia. Small lesions may affect the system most consistently where pathways converge. Dotted lines represent alternate routes that may become active with recovery. (From Roy, EA [Ed.]. Neuropsychological Studies of Apraxia and Related Disorders. New York: North-Holland, 1985, p. 175.)

ASSOCIATED IMPAIRMENTS

Referral

Primary impairments are the first signs of problems that result from the primary pathophysiology and that assist in making an eventual diagnosis or identification of dysfunction (see Box 18-1). The first signs of DCD are often not identified until the child reaches school age. Gubbay (1975) stated that clumsiness is usually only a problem between ages 6 and 12 years when functional limitations appear. Gubbay reported that in the younger age groups the environment tends to be less reactive and generally kinder because of the wider range of normal variation. The early signs of clumsiness are often viewed as part of normal developmental awkwardness or normal delay for premature infants. Parents often report that their children were overly messy when eating and dressing, started walking later than other children and are still awkward, were late talkers, had excessive levels of frustration and crying, and demanded continual adult attention. Laszlo and colleagues (1988) concluded that parents were poor judges of motor competence because although many described their child as "messy," "slow," and "unco-

ordinated," they were certain that this was "normal."

Parents, preschool teachers, or early elementary school teachers are usually the first to raise a concern related to impairments and functional limitations associated with DCD. If the concern is taken to a pediatrician or family doctor, a preliminary neurologic examination might reveal soft neurologic signs, such as muscle weakness, especially of the hands; poor coordination, especially in finger-to-nose movement and finger-thumb opposition; and possible choreiform movements seen as small jerky twitches of the upper extremities. But not all children with DCD have detectable soft signs, and initially the impairments associated with DCD may not be identified. In fact, some researchers believe that neurologic soft signs are an assortment of poorly related behaviors that have poor reliability as indicators of impairments related to DCD (Henderson, 1987). In spite of these criticisms, a neurologic evaluation serves the important function of ruling out the existence of more serious neurologic causes of motor incoordination.

As children with DCD reach school age, a set of behavioral and emotional limitations can become apparent and warrant another referral to a physician. Problems with distractibility have been identified in children with DCD (Hulme & Lord, 1986). Gubbay (1975) cited temper tantrums, frustration, poor self-esteem, depression, and rejection as possible problems. Shaw and colleagues (1982) concluded that children with learning disability and clumsiness had significantly lowered self-esteem and were less happy than other children. If depression is serious, psychiatric intervention or counseling might be needed. These emotional symptoms might also be signs of attention deficit hyperactivity disorder (ADHD) because clumsiness is an overlapping characteristic. A diagnosis of ADHD would influence future medical and educational programming decisions. Additional physical symptoms of abdominal pain, loss of bowel or bladder control unrelated to any physical problems, or headaches are often seen as children with DCD grow older (Levine, 1987). These complaints should be taken seriously, and previously unidentified medical conditions should be ruled out before other approaches to deal with the symptoms are implemented.

Physical Therapy Examination Findings

An examination by the physical therapist should rule out other possible diagnoses for the child's referring problems before concluding that DCD may be present. Children with DCD often exhibit impairments such as immature movement patterns and inconsistent motor responses, and postural reactions can be delayed or absent in some positions. It is not uncommon to find absent or poorly developed backward protective extension in ambulatory children with DCD. Joint laxity with scapular winging, elbow hyperextension, hypermobile fingers, and poor trunk extension, especially in sitting, can sometimes be identified. Static balance tasks are often difficult for the child to perform. By carefully observing associated areas of performance, the therapist may be able to relate the most striking impairments to difficulties in following directions when asked to perform a motor task or to poor attention-to-task. Children with DCD often cannot imitate body postures or follow two- or three-step motor commands. Frequent demonstration and actual physical assistance may be needed to accomplish items on standardized tests. Physical therapists must make evaluation hypotheses regarding the origin of a child's impairments.

As Roy and Square (1985) point out, apraxia can involve dysfunction of either the cognitive-linguistic (information processing) system or the motor-production system. Others have concluded that children with verbal sequencing deficits also have difficulty with sequential limb and oral gestures, suggesting an underlying motor disorder (Dewey et al., 1988). As experts in the motor-production system, physical therapists must distinguish the motor-production component of DCD from other sources of dysfunction. Referral to other team members with expertise in cognitive-linguistic functioning (e.g., psychologist, speech and language pathologist) should be made when deficits in these areas are hypothesized to be associated with a child's motor functioning problems.

Problem Definition

An information processing model has been used to explain some of the possible motor control impairments of DCD. Various abnormalities within and among the processing stages of stimulus identification, response selection, and response programming and within motor memory have been examined with respect to DCD.

While applying this information processing model to learning disabilities, Silver (1988) formed hypotheses regarding how different types of processing problems might result in motor incoordination. Using visual perception as an example of stimulus identification, Silver hypothesized that when children are impaired in judging distances, they will exhibit functional limitations such as bumping into things, falling off chairs, or knocking over drinks. Children with DCD also can be functionally limited by becoming disoriented on the playground or during physical education class because they have impairments related to organization of their position in space in relation to other persons and objects. Any activity that requires the eyes to tell the hands what to do (such as ball catching, rope jumping, completing puzzles) will be a functional limitation for these children. O'Brien and colleagues (1988) concluded that the degree of clumsiness was significantly related to the degree of visuoperceptual and visuomotor impairment.

Response selection is the next step in the information processing model. Van Dellan and Geuze (1988) used a fine motor task to compare reaction time and movement time. They concluded that the impaired cognitive decision process of response selection contributed to the functional limitation of slow performance in the children identified as clumsy.

Response timing problems also contribute to DCD impairments. Henderson and colleagues (1992) concluded that the principal source of prolonged response latency in children with DCD is within the process of searching for and retrieval of the correct responses with reliable timing. Lundy-Ekman and colleagues (1991) also concluded that timing and force control were separate response components associated with poor motor skills in children with DCD. The timing problems identified in clumsy children are believed to be caused by a central timekeeping mechanism, possibly the cerebellum (Williams et al., 1992).

Response selection requires memory skills. Forgetting which way to stand when preparing to hit a baseball and how to hold your hands on the bat can result in the appearance of clumsiness. Knowing how to cross your legs to assume a sitting posture is something parents, therapists, and teachers take for granted (Fig. 18–2). Children who have DCD and have an impairment related to response selection can be functionally limited because they have to figure out how to position their body every time they are asked to sit on the floor for group activities.

Considerable research exists regarding young children's use of memory strategies, especially for cognitive tasks. In a 1985 study, I found that even though 76% of normal 8-year-old children used verbal rehearsal to remember a cognitive sequencing task, only 33% used the same strategy to help them remember a motor sequencing task (David, 1985). Murphy and Gliner (1988) found that 6- to 9-year-old children designated as clumsy have even more trouble than their peers with visual and motor sequencing tasks requiring short- and long-term recall. In addition, some children with DCD have impaired visual memory when compared with their peers (Dwyer & McKenzie, 1994). Skorji and McKenzie (1997) found that children with DCD are more

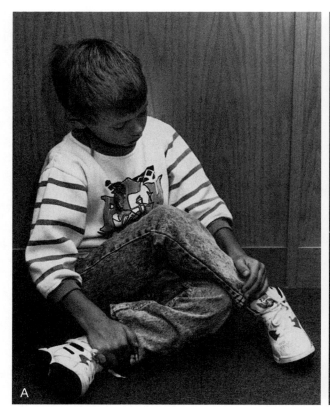 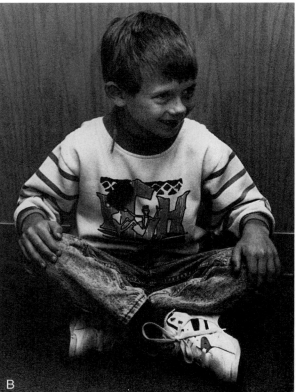

FIGURE 18–2. *A,* After many therapy sessions with verbal and physical prompts, this child is still unable to sit on the floor and cross his legs independently. *B,* After being reminded of the verbal cues he needs to say to himself, he now successfully crosses his legs.

dependent on visuospatial rehearsal to memorize a modeled movement than their peers.

Response programming requires sequencing of movement parameters. Children with impairments in sequencing skills cannot correctly sequence the steps in shoe-tying even though they have practiced it many times before. When children with DCD make a mistake in one step of the sequence, they have to start over again rather than simply redo the last step, or they may omit a different step in the sequence each time they try to tie their shoes (Fig. 18–3). This results in functional limitations related to slow and laborious movements and sometimes messy outcomes for certain tasks. The reliance on information feedback rather than feedforward programming may also contribute to slow performance (Rösblad & van Hofsten, 1994; Smyth, 1991).

Appropriate use of feedback loops to increase knowledge of performance or knowledge of results is one way learners receive information about their performance. The impact that impairments in kinesthetic feedback may have on the performance of motor skills by children with DCD is open to question. Hoare and Larkin (1991) found that children with DCD demonstrated impaired performance compared with their peers on only three of seven kinesthetic tasks tested: kinesthetic acuity, linear positioning, and weight discrimination. They concluded that caution should be used when labeling children as kinesthetically impaired on the basis of their performance on only a few tasks. Kinesthetic intervention must be individualized and task specific to improve motor performance for children with developmental clumsiness.

Other methods of performance feedback were studied by Lord and Hulme (1987), who found that children with motor clumsiness demonstrated impairments of size-constancy judgments, spatial position, and visual discrimination tasks. Inefficient use of visual feedback was also cited as a possible cause for poor performance by children identified as clumsy when they attempted a fast, goal-directed arm movement (van der Meulen et al., 1991a), but visual feedback was not a discriminating factor when

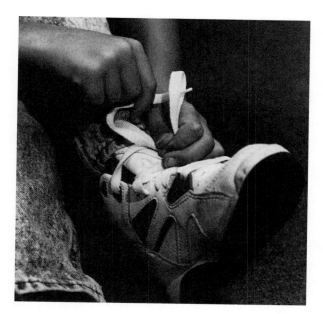

FIGURE 18–3. This 8-year-old boy still cannot independently tie his shoes. His verbal cues were "loop around and go through." He forgot to "loop around" and forgot to make a second loop.

an arm-tracking task was studied (van der Meulen et al., 1991b).

Although the recent research from an information processing framework adds to the knowledge base about children with DCD, physical therapists should remember that most of these studies have used motor learning tasks that are specific to an experimental paradigm and performed inside a laboratory environment. Whether the performance on these types of tasks is related to functional motor tasks in natural environments has not been studied. Future research should focus on functional tasks in natural environments, such as measurements of movement times when completing a writing sample, reaction times when asked to stand up from a classroom desk, or sequencing errors when tying shoes after physical education class.

As stated earlier, unless a child is receiving physical therapy for some other problem or being closely followed by a high-risk infant program, referral due to processing impairments such as diminished visual perception, limited motor memory, poor motor sequencing, excessive use of feedback, or poor spatial organization is often not made before kindergarten or early elementary school. Even when referred, standardized evaluations that assess information processing impairments are not currently available, except as part of some neuropsychologic examinations (Kaufman & Kaufman, 1983; Reitan & Wolfson,

1985; Rourke et al., 1986) or as a very specific, nonfunctional, and nonenvironmentally referenced kinesthetic task (Laszlo & Bairstow, 1985).

Prevention

Prevention of the impairments related to DCD has not been well addressed. General early intervention programs for infants at risk are becoming more common in the United States, especially as a result of the legislative mandates associated with Part C of the Individuals with Disabilities Education Act Amendments of 1997 (previously Part H). To date, most studies on the effects of early intervention have focused on improvements in cognitive development but not specifically on motor development (Mastropieri, 1988). Interestingly, some of the characteristics described by parents of children with DCD are similar to those used by Als and colleagues (1986, 1988) to describe preterm infants who display state disorganization.

Als (1986) has suggested the use of specific positioning and handling techniques to improve state regulation and diminish disorganized behavior to encourage more normal development in infants, toddlers, and preschoolers. This can be a significant contribution that physical therapists make to prevent or minimize future motor problems. Physical therapists must take advantage of single-subject research designs and systematic case studies with data-based progress monitoring to determine the efficacy of early intervention for at-risk infants and young children in reducing the impairments associated with DCD.

Referral to Other Disciplines

There is another group of young children seen by physical therapists who should be considered at risk for DCD. These are the children who were premature and were subsequently diagnosed with spastic diplegic cerebral palsy. Some of these children enter school and have increasing academic difficulties that eventually lead to an educational diagnosis of learning disability. When treating a preschool child with spastic diplegia and a birth history of prematurity and perinatal complications, physical therapists must be aware of early signs of motor incoordination.

The physical therapist can be the first to identify DCD and is therefore responsible for making appropriate referrals to other disciplines. Inconsistencies and abnormal functioning may be noticed in fine motor areas that are unrelated to impairments from cerebral palsy, such as abnormal muscle tone, postural control, muscle strength, and endurance. These findings may suggest that problems are not due to a motor-production component of the incoordination, leading the therapist to suspect a cognitive-linguistic component. For example, an 18-month-old child's poor visuomotor perception can be the reason the child cannot remove large pegs from a pegboard when other fine motor skills are age appropriate, visual acuity is normal, and abnormal muscle tone or strength is not interfering. Motor memory problems might explain why movement patterns that have been practiced repeatedly during past therapy sessions seem totally unfamiliar at the beginning of a subsequent session and have to be retaught each time with extensive verbal, visual, and physical cues. An observant physical therapist may notice that auditory memory is highly developed, especially for television commercials and songs, but conversational language is stereotypical and eye contact is difficult to achieve.

Research has found an increased incidence of DCD in combination with ocular motor and oral motor apraxia (Dewey et al., 1988; Rappaport et al., 1987). A follow-up study of adolescents who had been identified as having DCD when they were in elementary school documented associated problems of lower academic attainment, fewer social contacts, and poorer classroom concentration and behavior than in other children (Geuze & Borger, 1993). It should not be assumed that DCD is an isolated motor problem. If a child's overall developmental profile is age appropriate but unexplained gaps in performance or atypical behaviors unrelated to motor-production problems are present, physical therapists should consider the possibility of cognitive-linguistic components of DCD. Referrals to other disciplines (e.g., occupational therapy, speech and language pathology, early childhood education) should be made. If a child with spastic diplegia has academic problems, the physical therapist, as a member of the educational team, can help distinguish motor-production problems from other possible learning problems. Additional special or general education services may need to be recommended.

Summary

In conclusion, physical therapists have typically not treated the underlying impairments of DCD. However, when young children are referred to physical therapy for evaluation and movement dysfunction is identified as a possible impairment associated with DCD, intervention with progress monitoring techniques using objective outcome measures should be initiated. Often consultative services in conjunction with day care or preschool gross motor play programs is the most appropriate recommendation. Physical therapists can help educate parents and teachers concerning the progression of normal motor milestones and assist in the development of motor curricula for preschools, day care settings, and community recreation programs. Continued research to identify additional motor-production impairments using a motor control perspective may lead to new implications for physical therapy for the impairments related to developmental clumsiness.

TEAM EVALUATION AND MANAGEMENT OF DISABILITY

School-Age Period

Performance in Natural Environments and Typical Disabilities

Parent and teacher behavior checklists have been developed and used to screen children before a full examination to identify DCD (Henderson & Sugden, 1992; Laszlo et al., 1988; van der Meulen et al., 1991a). Parents know their child's developmental history and have observed his or her functioning in multiple environments. They have the best composite of diagnostic information. A thorough parental interview is therefore essential to any understanding of DCD. Parents identify disabilities that include ongoing problems with everyday activities of dressing, eating, grooming, and speech (see Box 18-1). When their children were preschoolers, these disabilities were excused as "slow development" or temperamental differences. Poor performance on everyday activities is tolerated less and less as children with DCD reach school age. Impairments mentioned earlier, including slow movement times, poor motor sequencing, poor motor memory, and perceptual problems, and resulting functional limitations of delayed motor skills make dressing, eating, and grooming painfully slow, messy, and dependent skills.

Teachers are the next most likely individuals to identify disabilities related to DCD. Often, the structured demands of the classroom with expectations of increasingly precise motor skills and shorter time frames for performance stress a child with DCD to his or her limit. Teachers are able to compare the performance of children with incoordination to that of their peers, something parents do not have as many opportunities to do.

Poor written communication is frequently the first disability educators identify (Fig. 18-4). There are many reasons for poor written communication, and the functional limitation of poor handwriting associated with DCD is only one of them. Treating handwriting as a motor-production problem when

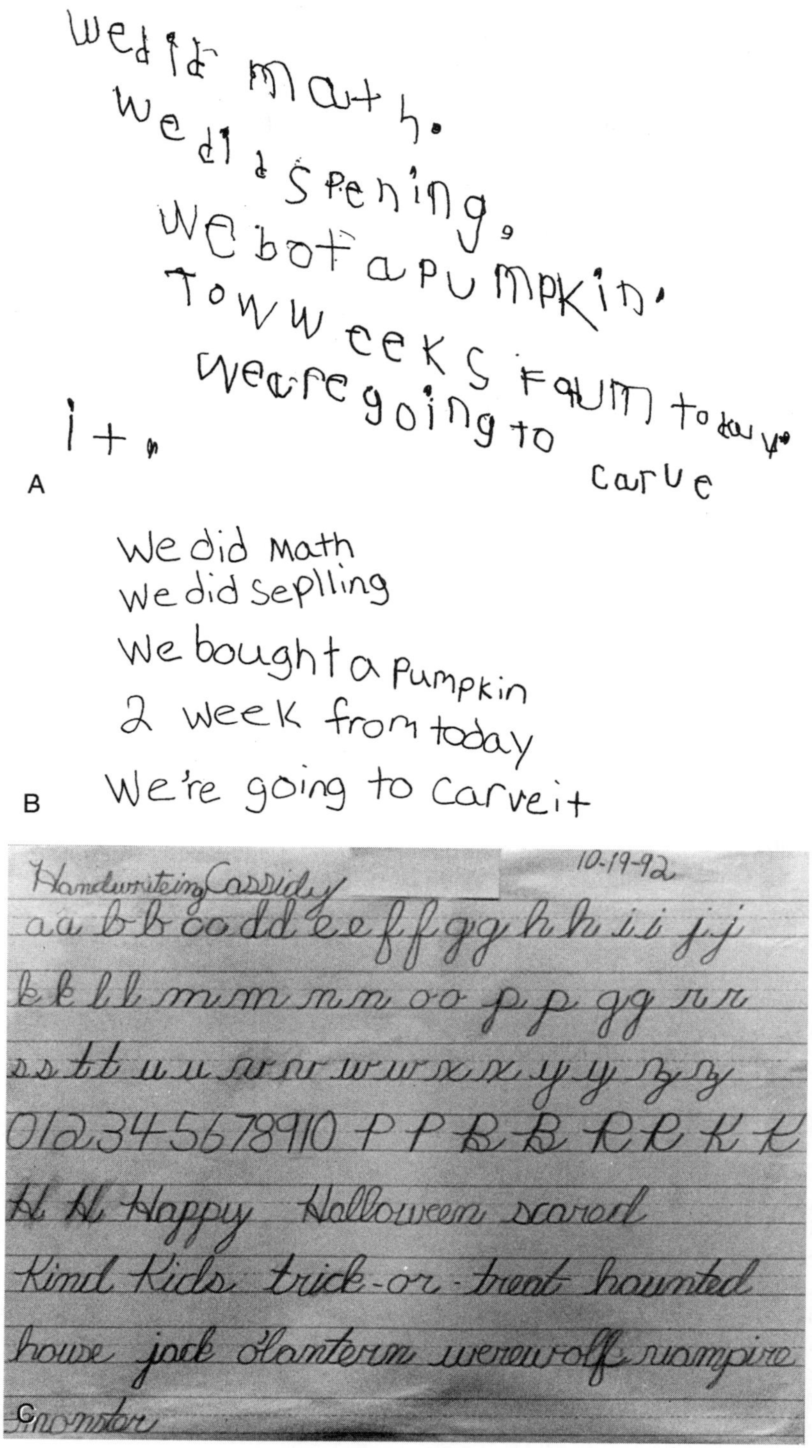

We did Math.
We did Spening,
We bot a pumpkin.
Tow weeks faum today
weare going to carve
it.

A

We did Math
We did Seplling

We bought a pumpkin
2 week from today
We're going to carveit

B

Handwriting Cassidy   10-19-92

aa bb oo dd e ff gg hh ii jj
kk ll mm nn oo p p gg rr
ss tt uu vr w w x x yy zz
0123456789 10 P P B B R R K K
H H Happy Halloween scared
Kind Kids trick-or-treat haunted
house jack o lantern werewolf vampire
monster

C

FIGURE 18–4. *A,* Handwriting sample of a third-grade child with a developmental coordination disorder and a learning disability. *B,* Handwriting sample obtained for comparison from a randomly selected third-grade peer without motor dysfunction. *C,* Sample of cursive writing from another peer without motor dysfunction demonstrates an even more advanced expectation of third graders.

the real issue is poor visual form recognition will only frustrate the child and the teacher. Whether the underlying processing impairments or the functional motor limitation should be treated is a question the family and the entire educational team should address.

Another common disability identified in early elementary school is poor performance in physical education class. Simple delayed maturation, limited gross motor play experience, poor motivation, or significant health or medical disorders, as well as DCD, should be considered as possible reasons for problems in physical education class.

Some evidence suggests that caution should be used when relying on the judgment of classroom or physical education teachers to identify children with DCD. Piek and Edwards (1997) compared the Movement Assessment Battery for Children (ABC) checklist results with actual performance on the Movement ABC examination (Henderson & Sugden, 1992). They found that classroom teachers identified only 25% of the children with DCD and physical education teachers identified only 49%. This discrepancy is partially explained by the different environments on which the two types of teachers based their observations. An accurate identification of children with DCD requires examinations that occur in multiple environments with diverse activities.

Functional Limitations

Functional limitations associated with the disabilities related to DCD (see Box 18–1) are typically examined by administering standardized and norm-referenced tests composed of discrete items of motor performance. One of the first test batteries designed to identify children with DCD is the Gubbay Tests of Motor Proficiency (Gubbay, 1975), which is reproduced in Appendix II at the end of this chapter. The test items Gubbay found to discriminate between children with and without clumsiness include whistling, skipping, rolling a ball with their foot, clapping while throwing a ball in the air, shoe-tying, threading beads, piercing holes in paper, and placing shapes in a form board. In a later study of 39 children with clumsiness, Gubbay (1978) found that the battery could be shortened to four items: throwing a ball in the air and clapping before it is caught, using a foot to roll a ball along a path, threading beads, and inserting shapes in slots. In addition to his Tests of Motor Proficiency, Gubbay believed that a full examination for DCD should include eight items related to the general history of the child; six items related to a physical examination; a supplementary neurologic examination; academic testing in the areas of reading, writing, and drawing; an electroen-

cephalogram; a skull radiograph; and psychologic testing.

A more current examination for DCD is the Movement ABC (Henderson & Sugden, 1992) normed for children 4 to 10 years old. It includes a screening checklist to be used by teachers and a norm-referenced examination. The checklist has four sections with 12 questions in each section and a fifth section with questions about the child's behaviors related to motor activities. Each of the first four sections has questions regarding the child's performance in one of the following environments: child stationary, environment stable (e.g., cutting); child moving, environment stable (e.g., walking); child stationary, environment changing (e.g., catching); and child moving, environment changing (e.g., kicking a ball). A total score is calculated and used to determine whether the child is at risk for (below 15% but above 5% cutoff) or has (below the 5% cutoff) movement problems.

The actual examination was developed from previous examinations, including the Test of Motor Impairment (TOMI) (Stott, Moyes, & Henderson, 1972) and The Henderson Revision of the Test of Motor Impairment (Stott, Moyes, & Henderson, 1984). It has three sections, each section containing items for each of three age bands—4 to 6 years, 7 to 8 years, and 9 to 10 years. Items are divided into manual dexterity, ball skills, and static and dynamic balance sections, including activities such as threading beads, putting pegs in a peg board, catching and throwing a bean bag, balancing on one leg, jumping, hopping, and heel-to-toe walking. A total score is used to determine if performance is within normal ranges, if a motor impairment is present, or if the impairment is serious.

Standardized tests of developmentally sequenced gross and fine motor items can be used to identify the motor delay associated with DCD. The Bayley Scales of Infant Development (Bayley, 1993), Alberta Infant Motor Scale (AIMS) (Piper & Darrah, 1994), Peabody Developmental Motor Scales (Folio & Fewell, 1983), and Miller Assessment for Preschoolers (Miller, 1982) are examples of developmental motor examinations used to identify motor delay in infants and preschool children. The Bruininks-Oseretsky Test of Motor Proficiency is designed to identify motor delay in older children (Bruininks, 1978). These are examples of tests to determine developmental motor delay, and they are *not* designed to be used for the identification of DCD.

Societal Limitations

When peers, parents, teachers, or communities place unwarranted restrictions, artificial barriers, or rigid expectations on individuals with DCD, a functional limitation or disability becomes a societal limitation. This can happen at any age. Rules may prevent a child from playing with his or her friends, restaurants may prevent families from eating out together, and police departments may prevent adolescents or adults from driving a car.

Poor gross motor skills of running, skipping, hopping, or jumping may create a functional limitation or disability for a child with DCD. However, if a physical education class or community recreation program strictly adheres to performance criteria for group activities such as baseball, basketball, or dance class, a child with DCD has been artificially prevented from participating with peers. If parents prevent their child from going down the street to play at a neighborhood park because they are unduly afraid the child will be hurt or will get lost, a barrier has been established and peer relationships have been limited.

Indoor manipulative play can pose just as much of a problem. When functional limitations exist in fine motor skills of coloring, cutting, and stacking objects, imaginative play with paper, small toy people, or building blocks is very difficult. Again, this becomes a societal limitation when materials and play expectations are not modified. By not allowing children to play with modified toys or when individualized expectations are not permitted, a child's experiences are artificially limited and the lack of practice prevents ongoing skill development. Manipulative games are soon avoided, and random, nonconstructive activities may take their place (Fig. 18–5). Isolation imposed by society becomes a self-perpetuating cycle of poor skill development, limited skill practice, poor performance, and further isolation. This cycle and its many negative consequences may all be due to an initial limitation created by teachers, parents, or peers.

If a community police department refuses to recognize that an adolescent or adult cannot pass a field sobriety test owing to inherent coordination problems, the individual with DCD may be mistakenly arrested for drunken driving. In this case, society may unnecessarily limit the person's freedom to drive and restrict community mobility and vocational options.

If a restaurant makes a family feel uncomfortable or asks them to leave because their child spills drinks or drops food on the floor, eating out will occur less often or may be limited to certain environments. When excessive cultural expectations related to independence or proper manners are not met and restrictions are created, a disability has become a societal limitation (see Box 18–1). Helping families and individuals with DCD to know their rights and identify compensatory means for full participation in meaningful activities is one of the physical therapist's most important roles.

Physical Therapy Referral, Examination, and Evaluation

With the passage of the Education of the Handicapped Act in 1975 (amended in 1990 and 1997 and now titled Individuals with Disabilities Education Act [IDEA]), physical therapists working in educational environments in the United States are often asked to assess children demonstrating problems with motor skills at school. Some of these children display the impairments and functional limitations described previously. The physical therapist in educational environments has the advantage of observing and examining children in their natural environments while the children participate in everyday, functional activities. Immediate collaborative consultation can occur with the classroom or physical education teacher to problem solve some of the concerns. Often, an initial collection of specific data can solve the problem without a complete physical therapy evaluation. Perhaps data collected during recess would reveal that the child in question really does not fall more frequently than two randomly chosen peers; the child may just come to the teacher more often for help. In this case the problem is not motoric, but behavioral, and an examination by a physical therapist is not needed. When data reveal that the child does indeed fall three times more often than other children during recess, an appropriate physical therapy examination can begin with already collected baseline data related to function. When children with possible DCD are examined in a clinical setting, in-depth interviewing of the parents and teachers and simulation of functional activities are needed to accurately identify true functional limitations and disabilities.

When a child's specific motor problem has been defined and it has been determined that an examination is indicated, the physical therapist should avoid repeating examinations already performed by other disciplines. When possible, an arena or transdisciplinary examination and evaluation should be considered. The "Guide to Physical Therapist Practice" (American Physical Therapy Association, 1997) outlines the following examination and evaluation framework. Initial determination of what practice pattern best describes a child's motor problems begins with the collection of historical information. The following types of information would be pertinent for a child suspected of having a DCD: a medical history, including pregnancy, delivery, and past and current health status; developmental history;

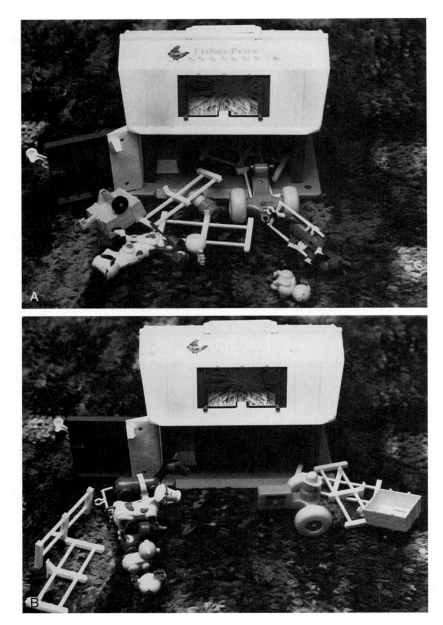

FIGURE 18–5. *A*, Arrangement of toys by a 4-year-old, who was later identified as having a developmental coordination disorder and a learning disability, after he was told to "Show me what you can do with these toys." *B*, A 4-year-old with normal development and given the same instructions arranged the toys like this.

previous musculoskeletal and neuromuscular examinations; and history of the current functional status from the family and school personnel. A physical therapy examination can begin with the same test and measures previously mentioned for the younger child. Referral to Preferred Practice Pattern 5A would prompt a physical therapist to choose tests of neuromotor development and sensory integration to ob-

tain a current level of motor and sensory functioning. Depending on the age of the child, the Peabody Developmental Motor Scales (Folio & Fewell, 1983) and the Bruininks-Oseretsky Test of Motor Proficiency (Bruininks, 1978) are possible choices. The Movement ABC (Henderson & Sugden, 1992) can be administered as a more direct examination of dexterity, agility, and coordination. To rule out abnormal movement patterns and motor control problems (related to neuromuscular or musculoskeletal disorders such as cerebral palsy, polyneuropathies, or muscular dystrophy), typical muscle performance and motor function examinations are administered, including muscle strength and endurance; muscle tone; joint mobility and spinal alignment; postural control and balance; righting, protective, and equilibrium responses; quality of movement during postural transitions; and gait analysis.

Throughout the examination, the physical therapist should note possible signs of related motor control and motor learning problems that might be contributing to motor incoordination. If the functional motor skills of dressing, eating, grooming, drawing, writing, or cutting have not been directly observed in their natural environments, simulations of these natural environmental conditions must be examined. Putting a coat on surrounded by 25 other 7-year-old children, all struggling in a small space to get dressed and get outside first, is much different than putting on a coat in a quiet room with one adult giving positive encouragement. If examinations must be performed in a hospital or clinic setting, behavior might need to be observed in a noisy, distracting, fast-paced environment such as a busy waiting room or children's play area.

An evaluation (analysis and synthesis of examination results), diagnosis, and prognosis by the physical therapist will then determine whether intervention or further examinations by other professionals is warranted. An examination may be needed by any of the following individuals: (1) a family physician or neurologist when neuromuscular or musculoskeletal concerns are identified; (2) an occupational therapist when fine motor, self-help, or motor planning areas need further examination; (3) a speech and language pathologist when speech, oral-motor dysfunction, or possible cognitive-linguistic problems are observed; (4) a psychologist when intellectual or behavioral issues have surfaced; or (5) an adapted physical education teacher when more thorough gross motor skill training is needed.

Decisions related to the need for physical therapy intervention must then be made. When an examination is performed by a physical therapist in an educational setting, the results are shared with the parents and other educational team members at a school conference or an individualized education program (IEP) meeting for a student in special education. When an examination is performed in a clinic, the clinical judgments and proposed therapy needs are discussed with the family and appropriate medical staff. In both instances, the need to share information with other service agencies is considered. If indicated, parental permission to release reports is ob-

tained. Interagency service coordination is extremely important.

Physical Therapy Intervention

Once impairments, functional limitations, and disabilities are identified, physical therapy goals and outcomes must be discussed with the child's team. This discussion should include an anticipated frequency and duration of therapy sessions needed for this episode of care. Specific and measurable goals and outcomes should be identified because little research evidence exists that substantiates the successful remediation of developmental incoordination. A few studies have shown that children with DCD improve in motor skills even without intervention (Knuckey & Gubbay, 1983; Roussounis et al., 1987). These studies, however, have been short term or have used only isolated tasks normed for younger children, or the children have improved but still demonstrate deficits compared with their peers. Losse and colleagues (1991) found that even with a year of intervention at age 6, children with DCD still had significant motor problems when they were 16 years old.

Additional short-term intervention studies have been reported. Schoemaker and colleagues (1994) identified 17 students (6 to 9 years old) who demonstrated clumsiness as measured on the Henderson revision of the TOMI (Stott et al., 1984). Physical therapy intervention lasted 3 months and consisted of 45-minute visits twice a week. The physical therapist performed her own evaluation and devised an individual intervention plan. The intervention was described as eclectic with a combination of sensorimotor training and Bobath neurodevelopmental techniques. The TOMI and Movement ABC were used to compare preintervention status with postintervention and 3 months postintervention status. Three TOMI items revealed a significant improvement: moving both hands rapidly during a fine motor skill, catching a ball, and static balance. Improvements were maintained for 3 months. The authors concluded that the effects of the intervention transferred to similar skills. However, they acknowledged that improvement was measured in a stable, restricted laboratory setting and that motor activity in natural environments is more complex.

Polatajko and colleagues (1995) used a process-oriented treatment approach to treat children with DCD. Process-oriented treatment was defined as kinesthetic training using a protocol created by Laszlo and Bairstow (1985), which used a special apparatus for arm movements on a runway. Three sets of children, 7 to 12 years old, with mild motor problems participated. They were randomly assigned to one of three groups. The process-oriented group was trained with activities designed to increase kinesthetic acuity, kinesthetic perception, and memory. Training by occupational therapists took place in 20-minute sessions two to three times a week. Each child participated in 5 to 12 training sessions depending on how quickly the child learned the task. Another group participated in what was defined as traditional occupational therapy sessions. Intervention consisted of a combination of sensory integrative, gross motor, fine motor, and perceptual-motor activities individually designed for each child. This group was seen for 45 minutes two to three times a week for a total of 24 sessions over 15 weeks. There was also a no-treatment group whose members were not seen by their therapist for 11 weeks. Multiple outcome measurements were used. The authors concluded that the children receiving the process-oriented intervention did not perform differently than the other groups except for kinesthetic acuity, the task they were trained on. It was concluded that increased kinesthetic acuity does not immediately transfer to increased motor performance in children with DCD. In addition, these children did not "spontaneously apply and generalize new-found skills… the data from the traditional group suggest that the motor problems of these children are very resistant to treatment, at least in the short term…all of the current treatment approaches warrant careful examination if they are to be continued to be used with children with DCD" (Polatajko et al., 1995, p. 317).

Some researchers believe that an important (Fisher & Murray, 1991) or even the primary (Gubbay, 1978) benefit of an evaluation for DCD is not subsequent intervention but rather the follow-up consultation that provides an explanation of the dysfunction to the child, the parents, and school personnel. Appendix I contains some resources for parents that may be useful in planning a program for family education.

When a decision is made to proceed with physical therapy, the physical therapist must determine the specific content of the intervention. Intervention for coordination, communication, and documentation of services and for child, family, and school personnel instruction should always be identified. Controversy exists regarding the need for direct intervention and whether direct intervention should be focused toward the underlying impairments, toward the functional limitations, or toward the actual disability or encompass a combination of all of these areas. Motor learning research would suggest that to decrease the functional limitation associated with DCD, direct intervention must include the specific functional task or motor skill training practiced in its appropriate functional environment (Gentile, 1987; Schmidt, 1988).

For example, to improve functional limitations related to static balance (standing on one foot to put on a boot, kicking a stationary ball, or standing in line without touching the people or objects around you), the skills have to be practiced repeatedly with slight variation so that underlying motor and cognitive strategies are learned. These skills also need to be practiced in an environment complete with multiple distractions and simultaneous activities occurring. The same is true for practicing handwriting or self-help skills such as putting on a jacket.

When underlying impairments are the target of remediation, therapeutic exercise should include activities such as the following: (1) increasing muscle strength in hand muscles needed for handwriting; (2) motor learning training to verbally identify and remember sequences for a task such as shoe-tying; (3) improving visual perception used for cutting skills; and (4) practicing attending to visual, auditory, or kinesthetic performance feedback information, such as watching in a mirror or trying to listen to the sounds generated when skipping and using this information to make a different response next time.

One can easily see how these approaches can be combined, especially when consultative physical therapy interventions for family and school instruction are integrated with more direct intervention and a variety of natural environments are used. If, for example, the problem is the inability to quickly and safely climb stairs between classes at school, isolated time with the physical therapist can initially be used to improve strength and endurance of hip and knee extensor muscles by repeatedly practicing going up and down stairs. The therapist can assist the student to verbally identify and rehearse the motor sequence needed to reciprocally climb up a flight of stairs and then practice the timing and order of the sequence in isolation until stair climbing can be performed faster and safely (Fig. 18-6A). The physical therapist would then instruct others so that the task can be repeated during the school day, but with extra time allowances, modified disturbances from other students, and prompted feedback by an educational associate or teacher (Fig. 18-6B). This can be combined with additional practice at home in a quieter environment and with prompting from a parent. Finally, reciprocal stair climbing would be performed during normal transition times between classes with typical numbers of other students, without prompts, and without adult guidance (Fig. 18-6C).

Whatever intervention approach is used, ongoing reexamination including careful monitoring of outcomes related to the remediation of the identified functional limitation or disability is imperative to be sure that the child is benefiting from the service. There are few standardized examinations that are useful to monitor and document change in

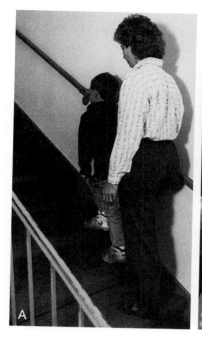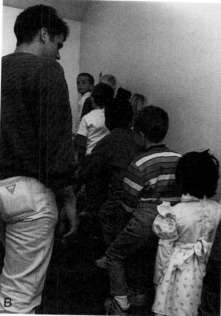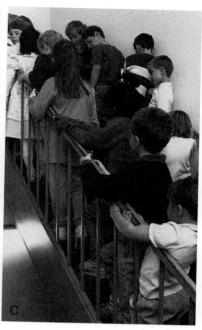

FIGURE 18–6. *A,* During the first stages of learning, natural environments are used with direct instruction from the physical therapist. *B,* During later stages of learning, natural environments and modified distractions are used with faded feedback from the classroom associate. *C,* Stair climbing is now performed in its natural environment with typical environmental distractions. The child is expected to monitor his own performance and make corrections as needed.

performance of functional skills in children. Haley and colleagues (1991) describe six different pediatric functional outcome measures, including the Gross Motor Function Measure (Russell et al., 1989), the Wee-Functional Independence Measure (Granger et al., 1989), and the Pediatric Evaluation of Disability Inventory (Haley et al., 1989). Unfortunately these instruments were designed for use in clinical settings and therefore are not individualized to a specific environmental context for a specific student. The School Function Assessment (Coster et al., 1998) was recently designed to meet this need for elementary school children. It contains three parts: a rating scale for participation in school activities in multiple environments, a rating of the physical and behavioral assistance and supports the student needs, and examination of performance on typical school activities.

IEPs, with measurable, annual goals written in behavioral terms with specific performance criteria and evaluation schedules, are designed to be used to monitor individual function within a school setting. Another alternative is the use of goal attainment scaling (Palisano et al., 1992). Five possible levels of specific functional attainment are individualized for a child to create a criterion-referenced measurement. (See Chapter 19 for additional information on goal attainment scaling.)

Reexamination should include the discussion of the prevention of secondary problems. If theories that propose that DCD is related to MBD are correct, one can assume that the primary neurologic problem is still present in older children and adults, even though compensatory mechanisms have developed. The identification of ways to prevent functional limitations from becoming disabilities can be one of the most important outcomes of physical therapy intervention.

Factors that would signal the need for a new episode of care should also be discussed. Continued physical therapy screening or examination throughout the elementary school years may be needed to help the educational team identify changes in motor development related to the child with DCD and to his or her peers. Environmental demands and variables related to growth are always changing, and levels of peer performance are continuing to improve typically at a faster rate than that of the child with a DCD. Additional episodes of physical therapy consultative services can help the educational team, which includes the parents, identify the appropriate balance between interventions to improve underlying motor impairments and appropriate functional compensations. Physical therapists can analyze movements required for play during recess and suggest ways to include children with DCD in group play or suggest alternative equipment for safer play so that accidents are prevented. Promoting peer interactions during motor play or altering play settings to lessen the motor demands of an activity can break the avoidance cycles that may be present.

Helping parents to understand their child's motor limitations is an important outcome of physical therapy and is a component of secondary prevention. Family and cultural expectations can be inconsistent with a child's motor abilities. Expecting proficiency in competitive sports or dance or valuing perfect penmanship can lead to frustration and unhappiness for everyone. Therapists can help families and children match interests and skills with expectations that lead to success. When parents can analyze a play situation in their neighborhood or community recreation program to determine which motor skills are interfering with their child's ability to participate, the play situation can be adapted to minimize their child's disability and help prevent the imposition of societal limitations on full participation in community activities.

Management of Developmental Coordination Disorders by Other Disciplines and Family Members

Coordination and communication with other disciplines are important physical therapy interventions. If delays in speech and poor social language skills are functional limitations and disabilities associated with developmental incoordination, intervention by speech and language pathologists is appropriate. As mentioned earlier, DCD is hypothesized to be related to processing problems that can be cognitive or linguistic in addition to, or instead of, motor-production problems. If linguistic concerns are identified, goals related to improved word recall and retrieval or verbal sequencing of multiple-step instructions are appropriate. If oral-motor impairments are related to motor production, goals are directed at improving articulation and fluency of speech.

Occupational therapists often use sensory integrative therapy to treat sensory impairments associated with motor incoordination. According to Fisher and Murray (1991), sensory integration theory is intended to explain mild-to-moderate problems in learning and behavior in children, especially those problems associated with motor incoordination and poor sensory processing that cannot be attributed to frank central nervous system damage or abnormalities. They also state that sensory integration intervention is hypothesized to improve the ability of the central nervous system to process and integrate sensory inputs and, through this process, to enhance conceptual and motor learning. However, Ottenbacher (1991) believes that clear empiric consensus does not exist regarding the validity of sensory integration theory or the effectiveness of sensory integration practice.

Adapted physical education teachers can consult with regular physical education teachers to help modify the curriculum so that the child with DCD can participate and be successful. Children with DCD have a lower activity level than their peers (Bouffard et al., 1996), decreased anaerobic power, and decreased muscle strength (O'Beirne et al., 1994). If a child cannot run fast enough or safely without falling, games such as baseball can be modified so that a designated runner is used or players are grouped in teams for all activities with one person hitting and one person running or one person catching and one person throwing. In addition, peer helpers can be identified to help the child with DCD practice basic motor skills such as hopping, jumping, or skipping.

If distractibility and organizational problems are identified, a school psychologist might consult with the classroom teacher to identify ways that classroom materials can be modified to minimize the number of separate pieces of paper, books, and pencils needed to complete a project. A behavior modification program might be started to reinforce classwork that is turned in on time and completed consistent with the instructions given. The psychologist can also assist the physical therapist in managing disruptive or otherwise negative behaviors that interfere with therapy.

When concerns regarding distractibility and hyperactivity arise, a referral to a physician should be considered for evaluation of possible attention deficit disorder or ADHD and to consider the appropriateness of stimulant medication. Although there is no evidence that drug therapy is indicated for motor-production components of DCD (Gubbay, 1975), when children who attend poorly bump into and trip over objects in their environment, medication might have the secondary effect of decreasing clumsiness (Conte, 1991). A physician can also determine if medication is indicated when prolonged unhappiness or depression is suspected.

When a child is receiving services from many disciplines, professionals must work with the family to jointly identify and prioritize problems and to set mutual goals and objectives. When using handwriting as an example of a functional limitation identified as a priority for intervention, a number of cooperative activities might take place. The physical therapist determines that proper positioning in the classroom can be facilitated by changing the height of the chair and position of the desk. The occupational therapist chooses the appropriate writing utensil and paper modifications so that the teacher can expect some written penmanship during selected school activities. At the same time, the occupational therapist has identified an appropriate computer program and keyboard modifications so that word processing skills can be taught and used for other written assignments during the class day. The parents may decide that they will devote time at home to practice the keyboarding skills in a nondistracting, low-demand environment. Classroom activities that cannot be accomplished quickly enough with penmanship or keyboarding are adapted by the teacher to minimize written demands. Tests are given with multiple-choice answers or lines connecting the matching pairs. Some assignments can be dictated and retained as an audio response, or an educational associate can transcribe the assignment, including mistakes, so that the student can practice proofreading skills. With a team effort, the child with DCD can become an adolescent who is better able to cope with environmental demands at home and at school.

Adolescence and Transition to Adulthood

Typical Disabilities

Although Gubbay (1975) believed that clumsiness was usually not a problem after age 12 years because intellectually the older child usually has matured sufficiently to compensate for these problems either by avoidance or concealment, many parents report that adolescence is especially difficult for children with DCD. Teenagers can be verbally and emotionally unaccepting of differences. Even though general motor clumsiness is a developmental characteristic for many adolescents as their body proportions change, motor proficiency is valued because competitive sports play an important role in peer interactions and expectations of some families. Academic demands increase in middle school and high school, and poor written communication skills can seriously interfere with academic achievement.

Increasing numbers of longitudinal studies now exist to support the existence of ongoing motor disability in adolescents (Cantell et al., 1994; Cermak et al., 1990; Geuze & Borger, 1993; Losse et al., 1991). Losse and colleagues (1991) conducted a 10-year follow-up study of 32 children, including 16 who had been identified as clumsy when they were around 6 years old. Although the 6-year-olds who had been identified as clumsy participated in 1 year of intervention (the specific type and amount of intervention were not identified) to promote learning of motor skills, the gains that were made were not maintained. After extensive retesting, Losse and col-

leagues concluded that the children with DCD continued to have significant motor difficulties at 16 years of age, with qualitative differences greater than quantitative measures indicated. These children also demonstrated significantly lower academic scores and handwriting problems and had difficulty organizing materials. The teenagers with continued DCD had more behavior problems, including being bullied, poor school attendance, and easy distractibility. Emotional problems such as low self-esteem, depression, and being shy or timid were also found. Losse and colleagues concluded that other studies reporting that some children apparently "outgrew" their clumsiness had used clinical or laboratory-based tests that underestimated qualitative problems and did not reflect competence in natural environments. Not all of the children identified as clumsy at age 6 were having problems at age 16, however. Losse and colleagues found that some bright and well-adjusted children seemed to have come to terms with their ineptitude and appeared to cope well with their school experiences, were able to talk freely about their problems, and evidently enjoyed other aspects of life.

Physical Therapy Evaluation

Adolescents with DCD would not typically reach middle school without previous identification of impairments, functional limitations, and disabilities. However, these problems could have been misinterpreted or misidentified in the past, and evaluation from a physical therapist at this time can still help clarify the problem. An initial evaluation or reevaluation would include the same areas mentioned for the younger school-age child. The use of standardized tests is limited by the lack of norms for teenagers. The Bruininks-Oseretsky Test of Motor Proficiency (Bruininks, 1978) is one of the few developmental tests normed for adolescents up to age 14 years 6 months. Beyond this age the best alternative is to use criterion-referenced functional outcome measures (Haley et al., 1991) or ecologic, data-based, direct observation of individual function.

Physical Therapy Intervention

Direct intervention would probably not be indicated except on a trial basis because compensatory skills are usually well established by now. Physical therapy consultation can provide information to school personnel and help establish a new set of expectations and accommodations to a new school environment. If avoidance tactics have been used in early years, these tactics can be interpreted by a new set of middle school teachers as laziness or low motivation. Demands on written communication increase, and new strategies and advanced keyboarding skills may be needed. If DCD is interfering with physical organizational skills needed to move from class to class without losing books and papers, physical therapists can analyze the environmental demands placed on changing postures and mobility. Suggestions can be made to strategically place a student's desk or books or shorten the distance between classes so that functional limitations related to impairments of poor spatial orientation or motor sequencing do not become an educational disability. Physical therapists can consult with families and physical educators to jointly identify leisure activities that promote fitness and lifelong skills rather than competitive sports that might lower self-esteem and increase risk of injury.

High school classes, learning to drive a car, and vocational exploration present new challenges for the student with DCD. The need for new strategies again arises. Physical therapy rescreening or reevaluation can help determine whether basic motor skill development is still changing or has reached a plateau. High schools have to provide individualized evaluation and modifications in driver's education instruction for students with DCD when driver's education is offered as part of the general high school curriculum. Referral to the state vocational rehabilitation agency for evaluation and future service provision can also be pursued before graduation from high school. If a student is in special education, the 1997 amendments of IDEA (PL 105-17) state that a student's future needs must be assessed by age 14 and that a transition plan must be created that includes the identification of needed vocational services by the time the student is 16 years old.

Although little research exists on adult outcomes for children with DCD, some inferences can be drawn from follow-up studies with adults who have a learning disability. Spreen (1988) followed 303 eight- to 12-year-old students with learning disabilities until they were in their twenties. A subset of these children had soft neurologic signs. This long-term follow-up study revealed that the learning problems did not disappear and that the learning problems put these adults at a disadvantage for advanced education and vocational opportunities. In addition, the subset of students with neurologic soft signs still had soft neurologic signs as adults. There was a strong direct relationship between overall achievement and integrity of motor skills. Spreen (1988) concluded that "soft" neurologic signs were not maturational inconsistencies or due to inattention but represented a persistent, probably lifelong impairment. The following quote from a 26-year-old

woman with a learning disability supports this conclusion (Cermak & Henderson, 1985, p. 235):

> Motor activities are also a problem; my muscles don't seem to remember past motions. Despite the many times I've walked down steps and through doors, I still have to think about how high to lift my foot and about planning my movements...I'm physically inept; I can bump into the same table ten times running. I'm always bruised and as a child people constantly labeled me as clumsy. Physical education courses were hell as a child, especially gymnastics...I cannot begin to explain the terror or disorientation.

For individuals with DCD, developing ongoing compensatory strategies for activities requiring motor skills is a lifelong endeavor.

CASE HISTORY
EVAN

Evan is currently 12 years old. At the adjusted age of 19 months, Evan's pediatrician referred him to a developmental disabilities clinic at a university-affiliated facility. As a part of this evaluation, Evan was seen by a physical therapist. This initial point in the decision-making process would correspond to step 1, the collection of initial data, of the hypothesis-oriented algorithm for clinicians (HOAC) by Rothstein and Echternach (1986). The physical therapist reviewed Evan's medical history and interviewed his parents to gather the following information. Evan was born at 32 weeks of gestation and was treated at a neonatal intensive care unit for respiratory distress syndrome and cardiac enlargement. At the adjusted age of 16 months, eye surgery was performed to correct a persistent strabismus on the left. Evan lives with his parents and was enrolled in a community day care program. Evan sat alone at 7 months, creeped on hands and knees at 10 months, and started walking at 16 months (all ages adjusted for prematurity).

The second step in HOAC is to generate a problem statement. The initial problem statements by Evan's family, with the physical therapy–related problem stated in parentheses, were as follows: Does Evan have significant motor delays (impairments or functional limitations)? If so, can he catch up to his age expectations and continue to develop normally (can they be remediated by physical therapy intervention)? What can we, his parents, do to help him (can future motor disabilities and societal limitations be prevented by training and education)? Although Evan's goals were not identified until his first IEP meeting, HOAC suggests establishing initial goals before the examination.

A possible initial goal for Evan could have been, Evan will demonstrate the motor skills of a 2-year-old by the time his adjusted age is 24 months.

The physical therapy examination results when Evan was 19 months old (adjusted age) included the following: joint range of motion within normal limits, posture normal except for a slightly rounded back in sitting, and low muscle tone in Evan's trunk, but slightly increased muscle tone in the lower extremities on physical exertion, especially when Evan tried to move from a back-lying position to sitting. Backward protective extension response in sitting could not be elicited, and asymmetric weight bearing was present in standing with the right leg internally rotated and the pelvis retracted on the right. Gross motor skills on the Motor Scale of the Bayley Scales of Infant Development (Bayley, 1969) were around the 13-month level (a raw score of 48 and a Psychomotor Developmental Index of 66). Evan could throw a ball but could not walk sideways or backward. Speech and language and cognitive scores were also around the 13- to 15-month level. Step 3 of HOAC is the examination as just described. A working hypothesis about the feasibility of the preestablished goal can now be made. At this point, due to Evan's young age, the examination resulted in an evaluation diagnosis of developmental delay, not developmental coordination disorder. Referrals to other disciplines included a referral to the local early childhood special education program.

This evaluation represented a crucial point in decision making for the physical therapist. Are Evan's slightly abnormal physical findings and motor delay significant enough to warrant (1) outpatient physical therapy, (2) physical therapy consultation with the family and day care personnel, or (3) recommendations for regular gross motor experiences through the day care? In this case, this decision was left up to the local physical therapist employed by the early childhood special education program. (In the state in which Evan lived, special education programs were available to all eligible children beginning at birth. With the passage of the IDEA amendments of 1997, Part C, Evan's early intervention needs would now be evaluated and served through the development of an Individualized Family Service Plan [IFSP]). A follow-up evaluation appointment at the clinic (including physical therapy) was made for 1 year later.

The local physical therapist evaluated Evan at his day care setting and interviewed the day care personnel and Evan's parents. Procedures performed at the developmental disabilities clinic 2 months previously were not repeated. Some gains in gross motor skills were noted. Evan could now walk sideways and backward and up and down stairs with help but still could not stand on one foot alone or jump. Gross motor

scores were scattered from 18 to 21 months (chronologic age = 23 months, adjusted to 21 months) on the Early Learning Accomplishment Profile for Young Children (Glover et al., 1978), which was administered by the early intervention preschool teacher. (Note: It is not uncommon to see a significant change in gross motor scores in a short time, especially when different examinations are used or when only a few items per age level appear on a test. The achievement of only a few new skills can move a motor score to a higher developmental-age level. For example, within a short time span of a few weeks, a 24-month-old child successfully passes items 56 and 57 on the Motor Scale of the Bayley Scales of Infant Development, "Walks with one foot on walking board" and "Stands up: II" [Bayley, 1969]. The Psychomotor Developmental Index then changes from 77 to 87 with age placement changing from 17.8 months to 21.9 months.)

Movement quality remained a concern, however. During play, Evan was observed to prefer to W-sit and would bunny-hop at times rather than creeping reciprocally. Movements lacked trunk rotation, and his gait still had awkward characteristics that included a wide base, low arm guard, and slightly bent hips and knees. No asymmetries were noted during the observation, but day care staff confirmed that asymmetries were sometimes present. Working hypotheses by the local physical therapist were as follows:

1. Delays can be remediated by normal preschool motor experiences.

2. Abnormal movement patterns are a concern and could interfere with future motor development.

Therefore, intervention consisting of consultative physical therapy services is warranted to train family members and day care providers to provide specific motor experiences for Evan so that future problems are prevented. Evan's IEP objectives included the following:

1. When playing spontaneously at day care, Evan will use three different sitting positions during a 20-minute free-play session on three consecutive observations. Day care staff will observe play and record the number and type of sitting positions used during three randomly chosen times per week.

2. When participating in structured gross motor play experiences, Evan will use a walking pattern that includes reciprocal arm swing when observed on three of four occasions per play session. Day care staff will observe and record data once a week.

3. Evan will be able to walk up and down his stairs at home without assistance. His parents will observe this once a week and record Evan's stair climbing pattern on data sheets provided by the physical

therapist. (These objectives would now appear as outcomes in Evan's IFSP, but, when written, Part C of the IDEA amendments of 1997 was not in effect.)

A home and day care program stressing positioning during play, games to promote trunk rotation, smooth transitions between postures, and general gross motor skills for 2-year-old children was written. Progress monitoring procedures were initiated (Fig. 18-7). The preschool teachers collected periodic data, and the early childhood special education teacher monitored the program every week during her visits. Physical therapy reevaluation took place every 3 months (steps 5 and 6 of HOAC). Program modifications were made periodically, and the initial episode of intervention consisted of seven visits over 19 months. The return visit to the developmental disabilities clinic was eventually canceled because Evan's parents did not believe that another evaluation was necessary and did not want to take the extra time off work.

After 9 months of service (when Evan was 32 months old) the physical therapist employed by the early childhood education program noted that backward protective extension was observed spontaneously during play and movements with trunk rotation were seen more frequently. W-sitting was still occasionally observed, but so were other types of sitting postures. Evan's gross motor skills as measured on the Brigance Diagnostic Inventory of Early Development (Brigance, 1978) were scattered from a 2-year (jumping off floor) to a 3-year age level (alternated feet going up stairs with railing). (This may seem like a large range in

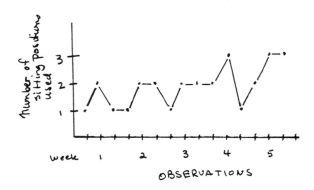

Week	Date	Type of sitting	Total positions used
1	9-10	w-sit	1
	9-12	w-sit, ring sit	2
	9-13	w-sit	1
2	9-17	w-sit	1
	9-18	w-sit, long sit	2
	9-21	w-sit, ring sit	2
3	9-25	w-sit	1
	9-27	w-sit, ring sit	2
	9-28	w-sit, modified ring	2
4	10-1	w-sit, modified ring	2
	10-4	w-sit, long sit, ring	3
	10-5	w-sit	1
5	10-9	w-sit, cross-leg	2
	10-10	w-sit, long, ring	3
	10-12	w-sit, cross-leg, long	3

FIGURE 18-7. Progress monitoring chart and graph for Evan.

developmental levels, but it is common, especially between 2 and 3 years of age when there are, again, very few items on most motor scales. In addition to wide ranges in motor levels due to test characteristics, clinical experience would support the finding that children with developmental clumsiness often display scattered motor skill profiles.)

Evan's gait pattern still reflected some internal rotation on the right and some toe dragging. Asymmetries inconsistently appeared and then disappeared but were never significant enough to warrant consideration of other diagnoses, such as hemiplegia from cerebral palsy. Day care staff reported that Evan disliked walking outside in the sand and strongly disliked having his socks removed. The day care and home programs were modified to reflect Evan's new skills and to include activities that encouraged sensory experiences, especially involving Evan's hands and feet.

When Evan was 3 years 6 months old, an educational staffing was held. Reassessment, step 9 of HOAC, revealed that Evan had met his IEP objectives and that no new functional motor goals requiring physical therapy services were identified. Therefore, physical therapy was discontinued.

This is a critical point in the decision-making process for the physical therapist and the IEP team. The primary criteria for discharge, as described in the "Guide to Physical Therapist Practice" (American Physical Therapy Association, 1997), is achievement of anticipated goals and desired outcomes. Continuing physical therapy services beyond a beneficial level would be an overutilization of service and a violation of some state licensure laws and the American Physical Therapy Association Standards of Practice for Physical Therapy (American Physical Therapy Association, 1996). Physical therapy should continue only when the skilled expertise of a physical therapist is needed. In this case, the IEP team, including the physical therapist, determined that the early childhood special education teacher had the skills needed to monitor Evan's motor behaviors.

Some concerns still existed because Evan would occasionally bump into objects and at times seemed oblivious to his surroundings. He was starting to avoid some gross motor play experiences, but day care staff believed that this was not yet a significant problem and were aware that the physical therapist could always be asked to consult again, if needed. Other areas of development continued to be slightly delayed, and inconsistencies in performance were increasing. For example, with a chronologic age of 3 years 6 months, Evan's intelligence quotient (IQ) score on the Stanford-Binet Intelligence Scale Form L-M (Terman & Merrill, 1973) was 91 plus or minus 3. Four subtests from the Illinois Test of Psycholinguistic Abilities (Kirk et al., 1968) indicated that Evan's auditory reception

and association were at or slightly above age level, but his scores for visual reception and association were delayed 1 to 1.5 years. The occupational therapist reported that Evan could not imitate block designs, but when given verbal guidance, he repeated the directions to himself and successfully completed the design. The team decided that Evan would benefit from a half-day preschool special education program. He returned to the day care program in the afternoon.

Evan's educational program was reviewed when he was 4 years old, and referrals for an occupational therapy and adapted physical education evaluation were made. The occupational therapy evaluation revealed joint laxity, especially in Evan's fingers and hands. His fine motor scores were around the 3-year level on the Peabody Developmental Motor Scales (Folio & Fewell, 1983). Dressing skills, as measured by a few items on the Peabody Fine Motor Scales, were also delayed. He was able to remove socks and a cap and lace a shoe through three holes but could not unbutton buttons. Functionally, Evan could not put on his jacket or a pullover shirt. A 6-month trial period of occupational therapy service was recommended. Individual weekly sessions with the physical education teacher were offered in addition to the group gross motor experience he was already receiving.

Evan's parents and preschool teacher were especially concerned about his poor visual skills. An evaluation was requested at the vision clinic at the university-affiliated facility where he was initially evaluated. A computed tomographic scan and electroretinogram were performed with normal results. Slightly decreased visual acuity was identified, as well as persistent "lazy eye" syndrome. Eye patching was recommended. Problems with visual perception were noted, and the ophthalmologist anticipated that Evan would have difficulty with depth perception.

After 6 months of occupational therapy, Evan's IEP objectives related to dressing and fine motor skills were implemented by the teacher of the preschool special education class. Occupational therapy was discontinued because the IEP team decided that the early childhood special education teacher could appropriately meet Evan's short-term objectives without the additional expertise of the occupational therapist. The logic behind this decision was similar to the decision to discontinue physical therapy when Evan was 3.5 years old.

This cycle of hypothesis-oriented problem solving was repeated when Evan was 6 years old. A reevaluation by special education personnel identified him as learning disabled, and a special class with integration into first grade was recommended for the next school year. Adapted physical education services were continued, and new occupational and physical therapy evaluations were recommended for the following fall.

Shortly after beginning first grade (at age 6.5), Evan was reevaluated by the physical therapist employed by the educational system. Evan's mother, his kindergarten teacher, and his special education consulting teacher were interviewed, and past medical and educational evaluations were read. Evan's teacher was especially concerned about his walking pattern. When walking down the hall, he often "bounced" from step to step, landing on his toes. He could walk appropriately on command but soon returned to this atypical pattern. A screening of gross motor skills using the Brigance Diagnostic Inventory of Early Development (Brigance, 1978) was performed by the adapted physical education teacher and revealed that Evan's skills were generally around the 5-year level, but some skills were scattered up to his age level. Evan's mother was pleased with the progress he had made over the years and had no concerns related to his walking or outdoor play.

The physical therapist observed Evan in the classroom, walking down the school hallway, at recess, and in physical education class. Playground skills were observed to be safe and generally consistent with Evan's peer group. Evan's mother was asked to send summer shorts and a tank top to school, and an individual evaluation was performed in the school gymnasium. A postural examination revealed scapular winging (right greater than left), a functional kyphosis, and diminished lordosis when standing. Subjectively, muscle tone appeared to be slightly low with elbow and knee hyperextension bilaterally. The Hughes Basic Gross Motor Assessment (Hughes, 1979) was administered, and Evan's overall score was 12 of an expected score of 33 for a 6-year-old. (The Hughes Basic Gross Motor Assessment is now out of print, and the Movement Assessment Battery for Children [Henderson & Sugden, 1992] would be an appropriate substitution.) Considerable difficulties were noted with any skill requiring motor planning. Movement quality was questionable with awkward, slow, and sometimes jerky responses in attempts at new skills and skills requiring dynamic balance (especially heel-to-toe walking, skipping, hopping, and ball-handling skills). The physical therapist noticed that Evan had difficulty imitating postures and following verbal directions.*

---

*The apparent discrepancy between Evan's score of approximately 5 years on the Brigance Inventory (Brigance, 1978) and the low score on the Hughes Basic Gross Motor Assessment (Hughes, 1979) is not surprising. These two tests are designed for different purposes. The Brigance (Brigance, 1978) is a criterion-referenced, developmental inventory sequenced for task analysis of motor behaviors without rigid administration procedures. The Hughes Gross Motor Assessment (Hughes, 1979) is a test designed specifically to identify minor motor dysfunction in children who appear to perform motor skills reasonably well. Children with DCD would be expected to perform better on a general inventory of skills than on a test with items specifically designed to identify the qualitative factors of performance.

This time the cycle of hypothesis-oriented problem solving generated a problem statement related to Evan's walking pattern and performance in physical education. Although the term *developmental coordination disorder* had not yet appeared in the *Diagnostic and Statistical Manual of Mental Disorders,* the description of motor problems by Evan's teacher met the criteria for clumsy child syndrome. The problem statement in essence was, Can physical therapy improve Evan's coordination and make his walking look normal? The results of the physical therapy examination were consistent with the current definition of DCD, and the physical therapist's working hypothesis was that Evan does have a motor disability that cannot be easily remediated but can be lessened by modifying the environment in the classroom and by removing societal limitations so that Evan can participate in a modified physical education class with peers. Physical therapy intervention beyond an initial consultation was not provided because Evan had safe and functional mobility skills at school. Family and education personnel were made aware of factors that may require a new episode of care.

The collaboration between the physical therapist and the adapted physical education teacher led to the identification of appropriate activities to promote static balance, improve erect postures, and increase shoulder girdle stability and general upper extremity and hand strength. The physical education class was already participating in a unit on general fitness, so the physical education teacher added wheelbarrow walking, crab-walking, and modified push-ups to the other activities the entire class performed. During their next unit on ball skills, the physical education teacher planned to use a variety of different sizes and weights of balls to increase grip strength and two-handed throwing. Students in a fifth-grade peer-helper program helped Evan practice balance skills such as one-foot standing, "Simon-says" games, and "stop-and-go" movements to music to encourage static posture imitation. Strategies to improve motor planning such as verbal labeling and rehearsing of motor sequences before skill performance were also implemented.

The classroom teacher was asked to monitor Evan's walking pattern and to notify the physical therapist if there was an increase in the number of times Evan fell or tripped. Evan's teacher, with the assistance of the school psychologist, also decided to try a behavior modification system of verbal or visual prompts to change Evan's walking pattern if it did not improve with the added emphasis on motor skills in physical education class. Suggestions were also given to the classroom teacher to modify Evan's desk and chair height to improve his sitting posture in class, especially for written work. A straight, wooden chair was found that allowed Evan's feet to rest flat on the floor. Nonslip material was added to his chair to prevent him from slipping forward. (Evan's previous chair was molded plastic and was very slippery.) These changes also helped promote an anterior pelvic tilt and back extension (Fig. 18–8).

Evan's fine motor skills in the classroom were becoming more of a concern and, following a reevaluation by occupational therapy, an IEP meeting was held to add occupational therapy consultation. IEP objectives were identified for Evan to promote the use of new learning strategies when writing and when using scissors and to improve Evan's ability to button, snap, and zip clothing. The entire IEP team, including Evan's parents, identified strategies to improve visual and motor sequencing during classroom activities and agreed to use the same strategies when Evan dressed at school or home.

At the end of first grade, the occupational therapist reported that Evan could button and unbutton medium-sized buttons on a "dressing vest" he used for practice. He was able to unbutton his own shirt, which had small buttons, but he still needed assis-

tance with the two upper buttons. Evan now understood the placement of each of his hands for buttoning and how the button must be manipulated. The occupational therapist reported that much of Evan's improvement was related to his increased attention span and concentration skills. Evan's mother was asked if she could come to school to observe these new dressing skills so that they could be practiced over the summer.

When Evan was in second grade, occupational therapy was discontinued because Evan's dressing skills were functional. Consultation was offered to the classroom teacher to assist with ongoing visuoperceptual problems during academic tasks such as writing. Evan continued to receive instruction in a special class with other students also identified as learning disabled, but he spent 2 hours a day in regular second grade and attended music, art, physical education, lunch, and recess with his second-grade peers. Adapted physical education collaborative consultation with the regular physical education teacher was continued.

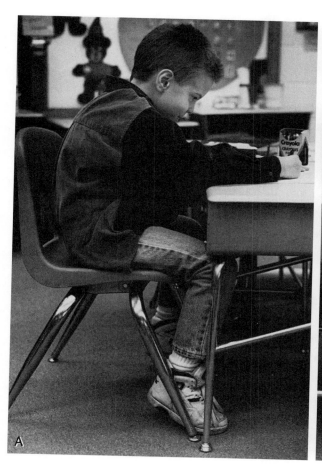
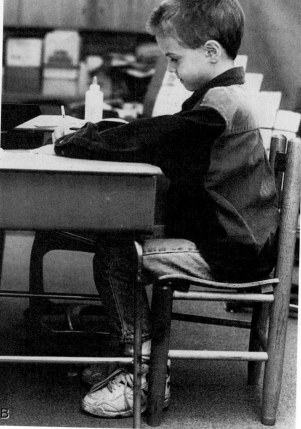

FIGURE 18–8. *A,* This child demonstrates poor posture that interferes with fine motor classroom activities. *B,* A different desk and chair improve this child's posture and improve the precision of his fine motor activities.

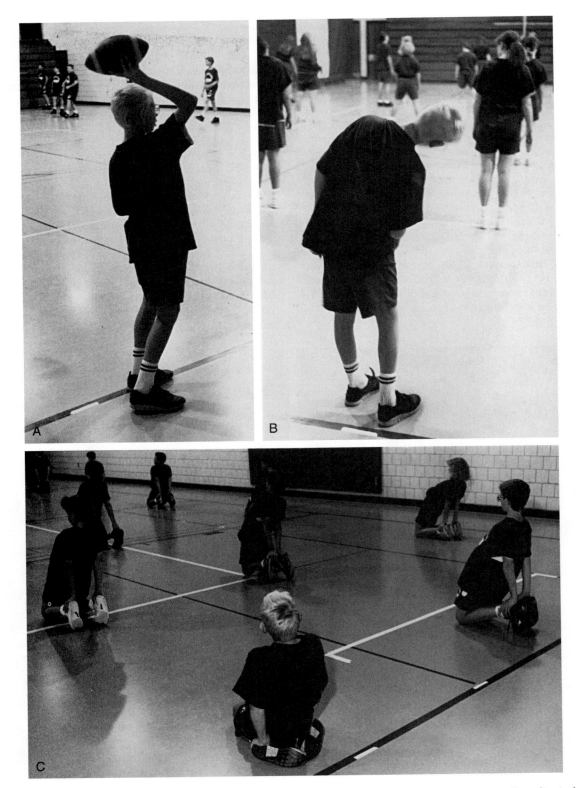

FIGURE 18–9. Evan participates in regular physical education classes, but his motor performance is still qualitatively and quantitatively below his peers. *A*, Evan and his peers are throwing footballs. His poor form contributes to decreased distance and accuracy. *B*, During warm-up exercises, Evan moves his entire body instead of isolating "neck circles." *C*, Evan has difficulty following instructions for a stretching exercise.

BRUININKS-OSERETSKY TEST OF MOTOR PROFICIENCY / Robert H. Bruininks, Ph.D.

INDIVIDUAL RECORD FORM
COMPLETE BATTERY AND SHORT FORM

NAME _Evan_   SEX: Boy ☒ Girl ☐   GRADE _7_

SCHOOL/AGENCY _Middle School_ CITY _____ STATE _____

EXAMINER _____ REFERRED BY _____

PURPOSE OF TESTING _re-evaluation_

Arm Preference: (circle one)		
(RIGHT)	LEFT	MIXED
Leg Preference: (circle one)		
RIGHT	(LEFT)	MIXED

	Year	Month	Day
Date Tested	___	___	___
Date of Birth	___	___	___
Chronological Age	12	9	9

Complete Battery:

SUBTEST	POINT SCORE Maximum	POINT SCORE Subject's	STANDARD SCORE Test (Table 23)	STANDARD SCORE Composite (Table 24)	PERCENTILE RANK (Table 25)	STANINE (Table 25)	OTHER Age equiv.
GROSS MOTOR SUBTESTS:							
1. Running Speed and Agility	15	6	2				5-11
2. Balance	32	19	3				5-8
3. Bilateral Coordination	20	9	6				7-11
4. Strength	42	16	5				4-11
GROSS MOTOR COMPOSITE		16 SUM		20-	1-	1	59
5. Upper-Limb Coordination	21	7	1				5-2
FINE MOTOR SUBTESTS:							
6. Response Speed	17	6	5				6-11
7. Visual-Motor Control	24	11	1				5-8
8. Upper-Limb Speed and Dexterity	72	21	1				5-8
FINE MOTOR COMPOSITE		7 SUM		20-	1-	1	58
BATTERY COMPOSITE		24 SUM		20-	1-	1	58

*To obtain Battery Composite: Add Gross Motor Composite, Subtest 5 Standard Score, and Fine Motor Composite. Check result by adding Standard Scores on Subtests 1-8.

Short Form:

	POINT SCORE Maximum	POINT SCORE Subject's	STANDARD SCORE (Table 27)	PERCENTILE RANK (Table 27)	STANINE (Table 27)
SHORT FORM	98	___			

DIRECTIONS

Complete Battery:

1. During test administration, record subject's response for each trial.

2. After test administration, convert performance on each item (item raw score) to a point score, using scale provided. For an item with more than one trial, choose best performance. Record item point score in circle to right of scale.

3. For each subtest, add item point scores; record total in circle provided at end of each subtest and in Test Score Summary section. Consult Examiner's Manual for norms tables.

Short Form:

1. Follow Steps 1 and 2 for Complete Battery, except record each point score in box to right of scale.

2. Add point scores for all 14 Short Form items and record total in Test Score Summary section. Consult Examiner's Manual for norms tables.

AGS Published by American Guidance Service, Inc., Circle Pines, MN 55014

FIGURE 18-10. Cover page from Evan's current Bruininks-Oseretsky Test of Motor Proficiency. (From Bruininks-Oseretsky Test of Motor Proficiency: Individual Record Form by Robert H. Bruininks © 1978 American Guidance Service, Inc., 4201 Woodland Road, Circle Pines, MN 55014-1796. All rights reserved.)

Throughout elementary school Evan's parents and his educational team knew that a physical therapist was available to answer questions, but no new concerns arose. Evan's ongoing problems related to DCD (difficulty planning and sequencing new motor activities, poor balance in environments with changing surfaces and many obstacles, and occasional falls) were managed by other members of his educational team.

Evan is now in seventh grade at a middle school. He continues to receive resource instructional assistance and consultative adapted physical education. Evan still stands with his knees slightly bent (right more than left) and demonstrates a "bouncy" gait without a heel-strike. However, he has no difficulty moving around the larger school building. He attends physical education class with other seventh graders (Fig. 18–9). His physical education teacher reports that Evan is weak and small compared with his peers. He participates in all the activities but performs them at his own rate and performance level. Evan is on task 80 to 90% of the time during warm-up activities. The only difficulties so far are frequent conflicts with the other boys. The physical education teacher believes that sometimes Evan solicits the conflict but that other times Evan is "picked on" by the other boys.

The adapted physical education teacher repeated an examination using the Bruininks-Oseretsky Test of Motor Proficiency (Bruininks, 1978) (Fig. 18–10). Evan's composite gross motor score yielded an age equivalency of 5 years 9 months (standard score of 16), and his composite fine motor score age equivalency was 5 years 8 months (standard score of 7). Although this test identifies Evan's developmental motor level, it is inappropriate for Evan to engage in 5- to 6-year-old gross motor activities when he is 12 years old. This information is used, instead, to modify regular middle school physical education activities.

No new motor concerns are expected to arise while Evan is attending middle school. Before the beginning of high school, when Evan will move to an even larger building, the physical therapist, special education consultant, and adapted physical education teacher will discuss the transition issues related to Evan's DCD.

Epilogue

Evan has just graduated from high school with his peers. He considers his high school experience to be very positive and enjoyed participating in the choir. He was especially excited to have the opportunity to sing the national anthem at the Special Olympics and at the State Fair. Evan's parents are very proud of his 3.2 grade point average. He was integrated into all classes except math. Evan will attend a community college in the fall and hopes to eventually enter a recording engineering program at a state university.

SUMMARY

DCD represents a cluster of characteristics affecting approximately 5% of the regular school-age population. The exact etiology is unknown, but DCD appears to have both motor-production and cognitive-linguistic components. Physical therapists play a role both in identifying the motor impairments and functional limitations associated with DCD and in providing intervention to prevent or minimize the disabilities and societal limitations that might otherwise occur. Physical therapists function as members of the comprehensive team needed to manage the multiple ramifications of DCD and its many associated learning and medical problems. DCD is a lifelong impairment that presents challenges for both adults and children.

Recommended Resources

Gubbay, SS. The management of developmental apraxia. Developmental Medicine and Child Neurology, *20*:643–646, 1978.

Henderson, SE. Motor development and minor handicap. In Kalverboer, AF, Hopkins, B, & Geuze, R (Eds.), Motor Development in Early and Later Childhood: Longitudinal Approaches. Cambridge, Great Britain: University Press, 1993, pp. 286–306.

Henderson, SE. Special issue: Developmental Coordination Disorder. Adapted Physical Activity Quarterly, *11*(2):111–235, 1994.

Roy, EA. Neuropsychological Studies of Apraxia and Related Disorders. New York: North-Holland, 1985.

Sellers, JS. Clumsiness: Review of causes, treatments, and outlook. Physical and Occupational Therapy in Pediatrics, *15*(4):39–55, 1995.

References

Als, H. A synactive model of neonatal behavioral organization: Framework for the assessment of neurobehavioral development in the premature infant and for support of infants and parents in the neonatal intensive care environment. In Sweeney, J (Ed.), The High-Risk Neonate: Developmental Therapy Perspectives. New York: Haworth Press, 1986, pp. 3–55.

Als, H, Duffy, FH, & McAnulty, G. Behavioral differences between preterm and full-term newborns as measured with the APIB system scores: I. Infant Behavior and Development, *11*:305–318, 1988.

American Physical Therapy Association. Standards of Practice for Physical Therapy (Amended). Alexandria, VA: American Physical Therapy Association, 1996.

American Physical Therapy Association. Guide to physical therapist practice. Physical Therapy, *77*(11):1163–1650, 1997.

American Psychiatric Association. Diagnostic and Statistical Manual of Mental Disorders—DSM-IV. Washington, DC: American Psychiatric Association, 1994.

Bayley, N. Bayley Scales of Infant Development. San Antonio, TX: Psychological Corporation, 1969.

Bayley, N. Bayley Scales of Infant Development, 2nd ed. San Antonio, TX: Psychological Corporation, 1993.

Bouffard, M, Watkinson, EJ, Thompson, LP, Dunn, JLC, & Romanow, SKE. A test of the activity deficit hypothesis with children with movement difficulties. Adapted Physical Activity Quarterly, *13*:61–73, 1996.

Brigance, AH. Inventory of Early Development. North Billerica, MA: Curriculum Associates, 1978.

Bruininks, R. Bruininks-Oseretsky Test of Motor Proficiency. Circle Pines, MN: American Guidance Services, 1978.

Cantell, MH, Smyth, MM, & Ahonen, TP. Clumsiness in Adolescence: Educational, motor, and social outcomes of motor delay detected at 5 years. Adapted Physical Activity Quarterly, 11(2):115–129, 1994.

Cermak, S. Developmental dyspraxia. In Roy, EA (Ed.), Neuropsychologic Studies of Apraxia and Related Disorders. Amsterdam: North-Holland, 1985, pp. 225–250.

Cermak, S, & Henderson, A. Learning disabilities. In Umphred, D (Ed.), Neurological Rehabilitation. St. Louis: Mosby, 1985, pp. 207–249.

Cermak, S, Trimble, J, Coryell, J, & Drake, C. Bilateral motor coordination in adolescents with and without learning disabilities. Physical and Occupational Therapy in Pediatrics, 10(1):5–17, 1990.

Clements, SD, David, JS, Edgington, R, Goolsby, CM, & Peters, JE. Two cases of learning disabilities. In Tarnopol, L (Ed.), Learning Disorders in Children: Diagnosis, Medication, Education. Boston: Little, Brown, 1971.

Conte, R. Attention disorders. In Wong, B (Ed.), Learning About Learning Disorders. San Diego: Academic Press, 1991, pp. 60–103.

Coster, W, Deeney, T, Haltiwanger, J, & Haley S. School Function Assessment. San Antonio: The Psychological Corporation, 1998.

David, KS. Motor sequencing strategies in school-aged children. Physical Therapy, 65:883–889, 1985.

Dewey, D, Roy, E, Square-Storer, PA, & Hayden, D. Limb and oral praxic abilities of children with verbal sequencing deficits. Developmental Medicine and Child Neurology, 30:743–751, 1988.

Dwyer, C, & McKenzie, BE. Impairment of visual memory in children who are clumsy. Adapted Physical Activity Quarterly, 11(2):179–189, 1994.

Faglioni, P, & Basso, A. Historical perspectives on neuroanatomical correlates of limb apraxia. In Roy, E (Ed.), Neuropsychological Studies of Apraxia and Related Disorders. Amsterdam: North-Holland, 1985, pp. 3–44.

Fisher, A, & Murray, E. Introduction to sensory integration theory. In Fisher, A, Murray, E, & Bundy, A (Eds.), Sensory Integration: Theory and Practice. Philadelphia: FA Davis, 1991, pp. 3–26.

Folio, MR, & Fewell, RR. Peabody Developmental Motor Scales and Activity Cards Manual. Allen, TX: DLM Teaching Resources, 1983.

Gaddes, W. Learning Disabilities and Brain Function: A Neuropsychological Approach. New York: Springer-Verlag, 1985.

Gentile, AM. Skill acquisition: Action, movement, and neuromotor processes. In Carr, JH, & Shepherd, RB (Eds.), Movement Science: Foundations for Physical Therapy in Rehabilitation. Rockville, MD: Aspen, 1987, pp. 93–154.

Georgieff, MK, Bernbaum, JC, Hoffman-Williamson, M, & Daft, A. Abnormal truncal muscle tone as a useful early marker for developmental delay in low birth weight infants. Pediatrics, 77:659–663, 1986.

Geschwind, N. The apraxias: Neural mechanisms of disorder of learned movements. American Scientist, 63:188–195, 1975.

Geuze, R, & Borger, H. Children who are clumsy: Five years later. Adapted Physical Activity Quarterly, 10:10–21, 1993.

Gillberg, C, Rasmussen, P, Carlstrom, G, Svenson, B, & Waldenstrom, E. Perceptual, motor and attentional deficits in six-year-old children: Epidemiological aspects. Journal of Child Psychology and Psychiatry, 23:131–144, 1982.

Glover, ME, Preminger, JL, & Sanford, AR. The Early Learning Accomplishment Profile for Young Children: Birth to 36 Months. Chapel Hill, NC: Chapel Hill Training-Outreach Project, 1978.

Granger, CV, Hamilton BB, & Kayton, R. Guide for the use of the functional independence measure (WeeFIM) of the Uniform Data Set for Medical Rehabilitation. Buffalo: Research Foundation, State University of New York, 1989.

Gubbay, SS. The Clumsy Child: A Study of Developmental Apraxic and Agnosic Ataxia. London: WB Saunders, 1975.

Gubbay, SS. The management of developmental apraxia. Developmental Medicine and Child Neurology, 20:643–646, 1978.

Haley, SM, Coster, WJ, & Ludlow, LH. Pediatric functional outcome measures. Physical Medicine and Rehabilitation Clinics of North America, 2(4):689–723, 1991.

Haley, SM, Faas, RM, Coster, WJ, Gans, BM, & Webster, HM. Pediatric Evaluation of Disability Inventory (PEDI). Boston: New England Medical Center, 1989.

Henderson, L, Rose, P, & Henderson, S. Reaction time and movement time in children with a developmental coordination disorder. Journal of Child Psychology and Psychiatry, 33:895–905, 1992.

Henderson, SE. The assessment of "clumsy" children: Old and new approaches. Journal of Child Psychology and Psychiatry and Allied Disciplines, 28:511–527, 1987.

Henderson, SE, & Sugden, D. Movement Assessment Battery for Children. London: The Psychological Corporation, 1992.

Hertzig, ME. Neurological soft signs in low birthweight children. Developmental Medicine and Child Neurology, 23:778–791, 1981.

Hoare, D, & Larkin, D. Kinaesthetic abilities of clumsy children. Developmental Medicine and Child Neurology, 33:671–678, 1991.

Hulme, C, & Lord, R. Clumsy children: A review of recent research. Child: Care, Health and Development, 12(4):257–269, 1986.

Hughes, J. Hughes Basic Gross Motor Assessment. Yonkers, NY: GE Miller, 1979.

Jongman, M, Henderson, S, de Vries, L, & Dubowitz, L. Duration of periventricular densities in preterm infants and neurological outcome at 6 years of age. Archives of Disease in Childhood, 69:9–13, 1993.

Kaufman, AS, & Kaufman, NL. Kaufman Assessment Battery for Children: Interpretive Manual. Circle Pines, MN: American Guidance Service, 1983.

Kertesz, A. Apraxia and aphasia: Anatomical and clinical relationship. In Roy, EA (Ed.), Neuropsychological Studies of Apraxia and Related Disorders. Amsterdam: North-Holland, 1985, pp. 163–178.

Kirk, SA, McCarthy, JJ, & Kirk, WD. Illinois Test of Psycholinguistic Abilities, Rev. ed. Urbana, IL: University of Illinois Press, 1968.

Knuckey, N, Apsimon, T, & Gubbay, S. Computerized axial tomography in clumsy children with developmental apraxia and agnosia. Brain and Development, 5:14–20, 1983.

Knuckey, N, & Gubbay, S. Clumsy children: A prognostic study. Australian Pediatric Journal, 19:9–13, 1983.

Laszlo, JI, & Bairstow, PJ. The measurement of kinaesthetic sensitivity in children and adults. Developmental Medicine and Child Neurology, 22:454–464, 1985.

Laszlo, JI, Bairstow, PJ, Bartrip, J, & Rolfe, UT. Clumsiness or perceptuo-motor dysfunction? In Colley, AM, & Beech, JR (Eds.), Cognition and Action in Skilled Behavior. Amsterdam: North-Holland, 1988, pp. 293–310.

Levine, M. Developmental pediatrics: Developmental dysfunction in the school-age child. In Behrman, R, & Vaughen, V (Eds.), Nelson Textbook of Pediatrics, 13th ed. Philadelphia: WB Saunders, 1987, pp. 84–95.

Lord, R, & Hulme, C. Kinesthetic sensitivity of normal and clumsy children. Developmental Medicine and Child Neurology, 29:720–725, 1987.

Losse, A, Henderson, SE, Ellimna, D, Hall, D, Knight, E, & Jongmans, M. Clumsiness in children—Do they grow out of it? A 10-year follow-up study. Developmental Medicine and Child Neurology, 33:55–68, 1991.

Lundy-Ekman, L, Ivry, R, Keele, S, & Woollacott, M. Timing and force control deficits in clumsy children. Journal of Cognitive Neuroscience, 3:367–376, 1991.

Luria, AR. Higher Cortical Functions in Man. New York: Basic Books, 1966.

Mastropieri, M. Learning disabilities in early childhood. In Kavale, K (Ed.), Learning Disabilities: State of the Art and Practice. Boston: College-Hill Publication, 1988, pp. 161–179.

Miller, LJ. Miller Assessment for Preschoolers. Littleton, CO: Foundation for Knowledge in Development, 1982.

Missiuna, C, & Polatajko, H. Developmental dyspraxia by any other name: Are they all just clumsy children? The American Journal of Occupational Therapy, 49(7):619–627, 1994.

Murphy, J, & Gliner, J. Visual and motor sequencing in normal and clumsy children. Occupational Therapy Journal, 8:89–103, 1988.

O'Beirne, C, Larkin, D, & Cable, T. Coordination problems and anaerobic performance in children. Adapted Physical Activity Quarterly, 11(2):141–149, 1994.

O'Brien, V, Cermak, S, & Murray, E. The relationship between visual-perceptual motor abilities and clumsiness in children with and without learning disabilities. American Journal of Occupational Therapy, 42:359–363, 1988.

Ottenbacher, KJ. Research in sensory integration: Empirical perceptions. In Fisher, A, Murray, E, & Bundy, A (Eds.), Sensory Integration: Theory and Practice. Philadelphia: FA Davis, 1991, pp. 387–401.

Palisano, RJ, Haley, SM, & Brown, DA. Goal attainment scaling as a measure of change in infants with motor delays. Physical Therapy, 72:432–448, 1992.

Piek, JP, & Edwards, K. The identification of children with developmental coordination disorder by class and physical education teachers. British Journal of Educational Psychology, 67:55–67, 1997.

Piper, MC, & Darrah, J. Motor Assessment of the Developing Infant. Philadelphia: WB Saunders, 1994.

Polatajko, HJ, Macnab, JJ, Anstett, B, Mallow-Miller, T, Murphy, K, & Noh, S. A clinical trial of the process-oriented treatment approach for children with developmental co-ordination disorder. Developmental Medicine and Child Neurology, 37:310–319, 1995.

Rappaport, L, Urion, D, Strand, K, & Fulton, A. Concurrence of congenital ocular motor apraxia and motor problems: An expanded syndrome. Developmental Medicine and Child Neurology, 29:85–90, 1987.

Reitan, RM, & Wolfson, D. The Hallstead-Reitan Neuropsychological Test Battery: Theory and Clinical Interpretation. Tucson, AZ: Neuropsychology Press, 1985.

Rösblad, B, & von Hofsten, C. Repetitive Goal-Directed Arm Movements in Children with Developmental Coordination Disorders: Role of Visual Information. Adapted Physical Activity Quarterly, 11:190–202, 1994.

Rothstein, JM, & Echternach, JL. Hypothesis-oriented algorithm for clinicians: A method for evaluation and treatment planning. Physical Therapy, 66:1388, 1986.

Rourke, BP, Bakker, D, Fisk, JL, & Strang, JD. The Neuropsychological Assessment of Children: A Treatment-Oriented Approach. New York: Guilford Press, 1986.

Roussounis, S, Gaussen, T, & Stratton, P. A 2-year follow-up study of children with motor coordination problems identified at school entry age. Child: Care, Health and Development, 13:77–391, 1987.

Roy, EA, & Square, P. Common considerations in the study of limb, verbal and oral apraxia. In Roy, EA (Ed.), Neuropsychological Studies of Apraxia and Related Disorders. New York: North-Holland, 1985, pp. 111–162.

Russell, DJ, Rosenbaum, PL, Cadman, DT, Gowland, C, Hardy, S, & Jarvis, S. The Gross Motor Function Measure: Reliability, validity and responsiveness of an evaluative instrument. Developmental Medicine and Child Neurology, 31:341–352, 1989.

Schmidt, R. Motor Control and Learning: A Behavioral Emphasis. Champaign, IL: Human Kinetics, 1988.

Schoemaker, MM, Hijlkema, MGJ, & Kalverboer, AF. Physiotherapy for clumsy children: An evaluation study. Developmental Medicine and Child Neurology, 36:143–155, 1994.

Shaw, L, Levine, MD, & Belfer, M. Developmental double jeopardy: A study of clumsiness and self-esteem in children with learning problems. Developmental and Behavioral Pediatrics, 3:191–196, 1982.

Silver, L. The Misunderstood Child: A Guide for Parents of Learning Disabled Children. New York: McGraw-Hill, 1988.

Skorji, V, & McKenzie, B. How do children who are clumsy remember modeled movements? Developmental Medicine and Child Neurology, 39:404–408, 1997.

Smyth, TR. Abnormal clumsiness in children: A defect of motor programming? Child: Care, Health and Development, 17:283–294, 1991.

Soltesz, M, & Brockway, N. The high-risk infant. In Tecklin, J (Ed.), Pediatric Physical Therapy. Philadelphia: JB Lippincott, 1989, pp. 40–67.

Spreen, O. Learning Disabled Children Growing Up: A Follow-up into Adulthood. New York: Oxford University Press, 1988.

Stott, DH, Moyes, FA, & Henderson, SE. Test of Motor Impairment. Guelph, Ontario: Brook Educational Publishing Limited, 1972.

Stott, DH, Moyes, FA, & Henderson, SE. The Henderson Revision of The Test of Motor Impairment. San Antonio: Psychological Corporation, 1984.

Tarnopol, L, & Tarnopol, M. Brain Function and Reading Disabilities. Baltimore: University Park Press, 1977.

Terman, LM, & Merrill, MA. Stanford-Binet Intelligence Scale: Form L-M. Chicago: Riverside Publishing, 1973.

U.S. Department of Education. Nineteenth Annual Report to Congress on the Implementation of The Individuals with Disabilities Education Act. Washington, DC: U.S. Government Printing Office, 1997.

Van Dellen, T, & Geuze, R. Motor response processing in clumsy children. Journal of Child Psychology and Psychiatry and Allied Disciplines, 29:489–500, 1988.

van der Meulen, JHP, Denier van der Gon, JJ, Gielen, CCAM, Gooskens, RHJM, & Willemse, J. Visuomotor performance of normal and clumsy children: I. Fast goal-directed arm movements with and without visual feedback. Developmental Medicine and Child Neurology, 33:40–54, 1991a.

van der Meulen, JHP, Denier van der Gon, JJ, Gielen, CCAM, Gooskens, RHJM, & Willemse, J. Visuomotor performance of normal and clumsy children: II. Arm-tracking with and without visual feedback. Developmental Medicine and Child Neurology, 33:118–129, 1991b.

Volpe, B, Sidtis, J, Holtzman, J, Wilson, D, & Gazzaniga, M. Cortical mechanisms involved in praxis: Observations following partial and complete section of the corpus callosum in man. Neurology, 32:645–650, 1982.

Watson, R, Fleet, W, Gonzalez-Rothi, L, & Heilman, K. Apraxia and the supplemental motor area. Archives of Neurology, 43:787–792, 1986.

Williams, HG, Woollacott, MH, & Ivry, R. Timing and motor control in clumsy children. Journal of Motor Behavior, 24(2):165–172, 1992.

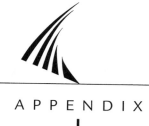

Resources for Parents of Children with Developmental Coordination Disorders

None of the following resources was written specifically for parents of children with developmental coordination disorders. There is a significant void in this area. The following resources contain information that can be adapted to specific children, especially if parents have the ability to consult with professionals who know their child's strengths and needs.

Barlin, AL, & Kalev, N. Hello Toes! Movement Games for Children. Pennington, NJ: Princeton Book Co, 1989.

Activities that parents can do with children 2 to 5 years old to enhance physical development are discussed in this book. It is a book of movement and dance games for adults and children to perform together.

Fish, HT, Fish, RB, & Golding, LA. Starting Out Well: A Parents' Approach to Physical Activity and Nutrition. Champaign, IL: Leisure Press, 1989.

Part I of this book is designed to give parents and educators concrete ways to enhance physical activity from birth through kindergarten age. Part II discusses nutritional choices for children.

Grosse, SJ, & Thompson, D. Play and Recreation for Individuals with Disabilities: Practical Pointers. Reston, VA: American Alliance for Health, Physical Education, Recreation and Dance, 1993.

This book includes activities across the life span, including outdoor environments, safe and appropriate play and play equipment, and active leisure such as dance and water exercise.

Lichtman, B. Innovative Games. Champaign, IL: Human Kinetics, 1993.

This paperback book includes games for students in grades 6 through 12. Games are organized into 35 activities with complete instructions and material suggestions.

Sellers, JS. Motor Development Program for School-Age Children. Arizona: Therapy Skill Builders, 1994.

A variety of resources for children ages 4 to 12 years are included in this 160-page book. There are instructions for making your own equipment, checklists of motor activities, and a description of eight motor stations with sequenced activities.

APPENDIX

II

Gubbay Tests of Motor Proficiency (Standardized for Children between Ages 8 and 12 Years)

THE ASSESSMENT OF THE CLUMSY CHILD

Test 1

Whistle through pouted lips.

The child is required to make a musical note of any pitch and intensity by blowing air through pouted lips.

Score: Pass or fail.

Test 2

Skip forward five steps.

Three attempts are allowed after demonstration of the test by the examiner (e.g., single hop on left leg, step, single hop on right leg, etc.—without skipping rope).

Score: Pass or fail.

Test 3

Roll ball with foot.

The child is required to roll a tennis ball under the sole of the preferred foot (with or without footwear) in spiral fashion around six matchboxes placed 30 cm apart. The ball is permitted to touch a maximum of three matchboxes before disqualification. Three attempts are allowed before failure.

Score: Expressed in time (seconds) or as failure.

Test 4

Throw, clap hands, then catch tennis ball.

The child is required to clap his or her hands to a maximum of 4 times after throwing a tennis ball upward and catching the ball with both hands. If able to catch the ball after 4 claps, the child is then required to catch the ball with one (either) hand after 4 claps. Three attempts are allowed before failure at any point.

Score: Expressed in one of the following seven categories:

1. Cannot catch the ball with both hands
2. Can catch the ball with both hands after 0 claps
3. Can catch the ball with both hands after 1 clap
4. Can catch the ball with both hands after 2 claps
5. Can catch the ball with both hands after 3 claps
6. Can catch the ball with both hands after 4 claps
7. Can catch the ball with preferred hand after 4 claps

Test 5

Tie one shoelace with double bow (single knot).

The examiner's right shoelace with approximately 20 cm lengths protruding from the shoe is offered.

Score: Expressed in time (seconds) or failure if greater than 60 seconds.

Test 6

Thread 10 beads.

The wooden beads are 3 cm in diameter with a bore of 0.8 cm, and the terminal 6 cm of the string is stiffened. (The beads are patented Kiddicraft toys that can be readily purchased.)

Score: Expressed in time (seconds).

Test 7

Pierce 20 pinholes.

The child is supplied with a stylus (long hatpin) and asked to pierce two successive rows of 0.1 inch × 0.1 inch (2.5 mm × 2.5 mm) squares on graph paper.

Score: Expressed in time (seconds).

Test 8

Posting box.

The child is required to fit six different plastic shapes in appropriate slots. (The posting box is a patented Kiddicraft toy that can be readily purchased.)

Score: Expressed in time (seconds) or failure if greater than 60 seconds.

Gubbay, SS. The Clumsy Child: A Study of Developmental Apraxic and Agnosic Ataxia. London: WB Saunders, 1975, pp. 155–156.

CHAPTER
19

Children with Cognitive Impairments

IRENE R. McEWEN, PT, PhD

Children with cognitive impairments often have secondary or associated delays in motor development and may have problems with motor learning and motor control. This is especially true of children whose cognitive functioning is moderately or severely limited. Some children's motor problems are minimal, requiring little, if any, physical therapy. Other children have cerebral palsy and other neurologic, musculoskeletal, and cardiopulmonary impairments that require considerable attention by physical therapists and other members of service delivery teams.

Many of the physical therapy evaluation and intervention strategies used with children who have cognitive impairments differ little from approaches employed with any child who has similar motor characteristics, as described in other chapters of this

volume. The learning characteristics of children with cognitive impairments, however, can make it necessary to modify or supplement these approaches. These aspects of evaluation and intervention, along with current "best practices" in educational programs for children with cognitive impairments, are the foci of this chapter. This chapter will cover the definition, incidence, prevalence, etiology, pathophysiology, and prevention of cognitive impairments in children; intervention to limit impairments and functional limitations and to prevent secondary impairments; the role of other disciplines; determinants of outcomes; team assessment of disability; determining goals and intervention; and considerations for transition to adulthood. The chapter ends with three case histories that illustrate the chapter content. One case also illustrates application of the

Guide to Physical Therapist Practice (American Physical Therapy Association, 1997).

DEFINITION OF COGNITIVE IMPAIRMENTS

The definition of cognitive impairments and the means by which children are identified as having cognitive impairments are, and have been, highly controversial (Evans, 1991; Zucker & Polloway, 1987). Much of the controversy surrounds the risk of inappropriately classifying children of cultural and linguistic minorities as having cognitive impairments. The validity of this concern is supported by overrepresentation of children from cultural and linguistic minorities among children who have been labeled as having cognitive impairments and children placed in special education (Jones & Payne, 1986).

Children with motor and sensory impairments also are at risk for being labeled as having cognitive limitations when they do not or for being classified as having a greater degree of cognitive impairment than actually exists (Chinitz & Feder, 1992). This is especially true if the evaluator has neither experience nor skill in examining children who require alternative input modes, such as manual signs, or alternative response modes, such as a communication board.

The term *mental retardation* is often used by organizations and education and social service agencies to refer to the condition of people whose cognitive impairments were acquired before age 18 (American Association on Mental Retardation, 1992). The definition of the term has evolved over the years from primary emphasis on intelligence test scores to an emphasis on functional abilities within natural environments. The most widely accepted definitions of mental retardation have been proposed by the American Association on Mental Retardation (AAMR), formerly the American Association on Mental Deficiency (AAMD). These have served as a basis for many other definitions, including those used by school districts for placement of students in special education (Evans, 1991; Jones & Payne, 1986; Zucker & Polloway, 1987).

In 1992, the AAMR board of directors adopted a new definition of mental retardation, which was intended to help change the way people with cognitive impairments are viewed. The definition is based on the supports people need within their own environments, rather than on an intelligence quotient (IQ)–derived level of cognitive functioning:

> Mental retardation refers to substantial limitations in present functioning. It is characterized by significantly subaverage intellectual functioning, ex-

isting concurrently with related limitations in two or more of the following applicable adaptive skills areas: communication, self-care, home living, social skills, community use, self-direction, health and safety, functional academics, leisure, and work. Mental retardation manifests before age 18 (American Association on Mental Retardation, 1992, p. 1).

Although an IQ of 70 to 75 or below still is required for a diagnosis of mental retardation, the 1992 definition emphasizes identification of the changing supports one needs over a lifetime to live successfully in the community, rather than simply on classification of the individual.

Other definitions of cognitive impairment or mental retardation have coexisted with the AAMR definition, including those used in the United States to qualify students for special education and for services for individuals with developmental disabilities. In the United States, Public Law 98-527, the Developmental Disabilities Act of 1984, authorized states to provide habilitation, medical, and social services for children and adults with cognitive impairments and, in some states, for people with other disabilities.

Because of the varying definitions of cognitive impairment and eligibility criteria, confusion can exist both within and between states as to who is considered to have cognitive impairment and who qualifies for which services. For this reason, physical therapists often need to seek information about programs in their own areas, the criteria for eligibility, and who is qualified to classify a child as having a cognitive impairment. Some programs provide wheelchairs, splints, and other equipment for children with cognitive impairments; other programs pay for services, such as physical therapy, respite care, and recreational activities.

For any child, a label of cognitive impairment primarily is useful as a "passport" to early intervention, special education, and other educational, social, and medical programs. Such a label provides little, if any, insight into the strengths of the individual or the services that are needed (Evans, 1991; Grossman, 1983; McCall, 1982) and may limit a child's opportunities if the label causes others to have inappropriate or inadequate expectations of the child's capabilities.

Assessment of Intellectual Functioning

Determining if a child has a cognitive impairment requires a standardized, norm-referenced measure of intelligence, which usually is administered by a psychologist or psychometrist. Even though most physical therapists do not administer intelligence tests, they are often able to promote an environment in which children with motor impairments can perform optimally, such as by providing positioning to enhance a child's communication and eye and hand use (Sents & Marks, 1989) or by assisting the examiner to determine alternative response modes for use by children who have motor impairments.

ASSESSMENT OF INFANTS

Physical therapists may be involved in the administration of tests designed to assess the cognitive abilities of infants, because many of these tests focus on an infant's sensorimotor development, such as accomplishment of motor developmental milestones or coordination of vision and hearing with body movement (Chinitz & Feder, 1992; Gibbs, 1990). These tests include instruments described by Campbell in Chapter 1 of this volume.

Unfortunately, sensorimotor-based infant evaluations are poor predictors of cognitive ability at later ages, with little, if any, relationship found between scores on infant tests and children's subsequent scores on intelligence tests for preschool or school-age children (Gibbs, 1990; Zelazo & Weiss, 1990). The most common error is identification of infants as having cognitive delays who later demonstrate normal intelligence (McCall, 1982). Better predictability has been found with children who have severe cognitive delays and multiple disabilities (Kopp & McCall, 1982), with most children who have severe cognitive delays being identified before they are 1 year old (Jones & Payne, 1986). Gibbs (1990) proposed that this is a result of the limited capacity of infants with severe impairments to be influenced by positive environmental circumstances; thus their range of possible outcomes is more restricted and their test scores are more stable over time.

Some recent tests of infant cognitive abilities have attempted to determine infants' intellectual functioning through evaluation of their information processing capacity rather than their sensorimotor skills. These tests use infants' behavioral responses to novel and previously presented stimuli to assess their visual or auditory memory and their ability to discriminate among stimuli (Chinitz & Feder, 1992; Zelazo & Weiss, 1990). These tests are based on the tendency of infants, almost from birth, to respond for shorter periods of time to stimuli to which they have been previously exposed. Thus, if an infant has a longer response to a new stimulus than to one presented previously, memory for the familiar stimulus and discrimination of the two stimuli are demonstrated. Visual attention to stimuli is often assessed, as with the Fagan Test of Infant Intelligence (FTII) (Fagan & Shepherd, 1987), but changes in heart rate, smiling, and other responses can also indicate an infant's processing of information (Zelazo & Weiss, 1990).

One advantage of information processing tests for infants is that they are essentially motor and language free, making them more appropriate for infants with motor and hearing impairments than many other tests (Drotar et al., 1989). Another advantage is that their predictive validity is much better than that of the tests that focus on sensorimotor behaviors (Zelazo & Weiss, 1990). This probably is because they tap information processing capacities that are more similar to requirements of intelligence tests for older children than are the qualities assessed by sensorimotor-based tests (Chinitz & Feder, 1992; Gibbs, 1990).

ASSESSMENT OF CHILDREN

According to Zucker and Polloway (1987), the most widely used IQ tests for children are the Stanford-Binet Intelligence Scale (Terman & Merrill, 1973), the Wechsler Intelligence Scale for Children, Revised (WISC-R) (Wechsler, 1974), and the Kaufman Assessment Battery for Children (Kaufman & Kaufman, 1983). Standardized administration of these and most other intelligence tests requires spoken and motor responses that seriously limit their usefulness with children who have communication and motor impairments.

A few intelligence tests have been developed that require children only to indicate a choice from among an array of alternatives. The Columbia Mental Maturity Scale (Burgemeister et al., 1972) is one such test, which was developed specifically to assess the intelligence of children with cerebral palsy and requires only that a child be capable of indicating which pictures are unrelated to others.

Raven's Progressive Matrices (Raven, 1958), requiring selection of missing elements of abstract designs, and the Leiter International Performance Scale (Leiter, 1969) are other non–language-based tests with minimal motor requirements. They may, however, suggest spuriously low cognitive abilities in children who have visuoperceptual deficits or visual impairments. It is also important to be aware that all of the tests with limited motor and language requirements sample only a narrow range of abilities compared with more traditional tests of intelligence, so they may either overestimate or underestimate more global aspects of a child's intelligence (Chinitz & Feder, 1992). For children with profound multiple disabilities, whose cognitive abilities are the most difficult to assess, tests of visual memory, similar to those developed for evaluation of infants, could provide some of the elusive information about their capacities to store and process information (Switzky et al., 1979).

Assessment of Adaptive Behaviors

Although examiners often emphasize intelligence test scores in the diagnosis of cognitive impairment (Evans, 1991), adaptive behaviors play an equal role. Assessment of adaptive behavior relies heavily on professional judgment, in both the selection of means to assess adaptive behaviors and in their interpretation. Physical therapists often can provide information about a child's adaptive behaviors, such as self-help and mobility skills, and may also be instrumental in provision of assistive devices that can help improve a child's adaptive skills.

Instruments to measure adaptive behaviors have been developed, but they are of more recent vintage than many of the intelligence tests and there are fewer of them. Tests that are commonly used include the AAMD Adaptive Behavior Scales (Nihira et al., 1974) and the Vineland Adaptive Behavior Scales (Sparrow et al., 1984).

Classification of Cognitive Impairment

Although the 1992 AAMR definition of mental retardation no longer uses subcategories of cognitive impairment, four levels of mental retardation were included in the 1983 AAMD definition (Grossman, 1983) and are still used in many programs. Mild, moderate, severe, and profound levels of retardation are based on intelligence test scores, even though deficits in adaptive behaviors also are required for a diagnosis of mental retardation. School districts in many states also use intelligence test scores to categorize students for special education services (Zucker & Polloway, 1987). Table 19–1 compares the 1983 AAMD classification by intelligence test

score with the classifications often used by school districts to categorize students for special education purposes.

INCIDENCE AND PREVALENCE OF COGNITIVE IMPAIRMENTS

Reported estimates of incidence and prevalence of cognitive impairments vary widely. The differences are thought to be due to a number of factors, including variations in the definition; the methodologies employed; the sex, age, and communities of the samples; and the sociopolitical factors affecting the design and interpretation of the studies (Jones & Payne, 1986).

The President's Committee on Mental Retardation estimated that 3% of the population has cognitive impairment acquired before age 18, an estimate that some have challenged as being too high (Tarjan et al., 1973). They believe not only that members of cultural and ethnic minorities have been inaccurately classified as having cognitive impairments but also that schools tend to identify students as having cognitive impairments who were not considered to have impairments before starting school and are not so identified as adults. Children who are classified as having mild cognitive impairments often are not identified until age 6 or older (Jones & Payne, 1986).

Among people with cognitive impairments, estimates are that 70 to 89% have mild limitation, 20% have moderate limitation, 5% have severe limitation, and 1% have profound limitation of cognitive functioning (Jones & Payne, 1986). Approximately 2% of all school-age children have been identified for educational purposes as having a severe disability (Evans, 1991).

ETIOLOGY AND PATHOPHYSIOLOGY OF COGNITIVE IMPAIRMENTS

Multiple causes of cognitive impairments exist, many of which have been identified and many of which have not. McLaren and Bryson (1987) reviewed 13 epidemiologic studies of cognitive impairments and concluded that causes could be identified for approximately 70% of those with severe impairments and 50% of those with mild impairments.

Over 350 etiologies for cognitive impairments have been identified that can be broadly categorized into prenatal, perinatal, and postnatal causes. Prenatal etiologies have been further classified as chromosomal disorders, syndromes, inborn errors of metabolism, developmental disorders of brain formation, and environmental influences. Perinatal causes include intrauterine disorders and neonatal disorders.

TABLE 19–1. Comparison of 1983 American Association on Mental Deficiency (AAMD) Levels of Retardation and Traditional Special Education Categories

AAMD Level of Retardation	Intelligence Test Score	Educational Category	Intelligence Test Score
Mild	55 to 70	Educable	50 to 75
Moderate	40 to 55	Trainable	25 to 50
Severe	25 to 40		
Profound	Below 25		

Classifications of postnatal causes include head injuries, infections, demyelinating disorders, degenerative disorders, seizure disorders, toxic-metabolic disorders, malnutrition, environmental deprivation, and hypoconnection syndrome (American Association on Mental Retardation, 1992).

Movement dysfunction is more often associated with some etiologies than with others, and, in general, children with more severe cognitive impairments are likely to have more severe motor delays and impairments (Anwar, 1986; Chinitz & Feder, 1992). Ellis (1963) proposed that the relatively poor motor performance of people with cognitive impairments is the result of their limited capacity to process information and the rapid decay of that information over time. Such cognitive deficits impede motor learning (Anwar, 1986), leading to the slow and clumsy movements that children with cognitive impairments often have, even when they do not have cerebral palsy or another movement-related diagnosis. Many children also have associated problems, such as vision and hearing impairments, cerebral palsy, low levels of arousal, seizure disorders, cardiopulmonary dysfunction, and various other medical problems that can further influence motor development, motor learning, and motor performance (Anwar, 1986).

Prevention

Some forms of cognitive impairment and associated disorders can now be prevented, such as those resulting from phenylketonuria, rubella, and lead poisoning. In addition, amniocentesis, ultrasound, and other techniques have enabled prenatal diagnosis of many conditions, which may help decrease morbidity, such as delivery of a child with myelodysplasia by cesarean section. Genetic counseling also can be offered.

Although the etiologic factors known to cause cognitive impairments may be present in a given child, complex and powerful interactions between those factors and later environmental events can alter the actuality or the severity of cognitive limitations and associated impairments. Some infants, for example, who have severe medical problems during the postnatal course, with documented neuroanatomic pathology during this period, have few if any sequelae. On the other hand, children with no known pathology but who experience one or more environmental risk factors may eventually be classified as having cognitive impairment, usually mild cognitive impairment (Campbell & Ramey, 1985).

Campbell and Ramey (1985) identified four important environmental factors that contribute to cognitive impairment: (1) malnutrition, (2) teratogens, (3) accidents and injuries, and (4) a poor psychologic environment. These environmental factors are likely to be related to socioeconomic status, which has been found to be one of the most powerful predictors of childhood intellectual functioning (Gibbs, 1990). Kochanek and colleagues (1990) found that, in children from birth to age 3 years, characteristics of their parents, such as the mother's education, more accurately predict whether a child will have a disability as an adolescent than the child's own characteristics.

In the United States, the family-centered services directed by Part C of the Individuals with Disabilities Education Act (IDEA), described in Chapters 31 and 32 of this volume, reflect a belief in the power of early social and physical environments to influence a child's development. It also implies confidence in the capability of physical therapists and other service providers to assist families to provide environments that both prevent unnecessary disability and promote the achievement of a child's potential. Ramey & Ramey (1992) found six components of early intervention programs to be the most critical for children's intellectual development and learning: (1) encouragement to explore and learn from the environment; (2) mentoring by trusted adults in basic cognitive skills; (3) celebration of the child's developmental accomplishments by others; (4) guided rehearsal and elaboration of new skills; (5) protection from inappropriate disapproval, teasing, and punishment; and (6) provision of a rich and responsive language environment.

PRIMARY IMPAIRMENT

Diagnosis/Problem Identification

The time at which impairments in intellectual functioning and movement become recognized varies widely, both within and between medical diagnoses. In some cases, prenatal or neonatal diagnosis can predict impairments that may not yet be apparent, such as with Down syndrome or myelodysplasia. In other cases, a medical diagnosis will not be made until after impaired functioning is noted, perhaps not until months or years after birth.

Delay in achievement of developmental motor milestones is often the first indication of cognitive impairment that was present prenatally or perinatally (Chinitz & Feder, 1992). This is particularly true for children with greater than mild cognitive impairments. Some children will develop normally for a period of time and then regress, such as those with Rett syndrome or Tay-Sachs disease. In these cases, too, motor manifestations of the condition often are the first indication of a more global developmental problem (Nomura & Segawa, 1990).

NEUROMOTOR IMPAIRMENTS OF CHILDREN WITH COGNITIVE IMPAIRMENTS

The movement impairments of children with limited cognitive functioning are as diverse as the pathophysiology of their primary and associated conditions. Most of the movement problems, however, have their bases in central nervous system pathology that most often leads to impairments in flexibility, force production, coordination, postural control, balance, endurance, and efficiency (Campbell SK, 1991). Cardiopulmonary and musculoskeletal impairments also may contribute to the movement problems.

Although the type and degree of movement and related problems vary greatly, certain medical diagnoses are likely to be associated with specific constellations of neuromuscular, musculoskeletal, and cardiopulmonary impairments. Table 19–2 summarizes impairments that are common among children with selected diagnoses who often are seen by physical therapists.

Physical therapy examination of the movement impairments of children who have cognitive impairments is similar to that of other children who have problems addressed by physical therapists. Observation, criterion-referenced instruments, norm-referenced tests, and other formats are used, depending on the age of the child, the problem being assessed, and the purpose of the assessment (see other chapters of this volume).

Although the same examination methods and tools may be used for children with and without cognitive impairments, it is important to recognize that a child's intellectual impairment may affect performance of motor activities. This is especially the case when a child has to follow directions or perform motor tasks that have major cognitive components. Examination of infants and young children may be less affected by intellectual abilities than that of older children and adolescents, and cognitive function probably will affect examination of impairments less than examination of functional limitations or disabilities.

LEARNING IN CHILDREN WITH COGNITIVE IMPAIRMENTS

By definition, impaired learning is what distinguishes children with cognitive impairments from other children. Although their motor problems often are similar to those of children without cognitive impairments and they respond to intervention based on the same physical therapy principles, the application of those principles must be sensitive to the children's learning characteristics. Research demonstrating that physical therapy is less effective with children who have cognitive impairments (Parette & Hourcade, 1984) may at least partially relate to inadequate modification of therapeutic approaches to enhance their learning.

The degree and types of learning impairments of children with cognitive limitations vary considerably, but several common learning characteristics have been identified. Compared with normally developing children, children with cognitive impairments have been found (1) to be capable of learning a fewer number of things; (2) to need a greater number of repetitions to learn; (3) to have greater difficulty generalizing skills; (4) to have greater difficulty maintaining skills that are not practiced regularly; (5) to have slower response times; and (6) to have a more limited repertoire of responses (Brown et al., 1979; Falvey, 1989; Orelove & Sobsey, 1996). Implications of these learning characteristics for physical therapy are described in later sections of this chapter.

Intervention to Limit Impairments and Functional Limitations and Prevent Secondary Impairment

Pediatric physical therapists have traditionally focused their efforts on interventions designed to limit musculoskeletal, neuromuscular, and cardiopulmonary impairments; reduce functional limitations; and prevent secondary impairments. Less emphasis has been placed on the potentially important role of physical therapy in limiting or preventing secondary cognitive, communication, and social-emotional impairments, which may result from motor disorders and restrictions.

LIMITING PHYSICAL IMPAIRMENTS AND FUNCTIONAL LIMITATIONS OF CHILDREN WITH COGNITIVE IMPAIRMENTS

Early identification of neuromuscular, musculoskeletal, and cardiopulmonary problems, at whatever age they occur, allows for intervention designed to limit the impairments, thus restricting the development of secondary impairments and functional limitations. Specific intervention will depend on the identified problems and on consequences that can be predicted to follow from the natural history of the condition. Children with Down syndrome and other relatively mild movement impairments, for example, often benefit from activities designed to enhance postural control and force production and

TABLE 19–2. **Neuromuscular, Musculoskeletal, and Cardiopulmonary Impairments Described in Children with Cognitive Impairments Caused by Selected Conditions***

Condition (Source)	Neuromuscular	Musculoskeletal	Cardiopulmonary
Cri-du-chat syndrome (Nyhan & Sakati, 1976)	Hypotonia in early childhood, sometimes hypertonia later	Minor upper extremity anomalies, scoliosis	Congenital heart disease is common
Cytomegalovirus infection (prenatal) (Bergsma, 1973)	Hypertonia, seizure disorder, microcephaly	Secondary to neuromuscular problems	Pulmonary valvular stenosis, mitral stenosis, atrial septal defect
de Lange syndrome (Berg et al., 1970; Jones, 1997)	Spasticity, intention tremor, seizure disorder (10–20%), microcephaly	Decreased bone age, small stature, small hands and feet, short digits, proximal thumb placement, clinodactyly of fifth fingers, other arm and hand defects, limited elbow extension	Neonatal respiratory problems, cardiac malformations, recurrent upper respiratory tract infections
Down syndrome (Harris & Shea, 1991; Shumway-Cook & Woollacott, 1985)	Hypotonia, low muscle force production, slow automatic postural reactions, slow reaction time, motor delays increase with age	Joint hyperflexibility, ligamentous laxity, foot deformities, scoliosis, atlantoaxial instability (20%)	Congenital heart disease (40%), lung hypoplasia with pulmonary hypertension
Fetal alcohol syndrome (Jones, 1997)	Fine motor dysfunction, weak grasp, visual motor deficits, ptosis	Joint anomalies with abnormal position or function, maxillary hypoplasia	Heart murmur, often disappears after the first year
Fragile X syndrome (Keenan et al., 1992; Rinck, 1992)	Hypotonia, poor coordination and motor planning, seizures	Hyperextensible finger joints, prominent jaw, scoliosis	Mitral valve prolapse
Hurler's syndrome (Carter, 1970; Jones, 1997)	Hydrocephalus	Joint contractures, claw-like deformities of hands, short fingers, thoracolumbar kyphosis, shallow acetabular and glenoid fossae, irregularly shaped bones	Cardiac deformities, including cardiac enlargement because of right ventricular hypertension; death frequently from cardiac failure
Lesch-Nyhan syndrome (Jankovic et al., 1988)	Hypotonia followed by spasticity and chorea, athetosis, or dystonia; compulsive self-injurious behavior	Secondary to neuromuscular problems	
Prader-Willi syndrome (Aughton & Cassidy, 1990; Laurance et al., 1981)	Severe hypotonia and feeding problems in infancy, excessive eating and obesity in childhood; poor fine and gross motor coordination	Short stature, small hands and feet	May be associated with cor pulmonale (most common cause of death)
Rett syndrome (Holm & King, 1990; Nomura & Segawa, 1990; Stewart et al., 1989)	Hypotonia in infancy, then gradually increasing hypertonia and loss of acquired skills; ataxia, apraxia, choreothestosis, or dystonia; progression from hyperkinesia to bradykinesia with age; slow reaction time; stereotypic hand movements (clapping, wringing, clenching); drooling; involuntary, rhythmic tongue movement and deviation; seizure disorder	Scoliosis, kyphosis, joint contractures, hip subluxation or dislocation, equinovarus deformities	Immature respiratory patterns; breathing irregularities, such as hyperventilation and apnea
Williams (elfin facies) syndrome (Jones, 1997)	Mild neurologic dysfunction; poor motor coordination	Hallux valgus	Variable congenital heart disease

*Some impairments are not exhibited by all children with the condition.

accomplishment of motor milestones (Harris & Shea, 1991). Other children with more severe impairments may benefit from positioning and other activities designed to maintain flexibility, prevent musculoskeletal malalignments and deformities, and enhance motor development and control. Such intervention is described in other chapters of this volume.

LIMITING COGNITIVE, COMMUNICATION, AND PSYCHOSOCIAL IMPAIRMENTS AND FUNCTIONAL LIMITATIONS

Children who have motor impairments that restrict or prevent exploration of their environments may be at risk for secondary delays in domains that are not primarily affected (Campbell SK, 1991), especially cognition, communication, and psychosocial development (Kermoian & Campos, 1988; Telzrow et al., 1987). Campos and Bertenthal (1987) believe that independent mobility is an organizer of psychologic changes in normally developing infants, especially developmental changes in social understanding, spatial cognition, and emotions. They also propose theoretic links between independent mobility and the growth of brain structures, self-awareness, attachment to others, and the ability to cope with the environment.

Most of the theoretic links have not been examined empirically, but relations between mobility and spatial cognition have received considerable research attention. Several studies have demonstrated that locomotion, not age per se, is related to changes in such spatial cognitive tasks as recognition of heights (Bertenthal et al., 1984), retrieving hidden toys (Benson & Uzgiris, 1985), and performance on Piagetian spatial search tasks by typical infants and infants with meningomyelocele (Kermoian & Campos, 1988; Telzrow et al., 1987). Self-produced locomotion also has been shown to influence social-communicative behaviors of infants (Gustafson, 1984), and the proposed theoretic link between mobility and development of brain structures has been supported by studies demonstrating that experience shapes the brains of animals (for a review see Kolb et al., 1998). New imaging techniques are showing similar effects of experience on the structure of infants' brains (Chugani, 1998).

Although much of the research has demonstrated an association between motor and cognitive development, other research suggests that the links are indirect, with motor and cognitive abilities facilitating each other but capable of relatively independent development. One study, for example, found that the object permanence task performance of children with cerebral palsy was more closely related to their

mental age than to the severity of their motor impairments (Eagle, 1985). This finding is consistent with the well-known capacity for some people to develop average or superior mental abilities in spite of severe motor impairments.

Further research is needed to determine the relative contributions of innate mental capability and sensorimotor experiences on various aspects of cognitive development. It may be that the inborn intelligence of some children enables them to compensate for their motor limitations, thus making them less vulnerable to effects of sensorimotor deprivation than children whose intellectual capacities are more limited.

Assuming that exploration and manipulation of the environment do influence cognitive, communication, and social-emotional development, physical therapy has an obvious role in the development of these nonmotor domains of children who have motor impairments. One means is through treatment strategies designed to improve motor performance, as described in other chapters of this volume. Two other potentially important means are providing alternative means of mobility when children's motor impairments prevent exploration of the environment at an age when other children are crawling and walking and the use of postural support systems to promote interaction with the environment.

USE OF POWER MOBILITY TO PREVENT SECONDARY IMPAIRMENTS

Butler (1991) asserts that self-produced locomotion can have such a powerful impact on development that functional means of mobility should be provided for all young children who have mobility restrictions, regardless of whether or not the child is expected to walk eventually. She proposes the concept of augmentative mobility, which, like augmentative communication, supports a child's own capabilities, allowing the child to select a means of mobility that is most convenient and efficient for a particular situation. Aided mobility is not seen as "giving up" on walking for young children, but as providing critical assistance at a time when it is needed for optimal development.

Several studies have demonstrated that very young children can learn to use power mobility devices. Zazula and Foulds (1983) reported that an 11-month-old child with congenital limb deformities learned to activate the controls of a motorized cart within 4 hours and controlled all aspects of the cart by 17 months. In another study, 12 of 13 children between ages 20 and 37 months, with various disabilities, became competent motorized wheelchair drivers within their homes after an average of 16.4 days (Butler et al., 1983).

Although these young children were believed to have normal intelligence, other studies have demonstrated that older children with cognitive impairments also can become independent users of power mobility devices (Verburg et al., 1990). It is reasonable to assume that certain cognitive abilities are necessary to achieve independent aided mobility, but the specific abilities that are necessary and the means to assess them have not been determined. Because normally developing children learn to crawl and become independently mobile well before their first birthday, and because children have become independently mobile using power mobility devices before age 2, children with cognitive impairments who have adequate vision and the cognitive skills typical of an 18-month-old (or perhaps younger) are likely to be capable of learning to use powered means of mobility, given appropriate equipment and opportunities.

USE OF ASSISTIVE POSITIONING TO PROMOTE ENVIRONMENTAL INTERACTION

Seating and other assistive positioning devices, as described in Chapter 24, also can influence children's interactions with their physical and social environments through their effects on such variables as hand function (Nwaobi, 1987), switch activation (McEwen & Karlan, 1989), and respiration (Nwaobi & Smith, 1986). One of the most important environmental interactions is communication with others, because it affects not only a child's own communication development but also cognitive and social-emotional development (Campbell PH, 1989; Siegel-Causey & Downing, 1987).

To learn to communicate, children must have opportunities to communicate. One study found that teachers initiated interactions at higher rates when children were positioned in wheelchairs than when they were in sidelyers or supine on a mat (McEwen, 1992). Observations suggested that wheelchairs promoted interaction by placing students nearer the normal interaction level of adults than positioning on the floor. The adults who participated in the study rarely sat on the floor to interact with children, unless they were involved in structured programming, a finding that is consistent with other investigations (Houghton et al., 1987).

In addition to providing opportunities for interaction with other persons in the environment, research suggests that positioning can also influence children's own communicative behaviors. Normally developing 3- to 6-month-old infants looked at their mothers for longer periods of time when they were supine than when reclined 45° or seated upright (Fogel et al., 1992). Similarly, children with profound cognitive impairments and physical disabilities interacted with attentive teachers and classroom assistants for longer periods of time when they were in the supine position than when they were seated in their wheelchairs or in a sidelyer (McEwen, 1992).

Positioning also may influence children's interactions with their environments through the effect of position on their behavioral state or arousal. Low levels of arousal and behavioral states that interfere with attention to environmental stimuli are common among children with the most severe multiple cognitive and motor impairments (Guess et al., 1988). Guess and colleagues found that when children with multiple disabilities were positioned upright their behavioral states were more compatible with learning than when they were placed in recumbent positions. Similarly, Landesman-Dwyer and Sackett (1978) found that children's activity levels and receptivity to environmental stimuli were improved when intervention included an upright position. Other studies suggest that oxygenation is improved in the upright position (Navajas et al., 1988), and inadequate oxygenation has been proposed as a factor contributing to the lethargy of children with profound multiple disabilities (Guess et al., 1988).

Although research concerning effects of positioning with children who have multiple disabilities is limited, it does suggest that positioning may influence children's interactions with their environments through a variety of mechanisms. The upright position is more likely to enhance children's receptivity to and opportunities for interaction with the environment than recumbent positions (Campbell PH, 1989; McEwen, 1992) and thus may help limit or prevent secondary cognitive, emotional, and communication impairments and functional limitations. There are some children, however, especially those functioning at very low levels of communication development, whose own communication may be facilitated by the supine position. Because supine may be socially isolating and physically detrimental, it should be monitored carefully and used only while the child is actively engaged in social interaction.

Role of Other Disciplines

The number of disciplines represented in the care of a child with cognitive impairments is often directly proportional to the severity of the child's cognitive limitations and to the number and severity of any associated disorders. All of a child's problems are usually not identified at the same time, so increasing numbers of disciplines may become involved as a child grows older. Because motor delays and movement disorders are often recognized relatively early, a physical therapist is likely to be one of the first members of an intervention team and so be in a position to recognize the need for input by other disciplines and refer the family to physicians and other service providers.

It has been estimated that nearly 50% of people with cognitive impairments have at least one other impairment (Kelleher & Mulcahy, 1985), each of which is likely to require the services of several different service providers. The prevalence of additional impairments is positively related to the severity of the cognitive impairment, with many children with cognitive and motor impairments having such problems as impaired hearing and vision, seizure disorders, and cardiopulmonary dysfunction (Kelleher & Mulcahy, 1985).

Some of the service providers who may need to be involved with children who have both cognitive and motor impairments are suggested by the 14 early intervention services named in Part C of IDEA: audiology; case management services; family training, counseling, and home visits; health service; medical services for diagnostic or evaluation purposes; nursing; nutrition services; occupational therapy; physical therapy; psychologic services; social work; special instruction; speech-language pathology; and transportation. Many children also require the services of several physicians and surgeons, orthotists, and vendors of assistive technology.

As children with cognitive impairments grow older and their impairments lead to functional limitations and disabilities, the number of involved disciplines often expands to include a variety of teachers, vocational counselors, and personnel of health and social service agencies. Young adults may need job coaches, group home supervisors, personal care assistants, and others who can provide the supports necessary to enable them to live as independently and successfully as possible in their communities.

Determinants of Outcomes

The determinants of outcomes for children with cognitive impairments or who are at risk for cognitive impairments usually are numerous and complex. From a dynamic systems point of view, described by Campbell in Chapter 1, the internal capacity of the child and the virtually unlimited environmental influences are logically equivalent and capable of affecting outcomes. The natural history of cognitive impairments and associated problems resulting from some etiologies, particularly those that are progressive, are relatively well described. Scoliosis, for example, nearly always develops in children with Rett syndrome (Holm & King, 1990). For others, especially infants and very young children, many complex endogenous and exogenous factors contribute to the ultimate impact of the initial insult and resulting pathophysiology, which makes prediction of outcome difficult. As discussed previously in this chapter, family environment has been found to be the best predictor of outcome, especially with children who have mild cognitive impairments (Gibbs, 1990; Ramey & Ramey, 1992).

TEAM ASSESSMENT OF DISABILITY

The complex problems of children with both cognitive and motor impairments usually require a team approach for assessment of disability and for planning, implementation, and evaluation of intervention (Foley, 1990; Orelove & Sobsey, 1996; Rainforth & York-Barr, 1997). The team always will include the child's family or other caregiver, with other team members as required by the nature and severity of the child's problems, the child's age, and the service delivery setting. Many children need the services of two or more teams at the same time, such as a clinically based health care team and an early intervention or public school team. Usually, the health care team is primarily responsible for assessment of the child's impairment-level needs, with the early intervention or school-based team responsible for limiting impairments and ongoing efforts to promote the highest possible level of functioning in the community. When the teams have mutual responsibilities and concerns, overlapping or conflicting services can result, with confusion for the family and unnecessary expenditure of limited resources. To avoid such problems, it is essential that the teams communicate well and that the roles and responsibilities of the members of each team are clear to all (Rainforth & York-Barr, 1997).

Because the nature and severity of a child's impairments often play a greater role in the foci of assessment and intervention than a child's age, this chapter is not organized chronologically, as are several other chapters of this volume that describe conditions in which age-related progressions can be identified. Age-related needs that occur during the transition to adulthood and are common to most children with cognitive impairments are discussed separately. The case histories at the end of the chapter describe application of evaluation and intervention principles for children of different ages with cognitive impairments and various mental and motor characteristics.

Models of Team Functioning

Each team must decide on a model of service delivery that will enable comprehensive evaluation of a child's disabilities and provide the most effective intervention. The transdisciplinary model of service delivery, developed in the mid-1970s by the United Cerebral Palsy National Collaborative Infant Project (1976), is increasingly being recommended as best practice in early intervention programs and in special education programs for children with severe and multiple disabilities (Foley, 1990; Orelove & Sobsey, 1996; Rainforth & York-Barr, 1997).

The transdisciplinary model permits greater coordination of comprehensive services for individuals with complex health, educational, and social needs than most other approaches. Two of the distinguishing features of the model are that assessments are conducted collaboratively by team members and a single, discipline-free service plan is developed to meet the highest-priority needs of the child and family. This mode of operation contrasts with other service delivery models in which service providers conduct separate assessments and develop separate, discipline-referenced intervention plans (McGonigel et al., 1994).

Another distinguishing feature of the transdisciplinary model is that one team member is designated as the primary service provider, usually the person who spends the greatest amount of time with the child or the person who has the skills necessary to address the child's greatest areas of need (McGonigel et al., 1994; Orelove & Sobsey, 1996). The primary service provider will change over time as the child's needs and environments change. A parent or physical therapist may be the primary service provider for an infant or young child, a teacher the primary service provider for an older child, and a personal care assistant the primary service provider for a young adult.

When employing a transdisciplinary approach, team members are responsible for determining which of their own disciplinary knowledge and skills are needed by the child, for consulting with and teaching the necessary knowledge and skills to the primary service provider and for monitoring outcomes. The primary service provider incorporates the knowledge and strategies of other disciplines into ongoing intervention with the child. In effect, team members "release" part of their roles to the primary service provider (McGonigel et al., 1994; Orelove & Sobsey, 1996).

Assessment of Disability

Assessment of a child's disability is best conducted in the environments in which the child actually participates or environments in which children of similar age and social background participate. Assessment in natural environments is increasingly advocated for all children who have disabilities, but especially for children with cognitive impairments who have difficulty generalizing skills from one setting to another. Such environmentally based assessment also is far more likely to lead to intervention that results in age-appropriate, functional outcomes than assessment that takes place in isolated or clinical settings, assessments that are based on a normal developmental sequence, or assessments that focus primarily on identification of impairments, such as range of motion, postural responses, or retention of primitive reflexes (Brown et al., 1979; Harris, 1991; McEwen & Shelden, 1995; Rainforth & York-Barr, 1997).

ECOLOGICAL OR ENVIRONMENTAL ASSESSMENTS

Brown and associates (1979) described an ecological or environmental approach to assessment that has subsequently been promoted by many others as a means to determine functional outcomes and plan programs for people who have cognitive impairments and, more recently, for children in early intervention programs (Falvey, 1989; Orelove & Sobsey, 1996; Rainforth & York-Barr, 1997; Thurman & Widerstrom, 1990). Functional outcomes have been emphasized in special education for a number of years and are increasingly being supported by pediatric physical therapists and therapists in other areas of practice (Harris, 1991; McEwen & Shelden, 1995; Rainforth & York-Barr, 1997). Functional skills have been defined as those activities or tasks that someone else will have to do if the child does not (Brown et al., 1979), that are age appropriate (Falvey, 1989), and that reflect the needs and interests of the child and family (Orelove & Sobsey, 1996). Some children can learn to complete a task or activity, others will be capable of learning to carry out only a part of it. Partial participation, or completion of only part of a task, is a legitimate outcome for some children who have severe disabilities (Ferguson & Baumgart, 1991). A child may, for example, be unable to transfer independently but can learn to unbuckle a seat belt and support his or her weight in standing. Another child may be unable to put a tape into a tape recorder but can learn to turn it on using a switch.

An ecological assessment is an approach or format, rather than a specific assessment instrument. There are four major steps in an ecological assessment, as described by Orelove and Sobsey (1996):

1. *Determine the domains to be included in the child's program.* Four domains are considered to be primary: home, community (e.g., school, stores, and church), vocational, and recreation-leisure. Certain critical skills, such as mobility, communication, and hand use, are required for functioning in all domains.

2. *Determine the environments and subenvironments within each domain in which the child currently functions or could function in the future.* A child's team might identify the home, school, and restaurant as especially important. Subenvironments could be the bedroom at home, the cafeteria at school, and the restroom in a restaurant.

3. *Determine the activities the child needs to function in each of the subenvironments.* Activities could include getting out of bed at home, obtaining and eating lunch at school, and using the toilet in a restaurant.

4. *Determine the skills the child needs for each activity.* Skills are determined through task analysis of the activities and identifying the components the child needs to be able to do to accomplish each of them. To get out of bed, for example, one child may need to respond to the alarm, remove the covers, assume a sitting position, and transfer to a wheelchair. A child with less ability could learn to do other components of the task, such as rolling over to sit up after the covers have been removed and assisting with the transfer.

An example of an ecological assessment is included in the case history of Jeff at the end of the chapter.

ARENA ASSESSMENT

An arena assessment is another type of assessment format that has been recommended for children with severe disabilities (Wolery & Dyk, 1984) and is widely used by transdisciplinary teams in early intervention programs (Foley, 1990; McGonigel et al., 1994). In an arena assessment, all team members observe the child at the same time and write an integrated report of their observations. This approach not only provides a more holistic and focused picture of the child than occurs when each discipline assesses the child separately, but also both parents and professional team members have perceived the arena approach to give a truer picture of the child's abilities, lead to more parent involvement, and promote greater team interaction and consensus (Wolery & Dyk, 1984).

During an arena assessment, one family member or professional interacts with the child and directs preplanned activities while the other team members sit at the periphery of the interaction and record their observations of the child's behaviors. These observations often focus on discipline-specific concerns, including discipline-related portions of comprehensive developmental tests, but observations are made within the context of the overall flow of behaviors exhibited as the child and facilitator interact. Team members are encouraged to record observa-

tions that may not be considered part of their disciplinary expertise.

Following the assessment, the team meets to discuss their observations, consider other available information, and collaboratively plan the intervention. In this way each team member can gain an understanding of the child's overall capabilities and limitations and recognize relationships among motor, communication, cognitive, social-emotional, and other behaviors. One criticism of the arena assessment is that it is conducted under artificial conditions using contrived tasks, so it does not provide as accurate a picture of a child's functional capabilities and limitations within the natural environment as does an ecological assessment (Rainforth & York-Barr, 1997).

Determining Intervention Goals and Outcomes

Outcomes of intervention to reduce a child's disability must represent specific functional skills that the child will acquire. Team members cannot assume that goals directed toward remediation of impairments, such as improving postural responses, range of motion, or strength, or toward reducing the degree of functional limitations indicated by failed items on a developmental test, will necessarily lead to meaningful outcomes (Harris, 1991; McEwen & Shelden, 1995; Rainforth & York-Barr, 1997). This is especially true of children with cognitive impairments who need many repetitions to learn, forget easily, and generalize poorly. This makes it unlikely that a child with cognitive impairments will be able to synthesize isolated activities or components of movement into meaningful skills.

P.H. Campbell (1991) proposed a "top-down" approach to determining outcomes, in which the desired functional outcomes are determined first, then obstacles to their accomplishment are identified, and then intervention to overcome the obstacles is planned and implemented (Fig. 19-1). This process in similar to the decision-making process of the hypothesis-oriented algorithm for clinicians (HOAC) (Rothstein & Echternach, 1986) described in Chapter 7 of this volume, in which the goals or outcomes for intervention are determined first, then the child is examined to generate a hypothesis about why they can or cannot be met at the present time.

As described earlier as a component of an ecological assessment, functional outcomes can be anything that are high priority and meaningful to the child and family, are age appropriate, and are, or could be, a home, community, recreation-leisure, or vocational activity. Giangreco and colleagues (1998, p. 13) pro-

TOP-DOWN APPROACH

BOTTOM-UP APPROACH

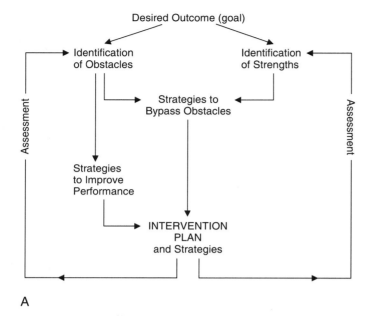

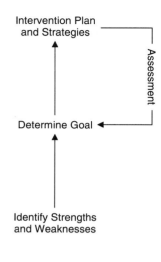

A   B

FIGURE 19–1. Comparison of a top-down approach *(A)*, in which assessments identify means to achieve desired outcomes, and a bottom-up approach *(B)*, in which assessment results determine outcomes. (From Campbell, PH. Evaluation and assessment in early intervention for infants and toddlers. Journal of Early Intervention, *15*:42, 1991. Copyright 1991 by Division for Early Childhood, the Council for Exceptional Children.)

posed five valued life outcomes for all children, including those with severe disabilities:

1. Having a safe, stable home in which to live now or in the future
2. Having access to a variety of places and engaging in meaningful activities
3. Having a social network of personally meaningful relationships
4. Having a level of personal choice and control that matches one's age
5. Being safe and healthy

Teams usually have the most difficulty determining meaningful outcomes for children with profound multiple disabilities who often have extremely limited repertoires of behavior. Evans and Scotti (1989) maintain that even these children can accomplish outcomes that require active behavioral changes, such as indicating a choice of food or activity or increasing body movements used to activate switches. Such active outcomes lead to acquisition of skills that reduce disability and are in contrast to passive activities that are done to the child, such as sensory stimulation, range-of-motion exercises, and positioning (often stated as something the child will "tolerate"). Passive activities may be part of the

intervention to help a child accomplish a skill, but only the child's active behavior can reduce disability (Downing, 1988).

One helpful tool for assisting families to identify meaningful outcomes and to measure whether they have been accomplished is the Canadian Occupational Performance Measure (COPM) (Law et al., 1994). The COPM was designed as an individualized measure of performance and satisfaction in self-care, productivity (work, household management, play/school), and leisure. Although the COPM was intended for occupational therapists, it is an equally useful tool for physical therapists. This chapter's section on Assessment of Outcomes for All Age Groups gives more information about the COPM.

When desired outcomes are determined first, as with Campbell's (1991) top-down approach, they are discipline free; that is, they describe the skills the child will accomplish without regard for discipline-related concerns. Only after team members identify the highest-priority outcomes do they decide which disciplines will be needed to help the child accomplish each one (Rainforth & York-Barr, 1997). This team-oriented process for determining outcomes is not necessarily inconsistent with the processes described in the HOAC (Rothstein & Echternach,

1986) or the *Guide to Physical Therapist Practice (Guide)* (American Physical Therapy Association, 1997), although both the HOAC and the *Guide* describe a unidisciplinary approach in which the physical therapist makes decisions in collaboration with only the patient and perhaps the patient's family. When working with children whose complex problems require teams of professionals, the process must include other professionals as well. Amy's case history at the end of this chapter provides an example of application of the *Guide* to the decision-making process of a school-based team.

INTERVENTION

During planning and implementation of intervention for children with cognitive impairments, it is important to keep in mind what are widely regarded as best practices for working with children who have cognitive impairments and other developmental disabilities. Some of these practices have been discussed previously and include families and children as full and equal team members, assessment in natural environments, and an emphasis on functional outcomes with active participation by children (McEwen & Shelden, 1995).

Other considerations that influence whether and how intervention is provided for children with cognitive impairments include use of cognitive referencing as a means to determine who will receive physical therapy services, full inclusion of children with cognitive impairments in least restrictive environments, use of teaching methods that are most likely to result in acquisition of motor skills by children with cognitive impairments, and the role of physical therapists in promoting development in nonmotor domains. Each of these considerations, which are discussed in the following sections, involve one or more of the three components of intervention included in the *Guide to Physical Therapist Practice* (1997): coordination, communication, and documentation; patient/client-related instruction; and direct intervention.

Cognitive Referencing

Cognitive referencing is an approach that has been used to determine whether children are eligible for services, especially for physical therapy, occupational therapy, and speech pathology in public schools (Carr, 1989). The approach is based on an assumption that children's potentials for gains in motor and communication development are related to their cognitive abilities and that children whose cognitive abilities are lower than or equal to their motor or communication abilities cannot benefit from services, so are not eligible for them.

Obviously, many children with cognitive impairments could be declared ineligible for physical therapy services under such an assumption, so the use of cognitive referencing has been highly controversial (Giangreco, 1990). Critics have been supported by at least one retrospective study that casts doubt on the validity of cognitive referencing as a means to predict which children will make gains in motor development (Cole et al., 1991) and by the U.S. Department of Education, Office of Special Programs (OSEP), which declared cognitive referencing to be an unlawful means to determine whether a child should receive related services in public schools (Rainforth, 1991). The OSEP statement reiterated the authority of each child's educational team to decide on the services necessary for that child to meet individualized educational goals. When goals of children with cognitive and neuromotor impairments focus on functional outcomes, some type of physical therapy often is needed, as determined through coordination and communication with other team members.

Inclusion of Children with Cognitive Impairments

The concept of least restrictive environments has its roots in the United States Constitution, which affirms that the government shall intrude into peoples' lives in the least restrictive manner possible (Witkin & Fox, 1992). Since the 1960s, this concept has been incorporated into state and federal laws affecting services for people with cognitive impairments, mandating that, to the extent possible, people with disabilities will go to school, live, and work in environments with people who do not have disabilities.

The definition of the least restrictive environment for people with cognitive impairments has been moving steadily away from segregated services and toward full inclusion in community-based settings, as evidenced by closure of many institutions for people with cognitive impairments and court-ordered inclusion of children with cognitive impairments in general education classrooms. In 1992, for example, a judge of the U.S. Court for the District of New Jersey ordered a New Jersey school district to develop a plan to include an 8-year-old boy with Down syndrome in his neighborhood elementary school, with any needed supplementary aids and services. One of the court's findings was that "school districts... must consider placing children with disabilities in regular classroom settings, with the use of supplementary aids and services...., before exploring other, more restrictive, alternatives" (TASH Force Strikes Again, 1992, p. 2). The IDEA amendments of 1997 placed additional emphasis on the need for individualized education program (IEP) teams to consider whether a child's needs can be addressed in the general education classroom with supplementary aids and services. Physical therapists often are involved in coordination and communication with other team members to decide on a child's educational placement.

Physical therapy is one of the services that must follow children with disabilities as they move into their communities and neighborhood schools. Physical therapists must provide all three components of intervention in these settings to promote children's accomplishment of functional outcomes that will enable them to participate as successfully as possible in inclusive environments (Rainforth & York-Barr, 1997). Giangreco and colleagues (1998) have written a helpful "how-to" manual for inclusion of children with severe disabilities in general education classrooms that addresses provision of physical therapy and other related services.

Teaching and Learning Considerations

Much of what physical therapists do is teach children to move more effectively and efficiently. A number of teaching strategies have been identified by educational researchers that optimize the learning of students with cognitive impairments and can be helpful to physical therapists when designing and implementing intervention plans. Although most of the strategies were designed for educational programming of students with cognitive impairments, they can be applied to motor learning as well as academic learning. Many of the strategies are closely related to current motor learning principles (see Chapter 6). Physical therapists should coordinate and communicate with other team members to identify opportunities for students to practice motor skills and should instruct parents, teachers, and other people in children's lives how to use the methods to promote learning during those opportunities. Physical therapists also may apply the principles during direct intervention with children.

INSTRUCTION IN NATURAL ENVIRONMENTS

One strategy that has received considerable attention over the past two decades and is intended to address several of the learning problems of students with cognitive impairments, especially severe cognitive impairments, is a focus on teaching functional skills in natural environments (Brown et al., 1979; Falvey, 1989). Because it takes students with cognitive impairments a long time to learn a few things,

and because they have difficulty generalizing and maintaining skills, traditional curricula that build sequentially on fundamental, nonfunctional skills have not generally led to meaningful gains. Children are often unable to generalize such nonfunctional activities as putting pegs in pegboards, for example, to functional activities such as putting coins in a machine to get a soft drink. Practicing "prerequisite" skills, such as writing the letters of the alphabet, also often fails to result in such functional outcomes as the ability to sign one's name or select the correct restroom in a public place.

Similar difficulties often are encountered by children with severe motor impairments when nonfunctional or presumed prerequisite skills are the focus of physical therapy. Research has largely failed to support children's generalization (carryover) of skills demonstrated during physical therapy sessions to other settings or synthesis of presumed components and prerequisites of movement into measurable functional motor activities (Brown et al., 1998; Horn, 1991).

When the emphasis is on acquisition of specific functional skills in natural environments, generalization is unnecessary or less difficult and skills are likely to be maintained by natural reinforcers and ongoing occasions for practice (Orelove & Sobsey, 1996). If several people work with the child on the same skills, learning may be enhanced by providing more opportunities to learn (repetitions) and by varying the stimulus conditions under which the skill is practiced, thus promoting generalization. These principles serve as a basis for integrated models of service delivery that have been advocated for physical therapists and occupational therapists working in early intervention and public school programs (Orelove & Sobsey, 1996; Rainforth & York-Barr, 1997). Although limited research has been conducted to support the effectiveness of teaching motor skills in natural environments, research in other areas, such as life skills, language, and social interaction, suggests that such an approach would be valuable.

BEHAVIORAL PROGRAMMING INTERVENTION

Behavioral programming is based on the assumption that behaviors are learned through interactions with the social, physical, and biologic environments, so, by manipulating the environment, behaviors can be taught (Bijou, 1966). Following a review of research on the effectiveness of motor skills instruction for children with neuromotor impairments, Horn (1991) concluded that physical therapists and occupational therapists should develop procedures to incorporate behavioral techniques into their intervention programs. She made this recommendation because of the relative success of interventions using behavioral techniques compared with the neuromotor and sensory stimulation techniques commonly used by occupational therapists and physical therapists. By incorporating behavioral techniques into other intervention strategies, physical therapists may not only be able to increase the rate at which children with cognitive impairments acquire motor skills and the number of skills they acquire but may also promote generalization and maintenance of motor behaviors.

POSITIVE REINFORCEMENT

A child is positively reinforced by a stimulus if a behavior that preceded the stimulus increases (Lutzker et al., 1983). Possible reinforcing stimuli are unlimited, ranging from tangible items, such as food and stickers, to social reinforcers, such as attention or praise, and abstract reinforcers, such as self-approval (Snell & Zirpoli, 1987). With children who have cognitive impairments, especially severe or profound retardation, common reinforcers such as praise, access to activities, and food often fail to lead to increases in behaviors, and identification of reinforcers can be a challenge (Orelove & Sobsey, 1996). To identify potential reinforcers, Haney and Falvey (1989) suggest (1) identifying natural consequences of the behavior, such as playing in water as a consequence of walking to the sink; (2) surveying the child's likes and dislikes by observing the child, or asking the child, parents, or teachers; and (3) offering paired choices to determine which of several potential reinforcers the child considers to be the most desirable. It is important that reinforcers not be overused, because children can become satiated and the stimuli will no longer have reinforcement value (Snell & Zirpoli, 1987).

Reinforcers have been effective in increasing motor behaviors, such as use of music as biofeedback to increase an erect head position (Maloney & Kurtz, 1982), and a combination of music and food to increase the distance that a child walked independently (Chandler & Adams, 1972). A common limitation of such studies, however, is that few have examined generalization to nonexperimental settings or maintenance of the behaviors beyond the period of intervention. Also, reinforcement has not been shown to result in acquisition of behaviors not previously in the child's repertoire. A combination of reinforcement with antecedent techniques and modification of consequences has, however, resulted in new behavioral responses (Horn, 1991; Reid et al., 1991).

ANTECEDENT TECHNIQUES

The first step in shaping a new behavior is to prompt the desired behavior or an approximation by providing instructions, models, cues, or physical prompts (Snell & Zirpoli, 1987). Instructions can take a variety of forms, such as verbal or gestural instructions (e.g., "Reach for the toy") or verbal instructions paired with models, cues, or physical prompts (e.g., "Reach for the toy," paired with facilitation of movement at the shoulder). Modeling provides a demonstration of a behavior that the child attempts to imitate. Cues direct a child's attention to a task that can result in the desired behavior, without a physical prompt. To cue the child to reach for the toy, the toy could be tapped on the table or held above the child to encourage an erect posture, reaching, or assuming a standing position. Many of the handling techniques used by physical therapists provide physical prompts for motor behaviors.

For optimal learning to occur, the type and amount of prompting must be matched to the skills of the child, with the least amount of help necessary being the most conducive to the child's learning (Snell & Zirpoli, 1987). Prompting should be faded as the child responds, so that natural cues eventually provide the stimulus for response. A natural cue is the least intrusive prompt (e.g., the presence of a friend serving as a cue for a child to lift the head) and is the level of prompt required for independent behaviors. Physical prompts, often used by physical therapists, are the most intrusive.

PROVIDING CONSEQUENCES

Once a behavior has been prompted, it can be improved or expanded through shaping or chaining techniques. Shaping and chaining can also be used to build new behaviors (Snell & Zirpoli, 1987) through reinforcement of behaviors that successively approximate the desired behavior.

New behaviors can be shaped by reinforcing behaviors that are increasingly similar to the target behavior, such as reinforcing components of standing up from a chair, or chaining to link standing, walking, opening doors, and other behaviors necessary to accomplish a goal of walking to lunch. Backward chaining, in which the last step in the sequence is learned first, is often a useful technique because children receive the reward of task completion, often a natural reinforcer, throughout the process of learning the skill (Lutzker et al., 1983; Snell & Zirpoli, 1987).

Behavioral intervention is one of the areas in which physical therapists should take advantage of the expertise of other members of service delivery teams, such as teachers and psychologists. Physical therapy educational prerequisites and curricula rarely provide more than superficial information about behavioral strategies, which limits the extent to which many physical therapists can use them effectively to promote the development of motor skills by children with cognitive impairments.

Promoting Children's Communication Development

When working with children who have cognitive impairments, all team members are responsible for promoting development in areas often not considered part of their disciplinary domains. One of the most effective ways physical therapists can contribute to the overall development of children with cognitive impairments is to assist efforts to improve their communication abilities. At its most basic level, communication enables children to influence their social and physical environments to control what happens to themselves. All children, even those with the most profound multiple disabilities, can communicate. Some communicate in many of the same ways as infants, such as looking at a person, crying, or smiling; others can learn to communicate using signs, communication boards, or electronic voice-output communication aids (Siegel-Causey & Downing; 1987; see also Chapter 24). Ability to control what happens to themselves is often said to be the key to prevention or reduction of these children's pervasive passivity or "learned helplessness," a condition that can effectively block educational efforts and be extremely resistant to change (Campbell PH, 1989).

The critical importance of communication and the need for all team members to participate in communication development was recognized by creation in the United States of the National Joint Committee for the Communicative Needs of Persons with Severe Disabilities in 1986. Representatives of seven organizations, including the American Physical Therapy Association, served on the joint committee and developed guidelines that crossed traditional disciplinary boundaries and reflect a "shared commitment to promoting effective communication by persons with severe disabilities thus providing a common ground on which the disciplines of the member organizations can unite their efforts to improve the quality of life of such persons" (National Joint Committee for the Communicative Needs of Persons with Severe Disabilities, 1992, pp. 1–2). This means that physical therapists are responsible for promoting effective communication, not only through such traditional means as positioning and improving motor skills to enable access to communication aids but also through provision of environments that acknowledge and address the Communication Bill of Rights (Fig. 19–2) of children who have communication impairments (National Joint Committee for the

Communicative Needs of Persons with Severe Disabilities, 1992).

Assessment of Outcomes for All Age Groups

Because children and young adults with cognitive impairments often progress slowly, particularly those with severe disabilities, it is important to use assessment methods that can be sensitive to small changes. This is necessary not only to document progress but also to prevent expenditure of time and effort on intervention strategies that are not leading to meaningful outcomes. Three related methods that are especially useful for assessing outcomes of physical therapy intervention for children with cognitive impairments are (1) accomplishment of behavioral objectives, (2) use of the Canadian Occupational Performance Measure (Law et al., 1994), and (3) single-subject research methodologies.

USE OF BEHAVIORAL OBJECTIVES

Assessment of outcomes can be relatively straightforward if functional goals and behavioral objectives leading to them are identified before intervention. As described by O'Neill and Harris (1982), the components of a behavioral objective enable therapists to monitor a child's progress toward accomplishment of a goal, to determine if it is necessary to modify an intervention, and to establish that goals have been met. Once a goal has been identified, such as "David will go to the kitchen and make himself a peanut butter sandwich," behavioral objectives leading to achievement of the goal can be developed by comparing David's abilities with the goal's requirements.

There are five components of a behavioral objective: *Who* will do *what*, under what *conditions, how well*, by *when*. These components permit an objective assessment of whether the goal is being met within the projected time frame. One of David's behavioral objectives, leading to the sandwich-making goal, may be to move himself from the living room to the kitchen, which could be written, "David will walk using his reverse walker from the living room to the kitchen in less than 2 minutes on four of five consecutive days after school by December 14, 20__." It should not be difficult to assess whether this objective, or part of it, is accomplished, regardless of the intervention methods used.

CANADIAN OCCUPATIONAL PERFORMANCE MEASURE

The COPM (Law et al., 1994) was designed to help identify and measure individually meaningful goals for people in the areas of self-care, productivity

All persons, regardless of the extent or severity of their disabilities, have a basic right to affect, through communication, the conditions of their own existence. Beyond this general right, a number of specific communication rights should be ensured in all daily interactions and interventions involving persons who have severe disabilities. These basic communication rights are as follows:

1. The right to request desired objects, actions, events, and persons and to express personal preferences or feelings.

2. The right to be offered choices and alternatives.

3. The right to reject or refuse undesired objects, events, or actions, including the right to decline or reject all proffered choices.

4. The right to request, and be given, attention from and interaction with another person.

5. The right to request feedback or information about a state, an object, a person, or an event of interest.

6. The right to active treatment and intervention efforts to enable people with severe disabilities to communicate messages in whatever modes and as effectively and efficiently as their specific abilities will allow.

7. The right to have communication acts acknowledged and responded to, even when the intent of these acts cannot be fulfilled by the responder.

8. The right to have access at all times to any needed augmentative and alternative communication devices and other assistive devices and to have those devices in good working order.

9. The right to environmental contexts, interactions, and opportunities that expect and encourage persons with disabilities to participate as full communicative partners with other people, including peers.

10. The right to be informed about the people, things, and events in one's immediate environment.

11. The right to be communicated with in a manner that recognizes and acknowledges the inherent dignity of the person being addressed, including the right to be part of communication exchanges about individuals that are conducted in his or her presence.

12. The right to be communicated with in ways that are meaningful, understandable, and culturally and linguistically appropriate.

FIGURE 19–2. Communication bill of rights. (From *Guidelines for Meeting the Communication Needs of Persons with Severe Disabilities* by the National Joint Committee for the Communication Needs of Persons with Severe Disabilities, 1992.)

(work, household management, and play/school), and leisure. An interviewer asks patients or caregivers to think about a typical day to identify activities in these areas that they want to do, need to do, or are expected to do. The interviewer then asks which of the activities the person is able to do satisfactorily and to rate the importance of these activities on a 10-point scale. Using the importance ratings, the interviewer asks the patient or caregiver to select the five problems that seem to be the most important and asks if the activities should be the focus of intervention. After the patient or caregiver selects activities for intervention, the person rates the current performance of each on a 10-point scale, from "not able to do it at all" to "able to do it extremely well," and rates satisfaction on a 10-point scale, from "not satisfied at all" to "extremely satisfied." Performance, satisfaction, and total scores are then calculated for each activity. Following a period of intervention,

outcomes can be measured by asking the patient or caregiver to again rate performance and satisfaction of each activity, and change scores can be calculated. Change scores are a useful measure of change across all goals for one child or as a measure of change across children.

SINGLE-SUBJECT RESEARCH METHODOLOGIES

Single-subject research methodologies are another useful means to assess intervention outcomes in clinical, educational, and other service settings. As described in Chapter 7 of this volume, these methodologies can be used to assess the outcomes for a single child or can assess effects of intervention across several children (Harris, 1991). McEwen and Karlan (1989) used an alternating treatment single-subject design to compare the effect of positioning in a chair, stander, prone wedge, and sidelyer on the ability of two preschool children to access a switch placed in several locations on a communication board–like grid. As shown in Figure 19–3, the data revealed that it took longer for both of the children to press the switch when they were in the sidelyer than when in the other three positions.

TRANSITION TO ADULTHOOD

Some children with cognitive impairments, especially those with severe and profound multiple disabilities, have need for physical therapy throughout their childhood years and during their transition to adulthood. The type of services provided will change with the needs of the child, as will the intensity of services and the service delivery model employed. Therapists working in public schools are especially likely to be involved in the transition to adulthood because Part B of the Individuals with Disabilities Education Act now requires that transition planning begin by at least age 14 for all students in special education.

The transition to adulthood is difficult for many young people, regardless of their abilities or disabilities. Until relatively recently, most young adults with cognitive impairments had few options available to them, and the greater their cognitive impairments, the fewer options they had. Employment options either did not exist or were limited to sheltered work-shops or activity centers. Residential options usually included staying at home with aging parents or moving into a large residential facility. They also had few choices about how they spent their time, with whom they spent time, or where they could go.

In recent years more employment and community life options have become available for people with cognitive impairments, including those with the most severe multiple disabilities. To be able to take full advantage of these options, young people need to prepare for transition to adult life throughout their years in school and then continue to receive support as the transition takes place and the new life begins. Physical therapy services can often make a critical difference in the options available to young people with both cognitive and neuromotor impairments as they make the transition to adult life and in the success of their transitions. Employment and residential options are especially important for most young people.

Employment

Employment options in the United States for people with cognitive impairments and multiple disabilities have expanded greatly over the past several years, particularly in some parts of the country. There are still many places in which sheltered work-shops, activity centers, and unemployment are the only alternatives, but progress is being made nation-

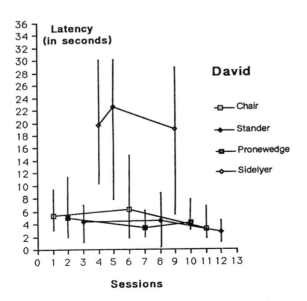

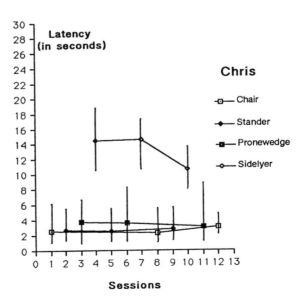

FIGURE 19–3. A single-subject alternating treatment design assessing means and ranges of switch-activation latency when two children were positioned in a chair, stander, prone wedge, and sidelyer. (From McEwen, IR, & Karlan, GR. Assessment of the effects of position on communication board access by individuals with cerebral palsy. Augmentative and Alternative Communication, 5:238–239, 1989. Copyright 1989 by the International Society for Augmentative and Alternative Communication.)

wide as federal, state, and other public and private initiatives support development and expansion of employment opportunities for people with disabilities (Bates, 1989; Cimera, 1998).

Supported employment, one model of employment services, has been responsible for increasing the employment options for those who have severe disabilities. Supported employment not only provides assistance to identify and acquire a job but also provides a person with ongoing support to learn how to do the job and to keep the job. There is no need to wait until a person is "ready" to do a job through sheltered training or "prevocational" activities, which usually fail to lead to meaningful, integrated employment even after long periods of time.

Since the early 1980s, supported employment has been gaining credibility as a viable employment option and received significant support from the Vocational Rehabilitation Act Amendments of 1986 (PL 99-506), which authorized new funds for states to provide supported employment services to people with severe disabilities. As yet, however, few communities offer a supported employment alternative to sheltered workshops and day activity centers for those with the most severe disabilities. The economic value of supported employment was indicated by Cimera (1998), who studied the cost-efficiency of supported employment programs and found that (1) supported employment is a cost-efficient way to serve people with severe mental retardation and multiple disabilities; (2) supported employment is cost-efficient from the cost-accounting perspective of the client, the taxpayer, and society; and (3) projections of lifelong benefits suggested that all individuals, regardless of the severity or number of disabilities, can be served cost-effectively in supported employment.

Physical therapy can often have a pivotal role in the successful employment of individuals who have both cognitive impairments and limited motor skills. Physical therapists can assist employment specialists to assess an individual's abilities to perform job-related motor skills and to identify jobs that are compatible with those skills. They can also identify assistive technology and environmental modifications that may enable the person to perform a job that might not be possible otherwise. Physical therapists can also help develop training for job-related motor skills and for self-care and mobility during working hours.

Residential Options

Most children with cognitive impairments live with their birth parents or with foster families. Some live in congregate residential facilities, such as state institutions for people with cognitive impairments, but many states have limited admission of children to such facilities in recent years (Willer & Intagliata, 1984). Although it was once believed that placement outside the home was the best alternative for children with cognitive impairments, public policy, education, and professional opinion now promote inclusion of most children in their natural homes (Blacher et al., 1992; Brown et al., 1989).

The factors associated with out-of-home placement of children with disabilities have been of concern to a number of researchers in recent years. Degree of cognitive impairment, maladaptive behaviors, and physical disability are variables that have been shown to predict whether children with cognitive impairments will be placed out of their homes (Meyers et al., 1985; Sherman, 1988). Other research suggests that ethnic background also may play a role in placement decisions, with more Anglo children being placed than African-American, Hispanic, or other ethnic groups (Blacher et al., 1992). Family characteristics, such as needs and resources, are also likely to influence whether a child is placed out of the home (Cole & Meyer, 1989).

With the current emphasis on deinstitutionalization and providing supports needed by families to keep their children with disabilities at home, planning for residential transitions has become an important part of their service programs as children with disabilities approach adulthood. The available residential options depend largely on the philosophies of those providing residential services; funding from state, federal, and other agencies; and the needs of the individual (Brown et al., 1989).

Large institutions are rarely considered a viable residential option today. Group homes for three to six people, located among other homes in residential neighborhoods, are about as large as facilities can be and still provide opportunities for integration into the neighborhood and community (Brown et al., 1989). Such living arrangements in the United States can be designated as an intermediate care facility for the mentally retarded, thus qualifying for Medicaid funds to provide the necessary staff and services. Residential options can also include living alone, or with one to three others in a house, apartment, or duplex, with the necessary support services.

Although community-living options for people with severe disabilities have increased steadily over the past decade, they still are limited in most communities, and necessary support services often are not available, either because of lack of funds or personnel shortages (Smull & Bellamy, 1991). Whatever the residential future of children with cognitive and neuromotor impairments, physical therapy services can often help expand the options, ease the transition, and promote independence within the residential environment.

CASE HISTORY
ALISE

Alise is 32 months old and has received home-based early intervention services since age 8 months. She has lissencephaly (also known as smooth brain syndrome), which was identified when she was 5 months old and had a seizure. Alise lives with her parents and 12-year-old brother in a suburb of a large city.

When Alise was 8 months old she did very little. She had great difficulty moving against the force of gravity, did not have head control, and could not roll over, sit, reach for objects, or grasp objects placed in her hands. She did not appear to make eye contact with people or objects and had difficulty sucking from a bottle and swallowing. The evaluation team conducted an arena assessment to document Alise's eligibility for early intervention services, including administration of the Battelle Developmental Inventory (BDI) (Newborg et al., 1984). At age 8 months, Alise's age-equivalent scores were in the birth to 2-month range in all developmental areas.

During the meeting to develop the Individualized Family Service Plan (IFSP), a top-down approach was used to first identify outcomes of intervention and then the strategies to achieve them. Alise's parents said that what they wanted most for Alise was for her to be able to roll over and sit by herself. They were also concerned about her vision and the difficulty she had swallowing without choking while drinking from her bottle.

A transdisciplinary model of service delivery was used by the early intervention program, and the team selected the physical therapist to be the primary service provider because Alise's parents were primarily concerned about her motor problems. The occupational therapist and a vision specialist would consult with the physical therapist to address the feeding and vision concerns, and other team members would be available for consultation as other needs were identified.

The physical therapist made weekly visits to Alise's home, working with Alise, her parents, and her brother to promote Alise's ability to move in opposition to the force of gravity, to eat more effectively, and to attend visually to people and objects in her environment (Figs. 19-4 and 19-5). A plastic booster chair with a tray, which is widely available for typical infants, was modified to enable Alise to maintain a seated position while on the floor or at the table. A stroller was also adapted for her.

Two years later, at 2 years 8 months, Alise can now maintain a sitting position when placed on the floor, drink liquids and eat ground foods without difficulty, and easily focus on and track objects and people. She is still unable to assume a sitting position, roll, or move about on the floor. She has particular difficulty using her hands and holds only her bottle, if it is placed in her hands, and will occasionally reach for her favorite fuzzy rubber ball. She sometimes uses her mouth to get things that she wants and will raise her legs when she is on her back in bed and wants to be picked up. She says approximately 10 words, including "no," "ahm"

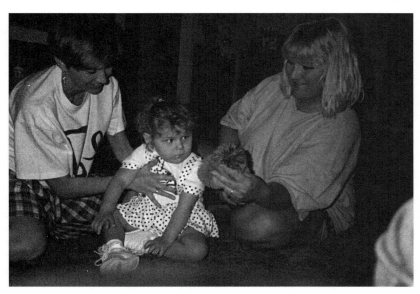

FIGURE 19-4. Physical therapist showing Alise's mother how to help her learn to move from a sitting position.

(mom), "da" (dad), and an approximation of her brother's name. Assistive equipment she now uses includes an adapted high chair, booster chair, and stroller; a prone stander; a walker with a tray; and a bath seat.

Two months ago, when Alise was 30 months old, her IFSP was updated. The desired outcomes identified by her parents were (1) that Alise would learn to get into and out of sitting by herself, (2) that she would learn to move around on the floor, and (3) that she would be able to play with toys with her hands. Because Alise's family continued to be primarily concerned about her motor development, the physical therapist remained the primary service provider. The IFSP also included a plan to prepare for Alise's transition from the early intervention program when she turns 3. Her mother wants Alise to stay at home until she is 5, so the early intervention team must identify the services that Alise and her family will need and determine how they can be obtained through other community agencies, such as the local education agency or developmental disabilities services.

CASE HISTORY
AMY

Amy's case illustrates an application of the *Guide to Physical Therapist Practice (Guide)* (American Physical Therapy Association, 1997) for a child with cognitive impairment in a public school setting. The process for "patient/client management" described in the *Guide* is

not always consistent with the team-oriented process used for making decisions about physical therapy services in schools. The terms *patient* and *client* also are inappropriate for school-based practice, where physical therapists usually refer to children as "students" or "children." Notes throughout the case example indicate other variations in the process described in the *Guide* that are necessary to provide appropriate school-based services.

Based on prior knowledge of Amy, the physical therapist identified the preferred practice patten as Neuromuscular Pattern A: Impaired Motor Function and Sensory Integrity Associated with Congenital or Acquired Disorders of the Central Nervous System in Infancy, Childhood, and Adolescence. Information about Amy and the process that her school team used to develop her IEP are summarized as follows, according to the *Guide's* five elements of patient/client (student) management.

Examination

History

General demographics. Amy is an 8-year-old girl. English is her family's native language.

Social history. Amy lives with her mother, father, and 12-year-old brother. Her mother is a nurse and her father owns a heating and air conditioning company. Amy participates in many family activities, such as church, camping, and car trips during the summer.

Occupation/employment. Amy is in a general third-grade class in her neighborhood elementary school, where she, her teacher, and a classroom assistant receive supports and services from a special education teacher, physical therapist, occupational therapist,

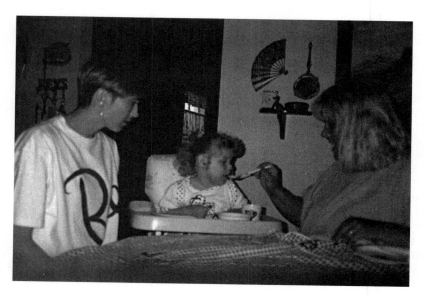

FIGURE 19–5. Physical therapist doing an ecological assessment of Alise's mealtime in her home.

and speech-language pathologist. For special education eligibility purposes, Amy is classified as having multiple disabilities.

Growth and development. When Amy was about 6 months old her mother became concerned because she did not seem to look at people and objects, did not reach for objects, and could not roll over. When she was 8 months old she was diagnosed with spastic quadriplegic cerebral palsy. The most recent norm-referenced developmental test was administered when she was 6 years old. At that time her age-equivalent scores on the Battelle Developmental Inventory (Newborg et al., 1984) were personal-social, 7 months; adaptive, 5 months; motor, 4 months; communication, 6 months; and cognitive, 5 months. Her school team believes that further norm-referenced testing would not be helpful.

Living environment. Amy lives with her parents and brother in a one-story house. The family has a van with a lift for Amy's wheelchair.

History of current condition. Note: The *Guide* states that the ''history of current condition'' should include ''patient/client, family, significant other, and caregiver expectation and goals for the therapeutic intervention.'' Although families may have expectations for physical therapy at this step in the process, a more appropriate process is for the child's team, including the family, to identify overall educational goals for the child, then later determine if physical therapy is necessary to achieve the goals (Giangreco et al., 1998).

Amy's parents said that they were concerned because Amy is so passive, does so little, and seems interested in so few things. They have three priorities for her education (1) that she learn to choose things, people, and activities that she wants; (2) that she become someone that other people like to be with because one of the things she seems to enjoy is being with other children; and (3) that she learn to help more during caregiving activities because she is becoming heavier and more difficult to handle and move.

Functional status and activity level. Amy will look when her name is called, smiles when people she likes talk with her, and enjoys being around other children. She often will close her eyes and drop her head when she does not have the attention of other people. Amy cannot grasp objects, but occasionally will reach toward objects. She eats ground foods fed from a spoon and drinks liquids from a cup. She is dependent on others for all self-care and mobility.

Medications. She takes Dilantin twice a day for seizures.

Other tests and measures. Amy is below the 99th percentile for weight and height. A report of a nutrition evaluation 6 months ago indicated that Amy was adequately nourished but recommended increasing the amount of calcium and protein in her diet.

Past history of current condition. Amy received home-based early intervention services, including physical therapy, from age 9 months to 3 years. From age 3 to 5 years she was in a half-day neighborhood preschool program, where she received physical therapy, occupational therapy, special education, and speech-language pathology services provided by her school district. When she was 5 years old she entered her neighborhood kindergarten, and since that time she has been included in general education classes.

Past Medical/Surgical History. When Amy was 5 years old she had bilateral achilles tendon and adductor lengthening. Two years later, she had a right varus derotation osteotomy for a subluxed hip.

Family history. Not known.

Health status. Amy's health generally is good, although she usually gets pneumonia at last once a year. Her seizure disorder is well controlled with medication. She usually sleeps through the night if someone turns her once.

Social habits. Amy moves very little, leading to a low level of physical fitness, which puts her at risk for cardiopulmonary disease as she grows older.

Systems review

Physiologic and anatomic status. Amy's severe neuromuscular impairments are likely to influence her cardiopulmonary, integumentary, and musculoskeletal status, which must be kept in mind when identifying goals and interventions. Her physiologic and anatomic status also may require consultation with or referral to a physician.

Communication, affect, cognition, language, and learning style. Amy is a passive child whose communication and cognitive development are far below those of typical 8-year-olds.

Tests and measures. Note: In a school environment, members of students' educational teams other than the physical therapist often administer tests and measures to examine some of the areas listed in the *Guide*. All team members then share results when developing the IEP. Some information was gathered formally using standardized methods or tools; other information was based on observation or prior knowledge. Other students' teams might have different expertise and be responsible for different areas. An occupational therapist on another team, for example, may know more about swallowing than a speech-language pathologist, or a physical therapist may know more about sensory integration than an occupational therapist.

Evaluation

The team met to discuss the information that each contributed to the development of Amy's IEP. Amy has many impairments, functional limitations, and disabilities, most of which the team agreed will not improve with intervention. The team also agreed that Amy's parents' concerns should be priorities in determining Amy's IEP goals. The physical therapist expressed concern that range-of-motion examination indicated that Amy's hip and knee range of motion had decreased since the last measurements 3 months previously.

Diagnosis. The physical therapist decided to use the Gross Motor Function Classification System (Palisano et al., 1997) to identify a diagnosis. Amy was functioning at the most limited level, Level V: Self-Mobility Is Severely Limited Even with the Use of Assistive Technology. This diagnosis is not used for special education and related services purposes.

Prognosis. The physical therapist and the rest of the team agreed that the prognosis for improving Amy's primary neuromuscular impairments was poor, but the prognosis for preventing secondary musculoskeletal impairments was more hopeful. The prognosis for improvement of functional limitations and disabilities also was poor, but the team agreed that with consistent and appropriate instruction, Amy probably could learn to help herself more, as her parents wished.

Note: The *Guide* states that as the next step in the prognostic process, the physical therapist should develop the plan of care, which includes the goals and outcomes, the specific direct interventions, and the frequency of visits and duration of the episode of care. In the educational environment, physical therapists do not make these decisions unilaterally. With the physical therapist's input, the team, including the student when appropriate, determines a student's goals. The *Guide* defines "goals" as remediation of impairments and "outcomes" as remediation of functional limitation, secondary or primary prevention of disability, and optimization of patient/client satisfaction. In Part B of IDEA, goals are the functional skills the student is expected to be able to achieve (reduction of functional limitations and disabilities). Part B does not use the term *outcomes.*

Plan of care. Note: In schools, the term *plan of care* is not used, but the IEP serves a similar purpose.

Amy's team wrote the following goals for her IEP:

1. Amy will indicate her choice of a person, activity, or object at least 10 times each day at school and 10 times at home for 5 consecutive days by May 20__.

2. When engaged in an activity with her classmates, Amy will interact with them by such means as looking at them, smiling, reaching, or vocalizing for at least 3 of 10 minutes during two activities on 5 consecutive school days by May 20__.

3. Amy will assist in transferring from her wheelchair by leaning forward when touched on the shoulder and asked to stand up and then bear her full weight after being assisted to a standing position during 10 consecutive transfers from her wheelchair by May 20__.

The team then wrote a sequence of benchmarks or short-term instructional objectives leading to each goal (not mentioned in the *Guide,* but required by IDEA). After writing the objectives, the team decided who would be necessary to help Amy achieve each objective and what each would contribute. The team also identified the general supports that Amy needs to attend school and to achieve her goals. Giangreco and associates (1998) described five categories of general supports, including supports needed to meet personal, physical, and sensory needs; to teach others about the student; and to provide the student with access and opportunities. The supports identified for Amy were as follows:

1. Personal: feeding, diaper changing, and other self-care
2. Physical: positioning and mobility
3. Sensory: avoiding intense stimuli, which cause Amy to withdraw
4. Teaching: teaching other children about Amy, her means of communication, and how to help her participate in activities
5. Access: promoting hand use during classroom activities

The team decided that her educational goals could best be met in a general education classroom, with supplemental aids and services. They agreed that a segregated special education setting was not only unnecessarily restrictive but that a general education classroom was more likely to provide the social and educational environment necessary to help Amy accomplish her goals. Supplemental aids and services in the general education classroom include a half-time assistant assigned to the classroom and ongoing consultation between Amy's classroom teacher and her special education team (a resource teacher, an occupational therapist, a physical therapist, and a speech-language pathologist).

The team decided that Amy's physical therapist was needed to help her achieve the third goal, involving transfers, and with the physical supports of positioning and mobility. The therapist also would help with motor aspects of other goals and consult with the physical education teacher about how to include Amy in activities that are meaningful for her. The physical therapist proposed and the team agreed that the physical therapist would see Amy and her classroom staff (teachers and classroom assistant) for 1 hour three times a week for the first 2 weeks of school, twice a week for the next 2 weeks, then once a week for 3 months, and then twice a month until the end of the school year. Over the school year, the physical therapist would provide 32 hours of service, or 32 "visits" (a term not used on an IEP).

Intervention

Physical therapists working in schools provide (1) coordination, communication, and consultation; (2) student-related instruction; and (3) direct intervention, as delineated in the *Guide*. To provide the necessary positioning and mobility supports, the physical therapist first determined that Amy's wheelchair was adequate for her needs (direct intervention). She also consulted with Amy's classroom teacher to determine which alternatives to wheelchair positioning would be used during which activities and who would be responsible for position changes. Positions and activities were matched to enable Amy to function as well as possible throughout the day. She uses a supine stander, for example, during a morning science class, which usually involves groups of students standing around tables as they work on a project together. She also stands in the afternoon during art class because her hand use seems to be better when she is standing.

The therapist taught the teacher and assistant how to place Amy in her wheelchair and other positioning devices (student-related instruction), about some of the basic mechanics of the wheelchair, and how to push the chair safely. She also taught Amy's classmates how to push Amy safely and issued wheelchair pushing licenses to those who demonstrated safe pushing techniques (student-related instruction). Other supports provided by the physical therapist were to teach Amy's teacher, the assistant, and her classmates some ways to encourage Amy to raise her head and use her hands during classroom activities, and to teach the assistant methods to use during caregiving activities, especially diaper changing, to help maintain Amy's joint flexibility (student-related instruction). The assistant also used diaper changing, when Amy was supine, as an opportunity to teach basic social interaction skills.

To help Amy achieve the goal of assisting with transfers, the physical therapist first worked with Amy to identify how best to help her to learn (direct intervention). She found that, although Amy could perform some aspects of a transfer, such as lean forward to prepare to stand, she usually would not, either spontaneously or when asked. She also did not place her feet on the floor as she was moved toward a standing position and did not bear her weight when placed on her feet. To teach Amy to assist with these components of the transfer, the physical therapist consulted with the special education resource teacher to develop a behavioral program. The program included (1) providing verbal and natural cues for a transfer (such as the presence of the supine stander), physical prompts, and reinforcement for leaning forward in her wheelchair, a motor behavior that was already within Amy's repertoire; (2) providing cues, physical prompts, and reinforcement during practice to learn to place her feet on

the floor and bear increasing amounts of weight, during transfers and other activities, to shape these skills, which were not yet within Amy's repertoire; (3) chaining the various components of the transfer, as Amy began to learn each one; and (4) eventually fading the verbal cues and physical prompts to permit the natural cues surrounding transfers to prompt Amy's participation.

After she was reasonably sure that the program developed to teach Amy to lean forward was effective, the physical therapist taught Amy's teacher, the classroom assistant, and her parents to implement the techniques whenever Amy transferred (student-related instruction). Because Amy had not demonstrated the ability to place her feet on the floor and bear her weight in standing, the physical therapist worked with Amy during transfers and other classroom activities to determine how best to provide physical prompts and other cues and to teach Amy to begin to learn to stand (direct intervention). She then taught Amy's teacher, the assistant, and her parents how to help Amy continue to develop this skill (student-related instruction).

Reexamination. Part B of IDEA requires that each short-term objective have an evaluation procedure and a schedule for evaluation to determine progress toward the goals and objectives. This is consistent with the "reexamination" step of the *Guide*. The physical therapist and the rest of Amy's team continuously observed her performance to evaluate her progress, and they modified or redirected the intervention, as necessary. Her progress toward meeting each of the IEP objectives was evaluated according to the timelines specified on the IEP.

Criteria for discharge. Note: The *Guide* says that discharge (a term not used in schools) is "based on the physical therapist's analysis of the achievement of anticipated goals . . . and desired outcomes." Reasons for discontinuing services in schools are consistent with the reasons outlined in the *Guide,* except that the physical therapist does not independently make the decision to discontinue services. The physical therapist may give the rest of the team rationale for discontinuing, but the team makes the decision, based on the student's need for physical therapy to achieve goals and provide necessary supports.

C A S E   H I S T O R Y
JEFF

Jeff is a 20-year-old who recently moved from Sunnyvale, a state residential facility for people with developmental disabilities, to a boarding house in the small town where his parents live. Three other young adults with disabilities live at the boarding house, and

TABLE 19–3. Example of an Ecological Assessment

Name: Jeff
Activity: Shopping
Environment: Dan's One-Stop

Steps Required	Jeff's Current Performance	Steps Can Acquire	Steps May Not Acquire	Compensatory Strategies	Intervention*
1. Go from home to Dan's and back using electric wheelchair.	Can open front door (outward), go down ramp and drive to the corner. Cannot go down curb (no curb cut), cross street safely, or go up curb. Once on the sidewalk, can drive to Dan's. Cannot open store door from outside. Can maneuver inside store and open door when leaving (outward). Cannot open door of home when returning.	1. Open doors of home and store when the door opens toward him; 2. go down curb; 3. ask for assistance and tell someone how to help him up a curb; and 4. cross the street safely.	Go up a curb without assistance.	Curb cuts.	1. Teach Jeff to open doors, go down curbs, and cross streets safely (PT, PCA). 2. Talk with city about making curb cuts and with store and house manager about modifying doors (Jeff, CM). 3. Program communication aid to request help with curbs and give instructions (mother, PT).
2. Select items in the store.	Does not always remember what he needs to get and cannot make or read a shopping list. Can get items that are at hand level, cannot shift weight or extend arm to reach low or high items.	1. Make and use shopping list; 2. improve ability to reach high and low items; and 3. ask for assistance to get out-of-reach items.	Reach items that are very high or very low.	A reacher?	Teach Jeff 1. to make and use a shopping list (OT, PCA); 2. to use a reacher, if it seems feasible (OT, PCA); and 3. to reach to higher and lower shelves (PT, PCA).
3. Carry items to checkout stand.	Cannot maneuver shopping cart. Items slide off lap, does not want to use tray.	Carry items in a bag or other container on lap or chair.	Push a grocery cart without endangering store and other people	Bag or other container that is accessible to Jeff.	Find container and teach Jeff to use it (OT and PCA).

*Note: Those involved with each intervention are determined after the intervention is identified. At this time, Jeff has the assistance of his personal care assistant (PCA), case manager (CM), mother, occupational therapist (OT), and physical therapist (PT).

Continued

TABLE 19-3. Example of an Ecological Assessment—cont'd

Steps Required	Jeff's Current Performance	Steps Can Acquire	Steps May Not Acquire	Compensatory Strategies	Intervention*
4. Put items on counter.	Can put items on counter, but is very slow, which annoys people in line behind him.	1. Put container on counter so clerk can remove items; or 2. ask for assistance	1. Increase speed sufficiently; or 2. lift full container to counter.	None.	1. Try to improve speed and lifting of container (PT, PCA); and program communication aid and teach Jeff to ask for assistance (mother and PCA).
5. Pay for purchases.	Cannot get wallet out of pocket, cannot get money out of wallet. Does not recognize denominations of bills or coins, cannot pay correct amount or check change.	1. Get money out of suitable container; 2. recognize bills and coins; and 3. give sufficient money to cover the purchase.	1. Get wallet out of pocket or money out of wallet; and 2. determine if change is accurate.	1. Use an accessible container for money; and 2. ask personal care assistant to compare bill and change occasionally.	1. Find accessible container for money and teach Jeff to use it (OT, PCA); and 2. teach Jeff to use money (OT, mother, PCA).
6. Carry purchases home.	Can carry small bag on lap, cannot carry large bag(s).	Carry purchases in container attached to chair.	Carry large or multiple bags on lap.	Alternate container (probably the same as in 3, above).	Find appropriate container for purchases (OT, PCA).
7. Put purchases away.	Can open cupboards with flat surfaces or knobs, drawers with knobs, and the refrigerator. Cannot open high or low cupboards or drawers with flat surfaces. Can put purchases away in places he can open and reach.	1. Open all drawers he can reach; and 2. put items away in higher and lower places.	Put items in very high or low places.	1. Make adaptations to allow Jeff to open kitchen drawers he can reach. 2. Rearrange cupboards and drawers so items Jeff uses are accessible.	1. Discuss adaptations and rearrangement with house manager (OT); and 2. improve Jeff's reach (also in 2, above) (PT, PCA).

*Note: Those involved with each intervention are determined after the intervention is identified. At this time, Jeff has the assistance of his personal care assistant (PCA), case manager (CM), mother, occupational therapist (OT), and physical therapist (PT).

they invited Jeff to live with them after he visited with them several months ago.

Jeff has spastic quadriplegic cerebral palsy and moderate cognitive impairments and had lived at Sunnyvale since he was 7 years old. For the first 9 years he spent most of his time in bed, receiving basic care but little education or habilitative services other than passive range-of-motion exercises.

When Jeff was 18, physical therapy and other services were expanded as a result of a court order. Since then, Jeff acquired and learned to use an electronic communication aid and an electric wheelchair. The chair has a custom-contoured seat and back to accommodate his moderate scoliosis, pelvic asymmetry with windswept hips, and lower extremity flexion contractures, which developed in spite of the passive range-of-motion exercises. He also learned to assume a standing position and bear much of his weight during assisted transfers. Bilateral ankle-foot orthoses, improved positioning in bed and wheelchair, active participation during all transfers, and use of good alternative positioning appear to have helped limit progression of his musculoskeletal deformities.

In preparation for Jeff's transition to the boarding house, his physical therapist, occupational therapist, and mother took him there for an ecological assessment to determine what skills Jeff needed to live there successfully. He can get help with dressing, bathing, and laundry, if necessary, but he has to be able to use the toilet independently and transfer to and from his bed without assistance. He also has to be able to use the telephone, make his own breakfast and lunch, and go shopping in a nearby grocery-variety store (see ecological assessment in Table 19–3, format from Baumgart et al., 1982).

To prepare for his move, Jeff's physical therapist worked with him on the aspects of toilet transfers and shopping identified by the ecological assessment, simulating what he will encounter in the community. Before Jeff moved, he, his therapists, and his mother spent several days at the boarding house going through a typical day to help Jeff generalize skills he learned at Sunnyvale to the boarding house and to identify problems and the means to overcome them.

When he moved to the community, Jeff enrolled in the local high school and a new IEP was written. Two of Jeff's educational goals relate to improving his independence at home and obtaining, learning, and keeping a job. His school physical therapist works with Jeff and his personal care assistant to increase his independence in his home and is working with his job coach to identify a job that Jeff can learn. Once a job is found, his physical therapist will also help Jeff learn to use public transportation and to use the toilet at work and will provide ongoing consultation with the job coach to solve problems as they arise.

The physical therapist's involvement to help Jeff become more independent in his home and work environments is directed toward reducing his disabilities. Positioning and orthoses are used to reduce functional limitations and prevent the development of additional musculoskeletal impairments. For Jeff, it is also important that he maintain or increase his flexibility and endurance. For this reason, the physical therapist helped Jeff find a YMCA in his community that has an accessible swimming pool and a gym in which he can work out. In collaboration with YMCA staff, the therapist and Jeff developed an exercise program that is appropriate for Jeff's needs and that he can carry out with the assistance of YMCA personnel. The physical therapist is available to serve as a consultant as needed.

Recommended Resources

PUBLICATIONS

Brown, DA, Effgen, SK, & Palisano, RJ. Performance following ability-focused physical therapy intervention in individuals with severely limited physical and cognitive abilities. Physical Therapy, 78:934–950, 1998.

Downing, JE. Including Students with Severe and Multiple Disabilities in Typical Classrooms: Practical Strategies for Teachers. Baltimore: Paul H. Brookes, 1996.

Giangreco, MF, Cloninger, CH, & Iverson, VS. Choosing Options and Accommodations for Children: A Guide to Educational Planning for Students with Disabilities, 2nd ed. Baltimore: Paul H. Brookes, 1998.

McEwen, IR, & Shelden, ML. Pediatric physical therapy in the 1990s: The demise of the educational versus medical dichotomy. Physical and Occupational Therapy in Pediatrics, 15:33–45, 1995.

Orelove, FP, & Sobsey, D (Eds.). Educating Children with Multiple Disabilities: A Transdisciplinary Approach, 3rd ed. Baltimore: Paul H. Brookes, 1996.

Rainforth, B, & York-Barr, J. Collaborative Teams for Students with Severe Disabilities: Integrating Therapy and Educational Services, 2nd ed. Baltimore: Paul H. Brookes, 1997.

ORGANIZATIONS AND THEIR JOURNALS

American Association on Mental Retardation (AAMR)
444 North Capitol Street, NW
Suite 846
Washington, DC 20001-1512
Phone: 202-387-1968 or 800-424-3688
E-mail: info@aamr.org
Internet: http://www.aamr.org
Journals: *American Journal on Mental Retardation (AJMR)* is a scholarly research journal. *Mental Retardation (MR)* is a practitioner's journal of research, reviews, and opinions.

TASH
29 W. Susquehanna Avenue
Suite 210
Baltimore, MD 21204
Phone: 410-828-8274
E-mail: info@tash.org
Internet: http://www.tash.org
Journal: *Journal of the Association for Persons with Severe Handicaps*

References

American Association on Mental Retardation. Mental Retardation: Definition, Classification, and Systems of Supports, 9th ed. Washington, DC: American Association on Mental Retardation, 1992.

American Physical Therapy Association. Guide to Physical Therapist Practice. Alexandria, VA: American Physical Therapy Association, 1997.

Anwar, F. Cognitive deficit and motor skill. In Ellis, D (Ed.), Sensory Impairments in Mentally Handicapped People. San Diego: College-Hill Press, 1986, pp. 169–183.

Aughton, DJ, & Cassidy, SB. Physical features of Prader-Willi syndrome in neonates. American Journal of Diseases of Children, 144:1251–1254, 1990.

Bates, P. Vocational training for persons with profound disabilities. In Brown, F, & Lehr, DH (Eds.), Persons with Profound Disabilities: Issues and Practices. Baltimore: Paul H. Brookes, 1989, pp. 265–293.

Baumgart, D, Brown, L, Pumpian, I, Nisbet, J, Ford, A, Sweet, M, Messina, R, & Schroeder, J. Principle of partial participation and individualized adaptations in educational programs for severely handicapped students. The Journal of the Association for the Severely Handicapped, 7(2):17–27, 1982.

Benson, JB, & Uzgiris, IC. Effect of self-initiated locomotion on infant search activity. Developmental Psychology, 21:923–931, 1985.

Berg, JM, McCreary, BD, Ridler, MAC, & Smith, GF. The de Lange Syndrome. New York: Pergamon Press, 1970.

Bergsma, D. Birth Defects: Atlas and Compendium. Baltimore: Williams & Wilkins, 1973.

Bertenthal, BI, Campos, JJ, & Barrett, KC. Self-produced locomotion: An organizer of emotional, cognitive, and social development in infancy. In Emde, RN, & Harmon, RJ (Eds.), Continuities and Discontinuities in Development. New York: Plenum, 1984.

Bijou, SW. A functional analysis of retarded development. In Ellis, NR (Ed.), International Review of Research in Mental Retardation, Vol. 1. New York: Academic Press, 1966, pp. 1–19.

Blacher, JB, Hanneman, RA, & Rousey, AB. Out-of-home placement of children with severe handicaps: A comparison of approaches. American Journal of Mental Retardation, 96:607–616, 1992.

Brown, DA, Effgen, SK, & Palisano, RJ. Performance following ability-focused physical therapy intervention in individuals with severely limited physical and cognitive abilities. Physical Therapy, 78:934–950, 1998.

Brown, F, Davis, R, Richards, M, & Kelly, K. Residential services for adults with profound disabilities. In Brown, F, & Lehr, DH (Eds.), Persons with Profound Disabilities: Issues and Practices. Baltimore: Paul H. Brookes, 1989, pp. 295–331.

Brown, L, Branston, MB, Hamre-Nietupski, S, Pumpian, I, Certo, N, & Gruenewald, L. A strategy for developing chronological age appropriate and functional curricular content for severely handicapped adolescents and young adults. Journal of Special Education, 12:81–90, 1979.

Burgemeister, BB, Blum, LH, & Lorge, I. Manual: Columbia Mental Maturity Scale, 3rd ed. New York: Psychological Corporation, 1972.

Butler, C. Augmentative mobility: Why do it? Physical Medicine and Rehabilitation Clinics of North America, 2:801–815, 1991.

Butler, C, Okamoto, GA, & McKay, TM. Powered mobility for very young disabled children. Developmental Medicine and Child Neurology, 25:472–474, 1983.

Campbell, FA, & Ramey, CT. High risk infants: Environmental risk factors. In Berg, JM (Ed.), Science and Service in Mental Retardation: Proceedings of the Seventh Congress of the International Association for the Scientific Study of Mental Deficiency (IASSMD). New York: Methuen, 1985, pp. 23–33.

Campbell, PH. Dysfunction in posture and movement with individuals with profound disabilities. In Brown, F, and Lehr, DH (Eds.), Persons with Profound Disabilities: Issues and Practices. Baltimore: Paul H. Brookes, 1989, pp. 163–189.

Campbell, PH. Evaluation and assessment in early intervention for infants and toddlers. Journal of Early Intervention, 15:36–45, 1991.

Campbell, SK. Central nervous system dysfunction in children. In Campbell, SK (Ed.), Pediatric Neurologic Physical Therapy, 2nd ed. New York: Churchill Livingstone, 1991, pp. 1–17.

Campos, JJ, & Bertenthal, BI. Locomotion and psychological development in infancy. In Jaffe, KM (Ed.), Childhood Powered Mobility: Developmental, Technical and Clinical Perspectives: Proceedings of the RESNA First Northwest Regional Conference. Washington, DC: RESNA, 1987, pp. 11–42.

Carr, SH. Louisiana's criteria of eligibility for occupational therapy services in the public school system. American Journal of Occupational Therapy, 43:503–506, 1989.

Carter, CH. Handbook of Mental Retardation Syndromes, 2nd ed. Springfield, IL: Charles C. Thomas, 1970.

Chandler, LS, & Adams, MA. Multiply handicapped child motivated for ambulation through behavior modification. Physical Therapy, 52:339–401, 1972.

Chinitz, SP, & Feder, CZ. Psychological assessment. In Molnar, GE (Ed.), Pediatric Rehabilitation, 2nd ed. Baltimore: Williams & Wilkins, 1992, pp. 48–87.

Chugani, HT. A critical period of brain development: Studies of cerebral glucose utilization with PET. Preventive Medicine, 27:184–188, 1998.

Cimera, RE. Are individuals with severe mental retardation and multiple disabilities cost-efficient to serve via supported employment programs? Mental Retardation, 36:280–292, 1998.

Cole, DA, & Meyer, LH. Impact of needs and resources on family plans to seek out-of-home placement. American Journal on Mental Retardation, 93:380–387, 1989.

Cole, KN, Mills, PE, & Harris, SR. Retrospective analysis of physical and occupational therapy progress in young children: An examination of cognitive referencing. Pediatric Physical Therapy, 3:185–189, 1991.

Downing, J. Active versus passive programming: A critique of IEP objectives for students with the most severe disabilities. Journal of the Association for Persons with Severe Handicaps, 13:197–201, 1988.

Drotar, D, Mortimer, J, Shepherd, PA, & Fagan, JF. Recognition memory as a method of assessing intelligence of an infant with quadriplegia. Developmental Medicine and Child Neurology, 31:391–394, 1989.

Eagle, RS. Deprivation of early sensorimotor experience and cognition in the severely involved cerebral-palsied child. Journal of Autism and Developmental Disabilities, 15:269–283, 1985.

Ellis, NR. Handbook of Mental Deficiency: Psychological Theory and Research. London: McGraw-Hill, 1963.

Evans, IM. Testing and diagnosis: A review and evaluation. In Meyer, LH, Peck, CA, & Brown, L (Eds.), Critical Issues in the Lives of People with Severe Disabilities. Baltimore: Paul H. Brookes, 1991, pp. 25–43.

Evans, IM, & Scotti, JR. Defining meaningful outcomes for persons with profound disabilities. In Brown, F, & Lehr, DH (Eds.), Persons with Profound Disabilities: Issues and Practices. Baltimore: Paul H. Brookes, 1989, pp. 83–107.

Fagan, JF, & Shepherd, PA. The Fagan Test of Infant Intelligence Training Manual. Cleveland: Infatest Corporation, 1987.

Falvey, MA. Introduction. In Falvey, MA (Ed.), Community-Based Curriculum: Instructional Strategies for Students with Severe Handicaps. Baltimore: Paul H. Brookes, 1989, pp. 1–13.

Ferguson, DL, & Baumgart, D. Partial participation revisited. Journal of the Association for Persons with Severe Handicaps, 16:218–227, 1991.

Fogel, A, Dedo, JY, & McEwen, IR. Effect of postural position and reaching on gaze during mother-infant face-to-face interaction. Infant Behavior and Development, 15:231–244, 1992.

Foley, GM. Arena evaluation: Assessment in the transdisciplinary approach. In Gibbs, ED, & Teti, DM (Eds.), Interdisciplinary Assessment of Infants: A Guide for Early Intervention Professionals. Baltimore: Paul H. Brookes, 1990, pp. 271–286.

Giangreco, MF. Letter to the editor. American Journal of Occupational Therapy, 44:470, 1990.

Giangreco, MF, Cloninger, CH, & Iverson, VS. Choosing Options and Accommodations for Children: A Guide to Educational Planning for Students with Disabilities, 2nd ed. Baltimore: Paul H. Brookes, 1998.

Gibbs, ED. Assessment of infant mental ability: Conventional tests and issues of prediction. In Gibbs, ED, & Teti, DM (Eds.), Interdisciplinary Assessment of Infants: A Guide for Early Intervention Professionals. Baltimore: Paul H. Brookes, 1990, pp. 77–89.

Grossman, HJ. Classification in Mental Retardation. Washington, DC: American Association on Mental Retardation, 1983.

Guess, D, Mulligan-Ault, M, Roberts, S, Struth, J, Siegel-Causey, E, Thompson, B, Bronicki, GJB, & Guy, B. Implications of biobehavioral states for the education and treatment of students with the most profoundly handicapping conditions. Journal of the Association for Persons with Severe Handicaps, 13:163–174, 1988.

Gustafson, GE. Effects of the ability to locomote on infants' social and exploratory behaviors: An experimental study. Developmental Psychology, 20:397–405, 1984.

Haney, M, & Falvey, MA. Instructional strategies. In Falvey, MA (Ed.), Community-Based Curriculum: Instructional Strategies for Students with Severe Handicaps. Baltimore: Paul H. Brookes, 1989, pp. 63–90.

Harris, SR. Functional abilities in context. In Lister, MJ (Ed.), Contemporary Management of Motor Control Problems: Proceedings of the II Step Conference. Alexandria, VA: Foundation for Physical Therapy, 1991, pp. 253–259.

Harris, SR, & Shea, AM. Down syndrome. In Campbell, SK (Ed.), Pediatric Neurologic Physical Therapy, 2nd ed. New York: Churchill Livingstone, 1991, pp. 131–168.

Holm, VA, & King, HA. Scoliosis in the Rett syndrome. Brain Development, 12:151–153, 1990.

Horn, EM. Basic motor skills instruction for children with neuromotor delays: A critical review. Journal of Special Education, 25:168–197, 1991.

Houghton, J, Bronicki, GJB, & Guess, D. Opportunities to express preferences and make choices among students with severe disabilities in classroom settings. Journal of the Association for Persons with Severe Handicaps, 12:18–27, 1987.

Jankovic, J, Caskey, TC, Stout, JT, & Butler, IJ. Lesch-Nyhan syndrome: A study of motor behavior and cerebrospinal fluid neurotransmitters. Annals of Neurology, 23:466–469, 1988.

Jones, ED, & Payne, JS. Definition and prevalence. In Patton, JR, Payne, JS, & Beirne-Smith, M (Eds.), Mental Retardation, 2nd ed. Columbus, OH: Charles E. Merrill, 1986, pp. 33–75.

Jones, KL. Smith's Recognizable Patterns of Human Malformation, 5th ed. Philadelphia: WB Saunders, 1997.

Kaufman, A, & Kaufman, N. Kaufman Assessment Battery for Children. Circle Pines, MN: American Guidance Service, 1983.

Keenan, J, Kastner, T, Nathanson, R, Richardson, N, Hinton, J, & Cress, DA. A statewide public and professional education program on fragile X syndrome. Mental Retardation, 30:355–361, 1992.

Kelleher, A, & Mulcahy, M. Patterns of disability in the mentally handicapped. In Berg, JM (Ed.), Science and Service in Mental Retardation: Proceedings of the Seventh Congress of the International Association for the Scientific Study of Mental Deficiency (IASSMD). New York: Methuen, 1985, pp. 15–22.

Kermoian, R, & Campos, JJ. Locomotor experience: A facilitator of spatial cognitive development. Child Development, 59:908–917, 1988.

Kochanek, TT, Kabacoff, RI, & Lipsitt, LP. Early identification of developmentally disabled and at-risk preschool children. Exceptional Children, 56:528–538, 1990.

Kolb, B, Forgie, M, Gibb, R, Gorny, G, & Rowntree, S. Age, experience and the changing brain. Neuroscience and Biobehavioral Reviews, 22(2):143–159, 1998.

Kopp, CB, & McCall, RB. Predicting later mental performance for normal, at-risk, and handicapped infants. In Baltes, PB, & Brim, OG (Eds.), Life-Span Development and Behavior. New York: Academic Press, 1982, pp. 33–61.

Landesman-Dwyer, S, & Sackett, GP. Behavioral changes in nonambulatory, profoundly mentally retarded individuals. In Meyers, CE (Ed.), Quality of Life in Severely and Profoundly Mentally Retarded People: Research Foundations for Improvement. Washington, DC: American Association on Mental Deficiency, 1978, pp. 55–144.

Laurance, BM, Brito, A, & Wilkinson, J. Prader-Willi syndrome after age 15 years. Archives of Disease in Childhood, 56:181–186, 1981.

Law, M, Baptiste, S, Carswell, A, McColl, MA, Polatajko, H, & Pollock, N. Canadian Occupational Performance Measure, 2nd ed. Toronto: Canadian Association of Occupational Therapists, 1994.

Leiter, R. The Leiter International Performance Scale. Chicago: Stoelting, 1969.

Lutzker, JR, McGimsey-McRae, S, & McGimsey, JF. General description of behavioral approaches. In Hersen, M, Van Hasselt, VB, & Matson, JL (Eds.), Behavior Therapy for the Developmentally and Physically Disabled. New York: Academic Press, 1983, pp. 25–56.

Maloney, FP, & Kurtz, PA. The use of a mercury switch head control device in profoundly retarded, multiply handicapped children. Physical and Occupational Therapy in Pediatrics, 2(4):11–17, 1982.

McCall, RB. Issues in the early development of intelligence and its assessment. In Lewis, M, & Taft, L (Eds.), Developmental Disabilities: Theory, Assessment and Intervention. New York: SP Medical and Scientific Books, 1982, pp. 177–184.

McEwen, IR. Assistive positioning as a control parameter of social-communicative interactions between students with profound multiple disabilities and classroom staff. Physical Therapy, 72:634–647, 1992.

McEwen, IR, & Karlan, GR. Assessment of effects of position on communication board access by individuals with cerebral palsy. Augmentative and Alternative Communication, 5:235–242, 1989.

McEwen, IR, & Shelden, ML. Pediatric physical therapy in the 1990s: The demise of the educational versus medical dichotomy. Physical and Occupational Therapy in Pediatrics, 15:33–45, 1995.

McGonigel, MJ, Woodruff, G, & Roszmann-Millican, M. The transdisciplinary team: A model for family-centered early intervention. In Johnson, LJ, Gallagher, RJ, LaMontagne, MJ, Jordan, JB, Gallagher, JJ, Huntinger, PL, & Karnes, MB (Eds.), Meeting Early Intervention Challenges: Issues from Birth to Three, 2nd ed. Baltimore: Paul H. Brookes, 1994, pp. 95–131.

McLaren, J, & Bryson, SE. Review of recent epidemiological studies of mental retardation: Prevalence, associated disorders, and etiology. American Journal on Mental Retardation, 92:243–254, 1987.

Meyers, CE, Borthwick, SA, & Eyman, RK. Place of residency by age, ethnicity, and level of retardation of the mentally retarded/developmentally disabled population of California. American Journal on Mental Deficiency, 90:266–270, 1985.

National Joint Committee for the Communicative Needs of Persons with Severe Disabilities. Guidelines for meeting the communication needs of persons with severe disabilities. ASHA, 34(suppl 7):1–8, 1992.

Navajas, D, Farre, R, Mar Rotger, M, Milic-Emili, J, & Sanchis, J. Effect of body posture on respiratory impedance. Journal of Applied Physiology, 64:194–199, 1988.

Newborg, J, Stock, JR, Wnek, L, Guidubaldi, J, & Svinicki, J. Battelle Developmental Inventory. Chicago: Riverside Publishing, 1984.

Nihira, K, Foster, R, Shellhaas, M, & Leland, H. AAMD Adaptive Behavior Scale, rev. ed. Washington, DC: American Association on Mental Deficiency, 1974.

Nomura, Y, & Segawa, Y. Characteristics of motor disturbance in Rett syndrome. Brain Development, 12:27–30, 1990.

Nwaobi, OM. Seating orientations and upper extremity function in children with cerebral palsy. Physical Therapy, 67:1209–1212, 1987.

Nwaobi, OM, & Smith, PD. Effect of adaptive seating on pulmonary function of children with cerebral palsy. Developmental Medicine and Child Neurology, 28:351–354, 1986.

Nyhan, WL, & Sakati, NO. Genetic and Malformation Syndromes in Clinical Medicine. Chicago: Year Book Medical Publishers, 1976.

O'Neill, DL, & Harris, SR. Developing goals and objectives for handicapped children. Physical Therapy, 62:295–298, 1982.

Orelove, FP, & Sobsey, D. Designing transdisciplinary services. In Orelove, FP, & Sobsey, D (Eds.), Educating Children with Multiple Disabilities: A Transdisciplinary Approach, 3rd ed. Baltimore: Paul H. Brookes, 1996, pp. 1–33.

Palisano, R, Rosenbaum, P, Walter, S, Russell D, Wood E, & Galuppi, B. Gross Motor Function Classification System for Cerebral Palsy. Developmental Medicine and Child Neurology, 39:214–223, 1997.

Parette, HP, Jr, & Hourcade, JJ. How effective are physiotherapeutic programmes with young mentally retarded children who have cerebral palsy? Journal of Mental Deficiency Research, 28:167–175, 1984.

Rainforth, B. OSERS clarifies legality of related services eligibility criteria. TASH Newsletter, April 1991, p. 8.

Rainforth, B, & York-Barr, J. Collaborative Teams for Students with Severe Disabilities: Integrating Therapy and Educational Services, 2nd ed. Baltimore: Paul H. Brookes, 1997.

Ramey, CT, & Ramey, SL. Effective early intervention. Mental Retardation, 30:337–345, 1992.

Raven, J. Raven's Progressive Matrices. Dumfries, Scotland: Crichton Royal, 1958.

Reid, DH, Phillips, JF, & Green, CW. Teaching persons with profound multiple handicaps: A review of the effects of behavioral research. Journal of Applied Behavior Analysis, 24:319–336, 1991.

Rinck, C. Fragile X syndrome. Dialogue on Drugs, Behavior and Developmental Disabilities (University of Missouri), 4(3):1–4, 1992.

Rothstein, JR, & Echternach, JL. Hypothesis-oriented algorithm for clinicians: A method for evaluation and treatment planning. Physical Therapy, 66:1388–1394, 1986.

Sents, B, & Marks, H. Changes in preschool children's IQ scores as a function of positioning. American Journal of Occupational Therapy, 43:685–687, 1989.

Sherman, BR. Predictors of the decision to place developmentally disabled family members in residential care. American Journal on Mental Retardation, 92:344–351, 1988.

Shumway-Cook, A, & Woollacott, MH. Dynamics of postural control in the child with Down syndrome. Physical Therapy, 65:1315–1322, 1985.

Siegel-Causey, E, & Downing, J. Nonsymbolic communication development: Theoretical concepts and educational strategies. In Goetz, L, Guess, D, & Stremel-Campbell, K (Eds.), Innovative Program Design for Individuals with Dual Sensory Impairments. Baltimore: Paul H. Brookes, 1987, pp. 15–48.

Smull, MW, & Bellamy, GT. Community services for adults with disabilities: Policy challenges in the emerging support paradigm. In Meyer, LH, Peck, CA, & Brown, L (Eds.), Critical Issues in the Lives of People with Severe Disabilities. Baltimore: Paul H. Brookes, 1991, pp. 527–536.

Snell, ME, & Zirpoli, TJ. Intervention strategies. In Snell, ME (Ed.), Systematic Instruction of Persons with Severe Handicaps, 3rd ed. Columbus, OH: Charles E. Merrill, 1987, pp. 110–149.

Sparrow, SS, Balla, DA, & Cichetti, CV. Vineland Adaptive Behavior Scales. Circle Pines, MN: American Guidance Service, 1984.

Stewart, KB, Brady, DK, Crowe, TK, & Naganuma, GM. Rett syndrome: A literature review and survey of parents and therapists. Physical and Occupational Therapy in Pediatrics, 9(3):35–55, 1989.

Switzky, HN, Woolsey-Hill, J, & Quoss, T. Habituation of visual fixation responses: An assessment tool to measure visual sensory-perceptual cognitive processes in nonverbal profoundly handicapped children in the classroom. AAESPH Review, 4:136–147, 1979.

Tarjan, G, Wright, SW, Eyman, RK, & Keeran, DV. Natural history of mental retardation: Some aspects of epidemiology. American Journal on Mental Deficiency, 77:369–379, 1973.

TASH force strikes again: Laski and Boyd win Oberti case in New Jersey. TASH Newsletter, November 1992, pp. 1–2.

Telzrow, RW, Campos, JJ, Shepherd, A, Bertenthal, BI, & Atwater, S. Spatial understanding in infants with motor handicaps. In Jaffe, KM (Ed.), Childhood Powered Mobility: Developmental, Technical and Clinical Perspectives: Proceedings of the RESNA first Northwest Regional Conference. Washington, DC: RESNA, 1987, pp. 62–69.

Terman, LM, & Merrill, MA. Stanford-Binet Intelligence Scales, 3rd rev. Boston: Houghton Mifflin, 1973.

Thurman, SK, & Widerstrom, AH. Infants and Young Children with Special Needs: A Developmental and Ecological Approach. Baltimore: Paul H. Brookes, 1990.

United Cerebral Palsy National Infant Collaborative Project. Staff Development Handbook: A Resource for the Transdisciplinary Process. New York: United Cerebral Palsy Association, 1976.

Verburg, G, Naumann, S, Balfour, L, & Snell, E. Remote training of mobility skills in persons who are physically and developmentally disabled. Proceedings of the RESNA 13th Annual Conference. Washington, DC: RESNA, 1990, pp. 195–196.

Wechsler, D. Wechsler Intelligence Scale for Children—Revised. New York: Psychological Corporation, 1974.

Willer, B, & Intagliata, J. An overview of the social policy of deinstitutionalization. In Ellis, N, & Bray, N (Eds.), International Review of Research in Mental Retardation, Vol. 12. New York: Academic Press, 1984.

Witkin, SL, & Fox, L. Beyond the least restrictive environment. In Villa, RA, Thousand, JS, Stainback, W, & Stainback, S (Eds.), Restructuring for Caring and Effective Education. Baltimore: Paul H. Brookes, 1992, pp. 325–334.

Wolery, M, & Dyk, L. Arena assessment: Description and preliminary social validity data. Journal of the Association for Persons with Severe Handicaps, 9:231–234, 1984.

Zazula, JL, & Foulds, RA. Mobility device for a child with phocomelia. Archives of Physical Medicine and Rehabilitation, 64:137–139, 1983.

Zelazo, PR, & Weiss, MJ. Infant information processing: An alternative approach. In Gibbs, ED, & Teti, DM (Eds.), Interdisciplinary Assessment of Infants: A Guide for Early Intervention Professionals. Baltimore: Paul H. Brookes, 1990, pp. 129–143.

Zucker, SH, & Polloway, EA. Issues in identification and assessment in mental retardation. Education and Training in Mental Retardation, 22:69–76, 1987.

CHAPTER
20

Cerebral Palsy

SANDRA J. OLNEY, BSc(P&OT), MEd, PhD
MARILYN J. WRIGHT, BScPT, MEd

Cerebral palsy (CP) is the neurologic condition most frequently encountered by pediatric physical therapists. It is a permanent but not unchanging neurodevelopmental impairment caused by a nonprogressive defect or lesion in single or multiple locations in the immature brain. The defect or lesion can occur in utero or during or shortly after birth and produces motor impairment and possible sensory deficits that are usually evident in early infancy (Scherzer & Tscharnuter, 1990). CP involves one or more limbs and frequently the trunk. It causes disturbances of voluntary motor function and produces a variety of symptoms. Nevertheless, CP is itself an artificial concept, comprising several causes and clinical syndromes that have been lumped together because of a commonality of management. The impaired control and coordination of voluntary muscles is accompanied by mental retardation or learning disabilities in 50 to 75% of children and by disorders of speech (25%), auditory impairments (25%), seizure disorders (25–35%), or abnormalities of vision (40–50%) (Batshaw & Perret, 1992; Schanzenbacher, 1989). Social and family problems may occur secondary to the presence of primary deficits.

In few conditions do therapists play such a central role or have as much potential to influence the outcome of children's lives. Their interventions have not only immediate but also lifelong effects, and can be efficient and cost-effective. Treatment of children is specialized: therapists provide services that will help them reach their full potential in their homes and communities. Furthermore, decisions about many medical interventions such as orthopedic surgery and spasticity management usually rely on input from physical therapists. The therapist's influence is not restricted to the medical center and treatment gymnasium, but frequently includes consultation regarding the child's functioning in settings within the home, school, recreation, and community environments. Good therapy not only helps the child with CP but also can have a positive influence on the child's family and caregivers. In summary, parents of children with disabilities want services that provide general and specific information about their child, provide coordinated and comprehensive care, and are provided by respectful and supportive professionals (King et al., 1998). The pediatric physical therapist is ideally suited to fill these roles.

533

This chapter discusses the background of cerebral palsy—the classification, etiology, and pathophysiology; prevention; associated impairments; and determinants of outcomes. Physical therapy examination, evaluation, and intervention that are related to each age between infancy and adulthood are discussed. The chapter concludes with two case histories.

NATURE AND CHARACTERISTICS OF CEREBRAL PALSY

Classification, Etiology, and Pathophysiology

CP has been classified in a number of ways. A classification based on the area of the body exhibiting impairment yields the designations of monoplegia (one limb), diplegia (lower limbs), hemiplegia (upper and lower limbs on one side of the body), and quadriplegia (all limbs). Another classification, based on the most obvious movement abnormality resulting from common brain lesions, yields spastic, dyskinetic, and ataxic types. The spastic type, in which the muscles are perceived as excessively stiff and taut, especially during attempted movement, results from involvement of the motor cortex or white matter projections to and from cortical sensorimotor areas of the brain. Involvement of the basal ganglia is reflected in dyskinesia or athetosis and sometimes in intermittent muscular tension of the extremities or trunk and involuntary movement patterns. A cerebellar lesion produces ataxia, or general instability of movement. A hypotonic classification, not known to be related to a particular lesion, is characterized by diminished resting muscle tone and decreased ability to generate voluntary muscle force. Symptoms of spasticity and dyskinesia may both be present in a child, with the type of CP referred to as mixed. The degree of severity of CP varies greatly, and the designations mild, moderate, and severe are often applied within types. The Gross Motor Disability Classification System is a five-level, age-categorized system that places children with CP into categories of severity that represent clinically meaningful distinctions in motor function (Palisano et al., 1997). Although the proportions of the various subtypes of CP vary with the reporting source, a series from Sweden noted that hemiplegia accounted for 36.4%; diplegia, 41.5%; quadriplegia, 7.3%; dyskinesia or athetosis, 10%; and ataxic forms, 5% (Hagberg et al., 1989a).

CP is a condition with multiple causes leading to damage within the central nervous system. Although the causes are not completely understood, certain prenatal, perinatal, and postnatal factors have been associated with CP (Torfs et al., 1990). There is gen-eral agreement that the majority of cases of CP in term infants are due to prenatal or unknown causes, whereas in the vast majority of preterm infants the lesion causing CP develops during the perinatal period. Preterm birth, although not believed to be causative, is associated with up to 33% of all cases, including more than 50% of diplegia (Pharoah et al., 1990), 25% of hemiplegia (Uvebrandt, 1988), and 5% of quadriplegia (Edebol-Tysk, 1989). Prenatal malnutrition, intrinsic developmental problems of the fetus, poor maternal prenatal condition, and maternal infection are also associated with CP (Menkes, 1990). Intracranial hemorrhage, especially among premature infants, is a well-established causal factor. Neonatal asphyxia is a significant perinatal event, but only a small minority of cases result from such events (Nelson & Ellenberg, 1986). Infection in the perinatal period is also important. The effects of hyperbilirubinemia and other blood incompatibilities frequently resulting in athetoid CP are a concern, particularly in developing countries.

The statistics from developing countries are in sharp contrast to those of developed countries. Studies have suggested that up to 63% of cases in the former have preventable causes associated with shortage of care personnel and inadequate financing for effective services (Karumuna & Mgone, 1990; Nottidge & Okogbo, 1991).

The dramatic decrease in perinatal mortality in developed countries during the 1980s, largely a result of improved survival rates for low birth weight infants, has given rise to the fear of increased numbers of children with neurodevelopmental impairments. In fact, there was a steady-state incidence of CP of about 2.5 per 1000 live births until about the mid-1950s (Little, 1958), which was followed by a decrease in incidence to about 1.5 per 1000 for about 15 years. Since then, the incidence has increased to near mid-1950s levels, if Swedish statistics are typical (Hagberg et al., 1989b). The change in this trend mainly reflects changes in the live birth rate of preterm infants, especially in those with spastic diplegia. A study conducted between 1982 and 1994 of a cohort of 2076 consecutively born infants with birth weights of 500 to 1500 g (O'Shea et al., 1998) concluded that the increasing survival of very low birth weight infants has not resulted in an increased prevalence of cerebral palsy among survivors. The risk of CP increases sharply with decreasing birth weight (Atkinson & Stanley, 1983; Hagberg et al., 1989a; Pharoah et al., 1987) and has been reported to be as much as 40 times higher in infants weighing less than 1000 g (Hagberg et al., 1989b).

The increased risk of CP in preterm infants must be put in perspective, however. Reports of long-term outcome of extremely premature infants, that is, infants born between 24 and 28 weeks of gestational age, suggest about a 75% survival rate, with more than 50% of those who survive free of major neurodevelopmental impairments, about 25% with major impairments, and about 11% with CP (Msall et al., 1991).

Autopsies of infants have revealed three types of neuropathic lesions (Weinstein & Tharp, 1989): neuropathy resulting from hemorrhage below the lining of the ventricles (subependymal), encephalopathy caused by anoxia or hypoxia, and neuropathy resulting from malformations of the central nervous system.

Most subependymal hemorrhages occur in infants of less than 28 weeks of gestational age and those with low birth weight. Intraventricular hemorrhages, present in up to 46% of infants weighing less than 1500 g (Papile et al., 1978), are thought to develop secondary to lesions of ischemic origin. In most cases, blood ruptures into the lateral ventricle and the ensuing connective tissue blocks the cerebrospinal fluid flow, frequently resulting in hydrocephalus. Anoxic or hypoxic encephalopathy results in gray matter and white matter lesions. Gray matter lesions are diffusely present throughout the cortex, basal ganglia and thalamus, brainstem, and spinal cord, whereas lesions in the white matter are frequently in the periventricular zone. Periventricular atrophy has been identified as the most common abnormality found in preterm infants who developed hemiplegic CP, occurring in 50% of cases (Wiklund et al., 1991b). It is unclear, however, whether the lesions occur before, during, or after birth. Although periventricular atrophy is a bilateral lesion thought to be responsible for most cases of preterm spastic diplegia, it has also been reported as an asymmetric or unilateral lesion or one with bilateral lesions expressing only unilateral clinical symptoms (Wiklund et al., 1991b).

Malformations of the central nervous system may generate hemorrhagic and anoxic lesions. Many factors may be responsible, including drug ingestion, radiation, and infection by viruses such as herpes simplex and rubella.

Attempts to relate cerebral lesions to the extent of disability have had only limited success. With respect to the side of expression, in the small percentage of children with hemiplegia with bilateral morphologic findings, subtle physical abnormalities were sometimes seen on the nonhemiplegic side (Wiklund & Uvebrant, 1991a). Results suggest the existence of a continuum between hemiplegia and diplegia resulting from periventricular lesions. Magnetic resonance imaging showed that, of several measures, only the amount of white matter correlated with the severity of disability (Yokochi et al., 1991). In children with hemiplegia, no significant correlations between size of lesion and severity of impairment have been found, although trends toward the association of less impairment with smaller lesions have been reported (Molteni et al., 1987; Wiklund & Uvebrant, 1991a). Quadriplegia has been associated with brainstem and basal nuclei damage in addition to cortical and subcortical lesions (Wilson et al., 1982). Further discussion of the causes of the various types of CP can be found in works by Menkes (1990) and Weinstein and Tharp (1989).

Progress in Primary Prevention

The primary way to reduce the incidence of CP is through good socioeconomic health of the population coupled with maternal education. The role of poverty and low socioeconomic status in the prevalence of CP (Dowding & Barry, 1990) and in determining the need for special educational resources (Msall et al., 1991) has frequently been overlooked, yet there is empirical evidence of its importance.

Certain maternal prepregnancy and pregnancy-related risk factors are associated with delivery of a child with a disability (Holst et al., 1989). Studies have suggested that improved intrapartum diagnosis of risk factors, prevention of asphyxia, and medical treatment of children with low Apgar scores would reduce the incidence of disabilities, as would intervention to prevent premature rupture of membranes. However reasonable these hypotheses may seem, no studies are known to have tested them.

The role of the obstetrician in preventing CP before birth occurs is limited (Weinstein & Tharp, 1989). Attention is directed toward developing effective prevention of and intervention for premature delivery, fetal distress, neonatal asphyxia, and mechanical birth trauma. Methods of inhibiting labor have met with much success, although the effects on incidence of CP remain unclear. Methods of antepartum fetal evaluation, including sonographic measurement, electronic fetal monitoring, fetal pH monitoring, and intrauterine pressure monitoring, have provided the obstetrician with powerful tools for assessing the need for active intervention in the labor process. Delivery procedures using high forceps and certain presentations of breech deliveries that were found to be associated with increased perinatal morbidity have dramatically decreased in favor of cesarean section. This is partly due to the increased safety of cesarean birth for both the mother and the fetus.

Impairment

Early detection of CP facilitates optimal management by the family and the health care and educational community. Complicating the picture is the instability of diagnosis; CP is reported to disappear over time in many low birth weight infants (Kitchen et al., 1987). In a study designed to determine the accuracy of diagnosis of CP at 2 years of age (Kitchen et al., 1987), only 55% of those so diagnosed at age 2 were deemed to have CP at age 5, but the diagnosis of those with moderate or severe involvement did not change. Only 1% of children not diagnosed at age 2 were identified at age 5 to have CP. Of those children in whom the diagnosis was no longer accurate at age 5, most had minor neurologic abnormalities and left-hand preference, but their psychologic test scores were no different from those of children who had never been diagnosed as having CP.

Tests of neurologic status, motor function, primitive reflexes, and posture have been assessed for their ability to identify CP (Burns et al., 1989). Although assessments performed at age 1 month failed to identify several of the infants who later showed CP, assessments made at 4 months of age resulted in some overidentification. At 8 months of age, the presence of three or more abnormal signs was highly predictive of CP, and the authors concluded that all but the mildest cases of CP can be identified by that age. Formal tests have varying abilities to detect motor abnormalities (Harris, 1989). The sensitivity of the Movement Assessment of Infants (MAI) has been calculated to be 73.5% in a high-risk population (Harris, 1987). When compared with the Bayley motor scale (Bayley, 1993), the MAI identified more than 3 times as many children with diplegia at 4 months of age, more than 2 times as many children with hemiplegia, and about 1.5 times as many children with quadriplegia (Harris, 1989). In children at 1 year corrected age, however, the Bayley motor scale demonstrated sensitivities of 100% for both spastic diplegia and quadriplegia and 75% for spastic hemiplegia. Furthermore, the MAI has a lower rate of specificity than does the Bayley motor scale; that is, a greater percentage of children with normal outcomes are identified as being at risk.

Physical Therapy—Related Impairments

Impairments in CP are problems with the neuromuscular and skeletal systems that are either an immediate result of the existing pathophysiologic process or an indirect consequence that has developed over time. Impairments can be classified, somewhat artificially, into single-system impairments and multisystem impairments.

SINGLE-SYSTEM IMPAIRMENTS

Single-system impairments are expressed in the muscular system and the skeletal system, even though the pathophysiologic damage occurred in the central nervous system. Primary impairments such as insufficient force generation, spasticity, abnormal extensibility, and exaggerated or hyperactive reflexes are evident in the muscular system; malalignments such as femoral anteversion and femoral and tibial torsion (Cusick & Stuberg, 1992) are secondary impairments evident in the skeletal system.

CP is characterized by insufficient force generation by affected muscle groups, which is consistent with low levels of electromyographic (EMG) activity and decreased moment of force output (Berger et al., 1982). When an activity leads to an active contraction, this impairment may be expressed as a deficiency in power (Olney et al., 1990), or when considered over time, in work. The term *strength* may refer to any of these measurable factors. Strength measurement in neurologic conditions is problematic, but when measured, strength has frequently been intimately linked with functional capabilities such as speed of walking (Bohannon, 1989).

The clinical term *tone* is used to describe the impairments of spasticity and abnormal extensibility. A sensation of abnormally high tone may be caused by spasticity, a velocity-dependent overactivity that is proportional to the imposed velocity of limb movement. Spasticity is especially evident in children with clonus but is frequently mistaken for problems of extensibility. Supraspinal and interneuronal mechanisms appear to be responsible for spasticity, with increased "gain" in the muscle spindles and increased excitation of Ia afferents having been ruled out as a cause of spasticity (Young, 1994). There is experimental evidence for three pathophysiologic mechanisms: reduced reciprocal inhibition of antagonist motor neuron pools by Ia afferents, decreased presynaptic inhibition of Ia afferents, and decreased nonreciprocal inhibition by Ib afferents. There is considerable evidence indicating that reciprocal inhibition is reduced in cerebral palsy (Hallett & Alvarez, 1983; Leonard et al., 1991). Adding to this effect are recent elegant studies using transcranial magnetic cerebral stimulation that have provided evidence of simultaneous activation of antagonistic muscle groups through abnormal alpha motor neuron innervation (Brouwer & Ashby, 1991). The role of decreased presynaptic inhibition of Ia afferents in spasticity has been deduced from experiments showing that vibration-induced inhibition of the H-reflex is much less in spastic than in normal muscles, a phenomenon that has been shown to be mediated by a presynaptic mechanism in animal models. Finally, nonreciprocal inhibition has been reported to be reduced and even replaced by facilitation in persons exhibiting spasticity with sustained hypertonia (Young, 1994), which suggests that there may be a further mechanism responsible for abnormal alpha motor neuron excitability.

The sense of abnormally high tone can also result from hypoextensibility of the muscle because of abnormal mechanical characteristics. Comparing healthy children with children with CP, Berger and colleagues (1982) found that the EMG activity of leg muscles in nearly all children with CP was reduced in affected limbs and that there were no indications of pathologic reflex effects on muscle activity. A force transducer on the tendo Achilles measured tension that was disproportionate to muscle activity and could best be attributed to mechanical changes in the muscle rather than to increased stretch reflexes from spasticity. These muscles were also seen to be abnormally stiff; that is, they produced more force for a given length change than did muscles in non-disabled children (Tardieu et al., 1982). The most accurate term for this impairment is *hypoextensibility*. The muscle offers resistance to passive stretching at a shorter length than that expected in a normal muscle. In addition, if greater than normal amounts of force are required to produce a change in length, the muscle is said to have increased stiffness. This is represented as the passive tension curve for CP (p,CP) in Figure 20–1A, in contrast to the normal passive tension curve (p,N) in Figure 20–1D, when one moves the ankle from a position of plantar flexion to one of dorsiflexion. When a clinician finds that it is not possible to manually stretch the muscle through a normal range using reasonable amounts of manual force, the muscle group is deemed to have a contracture, represented in Figure 20–2 as "Contracture," the difference between the joint angle at which this extreme resistance is encountered in the CP muscle and that of the normal muscle.

Figure 20–1 shows hypothetical active force-length characteristics of spastic plantar flexors (a,CP; see Fig. 20–1B) and normal plantar flexors (a,N; see Fig. 20–1E), that is, the force generated by the contractile elements of the muscle over the range of muscle lengths from a shortened position (plantar flexed) to a longer position (dorsiflexed). Note that the maximal force is lower for the CP muscle and also that the peak force occurs at a more plantar-flexed position in the CP muscle than in the normal muscle. The sum of the combined effects of active force output and passive stiffness for the CP muscle is shown as total tension curve CP, and the corresponding curve for the normal muscle is shown as total tension curve N (see Fig. 20–2). The complexity of the representation in Figure 20–2 underlines the difficulty faced by a physical therapist or physician in correctly assessing the cause of increased tone through clinical methods such as passive manipulation of the limb and clinical assessment of muscle strength.

If a muscle complex has become overlengthened, which is usually a secondary impairment resulting from repeated mechanical stretch, it is termed *hyperextensible*. The overlengthened muscle complex may also have decreased force-generating capabilities.

Few studies of the histology and morphology of spastic muscle have been reported, but they have shown that differences are present when spastic muscle is compared with normal muscle (Romanini et al., 1989). The slowly contracting fibers of the spastic adductor muscles demonstrate hypertrophy, whereas the fast fibers show atrophy. Surprisingly, there has been no evidence of increase in endomysial or perimysial connective tissue at any age of child, regardless of the clinical picture. The authors concluded that joint restrictions are attributable to the atrophy of muscle fibers, which makes the muscle less elastic and extensible, and possibly to an increase of fibrous tissue in the periarticular structures, although the latter was not verified.

There are no universally accepted methods of measuring spasticity (Katz & Rymer, 1989), although techniques include measurement of forces in response to standard passive stretches (tonic) or standard hammer stimuli (phasic), Hoffmann's reflex recording (Jones & Mulley, 1982), and measurement of responses to sinusoidal cycling or ramp stretches (Lin et al., 1994; Price et al., 1991). The modified Ashworth scale, though commonly used in clinical situations, is really an undifferentiated measure of spasticity and extensibility. It has been shown to be reliable in adults with neurologic conditions, although reliability has not been established for children (Bohannon & Smith, 1987).

MULTISYSTEM IMPAIRMENTS

In the second group of impairments are three multisystem impairments expressed in the neuromuscular system: poor selective control of muscle activity, poor regulation of activity in muscle groups in anticipation of postural changes and body movement (referred to as anticipatory regulation), and decreased ability to learn unique movements.

In CP there is poor selective control of muscle activity. Normal movement is characterized by orderly phasing in and out of muscle activation, coactivation of muscles with similar biomechanical functions, and limited coactivation of antagonists during phasic or free movement. In CP there is abundant evidence of inappropriate sequencing (Nashner et al., 1983) and coactivation of synergists and antagonists (Knutsson & Martensson, 1980).

The reasons for poor selective control of muscle activity are unknown. Failure of the normal recipro-

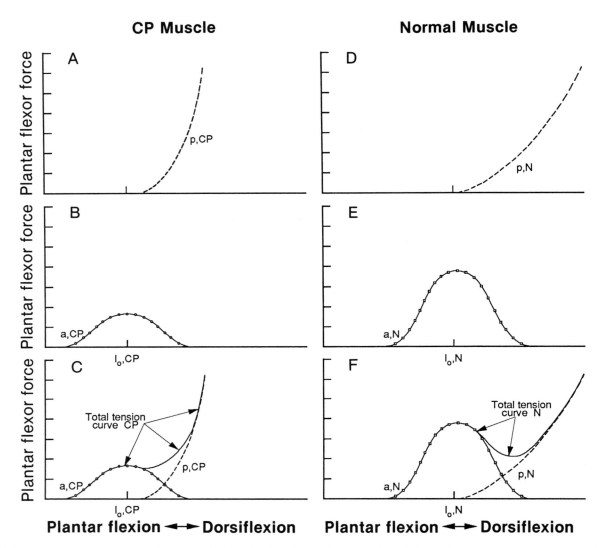

FIGURE 20–1. Representation of force capabilities of ankle plantar flexor muscle at different joint angles in normal muscle (N) and spastic muscle (CP). *A,* Resistance to passive stretch of spastic muscle (p,CP) increasing with more dorsiflexion. *B,* The force of active contraction (a,CP) varying with the joint angle, l_0 denoting resting length. *C,* The sum of the passive and active effects in spastic muscle. *D,* Resistance to passive stretch in normal muscle (p,N). *E,* Force of active contraction in normal muscle (a,N). *F,* The total tension curve comprising the sum of the passive and active effects in normal muscle. Note that 1) the slope (i.e., the stiffness) of p,CP in *A* is greater for the spastic muscle than for the normal muscles (p,N) in *D;* 2) the maximal active force achieved by the spastic muscle (a,CP) in *B* is less than the maximal active force of normal muscle (a,N) in *E;* and 3) the maximal active force for spastic muscle (a,CP) shown in *B* occurs at a more plantar-flexed position than that of the normal muscle (a,N) shown in *E.*

cal relationship of activity between agonist and antagonist muscles during voluntary movements has been observed (Berger et al., 1982; Hallett & Alvarez, 1983; Leonard et al., 1990), but whether segmental or supraspinal mechanisms or both are involved is unclear. Although Berbrayer and Ashby (1990) clearly demonstrated the presence of reciprocal inhibition in CP, it is not possible to exclude the possibility

that other spinal mechanisms may be impaired (Harrison, 1988). Direct evidence for a supraspinal origin is scant; however, researchers have concluded that in CP, the corticospinal projections are directed equally to the motoneurons of agonist and antagonist muscles of the ankle (Brouwer & Ashby, 1991). Reflex overflow to antagonist muscles in children with CP (Leonard et al., 1991) has been attributed

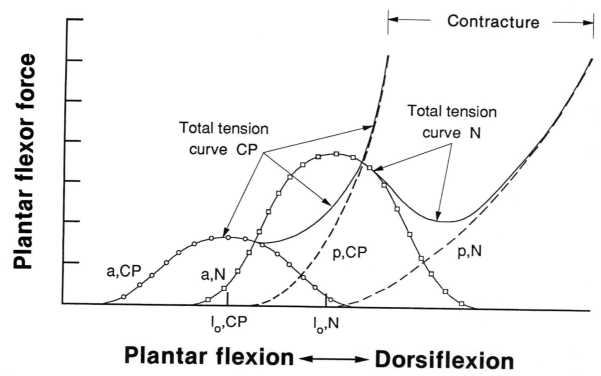

FIGURE 20–2. Complete representation of force capabilities of ankle plantar flexor muscle at different joint angles in normal muscle (N) and spastic muscle (CP) shown in Figure 20–1. a,CP = force of active contraction of spastic muscle; l_o,CP = resting length of spastic muscle; l_o,N = resting length of normal muscle; a,N = force of active contraction of normal muscle; p,CP = resistance to passive stretch of spastic muscle; p,N = resistance to passive stretch of normal muscle.

either to exuberant motoneuronal projections or to exuberant projections that extend to motoneurons innervating muscles other than the one being stimulated. From these studies, it appears certain that the neuronal "wiring" in CP is not normal.

Poor anticipatory regulation of muscle sequencing when postural correction is attempted has been reported by Nashner and colleagues (1983). In healthy individuals, changes in posture are preceded by preparatory muscle contractions that stabilize the body. In people with CP, the contraction that is needed to produce stability is frequently interrupted by destabilizing synergistic or antagonistic muscle activity.

There is some evidence that motor memory in children with CP is frequently impaired (Lesny et al., 1990). This finding is important in considering strategies for teaching movement, but it has received little attention to date.

Assessment of multisystem impairments usually involves measurement of a closely associated variable or number of variables and frequently involves dif-

ferent dimensions of the disabling process. Examination of the impairments of poor selective control of muscle activity, poor anticipatory regulation of muscle groups, and decreased ability to learn unique movements includes use of measures of balance, coordination, and motor control. Most are not in general clinical use. Two approaches to assessing balance are available: one is to disturb the supporting surface in a variety of ways (Nashner et al., 1983); the other is to perturb the subject or environment (Patla et al., 1989). In each case, kinematic, kinetic, and EMG responses are measured. Coordination has been documented with EMG records, which makes it possible to detect differences from normal records in timing of muscle activity onset and duration, in sequencing of agonists, and in co-contraction of antagonists. Gait has been the most commonly observed activity used to examine specific impairments of CP (Perry et al., 1976), and the potential for its wide clinical application has increased with the advent of fast and efficient computer systems.

Determinants of Prognosis or Outcome

About 90% of children with CP in developed countries survive to adulthood (Evans et al., 1990). Strauss and Shavelle (1998) found that the key predictors of a reduced life expectancy were lack of mobility and feeding difficulties. Survival of high-functioning adults was found to be close to that of the general population, but predictions of lifetime functional outcomes in CP are limited. A California study (Anonymous, 1991) reported that only 12 to 17% of people with CP registered with developmental services were competitively employed. Positive prognostic factors for employment included mild physical involvement, good family support, vocational training, and having good employment contacts. Mental retardation, seizures, and wheelchair dependency were factors reducing the likelihood of living independently. Senft and colleagues (1990) reported that more than 60% of registrants in a neuromuscular disability program were dependent on aging parents. In a review of the literature, Bleck (1987) included the following positive predictors of independence and employment of a person with CP: regular schooling, completion of secondary schooling, independence in mobility with the ability to travel beyond the home, good hand skills, living in a small rather than a large community, and having a diagnosis of spasticity rather than one of involuntary movements. Preliminary studies of life satisfaction suggest more positive outcomes, but few studies have included this important variable (Wacker et al., 1983).

Certain factors assist in predicting the ambulation potential of children with CP. Children with the hemiplegic type of CP usually have a good prognosis for ambulation, whereas the prognosis is less favorable for those with rigid or hypotonic types of CP (Crothers & Paine, 1988). Persistent tonic neck reflexes are associated with decreased likelihood of walking (Crothers & Paine, 1988). Some studies have reported that a remarkably large percentage of children who are able to sit independently by age 24 months eventually walk (Crothers & Paine, 1988) and that nearly all children with CP who eventually walk do so before 8 years of age (Bleck, 1975). Watt and colleagues (1989), examining all survivors of neonatal intensive care, have reported that nearly all who sat by 24 months of age walked 15 meters or more with or without assistive devices or orthoses by age 8 years. Independent sitting by 24 months remains the best predictor of ambulation, despite inclusion of neonatal variables, clinical types, primitive reflexes, and reactions (Watt et al., 1989).

EXAMINATION, EVALUATION, AND INTERVENTION

At all ages, the physical therapy examination of the child with CP will focus on the identification of disabilities, functional limitations, and impairments. In addition, physical therapy examination is used to measure change resulting from intervention at all levels of the disabling process and provide feedback to clients.

Physical therapists integrate information from the many aspects of their examination and evaluation with prognostic knowledge to predict the optimal level of improvement that can be expected. They then develop a plan of care that includes long-term and short-term goals and outcomes, specific interventions, and duration and frequency of intervention required to reach the goals and outcomes.

From infancy to adulthood, physical therapy goals for clients with CP should focus on the prevention of disability by minimizing the effects of functional limitations and impairments, preventing or limiting secondary impairments, maximizing the gross motor functions allowed by the organic deficits, and helping the child compensate for functions when necessary. Achieving these goals involves the promotion and maintenance of musculoskeletal integrity, the prevention of secondary impairment and deformity, the enhancement of optimal postures and movement to promote functional independence, and optimal levels of fitness.

The presence of impairments, such as low levels of force generation, spasticity, abnormal extensibility, and disturbed reflexes, can result in abnormal weight bearing and malalignment, which can, in turn, affect the orthopedic development of the spine and the extremities. The application of correct forces is required for optimal skeletal modeling before the skeleton ossifies (LeVeau & Bernhardt, 1984), although the research reported to date has offered little specific guidance. Of particular concern is the effect of increased hip flexion and adduction on acetabular development and hip joint stability. Neck and trunk asymmetry can result in torticollis or spinal deformities. At all ages, children with hypoextensibility and spasticity are prone to developing contractures. Although patterns of tightness vary, commonly at risk for contractures are the shoulder adductors; the elbow, wrist, and finger flexors; the hip flexors and adductors; the knee flexors; and the ankle plantar flexors (Massagli, 1991).

Furthermore, the physical therapist attempts to prevent environmental deprivation that could increase existing disabilities and attempts to provide support, guidance, and education for the child, the family, and the community. Goals are individualized for the particular child and family. They should be determined in collaboration with the family and based on the needs, expectations, and values of the whole family (Rosenbaum et al., 1998). Goal and outcome attainment should be regularly reassessed so that the therapy plan is adapted to reflect changes in the child's progress and the family's needs. An important component of therapy programs is education of the child and family about the disability to enable them to become capable of advocating and taking responsibility for their future.

The involvement of other health care professionals in the treatment of the infant with CP depends on the child's needs and the practices of the institution where the program occurs. Some facilities may have professionals from several disciplines working with the family, whereas at others it may be thought better to have a primary therapist initially, bringing in others for assessment or treatment as necessary. Regardless of practice approach, parents value coordination of care and consistency of service providers.

Increasing emphasis on the costs of provision of services and managed care have led some institutions to develop critical paths. This is a difficult task for CP due to the diversity of presentation and the chronic nature of the condition. An example of an outline of care for CP is the document *Cerebral Palsy—Critical Elements of Care*, which was developed by the Washington State Department of Health (1997).

Infancy

The life role of an infant is to grow and develop in response to being loved and nurtured by parents and caregivers in a home environment. Despite being dependent in most aspects of life, infants interact with, and develop an understanding of, the people in their lives, their surroundings, and themselves. From the time of birth, a child with CP may not experience the normal activities associated with infancy. As a result, the parents of an infant with CP may not receive the positive feedback of a normal nurturing experience and the satisfaction of observing the development of motor and social skills, that is, the normal rewards of caring for an infant. The parents must cope with the impact of the diagnosis and the grieving process that accompanies the awareness that their expectations of having a normal child will not be realized. They may be overwhelmed with the uncertainty that the future holds for them, their child, and their family. Many parents are also concerned with the immediate issues of providing basic infant care and are apprehensive about incorporating the specialized care necessary for their child's optimal development.

Movement is an important component in the learning and interactive processes of infancy. In infants who have CP, the nature and extent of their impairments affect their potential to develop and learn through movement. This may result in functional limitations in the development of gross motor skills and may affect their ability to interact with their parents, themselves, and their environment.

Physical Therapy Examination and Evaluation

Infant examination provides a baseline for the monitoring of improvement or deterioration, growth, maturation, and treatment effects. Therapists must determine the history, living environment, and social supports of an infant and the knowledge level and concerns of the family. Examination of impairment involves qualitative and, when possible, quantitative evaluation of the single-system and multisystem impairments. Observation of active range of motion (ROM) provides indirect assessment of the force-generating ability of muscle groups and some information about muscle extensibility. Determination of the passive ROM, using a slow, maintained stretch in a position that promotes relaxation, assesses muscle group extensibility and provides information about joints, such as the presence of dislocation. Normal maturational changes in joint range and alignment must be considered in evaluating the significance of measures.

Passive movement performed with greater velocity is used to assess spasticity and the sensitivity of the stretch reflex. Spasticity can be documented descriptively on the basis of resistance to movement and observations of spontaneous active movement and posturing. The severity of spasticity—whether it is mild, moderate, or severe—its distribution over the body and limbs, and its variations under different conditions should be noted. Frequently, there are variations in spasticity associated with positioning and the infant's effort and behavior. The modified Ashworth scale (Bohannon & Smith, 1987) or the muscle tone section of the MAI can be used (Chandler et al., 1980).

The presence or persistence of primitive reflexes and the development of the postural reactions of equilibrium, righting, and protective extension are assessed to determine their influence on selective control and anticipatory regulation of muscle group activity. The effects these reflexes and postural reactions have on positioning, handling, and the facilitation or inhibition of functional movement also need to be evaluated (Bly, 1991). The primitive reflex and the automatic reaction sections of the MAI

(Chandler et al., 1980) are appropriate to use when evaluating infants with CP.

Selective control and anticipatory regulation of muscle groups are assessed in the context of functional evaluation: for the infant, this is indicated by the assessment of gross motor skills. Standardized tests used by physical therapists when assessing infant movement include the MAI (Chandler & Harris, 1985), the Gross Motor Function Measure (Russell et al., 1989), the Peabody Developmental Motor Scales (Palisano et al., 1995), the Bayley Scales of Infant Development (Bayley, 1993), the Test of Infant Motor Performance (Murney & Campbell, 1998), and the Alberta Infant Motor Scale (Piper & Darrah, 1994). Various elements of movements and posture combine to produce functional gross motor skills. These include the ability to align one part of the body on another; to bear weight through different parts of the body; to shift weight; to move against gravity; to assume, maintain, and move into and out of different positions; and to perform graded, isolated, and variable movements with an appropriate degree of effort. When examining functional motor skills, proficiency in incorporating these elements into the achievement of purposeful and efficient movement must be evaluated.

Specific assessments of seating, feeding (Evans Morris & Dunn Klein, 1987), or respiratory problems may be necessary for infants with problems in these areas. Growth is often affected in children with CP; therefore, anthropometric measures, including head circumference, weight, and length, should be documented. Growth may influence, or be influenced by, feeding, exercise, and energy efficiency (Campbell et al., 1989). Other factors to be considered during assessment include the influence of an infant's temperament and behavior on performance; sensory, social, communication, and cognitive abilities; and support from the environment.

Physical Therapy Goals, Outcomes, and Intervention

Physical therapy in infancy is focused on educating the family, facilitating caregiving, and promoting optimal sensorimotor experiences and skills. Intervention must address current and potential problems. Early intervention for children with CP has been advocated to help infants organize potential abilities in the most normal way for them, although there is no definitive support for its efficacy (Barry, 1996; Campbell, 1990).

FAMILY EDUCATION

The foremost set of goals at all ages is to educate families about CP, to provide support in their accep-

tance of their child's problems, and to be of assistance when parents make decisions about managing both their own and their child's lives. Infancy is an important time to foster collaborative goal-setting and programming strategies with the parents and promote ongoing communication between families and service providers. These skills empower them to make decisions, solve problems, and set priorities, as well as to become effective advocates for their children and themselves. Although it is recognized that parents know their children best, at this stage, the parents' goals may be overly optimistic and hopeful. Therapists must be realistic about the prognosis and the efficacy of physical therapy while remaining hopeful and providing options for intervention. They can break down overall goals into objectives that are meaningful, obtainable, sequential, observable, and measurable (Kolobe, 1992).

HANDLING AND CARE

Abnormal postures and movements resulting from impairments can make an infant difficult to handle and position. These difficulties can affect an infant's interaction with the environment, reaction to caregiving activities, and development of gross motor skills. Therefore, a second physical therapy goal is to promote the parents' skill, ease, and confidence in handling and caring for their infant. These skills alleviate unnecessary stress for parents and child and also help reduce the influence of the impairments, thereby preventing unnecessary secondary impairments and limitations. Parents are taught positioning, carrying, feeding, and dressing techniques that promote symmetry, limit abnormal posturing and movement, and facilitate functional motor activity. The principles guiding these methods are 1) to use a variety of movements and postures to promote sensory variety, 2) to frequently include positions that promote the full lengthening of spastic or hypoextensible muscles, and 3) to use positions that promote functional voluntary movement of limbs.

FACILITATING OPTIMAL SENSORIMOTOR DEVELOPMENT

A third physical therapy goal in infancy is to facilitate optimal sensorimotor experiences and skills, thereby reducing functional limitations and disabilities. Therapy should focus on the development of well-aligned postural stability coupled with smooth mobility to allow the emergence of motor skills such as reaching, rolling, sitting, crawling, transitional movements, standing, and prewalking skills. These skills promote the development of spatial perception, body awareness, and mobility to facilitate play, social interaction, and exploration of the environment. Movements that include trunk rotation, dissociation of body segments, weight shifting, weight bearing, and isolated movements should be incorporated into gross motor exercises and activities. These movement components, if experienced with proper alignment, can give the sensory feedback of normal movement patterns and activities. Good sources for the handling and treatment of infants and children of other ages include the works of Finnie (1997), Jaeger (1987, 1989), Scherzer and Tscharnuter (1990), and Wilson (1991). A practical reference for parents is *Children with Cerebral Palsy* (Geralis, 1991). Careful instruction of the family in specific techniques and activities, ongoing reinforcement, encouragement, and support are essential. Clearly written, illustrated, and updated home programs can be beneficial. Computer-generated programs or videotaping can be used to produce personalized, effective, and efficient information regarding activities, positioning, and exercises.

The normal motor developmental sequence may assist in guiding the progression of motor activities, although research indicates that motor milestones and their components develop in overlapping sequences, with spurts of development interspersed with some plateaus and even regressions (Atwater, 1991). The child with CP does not always proceed along the normal developmental sequence, and therapy becomes more functionally oriented within the scope of the child's physical capabilities (Bly, 1991). The stage at which this happens depends on the severity of the impairments; in some children, it may occur early in life.

Activities or equipment may be used to allow attainment of functional skills when impairments otherwise prevent the development of certain skills. For example, the sitting position promotes visual attending, upper extremity use, and social interaction. Infants with CP may be unable to sit independently, may sit statically only with precarious balance, or may not even be able to be seated in commercially available infant equipment. Customized seating or adaptations to regular infant seats may be necessary to allow function in other areas of development to progress. Infants with limited upper extremity movement may be unable to bring their hands or toys to their mouths to provide normal oral-motor sensory input. In these cases, mouthing activities should be incorporated into therapy. Toys may need to be adapted to facilitate developmental activities.

The care of an infant exhibiting asymmetry, extensor posturing, and shoulder retraction illustrates these approaches. Such an infant should be carried, seated, and fed in a symmetric position that does not allow axial hyperextension and keeps the hips and knees flexed. Positioning of or playing with the upper extremities to allow the infant to see his or her hands, practice midline play, reach for his or her feet, or suck on fingers can promote sensorimotor awareness. Active movements, such as the handling of toys that require two hands and that encourage the infant to develop flexor control and symmetry, are incorporated into daily activities. These activities facilitate the use of the neck and trunk muscles, promoting anterior and posterior control. The introduction of lateral control is the next step in achieving functional head and trunk control. In some severely affected children, slight gains in head control may be a goal, whereas in minimally affected children a fairly normal progression of motor development is expected, even without intervention. These therapeutic interventions should not limit infants' spontaneous desires to move and play and explore their environments because even very young children need to be able to assert themselves and manipulate their world (Campbell, 1997).

Some physical therapists may adhere to specific treatment philosophies, although differing treatment approaches often have underlying similarities. Two approaches used with infants are neurodevelopmental treatment (NDT) and the Vojta approach. NDT has been widely used throughout North America and other parts of the world as a basis for the treatment of infants with CP. NDT is based on the theory that inhibiting or modifying impairments of spasticity and abnormal reflex patterns can improve movement. For infants, handling techniques encourage active movement, and thus they experience normal movement sensations. The ultimate aim of the treatment is the acquisition of functional movements that permit children the greatest degree of independence possible to prepare them for as normal an adolescence and adult life as can be achieved (Bobath & Bobath, 1984). The Vojta approach, a European-based practice, uses proprioceptive information from the trunk and extremities to activate the central nervous system and guide it toward normal motor ontogenesis by eliciting appropriate movement patterns (Vojta, 1984).

ROLE OF OTHER DISCIPLINES

Occupational therapists may be involved in upper extremity function, particularly as it relates to play. In addition, speech and language pathologists may be necessary if there are oral-motor problems interfering with feeding or early language development. Community infant development workers may be involved in home-based programs. Social workers may help the parents through the grieving process, explain programs, and direct them to appropriate resources. Likewise it may be helpful to join parent support groups or meet with parents who have been through similar experiences.

Preschool Period

During the preschool years, locomotor, cognitive, communication, fine motor, self-care, and social abilities develop to promote functional independence in children. The process is a dynamic one in which all these areas constantly interact with one another. The child's environment remains oriented toward the parents, family, and home during this period, but he or she begins to interact with the outside world. Child care centers, babysitters, nursery schools, and playmates thus become part of a preschooler's world.

For children with CP, the limitations in motor functioning may create disabilities in learning, socialization, and attainment of independence (Butler, 1991). Concerns of the parents include the impact of impaired performance on all areas of development: for example, their child's ability to participate in and become integrated into normal preschool activities, the development of cognition and language, and the long-term effect of disabilities on future life and independence.

During these years, the child's attainable level of motor skills can be predicted with a greater degree of accuracy, as the influences of motor impairments on functioning become apparent. A major area of concern for physical therapists is the child's ability to achieve independent mobility. In addition, skills in overall gross motor development continue to be a focus of physical therapy to minimize disabilities, such as the inability to learn and perform the self-care skills of toileting, dressing, grooming, and feeding, and the limitations in play, communication, social skills, and problem-solving behavior.

Physical Therapy Examination and Evaluation

Assessment of disability assumes a primary focus, but it is important to determine the role of function and impairment in the production of disability. Tests should be administered at regular intervals to document change that is due to treatment and/or maturation. Within the dimension of impairment, direct testing of the force-generating ability of muscle groups is not always appropriate because spasticity, abnormal extensibility, hyperactive reflexes, and poor selective control affect the assessment. In such cases, muscle strength should continue to be considered in a functional context. Observing activities such as moving between sitting and standing positions or ascending and descending stairs assess both concentric and eccentric power. Endurance should

be evaluated by observing the ability to walk age-appropriate distances or propel a wheelchair a comparable span. During these years, quantitative measures of joint ROM and skeletal alignment, including the rotational and torsional alignment of the pelvis and lower extremities (Cusick & Stuberg, 1992; see Chapter 15), should be documented using consistent and standardized procedures. Variations of 10 to 15° occur in intrarater goniometric measurement in children with CP (Stuberg et al., 1988), and caution must be used to avoid misinterpreting small changes. Noting the point at which initial resistance is met with passive range of motion is clinically relevant but difficult to accurately measure clinically.

Evaluation of function and disability are frequently included in the same assessments. The Gross Motor Function Measure (Russell et al., 1989) and the Peabody Developmental Motor Scales (Palisano et al., 1995) can continue to be used to monitor the child's motor progress. When assessing motor skills, the use of equipment to achieve an activity should be taken into consideration. For example, the use of orthoses in ambulation may substantially affect walking abilities.

Function and disability assessment should also include mobility and transfers, communication, social function, bowel and bladder control, self-care and the degree of reliance on caregivers, adaptive equipment, and environmental modifications in the performance of activities of daily living (ADL). The Pediatric Evaluation of Disability Inventory (Reid et al., 1993) assesses many of these functional skills in young children. The Functional Independence Measure for Children (WeeFIM), a pediatric version of the Functional Independence Measure (Msall et al., 1990), measures disability as quantified by burden of care. Other measures of ADL (Gowland et al., 1991) such as the Vineland Adaptive Behavior Scales (Sparrow et al., 1984) can be used. The Canadian Occupational Performance Measure (Law et al., 1990) can be used to ensure that goals are relevant to the family and to measure outcomes. Goal Attainment Scaling can be used to evaluate whether specific individualized treatment goals or outcomes have been met, but this form of assessment cannot replace standardized measures, particularly for research (Palisano, 1993). Disability measures also include attempts to assess health-related quality of life. These measures take into account age, specific disability, and the factors and values believed to be important by health care professionals, parents, and children themselves (Rosenbaum et al., 1990).

Assessments specific to certain activities or equipment may be indicated. These include evaluations of postural stability (Westcott et al., 1997), augmentative communication, mobility, and gait (Olney et al., 1990). Gait assessment measures ambulatory function, and if kinetic and EMG analyses are included, certain impairments are also evaluated (Fig. 20-3). The ROM of the hips, knees, and ankles in each phase of gait can be observed using a videotape. Particular attention should be paid to the propulsive movement of ankle plantar flexion during push-off and to the concurrent hip flexion. These two events are responsible for much of the forward movement of the body and are indirect measures of force generation of muscle groups. EMG recordings during walking show the general level of activation of each muscle group, the degree of co-contraction, and the

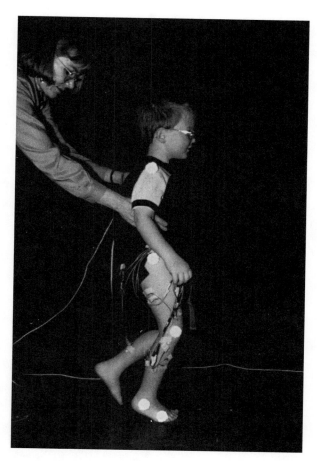

FIGURE 20-3. Child taking part in gait analysis. Electromyography shows patterns of muscle activities and aids identification of the presence of co-contraction of muscle groups. Markers at joints allow computer calculation of joint movements; force platforms embedded in floor permit measurement of individual muscle group contributions to the work of walking. (Courtesy of Human Motion Laboratory at School of Rehabilitation Therapy at Queen's University, Kingston, Ontario.)

selectivity and degree of sequencing of muscle-group activity—all indicators of impairment. Upper extremity activities such as reaching (Kluzik et al., 1990) have also been studied using videotaping and other sensing systems.

When assessing children in this age group, it is necessary to be aware of the effects of attention, cooperation, and the children's reaction to being assessed on the evaluation process. Parents or other caregivers can provide information on whether a child's performance is characteristic of his or her abilities.

Evaluation must take place at regular intervals to ensure that goals are still appropriate and therapy intervention is being appropriately directed.

Physical Therapy Goals, Outcomes, and Intervention

The impact and extent of the child's impairments become more established during the preschool years. Treatment focused specifically on reducing impairments and preventing secondary effects of impairment provides a backdrop for interventions aimed at higher levels of the disabling process to prevent isolation from the typical experiences of early childhood and family life. Optimal postural alignment and movements of the body that are conducive to musculoskeletal development, neurophysiologic control, and function, through exercise, positioning, and equipment, are the aims of many interventions. In many cases, physical therapy goals may serve as the building blocks for global interdisciplinary goals in communication, play, social interaction, and self-care activities. Therapists must be willing to respect the priorities of families and other professionals when determining goals, because it may not be possible to work on all areas at once. They must also be sure that treatment is conducive to the goals chosen and is motivating and fun for the child.

REDUCING PRIMARY IMPAIRMENT AND PREVENTING SECONDARY IMPAIRMENT

INCREASING FORCE GENERATION. Treatment to improve force generation of muscles in this age group is achieved through performing activities that create increased demands for production of both concentric and eccentric muscle force. Such activities include transitional movements, ball gymnastics, games, and practice of functional skills such as using stairs (Stern & Steidle, 1994).

SPASTICITY. Several options are available for the management of spasticity. Interventions have been directed toward decreasing the impairment of spasticity with the goals of prevention of secondary impairment, comfort and ease of positioning, and improved functional movement. Decreasing spasticity during the preschool years allows muscle lengthening and growth (Boyd & Graham, 1997; Rang, 1990) and may delay or eliminate the need for orthopedic surgery. Two interventions most appropriate for the preschool ages are selective dorsal rhizotomies and botulinum toxin A injections. These interventions are used if spasticity is interfering with function and conversely are not used if a child appears to be dependent on spasticity for function. Ideal candidates have fair to good trunk control and selective muscle control; good cognitive abilities, motivation, and parental support that are conducive to intensive postoperative therapy programs; and no fixed contractures or deformity. Severely affected patients, such as children with spastic quadriplegia, may be appropriate candidates; however, in these cases the goals are improved positioning, care, and comfort (McDonald, 1991). Selective dorsal rhizotomy is a surgical procedure in which the dorsal nerve rootlets supplying the lower extremity muscles are selectively cut. Prospective randomized controlled clinical trials have found spasticity to be substantially reduced. Function, as measured by the Gross Motor Performance Measure, has been shown to be improved in children who have received rhizotomies compared with those receiving equivalent physical therapy in some (Steinbok et al., 1997; Wright et al., 1998) but not in another (McLaughlin et al., 1998).

Gait analysis in children who have had rhizotomies has shown improved sagittal motion at the hip, knee, and ankle; however, abnormalities in patterns of muscle activation have persisted (Giuliani, 1991). This is attributed to continuing problems with motor control, which prohibit the proper sequencing of muscle action. Some gait improvements have been found to remain 10 years after surgery (Subramanian et al., 1998). Other positive effects that have been noted include improved oral-motor control, increased voice volume and endurance, improved temperament and concentration, improved bowel and bladder control, and improvement in growth parameters (McDonald, 1991).

Injections of small quantities of botulinum toxin A into muscles can prevent the presynaptic release of acetylcholine at the nerve-muscle junction. The effect peaks at 2 weeks and may last for 1 to 4 months. The drug is expensive but is often covered by insurance. Targeted muscles are those in which spasticity interferes with function and those that are most prone to developing contractures. These include the calf muscles, hamstrings, hip flexors, and adductors. Upper extremity muscles have also been successfully injected. Botox injections can also be used as a diagnostic measure before orthopedic or rhizotomy surgery or as an analgesic agent to reduce pain and

spasm postoperatively (Boyd & Graham, 1997). Injections in children with a dynamic component to calf equinus were successful in improving passive dorsiflexion, which may allow more opportunity for an increase in muscle length. The results were comparable with but longer lasting than those of a control group that received serial casting and also demonstrated fewer side effects (Corry et al., 1998).

Therapy focusing on functional outcomes, but also emphasizing muscle strengthening, is necessary after the spasticity intervention for optimal effectiveness, because the children's muscles are "weakened" without their spasticity (Fig. 20–4).

HYPOEXTENSIBILITY.   Various approaches are used to maintain muscle extensibility and joint mobility. Some therapists use manual stretching programs. The usefulness of these passive maneuvers is difficult to assess because active exercises, positioning programs, and equipment are usually used simultaneously. Research on the effectiveness of manual stretching on extensibility is inconclusive (Miedaner & Renander, 1987). Tremblay and colleagues (1990) found that a prolonged stretch of 30 minutes to the plantar flexors of children with CP reduced the impairment of spasticity and improved the voluntary activation of the plantar flexors but not the dorsiflexors. The effect lasted for as long as 35 minutes. In a parallel study, the stretching session did not produce a functional improvement in gait (Richards et al., 1991).

The effects of prolonged stretching programs have been studied (Tardieu et al., 1988), and it was found that contractures were prevented if the plantar flexor muscles were stretched beyond a minimum threshold length for at least 6 hours during daily

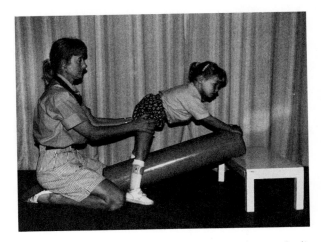

FIGURE 20–4. Exercises after rhizotomy are frequently directed toward increasing force generation of extensor muscles.

activity. The threshold length was the length at which the muscle began to resist a stretch. The data prompting this statement are suggestive rather than conclusive, however. Lespargot and colleagues (1994) found that physiotherapy and a moderate stretch imposed for 6 hours daily prevented muscle-body contracture but did not prevent shortening of the tendon.

CASTING AND ORTHOSES. Plaster or fiberglass casting has been used as an economical method of providing stretch and is commonly used in serial casting to lengthen hypoextensible calf muscles. Casting for a 3-week period was shown to be effective if the hypoextensibility was due to imbalance between the triceps surae and dorsiflexor muscles but not if the primary impairment was lack of appropriate muscle growth in response to bone growth (Tardieu et al., 1982). Serial casting has also been used for calf muscle and other muscle groups, such as the hamstrings and elbow flexors.

Lower extremity orthoses are used to reduce impairment, prevent secondary impairment, and facilitate function. The specific goals are prevention of contracture and deformity, provision of optimal joint alignment, provision of selective motion restriction, protection of weak muscles, control of tone and tonus-related deviations, enhancement of function, and postoperative protection of tissues (Cusick, 1990). Ricks and Eilert (1993) found that although casts and orthoses improved ambulation and preambulation skills, x-rays did not show significant changes in the bony alignment of the foot and ankle during weight bearing.

Many variations of ankle-foot orthoses (AFOs) are available, depending on the biomechanical and functional needs of the individual child (Knutsson & Clark, 1991). Solid AFOs are used if restriction of ankle movement is desired. Children who would benefit from freedom of movement at the joint can use hinged AFOs. Hinged AFOs frequently prevent plantar flexion but permit dorsiflexion, which allows stretching of the plantar flexor muscle group during walking. Hinged AFOs have been found to promote a more normal and efficient gait pattern than do rigid orthotics (Carmick, 1995; Middleton et al., 1988). Hainsworth and colleagues (1997) found that that the range of movement and gait deteriorated during the short periods without AFOs when compared with periods during which the AFOs were worn. Foot orthoses, or supramalleolar orthoses, may be used for children with pronation who do not require the ankle stabilization of an AFO (Knutsson & Clark, 1991). Supramalleolar orthoses, however, may not improve ankle motion in the sagittal plane (Carlson et al., 1997). Another variant is the posterior leaf spring orthosis, which is intended to prevent excessive equinus while mechanically augmenting push-off. A kinetic gait analysis of 31 children found that it reduced equinus in swing, permitted ankle dorsiflexion in stance, absorbed more energy during midstance, but reduced the desirable power-generating capabilities at push-off (Oonpuu et al., 1996).

Bivalved casts or therapist-fabricated splints have been used in place of AFOs as a less expensive alternative for children who are growing quickly, do not have access to funding, or require a period of evaluation. The bivalved casts, popular during the 1980s, incorporate design features such as toe extension support, which is purported to inhibit abnormal tone or reflex activity. Although clinicians have claimed that the splints reduce abnormal tone, improve positioning, and reduce unwanted reflexes, research has not substantiated the claims (Carlson, 1984).

Orthoses have also been used during sleep to prevent the secondary impairment of hypoextensibility, or contracture. Baumann and Zumstein (1985) found that the use of double-shell foot orthoses as night splints from age 3 years to the end of the skeletal growth period prevented calf muscle contractures from developing and made the need for surgery rare.

Other materials such as Lycra (Blair et al., 1995), neoprene, and tape have been used for splinting to assist children biomechanically and facilitate function. Caution must be taken concerning the skin tolerance of these materials.

ORTHOPEDIC SURGERY. Orthopedic surgery in preschoolers is usually performed to prevent secondary impairment by limiting the effects, but not the causes, of hypoextensibility and spasticity. For example, the lengthening of hypoextensible or spastic hip adductors (or both) may be performed to prevent subluxation or dislocation of the hip joint. Sometimes, however, surgery such as tendo Achilles lengthening is delayed because of the tendency for recurrence necessitating repeated surgery (Tardieu et al., 1982). Ideally, surgery is deferred until age 6 to 8 years, when multilevel corrections can be performed if necessary (DeLuca, 1996). Massagli (1991) has emphasized that musculoskeletal surgery does not alter the neurologically driven patterns of muscle activity, although lengthening, releasing, or transferring a muscle can alter its influence. Decreased force production is often a complication. Orthopedic surgery is sometimes combined with neurectomy if tonic activity of the muscle is present as a result of spasticity or other neurologic causes. A full discussion of the role of orthopedic surgery in CP can be found in the work of Rang (1990). Physical therapists play important roles in surgical decision making. They are also involved in the care of the child who is immobilized and in providing postoperative therapy (Harryman, 1992), particularly because decreased force production is a significant complication of surgery. Frequently forgotten is the importance of transporting children safely in motor vehicles when they are in casts, an activity for which various devices are available (Bull et al., 1989).

POSITIONING. Alignment of the body as a whole is important. Children should have a variety of positions in which they can optimally function, travel, and sleep. Varying the positions of children who are limited in movement also helps prevent the secondary impairments of positional contractures and deformity, as well as skin breakdown (Healy et al., 1997). Decreased ability to change body position during sleep can cause disrupted rest for children with CP (Kotagal et al., 1994).

Position changes can also contribute to pulmonary health. Severely involved children are at risk for chest complications because of chest wall biomechanics, feeding difficulties, immobility, and poor coughing abilities. Adaptive seating has also been shown to improve pulmonary functioning (Nwaobi & Smith, 1986). For the preschooler, sitting, standing, lying, and a position suitable for playing on the floor are important. When prescribing seating systems, it is necessary to be aware of not only the child's comfort and functional abilities but also the caregivers' concerns and needs and the child's environment. Seating inserts can be used in a variety of situations and with equipment such as strollers and wheelchairs, which are often needed to enable parents to transport their child easily. Specific suggestions are included in Chapter 24. Approved car seats and restraints are necessary for safe and comfortable vehicular transportation (Shaw, 1987).

Positioning in standing is thought to reduce or prevent secondary impairments by maintaining lower extremity muscle extensibility, maintaining or increasing bone mineral density, and promoting optimal musculoskeletal development (Stuberg, 1992), including acetabular development. A study of bone mineralization in children with hemiplegic CP concluded that bone size and density decrease with increasing neurologic involvement, and weight bearing may slightly lessen the effect (Lin & Henderson, 1996). Optimally, standing involves movement and activity to provide intermittent loading and muscle strain. Standing programs are often started at 1 year of age if children are not able to bear their weight effectively on their own. Stuberg (1992) recommended positioning in standing for 45 minutes two or three times a day to control lower extremity flexor contractures, and for 60 minutes four or five times per week to facilitate bone development, but notes

that there is no definite evidence to support these guidelines. Maintenance of the child's ability to bear full weight through the legs reduces the need to be lifted by caregivers.

TREATMENT OF FUNCTIONAL LIMITATIONS

Physical therapy for treatment of functional limitations is often intensive during the preschool years. The frequency of treatment varies, depending on the resources available, complementary programming, client goals, parental needs and desires, and the child's response to treatment. Optimal treatment frequency is unknown, but periods of increased frequencies have shown improvements in attainment of specific treatment goals at levels that were maintained when frequency decreased, provided the skills were incorporated into daily functional activities. Bower and McLellan (1992) found that bursts of intensive physiotherapy directed at achievable specific measurable goals accelerated the acquisition of motor skills compared with conventional physical therapy.

Therapy should be challenging and meaningful to the child and progress to integrating the skills learned into functional and cognitively directed skills for carryover. Movement tasks should be goal oriented and interesting to maintain motivation and arousal. For example, kicking a soccer ball may be a more functional and motivating method of developing balance skills than practicing standing on one foot. Children with CP are able to perform concrete perceptuomotor tasks much more readily than abstract ones, even if the same movements are involved (van der Weel et al., 1991), because more information is available from the environment to direct the task.

Motor control and motor-learning principles (see Chapter 6) can be used to develop treatment strategies for reducing functional limitations. Feedback is important in the process of learning skilled movement. Feedback through the child's sensory receptors provides intrinsic information, whereas extrinsic feedback through various forms of biofeedback provides information from external sources. Knowledge of results contributes information about movement outcome, and knowledge of performance supplies feedback about the nature of the movement (Poole, 1991).

Feedforward mechanisms must also be considered, because there is a cognitive component to movement skills. In some instances, cognitive strategies may be able to compensate for some of the inherent motor limitations.

Many children with CP do not have normal cognition and behavior, and activities must be adapted accordingly. If a child is unable to learn, training using memorization of solutions may be necessary, although limited transfer to novel situations will occur (Higgins, 1991). If behavioral factors are negatively affecting treatment, a behavioral approach using appropriate motivators may encourage children to work on certain skills (Horton & Taylor, 1989).

Improvements in functional movement of the preschool-age child are made by reducing the effects of the multisystem impairments of selective control, anticipatory regulation, and learning of unique movements. Although there is a growing literature on motor learning (see Chapter 6), on motor control in skill acquisition (see Chapter 2), and on the biomechanics of movement, the profession is still far from being able to provide optimal strategies for treatment that are known to be effective (Fetters, 1991). The therapist who treats children with CP should modify approaches as research produces new insights in the areas of motor learning and motor control.

FEEDING, DROOLING, AND TOILETING. Some children with CP, particularly those who are severely affected, may have oral-motor problems, such as poor mouth closure, retraction or thrusting of the tongue, poor tongue movements, and poor coordination in swallowing, which can make speech and feeding difficult. Feeding problems can be aggravated by other problems such as impaired self-feeding and difficulties in expressing hunger or food preferences that may result in inadequate nutritional intake and poor growth (Gisel & Patrick, 1988; Reilly & Skuse, 1992). Gastroesophageal reflux and aspiration also occur in children with severe CP. Oral-motor programs, proper positioning, and parent education and support are important issues to address (Evans Morris & Dunn Klein, 1987). In extreme cases, gastrostomy and antireflux procedures may be necessary to improve growth and enhance the quality of life for the child and the family (Rempel et al., 1988).

Drooling, a significant problem in about 10% of children with CP, can cause social embarrassment and affect the quality of social integration (Blasco et al., 1992). It can result from dysfunctional oral-motor activity, oral sensory problems, or inefficient and infrequent swallowing. Management may include waiting for further neurologic maturation, feeding and oral stimulation programs, behavior modification programs, medications, or surgery.

Failure to develop an appropriate toileting routine during the preschool years can result in an ongoing disability, because incontinence can provoke negative reactions from caregivers and peers. Expectations of toileting in children with CP should be similar to those for children of comparable cognitive abilities, and therapists should encourage training at

a comparable age and recommend appropriate adaptive equipment as necessary (Shaw, 1990).

MOBILITY

Ambulation is a major concern of physical therapists during these years. Emphasis in treatment is initially on prewalking skills, such as attaining effective and well-aligned weight bearing, promoting dissociation and weight shifting, and improving balance. Ambulatory aids, such as walkers and crutches, may be used, either temporarily while the child is progressing to more advanced gait skills or as long-term aids for independent mobility. The use of posterior walkers has been found to encourage a more upright posture during gait and to promote better gait characteristics than does the use of anterior walkers (Fig. 20–5) (Logan et al., 1990).

Children in this age group are becoming aware of the concept of achievement, and although ambulation is a coveted skill, it should not become an all-consuming goal, particularly if it may not be attainable. When interviewing adults with significant

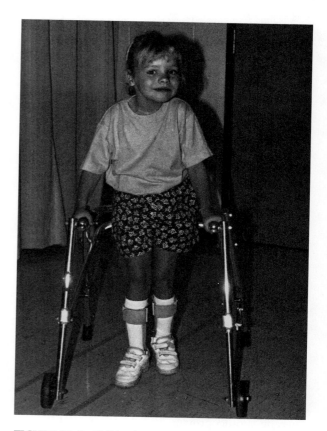

FIGURE 20–5. Child using a posterior walker, reported to promote upright posture and higher walking speeds than an anterior walker.

impairment, Kibele (1989) found that they remembered walking as the most important goal set for them by their parents and therapists. This resulted in feelings of failure from an early age and also in a loss of faith in rehabilitation professionals.

The provision of alternative means to allow children functional, independent mobility when ambulation is impossible or inefficient is recommended. Sometimes this need is met with an adapted tricycle (Fig. 20-6) or manual wheelchair; other children require one of a wide variety of power mobility devices available (Jones, 1990) and may need special controls (Fig. 20-7). These enable children with CP to explore their environment and achieve a sense of independence and competence. Power mobility may also promote the development of initiative (Butler, 1991) and the acquisition of spatial concepts. The lack of self-propelled locomotion can result in apathy, withdrawal, passivity, and dependent behavior that can persist into later life (Butler, 1991).

If power mobility is being considered, fine motor control, cognitive abilities, behavior, environment, visual and auditory abilities, and financial resources must all be taken into account. Children with motor limitations have become safely and effectively mobile in power wheelchairs at as young as 17 months of age (Butler, 1991). Parents may initially be hesitant about introducing power mobility to young children, fearing that it signifies giving up on walking. Power mobility does not preclude ambulation-oriented therapy but provides the child with a method of moving about independently in the meantime. For children who will continue to be wholly dependent on power mobility for independence, it provides mobility at an appropriate age and gives the families an indication of the implications of power mobility on housing and transportation needs. For more information, see Chapter 24.

PLAY

Play, the primary productive activity for children, should be intrinsically motivating and pleasurable. The benefits of play include the children's discovering the effects they can have on objects and people in their environment; developing social skills; and promoting the development of perceptual, conceptual, intellectual, and language skills. Limitations in the play of children with physical disabilities may affect their experiential learning derived from play and result in decreased independence, motivation, imagination, creativity, assertiveness, social skills, and self-esteem (Blanche, 1997; Missiuna & Pollock, 1991). Therapy should provide and demonstrate play opportunities (Fig. 20-8). Appropriate toys and play methods should be suggested to parents and caregivers. If children are physically unable to play with

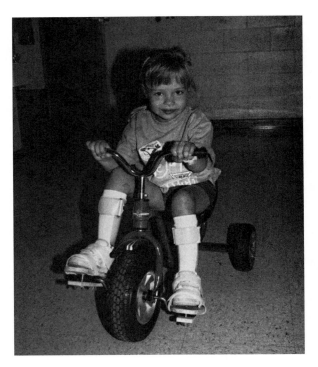

FIGURE 20-6. An adapted tricycle may meet a child's needs for mobility.

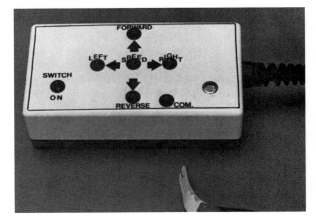

FIGURE 20-7. Single-switch scanning computer controller for power wheelchair permits independent mobility for children with very limited motor control. Developed at Hugh MacMillan Rehabilitation Centre, Toronto, Ontario.

regular toys, a variety of adaptations, such as switch accessing, can make their toys usable (Langley, 1990). Environmental control equipment also can be introduced to preschoolers.

It is important that children are not overprotected in their attempts to play. Parents should be

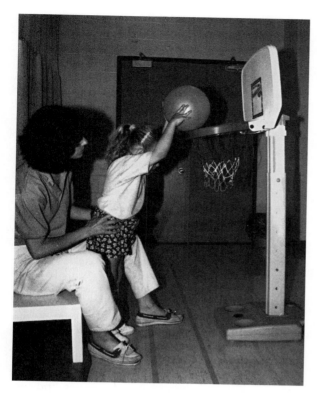

FIGURE 20–8. Therapeutic exercise programs can include highly motivating play activities. Throwing a basketball may be more motivating than trunk extension exercises.

encouraged to let their children enjoy typical play activities, such as rolling down hills and getting dirty in the mud. Therapists must ensure that therapy and home programs promote, rather than interfere with, the normal play experiences parents have with their children.

INTERVENTION APPROACHES

NDT is a treatment approach that is used with the age group and that continues to evolve with advances in the field (Bly, 1991). Research studies on the effectiveness of NDT are available but controversial and reflect the difficulty in conducting clinical research (Palisano, 1991). However, NDT strategies incorporated into treatment have been shown to improve control of functional movements (Kluzik et al., 1990). Strategies such as practice may need to be integrated into NDT for optimal improvement in specific skills (Jonsdottir et al., 1997).

Conductive Education (CE), an approach originated by Andras Peto in Hungary, is based on the theory that the difficulties of the child with motor dysfunction are problems of learning. The goal of treatment is the ability to function independently in the world without aids, an important objective in Hungary, where schools are not adapted for children with disabilities. Participants are selected for their ability to learn, which may make some children ineligible for the program. They are usually treated in group settings that provide the incentive of competition and allow more time in therapy than does individual treatment. Functional goals are broken down into small steps. Children initiate the activities on their own, with direct conscious action aided by mental preparation (Bairstow et al., 1991). Research on CE is limited; however, a study by Reddihough and colleagues (1997) found that children in a CE program made progress similar to that of children involved in neurodevelopmental programs.

Knowledge of a variety of theoretic models, not necessarily pediatric in origin, can help form a therapist's approach to treating children with cerebral palsy. Carr and Shepherd's task-related movement science–based approach (Shepherd, 1995), the motor control theories of Shumway-Cook and Woollacott (1995), and the dynamic systems theory (Darrah & Bartlett, 1995) can be integrated into physical therapy interventions for children with CP. The family-centered service philosophy of service provision can be applied to all treatment approaches.

It is difficult to compare the effectiveness of different approaches because there are also discrepancies in parameters such as frequency, skill level of individual therapists, compliance of families, and age and abilities of the patients. In a study comparing four treatment approaches, Bower and colleagues (1996) found that parents were most pleased with therapy when they requested the services, when they were present during treatment, and when targeted goals were met. They concluded that the most appropriate approach for a child would be one that would meet the needs of the particular child. Parents of children with CP often consider alternative therapies that may not be accepted by some professionals and are usually expensive. If families choose to take an approach other than the one offered by the therapist, it is necessary to respect their choice. Reasons for seeking alternatives include a desire for more therapy, dissatisfaction with present therapy, and belief that their child could do better (Milo-Manson et al., 1997). Therapists should not react defensively but should provide impartial information about the therapies in question.

FAMILY INVOLVEMENT

The importance of providing family-centered service continues. Planning of interventions should take into account the child within the context of the family. Therapists should be sensitive to the family's stresses, dynamics, child-rearing practices, coping mechanisms, privacy, values, and cultural variations. Therapists should be flexible in their approach and programming (Kolobe, 1992). Special efforts must be made to deal with the effects of a child with CP on the siblings (Powell & Ogle, 1985).

Family involvement is crucial for integrating treatment into everyday life. Home programs are important for optimal results from therapy programs because strengthening, extensibility, and motor learning often require more input than can be provided by limited treatment resources. It is necessary to find a balance between providing parents with home programs that make them an integral part of their child's therapy and burdening them with activities they cannot realistically be expected to carry out. Obstacles may include constraints on time, energy, skills, or resources or negative effects on the parent-child relationship. Hinojosa and Anderson (1991) found that although mothers of preschoolers with CP did not carry out specific home programs designed by therapists, they did activities that could be integrated into their daily routines and interactions and that were not stressful for the child or the caregiver.

Siblings can be included in home programs. Craft and colleagues (1990) studied a group of children with CP whose siblings had been educated about the condition and ways in which they could encourage their brother or sister to be more independent. As a result of this, the children with CP showed increases in ROM and in functional independence.

ROLE OF OTHER DISCIPLINES

Occupational therapists work closely with the children at this age to develop independence in activities such as dressing, feeding, toileting, and playing. Speech and language pathologists continue to develop efficient methods of communication in children with CP. Psychologists assess cognitive skills and advise on the interaction of intellectual abilities with the other areas of development. Social workers and behavior therapists continue to provide ongoing support to the families, because the stresses involved in parenting a child with a disability persist (Sternisha et al., 1992). Team assessment and intervention are imperative for addressing issues such as feeding problems, augmentative communication, and transition to school.

School-Age and Adolescent Period

During the school-age and adolescent years, children typically become more involved in school and community life while remaining dependent on their families and living in their parental homes. They refine and augment the basic functional skills they have learned and develop life skills that will enable them to cope effectively with the demands of daily living and, it is hoped, independent adult life.

These can be difficult years for children with CP. They become more aware of the reality, extent, and impact of their disabilities on themselves and their families. As they strive to contend with the normal stresses of growing up, particularly those of adolescence, they must also cope with being different, acknowledge the potential obstacles to attaining independence, and work to overcome them.

Parents remain anxious about how their child's disabilities will affect their participation in educational environments and in social situations. They may worry about their child's future as an adult (Hallum, 1995). While continuing to be naturally attentive, they have to avoid being overprotective and begin to allow their child to take risks and become independent in the outside world. In some cases, there may be financial concerns regarding the need for special equipment, transportation, and home renovations. Parents of children who are dependent in ADL and transfers may suffer from physical stresses, such as back problems.

Typical disabilities encountered during these years include a lack of independent mobility, poor endurance in performing routine activities, and continued difficulty and slowness with self-care and hygiene skills at a time when privacy is becoming increasingly important. Adolescents may also not have the opportunity to develop socially and sexually and may lack the ability to acquire age-appropriate levels of independence from the family. Societal barriers may reduce access to community and school facilities, thus limiting opportunities for participation in social, cultural, and athletic activities.

Physical Therapy Examination and Evaluation

Assessment of impairments that could interfere with function, or lead to further secondary impairment, such as scoliosis, continues to be important. Children in this age group may be able to participate in measurement of force production using dynamometry. Assessment of gross motor function is appropriate, because children are often making gross motor progress during their school years. They may also change as a result of interventions such as surgery, the use of orthoses, and periods of intensive therapy. The development of the Gross Motor Performance Measure (Boyce et al., 1995) may help in detecting the fine increments of motor skill gains that are characteristic of children who are severely affected. For children with mild degrees of involvement, the Bruininks-Oseretsky Test of Motor Proficiency (Bruininks, 1978) may be useful in measuring specific components of higher levels of motor function. Tools such as the School Function Assessment may be used in educational settings (Coster et al., 1994).

Gait analysis continues to be helpful in assessing ambulatory children, particularly when decisions about surgery are being made (Lee et al., 1992), although this opinion is not held by all (Abel, 1995). Endurance and efficiency of movement become increasingly important during these years as the children venture into the community on their own or with their peers. Mechanical energy costs can be assessed with motion analysis equipment (Olney et al., 1987). In the clinical setting, physiologic measures such as the physiologic cost index for activities such as ambulation can give energy cost estimates (Butler, 1991; Mossberg et al., 1990) or assist in selecting assistive devices (Rose et al., 1985). In a laboratory setting, ergometer assessment can analyze other aspects of endurance (Parker et al., 1992). An important consideration in maximizing endurance for daily activities is the effect of excessive weight gain, because it can compromise optimal function and efficiency.

Privacy of individuals at all ages should be respected, but it is particularly important during these years when children are becoming more aware of their bodies and their sexuality. Children should be appropriately dressed when attending therapy sessions and clinics, particularly if they are being seen by unfamiliar people or are being photographed or videotaped. If it is necessary for children to remove their clothing, their permission should be asked and a reason given for doing so. It is important to include the clients in conversations that involve them and not to converse only with caregivers or other professional staff.

Physical Therapy Goals, Outcomes, and Interventions

As goals become oriented toward the child's or adolescent's lifestyle, emphasis is on maintaining or improving the level of function while considering the stresses of growth, maturation, and increasing demands in life skills and participation in community activities. Although the pathophysiologic impairment of CP is nonprogressive, there are changes related to the stresses of increasing size, accumulative physical overuse, and a more competitive lifestyle. For example, as children advance to higher grades in school, there may be longer distances to walk between classes. Contractures may rapidly develop during periods when bones are growing faster than muscles (Tardieu et al., 1982). Secondary orthopedic and functional problems must be anticipated and avoided. The maintenance of muscle ex-

tensibility and force generation, joint integrity, and fitness is important in preventing secondary impairments that can result from the stresses of aging. This age group also needs to develop problem-solving strategies to overcome environmental and societal barriers to become as independent and active as possible in home, school, recreational, social, and community life.

In many cases, adolescents can and should be involved in setting goals and determining programming. It is important during these years to encourage them to take responsibility for their own health, care, and decision making so that they are prepared to assume these responsibilities in adulthood (Fox et al., 1992). It is also important to look ahead and set goals that are appropriate for their later life situations and independence. Therapists should strive to foster self-esteem and assertiveness in children and adolescents by emphasizing their abilities, finding areas and activities in which they can excel, and helping them to acknowledge their difficulties with a view toward identifying appropriate compensations and use of attendant care. In the case of children with severe (multiple) disorder, goals are oriented toward minimizing impairments to facilitate caregiving and comfort.

REDUCING PRIMARY IMPAIRMENT AND PREVENTING SECONDARY IMPAIRMENT

The impairment of deficient muscle force generation that may result in functional limitations and disabilities is important to address in this age group. Damiano and co-workers (1995) used ankle weights in a 6-week progressive resistive strengthening program for the quadriceps in 14 children with spastic diplegia. Stride length increased, and knee flexion at initial contact decreased. An 8-week isokinetic strengthening program for mildly affected adolescents effected strength gains of 12 to 30% in knee extensors and flexors but no increase in spasticity (MacPhail & Kramer, 1995). Nine of the seventeen subjects showed improvements in the standing and walking, running, and jumping dimensions of the Gross Motor Function Measure. Using free weights in a home program supervised by a family member, Damiano and Abel (1998) reported average strength gains of 69% when the two weakest muscle groups were trained in children with spastic diplegia or hemiplegia. The gains were associated with positive functional outcomes, although, as with the MacPhail and Kramer study, it is not clear whether increasing strength alters gait efficiency.

Various methods of electrical stimulation have been used as an adjunct to the treatment of CP to reduce spasticity, to increase force production and extensibility, and to improve function activities such as gait (Stanger & Bertoti, 1997). This treatment adjunct is particularly useful in postoperative muscle training and strengthening. Protocols should be individualized for patients following careful analysis of movement, and application should be closely monitored.

It was once thought that individuals had no control of their spasticity. Subjects with CP, however, have been able to reduce their responsiveness to a stretch reflex stimulus imposed during a lower limb activity (O'Dwyer et al., 1994). These findings encourage further exploration of the possibilities of reducing spastic responses.

Pharmacologic intervention can be used to control the impairment of spasticity. The use of oral medications has been poorly studied, but medication may be appropriate for some children (Pranzatelli, 1996). Children must be carefully assessed for appropriateness and monitored closely for side effects. Baclofen, a synthetic agonist of aminobutyric acid, has an inhibitory effect on the presynaptic excitatory neurotransmitter release. It has been shown to reduce spasticity in individuals with CP (Campbell et al., 1995). If taken orally, doses high enough to give the proper concentration in the cerebrospinal fluid can cause side effects such as drowsiness. To circumvent this problem, baclofen is most effective if given intrathecally by a continuous infusion pump implanted in the abdomen that releases the drug at a slow, constant rate into the subarachnoid space. The use of intrathecal baclofen has been postulated to reduce the need for orthopedic surgery (Gerszten et al., 1998).

Biofeedback is a useful tool in addressing single-system and multisystem impairments during these years (Fig. 20–9) because by this time children have usually developed abstract thinking and sufficient cognitive ability to use it optimally. Positive results have been reported, but carryover is often limited, generalization to real-life situations is not readily demonstrated, and treatment is time consuming (James, 1992). Toner and colleagues (1998) found that a program of biofeedback improved active range of motion and strength and motor control in dorsiflexion in a group of children with CP.

The secondary impairment of joint or muscle contracture may occur in this age group, particularly in the more severely affected patients. This can be a result of chronic muscle imbalance, abnormal posturing, or static positioning. Casting may be used to increase the range of joint movement by lengthening muscles or tendons or both with no associated loss in strength (Brouwer et al., 1998; Cusick, 1990; O'Dwyer et al., 1989; Tardieu et al., 1982). Interventions of botulinum toxin A and casting may comple-

ment each other in children with spasticity and contractures. Anderson and colleagues (1988) found that soft splints made of polyurethane foam were effective in reducing severe knee flexor contractures; this may be an attractive alternative for low-income families.

Orthopedic surgery continues to be used to reduce the effects of primary and secondary impairment on mobility, posture, cosmesis, and hygiene and to prevent further secondary impairment. Possible surgical procedures include muscle lengthenings or transfers, tenotomies, neurectomies, osteotomies, and fusions.

Surgery may improve posture and gait, but outcomes can be unpredictable because muscle weakness often results. As children get older, they should be active participants in surgical decision making that may be influenced by their interests, priorities, and concerns about interruptions in their lives as a result of hospitalizations, immobilizations, and recovery periods.

The secondary impairment of joint hypomobility resulting from capsular or ligamentous tightness can be treated with manual therapy techniques (Brooks-Scott, 1995). Joint mobilizations may be used to regain joint mobility, particularly after immobilization. Therapists must ascertain whether joint structures are causing movement restriction and must also be aware of the contraindications and precautions relevant to using mobilizations in growing and neurologically involved patients (Harris & Lundgren, 1991).

Spasticity, abnormal extensibility of muscles, muscular imbalance, and decreased force generation can result in scoliosis, which, in turn, can affect

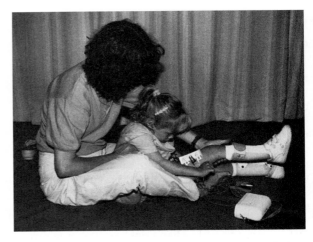

FIGURE 20–9. Biofeedback is a useful treatment tool when precise objectives can be identified.

positioning and respiratory status. Spinal deformity can be a particularly difficult problem in the severely affected patient. Rigid orthoses can result in skin breakdown and patient intolerance; by contrast, the use of a soft orthosis has been found to be beneficial in the management of scoliosis in patients with CP (Letts et al., 1992). In some cases, surgical intervention may be necessary (see Chapter 10).

MOBILITY AND ENDURANCE

Many compensatory strategies can be implemented to promote function and circumvent disability during the school years. The continued use of power mobility devices is important for independent mobility. Often children who are able to walk independently need an alternative form of mobility, such as a manual wheelchair or a power scooter, as they become larger and need to travel greater distances to meet their social and educational objectives. Ambulant children with cerebral palsy are less active than their peers (van den Berg–Emons et al., 1995). Availability of power mobility should not preclude activity to the point of decreased musculoskeletal integrity or physical fitness. Mobility devices may require modifications, such as ramps to buildings or washroom renovations, for accessibility. Driver training offers the freedom to travel independently. For those unable to drive, instruction in the use of public or special transportation should be provided.

The functional limitation of low endurance levels, frequently related to inefficiency of movement, has been identified in children with CP. Rose and colleagues (1990) found that energy expenditure indices based on oxygen uptake and heart rate measured at a given walking speed were 3 times higher in children with CP than in normal control children. Findings that were similar, but based on mechanical energy analyses, were reported for children with hemiplegia (Olney et al., 1987). Rose and colleagues (1985) also found that children who were ambulatory with wheeled walkers or quadruped canes had high physiologic workloads when walking for 5 minutes, suggesting that it is impractical for such children to walk long distances. Orthoses may also influence energy expenditure. Mossberg and colleagues (1990) showed that the use of AFOs significantly reduced the energy demands of walking in children with spastic diplegia.

SCHOOL AND COMMUNITY

Many children are involved in school-based programs, particularly with continuing application of the Education for All Handicapped Children Act in 1975 in the United States (Poirier et al., 1988) and the Charter of Rights and Freedoms in Canada in 1982 (Poirier et al., 1988). In most jurisdictions, the educational program must be implemented in the least restrictive environment for that child, and "the child . . . mainstreamed to the fullest possible extent" (Clune & Van Pelt, 1985). Facilities and resources such as support personnel, equipment for accessibility, and computer-based systems (Fig. 20–10) are necessary to meet the physical needs of children in the school system. Therapists working with school personnel may instruct assistants and teachers in positioning, lifting, and transferring the children; carrying out exercise programs; and adapting and developing physical education programs (Wilcox, 1988). Therapists may also be involved in accessibility, transportation, evacuation, and other safety

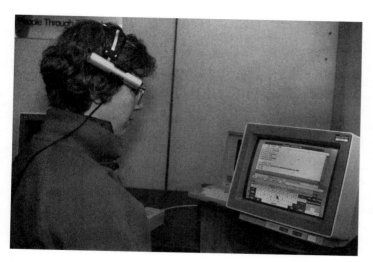

FIGURE 20–10. Computer-based communication system with visual keyboard on computer screen and head pointer acting as controller. Developed at Hugh MacMillan Rehabilitation Centre, Toronto, Ontario.

issues. Therapists working in school settings must be sensitive to the physical and scheduling constraints of the educational environment and be willing to compromise to meet the educational priorities of the students. Therapy may range from consultation and monitoring for students who are thought to have reached their maximal level of functioning, to active therapy for children who have specific treatment goals. When children are primarily seen through the educational system, effort must be made to keep the family involved in all aspects of care and treatment. See Chapter 32 for further information on this subject based on experiences in the United States.

In addition to educating school staff about children with CP, therapists can help educate the other children in the classroom. Knowledge about, and positive interactions with, people with disabilities can create positive attitudes, particularly when children are between 7 and 9 years of age, because their attitudes about people with disabilities are flexible at this age (Morrison & Ursprung, 1987).

It is important for children with disabilities to be involved in community and recreational activities that provide social as well as therapeutic opportunities. Many adapted or integrated sports activities are suitable for people with CP, including horseback riding (MacKinnon et al., 1995), swimming, skiing, sailing, canoeing, camping, kayaking, fishing, bungee jumping, yoga, and tai chi. Adapted games can provide athletic competition and participation in team experiences and can facilitate the social aspects of sports (Jones, 1988).

All athletes are at risk for sports-related injuries, but relatively minor injuries can incapacitate people with CP. They should be encouraged to be responsible for their bodies during sports activities by following appropriate conditioning, warm-up, and cool-down routines; following comprehensive injury prevention programs, which include strengthening, flexibility, and aerobic and anaerobic training activities; and using appropriate protective and orthotic equipment. Injuries should be treated promptly. The knee is the most frequently injured body part in athletes with CP. Shoulders, hands, and ankles are also vulnerable (Ferrara et al., 1992). For more information, see Chapter 17.

During these years, children learn about their bodies, their sexuality, and appropriate interactions with other people. Children and adults with disabilities have an increased risk of suffering abuse, including sexual abuse, which can result in physical, social, emotional, and behavioral consequences (Hallum, 1995; Sobsey & Doe, 1991). Many of the perpetrators have relationships with the victims that are similar to those commonly found among nondisabled victims; however, some abusers have relationships spe-cifically related to the victim's disability. These people can be personal care attendants, transportation providers, residential care staff, and other disabled individuals. Abuse is a serious matter that must be guarded against at all times. Physical therapists must know how to detect the signs of abuse, be sensitive and receptive to clients who may choose to confide in them, and know the proper procedures to follow if they suspect abuse. They must work with other professionals to promote assertiveness and positive self-esteem in their clients.

All professionals involved with patients who have CP must educate them in being streetwise. Their physical and sometimes cognitive limitations can make them particularly vulnerable to crime. Children and adolescents with disabilities should be taught to avoid threatening situations. They should be warned about carrying valuables (large sums of money or important medications) with them, particularly in a purse that attracts attention and is easy to grab, such as one slung over a wheelchair handle. Attendance at self-defense courses should be encouraged; some that are specifically designed for people with disabilities are becoming available.

Health care professionals must realize that although parents have been coping with their children's needs for a number of years, parent education is still important: their children and their needs are constantly changing. Continued attention to education in lifting and transferring is necessary to prevent injury to caregivers as their children grow larger and heavier and they themselves are aging.

ROLE OF OTHER DISCIPLINES

Occupational therapists may be involved in promoting independence in ADL. Multidisciplinary life-skills training may be offered to focus on self-care, community living, and interpersonal relationships. Prevocational training and related activities, such as money management and employment searching, may be necessary. Psychologists or social workers may be involved in social and sexual counseling.

Transition to Adulthood

The life role of an adult is to be an independently functioning and self-sufficient individual who has a satisfying social and emotional life and is a contributing member of society. The natural environment for adults is living independently in the community, alone or with others, with employment to support them.

The extent to which people with CP can realize these goals depends on factors such as level of cognition, available resources and support, and independence in self-care activities and mobility. Many adults with CP continue to live with their families, in group homes, or in institutions, and a small proportion of them are employed. In Finland, a study of young adults who had been followed since childhood revealed that 31% of those older than 19 years were competitively employed, but an additional 21% who were judged to be employable were unemployed (Sillanpaa et al., 1982). Finding employment can be particularly difficult when there is considerable unemployment in the able-bodied population.

At a time when most parents are experiencing freedom from caregiving responsibilities, many parents of children with CP continue to have these obligations and have to cope with many anxieties (Hallum, 1995). Their concerns focus on how their child can function as an independent adult, how they can continue to care for their child as they themselves age, and who will care for the child when they are unable to do so. They, and their child, may also be coping with a decrease in the number of relatively organized and available programs that were available for the younger child.

Physical therapy involvement continues to address all levels of the disabling process; however, there is an emphasis on working together with the individual, the family, and the health care team to provide comprehensive planning to ease the transition to adulthood.

Physical Therapy Examination and Evaluation

Although there is a continuing need to assess impairment, adult assessments focus on function and disability, particularly on the level of independent functioning. A variety of functional disability scales, such as the Barthel Index, have been developed for adults in general rather than for adults with a particular disability (Mahoney & Barthel, 1965). These measure performance in various self-care, independence, and mobility functions (Spector, 1990).

Physical Therapy Goals, Outcomes, and Interventions

The major goal during this period of transition is to maximize the client's capabilities to achieve optimal independence and happiness as an adult. Ideally, the medical, therapeutic, and educational goals of childhood have had this as a long-term goal in earlier intervention. In a study of adults with CP health in terms of acute illnesses was not a problem, but 76% had multiple musculoskeletal problems, and many nonambulatory adults had urinary complaints. Equipment and therapy needs were poorly met (Murphy et al., 1995). In many situations, professionals, the client, and the family are dealing with

external environmental forces that make it difficult for a person to overcome disabilities.

REDUCING PRIMARY IMPAIRMENT AND PREVENTING SECONDARY IMPAIRMENT

Although there is a focus on overall disability, therapists must still be cognizant of the impact of impairment on function. Adults with CP must deal with the normal effects of aging in addition to their existing impairments (Overeynder & Turk, 1998). Insufficient force generation and hypoextensibility can still respond to therapy. Although secondary impairments such as contracture may appear to be static, there can still be deterioration, so monitoring and treatment, if necessary, should be available. If significant deformity occurs, aggressive salvage surgery may be necessary for comfort and ease of care. One example is proximal femoral resection if a hip is painful or if hip mobility is limited to the extent that sitting and perineal care are affected; however, this surgery has a high complication rate (Perlmutter, 1993).

Of particular importance is the prevention of overuse syndromes, joint degeneration, progression of contractures, osteoporosis, poor endurance, and pathologic fractures. Cervical and back pain, nerve entrapment syndromes, or tendinitis can occur as a result of excessive and repetitive physical stresses (Bergman, 1994; Murphy et al., 1995). Such injuries should be treated with orthopedic therapy techniques, as they would be in the general population. Preventive treatment to minimize the long-term effects of the neuromuscular dysfunction may be beneficial. This may include use of additional mobility aids or devices, orthoses, or surgery. Changes to the adult's environment may be necessary to maintain optimal independence (Overeynder & Turk, 1998).

LIFE SKILLS

Ongoing involvement in fitness and recreational activities should be planned. This will provide social opportunities, as well as maintain or improve cardiovascular fitness, weight control, and integrity of joints and muscles; help prevent osteoporosis; and generally promote the optimal health that contributes to independent functioning. Fitness clubs, swimming, wheelchair aerobics, and adapted sports are options. Endurance continues to be an important concern. Fernandez and Pitetti (1993) found that the values for physical work capacity of ambulatory adults with CP were significantly lower than normal values and concluded that adults with CP would possibly experience fatigue before completing a normal workday. However, physical work capacity and work-related activities improved with training.

Technology is providing adults with CP many options that were not previously available. These include computers for communication, artificial speech devices, environmental control devices, and mobility devices. For more information, see Chapter 24.

Society is becoming more conscious of the rights and needs of the disabled (Bickenbach, 1993). Human rights legislation now exists to accommodate people with disabilities and to prevent discrimination against them in areas such as employment, accessibility, the legal system, and education. Government programs and services are available to people with disabilities. Theaters, restaurants, libraries, museums, government buildings, educational facilities, shopping areas, parks, campground facilities, and parking lots are becoming accessible, where possible, through the provision of ramps, appropriate washroom facilities, and other modifications. Air and rail travel is also becoming more accessible to people with special mobility needs, and there are now travel organizations that cater to people with disabilities. In some situations, funding for assistive devices, living allowances, and housing and tax exemptions help prevent undue hardship. Therapists should be aware of the facilities available to the disabled and the political policies and issues concerning the disabled and should advocate their advancement.

TRANSITION PLANNING

Ideally, the planning for the transition to adult services and lifestyle takes place before the actual major life changes. Areas to be addressed when planning for the transition include the following: vocational training or postsecondary educational placement, which may range from higher education to supported work models; living arrangements (independent, with family, institutional, or other supportive care); leisure and recreation (religious groups, community programs, and recreational centers); personal management, including birth control; social skills; and household management. The continuation of professional health services must also be dealt with (Fox et al., 1992). This includes the provision of therapy when needed, medical consultation, primary care, and equipment needs and maintenance. Financial planning and education about budgeting, tax and other governmental benefits, advocacy and legal services, guardianship, conservatorship, wills, and trusts must be addressed (Hallum, 1995).

RESEARCH NEEDS

Research in CP is urgently needed. The selection of treatment for an individual with CP requires predictive information about the effects of interventions, if any, on the pathophysiology, impairments, functional limitations, and disabilities of the person throughout the life span, yet even descriptive information is limited. To take a simple example, to decide whether orthoses are appropriate for a particular child, we should know whether the impairment of hypoextensibility is preventable by orthoses, as some studies suggest (Tardieu et al., 1988), and, if so, under what conditions. Furthermore, we should know if force generation capability is changed with orthotic wear, how force output changes with growth, and what conditions favor successful long-term outcomes. The multisystem impairments of poor selective control of muscles, poor anticipatory regulation of movement, and decreased ability to learn unique movements have received little attention.

We need better information about the relationships between measures at each level of the disabling process. This will facilitate specificity of treatment. There is a need for research that predicts long-term outcomes. Finally, there are needs for specific and sensitive measurements of all dimensions of the disabling process to be developed within a focused research program.

GLOBAL ISSUES

The treatment of children with CP varies throughout the world. Physical therapists use many different approaches and combinations of approaches, depending on the facilities available, the child's and the family's needs, the therapist's training and background, and the diversity of client values, beliefs, and priorities. Many of the treatments and technologies discussed are practiced in developed countries, where services, although variable in their extent, quality, and funding, are available and accessible. However, much of the world's population lives in underserviced areas, particularly in developing nations or in remote areas of developed nations. Often, many of the principles and equipment ideas developed elsewhere can be adapted to the various situations (Werner, 1987). Using indigenous materials to fabricate effective and affordable equipment, recycling used equipment, and training local personnel or fostering exchange programs can help provide resources to underserviced areas.

It is important to be sensitive to local customs, cultures, and environmental situations when adapting programs for different settings. Often, the direct application of a certain method is impractical or inappropriate because of economic, geographic, or cultural differences. There is an increasing emphasis on community-based rehabilitation, which promotes interventions that are practical and functional for the particular settings, lifestyles, and cultures.

PROFESSIONAL ISSUES

Therapists who care for children with CP must realize that the work can be physically demanding. They must practice appropriate lifting and handling precautions and should maintain a suitable level of fitness if they are actively treating patients. Working with children and their families can also be emotionally stressful. Therapists may often be challenged with ethical issues, unrealistic expectations and demands, limited resources, and the pressures of dealing with families during the grieving period and other times of crisis. Therapists need to concentrate on what is positive and realize that they cannot control all the variables in their patients' conditions and lives. Professionals must acknowledge their own needs and reactions and feel comfortable in seeking assistance and support from others.

This chapter concludes with two case histories that illustrate some of the management principles discussed in this chapter.

CASE HISTORY
JAMIE

Jamie is an 8-year-old boy with spastic diplegia and microcephaly. After a pregnancy complicated by preeclamptic toxemia, labor began at 37 weeks of gestation, and an emergency cesarean section became necessary when fetal distress occurred. Treatment was begun in the hospital. On returning home with their child, the parents performed routine stretches daily, and a therapist visited every other week. A mothers' support group met every 2 weeks, which provided general information and guidance, as well as support.

When Jamie was about 1.5 years of age, the family moved to a town in another province where coordinated services were provided. Jamie took part in physical therapy, occupational therapy, and speech therapy and was assessed routinely by the psychologic services. When he began attending day care, he received services from the same therapists, and the parents, teachers, and therapists worked together on his treatment.

When Jamie was 3.5 years old, the impairment of hypoextensibility of the hamstrings and heel cords was present. Functionally, he was able to walk independently, although he fatigued easily. Toe-walking was common and accompanied by slight knee flexion and adduction and internal rotation of the hips. His right limb showed more impairment than his left. Bivalved short leg casts were worn for 2 hours three times a day, the goal being to prevent further hypoextensibility of the ankle plantar flexors.

At age 4.5 years, Jamie's gait was examined in the Motion Analysis Laboratory at the School of Rehabilitation Therapy at Queen's University in Kingston, Ontario. He walked at an average of 0.71 m/s, compared with the normal value for his age of about 1.00 m/s (Sutherland et al., 1980). Joint excursions were reduced (Fig. 20–11). He walked with marked plantar flexion of the right foot and with slight flexion and reduced excursion of both knees, and he had reduced power generation of the ankle plantar flexors on both sides (A2-PF, Fig. 20–12), which was evidence of low force-generating capability, hypoextensibility, or both. He was compensating for these deficiencies with larger than normal pull-off by hip flexors on the left side (H3-F, Fig. 20–12). The family engaged Jamie in an electrostimulation program from an outside clinic in which the quadriceps and ankle dorsiflexors were stimulated overnight at a level below that required to produce muscle contraction. During the next few months, while electrostimulation and weekly therapy were continued but the use of casts was not, Jamie's ankle plantar flexors became much more hypoextensible. The use of bivalved casts was reintroduced, and the previous range was regained rapidly.

Clinical examination when Jamie was 5.5 years old revealed that his hip adductors, knee flexors, and ankle plantar flexors were more hypoextensible; functionally, he was walking on his toes with reduced excursions of his ankles. Although a number of surgical alternatives were considered, including rhizotomy, the family decided on a lengthening of the right heel cord. The goals of gait reeducation were toward attaining initial contact with the heel and an extended knee and achieving effective push-off with the ankle plantar flexors. His electrical stimulator was used in treatment postoperatively to strengthen the ankle dorsiflexors and the surgically weakened plantar flexors. Other treatment goals and activities included climbing and descending stairs with one foot per stair and stepping off a stair or curb without hand support. Because Jamie had a keen interest in sports, movement components such as weight shifting, balancing, and eye-hand-foot coordination and skills such as running, starting and stopping, changing direction, and throwing were incorporated into sports activities such as baseball, soccer, and badminton. The improvement noted at a 6-month postsurgical gait analysis (see Fig. 20–11) was more marked on the right side, but several improvements were noted on the left. On the right side, initial contact was made with the heel, and ankle dorsiflexion during late stance reached about 15°. The knees on both sides were more extended at initial contact and extended more in late stance than was the case before surgery. The push-off power of the right ankle was greater after surgery (A2-PF, Fig. 20–12) than before surgery, and right hip power was more effective (H1-E, hip extensors in early stance; H3-F, hip flexors at pull-off; Fig. 20–12). Average walking velocity was

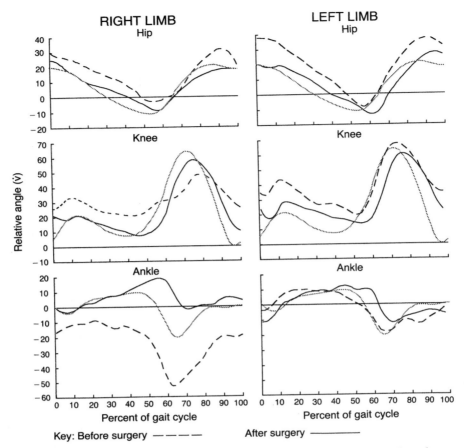

FIGURE 20–11. Plots of joint angles from gait analysis of one stride for Jamie, shown presurgically and postsurgically and with normal values (dotted line). Each plot represents one stride beginning and ending with initial contact of the foot on the floor. Plotted upward (positively) are hip flexion, knee flexion, and ankle dorsiflexion. Note limited knee extension on both sides, extreme limitation of ankle dorsiflexion on the right, and normalization of postsurgical values.

0.82 m/s. Jamie was able to join the community soccer league the following summer.

Jamie attends school in a regular classroom, although he has some cognitive limitations. He is visited by a familiar therapist from the treatment center every 2 or 3 weeks and attends speech therapy weekly. The main problem the parents have encountered within the school system is a practice of inflexibly classifying the children according to their chronologic age only. Although Jamie is cognitively young and physically small for his age, there has been considerable reluctance to permit him to join younger groups, even for sports. Outside of school, Jamie takes part in a number of athletic activities. He is interested in team sports, and the family has been pleased with the efforts of coaches and managers to include him in organized teams.

Update: 5 years later

Jamie is now a happy and likeable 13-year-old about to face the challenges of adolescence. He is completing his last year of school at the intermediate level and will be entering a public high school next year. The family is very happy with his education to date, and is trying to help him prepare for the challenges of a large school in which the children are expected to be independent. His cognitive impairments are more limiting than his physical situation. Still small for his age, he has not been able to continue in team sports. His greatest joy is karate, which he attends 3 days a week. He expects to receive his violet belt soon. This activity has helped him with self-discipline, balance, and coordination. Jamie attends physical therapy about every 3 weeks, where he concentrates on stretching and functional activities that

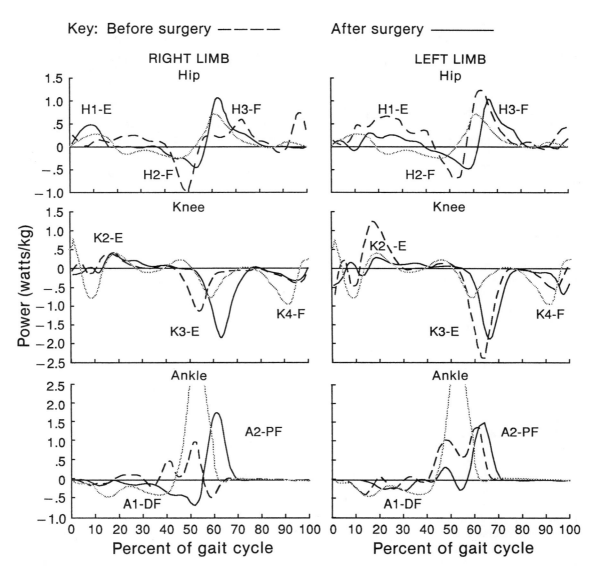

FIGURE 20–12. Plots of joint power from gait analysis of one stride for Jamie, shown presurgically and postsurgically and with normal values (dotted line). Each plot represents one stride beginning and ending with initial contact of the foot on the floor. Plotted upward (positively) are muscle power generations (concentric contractions), and downward (negatively) are muscle power absorptions (eccentric contractions). Plots of Jamie's right side show low force generation of right hip extensors in early stance (H1-E), of hip flexors at pull-off (H3-F), and of ankle plantar flexors (A2-PF) presurgically, and increases in all of these after surgery. Plots of Jamie's left side show compensatory increase in H3-F (pull-off of hip flexors) presurgically, and normalization after surgery.

are complementary to his karate practice. About once a year, the hypoextensibility of his left calf group is treated with about 3 weeks of serial casting.

CASE HISTORY
NICOLE

Nicole has moderate to severe spastic diplegia. She was born at 29.5 weeks of gestation after placental separation. She weighed 1300 g and had an Apgar score of 8 at 5 minutes. She was treated with ventilation for 8 hours and then was weaned off the ventilator onto continuous positive airway pressure, and then to oxygen. She received phototherapy for 3 days for an increased bilirubin level and was administered theophylline for apnea. Nicole remained in the neonatal intensive care unit for 6 weeks and then went home to live with her parents and 3-year-old sister.

Nicole was followed up at the screening clinic for high-risk infants. At 3 months of age corrected for prematurity, she exhibited extensor positioning of her neck and trunk and hypertonicity was emerging in her legs, but her family did not have any concerns. At 4 months of corrected age, these findings were discussed with her mother, and positioning and handling recommendations were made. At 5 months of corrected age, the diagnosis of CP was made on the basis of hypertonicity in her extremities, affecting lower extremities more than upper; strong, persisting primitive reflex activity; and delayed development of head and trunk control. An ultrasound scan at this time showed the left lateral ventricle to be slightly enlarged and the right lateral ventricle to be at the upper limits of normal in size. The periventricular brain parenchyma appeared normal.

Management by a developmental pediatrician, a social worker, an orthopedic surgeon, a physical therapist, and later an occupational therapist was coordinated at the local children's treatment center. Nicole attended physical therapy sessions weekly. The basic therapy was based on NDT and encouraged active control of movement and play. Positions that reduced the influence of her extensor posturing were used to encourage active control of movements and functional skills. Bivalved casts were introduced early to maintain muscle extensibility and provide optimal alignment of her feet when she was working on standing activities. The casts also reduced some of the extensor posturing in her lower extremities, resulting in improvements in her alignment in sitting and standing and improvements in the quality of functional activities in these positions. These casts were later replaced with solid AFOs when growth slowed down, and Nicole was

eager to wear regular shoes. Customized seating and a standing frame gave her a variety of positions that offered opportunities to interact with others and use her hands and provided some weight bearing with her body optimally aligned.

At 2 years of age, the impairments of adductor hypoextensibility and spasticity were treated surgically with bilateral adductor muscle releases and anterior obturator neurectomies. The purpose of the surgery was to give her more functional motion at her hips and to put her hip joints in an optimal position for acetabular development; it was also intended to avoid the potential secondary impairment of hip subluxation or dislocation.

During her preschool years, Nicole attended an integrated child care program with government-subsidized funding for children with special needs. This setting allowed for integration with able-bodied children and also gave Nicole and her family opportunities to meet other children with special needs and their families. Nicole's physical and occupational therapists visited the center regularly to discuss Nicole's abilities, programs, handling, and equipment. Her resource teacher was invaluable in coordinating care, supporting the family, and adapting or acquiring equipment.

When Nicole was 5 years of age, she was progressing slowly in her gross and fine motor skills. However, spasticity in her lower extremities that was clinically apparent was affecting her ability to maintain well-aligned postural stability, and she could not move easily using optimal patterns of movement. These restrictions resulted in functional limitations in sitting, standing, transitional movements, fine motor activities, and ADL and limited her potential for independence. Ambulation was not functional, but she could move about independently in a power chair and had some limited mobility in a manual wheelchair. The prominence of spasticity and the generally good force-generating capabilities of her musculature prompted the decision to have a selective dorsal rhizotomy.

After the rhizotomy, Nicole's lower extremity tone was greatly reduced, and Nicole participated in daily inpatient physical therapy and occupational therapy sessions for 8 weeks postoperatively and then had sessions twice a week for the next year (Figs. 20–13 and 20–14).

A Gross Motor Function Measure evaluation was done preoperatively and 1 year after the surgery. Her scores improved from 88 to 96% in lying and rolling; from 78 to 87% in sitting; from 19 to 57% in crawling and kneeling; from 13 to 32% in standing (with AFOs); and from 7 to 10% in walking, running, and jumping (with AFOs). She had been able to walk 10 m at 0.04 m/s preoperatively but could walk 30 m at 0.15 m/s at her 1-year follow-up. Although these findings indicated that there had been improvements in her gait,

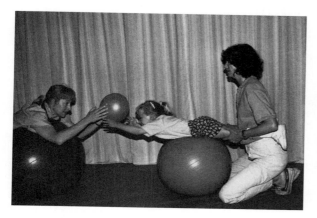

FIGURE 20–13. Mother and therapist with Nicole, encouraging force generation of trunk and hip extensors.

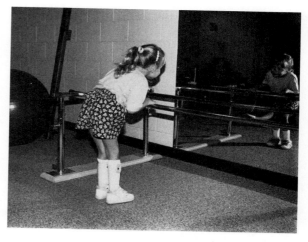

FIGURE 20–15. Despite many improvements after posterior rhizotomy, Nicole still shows diminished force-generating ability in hip and knee muscles.

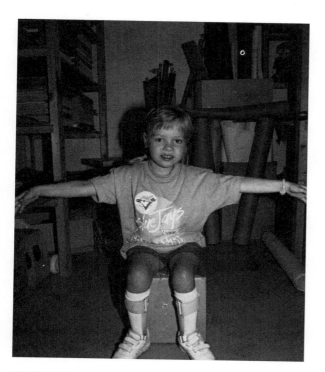

FIGURE 20–14. Nicole, wearing ankle-foot orthoses, doing exercises at school.

the distance and velocity of her walking were still much below age norms and did not result in functional ambulation. She had improved isolated muscle control, which was demonstrated by improved active ROM of her quadriceps, dorsiflexors, and plantar flexors. Her passive ROM improved in her hips, knees, and ankles, particularly in motions involving the hamstring muscles. Nicole continues to have decreased muscle force production, particularly in her hip and knee extensor muscles (Fig. 20–15).

Nicole showed improvements in her self-care skills, particularly in dressing her lower extremities, because she was able to move one leg independently of the other. On a modified Klein-Bell test of ADL, she achieved 9/33 before surgery and 19/33 when tested 1 year later. She was able to function better with her hands in activities such as opening jars, printing, and propelling her manual wheelchair. The improvements were believed to be the result of better trunk control and co-contraction in the shoulder musculature rather than of changes in the intrinsic muscles of her hands, motor planning, or visuoperceptual skills—areas that continue to be problems for Nicole. The Beery Developmental Test of visuomotor integration score was at an age equivalency of 4.1 both preoperatively and postoperatively.

Nicole now attended her neighborhood school. Transportation was provided by the school board in a school bus with a wheelchair lift so that she could travel to school with her peers. The educational system also provided a full-time educational assistant to help Nicole with transfers, toileting, schoolwork, and exercise and sports programs. She played with her friends on the playground at lunch and recess in her power chair. She used a typewriter to increase the speed at which she could put information down on paper.

Nicole's family has worked with medical, educational, governmental, and community organizations to gain access to services and programs that provide her with normal childhood experiences and minimize disabilities. Nicole has been involved with horseback riding, swimming programs, and adapted games. She rides in her family's boat using a Tumble Form seat, goes on an annual vacation to Florida, and traveled to England to be a flower girl at her aunt's wedding. She attends her peers' birthday parties, where her friends or their parents help her as necessary. She has modeled in fashion shows in her wheelchair. Nicole has attended the community day camp, Brownies, and the Easter Seals family camp in the summer.

Resources her family has found useful include the Easter Seals Society; the Ontario government's Assistive Devices Program; parent support groups; and the Community and Social Services Respite Care Program, which provides funds for students to work with Nicole and provide parent relief. The Canadian railroad, VIA Rail, which allows wheelchair escorts to ride free and offers reduced rates for Nicole, is useful for traveling to out-of-town appointments.

Nicole and her family face barriers. The family home is in the country and has a gravel driveway. The house is not wheelchair accessible because there are stairs into the house, stairs inside, and narrow doorways. Thick carpeting makes manual wheelchair pushing and walker maneuvering difficult. When Nicole visits friends, their homes have similar obstacles. Renovations have been made to the school washroom, and equipment has been provided, but the entrance doors are too heavy to open, playground equipment is inaccessible, and classroom door handles are difficult to turn. There is no public wheelchair transportation in their township community. Although obstacles are becoming less common as society becomes more aware of accommodations necessary for people with disabilities, barriers such as buildings without ramps, inadequate parking, and inaccessible washrooms still exist.

Nicole's parents have found regular family conferences invaluable in helping to facilitate effective family and school involvement in therapy programs. In these conferences, all the team members meet to discuss short- and long-term goals. Agendas and minutes clarify the objectives of the meetings and document the decisions that are made. Such conferences help empower parents and allow them to become effective advocates for their children. They also reinforce the philosophy of teamwork and partnership with the therapists and the treatment center.

Nicole's parents have found Craig Shield's book *Strategies: A Practical Guide for Dealing with Professionals and Human Service Systems* to be helpful (Shields, 1987). They believe that home visits designed to deal with issues of daily routines, integrate treatment goals into home life, and involve all family members are important. Similarly, school visits are important. Nicole's parents believe that it is particularly important not to withhold any information from the family. They also emphasize the need for feedback and encouragement to the family, especially to the primary caregiver.

Update: 5 years later

Nicole is now a warm and friendly 13-year-old who will be entering high school next year. Her parents have worked closely with teachers and administrators of the school, where she has a half-day educational attendant who helps with her schoolwork and gives personal assistance. Her above average knowledge of computer functions allows her to develop more efficient ways of completing her school assignments and communicating with others. Nicole uses a taxi fitted for wheelchair transport when she travels by herself to school and to the shopping mall. She uses a power wheelchair in most places other than her own home, where she uses a manual wheelchair. For recreation, Nicole swims at a local pool, and, in the summer, attends a camp. Like many teenagers, she uses a chat line on the Internet, and she speaks with her friends on the telephone.

Because Nicole had received some professional services (notably the dorsal rhizotomy) from a nearby city, it was difficult for the family to obtain a consensus of prognostic information that would help them make decisions about their home and lifestyle. Nicole's mother arranged a telephone conference between all of the relevant professionals in the two cities and Nicole and herself, which she felt was the single most important event in the past several years. As a result, Nicole's family has built an addition to their home, which makes the downstairs fully accessible. It also has a large deck that allows Nicole to go outdoors on her own and gives a second entrance to the house. The driveway is paved to enable her to reach her taxi or bus. She needs one-person assistance with transfers, toileting, and dressing, but she showers and washes her own hair independently using a commode chair in a wheel-in shower. Nicole eats independently.

Nicole is seen by a physical therapist working in the school system about once a month, and she attends a teen group for girls organized by the professionals of the Child Development Centre. Stressing life skills, the meetings also provide opportunities for the teens to discuss items of mutual interest. Her mother thinks physical therapy may be needed to maintain the range of motion in her hamstrings, which is needed for upright standing during transfers.

Nicole's parents are very active advocates for changes that will provide people with disabilities with a full range of life's opportunities. They believe parents must be prepared to play central, responsible leadership roles within groups and agencies that can assist in these endeavors.

ACKNOWLEDGMENTS

Acknowledgments are extended to the Child Development Centre of the Hotel Dieu Hospital, Kingston, Ontario; the Motion Analysis Laboratory at the School of Rehabilitation Therapy at Queen's University, Kingston, Ontario; the

Bloorview-MacMillan Rehabilitation Centre, Toronto, Ontario, for assistance in providing data and photographs; and to the parents of Jamie and Nicole for their support of and contributions to the case histories.

Recommended Resources

Barry, MJ. Physical therapy interventions for patients with movement disorders due to cerebral palsy. Journal of Child Neurology, 11(suppl 1):S51–S60, 1996.

Campbell, SK. Therapy programs for children that last a lifetime. Physical and Occupational Therapy in Pediatrics, 17(1):1–15, 1997.

Geralis, E (Ed.). Children with Cerebral Palsy. Rockville, MD: Woodbine House, 1991. Available from Ingram, 1125 Heilquaker Boulevard, Leverane, TN 37086-1986.

Gowland, C, King, G, King, S, Law, M, Letts, L, MacKinnon, L, Rosenbaum, P, & Russell, D. Review of Selected Measures in Neurodevelopmental Rehabilitation. Research Report 91-2, Neurodevelopmental Clinical Research Unit, Chedoke-McMaster Hospitals, 1991. Available from Chedoke-McMaster Hospitals, PO Box 2000, Station A, Hamilton, Ontario, Canada, L8N 3Z5.

Jaeger, DL. Transferring and Lifting Children and Adolescents: Home Instruction Sheets. Tucson, AZ: Therapy Skill Builders, 1989. Available from Therapy Skill Builders, 555 Academic Court, San Antonio, TX, 78204-2498.

Jaeger, L. Home Program Instruction Sheets for Infants and Young Children. Tucson, AZ: Therapy Skill Builders, 1987. Available from Therapy Skill Builders, 555 Academic Court, San Antonio, TX, 78204-2498.

Law, M, King, G, MacKinnon, E, Russell, D, Murphy, C, Harley, P, & Bosch, E. All About Outcomes: A Program to Help You Organize Your Thinking About Outcome Measures (CD-ROM). Thoroughfare, NJ: Slack, Inc.

Lollar, DJ (Ed.). Preventing Secondary Conditions Associated with Spina Bifida or Cerebral Palsy. Washington, DC: Spina Bifida Association of America, 1994, pp. 54–64.

Washington State Department of Health. Cerebral Palsy—Critical Elements of Care. Seattle, WA: Washington State Department of Health, 1997. Phone: 206-517-2462.

Wilcox, C. Hey, What About Me! Activities for Disabled Children. Toronto: Doubleday Canada, 1988. Available from Doubleday, 105 Bond Street, Toronto, Ontario, Canada, M5B 1Y3.

WEB SITES

American Academy for Cerebral Palsy and Developmental Medicine: http://aacpdm.org/

United Cerebral Palsy: http://www.ucpa.org/

Ontario Federation for Cerebral Palsy: http://www.ofcp.on.ca/

References

Abel, MF. Gait laboratory analysis for pre-operative decision making in spastic cerebral palsy: Is it all that it is cracked up to be? (Letter; Comment). Journal of Pediatric Orthopedics, 15:698–700, 1995.

Anderson, JP, Snow, B, Dorey, FJ, & Kabo, JM. Efficacy of soft splints in reducing severe knee-flexion contractures. Developmental Medicine and Child Neurology, 30:502–508, 1988.

Anonymous. Residential arrangements for adults with cerebral palsy—California, 1988. Morbidity & Mortality Weekly Report, 40(1):16–18, 1991.

Atkinson, S, & Stanley, FJ. Spastic diplegia among children of low and normal birthweight. Developmental Medicine and Child Neurology, 25:693–708, 1983.

Atwater, SW. Should the normal motor developmental sequence be used as a theoretical model in pediatric physical therapy? In Lister, MJ (Ed.), Contemporary Management of Motor Control Problems: Proceedings of the II STEP Conference. Alexandria, VA: Foundation for Physical Therapy, 1991, pp. 89–93.

Bairstow, P, Cochrane, R, & Rusk, I. Selection of children with cerebral palsy for conductive education and the characteristics of children judged suitable and unsuitable. Developmental Medicine and Child Neurology, 33:984–992, 1991.

Barry, MJ. Physical therapy interventions for patients with movement disorders due to cerebral palsy. Journal of Child Neurology, 11(suppl 1):S51–S60, 1996.

Batshaw, MI, & Perret, YM. Children with Disabilities: A Medical Primer, 3rd ed. Toronto: Paul H. Brookes, 1992.

Baumann, JU, & Zumstein, M. Experience with a plastic ankle-foot orthosis for prevention of muscle contracture. Developmental Medicine and Child Neurology, 27:83, 1985.

Bayley, N. Bayley II. San Antonio: Psychological Corporation, 1993.

Berbrayer, D, & Ashby, P. Reciprocal inhibition in cerebral palsy. Neurology, 40:653–656, 1990.

Berger, W, Quintern, J, & Deitz, V. Pathophysiology of gait in children with cerebral palsy. Electroencephalography and Clinical Neurophysiology, 53:538–548, 1982.

Bergman, JS. Protecting the mobility of the aging person with spina bifida or cerebral palsy. In Lollar, DJ (Ed.), Preventing Secondary Conditions Associated with Spina Bifida or Cerebral Palsy. Washington, DC: Spina Bifida Association of America, 1994, pp. 54–64.

Bickenbach, J. Physical Disability and Social Policy. Toronto: University of Toronto Press, 1993.

Blair, E, Ballantyne, J, Horsman, S, & Chauvel, P. A study of a dynamic proximal stability splint in the management of children with cerebral palsy. Developmental Medicine and Child Neurology, 37:544–554, 1995.

Blanche, EI. Doing with—Not doing to: Play and the child with cerebral palsy. In Parham, LD, & Fazio, LS (Eds.), Play in Occupational Therapy for Children. St. Louis: Mosby, 1997, pp. 202–218.

Blasco, PA, Allaire, JH, and participants of the Consortium on Drooling. Drooling in the developmentally disabled: Management practices and recommendations. Developmental Medicine and Child Neurology, 34:849–862, 1992.

Bleck, EE. Locomotor prognosis in cerebral palsy. Developmental Medicine and Child Neurology, 17:18–25, 1975.

Bleck, EE. Orthopedic Management in Cerebral Palsy. Philadelphia: JB Lippincott, 1987.

Bly, L. A historical and current view of the basis of NDT. Pediatric Physical Therapy, 3:131–135, 1991.

Bobath, K, & Bobath, B. The neuro-developmental treatment. In Scrutton, D (Ed.), Management of the Motor Disorders of Children with Cerebral Palsy. Clinics in Developmental Medicine (No. 90). Philadelphia: JB Lippincott, 1984, pp. 6–18.

Bohannon, RW. Is the measurement of muscle strength appropriate in patients with brain lesions? Physical Therapy, 69:225–236, 1989.

Bohannon, RW, & Smith, MB. Interrater reliability of a modified Ashworth scale of muscle spasticity. Physical Therapy, 67:206–207, 1987.

Bower, E, & McLellan, DL. Effect of increased exposure to physiotherapy on skill acquisition of children with cerebral palsy. Developmental Medicine and Child Neurology, 34:25–39, 1992.

Bower, E, McLellan, DL, Arney, J, & Campbell, MJ. A randomised controlled trial of different intensities of physiotherapy and different goal-setting procedures in 44 children with cerebral palsy. Developmental Medicine and Child Neurology, 38:226–237, 1996.

Boyce, W, Gowland, C, Rosenbaum, P, Lane, M, Plews, N, Goldsmith, C, Russell, D, Wright, V, Zdrobov, S, & Harding, D. The Gross Motor Performance Measure: Validity and responsiveness of a measure of quality of movement. Physical Therapy, 75:603–613, 1995.

Boyd, R, & Graham, HK. Botulinum toxin A in the management of children with cerebral palsy: Indications and outcome. European Journal of Neurology, 4(suppl 2):S15–S22, 1997.

Brooks-Scott, S. Mobilization for the Neurologically Involved Child. Tucson, AZ: Therapy Skill Builders, 1995.

Brouwer, B, & Ashby, P. Altered corticospinal projections to lower limb motoneurons in subjects with cerebral palsy. Brain, 114:1395–1407, 1991.

Brouwer, B, Wheeldon, RK, Stradiotto-Parker, N, & Allum, J. Reflex excitability and isometric force production in cerebral palsy: The effect of serial casting. Developmental Medicine and Child Neurology, 40:168–175, 1998.

Bruininks, RH. Bruininks-Oseretsky Test of Motor Proficiency: Examiner's Manual. Circle Pines, MN: American Guidance Service, 1978.

Bull, MJ, Weber, KL, DeRosa, GP, & Bruner Stroup, K. Transporting children in body casts. Journal of Pediatric Orthopedics, 9:280–284, 1989.

Burns, YR, O'Callaghan, M, & Tudehope, DI. Early identification of cerebral palsy in high risk infants. Australian Paediatric Journal, 25:215–219, 1989.

Butler, C. Augmentative mobility: Why do it? Physical Medicine and Rehabilitation Clinics of North America, 2(4):801–815, 1991.

Campbell, SK. Introduction to the special issue. Pediatric Physical Therapy, 2:123–125, 1990.

Campbell, SK. Therapy programs for children that last a lifetime. Physical and Occupational Therapy in Pediatrics, 17(1):1–15, 1997.

Campbell, SK, Almeida, GL, Penn, RD, & Corcos, DM. The effects of intrathecally administered baclofen in patients with spasticity. Physical Therapy, 75:352–362, 1995.

Campbell, SK, Wilhelm, IJ, & Slaton, DS. Anthropometric characteristics of young children with cerebral palsy. Pediatric Physical Therapy, 1:105–108, 1989.

Carlson, SJ. A neurophysiological analysis of inhibitive casting. Physical and Occupational Therapy in Pediatrics, 4(4):31–42, 1984.

Carlson, WE, Vaughan, CL, Damiano, DL, & Abel, MF. Orthotic management of gait in spastic diplegia. American Journal of Physical Medicine and Rehabilitation, 76:219–224, 1997.

Carmick, J. Managing equinus in a child with cerebral palsy: Merits of hinged ankle-foot orthosis. Developmental Medicine and Child Neurology, 37:1006–1019, 1995.

Chandler, L, & Harris, S. Movement assessment of infants. Workshop Presentation, Northeastern District of the Section on Pediatrics of the American Physical Therapy Association, Amherst, MA. Cited in Campbell, SK. Assessment of the child with CNS dysfunction. In Rothstein, JM (Ed.), Measurement in Physical Therapy. New York: Churchill Livingstone, 1985.

Chandler, LS, Andrew, MS, & Swanson, MW. Movement Assessment of Infants: A Manual. Rolling Bay, WA: Infant Movement Research, 1980.

Clune, WH, & Van Pelt, MH. A political method of evaluating the Education for All Handicapped Children Act of 1975. Law and Contemporary Problems, 48(1):7–62, 1985.

Corry, IS, Cosgrove, AP, Duffy, CM, McNeill, S, Taylor, TC, & Graham, HK. Botulinum toxin A compared with stretching casts in the treatment of spastic equinus: A randomised prospective trial. Journal of Pediatric Orthopedics, 18:304–311, 1998.

Coster, WJ, Deeney, TA, Haltiwanger, JT, & Haley, SM. School Function Assessment. Boston University, 1994.

Craft, MJ, Lakin, JA, Oppliger, RA, Clancy, GM, & Vanderlinden, DW. Siblings as change agents for promoting the functional status of children with cerebral palsy. Developmental Medicine and Child Neurology, 32:1049–1057, 1990.

Crothers, B, & Paine, RS. The Natural History of Cerebral Palsy (2nd ed.). Philadelphia: Lippincott, 1988.

Cusick, BD. Progressive Casting and Splinting for Lower Extremity Deformities in Children with Neuromotor Dysfunction. Tucson, AZ: Therapy Skill Builders, 1990.

Cusick, BD, & Stuberg, WA. Assessment of lower extremity alignment in the transverse plane: Implications for management of children with neuromotor dysfunction. Physical Therapy, 72:3–15, 1992.

Damiano, DL, & Abel, MF. Functional outcomes of strength training in spastic cerebral palsy. Archives of Physical Medicine and Rehabilitation, 79:119–125, 1998.

Damiano, DL, Kelly, LE, & Vaughn, CL. Effects of quadriceps femoris muscle strengthening on crouch gait in children with spastic diplegia. Physical Therapy, 75:658–671, 1995.

Darrah, J, & Bartlett, D. Dynamic systems theory and management of children with cerebral palsy: Unresolved issues. Infants and Young Children, 8:52–59, 1995.

DeLuca, PA. The musculoskeletal management of children with cerebral palsy. Pediatric Clinics of North America, 43:1135–1150, 1996.

Dowding, VM, & Barry, C. Cerebral palsy: Social class differences in prevalence in relation to birthweight and severity of disability. Journal of Epidemiology and Community Health, 44:191–195, 1990.

Edebol-Tysk, K. Epidemiology of spastic tetraplegic cerebral palsy in Sweden. I: Impairments and disabilities. Neuropediatrics, 20:41–45, 1989.

Evans, PM, Evans, SJW, & Alberman, E. Cerebral palsy: Why we must plan for survival. Archives of Disease in Childhood, 65:1329–1333, 1990.

Evans Morris, S, & Dunn Klein, M. Pre-feeding Skills: A Comprehensive Resource for Feeding Development. San Antonio, TX: Therapy Skill Builders, 1987.

Fernandez, JE, & Pitetti, KH. Training of ambulatory individuals with cerebral palsy. Archives of Physical Medicine and Rehabilitation, 74:468–472, 1993.

Ferrara, MS, Buckley, WE, McCann, BC, Limbird, TJ, Powell, JW, & Robl, R. The injury experience of a competitive athlete with a disability: Prevention implications. Medicine and Science in Sports and Exercise, 24:184–188, 1992.

Fetters, L. Measurement and treatment in cerebral palsy: An argument for a new approach. Physical Therapy, 71:244–247, 1991.

Finnie, NR. Handling the Young Cerebral Palsied Child at Home, 3rd ed. Oxford: Butterworth-Heinemann, 1997.

Fox, AM, Gillett, JM, & Goldberg, B. Adults with cerebral palsy: Who provides medical care? Annals of the Royal College of Physicians and Surgeons of Canada, 25:206–209, 1992.

Geralis, E (Ed.). Children with Cerebral Palsy. Rockville, MD: Woodbine House, 1991.

Gerszten, PC, Albright, AL, & Johnstone, GF. Intrathecal baclofen infusion and subsequent orthopedic surgery in patients with spastic cerebral palsy. Journal of Neurosurgery, 88:1009–1013, 1998.

Gisel, EG, & Patrick, J. Identification of children with cerebral palsy unable to maintain a normal nutritional state. Lancet, 1:283–286, 1988.

Giuliani, CA. Dorsal rhizotomy for children with cerebral palsy: Support for concepts of motor control. Physical Therapy, 71:248–259, 1991.

Gowland, C, King, G, King, S, Law, M, Letts, L, MacKinnon, L, Rosenbaum, P, & Russell, D. Review of Selected Measures in Neurodevelopmental Rehabilitation. Research Report 91-2, Neurodevelopmental Clinical Research Unit, Chedoke-McMaster Hospitals, 1991.

Hagberg, B, Hagberg, G, Olow, I, & vonWendt, L. The changing panorama of cerebral palsy in Sweden. V. The birth year period 1979–82. Acta Paediatrica Scandinavica, 78:283–290, 1989a.

Hagberg, B, Hagberg, G, & Zetterstrom, R. Decreasing perinatal mortality—Increase in cerebral palsy morbidity? Acta Paediatrica Scandinavica, 78:664–670, 1989b.

Hainsworth, F, Harrison, MJ, Sheldon, TA, & Roussunis, SHP. Preliminary evaluation of ankle orthoses in the management of children with cerebral palsy. Developmental Medicine and Child Neurology, 39:243–247, 1997.

Hallett, M, & Alvarez, N. Attempted rapid elbow flexion movements in patients with athetosis. Journal of Neurology, Neurosurgery and Psychiatry, 46:745–750, 1983.

Hallum, A. Disability and the transition to adulthood: Issues for the disabled child, the family, and the pediatrician. Current Problems in Pediatrics, 25:12–50, 1995.

Harris, SR. Early detection of cerebral palsy: Sensitivity and specificity of two motor assessment tools. Journal of Perinatology, 7:11–15, 1987.

Harris, SR. Early diagnosis of spastic diplegia, spastic hemiplegia, and quadriplegia. American Journal of Diseases of Children, *143*:1356–1360, 1989.

Harris, SR, & Lundgren, BD. Joint mobilization for children with central nervous system disorders: Indications and precautions. Physical Therapy, *71*:890–896, 1991.

Harrison, A. Spastic cerebral palsy: Possible spinal interneuronal contributions. Developmental Medicine and Child Neurology, *30*:769–780, 1988.

Harryman, SE. Lower-extremity surgery for children with cerebral palsy: Physical therapy management. Physical Therapy, *72*:16–24, 1992.

Healy, A, Ramsey, C, & Sexsemith, E. Postural support systems: Their fabrication and functional use. Developmental Medicine and Child Neurology, *39*:706–710, 1997.

Higgins, S. Motor skill acquisition. Physical Therapy, *71*:123–139, 1991.

Hinojosa, J, & Anderson, J. Mothers' perceptions of home treatment programs for their preschool children with cerebral palsy. The American Journal of Occupational Therapy, *45*:273–279, 1991.

Holst, K, Andersen, E, Philip, J, & Henningsen, I. Antenatal and perinatal conditions correlated to handicap among 4-year-old children. American Journal of Perinatology, *6*:258–267, 1989.

Horton, SV, & Taylor, DC. The use of behavior therapy and physical therapy to promote independent ambulation in a preschooler with mental retardation and cerebral palsy. Research in Developmental Disabilities, *10*(4):363–375, 1989.

Jaeger, DL. Transferring and Lifting Children and Adolescents: Home Instruction Sheets. San Antonio, TX: Therapy Skill Builders, 1989.

Jaeger, L. Home Program Instruction Sheets for Infants and Young Children. San Antonio, TX: Therapy Skill Builders, 1987.

James, R. Biofeedback treatment for cerebral palsy in children and adolescents: A review. Pediatric Exercise Science, *24*:198–212, 1992.

Jones, CK. In search of power for the pediatric client. Physical and Occupational Therapy in Pediatrics, *10*(2):47–68, 1990.

Jones, EW, & Mulley, GP. The measurement of spasticity. In Rose, FC (Ed.), Advances in Stroke Therapy. New York: Raven Press, 1982.

Jones, JA (Ed.). Training Guide to Cerebral Palsy Sports. Champaign, IL: Human Kinetics, 1988.

Jonsdottir, J, Fetters, L, & Kluzik, J. Effects of physical therapy on postural control in children with cerebral palsy. Pediatric Physical Therapy, *9*:68–75, 1997.

Karumuna, JMS, & Mgone, CS. Cerebral palsy in Dar es Salaam. Central African Journal of Medicine, *36*(1):8–10, 1990.

Katz, RT, & Rymer, WZ. Spastic hypertonia: Mechanisms and measurement. Archives of Physical Medicine and Rehabilitation, *70*:144–155, 1989.

Kibele, A. Occupational therapy's role in improving the quality of life for persons with cerebral palsy. American Journal of Occupational Therapy, *43*:371–377, 1989.

King, G, Law, M, King, S, & Rosenbaum, P. Parents' and service providers' perceptions of the family-centredness of children's rehabilitation services. Physical and Occupational Therapy in Pediatrics, *18*:21–40, 1998.

Kitchen, WH, Ford, GW, Rickards, AL, Lissenden, JV, & Ryan, MM. Children of birth weight <1000 g: Changing outcome between ages 2 and 5 years. Journal of Pediatrics, *110*:283–288, 1987.

Kluzik, J, Fetters, L, & Coryell, J. Quantification of control: A preliminary study of effects of neurodevelopmental treatment on reaching in children with spastic cerebral palsy. Physical Therapy, *70*:65–78, 1990.

Knutsson, LM, & Clark, DE. Orthotic devices for ambulation in children with cerebral palsy and myelomeningocele. Physical Therapy, *71*:947–960, 1991.

Knutsson, LM, & Martensson, A. Dynamic motor capacity in spastic paresis and its relation to prime mover dysfunction, spastic reflexes and antagonist co-activation. Scandinavian Journal of Rehabilitation Medicine, *12*:93–106, 1980.

Kolobe, THA. Working with families of children with disabilities. Pediatric Physical Therapy, *4*:57–63, 1992.

Kotagal, S, Gibbons, VP, & Stith, JA. Sleep abnormalities in patients with severe cerebral palsy. Developmental Medicine and Child Neurology, *36*:304–311, 1994.

Langley, MB. A developmental approach to the use of toys for facilitation of environmental control. Physical and Occupational Therapy in Pediatrics, *10*(2):69–91, 1990.

Law, M, Baptiste, S, McColl, MA, Opzoomer, A, Polatajko, H, & Pollock, N. The Canadian Occupational Performance Measure: An outcome measure for occupational therapy. Canadian Journal of Occupational Therapy, *57*:82–87, 1990.

Lee, EH, Goh, JCH, & Bose, K. Value of gait analysis in the assessment of surgery in cerebral palsy. Archives of Physical Medicine and Rehabilitation, *73*:642–646, 1992.

Leonard, CT, Hirschfeld, H, Moritani, T, & Forssberg, H. Myotatic reflex development in normal children and children with cerebral palsy. Experimental Neurology, *111*:379–382, 1991.

Leonard, CT, Moritani, T, Hirschfeld, H, & Forssberg, H. Deficits in reciprocal inhibition of children with cerebral palsy as revealed by H reflex testing. Developmental Medicine and Child Neurology, *32*:974–984, 1990.

Lesny, I, Nachtmann, M, Stehlik, A, Tomankova, A, & Zajidkova, J. Disorders of memory of motor sequences in cerebral palsied children. Brain and Development, *12*:339–341, 1990.

Lespargot, A, Renaudin, E, Khouri, N, & Robert, M. Extensibility of hip adductors in children with cerebral palsy. Developmental Medicine and Child Neurology, *36*:980–988, 1994.

Letts, M, Rathbone, D, Yamashita, T, Nichol, B, & Keeler, A. Soft Boston orthosis in management of neuromuscular scoliosis: A preliminary report. Journal of Pediatric Orthopedics, *12*:470–474, 1992.

LeVeau, BF, & Bernhardt, DB. Developmental biomechanics: Effects of forces on the growth, development and maintenance of the human body. Physical Therapy, *64*:1874–1882, 1984.

Lin, JP, Brown, JK, & Brotherstone, R. Assessment of spasticity in hemiplegic cerebral palsy. II. Distal lower-limb reflex excitability and function. Developmental Medicine and Child Neurology, *36*:290–303, 1994.

Lin, PP, & Henderson, RC. Bone mineralization in the affected extremities of children with spastic hemiplegia. Developmental Medicine and Child Neurology, *38*:782–786, 1996.

Little, WJ. On the influence of abnormal parturition, difficult labours, premature births and asphyxia neonatorum on the mental and physical condition of the child, especially in relation to deformities. Transactions of the Obstetrical Society of London 1862. Cerebral Palsy Bulletin, *1*:5–34, 1958.

Logan, L, Byers-Hinkley, K, & Ciccone, CD. Anterior versus posterior walkers: A gait analysis study. Developmental Medicine and Child Neurology, *32*:1044–1048, 1990.

MacKinnon, JR, Noh, S, Lariviere, J, MacPhail, A, Allan, DE, & Laliberte, D. A study of therapeutic effects of horseback riding for children with cerebral palsy. Physical and Occupational Therapy in Pediatrics, *15*(1):17–34, 1995.

MacPhail, HEA, & Kramer, JF. Effect of isokinetic strength-training on functional ability and walking efficiency in adolescents with cerebral palsy. Developmental Medicine and Child Neurology, *37*:763–775, 1995.

Mahoney, FI, & Barthel, DW. Functional evaluation: The Barthel Index. Maryland Medical Journal, *14*:61–65, 1965.

Massagli, TL. Spasticity and its management in children. Physical Medicine and Rehabilitation Clinics of North America, *2*:867–889, 1991.

McDonald, CM. Selective dorsal rhizotomy: A critical review. Physical Medicine and Rehabilitation Clinics of North America, *2*:891–915, 1991.

McLaughlin, JF, Bjornson, KF, Astley, SJ, Graubert, C, Hays, RM, Roberts, TS, Price, R, & Temkin, N. Selective dorsal rhizotomy: Efficacy and safety in an investigator-masked randomized clinical trial. Developmental Medicine and Child Neurology, 40:220–232, 1998.

Menkes, JH. Textbook of Child Neurology, 4th ed. Philadelphia: Lea & Febiger, 1990.

Middleton, EA, Hurley, GRB, & McIlwain, JS. The role of rigid and hinged polypropylene ankle-foot orthoses in the management of cerebral palsy: A case study. Prosthetics and Orthotics International, 12:129–135, 1988.

Miedaner, JA, & Renander, J. The effectiveness of classroom passive stretching programs for increasing or maintaining passive range of motion in non-ambulatory children: An evaluation of frequency. Physical and Occupational Therapy in Pediatrics, 7(3):35–43, 1987.

Milo-Manson, G, Rosenbaum, P, & Steele, C. Alternative therapies: Prevalence and pattern of use in pediatric rehabilitation. Developmental Medicine and Child Neurology, 39(suppl 75):19, 1997.

Missiuna, C, & Pollock, N. Play deprivation in children with physical disabilities: The roles of the occupational therapist in preventing secondary disability. American Journal of Occupational Therapy, 45:882–888, 1991.

Molteni, B, Oleari, G, Fedrizzi, E, & Bracchi, M. Relation between CT patterns, clinical findings and etiology in children born at term, affected by congenital hemiparesis. Neuropediatrics, 18:75–80, 1987.

Morrison, JM, & Ursprung, AW. Children's attitudes toward people with disabilities: A review of the literature. Journal of Rehabilitation, 53(1):45–49, 1987.

Mossberg, KA, Linton, KA, & Friske, K. Ankle-foot orthoses: Effect on energy expenditure of gait in spastic diplegic children. Archives of Physical Medicine and Rehabilitation, 71:490–494, 1990.

Msall, ME, Buck, GM, Rogers, BT, Merke, D, Catanzaro, NL, & Zorn, WA. Risk factors for major neurodevelopmental impairments and need for special education resources in extremely premature infants. Journal of Pediatrics, 119:606–614, 1991.

Msall, ME, Roseberg, S, DiGuadio, KM, Braun, SL, Duffy, L, & Granger, CV. Pilot test for the WeeFIM for children with motor impairments (Abstract). Developmental Medicine and Child Neurology, 32(9, suppl 62):41, 1990.

Murney, ME, & Campbell, SK. The ecological relevance of the Test of Motor Performance elicited scale items. Physical Therapy, 78:479–489, 1998.

Murphy, KP, Molnar, GE, & Lankasky, K. Medical and functional status of adults with cerebral palsy. Developmental Medicine and Child Neurology, 37:1075–1084, 1995.

Nashner, L, Shumway-Cooke, A, & Marin, O. Stance posture control in select groups of children with cerebal palsy: Deficits in sensory organization and muscular coordination. Experimental Brain Research, 49:393–409, 1983.

Nelson, KB, & Ellenberg, J. Antecedents of cerebral palsy. Multivariate analysis of risk. New England Journal of Medicine, 315:81–86, 1986.

Nottidge, VD, & Okogbo, ME. Cerebral palsy in Ibadan, Nigeria. Developmental Medicine and Child Neurology, 33:241–245, 1991.

Nwaobi, OM, & Smith, PD. Effect of adaptive seating on pulmonary function of children with cerebral palsy. Developmental Medicine and Child Neurology, 28:351–354, 1986.

O'Dwyer, NJ, Neilson, PD, & Nash, J. Mechanisms of muscle growth related to muscle contracture in cerebral palsy. Developmental Medicine and Child Neurology, 31:543–552, 1989.

O'Dwyer, N, Neilson, P, & Nash, J. Reduction of spasticity in cerebral palsy using feedback of the tonic stretch reflex: A controlled study. Developmental Medicine and Child Neurology, 36:770–786, 1994.

Olney, SJ, Costigan, PA, & Hedden, DM. Mechanical energy patterns in gait of cerebral palsied children. Physical Therapy, 67:1348–1354, 1987.

Olney, SJ, MacPhail, HEA, Hedden, DM, & Boyce, WF. Work and power in hemiplegic cerebral palsy gait. Physical Therapy, 70:431–438, 1990.

Oonpuu, S, Bell, KJ, Davis, RB, & DeLuca, PA. An evaluation of the posterior leaf spring orthosis using joint kinematics and kinetics. Journal of Pediatric Orthopedics, 16:378–384, 1996.

O'Shea, TM, Preisser, JS, Klinepeter, KL, & Dillard, RG. Trends in mortality and cerebral palsy in a geographically based cohort of very low birthweight neonates born between 1982 to 1994. Pediatrics 101:642–647, 1998.

Overeynder, JC, & Turk, MA. Cerebral palsy and aging: A framework for promoting the health of older persons with cerebral palsy. Topics in Geriatric Rehabilitation, 13(3):19–24, 1998.

Palisano, R. Research on the effectiveness of neurodevelopmental treatment. Pediatric Physical Therapy, 3:143–148, 1991.

Palisano, R. Validity of goal attainment scaling in infants with motor delays. Physical Therapy, 73:651–660, 1993.

Palisano, R, Kolobe, T, & Haley, S. Validity of the Peabody Developmental Gross Motor Scale as an evaluative measure of infants receiving physical therapy. Physical Therapy, 75:939–951, 1995.

Palisano, R, Rosenbaum, P, Walter, S, Russell, D, Wood, E, & Galuppi, B. Development and reliability of a system to classify gross motor function in children with cerebral palsy. Developmental Medicine and Child Neurology, 39:214–223, 1997.

Papile, L, Burstein, J, Burstein, R, & Koffler, H. Incidence and evolution of subependymal and intraventricular hemorrhage: A study of infants with birthweight of less than 1500 gms. Journal of Pediatrics, 92:529–534, 1978.

Parker, DF, Carriere, L, Hebestreit, H, & Bar-Or, O. Anaerobic endurance and peak muscle power in children with spastic cerebral palsy. American Journal of Diseases of Children, 146:1069–1073, 1992.

Patla, AE, Winter, DA, Frank, JS, Walt, JS, & Prasad, S. Identification of age-related changes in the balance control system. Proceedings of the APTA Forum on Balance. Nashville, TN: American Physical Therapy Association, 1989.

Perlmutter, MN, Snyder, M, Miller, F, & Bisbal, R. Proximal femoral resection for older children with spastic hip disease. Developmental Medicine and Child Neurology, 57:525–531, 1993.

Perry, J, Hoffer, M, Antonelli, D, Plut, J, Lewis, G, & Greenberg, R. Electromyography before and after surgery for hip deformity in children with cerebral palsy. Journal of Bone and Joint Surgery (American), 58:201–208, 1976.

Pharoah, POD, Cooke, T, Cooke, RWI, & Rosenbloom, L. Birthweight specific trends in cerebral palsy. Archives of Disease in Childhood, 65:602–606, 1990.

Pharoah, POD, Cooke, T, Rosenbloom, L, & Cooke, RWI. Trends in birth prevalence of cerebral palsy. Archives of Disease in Childhood, 62:379–384, 1987.

Piper, MC, & Darrah, J. Motor Assessment of the Developing Infant. Philadelphia: WB Saunders, 1994.

Poirier, D, Goguen, L, & Leslie, P. Educational Rights of Exceptional Children. Toronto: Carswell, 1988.

Poole, JL. Application of motor learning principles in occupational therapy. American Journal of Occupational Therapy, 45:531–537, 1991.

Powell, TH, & Ogle, PA. Brothers and Sisters—A Special Part of Exceptional Families. Baltimore: Paul H. Brookes, 1985.

Pranzatelli, MR. Oral pharmacology for the movement disorders of cerebral palsy. Journal of Child Neurology, 11(suppl 1):S13–S22, 1996.

Price, R, Bjornson, KF, Lehmann, JF, McLaughlin, JF, & Hays, RM. Quantitative measurement of spasticity in children with cerebral palsy. Developmental Medicine and Child Neurology, 33:585–595, 1991.

Rang, M. Cerebral palsy. In Morrissy, RT (Ed.), Lovell and Winter's Paediatric Orthopedics, 3rd ed. Philadelphia: JB Lippincott, 1990, pp. 465–506.

Reddihough, D, King J, Coleman, G, & Catanese, T. Efficacy of programs based on conductive education for young children with cerebral palsy. Developmental Medicine and Child Neurology, 39(suppl 75):20, 1997.

Reid, DT, Boschen, K, & Wright, V. Critique of the Pediatric Evaluation of Disability Inventory (PEDI). Physical and Occupational Therapy in Pediatrics, 13(4):57–87, 1993.

Reilly, S, & Skuse, D. Characteristics and management of feeding problems of young children with cerebral palsy. Developmental Medicine and Child Neurology, 34:379–388, 1992.

Rempel, GR, Colwell, SO, & Nelson, RP. Growth in children with cerebral palsy fed via gastrostomy. Pediatrics, 82:857–862, 1988.

Richards, CL, Malouin, F, & Dumas, F. Effects of a single session of prolonged stretch on muscle activations during gait in spastic cerebral palsy. Scandinavian Journal of Rehabilitation Medicine, 23:103–111, 1991.

Ricks, NR, & Eilert, RE. Effects of inhibitory casts and orthoses on bony alignment of foot and ankle during weight-bearing in children with spasticity. Developmental Medicine and Child Neurology, 35:11–16, 1993.

Romanini, L, Villani, C, Meloni, C, & Calvisi, V. Histological and morphological aspects of muscle in infantile cerebral palsy. Italian Journal of Orthopaedics and Traumatology, 15:87–93, 1989.

Rose, J, Gamble, JG, Burgos, A, Medeiros, J, & Haskell, WL. Energy expenditure index of walking for normal children and for children with cerebral palsy. Developmental Medicine and Child Neurology, 32:333–340, 1990.

Rose, J, Medeiros, JM, & Parker, R. Energy cost index as an estimate of energy expenditure of cerebral-palsied children during assisted ambulation. Developmental Medicine and Child Neurology, 27:485–490, 1985.

Rosenbaum, P, Cadman, D, & Kirpalani, H. Pediatrics: Assessing quality of life. In Spilker, B (Ed.), Quality of Life Assessment in Clinical Trials. New York: Raven Press, 1990, pp. 205–215.

Rosenbaum, P, King, S, Law, M, King, G, & Evans, J. Family-centred service: A conceptual framework and research review. Physical Therapy and Occupational Therapy in Pediatrics, 18(1):1–20, 1998.

Russell, D, Rosenbaum, P, Cadman, D, Gowland, C, Hardy, S, & Jarvis, S. The Gross Motor Function Measure: A means to evaluate the effects of physical therapy. Developmental Medicine and Child Neurology, 31:341–352, 1989.

Schanzenbacher, KE. Diagnostic problems in pediatrics. In Pratt, PN, & Allen, AS (Eds.), Occupational Therapy for Children. Toronto: Mosby, 1989, p. 97.

Scherzer, AL, & Tscharnuter, I. Early Diagnosis and Therapy in Cerebral Palsy: A Primer on Infant Developmental Problems, 2nd ed. New York: Marcel Dekker, 1990.

Senft, KE, Pueschel, SM, Robison, NA, & Kiessling, LS. Level of function of young adults with cerebral palsy. Physical and Occupational Therapy in Pediatrics, 10(1):19–25, 1990.

Shaw, G. Vehicular transport safety for the child with disabilities. American Journal of Occupational Therapy, 41:35–42, 1987.

Shaw, J. Continence in cerebral palsy. Health Visitor, 63:301–302, 1990.

Shepherd, RB. Training motor control and optimizing motor learning. In Shepherd, RB (Ed.), Physiotherapy in Paediatrics, 3rd ed. Oxford: Butterworth-Heinemann, 1995.

Shields, CV. Strategies: A Practical Guide for Dealing with Professionals and Human Service Systems. Richmond Hill, Ontario: Human Services Press, 1987.

Shumway-Cook, A, & Woolacott, M. Motor Control: Theory and Practical Applications. Baltimore: Williams & Wilkins, 1995.

Sillanpaa, M, Piekkala, P, & Pisirici, H. The young adult with cerebral palsy and his chances of employment. International Journal of Rehabilitation Research, 5:467–476, 1982.

Sobsey, D, & Doe, T. Patterns of sexual abuse and assault. Sexuality and Disability, 9:243–259, 1991.

Sparrow, SS, Balla, DA, & Ciccetti, DV. Vineland Adaptive Behavior Scales (Survey Form). Circle Pines, MN: American Guidance Service, 1984.

Spector, RC. Functional Disability Scales. In Spilker, B (Ed.), Quality of Life Assessments in Clinical Trials. New York: Raven Press, 1990, pp. 115–129.

Stanger, M, & Bertoti, D (Eds.), An overview of electrical stimulation for the pediatric population. Pediatric Physical Therapy, 9(3): 95–143, 1997.

Steinbok, P, Reiner, AM, Beauchamp, R, Armstrong, RW, & Cochrane, DD. A randomized clinical trial to compare selective posterior rhizotomy plus physiotherapy with physiotherapy alone in children with spastic diplegic cerebral palsy. Developmental Medicine and Child Neurology, 39:178–184, 1997.

Stern, L, & Steidle, K. Pediatric Strengthening Program Reproducible Exercises. Tuscon, AZ: Therapy Skill Builders, 1994.

Sternisha, C, Cays, M, & Campbell, L. Stress responses in families with handicapped children: An annotated bibliography. Physical and Occupational Therapy in Pediatrics, 12(1):89–103, 1992.

Strauss, D, & Shavelle, R. Life expectancy of adults with cerebral palsy. Developmental Medicine and Child Neurology, 40:369–375, 1998.

Stuberg, WA. Considerations related to weight-bearing programs in children with developmental disabilities. Physical Therapy, 72:35–40, 1992.

Stuberg, WA, Fuchs, RH, & Miedaner, JA. Reliability of goniometric measurements of children with cerebral palsy. Developmental Medicine and Child Neurology, 30:657–666, 1988.

Subramanian, J, Vaughan, CL, Peter, JC, & Arens, LJ. Gait before and 10 years after rhizotomy in children with cerebral palsy spasticity. Journal of Neurosurgery, 88:1014–1019, 1998.

Sutherland, DH, Olshen, R, Cooper, L, & Woo, SY. The development of mature gait. Journal of Bone and Joint Surgery (American), 62: 336–353, 1980.

Tardieu, C, Huet de la Tour, E, Bret, MD, & Tardieu, G. Muscle hypoextensibility in children with cerebral palsy: I. Clinical and experimental observations. Archives of Physical Medicine and Rehabilitation, 63:97–102, 1982.

Tardieu, C, Lespargot, A, Tabary, C, & Bret, MD. For how long must the soleus muscle be stretched each day to prevent contracture? Developmental Medicine and Child Neurology, 30:3–10, 1988.

Tardieu, G, Tardieu, C, Colbeau-Justin, P, & Lespargot, A. Muscle hypoextensibility in children with cerebral palsy: II. Therapeutic implications. Archives of Physical Medicine and Rehabilitation, 63:103–107, 1982.

Toner, LV, Cook, K, & Elder, GCB. Improved ankle function in children with cerebral palsy after computer assisted motor learning. Developmental Medicine and Child Neurology, 40:829–835, 1998.

Torfs, CP, van den Berg, BJ, & Oechsli, FW. Prenatal and perinatal factors in the etiology of cerebral palsy. Journal of Pediatrics, 116:615–619, 1990.

Tremblay, F, Malouin, F, Richards, CL, & Dumas, F. Effects of prolonged muscle stretch on reflex and voluntary muscle activations in children with spastic cerebral palsy. Scandinavian Journal of Rehabilitation Medicine, 22:171–180, 1990.

Uvebrandt, P. Hemiplegic cerebral palsy. Aetiology and outcome. Acta Paediatrica Scandinavica Supplement, 345:5–100, 1988.

van den Berg-Emons, HJG, Saris, WHM, de Barbanson, DC, Westerterp, KR, & can Baak, MA. Daily physical activity of schoolchildren with spastic diplegia and of health control subjects. Journal of Pediatrics, 127:578–584, 1995.

van der Weel, FR, van der Meer, ALH, & Lee, DN. Effect of task on movement control in cerebral palsy: Implications for assessment and therapy. Developmental Medicine and Child Neurology, 33: 419–426, 1991.

Vojta, V. The basic elements of treatment according to Vojta. In Scrutton, D (Ed.), Management of the Motor Disorders of Children with Cerebral Palsy. Philadelphia: JB Lippincott, 1984, pp. 75–85.

Wacker, DP, Harper, DC, Powell, WJ, & Healy, A. Life outcomes and satisfaction ratings of multihandicapped adults. Developmental Medicine and Child Neurology, 25:625–631, 1983.

Washington State Department of Health. Cerebral Palsy—Critical Elements of Care. Seattle, WA: Washington State Department of Health, 1997.

Watt, JM, Robertson, CMT, & Grace, MGA. Early prognosis for ambulation of neonatal intensive care survivors with cerebral palsy. Developmental Medicine and Child Neurology, 31:766–773, 1989.

Weinstein, SL, & Tharp, BR. Etiology and timing of static encephalopathies of childhood (cerebral palsy). In Stevenson, DK, & Sunshine, P (Eds.), Fetal and Neonatal Brain Injury. Toronto: BC Decker, 1989.

Werner, D. Disabled Village Children: A Guide for Community Health Workers, Rehabilitation Workers, and Families. Palo Alto, CA: Hesperian Foundation, 1987.

Westcott, SL, Paxhowes, L, & Richardson, PK. Evaluation of postural stability in children: Current theories and assessment. Physical Therapy, 77:629–643, 1997.

Wiklund, LM, & Uvebrant, P. Hemiplegic cerebral palsy: Correlation between CT morphology and clinical findings. Developmental Medicine and Child Neurology, 33:512–523, 1991a.

Wiklund, LM, Uvebrant, P, & Flodmark, O. Computed tomography as an adjunct in etiological analysis of hemiplegic cerebral palsy. I: Children born preterm. Neuropediatrics, 22:50–56, 1991b.

Wilcox, C. Hey, What About Me! Activities for Disabled Children. Toronto: Doubleday Canada, 1988.

Wilson, ER, Mirra, S, & Schwartz, JF. Congenital diencephalic and brain stem damage: Neuropathologic study of three cases. Acta Neuropathologica, 57:70–74, 1982.

Wilson, JM. Cerebral palsy. In Campbell, S (Ed.), Pediatric Neurologic Physical Therapy, 2nd ed. New York: Churchill Livingstone, 1991, pp. 301–360.

Wright, FV, Sheil, EMH, Drake, JM, Wedge, JH, & Naumann, S. Evaluation of selective dorsal rhizotomy for the reduction of spasticity in cerebral palsy: A randomized controlled trial. Developmental Medicine and Child Neurology, 40:239–247, 1998.

Yokochi, K, Aiba, K, Horie, M, Inukai, K, Fujimoto, S, Kodama, M, & Kodama, K. Magnetic resonance imaging in children with spastic diplegia: Correlation with severity of their motor and mental abnormality. Developmental Medicine and Child Neurology, 33:18–25, 1991.

Young, RR. Spasticity: A review. Neurology, 44(11 suppl 9):512–520, 1994.

C H A P T E R
21

Spinal Cord Injury

KRISTINE A. SHAKHAZIZIAN, PT
TERESA L. MASSAGLI, MD
TERESA L. SOUTHARD, PT

Acquired lesions of the spinal cord occur far less commonly in children than in adults, but the unique aspects of growth and development can make treatment of the rare child with spinal cord injury (SCI) a challenge for pediatric physical therapists. The rehabilitation process may take years because the young child requires time to achieve adequate upper body strength, adult body proportions, and cognitive skills for maximal independence. The child who is not skeletally mature may develop orthopedic problems during growth, which may result in altered function. Direct intervention, monitoring skill acquisition, and assessing equipment needs are important roles for the physical therapist.

This chapter describes the pathophysiology and resulting neurologic impairments, functional limitations, and disabilities of children with SCI. Examination, prognosis, goals and outcomes, and physical therapy intervention for the child with pediatric SCI are then discussed.

EPIDEMIOLOGY

The most common cause of SCI for all ages is trauma. The overall incidence is estimated to be 30 to 40 injuries per million persons per year, or around 10,000 new cases each year in the United States. Children younger than 16 years of age account for less than 5% of these cases. Motor vehicle crashes, sports, violence, and falls are the leading causes, and traumatic SCI more frequently occurs in boys, during the summer, and on weekends (Go et al., 1995). Traumatic SCI is more common in children 10 to 15 years old and from birth to 5 years old than in children who are 5 to 9 years old (Kewalramani et al., 1980). Violence as a cause of SCI is increasing in frequency, particularly in older teenagers of African-American race or Hispanic ethnicity (Go et al., 1995). Child abuse accounts for some cases of SCI, particularly in younger children, but its frequency as a cause of SCI is unknown. Developmental anomalies of the cervical vertebrae can place the spinal cord at increased risk of injury. These anomalies include instability of the atlantoaxial joint, as seen in Down syndrome or juvenile rheumatoid arthritis, and dysplasia of the base of the skull or upper cervical vertebrae, as seen in achondroplasia.

Nontraumatic causes of SCI in children often have an insidious onset and can be difficult to diagnose. Specific incidence data are not available for such causes, which include tumor, transverse myelitis, epidural abscess, arteriovenous malformation, and multiple sclerosis. Treating the child with SCI resulting from the presence of a tumor is especially challenging because the child's overall medical condition and the progression of disease dramatically influence the formulation of goals or attainment of outcomes.

PATHOPHYSIOLOGY

The site or level at which SCI occurs is often related to the cause of injury and the child's age. Most of the nontraumatic causes of SCI occur in the thoracic spinal cord. By contrast, vertebral dysplasias place the upper cervical spinal cord or lower brainstem at risk. Birth trauma due to traction and angulation of the spine at a breech delivery most commonly causes SCI at the cervicothoracic junction. In the child younger than 8 to 10 years old, the cervical spine has greater mobility than it does in adults because of ligamentous laxity, shallow angulation of the facets, incomplete ossification of vertebrae, and relative underdevelopment of the neck muscles for the size of the head (Wilberger, 1986). Young children are therefore more likely to experience injury at the upper cervical spine than are adults (Bohn et al., 1990), and SCI may occur without any signs of bone damage by radiography, a finding referred to as spinal cord injury without radiographic abnormality, or SCIWORA (Pang & Wilberger, 1982). In children, 55% of cases of traumatic SCI result in tetraplegia owing to injury between the first cervical and first thoracic root levels, and 45% result in paraplegia from injury below the first thoracic level (Go et al., 1995).

Most cases of traumatic SCI are caused by a blunt, nonpenetrating injury to the spinal cord in which the cord is not lacerated or transected. The direct effect of the trauma is immediate disruption of neural transmission in the gray and white matter of the spinal cord at and below the injury site, resulting in spinal shock. Reactive physiologic events evolve over a period of hours and induce secondary injury to the spinal cord (Faden, 1983). The exact sequence of events between transfer of kinetic energy to the cord and subsequent neuronal death is unknown. Animal models have shown that ischemia, hemorrhage, edema, calcium influx into cells, and generation of free radicals contribute to cell membrane degradation and death of neurons (Janssen & Hansebout, 1989). In gray matter, neurons that die are not replaced. In white matter, axonal segments distal to the injury degenerate and synapses no longer function. Although axonal sprouting does occur to a limited degree in the central nervous system, it appears to be functionally insignificant, and most of the recovery observed in patients with incomplete lesions is probably due to resolution of neurapraxic injury.

The zone of injury within the spinal cord is usually large enough to cause a transition in neurologic function from normal to abnormal or from normal to absent over several spinal root levels. Soon after SCI, the level of injury may appear to move cephalad as the secondary or indirect processes set in. Later, the level of injury may move caudally as these factors resolve, as sprouting develops (either within the spinal cord or peripherally to denervated muscles), or as hypertrophy of weak muscles occurs. Research has shown that the extent of injury may diminish for as long as 1 year (Wu et al., 1992), and it is obvious that until the natural history of SCI and recovery is delineated, experimental treatments may be inappropriately credited with enhancing recovery.

If some function below the zone of the spinal cord injury remains and motor function or sensation is present in the lowest sacral segment, the child has an incomplete SCI. After traumatic SCI, incomplete lesions are found in 40% of children with paraplegia and in 55% of those with tetraplegia (Go et al., 1995). Several distinct patterns of clinical syndromes have been described. Injury to the anterior spinal cord produces variable motor paralysis, with reduced sensation of pain and temperature but with preserved dorsal column function. Hemorrhage in the central part of the cervical spinal cord produces flaccid weakness of the arms and strong but spastic legs, with preservation of bladder and bowel function. Posterior cord lesions are rare and produce selective loss of proprioception. Stab wounds may produce a Brown-Sequard lesion with ipsilateral paralysis and proprioceptive loss and contralateral loss of pain and temperature sensation. Injury to the lumbosacral nerve roots results in cauda equina syndrome, with lower extremity weakness and areflexia of the legs and bladder.

Delayed cavitation (syringomyelia) within the

damaged spinal cord can occur in patients with complete or incomplete lesions. The occurrence of a cystic cavitation, or syrinx, appears to be common after SCI, occurring in 51% of one series of children (Backe et al., 1991). In a small number of such patients the cyst may progressively enlarge, resulting in further loss of neurologic function months to years after SCI. Signs and symptoms that may herald presence of a syrinx include loss of motor function, ascending sensory level, increased spasticity or sweating, and new onset of pain or dysesthesia.

PREVENTION

Efforts to prevent SCI have been undertaken by health care and education professionals. The National Spinal Cord Injury Database has been in existence since 1973. It collects data from about 15% of new SCI cases in the United States from 24 federally funded model SCI care systems. Information from this database has helped identify high-risk groups to guide development of prevention programs (Go et al., 1995). Pediatric health professionals play important roles in education regarding proper seat belt and car seat use. Lap seat belts must be placed across the pelvis, not across the waist, and shoulder harnesses should cross the clavicle, not the neck, to avoid lumbar or cervical spine injury in the event of a collision. Health care professionals and schools have supported cooperative programs to reduce diving injuries (the most common sports-related cause of SCI) and other high-risk activities (Richards et al., 1991). The Committee on Sports Medicine of the American Academy of Pediatrics (1984) has recommended screening programs to assess cervical spine stability for children known to be at risk of atlantoaxial instability (e.g., Down syndrome).

MEDICAL DIAGNOSIS AND MANAGEMENT

The early management of a child with SCI is focused on stabilization of the spine to prevent further damage to the intact but injured spinal cord. The spine is immobilized during transport and throughout all assessments and procedures. At the hospital, a thorough neurologic examination is performed to determine the motor and sensory level of SCI and the completeness of injury. Spinal shock is usually present, although occasionally it has resolved by the time the patient is treated in the emergency department. In spinal shock, the muscles are flaccid below the SCI and all cutaneous and deep tendon reflexes are absent. This state persists for hours to weeks and is said to be over when sacral reflexes, including the bulbocavernous and anal reflexes, are present.

Further evaluation is undertaken with plain radiographs of the whole spine from the first cervical to the sacral vertebrae to identify any fractures, facet subluxations, or dislocations. A small but significant number of patients may have more than one site of injury to the spine and spinal cord. Computed tomography and magnetic resonance imaging are used to diagnose root impingement, presence of bone fragments in the spinal canal, cord compression, and spinal cord hemorrhage.

Whether immediate surgical intervention to correct bone injury and decompress the spinal cord is effective in reducing paralysis is unknown because the numerous surgical procedures have never been subjected to randomized clinical trials. Surgery often allows a patient to be mobilized more quickly, but ultimate levels of independence or recovery do not appear to be altered (Murphy et al., 1990). The main goal of surgery is to prevent later deformity, pain, or loss of neurologic function. Surgery may not be necessary if spinal alignment can be achieved with traction and maintained with an orthosis. Surgery is indicated if there is a penetrating injury, if traction has failed to reduce a dislocation, if nerve root impingement exists, or if bone fragments are compressing the cauda equina. Regardless of whether surgery is performed, if bone injury has occurred patients usually wear an external orthosis until bone fusion is complete, often for 3 or more months. For some lower-level injuries, the surgeon may have the child wear an orthosis with a thigh piece (Fig. 21–1), which permits only limited hip flexion (e.g., to only 60°). This is done to reduce torque on the immature fusion mass, which could occur from pull of the hamstrings on the pelvis in a position of hip flexion.

Researchers have tried pharmacologic interventions to halt the chain of secondary events producing neural damage and to protect compromised but viable cells. Antioxidants, free radical scavengers, opiate antagonists, vitamins, thyrotropin-releasing hormone, and calcium channel blockers are a few of the agents that have been tested (Rhoney et al., 1996). It is a slow process to bring new pharmacotherapies into clinical practice, due to the necessary steps of animal trials, followed by preliminary and then larger-scale trials in humans. Human trials must be placebo controlled and have a sufficient period of follow-up to assess the efficacy of the treatment. Because spinal cord injury is not very common, clinical trials usually require collaboration among many medical centers. High doses of corticosteroids (methylprednisolone) administered within the first 8 hours and continued for 24 to 48 hours have been shown to slightly enhance motor recovery in humans (Bracken et al., 1997). Recently, administration of GM-1 ganglioside within the first 72 hours after SCI

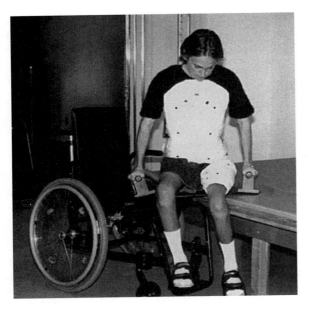

FIGURE 21–1. Teen wearing a TLSO with a thigh piece that restricts hip flexion uses a sliding board and push-up blocks to begin learning transfers.

was shown to enhance neurologic recovery, and further studies are in progress (Geisler, 1998). Gangliosides are glycolipids that form a major component of cell membranes and may act by blocking cell membrane degradation. At this time, methylprednisolone is the only medication used in standard clinical practice, but GM-1 ganglioside may also become widely used after clinical trials are completed and the drug is approved by the Food and Drug Administration.

Trauma to the spinal cord provokes the development of scar tissue, which includes both connective tissue elements and glial hyperplasia. Scientists have not yet determined why axons are unable to grow across this scar tissue area. Some researchers have proposed that the glial cells act as a surrogate target for the regrowing axons, whereas others have argued that the glial cells engender a nonpermissive substrate for axonal growth. Strategies to promote spinal cord regeneration have included use of neurotrophic factors, monoclonal antibodies directed against glial cells, and intraspinal transplants of peripheral nerve tissue, fetal spinal cord tissue, or omental tissue from the abdomen. Both in vitro techniques and animal models have been used to demonstrate that injured axons can survive and grow under certain environmental conditions, but the feat of effecting axonal growth across scar tissue and through appropriate myelin sheaths to reach and innervate appropriate muscles remains elusive. Significant progress has occurred in the last 5 to 10

years in understanding the inhibitory factors, as well as those promoting axonal sprouting. It is difficult to envision a timetable for a cure for SCI, but in the next decade there will likely be many clinical trials involving human subjects as in vitro or animal work on regeneration progresses. Clinical trials involving human subjects in the next several years will most likely involve antibodies against growth-inhibiting substances in the spinal cord, and building cellular bridges across injured spinal cord using fetal spinal cord or fetal glial transplants (Giovanini et al., 1997; Schwab, 1996).

Patients and families have been and will continue to be tempted by unproven therapies, often at considerable personal financial expense. Therapists can help patients and families evaluate the evidence regarding potential therapies. Any purported cure should be subjected to randomized clinical trial before being offered to hopeful but vulnerable patients. It is reasonable for patients and therapists to hold out hope for a cure for SCI. It is often just this hope that motivates patients and caregivers to be meticulous about preventing secondary complications.

With ongoing appropriate medical care, long-term survival after traumatic SCI is not only possible but likely. Life expectancy is approximately 85% of average for those with paraplegia and incomplete tetraplegia, and about 75% of average for those with tetraplegia (DeVivo & Stover, 1995).

IMPAIRMENTS AND FUNCTIONAL LIMITATIONS

Defining the Level of Spinal Cord Injury

A common terminology should be used by all professionals when describing the motor or sensory level of SCI. The most widely used standards are those published by the American Spinal Injury Association (ASIA) (1996). These standards have been developed by consensus of a multidisciplinary group of clinical experts and have been revised four times since their initial publication in 1982. The ASIA standards define right and left motor levels, right and left sensory levels, and incomplete and complete injuries.

The ASIA standards accept the widely used system of muscle grading: 0 = absence, total paralysis; 1 = trace, palpable, or visible contraction; 2 = poor, active movement through full range of motion (ROM) with gravity eliminated; 3 = fair, active movement through full ROM against gravity; 4 = good, active movement through full ROM against moderate resistance; and 5 = normal, active movement through full ROM against full resistance. Motor levels may differ for right and left sides of the

TABLE 21-1. Key Muscles for Motor Level Classification

C5	Elbow flexors (biceps, brachialis)
C6	Wrist extensors (extensor carpi radialis longus and brevis)
C7	Elbow extensors (triceps)
C8	Finger flexors to the middle finger (flexor digitorum profundus)
T1	Small finger abductors (aductor digiti minimi manus)
L2	Hip flexors (iliopsoas)
L3	Knee extensors (quadriceps)
L4	Ankle dorsiflexors (tibialis anterior)
L5	Long toe extensors (extensor hallucis longus)
S1	Ankle plantar flexors (gastrocnemius, soleus)

From American Spinal Injury Association. International Standards for Neurological and Functional Classification of Spinal Cord Injury. Chicago: American Spinal Injury Association, 1996.

body. The key muscles for determination of motor level are listed in Table 21-1. Because all muscles have innervation from more than one root level, the presence of innervation by one root level and the absence by the next lower level results in a weakened muscle. The ASIA-defined motor level is the most caudal root level in which muscle strength is grade 3 or more. By convention, if a muscle has grade 3 strength and the next most rostral muscle is grade 5, the grade 3 muscle is considered to have full innervation by the higher root level, for which it is named. For example, if there is no activity in the C8 key muscle, the C7 key muscle is grade 3, and the C6 key muscle is grade 5, the motor level is C7. In the 1996 revision of the ASIA standards, the requirement for the next most rostral key muscle to be grade 5 was added. Therefore, a patient with a grade 2 C8 key muscle, grade 3 C7 key muscle, grade 4 C6 key muscle, and grade 5 C5 key muscle is labeled C6, not C7. One disadvantage to using only the ASIA key muscles to define a level of function is the omission of examination of hip extensors, hip abductors, and knee flexors. These other L5 and S1 muscles play an important role in activities such as transfers, ambulation, and stair climbing. Strength grades of the key muscles can be added together for both sides of the body to create a composite ASIA motor score. This score has been used in research studies assessing efficacy of pharmacologic treatment of SCI. It can also be used to predict function and need for assistance (Saboe et al., 1997). Waters and colleagues (1994) found that if the sum of the key muscles from both lower extremities (L2-S1) is 30 or higher, the patients were community ambulators. Those with scores less than 20 were limited ambulators who required knee-ankle-foot orthoses (KAFOs) and crutches.

The sensory level may not correspond exactly to the motor level. Determining the sensory level is especially helpful in injuries above C5, or to the thoracic spinal cord, where there are no key muscles to define the level of SCI. Rather than relying on dermatome charts, which vary from one text to another, the ASIA standards rely on the presence of normal light touch and pinprick sensation at a key point in each of the 28 dermatomes on the right and left sides of the body (Fig. 21-2 and Table 21-2). Proprioception should also be assessed below the level of injury in patients with incomplete SCI to determine integrity of dorsal column function.

A patient is said to have an incomplete SCI only if motor or sensory function is present in the lowest sacral segment, implying voluntary control of the external anal sphincter or sensation at the mucocutaneous junction or both. Incomplete lesions are referred to in two ways: by the ASIA Impairment Scale (Table 21-3) and by neuroanatomic description. Distinct neuroanatomic patterns of incomplete lesions include the central cord syndrome, Brown-Sequard syndrome, anterior cord syndrome, and posterior cord syndrome previously described in the section on pathophysiology. The cauda equina syndrome may be complete or incomplete.

Precise description of the motor and sensory loss after SCI is important for two reasons. First, it helps predict the likelihood of further neurologic recovery in both complete and incomplete syndromes. For instance, in motor complete C5 tetraplegia, most if not all patients gain one full motor level, achieving grade 3 wrist extensor movement (a C6 muscle) during the first 8 months after injury (Ditunno et al., 1987). Researchers have also determined that in SCI above T11, preservation of pinprick sensation has predictive value for return of motor function and independent ambulation, probably because of the proximity of the ascending pain fibers and descending motor fibers in the spinal cord (Crozier et al., 1991).

Prognostic information is also available for the neuroanatomic incomplete syndromes. Anterior cord syndrome is usually due to damage to the anterior spinal artery, causing infarction in the spinal cord. Prognosis for return of function is poor. In posterior cord syndrome, motor function is preserved but the loss of proprioception means ambulation is unlikely. In Brown-Sequard and central cord syndromes, prognosis for ambulation and bladder and bowel control is very good but hand function may be impaired, depending on the level of injury. Lesions of the cauda equina are essentially lesions of the peripheral nerve or lower motoneuron and may show recovery over several years owing to resolution

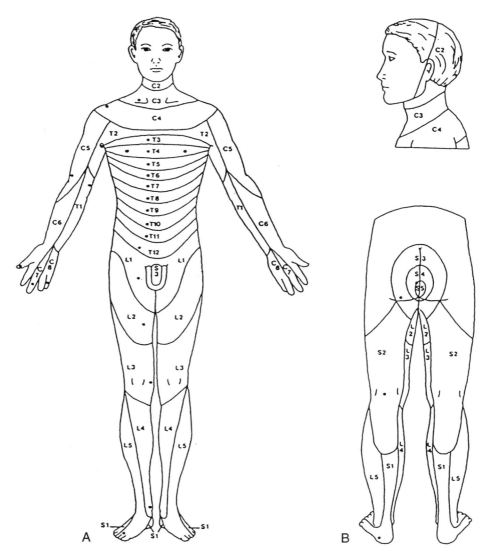

FIGURE 21–2. *A,* Anterior view of key sensory areas by dermatome. *B,* Posterior view of key sensory areas by dermatome. (From American Spinal Injury Association. International Standards for Neurological and Functional Classification of Spinal Cord Injury, Revised 1996. Chicago: American Spinal Injury Association, 1996.)

of neurapraxia or to regrowth of damaged axons, as well as to peripheral sprouting.

The second reason for the importance of precise definition of the level of SCI is that it helps predict the ultimate level of independence a patient can expect to achieve in the areas of mobility, self-care, and even communication. Tables 21–4 and 21–5 delineate the optimal functional abilities for each level of motor complete SCI. Patients with incomplete SCI may exceed the expectations for any given level of injury. Such expectations for independence must also be tempered by consideration of the child's age,

which influences developmental expectations. It can take years for a preschooler to reach the expected level of independence, or he or she may fall short if complications, particularly orthopedic, ensue.

Medical Complications

A host of medical complications can occur after SCI and may affect a child's ability to participate in physical therapy and rehabilitation (Massagli & Jaffe, 1990). With lesions of the cervical or thoracic spinal cord, altered respiratory function may occur, ranging

TABLE 21-2. Key Sensory Areas

C2	Occipital protuberance
C3	Supraclavicular fossa
C4	Top of the acromioclavicular joint
C5	Lateral side of the antecubital fossa
C6	Thumb
C7	Middle finger
C8	Little finger
T1	Medial (ulnar) side of the antecubital fossa
T2	Apex of the axilla
T3	Third intercostal space
T4	Fourth intercostal space (nipple line)
T5	Fifth intercostal space (midway between T4 and T6)
T6	Sixth intercostal space (level of xiphisternum)
T7	Seventh intercostal space (midway between T6 and T8)
T8	Eighth intercostal space (midway between T6 and T10)
T9	Ninth intercostal space (midway between T8 and T10)
T10	Tenth intercostal space (umbilicus)
T11	Eleventh intercostal space (midway between T10 and T12)
T12	Inguinal ligament at midpoint
L1	Half the distance between T12 and L2
L2	Midanterior thigh
L3	Medial femoral condyle
L4	Medial malleolus
L5	Dorsum of the foot at the third metatarsal phalangeal joint
S1	Lateral heel
S2	Popliteal fossa in the midline
S3	Ischial tuberosity
S4–S5	Perianal area (taken as one level)

From American Spinal Injury Association. International Standards for Neurological and Functional Classification of Spinal Cord Injury. Chicago: American Spinal Injury Association, 1996.

TABLE 21-3. ASIA Impairment Scale

A	**Complete**—No sensory or motor function in the sacral segments S4–S5.
B	**Incomplete**—Sensory but not motor function is preserved below the neurologic level and extends through the sacral segments S4–S5.
C	**Incomplete**—Motor function is preserved below the neurologic level, and more than half of key muscles below the neurologic level have a muscle grade less than 3.
D	**Incomplete**—Motor function is preserved below the neurologic level, and more than half of key muscles below the neurologic level have a muscle grade greater than or equal to 3.
E	**Normal**—Sensory and motor function is normal.

From American Spinal Injury Association. International Standards for Neurological and Functional Classification of Spinal Cord Injury. Chicago: American Spinal Injury Association, 1996.

from total paralysis of the diaphragm to diminished vital capacity or weakened forced expiration during coughing. SCI at a midthoracic level or above can interrupt sympathetic outflow, leading to orthostatic hypotension, impaired ability to sweat or shiver, and autonomic dysreflexia. Autonomic dysreflexia is a massive reflex sympathetic discharge that occurs after SCI above midthoracic levels in response to noxious stimuli. Clinical features include headache, flushing, sweating, pilomotor activity, rapid or reduced heart rate, and hypertension. The hypertensive crisis poses a danger to patients and can cause stroke, seizures, or even death. School-age children and adolescents are capable of reporting headaches, but younger children may have difficulty in verbalizing symptoms, and autonomic dysreflexia is often overlooked in these youngsters. Paralyzed and dependent lower extremities can develop edema and

deep vein thromboses. In the first weeks after SCI, gastrointestinal bleeding from stress ulcers may occur, but the frequency (20%) is no greater than that in patients with other acute serious medical conditions (Sugarman, 1985). Deep vein thrombosis occurs as frequently in children with SCI as it does in adults, or in about 13% of cases (Waring & Karunas, 1991). Neurogenic pain can occur after SCI at, above, or below the level of injury and is relatively more common with cauda equina lesions. Loss of descending input to the sacral spinal cord or damage to the sacral nerve roots leads to impairment of bladder and bowel emptying, loss of sexual response, and male infertility.

Almost unique to children is the problem of immobilization hypercalcemia. During the first year after SCI, approximately 40% of bone mineral density is lost via calcium excreted in the urine. Children are more likely to have rapid bone turnover, resulting in a larger load of calcium than the kidneys can excrete. This produces elevated serum calcium or hypercalcemia. Nonspecific symptoms include lethargy, nausea, altered mood, and anorexia. Remobilization is an important aspect of treatment in persons without SCI (e.g., the child with a femur fracture), but it is not known if this is effective in reducing hypercalcemia after SCI. The mainstays of treatment are primarily medical and aimed at reducing calcium loss from bones or at enhancing urinary excretion. Pathologic fractures, or osteoporosis, which occur at an increased rate in persons with bone mineral density below 40% of normal, are a potential complication of osteopenia. Deposition of new bone in periarticular soft tissue can also occur in paralyzed extremities. This heterotopic ossification can be asymptomatic, or it may interfere with ROM

TABLE 21–4. Mobility in Complete Tetraplegia: Expected Function and Necessary Equipment

Functional Skill	Mobility for Level of Injury			
	C1–C4	C5	C6	C7–T1
Bed mobility	D	A: Even with electric bed	I: May use equipment; electric bed helpful	I: Electric bed helpful
Transfers	D: May need mechanical lift	D: May need mechanical lift	Some I with or without sliding board	I: May need sliding board
Wheelchair	I: PWC, head, chin, mouth, or tongue control	I: PWC, hand control with splint	I: MWC, may use adapted rims; likely to use PWC in community	I: MWC
Pressure relief	D: Bed, MWC I: Power tilt PWC	D: Bed, MWC I: Power tilt PWC	I: Leaning to side	I: Push-up on open hands
Transportation	U: Driving; van with lift needed	I: Upper extremity controls; van with lift needed	I: Hand controls A: Load MWC	I: Hand controls I: Load MWC

Adapted from Massagli, TL, & Jaffe, KM. Pediatric spinal cord injury: Treatment and outcome. Pediatrician, *17*:244–254, 1990. Reprinted with permission of S. Karger, Basel.

A, Assistance required; *D*, dependent; *I*, independent; *MWC*, manual wheelchair; *PWC*, power wheelchair; *U*, unable.

TABLE 21–5. Mobility in Complete Paraplegia: Expected Function and Necessary Equipment

Functional Skill	Level of Injury		
	T2–T10	T11–L2	L3–S2
Manual wheelchair	I: Indoors and in community	I: Indoors and in community	May not need MWC except long distances, recreation
Ambulation	SBA: Exercise only; need KAFOs or RGOs and forearm crutches or walker; not practical for T2–T6	I: Indoors with KAFOs or RGOs and forearm crutches; some can do stairs with railing	I: Indoors and community with AFOs; may need forearm crutches or cane
Driving	I: Hand controls I: Load MWC	I: Hand controls I: Load MWC	Can drive automatic transmission; may prefer hand controls

Adapted from Massagli, TL, & Jaffe, KM. Pediatric spinal cord injury: Treatment and outcome. Pediatrician, *17*:244–254, 1990. Reprinted with permission of S. Karger, Basel.

AFOs, Ankle-foot orthoses; *I*, independent; *KAFOs*, knee-ankle-foot orthoses; *MWC*, manual wheelchair; *RGOs*, reciprocating gait orthoses; *SBA*, standby assistance.

around a joint or even cause ankylosis. The most commonly affected joints are hips, knees, shoulders, and elbows.

Spasticity is a frequent occurrence after SCI and usually evolves within a period of 1 to 2 years. Although initially the patient is flaccid, hypertonus gradually appears, and in the first 3 to 6 months after SCI the patient develops hyperreflexia, clonus, and flexor spasms. Later, extensor spasms usually predominate. Evolution of spasticity after central nervous system insult is common and is seen in other conditions such as cerebral palsy and stroke. In SCI, the immediate effects of loss of supraspinal inhibition and the later-developing effects of denervation

supersensitivity and sprouting by afferent and collateral neurons probably all contribute to the development of spasticity, but the sequence of events behind the evolution of clinical manifestations of spasticity is not known.

REHABILITATION MANAGEMENT

The acute rehabilitation and long-term treatment of children with SCI require a comprehensive interdisciplinary approach involving both hospital and school-based personnel. Team members typically include physicians, nurses, a dietitian, occupational therapists, therapeutic recreation specialists, a social worker, an orthotist, a clinical psychologist, and teachers, as well as physical therapists, the child, and the family.

A pediatric physiatrist provides medical management of the complications noted earlier and serves as a team leader. In some centers, this role may be filled by an orthopedist, a neurologist, or a pediatrician. Researchers, however, have shown that referral of patients with SCI to comprehensive, multidisciplinary SCI centers is more cost-effective, with improved patient outcomes, reduced hospital and long-term nursing care charges, and improved prospect for long-term patient earnings, compared with unspecialized care for SCI patients (Johnston & Keith, 1983). The lead physician may also request consultation by other physicians such as an orthopedic surgeon or neurosurgeon to monitor spine stability and alignment, a urologist to monitor urinary tract function, and a pulmonologist for ventilator management.

Physical therapists develop age-appropriate ROM and strengthening programs. They address functional mobility, including bed mobility, transfers, sitting balance, ambulation, and wheelchair skills. The physical therapist makes recommendations on lower extremity orthoses and plays a primary role in the ordering of the wheelchair.

Rehabilitation nurses manage bladder and bowel care, monitor skin for pressure ulcers, provide emotional support to patients, and train the patient and family to carry out these tasks at home. Children can be taught self-management of bladder and bowel emptying at about age 5 years but may need reminders or supervision for many more years. The dietitian educates the child and family in meal selection to avoid protein catabolism or, conversely, obesity and to choose high-fiber foods to facilitate bowel management.

Occupational therapists provide training in self-care management, in use of orthoses to aid hand function in tetraplegia, and in use of adaptive writing equipment. They often assist physical therapists with upper extremity strengthening and wheelchair prescriptions. Goals for self-care management must be set according to usual expectations for age. For the older teenager, the occupational therapist may also provide training in home and money management, prevocational skills, travel within the community, and use of adaptive equipment for driving. An orthotist is needed if either functional hand orthoses or lower extremity orthoses are necessary. Therapeutic recreation specialists find leisure activities, including sports, in which the child can be independent and explore function in the community.

Social workers are indispensable for working with funding agencies. Inpatient and outpatient rehabilitation funding may be determined by visit, day, or dollar amount. A child may be eligible for a combination of funding through private insurance, Medicaid, and state developmental disability programs. The social worker helps determine eligibility and benefits and works with the family, rehabilitation team, and third-party payers in making the best use of available rehabilitation resources. The social worker also assists with discharge planning and provides support to the patient and family. A team member skilled in mental health should monitor the child's adaptation to disability and be available to help the child verbally process the injury and rehabilitation treatment. This could be a skilled social worker, but if a behavior management program using reinforcers is needed, a clinical psychologist should be consulted. In some rare cases, the child may truly be clinically depressed, and a psychiatrist can be consulted if a medication trial is contemplated. As described by Fordyce (1981), acquisition of SCI accompanied by pain, medical complications, altered cosmesis and body image, and the new and challenging rehabilitation procedures can be expected to have a significant impact on the patient's affect, self-esteem, and behavior. The child's adjustment to SCI does not necessarily follow predictable stages of crisis response such as shock, denial, depression, and adaptation. Adjustment to SCI probably occurs over several years. The verbal or attitudinal expressions of children with new SCI are less predictive of outcome than are their behaviors. Physical therapists can facilitate adjustment by actively engaging the child in acquiring the skills needed to maximize independence.

The psychologist or psychiatrist may also need to confront issues of premorbid risk-taking behavior or even substance abuse. Psychologists, nurses, and pediatric physiatrists collaborate in discussing sexuality and changes in sexual functioning with teenagers who have had SCI.

Teachers are particularly important during the acute rehabilitation phase because the length of hospitalization after SCI is often 1 to 3 months and the child must keep up with his or her curriculum. The teacher can be instrumental in assisting the receiving school to prepare for the child's return. Schools and state agencies should be asked to participate in vocational planning and counseling with teenagers.

THE YOUNG CHILD WITH SPINAL CORD INJURY

Examination of Performance

Infants, toddlers, and preschoolers can incur SCI as a result of birth trauma, child abuse, motor vehicle crashes, tumor, or even transverse myelitis. In infants, determination of the motor and sensory levels of SCI can be challenging and may require multiple examinations to determine what movement is voluntary and what is reflex mediated. Examination of passive ROM should be performed, as for any infant. The therapist can determine functional limitations by comparing the infant's motor skills such as head control, rolling, sitting balance, transitional movements, crawling, and standing with expected developmental milestones. Very young children with SCI require careful follow-up over time to be sure they meet functional expectations and are not infantilized by caregivers.

Examination of the performance of preschool children with a recent SCI is rarely completed in one session. These children are commonly anxious in the presence of health care professionals. Trust must be established in the child and the parents. This means taking extra time to play and talk with the child and to interact with the parents. Some children are initially fearful of movement, whereas others act fearlessly. In the former case, it will take time to build their confidence. In the latter case, the child may attempt to remove the cervical collar or body jacket or may assume body positions that stress the healing fusion. Thus additional adult supervision may be necessary to comply with precautions during the healing phase.

Quantification of impairments in the young child is often unreliable because young children are unable to cooperate consistently with formal testing. Passive ROM measurement is possibly an exception to this, but its reliability in children with SCI has not been established. In children without SCI and in children with myelodysplasia, manual muscle testing is generally unreliable if the child is younger than 5 years old (McDonald et al., 1986; Molnar & Kaminer, 1992). In young children, strength testing is often estimated by encouraging and observing movement. Ideally, the therapist places the child in various positions and encourages him or her to reach for toys with a single extremity. This allows examination of gravity-eliminated and antigravity movements, as well as comparison of left and right extremities. Resistance can be provided with small wrap weights (0.25 lb) or the weight of handheld toys. In reality, the physical therapist is often forced to observe spontaneous play and record descriptions of available movements. This may include facilitating the child's basic postural responses, such as positive support of the lower extremities or protective extension of the upper extremities. Ruling out substitutions can be challenging. Muscle strength is recorded as 0 through 5, as with adults (rarely with the finer + or − gradations). Scores of 4 and 5 are subjective measures, particularly in growing children, but with experience, the therapist can become a more accurate evaluator.

Cardiorespiratory endurance is commonly diminished in children with recent SCI but is difficult to quantify because they cannot complete the available standardized tests requiring walking or running (see Chapter 5). Therapists can make clinical estimates of endurance by recording the length of time a child can engage in an activity or the number of repetitions of a movement completed before the child needs to rest. Accurate recording of these data can be used to document changes in endurance over time.

Both the Functional Independence Measure for Children (WeeFIM) (Granger et al., 1988; Ottenbacher et al., 1996) and the Pediatric Evaluation of Disability Inventory (PEDI) (Haley et al., 1992; Nichols et al., 1996) are used as measures of functional skills for patients with SCI. Regardless of which assessment tools are preferred, the physical therapist must establish a complete baseline of the child's abilities and determine whether limitations are due to the child's age, the neurologic impairment, the need to wear a spinal orthosis, or other causes. Any standard physical therapy examination includes testing of the child's ability to reach, roll, position in bed, come to sitting, balance in sitting, scoot, crawl, transfer, come to kneel, stand, and ambulate. Some or all of these may not be possible, so the type and amount of assistance needed are recorded, or the therapist may simply record "unable."

Physical therapists should include parents as active participants during the examination phase. Parents need to receive accurate, understandable information about their child's condition. Because they are trying to adapt to the sudden change in their child's health, they often are unable to generate therapy outcomes for their child beyond wanting the child "to walk again." The therapist and SCI team must assist the family and child in establishing realistic outcomes. One must consider the child's level of injury (see Tables 21–4 and 21–5), the completeness of injury, the age of the child, and the family's expectations for the child. If the wearing of a spinal orthosis limits some activities, some goals may need to be postponed until it is removed, which may be after discharge from inpatient rehabilitation.

Impairments and Functional Limitations

The child's anxiety with strangers and fear of movement often persist beyond the examination phase and affect treatment. The physical therapist should start with brief sessions that have low demand and high success and then gradually increase the duration and expectations of the therapy sessions. The therapist can provide predictability and promote trust by establishing routines for scheduling, treatment session locations, and safe play space, and whenever possible should give the child choices regarding play activities.

Parents should be included in treatment sessions whenever possible. Although many children work better in therapy sessions in the absence of parents, parents should be regularly included to see the new skills their child can independently accomplish and the emerging skills that require assistance. Parents must become experts in all aspects of their child's mobility and use of adaptive equipment. Parent education and training should be an ongoing process that begins soon after the initial examination and is completed in time for practice on day or overnight outings.

During physical therapy sessions with the child, it is nearly impossible to do isolated treatment of impairments, with the exception of ROM activities. The child's motivation for play gives overall structure for the sessions. Within that, the therapist designs activities that encourage strengthening, reaching, rolling, sitting, transitions, and mobility in various combinations.

Sitting balance is often one of the major goals of therapy. Balance is impaired by altered strength and sensation and often by the presence of a spinal orthosis. Conversely, a child with tetraplegia or high paraplegia may benefit from a soft orthosis to facilitate sitting, leaving hands free for other activities (Fig. 21-3). The seated child is encouraged to progress from therapist support to self-support at a table top or on a mat and to independent sitting if this is realistic given the level and completeness of injury. These goals may be achieved by distracting the child or engaging the child in play activities.

If some lower extremity function has been preserved, the therapist helps children progress to crawling, kneeling, and standing activities when the functioning lower extremity muscles can be appropriately strengthened. Some children require orthoses for distal weakness in the lower extremities. Table 21-5 outlines the expected functional ambulation by level of SCI. Preschool-age children can learn to use reciprocating gait orthoses and KAFOs, but they generally rely on a front-wheeled walker, as opposed to crutches, until age 7 to 8 years. Further discussion of gait training and use of orthoses is presented in the section on school-age and adolescent children.

Orthoses may also be needed by children with absent muscle function for maintaining ROM, for instance at the ankle or in the hands. As with any insensate area, the skin must be regularly examined to avoid pressure ulcers.

If community ambulation is not an expected outcome, the child needs a wheelchair for mobility. For young children with SCI at or above C6, a power wheelchair is needed for independent mobility.

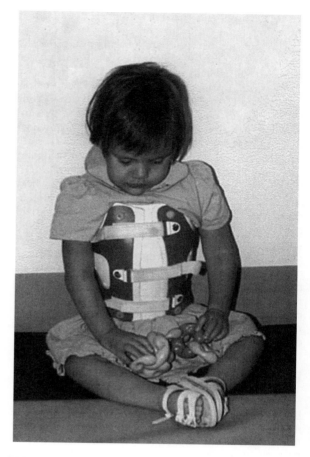

FIGURE 21-3. A soft orthosis provides external support, improving sitting balance and allowing this child with a high thoracic SCI to use both hands in play.

Some young children with lower levels of cervical SCI, or even high thoracic injuries, may be able to propel a manual wheelchair for only limited distances on smooth, level surfaces owing to lack of upper body strength and endurance. For these children to be exposed to a broader range of environments, such as preschool playgrounds or uneven or steep terrain around the family home, prescription of a power wheelchair is justifiable to promote age-appropriate functional mobility. A child as young as 18 to 24 months may be trained to use a power wheelchair but requires adult supervision for safety. In addition, a manual wheelchair is necessary to provide these children with a substitute when the power chair needs repairs. The manual wheelchair is also useful for transport and in places where the larger, heavier power chair is impractical. Many families do not have a home with hallways or doors large enough to accommodate a power wheelchair, so this wheelchair may be used primarily in community and school settings and the manual wheelchair used in the home.

The seating components of either a power or manual wheelchair are prescribed with skin protection and spinal alignment in mind. A level pelvis avoids undue pressure over the ischial tuberosities and facilitates a straight spine (Hobson & Tooms, 1992). A solid seat and back are preferred to sling upholstery in this age group. Several types of wheelchair cushions are available, but none is universally effective for all persons with SCI, and individual assessment is required to prevent pressure ulcers (Garber & Dylerly, 1991). Children who use a wheelchair and their parents must be trained to complete transfers. Children younger than 4 years often lack the upper body strength to transfer independently and typically require a one-person lift transfer. Use of a sliding board or pivot transfer is appropriate for older children (5 to 7 years). Pressure-relief techniques must also be taught. Younger children often rely on caregivers for tilt-back pressure relief. Older children may be able to complete one of the techniques independently, depending on the level and completeness of injury (see Table 21–4).

Prevention of Secondary Impairments

As discussed in the section on medical management, a number of secondary impairments can arise after SCI. Many of these can lead to functional limitations and disability. Physical therapists contribute to prevention, treatment, and monitoring of pressure ulcers, contractures, edema, spasticity, pathologic fractures, and scoliosis. Pressure ulcers occur as a result of improper positioning or inadequate pressure relief and can limit ability to sit. Very young children may not need frequent pressure relief because body weight is not great enough to impair tissue blood flow and they are often held and handled frequently enough that they do not remain in one position too long. As children grow older, however, it is often difficult for them to understand the importance of routine pressure-relief activities.

Contractures can arise as a result of static positioning, spasticity, or heterotopic bone formation and may interfere with positioning or voluntary movement. Hip subluxation and dislocation are common in children who have onset of SCI before age 5, so stretching of hip adductors and flexors is important. Dependent edema is more common in children with flaccid lower extremities. When it develops, it predisposes skin to breakdown by increasing fragility and by altering the fit of garments and braces. Spasticity may be present and cause no functional limitations, or it may impair positioning, transfers, or other voluntary movements. Conversely, spasticity may be helpful for those with incomplete SCI who use it to achieve or maintain standing. Pathologic fractures can occur to osteopenic extremities with improper transfers, falls, or forceful ROM exercises. Scoliosis occurs in virtually all children with SCI in this age group and can affect comfortable seating and respiratory function. Although family training and positioning needs are initially managed or determined by inpatient physical therapists, outpatient and school physical therapists have an important role in monitoring and maintaining ROM and in using stretching and positioning to minimize spasticity. They monitor and promote the upper body strength that allows the growing child to perform independent pressure relief. They also monitor positioning in seating devices and the fit of adaptive equipment, including wheelchairs and orthoses.

No treatment, including passive standing and electrical stimulation, has yet been found to prevent or reverse osteopenia in paralyzed extremities, so the presence of osteopenia and the risk of pathologic fractures should be assumed for all children with SCI, even for those with spasticity. Although it is important to provide proper pelvic alignment and trunk support in wheelchairs, external devices do not prevent the ultimate development of scoliosis, and many children require treatment with bracing and then spinal fusion after they have achieved the majority of their expected height. Both braces and spinal fusion can dramatically reduce trunk mobility, so it becomes imperative to maximize passive hip ROM.

Minimizing Disability and Disadvantage

While hospitalized, the child must practice mobility skills outside of structured therapy sessions. Thus children must be encouraged to partially or fully self-propel during daily activities. Family and other team members must be familiar with each child's skills and routines to maximize the child's independence across settings and activities. For instance, nurses should be updated on progress in mobility skills so that the child can be encouraged to incorporate these abilities into play activities or getting to meals.

The child must eventually be trained in using these new skills in the community. Community reentry activities are often the combined responsibility of physical therapists, occupational therapists, and therapeutic recreation specialists. Children must become familiar with common architectural barriers such as curbs, heavy doors, and high shelves and learn how to negotiate them or ask for help. Caregivers need to be trained in the type and amount of assistance to provide and cautioned against being overly helpful. Discharge planning and long-term management should address mobility issues in the child's home, school, and community. Whenever possible, a home evaluation should be conducted early in the child's hospital stay. If home modifications are necessary for wheelchair accessibility or safety, the family needs time to gather financial resources and complete modifications. These modifications can be evaluated during weekend passes. Public schools employ physical and occupational therapists who can provide accessibility information while the child is still hospitalized. Upon school entry, the child can be assisted with accommodations under the provisions of section 504 of the Vocational Rehabilitation Act of 1973. The therapist plays a major role as a consultant to the faculty, family, and student regarding accessibility issues and needed modifications to architectural barriers or curriculum. For children living great distances from the hospital, school and other community therapists can provide a local perspective and become a resource to the family. Another area of concern in community reentry is safe transportation. The physical therapist can assist the family with evaluating safe transportation of their child. If a van will be used, wheelchair tie-downs will be necessary. If the child can sit in a vehicle seat, appropriate car seats, booster seats, or restraints are needed, depending on the child's age and amount of trunk and neck control.

Ongoing Monitoring

The key to ensuring maximal function in young children with SCI is to provide ongoing examination of impairments and function and to regularly reestablish outcomes appropriate for the child's age. At least two mechanisms are available to accomplish this objective. Children who are discharged from rehabilitation centers are routinely seen in follow-up visits two or more times each year. These reevaluations include medical follow-up to reexamine the level and completeness of injury, to evaluate changes in bladder function or skin integrity, to monitor the spine for development of scoliosis, and to determine the need for medications to treat spasticity or bladder or bowel incontinence.

Reexamination by the physical therapist is an important part of these follow-up visits. For children who have developed sufficient upper extremity strength, a standard push-up for pressure relief in the wheelchair may be taught, and children should learn to check their skin each day. These children are often gaining more independence in self-propelling outdoors and on inclines. They may need instruction and training to participate more in transfers. The child's wheelchair should be reassessed and

adapted as needed to accommodate the child's growth and to ensure that any modifications enhance independence.

The physical therapy reexaminations at the rehabilitation facility follow a consultative model. The ongoing progress toward age-appropriate outcomes may occur in a hospital-based outpatient therapy program, but it is more typically accomplished through therapy services offered in early intervention programs or in publicly funded developmental preschools. Therapists in these programs ideally are in contact with the rehabilitation centers on a regular basis to update progress and goals and to identify new concerns and equipment needs.

A small number of children with SCI may actually experience progressive decline in function over time. These are usually children with SCI caused by progressive or metastatic tumor. It can be unsettling and challenging for rehabilitation professionals to care for such patients, but it is an important aspect of their work. Often such children need more equipment over time, such as more bracing or a wheelchair with more supportive seating. These children can often be very ill from ongoing chemotherapy or radiation treatments, and it may be more practical to rent equipment than to purchase it. Coordination of efforts among oncology and rehabilitation staff, the patient, and the family is crucial.

THE SCHOOL-AGE CHILD AND ADOLESCENT WITH SPINAL CORD INJURY

Examination of Performance

The examination of older children is usually more straightforward than that of preschoolers, toddlers, or infants and can be conducted as for an adult. ROM measurements and manual muscle testing are completed. As previously noted, endurance testing is limited because standardized testing requires lower extremity function. Research is needed in this area, particularly in standardization of upper extremity ergometry. The same basic mobility skills must be assessed as with younger children, that is, rolling, coming to sit, sitting balance, transfers, and locomotion. Functional examination may include the PEDI or Functional Independence Measure (FIM) (Hamilton et al., 1987). The FIM is a measure of functional limitations or disability for those older than 7 years. It can be used to assess the same categories of function (using the same seven-level scale) as the WeeFIM. The FIM is widely used in national databases of persons with SCI.

Parents may or may not be present during the actual examination. They should be provided with accurate, understandable information, and as previously noted, families and children in their early crisis phase often need the rehabilitation team to assist them with realistic outcome setting. The therapist must nevertheless keep in mind that these children may be confronting the potential permanence of their condition. The therapist may notice the adolescent being withdrawn or angry or in denial or even enthusiastic to begin therapy. These behaviors may fluctuate and change rapidly. Children who have returned to school may be better able to identify personal goals. Although age plays a smaller role in outcome development, level and completeness of injury must be considered.

Impairments and Functional Limitations

When planning physical therapy sessions, it is important to be sensitive to the child's current emotional status. Treatment session demands can be modified to most appropriately challenge the child. An issue commonly expressed by teenagers is that of not being able to trust their bodies. The altered motor and sensory processes and potential changes in bowel and bladder function can make their bodies feel foreign to them. In addition, teenagers are accustomed to privacy and independence in their lives. Both their injury and subsequent reliance on a hospital environment and adaptive equipment can disrupt their sense of control. The rehabilitation team should respect their privacy and allow them to participate in scheduling therapy, nursing care, and free time.

Parents need to be included regularly in sessions to observe their child's progress and receive updated training for transfers, wheelchair mobility, pressure relief, use of orthoses, and ambulation. It can be helpful to allow close friends to observe therapy and attend outings. If friends feel comfortable with the injured adolescent, their presence may help lessen social isolation.

Treatment sessions are more structured with older than with younger children. The first step is to get the child upright and out of bed. If orthostatic hypotension is a problem, this process may require several sessions and use of a wheelchair with a reclinable back to allow the child to gradually assume a fully upright posture. Protocols for remobilizing the newly injured older child or teenager with SCI often use a tilt table to gradually elevate the child's head, although use of this tactic has not yet been proved to hasten resolution of orthostatic hypotension. Other useful measures include support stockings, wrapping the legs with Ace bandages, and using abdominal binders to deter venous pooling. In addition, the therapist should be alert for any complaints of headaches that may signal autonomic dysreflexia, a problem described in the section on medical management. The therapist should monitor heart rate and blood pressure and, when appropriate, alert the medical staff.

Teenagers are familiar with the concept of exercise, so they can participate in progressive resistive exercises beginning with powder board and progressing to weight lifting. All innervated musculature must be strengthened. This includes muscles that have normal grade 5 strength because they will need to compensate for weakened or paralyzed muscles. Shoulders must maintain full ROM for ease of dressing. Patients with tetraplegia who have wrist extension but no hand function should be allowed to develop mild finger flexor tightness. This provides a tenodesis grasp, which occurs with wrist extension. Stretching the hamstrings to 100 to 110° and having adequate hip external rotation is necessary for dressing and self-care. It is important to have excessively flexible hamstrings to prevent overstretching of the low back. Maintaining a tight low back is crucial for transfers and bed mobility to ensure that head and shoulder movements maximally effect lower body mobility. Ankle ROM must be maintained at neutral for proper placement on the wheelchair footrest.

A small number of children with tetraplegia have upper cervical injuries (C1–C3) that necessitate mechanical ventilation (see Chapter 25). Physical therapy intervention for these children and for those with C4 tetraplegia has a more narrow focus, because the child is dependent with bed mobility, transfers, and sitting balance (see Table 21–4). Spasticity tends to be more problematic with this population. Daily passive ROM can help reduce tone and facilitate positioning. The family must be thoroughly trained in all aspects of the child's mobility and care, and the child must be trained to instruct others in his or her care, including use and maintenance of the wheelchair and any other equipment. Caregivers need to learn pivot transfers and use of a mechanical lift. The child will need a power and a manual wheelchair. The wheelchairs must be ordered as soon as possible, but it is likely that they will not arrive before discharge, so rental wheelchairs may be necessary. Environmental controls and a more complex power wheelchair are needed for independent mobility. The joystick is replaced with head, tongue, or sip-and-puff controls, and the power tilt must allow for ventilator placement. The manual wheelchair should have tilt-in-space capability as well. All wheelchairs and environmental control systems should be chosen by the rehabilitation team, child, and family in consultation with a knowledgeable vendor (see Chapter 24). The therapist should be aware of available funding for wheelchairs and other durable medical equipment. There may be limitations in coverage, and the therapist can assist the family in prioritizing equipment needs.

For children and teenagers with C5 or lower tetraplegia, the focus of physical therapy is on maintaining ROM, upper extremity strengthening, bed mobility, sitting balance, transfer training, and the ordering and training in use of adaptive equipment. Those with tetraplegia at C5 and C6 or above (and even some at C7) need a power wheelchair in addition to a manual wheelchair. Pressure relief may be accomplished by lateral or forward weight shift. Those without adequate trunk control for weight shifting will need the addition of a power tilt-in-space feature on the wheelchair. Ordering the appropriate wheelchair can be challenging because approximately half these children have incomplete injuries and the extent of their recovery may not be clear for months.

For children with paraplegia, transfer training initially includes sliding board transfers. Push-up blocks can also be helpful when first learning transfers (see Fig. 21-1). As upper extremity strength increases, the child may be able to transfer without a sliding board. Older children must also practice car transfers and how to get up from and down to the floor with and without assistance. Wheelchair mobility must be practiced on even and uneven terrain and up and down ramps and curbs. Wheelies can be taught at about age 8 years to facilitate managing curbs and uneven terrain. Pressure-relief techniques must also be taught (see Table 21-4). The child with paraplegia can lift the buttocks off the seat for 20 to 60 seconds two or three times an hour. If the child with paraplegia is not able to ambulate long distances, a manual wheelchair should be prescribed. Lightweight components should be used, and if it is anticipated that the child will be very active or frequently traverse rough terrain, a rigid frame, as opposed to a folding frame, is more appropriate. If the teenager has completed most of his or her growth and has a low thoracic or lumbar level SCI, a low sling back with a taut sling seat may be used in place of the solid seat and back.

For teenagers with preserved or recovered lower extremity function, ambulation may be a realistic outcome. Often, an orthosis is needed (see Table 21-5). Donning and removing orthoses must be practiced, as well as controlled sit-to-stand maneuvers and finding the balance point in standing. As with most ambulation training, practice begins in the parallel bars and progresses to use of other assistive devices when the child gains enough control. Ambulation is most practical for those who have at least grade 3 strength in one set of quadriceps muscles. At higher injury levels, the child requires KAFOs and some type of upper extremity assistive device. A four-point gait is possible for those with strong hip flexors or with the use of reciprocating gait orthoses. The swing-through gait pattern is, however, much more efficient. Five to twelve times as much energy is expended walking with KAFOs compared with that required for normal gait on even terrain (Jaeger et al., 1989). Numerous follow-up studies of adults have found that more than half of patients who have reciprocating gait orthoses (RGOs) or KAFOs prescribed do not use them at all in the long term, and the majority of the rest of patients use them only for standing or exercise (Jaeger et al., 1989). The most common reasons for discontinuing use of the braces are the excessive energy costs and the need for assistance to don and remove them and to use them for ambulation. Given the significant expense of brace manufacture and ambulation training, it is often best to complete initial rehabilitation outcomes and master independent wheelchair mobility before ordering braces. Periodic reexamination of the child's physical abilities and outcomes as an outpatient can then be used to determine whether ambulation with braces is a reasonable goal. Many patients become less interested over time in ambulation requiring extensive bracing as the permanence of the injury becomes more apparent. Those who remain interested may have more specific needs for standing or limited walking that increase the likelihood of long-term use of the orthoses.

Functional Electrical Stimulation

Functional electrical stimulation (FES) has been applied in many areas in SCI, including muscle strengthening, cardiovascular conditioning, ambulation, and hand function. In all of these areas, research continues into the effectiveness, efficiency, and long-term outcome of FES. With all uses of FES, it is important that there be realistic expectations by the family and child.

FES for strengthening is useful only in cases of upper motoneuron paralysis where the intact peripheral nerve is stimulated, causing muscle contraction. In lower motoneuron injuries to the cauda equina, the peripheral nerve and its muscular branches undergo wallerian degeneration, so the muscle must be stimulated directly and larger pulse widths and current amplitudes are necessary to produce contractions. The whole muscle must be flooded with current, and the contraction response is often inadequate. The stimulation parameters can be painful in those who have some preservation of sensation.

FES has been used as a strengthening modality for partially paralyzed muscles. In crossover studies of FES-assisted exercise versus conventional resistive exercise, no significant increases in maximal strength have been found with use of FES (Seeger et al., 1989). However, FES-assisted exercise has been found to be more effective than upper extremity ergometry for strengthening the triceps muscles (Needham-Shropshire et al., 1997a). FES does improve strength, muscle mass, and endurance of totally paralyzed muscles and can improve aerobic capacity (Mohr et al., 1997). Because degenerative joint disease of the shoulder is a significant problem for aging persons with SCI, one advantage of FES over conventional exercise as an aerobic training strategy is that more muscle groups are exercised, placing less stress on the upper extremities.

Exercise must be performed regularly to maintain positive effects. Home bicycle ergometer units with FES are now available, but follow-up studies have shown that patients with SCI are often too busy to use this expensive equipment on a regular and long-term basis (Sipski et al., 1993). In patients who do exercise consistently, increase of muscle bulk occurs concomitantly with increase of strength in paralyzed muscles. In addition, blood flow to muscles is increased during stimulation, and the combination of increased bulk and improved circulatory flow may help prevent pressure ulcers (Levine et al., 1990). Researchers and clinicians hoped that FES could help reverse osteopenia after SCI, but to date, none of the protocols used, including those combined with ambulation (Needham-Shropshire et al., 1997b), has been able to increase bone mass. FES may actually be dangerous in those with the most severe osteopenia because it may cause pathologic fractures (Phillips, 1987).

FES has also been applied to facilitate standing and walking after SCI. Surface, percutaneous, or implanted electrodes are used to deliver current to lower extremity nerves innervating muscles such as the quadriceps and gluteals. The development of sensors to determine leg position, force, acceleration, and muscle fatigue has lagged behind progress in stimulation but is necessary to improve the quality and efficiency of movement. None of the currently available technologic methods permits standing or walking without upper extremity assistive devices. Hybrid systems using FES and orthoses have also been developed, and less expensive garments with surface electrodes sewn into them for easier application are available. The energy costs of walking with FES are comparable to those of using KAFOs but may be slightly reduced when FES is combined with reciprocating gait orthoses (Hirokawa et al., 1990; Yarkony et al., 1992). At present, this technology remains imperfect, expensive, and not widely available. Data on long-term use other than in a limited number of research subjects have not been published.

FES has been used in patients with tetraplegia to improve or restore hand function. For adolescents with C5 and C6 tetraplegia who are skeletally mature and who lack grasp and release, surgical reconstruction at the forearm and hand in conjunction with implanted electrodes can provide palmar and lateral grasp. An external unit is worn and small shoulder movements control hand movements. This may allow the child to perform activities such as basic hygiene, eating, and writing more independently and without the use of an orthosis (Mulcahey et al., 1997). As with other complex technologies, subjects have had variable patterns of long-term use because they need to rely on others to don the stimulator (Mulcahey et al., 1993).

Prevention of Secondary Impairments

The secondary impairments facing older children and adolescents with SCI are similar to those for younger children, with a few additions. In this older age group, cardiovascular fitness and overuse syndromes are important to consider. Studies of adults with chronic SCI have shown that physical work capacity inversely correlates with lesion level and that cardiovascular responses to exercise are abnormal because of a deficient sympathetic nervous system (Drory et al., 1990). Such persons may be at increased risk for cardiovascular compromise and disease. Clinicians should encourage regular aerobic exercise in older children and young adults with SCI to help them develop lifelong habits of health promotion. School therapists can facilitate participation in an adaptive physical education program, community-based recreational programs for people with disabilities, or competitive wheelchair sports. Stotts (1986) found that athletes with paraplegia were less likely to incur avoidable medical complications than nonathletes with paraplegia. Consideration of such participation must be balanced against the recognized propensity for overuse syndromes in these athletes, including such problems as carpal tunnel syndrome, tendinitis, rotator cuff impingement, and degenerative disease of shoulder joints. Patients with tetraplegia and wheelchair athletes at any level have a high incidence of impingement syndrome and rotator cuff tears. An imbalance of strength at the shoulder with relative weakness of humeral head depressors may be contributory, and patients should engage in a program of balanced shoulder exercises (Burnham et al., 1993).

Minimizing Disability and Disadvantage

Getting into the community as soon as is feasible is important for older children and adolescents with SCI. As is the case with younger children, outings are practice sessions for return to the community. In addition to the usual home and school assessments, the complex issue of transportation must be addressed. The teenager's friends may need to be trained in car transfers so that he or she can stay socially active. The teenager returning to driving needs to be independent with transfers and with loading and unloading the wheelchair. Above all, teenagers should be encouraged to problem solve the management of architectural barriers and ask for assistance if safety is jeopardized. On return to the community, the teenager's primary resource for mobility and seating issues is the school therapist. Some teenagers, especially those with higher levels of injury, may benefit from use of animal aids, such as dogs trained by the program Canine Companions for Independence (P.O. Box 446, Santa Rosa, CA 95402; www.caninecompanions.org/index.html).

Ongoing Monitoring and Transition to Adulthood

Unlike younger children, school-age children and adolescents with SCI are usually closer to their predicted function for level of injury by the time of discharge from the rehabilitation unit. As mentioned previously, however, neurologic changes may continue for some months; for example, children with C5 complete tetraplegia may develop antigravity wrist extension during the first 8 months after injury, and outpatient or school therapists may need to formulate new goals. In many children, upper body strength of intact muscles continues to improve, enabling smoother transfers or easier wheelchair propulsion up inclines. In general, however, the majority of physical therapy involvement after discharge eventually entails a consulting and monitoring role, for example, making sure that mobility skills learned in the hospital environment are generalized to the child's home and community, monitoring ROM or spasticity, and updating equipment. Any deterioration in motor strength should be referred for medical evaluation because it may signify development of a syrinx.

Older children and adolescents require reexamination similar to that of younger children in a rehabilitation center once or twice a year. The focus of these examinations is on medical issues, equipment needs, and efficacy of home or outpatient stretching or exercise programs. For teenagers, such visits should include discussions related to sexuality and reproduction (Haseltine et al., 1990). Young women need to know that their fertility is not impaired by spinal cord injury but that sexual response and orgasm may be. Pregnant women with SCI should be managed at high-risk centers to avoid respiratory and urinary tract complications, detect threatened preterm births, and prevent autonomic dysreflexia during delivery. Although the majority of males with SCI can have erections, these are often fleeting and not adequate for vaginal penetration. Few men with SCI have ejaculations, and sperm quality decreases over time for reasons that are not entirely clear. New techniques for retrieval of sperm and for artificial insemination have helped some men with SCI to father children. In addition to this physiologic information, it is important to include issues of intimacy and relationships in discussions of sexuality.

We have found that although the majority of young school-age children with SCI receive direct physical and occupational therapy services in school, few adolescents receive such services. The therapist works from a consultant model, using the faculty and student to carry out programs and recommendations. Issues may include supporting the teen to continue with regular pressure releases, stretching and other home programs, and progressing mobility skills to community distances. The physical and occupational therapist should also consult with the faculty and student regarding an appropriate physical education program; modification of classroom and desk setup; and accessibility to lockers, bathroom, and lunchroom. In reality, many adolescents with SCI have no physical education program, face problems of accessibility at school, and report that breakdown of wheelchairs (both power and manual) contributes to absences at school (Massagli et al., 1996). The fact that the number of years of education after injury is more significant than absolute amount of education in predicting employment after SCI (El Ghahit & Hanson, 1979) speaks to the importance of ensuring success in school for such children. Unfortunately, only 50% of teenagers with a ninth- to eleventh-grade education at the time of their SCI finish high school (DeVivo et al., 1991).

We have also found that few adolescents with SCI receive educational or vocational counseling beyond selection of classes each term (Massagli et al., 1996). Such students may qualify for transition planning under the Individuals with Disabilities Education Act, Public Law 101-476. School physical therapists might participate in a transition program by assessing functional mobility skills in the community or work-study setting. When the teenager with SCI becomes 18 years of age, she or he is eligible for state vocational counseling services. Such services are often important sources of funding for vocationally related education or even equipment.

Three case histories illustrate the application of the principles discussed in this chapter. The first describes the experiences of a child injured as an infant; the second, those of a young school-age child; and the third, those of a teenager.

CASE HISTORY
STACY

This case study demonstrates the physical therapy management of a very young child with complete tetraplegia and highlights the importance of parent education and training. The need to monitor the acquisition of skills is also discussed.

Stacy was injured at 9 months of age. She was an unrestrained passenger in a motor vehicle crash. Although she did not sustain bone injury to the spine, magnetic resonance imaging revealed a C6 to T1 intracord hemorrhage. Formal manual muscle testing could not be conducted because of her age, so gross estimates of muscle strength were made. Shoulder flexion was estimated at grade 4, elbow flexion at grade 3, and elbow extension at grade 2. Wrist extension was estimated at grade 3, with movements of the fingers graded at trace. Her sensory examination was difficult to interpret, but she did not appear to have reliable pinprick in the lowest sacral dermatome. Pinprick in the lower extremities induced triple flexion involuntary responses. She was diagnosed with C5 tetraplegia, ASIA Impairment Scale level A. Even though the key muscles for C6, wrist extensors, were grade 3, the next higher key muscle was not grade 5. Therefore, a level of C5 was assigned.

At her initial physical therapy examination, Stacy had normal passive ROM with the exception of tightness noted at the end range of shoulder flexion and abduction and elbow extension. Functionally, Stacy was unable to roll, and when placed in prone-on-elbows could sustain the position only very briefly. When placed in sitting with full trunk support, she could raise her head to within about 20° of vertical.

After approximately 2 weeks of acute medical care, Stacy was transferred to an inpatient pediatric rehabilitation facility. Considering her age and level of injury, physical therapy interventions and outcomes were targeted at three major areas (Fig. 21–4).

Within approximately 2 weeks, Stacy's caregivers had learned and demonstrated competence in all aspects of her care, and she was discharged to home. At that time, she continued to show good ROM and some increase in using her upper torso musculature.

From a functional standpoint, Stacy was able to reach against gravity when lying supine and to assist minimally in rolling herself to the side. When positioned in prone on her elbows, she was able to maintain her head upright intermittently for 1 to 2 minutes. She was unable to roll out of prone into supine. When in sitting, she was able to prop herself on the upper extremities with some success.

Therapy services were transitioned to a community Birth to Three program, and she began to receive physical therapy and occupational therapy two times per week with a focus on trunk control, upper extremity weight bearing, and the facilitation of developmental milestones.

By 1 year after SCI, her elbow extensor strength had improved to grade 3 and she had a pincer grasp bilaterally but weak finger flexion and no finger extension. She did not show substantial changes in ROM or tone, but demonstrated continued improvement in her functional skills. She was able to move from prone to supine independently. When placed in sitting she could sit but needed to use her hands for support. Stacy was able to move from sitting to prone by moving onto her forearms over her legs. She was able to "commando crawl" 5 to 10 feet by pulling with the upper extremities.

Her family reported two major concerns. The first was whether Stacy would eventually be able to walk with braces. Her prognosis was discussed and the concept of the use of a wheelchair was introduced. Benefits of increasing her strength and increasing her independence in mobility were emphasized. It was also emphasized that the use of the wheelchair would in no way hinder her potential ability to walk someday if she were to have neurologic return of function. The other concern was that of headaches and flushing of the face that the family had noted. This raised the question of autonomic dysreflexia. The family was instructed in taking Stacy's blood pressure when these episodes occurred. The visiting home nurse was also contacted to help assess this.

When Stacy was 2.5 years old, her examination revealed continued gains in finger flexion but no change in finger extension. Formal manual muscle testing was still not possible because of her age. Her sensory examination revealed no response to pinprick below the C7 dermatome. Her physical therapy examination revealed further improvements in function. Stacy was able to independently commando crawl and transition from prone to sit without difficulty. Her sitting balance had improved, and she could reach for and play with toys but needed to keep one hand on the floor for support. She was beginning to scoot backwards in sitting and pivot in prone. Her hand strength was notably improved, and overall hand function was better. Owing to her growth and improvements in

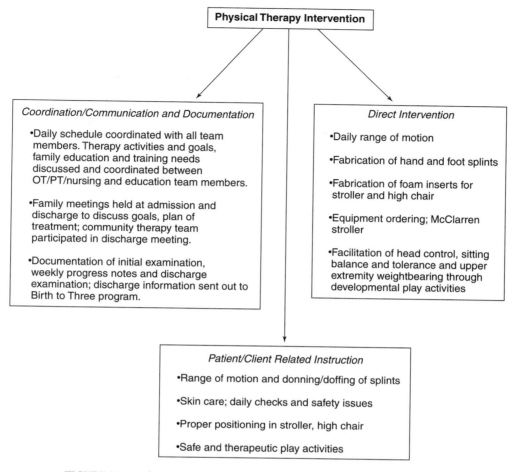

FIGURE 21-4. Physical therapy intervention for an infant with C5 tetraplegia.

upper extremity function, a trial use of a manual wheelchair was conducted. Stacy was able to sit well with hip pads and a hip belt on a solid seat with a solid back. She was able to propel only minimally during the initial trial. A wheelchair prescription was provided, with recommendations for a solid seat and back, hip supports and belt, and a headrest and knee adductors. Over the next months, Stacy learned to self-propel short distances with some difficulty.

By age 3.5, Stacy was receiving physical therapy once a week at school and once a week at a local hospital. Stacy was fitted for a pair of hip-knee-ankle-foot orthoses (HKAFOs) because her parents were very interested in a trial of standing and ambulation. It was explained that with Stacy's level of injury, this would probably only be a therapeutic activity and would not result in independent functional ambulation. Her community therapists provided gait training with the orthoses and a posture control walker.

The other issue discussed at the SCI clinic was prescription of a car seat. She had outgrown a standard car seat but had poor trunk control, necessitating an adapted car seat.

Stacy returned to the SCI clinic at age 4. Therapy services were unchanged. She was now able to sit briefly without upper extremity support. With moderate to maximal assistance she could walk a short distance with a walker and HKAFOs, employing a swing-through gait pattern. Although Stacy exhibited improving upper extremity function, it was discussed with her family that she would probably not attain enough strength in the upper extremities to keep up with her peers at school or in her rural home setting in a manual wheelchair and that a power wheelchair would be necessary. They agreed, and a power wheelchair mobility trial was done. Stacy enjoyed the independent movement and demonstrated good control of the chair using a proportional joystick with a small knob. A power wheelchair with head, trunk, and hip supports and belt was ordered for her. A wheelchair cushion was also ordered. Her school therapist supervised a power wheelchair training program. A sliding board was also ordered so she could begin transfer training.

When seen in the SCI clinic at age 6, Stacy was able to scoot in all directions independently. She was able to pull herself up onto furniture. She was able to walk a short distance using HKAFOs and a walker using a swing-through gait pattern, but with great effort and only in therapy. She was lifted for all transfers. She used her power wheelchair at school and used her manual wheelchair at home. She was often pushed in the chair and had difficulty with directionality and endurance. It was emphasized to her parents that it was important for Stacy to learn to do transfers and to improve her manual wheelchair skills in order to give her more independence.

Stacy was again seen in the clinic at age 7. At this visit, she was finally able to cooperate for formal manual muscle testing and sensory examination. She had grade 5 shoulder flexion and abduction, elbow flexion, and wrist extension and grade 4 elbow extension. Finger flexors were grade 3 and finger abductors grade 2. Grip strength was 1 kg bilaterally. She had intact sensation to C7. Her level of injury was redefined as C7 tetraplegia, ASIA Impairment Scale A. She was now receiving therapy only at school. She was able to transfer with moderate assistance using the sliding board. She used her HKAFOs infrequently and had become fearful of standing in them. She was able to propel her manual wheelchair only over level indoor surfaces and preferred the power wheelchair for mobility. Adjustments for growth were ordered for her manual wheelchair. It was recommended that therapy continue to focus on transfer training and wheelchair skills. Ambulation training was discussed, and the relative benefits of this for lower extremity ROM and upper extremity exercise were contrasted with the need to develop functional independence in transfers and wheelchair use. It was suggested that Stacy continue to use the orthoses if she was interested and motivated but that the main focus in therapy should be the goals mentioned previously.

Reflections on practice

Therapists will frequently encounter families who remain hopeful that their child will ambulate. In fact, even limited ambulation may be more practical than using a power wheelchair inside a small home. In setting outcomes, the therapist must also keep an eye to the future, to consider the functional environments a child will face in the home, school, community, and ultimately the workplace. The basic skills of transfers, wheelchair mobility, and being able to direct one's own care must be incorporated at appropriate developmental stages. In addition, whereas an adult with C7 tetraplegia would be expected to be independent with transfers and a manual wheelchair, a young child is unlikely to have the upper body strength to perform these tasks and will have greater independence at a young age in a power wheelchair. In the first year after SCI, Stacy would have benefited from the now available soft trunk orthosis (see Fig. 21–3) to facilitate sitting and to free her hands for play.

CASE HISTORY
ALEX

This case study illustrates the acquisition of skills with growth and development in a young school-age child with a spinal cord injury. Medical complications, both in the acute phase and over time, are also discussed because of their impact on function.

Alex was injured in a high-speed motor vehicle crash at age 5. He had an L3–L4 ligamentous tear with right facet dislocation and a right T10 pedicle fracture with cord damage. He was diagnosed with T10 paraplegia, ASIA Impairment Scale level A. He underwent L3–L4 open reduction and external fixation and a right posterior iliac bone graft. He had intestinal injuries and underwent small bowel resection and had a colostomy. A gastrostomy tube was placed several days later to help decompress his stomach. He was fitted with a thoracolumbar sacral orthosis with a cutout for his gastrostomy tube and colostomy. Two weeks after injury, Alex was transferred to a pediatric inpatient rehabilitation unit.

It took several sessions to complete tests and measures for the physical therapy examination. The therapist initially scheduled short sessions and spent much of the time playing, developing rapport, and employing strategies that helped decrease Alex's anxiety and improve participation. Upper extremity strength was within normal limits, although endurance for activities was decreased. Straight leg raise was 50°. All other ROM was within normal limits. Sensation and movement were absent below the T10 level. There was no lower extremity spasticity. Alex required maximal assistance for all of his mobility, including rolling, getting in and out of sitting, sitting balance, and transfers. He could not self-propel a wheelchair. He frequently complained of stomach pain, and pancreatitis was diagnosed.

Over the next month, Alex adjusted well to the hospital environment. His cooperation and participation improved. Therapy was done in the context of play. Skills were taught starting with small components, and therapy was structured to ensure maximal success. Intervention focused on sitting balance, bed mobility, and transfers. Sliding board, push-up blocks, and leg loops were used to facilitate transfers and bed mobility.

Range of motion was provided with a focus on hamstring stretching. Alex began learning basic wheelchair skills. Purchase of his own lightweight wheelchair with a pressure-relieving cushion was initiated. Plastic ankle-foot orthoses were fabricated for night wear. After 3.5 months, Alex met the discharge outcomes, which were set based on his age and level of injury, and was discharged home (Box 21–1).

Integration into school was carefully coordinated with his school district. He began half-day kindergarten and received occupational therapy two times per week at school. Physical therapy was initially provided on a consultative basis through the SCI clinic.

Alex was seen 1 year after injury in the clinic. Lower extremity spasticity had developed, and hip flexor tightness was noted. He was referred for outpatient physical therapy for upper extremity strengthening, lower extremity ROM, and more advanced wheelchair skills (Box 21–2).

In the first years after injury, Alex was introduced to adaptive sports, and he became an enthusiastic and talented skier, swimmer, and track competitor. Mild hip flexion contractures developed during these years, and scoliosis was diagnosed at age 7.

Three years after injury, Alex expressed interest in a walking trial. This was done over the summer and was an episode of more intense physical therapy at the regional children's hospital. KAFOs were fabricated initially and a pelvic piece was added later. Because of his hip flexion contractures and lower extremity spasticity, he had a difficult time donning the orthotics. He was unable to lock his hips into extension when standing. Thus, while able to walk in the parallel bars, he was unable to independently walk outside of them with a walker. He decided to continue to work on walking with his outpatient physical therapist during the school year. Nine months later, Alex stopped his ambulation attempts because of lack of progress. He asked about the use of FES for ambulation and after learning that the current state of technology did not result in functional ambulation, decided to not pursue this. He was discharged from outpatient physical therapy at age 10.

By age 12, wheelchair skills improved to include negotiating steeper inclines and higher curbs. Alex was fully independent in wheelchair mobility with the exception of loading his wheelchair into a vehicle. He competed in sports at the national level. At 12.5 years of age, he developed painful right forearm tendinitis. He used a rental power wheelchair for several months because propelling his manual wheelchair aggravated the tendinitis. Anti-inflammatories were prescribed along with outpatient physical therapy for strengthening. Later that same year at the SCI clinic, he described posterior axillary pain. Examination revealed muscular imbalance with weak external rotators as a likely cause. He was instructed in a home program of strengthening. Hip flexor tightness was worsening despite a program of active stretching and passive stretching using the prone position.

By age 14 his scoliosis had increased to 55°. A posterior spinal fusion was done. Postoperatively, Alex was restricted in his sports activities. At the SCI clinic that year, his hip flexion contractures were found to be tighter at −30° on the right and −20° on the left.

Alex was seen again in the SCI clinic at age 15. He was still not very active because of restrictions from his spinal surgery. Hip flexion contractures had increased to −45° on the right and −30° on the left. His right hip was subluxing. The physiatrist discussed hip management options. Alex also complained of upper back pain. Posterior shoulder and scapular strengthening and anterior shoulder stretching to avoid impingement syndrome were reviewed with him by the physical therapist.

Alex was then seen in clinic at age 16 to discuss management of his subluxed hip. Although he was now cleared for sports activities, his lumbar mobility had decreased significantly as a result of the spinal fusion and could no longer compensate for the limitation in hip extension. Although this did not affect his

---

BOX 21–1. Skills Acquired during Inpatient Rehabilitation at Age 5 in a Patient with T10 Paraplegia

- Independent bed mobility
- Independent short and long sitting balance
- Independent transfers from wheelchair to bed and back using a sliding board
- Independent push-up pressure releases with reminders
- Self-propel wheelchair over level terrain

BOX 21–2. Skills Acquired from Ages 6 to 9 in a Patient with T10 Paraplegia

- Independently perform self range of motion
- Perform all transfers without a sliding board independently, including from floor to wheelchair
- Independently assume, maintain, and move in a wheelie position
- Ascend and descend low curbs independently
- Self-propel over mild uneven terrain in a wheelie position
- Ascend and descend mild hills

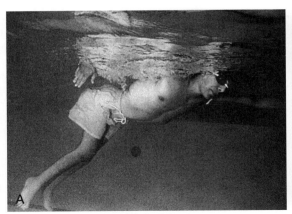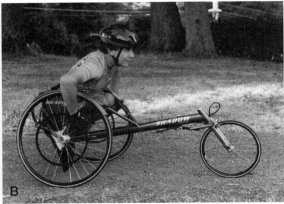

FIGURE 21–5. Decreased lumbar mobility resulting from back surgery for scoliosis significantly worsens positioning and performance in the water, but has no effect on positioning for track events. *A,* Position in water. *B,* No effect for track.

skiing or track skills, his position in the water changed because his hips were now in a much greater degree of flexion (Fig. 21–5). This caused him to swim more slowly and he sustained a significant loss in his competitive standing.

Reflections on practice

The need for episodic physical therapy can occur years after initial rehabilitation. The physical therapist must be knowledgeable about typical musculoskeletal problems such as overuse and shoulder impingement syndromes that can occur as a result of a spinal cord injury, paralysis, and resulting wheelchair usage. Wheelchair athletes propel their chairs with shoulders flexed and internally rotated, placing them at increased risk for impingement. They need to actively exercise humeral depressors, especially external rotators. Compared with adults, children who sustain SCI are at risk for unique orthopedic complications that may interfere with achieving maximal function.

CASE HISTORY
ADAM

This case demonstrates the long-term physical therapy management of a teenager with incomplete paraplegia caused by cauda equina injury. This teenager continued to experience long-term functional improvements owing to a combination of neurologic recovery and active strengthening programs. Four years of treatment and follow-up were needed before he reached a plateau of function.

Adam was injured at age 14 when he fell from a tree. He sustained a burst fracture of the L3 vertebra and a complete anterior dislocation of L3 on the L4 vertebra. On the day after his injury, he underwent surgery to reduce the dislocation, and instrumentation was placed across the two vertebrae for stabilization. Postoperatively, Adam was given a thoracolumbosacral orthosis (TLSO) to wear 24 hours a day for the next 3 to 4 months until fusion was complete. Owing to the instability of the initial injury and the short segment of fusion and instrumentation, a thigh piece was added to the TLSO to prevent hip flexion beyond 80° (see Fig. 21–1).

Eight days after his injury, Adam was admitted to a pediatric rehabilitation program. His cauda equina spinal cord injury was classified as L2 paraplegia, ASIA Impairment Scale level B. His impairments included deficits in motor and sensory functioning, loss of voluntary bladder and bowel control, and orthostatic hypotension. Motor examination, functional skills, and physical therapy intervention are outlined in Table 21–6. Range of motion was normal throughout, except straight leg raising was possible to only 30° bilaterally because of posterior thigh pain. His sensory examination to pinprick showed that he had lost normal sensation below the medial femoral condyles and had decreased sensation in the L4 and L5 dermatomes, absent sensation at S1, but preservation of pinprick at S4–S5, perianally. There were no problems with spasticity because cauda equina injuries result in lower motoneuron deficits with flaccid paralysis.

His sitting tolerance was limited by orthostatic hypotension, and he could only sit up with the wheelchair back reclined 45°. From such a position, he could not propel his wheelchair. Support stockings

TABLE 21–6. Physical Therapy Intervention during Inpatient Rehabilitation for Teen with Cauda Equina Spinal Cord Injury

Date	Lower Extremity Strength			Functional Status	Physical Therapy Intervention
Admission to rehabilitation unit	Grade 3 hip flexion and knee extension. Grade 0 for all other lower extremity muscles.			Assist needed for bed mobility and transfers. Unable to self-propel wheelchair, stand, or walk.	Direct intervention for bed mobility, transfers, wheelchair skills, and upper/lower extremity strengthening.
One month after SCI	Grade 3+ hip flexion and knee extension. Grade 0 for all other lower extremity muscles.			Independent bed mobility. Transfers with a sliding board. Independent wheelchair mobility. Beginning to stand in parallel bars.	Direct intervention with focus on upper and lower extremity strengthening and gait training. Referred for solid-ankle AFOs.
Four months after SCI: discharge from inpatient rehabilitation program		**Right**	**Left**	Ambulates independently with wheeled walker and AFOs up to 150 ft. Uses wheelchair for long distances.	Direct outpatient intervention for lower extremity strengthening and gait training. School-based consultation for adaptive physical education and mobility in school.
	Hip flexion	4−	4−		
	Hip abduction	0	2		
	Hip extension	1	1		
	Knee extension	4+	4+		
	Knee flexion	2	2		
	Ankle dorsiflexion	0	1		
	Long toe extensors	0	1		
	Ankle plantar flexion	0	1		

and Ace wraps around his legs were used in conjunction with progressively increasing his upright sitting. His FIM scores were complete independence (7) in communication and social cognition. In self-care, he was completely independent (7) for eating and grooming but needed moderate assistance (3) for bathing, set-up assistance (5) for upper body dressing, maximal assistance (2) for lower body dressing, and total assistance (1) for toileting and bladder and bowel management. For mobility and locomotion, he needed maximal assistance (2) for all transfers and total assistance (1) for locomotion, using a wheelchair. He was unable to ascend stairs.

His disabilities on admission included lack of independence in bed mobility, transfers, and indoor and community mobility. With his level of injury, realistic long-term outcomes were independence in bed mobility and transfers and ambulation at home and in the community using ankle-foot orthoses (AFOs) and crutches. Short-term goals included tolerance to the upright position, improved hamstring range of motion to allow long-sitting, improved upper extremity strength and endurance to allow independent transfers and wheelchair propulsion, and lower extremity strengthening of the weakened muscle groups.

After 2 weeks, he had only rare episodes of symptomatic orthostatic hypotension. A lighter-weight wheelchair was substituted for the recliner wheelchair.

One month after admission to rehabilitation, there was minimal change in lower extremity strength, but significant improvement with his functional skills (see Table 21–6). Hamstring ROM continued to be limited owing to complaints of pain with stretching. Upper body strength improved, so that Adam could lift his trunk to do independent pressure relief and could transfer himself without a sliding board to level heights.

Two months after injury, Adam had increased knee extensor strength to grade 4. Solid-ankle AFOs were fabricated, and he began to stand in the parallel bars. Within another month he had adequate standing balance to begin gait training with a walker. He had also begun to get return of hamstring function. Several weeks later he was independently ambulating with a walker and had met all of his inpatient discharge outcomes and so was discharged to home. Functional skills and lower extremity strength at discharge are shown in Table 21–6. He was reclassified as having L2 paraplegia, ASIA Impairment Scale level C. Straight leg raising was 85° bilaterally, and all other passive ROM was normal. Adam's FIM scores had improved to complete independence (7) in all areas of self-care except bathing; to modified independence (6) for bathing and bladder and bowel management; to complete independence (7) in transfers to bed, chair, wheelchair, and toilet; and to modified independence (6) for transfers to the bathtub chair and for locomotion using a wheelchair or ambulating with the walker and

AFOs. He needed moderate assistance (4) to ascend stairs.

At reexamination 1 year after SCI, Adam demonstrated improved strength, particularly in knee flexors, hip extensors, and hip abductors. These resulted in improved function, but his classification remained L2 paraplegia, ASIA Impairment Scale C, because he had weakness in the L4, L5, and S1 key muscles used by the ASIA scale. Adam had discontinued his participation in the outpatient physical therapy program the month before but was continuing to work on stretching and strengthening at home. He demonstrated significant improvements in strength and ambulation skills (Table 21-7). His left AFO was changed to one with a hinged ankle to allow free dorsiflexion but no plantar flexion past neutral to allow motion and the possibility of strengthening these muscle groups while walking. Continued home ROM and strengthening exercises were recommended.

Reexamination 2 years after his SCI demonstrated a grade increase in left hip extension and abduction and a half-grade increase in right hip extension. This additional strength allowed Adam to ambulate without crutches (see Table 21-7). His level of SCI was now L3 paraplegia, ASIA Impairment Scale C. He needed new AFOs because of wear and tear. He had developed skin breakdown on the lateral border of his left foot and on his right shin from rubbing against the AFO and the Velcro closure. He no longer used his forearm crutches. Range of motion was well maintained. He was provided with new AFOs and counseled regarding care of insensate skin. Because he was working out in a gym several times a week, specific exercises were recommended for strengthening hip girdle and knee flexor muscles.

At his last examination four years after SCI, Adam had shown some improvement in right lower extremity strength of the targeted muscle groups (see Table 21-7). He also demonstrated new plantar flexion at the right ankle. Bilateral hinged AFOs were prescribed. Adam was a senior in high school and worked after school in a gas station. He had returned

TABLE 21-7. **Physical Therapy Intervention and Consultation during Outpatient Rehabilitation for Teen with Cauda Equina Spinal Cord Injury**

Date	Lower Extremity Strength			Functional Status	Physical Therapy Intervention
One year after SCI		**Right**	**Left**	Ambulates with forearm crutches and AFOs using bilateral reciprocal gait pattern. Starting to walk without crutches. Wheelchair discontinued.	Outpatient physical therapy discontinued; instructed in home exercise program. Consultation through rehab clinic. Home exercise program updated at clinic visit. Hinged AFO on left recommended due to increased plantar-flexion strength.
	Hip flexion	4–	4		
	Hip abduction	3–	3		
	Hip extension	2	3		
	Knee extension	5	5		
	Knee flexion	3	4		
	Ankle dorsiflexion	0	2		
	Long toe extensors	0	3		
	Ankle plantar flexion	0	2		
Two years after SCI		**Right**	**Left**	Ambulates without forearm crutches and with AFOs. Works out at a gym several times per week.	Consultation through rehab clinic; instructed in specific exercises for right leg muscles.
	Hip flexion	4	4		
	Hip abduction	3–	4		
	Hip extension	3–	4		
	Knee extension	5	5		
	Knee flexion	3	4		
	Ankle dorsiflexion	0	2		
	Long toe extensors	0	3		
	Ankle plantar flexion	0	3		
Four years after SCI		**Right**	**Left**	Has returned to all preinjury recreational and leisure activities, including hiking, fishing, and hunting.	Consultation through rehab clinic. Recommended hinged AFO on right due to increase in plantar-flexion strength.
	Hip flexion	5	5		
	Hip abduction	4	4		
	Hip extension	3+	4		
	Knee extension	5	5		
	Knee flexion	4	4		
	Ankle dorsiflexion	0	2		
	Long toe extensors	0	3		
	Ankle plantar flexion	2	3		

to an outdoor lifestyle, hiking, fishing, and hunting on a regular basis. He planned to enroll in a community college to study forestry. He was advised of state vocational rehabilitation services available to him and was referred to an adult SCI rehabilitation program for long-term monitoring of renal function and prescription of orthoses.

Reflections on practice

At various points in his course of recovery, Adam demonstrated functional improvement, sometimes as a result of neurologic improvement and other times as a result of targeted functional skills training, strengthening, and gait training. Comprehensive reexaminations, including precise manual muscle testing, were critical in order to set new goals and implement appropriate interventions to meet these goals.

SUMMARY

Physical therapy for the child with SCI can, at first glance, appear straightforward. Preserving ROM and promoting strength and endurance are the cornerstones for the functional achievement predicted by the level of injury. Yet predicting realistic long-term outcomes and attaining them require respect for the broader and more complex picture. The physical therapist must consider the cause of the injury (progressive vs. stable), the completeness of the injury (preserved motor function, sensory function), and the potential for, or presence of, secondary complications (scoliosis, skin breakdown, contractures). The therapist must also be sensitive to the child's age, the child's adaptation to the disability, and the child's ability to meet age-appropriate expectations in the home, school, and community. Unlike adults with SCI, who may be very close to expected levels of independence at discharge from inpatient rehabilitation, children often require years of outpatient therapy to achieve optimal outcomes. Thus it becomes imperative to provide the child and the family with a team approach, incorporating multiple disciplines and settings to maximize the child's potential for functional independence.

Recommended Resources

Betz, RR, & Mulcahey, MJ (Eds.). *The Child with a Spinal Cord Injury.* Rosemont, IL: American Academy of Orthopedic Surgeons, 1996.

National Spinal Cord Injury Association (NSCIA)
600 West Cummings Park, Suite 2000
Woburn, MA 01801
http://www.spinalcord.org/

The Rehabilitation Learning Center
Harborview Medical Center
Seattle, WA
http://depts.washington.edu/rehab

Spinal Cord Injury Self-Care Manual. San Francisco: Shriners Hospital for Crippled Children, 1989.
Yes, You Can! Paralyzed Veterans of America, 1989
c/o Office Service, A01
18th Street NW
Washington, DC 20006

References

American Spinal Injury Association. International Standards for Neurological and Functional Classification of Spinal Cord Injury. Chicago: American Spinal Injury Association, 1996.

Backe, HA, Betz, RR, Mesgarzadeh, M, Beck, T, & Clancy, M. Posttraumatic spinal cord cysts evaluated by magnetic resonance imaging. Paraplegia, 29:607–612, 1991.

Bohn, D, Armstrong, D, Becker, L, & Humphreys, R. Cervical spine injuries in children. Journal of Trauma, 30:463–469, 1990.

Bracken, MB, Shepard, MJ, Holford, TR, Leo-Summers, L, Aldrich, EF, Fazl, M, Fehlings, M, Herr, DL, Hitchon, PW, Marshall, LF, Nockeb, RP, Pascale, V, Perot, PL, Piepmeier, J, Sonntag, VK, Wagner, F, Wilberger, JE, Winn, HR, & Young, W. Administration of methylprednisolone for 24 or 48 hours or tirilazad mesylate for 48 hours in the treatment of acute spinal cord injury. Results of the Third National Acute Spinal Cord Injury Randomized Controlled Trial; National Acute Spinal Cord Injury Study. Journal of the American Medical Association, 277:1597–1604, 1997.

Burnham, RS, May, L, Nelson, E, Steadward, R, & Reid, DC. Shoulder pain in wheelchair athletes; the role of muscle imbalance. American Journal of Sports Medicine, 21:238–242, 1993.

Committee on Sports Medicine, American Academy of Pediatrics. Atlantoaxial instability in Down syndrome. Pediatrics, 74:152–153, 1984.

Crozier, KS, Graziani, V, Ditunno, JF, & Herbison, GJ. Spinal cord injury: Prognosis for ambulation based on sensory examination of inpatients who are initially motor complete. Archives of Physical Medicine and Rehabilitation, 72:119–121, 1991.

DeVivo, MJ, Richards, JS, Stover, SL, & Go, BK. Spinal cord injury: Rehabilitation adds life to years. Western Journal of Medicine, 154:602–606, 1991.

DeVivo, MJ, & Stover, SL. Long term survival and causes of death. In Stover, SL, DeLisa, JA, & Whiteneck, GG (Eds.), Spinal Cord Injury: Clinical Outcomes from the Model Systems. Gaithersburg, MD: Aspen, 1995, pp. 289–316.

Ditunno, JF, Sipski, ML, Posuniak, EA, Chen, YT, Staas, WE, & Herbson, GJ. Wrist extensor recovery in traumatic quadriplegia. Archives of Physical Medicine and Rehabilitation, 68:287–290, 1987.

Drory, Y, Ohry, A, Brooks, ME, Dolphia, D, & Kellerman, JJ. Arm crank ergometry in chronic spinal cord injured patients. Archives of Physical Medicine and Rehabilitation, 71:389–392, 1990.

El Ghahit, AZ, & Hanson, RW. Educational and training levels and employment of the spinal cord injured patient. Archives of Physical Medicine and Rehabilitation, 60:405–406, 1979.

Fordyce, WE. Behavioral methods in medical rehabilitation. Neuroscience and Biobehavioral Reviews, 5:391–396, 1981.

Garber, SL, & Dyerly, LR. Wheelchair cushions for persons with spinal cord injury: An update. American Journal of Occupational Therapy, 45:550–554, 1991.

Geisler, FH. Clinical trials of pharmacotherapy for spinal cord injury. Annals of the New York Academy of Sciences, 845:374–381, 1998.

Giovanini, MA, Reier, PJ, Eskin, TA, Wirth, E, & Anderson, DK. Characteristics of human fetal spinal cord grafts in the adult rat spinal cord: Influences of lesion and grafting conditions. Experimental Neurology, 148:523–543, 1997.

Go, BK, DeVivo, MJ, & Richards, JS. The epidemiology of spinal cord injury. In Stover, SL, DeLisa, JA, & Whiteneck, GG (Eds.), Spinal Cord Injury: Clinical Outcomes from the Model Systems. Gaithersburg, MD: Aspen, 1995, pp. 21–25.

Granger, CV, Hamilton, BB, & Kayton, R. Guide for the Use of the Functional Independence Measure for Children (WeeFIM) of the Uniform Data Set for Medical Rehabilitation. Buffalo, NY: State University of New York, Research Foundation, 1988.

Haley, SM, Faas, RM, Coster, WJ, Webster, H, & Gans, BM. Pediatric Evaluation of Disability Inventory. Boston: New England Medical Center, 1992.

Hamilton, BB, Granger, CV, Sherwin, FS, Zielezny, M, & Tashman, JS. A uniform national data system for medical rehabilitation. In Fuhrer, MJ (Ed.), Rehabilitation Outcomes: Analysis and Measurement. Baltimore: Paul H. Brookes, 1987, pp. 137–147.

Haseltine, FP, Cole, SS, & Gray, DB (Eds.). Reproductive Issues for Persons with Physical Disabilities. Baltimore: Paul H. Brookes, 1990.

Hirokawa, S, Grimm, M, Le, T, Solomonow, M, Baratta, RV, Shoji, H, & D'Ambrosia, RD. Energy consumption in paraplegic ambulation using the reciprocating gait orthosis and electric stimulation of the thigh muscles. Archives of Physical Medicine and Rehabilitation, 71:687–694, 1990.

Hobson, DA, & Tooms, RE. Seated lumbar/pelvic alignment. A comparison between spinal cord injured and noninjured groups. Spine, 17:293–298, 1992.

Jaeger, RJ, Yarkony, GM, & Roth, EJ. Rehabilitation technology for standing and walking after spinal cord injury. American Journal of Physical Medicine and Rehabilitation, 68:128–133, 1989.

Janssen, L, & Hansebout, RR. Pathogenesis of spinal cord injury and newer treatments: A review. Spine, 14:23–32, 1989.

Johnston, MV, & Keith, RA. Cost benefits of medical rehabilitation: Review and critique. Archives of Physical Medicine and Rehabilitation, 64:147–154, 1983.

Kewalramani, LS, Krauss, JF, & Sterling, HM. Acute spinal-cord lesions in a pediatric population: Epidemiological and clinical features. Paraplegia, 18:206–219, 1980.

Levine, SP, Kett, RL, Gross, MD, Wilson, BA, Cederna, PS, & Juni, JE. Blood flow in the gluteus maximus of seated individuals during electrical muscle stimulation. Archives of Physical Medicine and Rehabilitation, 71:682–686, 1990.

Massagli, TL, Dudgeon, BJ, & Ross, BW. Educational performance and vocational participation after spinal cord injury in childhood. Archives of Physical Medicine and Rehabilitation, 77:995–999, 1996.

Massagli, TL, & Jaffe, KM. Pediatric spinal cord injury: Treatment and outcome. Pediatrician, 17:244–254, 1990.

McDonald, CM, Jaffe, KM, & Shurtleff, DB. Assessment of muscle strength in children with meningomyelocele: Accuracy and stability of measurements over time. Archives of Physical Medicine and Rehabilitation, 67:855–861, 1986.

Mohr, T, Andersen, JL, Biering-Sorensen, F, Galbo, H, Bangsbo, J, Wagner, A, & Kjaer, M. Long-term adaptation to electrically induced cycle training in severe spinal cord injured individuals. Spinal Cord, 35:1–16, 1997.

Molnar, GE, & Kaminer, RE. History and examination. In Molnar, GE (Ed.), Pediatric Rehabilitation, 2nd ed. Baltimore: Williams & Wilkins, 1992, pp. 1–18.

Mulcahey, MS, Betz, RR, Smith, BT, Weiss, AA, & Davis, SE. Implanted functional electrical stimulation hand system in adolescents with spinal injuries: An evaluation. Archives of Physical Medicine and Rehabilitation, 78:597–607, 1997.

Mulcahey, MS, Smith, BT, Betz, RR, Triolo, RJ, & Peckham, PH. Functional neuromuscular stimulation: Outcomes in young people with tetraplegia. Journal of the American Paraplegia Society, 17:20–35, 1993.

Murphy, KP, Opitz, JL, Cabanela, ME, & Ebersold, MJ. Cervical fractures and spinal cord injury: Outcome of surgical and nonsurgical management. Mayo Clinic Proceedings, 65:949–959, 1990.

Needham-Shropshire, BM, Broton, JG, Cameron, TL, & Klose, KJ. Improved motor function in tetraplegics following neuromuscular stimulation-assisted arm ergometry. Journal of Spinal Cord Medicine, 20:49–55, 1997a.

Needham-Shropshire, BM, Broton, JG, Klose, KJ, Lebwohl, N, Guest, RS, & Jacobs, PL. Evaluation of a training program for persons with SCI paraplegia using the Parastep 1 ambulation system: Part 3. Lack of effect on bone mineral density. Archives of Physical Medicine and Rehabilitation, 78:799–803, 1997b.

Nichols, DS, & Case-Smith, J. Reliability and validity of the Pediatric Evaluation of Disability Inventory. Pediatric Physical Therapy, 8:15–24, 1996.

Ottenbacher, KJ, Taylor, ET, Msall, ME, Braun, S, Lane, SJ, Granger, CV, Lyons, N, & Duffy, LC. The stability and equivalence reliability of the Functional Independence Measure for children (WeeFIM). Developmental Medicine and Child Neurology, 38:907–916, 1996.

Pang, D, & Wilberger, JE. Spinal cord injury without radiographic abnormalities in children. Journal of Neurosurgery, 57:114–129, 1982.

Phillips, CA. Medical criteria for active physical therapy: Physician guidelines for patient participation in a program of functional electrical stimulation. American Journal of Physical Medicine, 66:269–286, 1987.

Rhoney, DH, Luer, MS, Hughes, M, & Hatton, J. New pharmocologic approaches to acute spinal cord injury. Pharmacotherapy, 16:382–392, 1996.

Richards, JS, Hendricks, C, & Roberts, M. Prevention of spinal cord injury: An elementary education approach. Journal of Pediatric Psychology, 16:595–609, 1991.

Saboe, LA, Darrah, JM, Pain, KS, & Guthrie, J. Early predictors of functional independence 2 years after spinal cord injury. Archives of Physical Medicine and Rehabilitation, 78:644–650, 1997.

Schwab, ME. Molecules inhibiting neurite growth: A minireview. Neurochemical Research, 21:755–761, 1996.

Seeger, BR, Law, D, Creswell, JE, Stern, LM, & Potter, MB. Functional electrical stimulation for upper limb strengthening in traumatic quadriplegia. Archives of Physical Medicine and Rehabilitation, 70:663–667, 1989.

Sipski, ML, Alexander, CJ, & Harris, M. Long term use of computerized bicycle ergometry for spinal cord injured subjects. Archives of Physical Medicine and Rehabilitation, 74:238–241, 1993.

Stotts, KM. Health maintenance: Paraplegia athletes and nonathletes. Archives of Physical Medicine and Rehabilitation, 67:109–114, 1986.

Sugarman, B. Medical complications of spinal cord injury. Quarterly Journal of Medicine, 54:3–18, 1985.

Waring, WP, & Karunas, RS. Acute spinal cord injuries and the incidence of clinically occurring thromboembolic disease. Paraplegia, 29:8–16, 1991.

Waters, RL, Adkins, R, Yakura, J, & Vigil, D. Prediction of ambulatory performance based on motor scores derived from standards of the American Spinal Injury Association. Archives of Physical Medicine and Rehabilitation, 75:756–760, 1994.

Wilberger, JE. Spinal Cord Injuries in Children. New York: Futura, 1986.

Wu, L, Marino, R, Herbison, GJ, & Ditunno, JF. Recovery of zero-grade muscles in the zone of partial preservation in motor complete quadriplegia. Archives of Physical Medicine and Rehabilitation, 73:40–43, 1992.

Yarkony, GM, Roth, EJ, Cybulski, G, & Jaeger, RJ. Neuromuscular stimulation in spinal cord injury. I: Restoration of functional movement of the extremities. Archives of Physical Medicine and Rehabilitation, 73:78–86, 1992.

C H A P T E R
22

Brain Injuries: Traumatic Brain Injuries, Near-Drowning, and Brain Tumors

GINETTE A. KERKERING, PT
WENDY E. PHILLIPS, PT, PCS, MA, MS

Pediatric physical therapists see a large number of children with central nervous system (CNS) dysfunction. Many of these children have neurologic involvement from birth, but many acquire neurologic insults later in childhood. This chapter will focus on brain injuries acquired by children after birth. Three primary acquired brain injuries are traumatic brain injuries, near-drowning injuries, and brain tumors. Although these three etiologies of brain injury are different and will be discussed as such, physical therapy management of children with brain injury will be discussed as a whole. New guidelines of treatment using *The Guide to Physical Therapist Practice* will also be discussed.

It is important to remember that although all three forms of brain injury can occur in the adult population, children will be different in terms of medical management and rehabilitation management. These differences are based primarily on the physiologic differences in children and the developmental milestones achieved before injury.

TRAUMATIC BRAIN INJURY

Incidence

Traumatic brain injury is the leading cause of death and injury-related disability among children and young adults. More than 1 million children sustain traumatic brain injuries every year. Brain injuries are classified as severe, moderate, or mild using the Glasgow Coma Scale (GCS). Of the 1 million injuries, 5% of the children were pronounced dead on arrival, 6% were classified as severe brain injury (GCS of 8 or less), and 8% were classified as moderate brain injury (GCS of 9–12). The remaining 82% were classified as mild brain injuries (GCS of 13–15) (Kraus et al., 1990). According to the National Pediatric Trauma Registry, more than 30,000 children sustain permanent disability as a result of brain injury each year, with boys twice as likely as girls to suffer a traumatic brain injury. Children are especially at risk in the afternoon hours after they have been dismissed from school.

Etiology

There are numerous mechanisms of traumatic brain injury in the pediatric population. These causes may be differentiated by age. In the infant population, more than two thirds of the injuries sustained are from falls. In the preschool population, the primary injuries sustained are from falls (51%) and motor vehicle accidents (22%). School-age children, from 5 to 9 years, are equally divided among motor vehicle accidents (31%), falls (31%), and sports and recreation-related activities (32%). A greater percentage of sports and recreation injuries (43%) is found among 10- to 14-year-olds (Kraus et al., 1990).

Brain injury that results from closed head injury may be related to both primary and secondary factors. Primary injuries are related to the forces that occur at the time of initial impact. Secondary injuries are related to systemic response to the primary trauma.

Primary Injuries

Primary injuries, or those injuries related to the forces that occur at the time of initial impact, may be grouped with respect to the role played by acceleration factors. *Acceleration-dependent injuries* are related to the effects that occur when a force is applied to a movable head. They may be translational or rotational. In the case of translational injuries, a vector related to the force applied to the head passes approximately through the head's center of mass. In rotational injuries, the resultant force vector does not pass through the center of mass of the head, and angular acceleration results. For most force vectors, the result is not purely translational or rotational but a combination of the two.

In the case of a *translational injury,* the response to a force applied to the side of the skull is lateral movement of both the skull and the brain. As the skull contacts an immovable object such as the door frame of an automobile, it rapidly decelerates. The brain, however, continues to move laterally until it is stopped by the lateral aspect of the skull. The injury that results from the initial impact of the brain on the skull is translational and is termed a *coup* lesion. The lesion that occurs as the brain reacts secondarily to the initial force against the skull (moving in the opposite direction against the skull on the opposite side) is termed *contrecoup.* Countrecoup injuries may also cause significant brain injury.

Rotational injury occurs when the brain remains stationary while the skull rotates. The resultant forces are angular. Rotational injuries have been related to shearing trauma, which may be manifested as brain surface contusions and lacerations (Pang, 1985). Diffuse axonal injuries have also been related to shearing trauma.

Primary injuries can also result from factors not related to acceleration. Brain injury that results from skull depression into brain tissue is one example. Vibration coinciding with the application of an initial force to the skull has also been hypothesized as a cause of nonacceleration-related injury (Marcal & Nickell, 1973).

Secondary Injuries

Secondary injuries, or those that occur due to processes evoked in response to the initial trauma, account for a significant amount of the overall damage that occurs in traumatic brain injury. One of the most common causes of secondary injuries is *cerebral edema.* Unchecked cerebral edema and the resultant increase in intracranial pressure can lead to brain herniation, multiple cerebral infarctions, permanent brainstem necrosis, and irreversible coma (Pang, 1985). After a traumatic brain injury, cerebral edema is frequently a result of increased capillary permeability. Fluid leaks slowly out of the capillaries into the brain parenchyma, leading to clinically significant effects 4 to 6 hours after injury with peak effects at 24 to 36 hours after injury (Pang, 1985).

Epidural hematomas result when the middle meningeal artery, vein, or venous sinus bleeds into the epidural space between the dura and the skull. This usually follows a skull fracture or bending of the skull into the brain. As the skull recoils, the space between the skull and dura may fill with blood, creating the hematoma. The rate of blood collection, and the resultant increase in intracranial pressure, determines the prognosis. The prognosis for rapidly accumulating hematomas is grave. The location of the hematoma also affects outcome, with temporal or posterior fossa hematomas more likely to cause brain shift and brainstem compression than a hematoma in the frontoparietal area (Pang, 1985).

Acute subdural hematomas are related to extensive cortical injury and lacerated cortical vessels. Edema in the underlying brain tissue develops rapidly. Acute cerebral hematomas must be removed expediently. Their ultimate effect on recovery depends on both the time between development and evacuation of the hemorrhage and on the extent of damage to underlying brain tissue.

Increased intracranial pressure frequently occurs after brain injury as a result of edema and hematoma. Further damage to cerebral tissue from brainstem herniation may result. Initial increases in intracranial pressure are accommodated by expulsion of cerebrospinal fluid into the subarachnoid space and ventricles and by expulsion of cerebral venous blood into the jugular veins or scalp (Lofgren & Awetnow, 1973). At the point when compensatory mechanisms are no longer effective, a rise in intracranial pressure occurs. When the magnitude of increase in intracranial blood and fluid volume is compared with the resultant increase in intracranial pressure, the relation between the two increases exponentially (Pang, 1985). For these reasons, intracranial pressure is closely monitored in patients with brain injury.

Because of the traumatic nature of these brain injuries, there will frequently be other injuries to assess as well. These other injuries can be fractures, skin abrasions, and internal injuries. At times a child will suffer both a spinal cord injury and a brain injury during a traumatic event.

Medical and Surgical Management

Interventions for the child with traumatic brain injury may include surgery, the use of pharmacologic agents, and the use of mechanical ventilation. All of these interventions are aimed at sustaining life and preventing secondary injuries to the brain. Because a leading cause of secondary injury is the result of increased intracranial pressure, management is aimed primarily at controlling this pressure. Pressure is monitored by an intracranial pressure bolt. Surgical interventions include the evacuation of sub-

dural or intracerebral hematomas. These procedures are used to decrease intracranial pressure and reduce pressure-related secondary brain injuries.

Pharmacologic agents are also frequently used to decrease cerebral edema and pressure-related secondary injuries. Sedatives, paralytics, diuretics, and barbiturates can all be used to treat cerebral edema in children with appropriate physiologic monitoring (Ewing-Cobbs et al., 1995). Pharmacologic agents may also be used to induce paralysis in cases in which movement would interfere with the administration of other medical interventions.

Hyperventilation, or mechanically assisted ventilation at a rate greater than usual, may temporarily reduce intracranial pressure. Once hyperventilation is discontinued, intracranial pressure may increase again. Hyperventilation is, therefore, a temporary measure used until other interventions such as surgery are available.

Several medical complications are commonly found in children who have had a traumatic brain injury. Fever and infection are common responses to trauma. McLean and colleagues (1995) have suggested that children who sustain a traumatic brain injury may have a suppressed immune system as a result of the trauma. Neurologic complications consist of subdural fluid collections, posttraumatic hydrocephalus, posttraumatic seizures, visual dysfunction, auditory and vestibular dysfunction, motor deficits, peripheral nerve injuries, and a low incidence of associated spinal cord injury. Endocrine dysfunctions that can occur after traumatic brain injury in children include diabetes insipidus, syndrome of inappropriate antidiuretic hormone (SIADH), and precocious puberty. Skin and gastrointestinal disorders have also been noted in children who have suffered a traumatic brain injury. Orthopedic complications are generally fractures, including skull fractures, and heterotopic ossification (McLean et al., 1995).

Pediatric patients who sustain a traumatic brain injury are at risk of developing heterotopic ossification (HO), which is pathologic bone formation around a joint in the pericapsular space (Citta-Pietrolungo et al., 1992). It is frequently characterized by pain, decrease in range of motion, and swelling of the joint. The etiology of HO is still unclear, but it has been found to be related to an increased muscle tone around a joint, immobility, and coma (Citta-Pietrolungo et al., 1992). Research has shown that 3 to 20% of children who sustain a traumatic brain injury may develop HO (Hurvitz et al., 1992). A bone scan is the best method of detection of HO. Medical treatment ranges from management with indomethacin to surgical excision of the bone. Aggressive physical therapy aimed at maintaining range of motion and strength around the joint should be implemented if HO is suspected or diagnosed. Because some joints with HO may progress to ankyloses, splinting and casting may be necessary in severe cases to maintain the joint in a functional position.

Children are assessed for level of coma throughout the initial traumatic episode. Level of coma is monitored using criterion-based behavioral scales such as the Glasgow Coma Scale (Teasdale & Jennett, 1974) and the Rancho Los Amigos Scale (Hagen et al., 1979). Both of these scales assess a child's ability to respond to various stimuli ranging from a painful stimulus to a complex verbal command. A child's orientation to time and place is also assessed. An increase in summary score of the Glasgow Coma Scale on successive administrations is an indicator of improvement. The administration of the Rancho Los Amigos Scale results in classification of a child into one of eight cognitive levels. Progression to a numerically higher level is an indicator of progress. The Children's Orientation and Amnesia Test (COAT) (Ewing-Cobbs et al., 1989) is also used to evaluate level of coma in children. Test items of the COAT, particularly those that assess the appropriateness of verbal responses to orientation questions, are based on facts commonly known by children.

NEAR-DROWNING

Incidence

Drowning is the fourth leading cause of fatal childhood injuries between 0 and 19 years of age. The most common age groups affected are children younger than age 4 years and adolescents (Fields, 1992). Drowning occurs in a wide variety of aquatic and household environments, including pools, lakes, oceans, bathtubs, and buckets.

Near-drowning has been defined as an episode in which someone survives a period of underwater submersion (Fisher, 1993). Near-drowning may also be referred to as a submersion injury. Survivors may experience cardiac, CNS, or respiratory system complications and may require rehabilitation.

Etiology

To understand the injuries caused from a near-drowning incident, it is necessary to understand the pathophysiology that occurs with near-drowning. It is hypothesized that in the sequence of drowning, the victim undergoes a period of panic, struggling, and automatic swimming movements. Apnea occurs and water is aspirated. Once the person is unconscious, fluid is passively introduced into the airways and cardiac arrest follows shortly afterward (Fields, 1992).

Aspiration was once thought to alter the body's electrolyte balance depending on whether the drowning occurred in freshwater or salt water. However, few submersion victims who survive have been found to aspirate enough fluid to change their electrolyte balance significantly. The presence of chlorine is the water also does not appear to adversely affect the pulmonary pathophysiology (Fields, 1992).

Hypoxemia is the most important consequence associated with submersion injuries. In freshwater submersion injuries, the hypoxemia is primarily due to the inactivation of pulmonary surfactant, which leads to a decrease in lung compliance. In saltwater aspiration, hypoxemia occurs as a result of an osmotic gradient that is formed across the alveolar-capillary membrane. This gradient pulls fluid and protein from the capillaries into the alveoli, causing pulmonary edema (Fields, 1992).

The brain and the heart are the organs most susceptible to injury as a result of asphyxia related to near-drowning injuries. Even when resuscitation is successful, the period of anoxia that has occurred may cause irreversible hypoxic-ischemic brain injury, including brain death (Cohn et al., 1980). Cerebral edema and herniation are complications associated with hypoxic-ischemic injury. Several factors may make children less susceptible to hypoxic-ischemic insult than adults. These include the lower amount of subcutaneous fat, relatively large surface area, and increased mobility when they are immersed. This allows children to become hypothermic faster. This is significant because of the documented improved recovery of people submersed in cold water versus warmer water (Fields, 1992). Second, it is thought that children are more susceptible to the diving reflex. The diving reflex occurs with submersion and consists of bradycardia and preferential shunting of blood to the brain and heart, which leaves them less susceptible to the hypoxic-ischemic injuries of near-drowning episodes.

The factors that predict functional recovery in children who have experienced a near-drowning episode include the length of the period of submersion and the length of time before resuscitation is begun. More specifically, the length and severity of ischemia are important factors (Beyda, 1991). Coma, spasticity, and abnormal posturing are manifestations of CNS injury that may be present after near-drowning.

Medical and Surgical Management

In general, neuronal cells are not able to tolerate periods of complete ischemia lasting longer than 5 minutes without sustaining permanent injury; irreversible neuronal injury has been demonstrated to increase significantly after 10 minutes (Safar, 1988).

The magnitude of the neuronal injury that occurs is also related to both the level of blood flow during the complete ischemic interval and the total duration of the ischemia. The most important intervention at the site of the incident is immediate and effective cardiopulmonary resuscitation (Fields, 1992).

Once the patient is in the hospital, medical interventions are focused on supporting respiration and attempting to prevent further neurologic injury. Traditional and high-frequency mechanical ventilation are used to treat acquired respiratory distress syndrome and may indirectly prevent further CNS complications. Extracorporeal membrane oxygenation (ECMO) is a respiratory system intervention in which blood is oxygenated mechanically outside the body, allowing the lungs to "rest." Ventilation is frequently used in conjunction with pharmacologic paralysis of the musculoskeletal system, placing the child at risk for contractures, muscle weakness, and atrophy.

Cardiac function continues to be monitored in the initial phases if persistent myocardial dysfunction occurs after resuscitation. Therapies for the cardiac dysfunction are based on the specific hemodynamics and adequacy of oxygenation found.

Central nervous system management may involve intracranial pressure monitoring if there is risk of cerebral edema causing high intracranial pressures. Edema generally occurs within 24 hours, with the maximum occurring at approximately 72 hours. As in traumatic brain injury, monitoring may be done with an intracranial pressure bolt.

BRAIN TUMORS

Incidence

The reported incidence of brain tumors in children 15 years of age and younger in the general population has been estimated to be 2.5 to 3.5 per 100,000 (Lannering et al., 1990). Although this incidence in the general pediatric population is relatively low, physical therapists can expect to be involved in the treatment of some of these children.

Types of Pediatric Brain Tumors

Pediatric brain tumors are described as being either focal or diffuse. Diffuse tumors extend to a wider area of brain tissue than focal tumors. Diffuse tumors are associated with a short and rapidly declining clinical course and have a wide constellation of presenting signs and symptoms.

Tumors that are less than 2.5 cm in diameter are considered focal (Shiminsky-Maher et al., 1991). Focal tumors, unlike diffuse tumors, are not associated with edema. Focal tumors are slow growing

and typically have a long clinical history with symptoms evolving over a relatively long period of time. Clinical symptoms are more discrete and depend on the exact location of the tumor. Pediatric brain tumors may also be generally classified according to their location and include tumors occurring in the posterior fossa, the brainstem, or the midline region.

Posterior Fossa Tumors

Three of the most common cerebellar tumors that occur in childhood are cerebellar astrocytomas, medulloblastomas, and ependymomas. Astrocytomas are usually well circumscribed and may be cystic. Ten-year survival rates range from 29 to 96% depending on tumor subtypes (Menkes & Till, 1990). Medulloblastomas infiltrate the floor or lateral wall of the fourth ventricle and extend into its cavity. The prognosis for medulloblastomas is variable according to subtype as well. Ependymomas are slow growing and may be asymptomatic. Evidence of malignancy is found in approximately 5% of cases, mostly in infants (Menkes & Till, 1990).

Clinical symptoms of posterior fossa tumors are related to increased cranial pressure and involvement of cerebellar structures. Headaches that are nonlocalized or frontal are an early symptom. Vomiting is the most common sign of cerebellar tumors and may be related to increased intracranial pressure or to direct pressure on the medullary vagal nuclei.

Motor signs of cerebellar involvement are ataxia, dysmetria, dysdiadochokinesia, intention tremor, and hypotonia. Hemiplegia and oculomotor signs may be clinical manifestations of cerebellar astrocytoma. When tumors extend into the brainstem, unilateral hearing loss and facial weakness may be found (Epstein & Wisoff, 1987). When the tumor extends rostrally or caudally from the medulla, quadriparesis, neck pain, and torticollis may be present (Epstein & Wisoff, 1987, 1988).

Brainstem Tumors

Brainstem tumors most frequently arise from the pons and on radiographic examination appear as a symmetric enlargement of the brainstem (Menkes & Till, 1990). Because of their location and close association with the centers that regulate vital functions, the prognosis for children with such tumors is usually poor.

Clinical symptoms associated with brainstem tumors include cranial nerve palsies, pyramidal tract signs, and cerebellar signs that occur without evidence of increased intracranial pressure (Bray et al., 1958; Stroink, 1986). Vomiting and headache may also be present.

Motor signs of brainstem tumors include gait disturbances, dysarthria, torticollis, quadriparesis, and hemiparesis. Gait deviations may be related to coordination problems or spasticity. Progression of the tumor to include cerebellar or spinal cord involvement is likely to be related to impairments in gait.

Midline Tumors

Craniopharyngiomas, optic nerve gliomas, and pineal tumors are examples of tumors that occur in midline brain regions. Clinical signs and symptoms of midline tumors are determined by the tumor's size and location and its relationship to adjacent brain structures. In the case of craniopharyngiomas, progression of the tumor is related to symptoms of increasing intracranial pressure, visual complaints, and endocrine disturbances (Epstein & McCleary, 1986; Menkes & Till, 1990). In the case of optic nerve gliomas, visual disturbances are the predominant clinical symptom. Symptoms of pineal tumors are often related to increased intracranial pressure and include headache. The inability to direct eye movement outward bilaterally is sometimes also present.

Cerebral Hemisphere Tumors

Cerebral hemisphere tumors make up approximately 40% of pediatric brain tumors (Gjerris, 1978). Symptoms of increased intracranial pressure are frequently the initial signs and symptoms of cerebral hemisphere tumors. Headache is most typical of these and is often transitory, occurring in the morning or during the night. Vomiting is another common sign of increased intracranial pressure. Although vomiting may occur in conjunction with nausea, it is not usually projectile. It often occurs in the morning and is not related to the child's eating pattern. Seizures are also a common clinical sign of cerebral hemisphere tumors. Children who experience seizure often have no other neurologic deficit (Blume et al., 1982).

Medical and Surgical Management

Medical treatment of pediatric brain tumors includes surgery, radiation therapy, chemotherapy, or a combination of these therapies. The treatment selected depends on the type, location, and characteristics of the tumor.

Surgery

Surgical excision of a brain tumor may be performed as a primary treatment or may be performed in conjunction with other treatments such as radiation therapy or chemotherapy. In cases in which full surgical excision of the tumor is not possible, radiation therapy is administered after surgery in an attempt to eradicate residual tumor cells. When hydrocephalus is present secondary to the obstruction of cerebrospinal fluid by a tumor, surgical intervention may include the placement of a shunt (Cochrane et al., 1994).

Radiation Therapy

Radiation therapy is frequently administered as an adjunct to surgical intervention and is often begun a few weeks after surgery (Berry, 1981). A radiation beam is directed at the tumor as a predetermined dose of energy is administered. This process is repeated on a regular schedule for several days or weeks. The effect of the administration of the radiation is to slow or halt the proliferation of tumor cells. Adjacent cells and physiologic structures are often also affected, which results in various immediate and long-term side effects.

Acute radiation encephalopathy occurs when vascular damage caused by the radiation results in increased vessel wall permeability. Side effects noted in the patient who is undergoing radiation include lethargy, nausea, and vomiting. Neurologic signs that existed before surgical intervention may reappear. Corticosteroids are often administered to treat edema and related symptoms. A more frequent (daily) administration of less intense radiation has been suggested as an alternative that may prevent severe edema-related symptoms (Menkes & Till, 1990).

Chemotherapy

The aim of chemotherapy is to kill significant numbers of tumor cells in each of the successive administrations of the chemotherapy. Antineoplastic drugs are frequently administered together to act against the tumor cells at different biomechanical sites.

Antineoplastic drugs that affect tumor cells also affect other rapidly growing, normal tissues, such as bone marrow, gastrointestinal epithelium, and hair follicles. The toxic effect of antineoplastic drugs on normal tissues causes the frequently experienced side effects of hair loss, nausea and vomiting, and immune system depression.

Although medical interventions such as surgery, radiation therapy, and chemotherapy are often effective in the treatment of pediatric brain tumors, adjacent brain tissues and structures may be negatively affected. The side effects of commonly administered interventions have been related to toxicity to normal brain tissue (Castel & Caille, 1989). These effects have been classified as "acute," occurring within 1 to 6 weeks after treatment; "early delayed," occurring 3 weeks to 3 months after treatment; and "late delayed," occurring several months to years after treatment (Castel & Caille, 1989). Toxic treatment effects together with direct tumor effects have been associated with changes in neurologic status, including cognitive abilities (Cohen et al., 1983).

DIAGNOSTICS TESTS FOR CHILDREN WITH BRAIN INJURIES

Several diagnostic tests are commonly used in children with brain pathology. It is important for the physical therapist to have an understanding of these tests, because this will allow them a more complete understanding of the patient's injuries and clinical signs.

Magnetic resonance imaging (MRI) is a diagnostic tool based on signals emitted by protons when placed in a magnetic field. Different tissues in the body have different proton concentrations, which allows for a clear contrast between tissues. MRI is a frequently used diagnostic tool in the evaluation of pediatric CNS problems. In fact, MRI has been suggested to be superior to other diagnostic tools for this purpose (Gusnard & Zimmerman, 1990). For example, bone artifacts often noted on computed tomography (CT) of the posterior fossa are not a problem with MRI. MRI may also differentiate between benign structures such as a collection of cerebrospinal fluid and malignant masses such as cystic tumors. Additionally, MRI is very sensitive in the detection of blood and is particularly useful in the evaluation of hemorrhage.

Computed tomography is used to show thin slices though the brain on the basis of x-rays. Various planes of sectioning may be chosen by the examiner. CT is most successful in the assessment of areas of calcification, the evaluation of a foreign body in a sensitive location, and the identification of skull and bony abnormalities. CT may also be the evaluative tool of choice at times when a screening must be performed quickly. CT is less costly than MRI, and financial restraints may influence the selection of CT versus MRI diagnostic testing (Fig. 22–1).

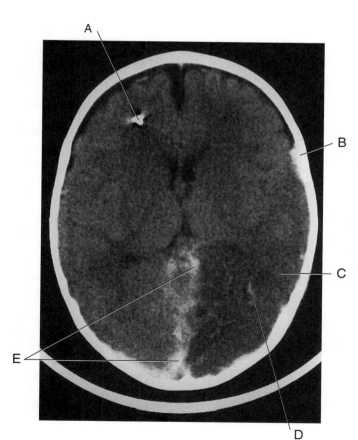

FIGURE 22–1. Computed tomography scan of a child with a traumatic brain injury sustained in a motor vehicle accident. The left border of the photo is the right hemisphere. Clockwise from the top: *A,* Intracranial pressure bolt placed in the right frontal cortex; *B,* small left subdural hematoma; *C* and *D,* area of ischemia in left parietal, temporal, and occipital lobes; *E,* subarachnoid hemorrhage.

Electroencephalography (EEG) is the recording of brain activity from externally applied electrodes. The EEG records waveforms representing brain activity. In a nonstimulated situation, the EEG primarily shows slow waves. With an increase in stimulation in the brain, the waveforms become faster with a lower amplitude. The evaluator notes frequency, amplitude, and organization of the waveform. Different neurologic conditions have characteristic EEG changes, and EEG plays a primary role in diagnosing seizure disorders.

The visually evoked response (VER) is another electrodiagnostic test used in brain injuries. This test uses electrical impulses with visual stimuli to detect abnormalities in the visual pathways. A similar test is the brainstem auditory evoked response (BAER). The BAER also uses electrical impulses to determine abnormalities along the auditory pathways and other abnormalities in the brainstem.

COGNITIVE CHANGES IN CHILDREN WITH BRAIN INJURIES

Children with brain injuries will probably have changes in cognitive functioning. An understanding of these areas of potential changes will allow the physical therapist to complete an appropriate and successful evaluation. Injuries from chemotherapy, radiation, anoxia, and hemorrhage will affect not only a child's motor patterns but also the ability to attend, follow directions, complete complicated motor tasks, and use executive functioning.

Memory Functioning

Memory is evaluated, particularly with respect to the child's ability to learn new material. Although the child may retain and remember material learned before a brain injury, learning new information may be problematic. Difficulties in the area of memory skills pose obvious problems for the child who will be returning to school. Less obvious are the influences of memory deficits on rehabilitative treatment.

The child who demonstrates difficulty learning new material may not progress as quickly as would be expected in learning an exercise program or in achieving independence in functional skills. For example, a child who demonstrates sufficient strength and coordination skills to perform a home exercise program may not be able to achieve the goal of independence in performing the program because of an inability to remember the component parts from one treatment session to the next.

Memory deficits may also be demonstrated by unsafe performance of functional skills. The omission of safety-related behaviors when performing transfers, for example, may limit the functional independence of a child whose balance and coordination skills are sufficient for the performance of the task.

The limiting effect of memory deficits may be particularly frustrating for parents. A change in memory skills may increase the child's level of dependence. Such an apparent developmental regression may be perceived by a parent as the child's unwillingness to "try hard" or as a behavior problem that is within the child's control to change. The results of an evaluation of a child's memory skills and capacity for new learning will be helpful in the development of an appropriate rehabilitation program and establishment of appropriate functional goals. Working with the family, the speech therapist, and the pediatric psychologist, the pediatric physical therapist may help determine the effect of memory and learning deficits on the child's functional abilities and the related need for assistance, environmental modification, or both.

Executive Skills

The ability to formulate and switch conceptual sets, the ability to use feedback to initiate behavioral change, and the ability to exercise judgment in social and community settings are included under the rubric of "executive skills." Deficits in executive functioning are often associated with frontal lobe injury and may be expressed as impulsive behavior resulting in failure to observe safety precautions or an inability to recognize socially appropriate behaviors.

The inability to change conceptual sets may be demonstrated in perseveration on a task or the inability to change activities without becoming disorganized. Difficulty switching conceptual sets may also influence the ability to perform reciprocal movements, alternating patterns of movement, or tasks with reciprocal or alternating components.

Arousal level and attentional ability may be impaired by frontal lobe lesions or lesions affecting the brainstem. A child's ability to follow commands or to benefit from feedback while learning motor and functional skills may be affected by level of arousal. A child who is able to maintain a level of arousal at which incoming environmental stimuli are neither overstimulating nor insufficient to elicit the child's attention is likely to benefit more from training or instruction than the child who is hypoaroused or hyperaroused.

When possible, a determination of the time of day at which arousal level is optimal or an alteration of therapeutic goals within a given treatment session in response to current arousal status may increase the effectiveness of intervention. Medications such as antiseizure or pain agents may also affect arousal. A knowledge of pharmacologic agents being used and time administered may assist in optimizing treatment.

Visuospatial Skills

Visuospatial and perceptual deficits can affect a child's perception of the environment. These deficits may influence cognitive tasks and motor performance and functional mobility skills (Fig. 22–2). Such deficits are frequently associated with lesions in the temporal or occipital lobes of the brain. A figure-ground deficit, or the inability to distinguish a given form from the background, may be related to difficulty with functional mobility skills. For example, problems with foot placement or the placement of an assistive device on a complex surface such as a step or a ramp may be related to visuospatial skills. Visuospatial deficits may also limit the level of functional independence achieved. For example, a child who is unable to put on an orthosis because of visuospatial deficits may ultimately be dependent in functional mobility even though he or she is able to ambulate on flat surfaces independently after the orthosis is on. A child with visuospatial deficits related to memory skills may demonstrate difficulty developing a cognitive map of his or her environment. Consequently, this child may have difficulty moving independently from place to place in the home, school, or community.

Language

Temporal lobe lesions may result in deficits in expressive or receptive language skills that can affect

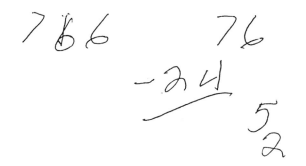

FIGURE 22–2. Math problem completed by a 12-year-old girl 2 days after removal of a brain tumor. The therapist asked the child to subtract 24 from 76. Note the correct answer, despite the perceptual difficulties with constructing the problem.

communication between therapist and patient, and can ultimately affect rehabilitation treatment. Language deficits are addressed in depth by speech and language pathologists. A basic understanding by the physical therapist will assist in communication during treatment sessions.

Receptive language deficits impair a child's ability to comprehend the instructions that are given for the performance of a task or activity. Determination of the extent of a child's receptive language impairment and the most effective means of communication will increase the results from treatment and decrease the therapist's and child's frustration.

Expressive language disorders impair a child's ability to communicate information to others. A child with an expressive disorder may fully comprehend verbally communicated information and successfully formulate a cognitive response. A breakdown occurs, however, between the formulation of the response and the execution or verbal expression of what was intended. In this case, the child may not be able to express a related idea or concern. In this situation, as in the case of the child with a receptive disorder, knowledge of the child's most efficient mode of communication may lessen frustration related to the inability to express an intended response.

PHYSICAL THERAPY MANAGEMENT

Campbell (1992) has described a theoretic framework for the measurement of motor performance in children with cerebral palsy that may be generalized to the population of children with other diagnoses and disabilities, including children with diagnosis of some insult to the brain. The framework incorporates the terminology of the World Health Organization as used in documents that address individuals with disabilities. According to this framework, motor dysfunction may be considered in three different dimensions: an organ/systems or impairment dimension, a functional limitations dimension, and a disability dimension. An extension of this model developed by the National Center for Medical Rehabilitation Research is presented in Chapter 7. This concept was utilized in the development of the *Guide to Physical Therapist Practice* (the *Guide*) (American Physical Therapy Association, 1997).

Physical therapy management of the child with an insult to the brain will be outlined according to the practice guidelines in the *Guide*. Examination and intervention of children with insults to the brain, regardless of the cause of the insult, will be similar in many respects. Differences specific to traumatic brain injury, near-drowning, and brain tumors will be discussed as appropriate.

Examination

The physical therapy examination is performed before any intervention. Many of the children described in this chapter will be transferred from one setting to another during the course of their recovery. These settings may include an acute care hospital, a rehabilitation center, an outpatient therapy center, or a school. A thorough examination should be performed on entry into each new setting. The examination includes three parts: history, systems review, and tests and measures.

A detailed history is the first component of the examination. In children with brain injury, it is important to carefully review the medical record. MRI, CT, and EEG reports provide the therapist with critical information regarding the anatomic and physiologic changes that have taken place as a result of the insult. Previous and current medications should be reviewed. In the acute care environment, for those patients on ventilator support, it is important to know if they are receiving paralytics. These drugs remove the child's ability to move actively in order to maximize the respiratory support. This puts the child at risk for muscle atrophy and loss of range of motion. If a child has demonstrated EEG changes consistent with seizures, the child will probably be administered antiseizure medication. These commonly have side effects of drowsiness and decreased level of alertness. Other medications may be given to the child who is still in an agitated state. These may help the child sleep, participate in therapies, and tolerate changes in stimulation.

The history should also record any other damage from the event. This could include orthopedic injuries sustained in a traumatic injury or cardiac changes from an anoxic event. Any surgical procedures should be noted in the history as well. If a child has received other therapy services before the examination, that should be noted, and ideally contact should be made with the therapists who provided those services. Any prior medical history that would affect physical therapy intervention should also be noted. An example of this is the child with a brain injury who had a premorbid diagnosis of developmental dyspraxia.

Including the child and family during the history process allows the family to express expectations and desired outcomes. This information will allow the therapist to more fully understand the family's perception of the extent of injuries and deficits present and will be utilized in setting functional goals.

The systems review is a brief screening that will allow the therapist to focus the physical examination. For a child with brain injury, this screening should include information that will allow referral to other disciplines as well. Screenings may include a gross assessment of activities of daily living, feeding, and cognitive issues. An example would be a child who had a submersion injury. A screening may quickly demonstrate that the child has no independent mobility, is unable to complete age-appropriate activities of daily living, and coughs when she drinks thin liquids. Because of the review of systems, an appropriate referral is made to both occupational therapy and speech therapy.

After completing the history and review of systems, the therapist then selects the appropriate tests and measures to complete the evaluation. If chosen appropriately, the tests and measures should allow the physical therapist to make an accurate evaluation, diagnosis, and prognosis. For children with brain injuries, a variety of tests and measures can be used. These may be broken down into tests for impairments, tests for functional limitations, and tests for disabilities. See Box 22-1 for common impairments, functional limitations, and disabilities seen in children with brain injuries.

Tests and Measures for Impairments

Loss of functional active or passive range of motion (ROM) may be a risk for the child who is unable

---

BOX 22-1. Common Impairments, Functional Limitations, and Disabilities in Children with Brain Injuries

Impairments	Functional Limitations	Disabilities
Abnormal muscle tone	Decreased age-appropriate mobility	Dependent mobility
Postural asymmetry	Delayed gross motor skills	Dependent self-help skills
Decreased muscle strength	Poor school performance	Social isolation
Loss of range of motion	Poor ability to follow directions	Limited play with peers
Ataxia	Decreased attention to environment	
Poor balance		
Behavior state changes		
Poor motor planning		
Poor visual perceptual skills		
Impaired cognition		

to continue with normal levels of activity either because of direct effects of the injury or because of the side effects of medical intervention. A child with a brainstem glioma may demonstrate limited volitional movement of the lower extremities related to spasticity and, without ROM exercises, may develop hypoextensibility or contractures. On the other hand, a child who does not demonstrate motor dysfunction directly related to the brain injury may experience limited mobility related to the general or specific side effects of medical treatment. Those children receiving respiratory support through a ventilator or ECMO may be paralyzed pharmacologically, which may lead to a loss of both ROM and strength. A child whose activity level is limited by nausea and vomiting or fatigue may also be at risk for loss of flexibility and ROM. Specific side effects of chemotherapy have also been related to limited ROM or flexibility. Vincristine, an antineoplastic agent used in the treatment of medulloblastoma and other tumors, has been associated with peripheral neuropathy, especially when levels approach toxicity (Kosmidis et al., 1991).

Passive range of motion may be assessed regardless of the cognitive abilities of the child. Changes in passive ROM should be documented and should include information as to why the change has occurred. Active ROM should be assessed frequently, with documentation of changes that are noted. With the child or adolescent who remains cognitively intact, this task is relatively straightforward. For the young infant or child, active ROM information is typically obtained by careful observation of the child's movement during play.

Changes in muscle tone may be noted at the same time as assessment for ROM. Passive movement at different velocities is used to examine muscle tone changes at rest. Active movements must be carefully observed to determine any differences in tone with volitional movement. Frequently, a child will be observed to have lower muscle tone at rest but, with activity, appears to have increased tone because of postural fixing in an attempt to stabilize the joint. Symmetry of tone is often disturbed with brain injuries; therefore, tone should be assessed thoroughly bilaterally.

Impairments in strength are also a common finding among children with brain insults. Muscle weakness that results from generally decreased activity may be present in children who are undergoing chemotherapy or radiation therapy. Less frequently administered treatments such as bone marrow transplant will also put children at risk for muscle weakness. After extended periods of bed rest or sedentary behavior, muscle atrophy may be expected. In the case of a child with a peripheral neuropathy related to vincristine chemotherapy, atrophy is also likely to result. Children whose tumors cause alterations in postural tone will also experience weakness. In the case of a child who has spasticity in agonist muscle groups, weakness can be expected in the antagonist groups. The child whose tumor caused hypotonia may also experience weakness related to less frequent functional use of muscle groups, especially antigravity muscles.

In the pediatric brain injury population, standardized manual muscle testing is difficult because of the need for the child to follow specific instructions. Because of age and cognitive deficits, many of these children are unable to accurately follow the instructions. Therefore, it is again necessary to complete a careful observation of the child's active movements. Documentation may report the child's ability to move against gravity, to support weight, to support an object, or to complete a movement requiring strength in a certain muscle group.

With increases in active movement and in positions against gravity, impairments in equilibrium and righting reactions may be observed. These reactions may be tested in a variety of positions and activities. Completion, symmetry, and speed of the reactions are qualitative information that should be noted when testing these reactions. In the young infant or the child who shows significant involvement, deep tendon reflexes and primitive reflexes should be assessed. These primitive reflexes may include the Babinski reflex, which, beyond age 7 months, is pathologic. Other reflexes such as the asymmetric tonic neck reflex and the tonic labyrinthine reflex should also be assessed.

Sensory testing in the pediatric brain injury population is challenging for a variety of reasons. First of all, by virtue of injury, these children may have cognitive deficits that impair their ability to be able to accurately respond to sensory input. Age may also lead to inability to accurately respond to sensory input.

Sensory inputs should be introduced selectively with careful observation to determine the response. Responses to input are noted as being either generalized, with a full-body response and physiologic changes with any input, or localized. Localized responses are more appropriate responses with the response specific to the system being stimulated. For example, if a nail bed is squeezed to assess for a pain response, a generalized response would be to see an increase in heart rate with a total body flexion withdrawal. A localized response to this same input is to observe withdrawal of the stimulated extremity, or the child may look toward the pain. As the child begins more active movement, sensory assessment can be completed in more depth, adding proprioception and kinesthesia to the systems assessed.

Coordination deficits may also be demonstrated in children who experience alterations of postural tone or weakness. A child demonstrating poor balance or motor control may be impaired by sensory integration disorders. This is characterized by either inadequate perception of sensory input or an inappropriate motor response to the input. Deficits in balance and coordination abilities may be anticipated in children whose tumors are located in the posterior fossa and affect the cerebellum (Menkes & Till, 1990). Visuoperceptual skills are commonly impaired in children with a brain insult. Deficits such as neglect and poor proprioception are also commonly noted. The classic "foam and dome" test, designed by Shumway-Cook and Horak (1986), is an excellent method of determining sensory integration deficits and their effect on balance in older children. For the young child and infant population, selective introduction of different sensory input and careful observation of the motor response is necessary to determine sensory integration difficulties.

Ataxia may become apparent as the child begins to initiate purposeful movement characterized by the loss of muscle coordination. Ataxia is a movement disorder that can be caused by damage to several different nervous system structures. Common causes of ataxia are damage to the cerebellum or to the sensory structures. These two types of ataxia are distinguishable because sensory ataxia worsens significantly when the child's eyes are closed (Bastian, 1997). Oscillations during movement will be observed with an increase in the oscillations as the tasks increase in difficulty. Limb ataxia will be observed in tasks such as active reaching and tying shoes. Proximal, or truncal, ataxia is more evident in upright postures with increasing antigravity demands. Assessment and documentation focus on movements and positions that affect ataxia.

Apraxia may also be present in children who have sustained a brain injury. Apraxia is an impairment in the child's ability to plan and execute a motor task. The child will be unable to demonstrate a requested task but may be able to complete the task automatically. For example, the child will be unable to lift his leg on demand, but if a ball were rolled to him, he would be able to kick the ball. Apraxia of speech may also be seen and is demonstrated by the child's inability to coordinate oral, laryngeal, and respiratory muscles for functional speech.

Particularly in the acute care setting, impairments may be noted in the cardiorespiratory system. For all three diagnoses, the cardiorespiratory system may be limited by a variety of factors. Children with brain trauma may also have thoracic trauma. They may also be limited by an overall state of lethargy that can occur with head trauma. Children who experience a submersion injury may have had damage to the myocardium, leaving them with limited endurance. Children with brain tumors may be limited by side effects from chemotherapy. The cardiorespiratory status should be assessed in the physical therapy examination by monitoring heart rate, respiratory rate, blood pressure, and oxygen saturation during activities. This is convenient in the pediatric intensive care setting because of the close nursing supervision and monitors available, but may also be done in other settings with the appropriate monitoring devices.

Assessment of arousal, attention, and cognition is another critical area. Children who have injuries to their brain will most likely show changes in one or all of these areas. Knowledge of a child's behavior states and what assists the child in reaching an optimal behavior state will increase the efficiency of physical therapy intervention. Position changes, motoric demands, and fatigue may affect arousal and attention and should be documented. Formal assessment of attention and cognition is generally completed by a speech-language pathologist or psychologist.

Physical therapists may also do a quick scan of cranial nerve integrity when evaluating children with brain injury. It is common to find that children with an insult to the brain often have difficulties with vestibular input. This may be evident from nausea and dizziness observed when moving to a sitting position. The use of swings, visual tracking, and functional reach tests will allow an assessment of the integrity of the vestibular system. If a child has difficulty swallowing and controlling secretions, a referral should be made to a speech pathologist.

Measures of Functional Limitation and Disability

Functional limitations are defined as potentially remediable inability to perform a task as a result of an impairment. For example, a child who has lost range of motion into dorsiflexion may be unable to ambulate because of poor ankle strategies. In the disability domain, a child's ability to function and be integrated into the community at large is a concern. Standardized tests are available for the physical therapist's use to determine both functional limitations and disabilities for children with brain injuries.

Two tests specifically assess functional skills. These tests were designed to be utilized for the pediatric rehabilitation population and work well for those children who have brain insults. The Pediatric Evaluation of Disability Inventory (Haley et al., 1992) and the WeeFIM (Braun & Granger, 1991) are both criterion-referenced indicators of change in functional skills such as mobility and self-care. The WeeFIM is the pediatric equivalent of the Functional

Independence Measure used for adult rehabilitation patients. The WeeFIM measures a child's independence in the areas of self-care, sphincter control, transfers, locomotion, communication, and social cognition. The PEDI is standardized for children ages 6 months to 7.5 years. It measures skills in three content domains: (1) self-care, (2) mobility, and (3) social function. The PEDI focuses on the function of specific tasks and also rates caregiver assistance and modification. This allows a good overall assessment of many skills. The use of standardized measures to monitor motoric and functional change is useful to document progress as required by third-party payers.

Neuromotor development is also important to assess in children with brain injury. Several standardized tests assess motor development. The Bayley Scales of Infant Development is appropriate to use for children from birth to 42 months of age. This test scores the children on a mental and motor scale and is useful for a full evaluation of all skills. It gives the examiner an index score, as well as an age equivalence score, which may be needed to qualify for funding and state programs. The Peabody Developmental Motor Scales (PDMS) is appropriate for children from birth to 83 months of age and assesses both gross and fine motor skills. The Bruininks-Oseretsky (Bruininks, 1978) is standardized for children from ages 4.5 to 14.5 years and also is used to assess fine and gross motor tasks. See Chapter 1 for more detailed information on these standardized tests.

Evaluation

After a thorough examination is complete, the therapist must then make several judgments based on the results. Included in these judgments is severity of impairment, functional limitation, and disability; system involvement; the living environment; and social supports.

When making decisions regarding the severity of impairment, there are several factors to address. First, of course, are the specific deficits noted in the examination. Knowledge of the pathophysiology of the various brain insults and other physiologic processes will help predict expected improvements in function. Length of time since the brain injury and any prior interventions should also be taken into account. If the impairment, such as muscle contracture or strength, is not expected to improve spontaneously, the therapist must decide what type, frequency, and duration of intervention is needed to address each identified impairment.

Functional limitations should be assessed relevant to age of the child and severity of the limitation. For instance, if an infant has significant motor deficits as a result of an insult, it may be reasonable to

discharge the child home with the family and provide both home and outpatient physical therapy intervention. On the other hand, if the child is an adolescent with significant mobility needs and poor judgment of safety issues, the family may not be able to care for the child at home, and the child may benefit from a rehabilitation stay to address these issues and to train the family in home management.

Disability may also be addressed in relation to the age of the child. As children grow and mature, their function in society expands. Their role increases from that of an infant, whose primary role is to grow and explore, to a child who interacts on an increasing basis with the world. Again, an infant may not necessarily show severe disability initially after an insult, but these deficits may appear as the child grows and matures. An adolescent who sustains an insult will generally demonstrate disability in the motor areas immediately, but it may not be until a return to school that some of the cognitive deficits become apparent.

Knowledge of the living environment and social supports should be considered in the evaluation process. A 10-year-old child with significant motor needs may be a perfect candidate for a power wheelchair. However, if that child lives in a single-wide trailer, a power wheelchair may not be a functional means of mobility. An infant with significant motor and feeding needs who is to be placed with a parent who has also sustained an injury may need significantly more intervention and training than the same infant who is cared for by an intact family unit, capable of carrying out some activities at home.

Diagnosis

From the information gained in the examination, the physical therapist develops a diagnosis for children with brain insults. This diagnosis is not a medical diagnosis, but rather a label that encompasses a cluster of signs, symptoms, syndromes, or categories. Additional information may be obtained from other professionals to assist the physical therapist in making a diagnosis. For example, a child with a traumatic brain injury who also has a fractured humerus may fit the diagnostic groups of skeletal deficits, impaired balance, impaired arousal and attention, and impaired motor function. The diagnosis is then used to guide the therapist in determining the most appropriate intervention.

Prognosis

Based on the diagnosis, the physical therapist must consider the likely outcomes of intervention. For children who have a brain injury, the prognosis will depend on the severity of their injury, the rate of recovery, and the social and physical supports available to them at home and at school. Determining prognosis and outcomes in children is more complex than in adults because children are growing and developing while they are recovering. A key component when determining the prognosis is to assess the child in relation to what age-appropriate activities the child would normally be participating in at home, at school, and in the community.

Plan of Care

The plan of care should be formulated once the physical therapist has determined the diagnosis and prognosis. The plan of care should include long- and short-term goals and outcomes, specific interventions, duration and frequency of intervention necessary to achieve the desired outcomes, and discharge criteria. Goals should be related to changes in impairments, and outcomes should be related to changes in functional limitations and disability. Goals and outcomes are determined based on the clinical evaluation, resources available, knowledge of pathophysiology, and the child's age. For infants, outcomes are focused on the infant being able to explore the environment with continuing progression in development. Because of dramatic changes in growth that an infant will undergo, goals and outcomes should be addressed for long-term needs as well. For the school-age child or adolescent, outcomes should focus on mobility in terms of interaction with peers and safe independence. For children with brain insults who are not involved in school at the time of examination, the plan of care should include goals related to integration back into the educational setting.

Intervention

Physical therapy intervention consists of purposeful and skillful interactions of the therapist with the child and family to produce changes that are consistent with the diagnosis and prognosis. The physical therapist provides direct intervention, as well as instruction and coordination, communication, and documentation.

Intervention interactions of coordination, communication, and documentation for the child with a brain insult consist of communication and coordination with all involved with the child's care. For this population, communication may be with the physician, other health care team members, third-party payers, and educational personnel. Participation in care conferences and discharge planning fall under this intervention. Communication and coordination relating to goals of integration or reintegration into

the school setting are vital to a child's successful return into the community.

Instruction is a cornerstone of physical therapy intervention. A child with brain insult may have many deficits, some obvious and others subtle. Children are often confused about their own deficits, and siblings have difficulty understanding why their brother or sister can no longer do the things that he or she used to be able to do. The family, including siblings when appropriate, and child need to be instructed in all areas that have changed as a result of the insult and how physical therapy will address these areas. Proper child and family instruction will lead to an increased carryover of therapeutic activities and a decreased level of frustration and helplessness for both the child and family.

Direct interventions, of course, will take up a major part of the time spent with the patient and should focus on addressing specific impairments, functional limitations, and disabilities. Direct interventions include but are not limited to therapeutic exercise, manual therapy techniques, selection of assistive or adaptive devises, electrotherapeutic modalities, physical agents, mechanical modalities, functional training in self-care, and functional training in community and school settings.

Intervention for Impairments

Traditional medical treatments of brain injury management address intervention at the impairment level. These treatments involve chemotherapy and radiation, respiratory support, surgical management, and cardiopulmonary support. Physical therapy management and evaluation at the impairment level focuses on specific component deficits. Examples are ataxia and hypotonia or related weakness, which may be considered manifestations of the brain pathology at the organ systems level.

Weakness is a common impairment in children with brain injury. Strengthening activities will therefore be a large part of the physical therapy intervention. Strength has been shown to be correlated with an increase in motor performance in children with cerebral palsy (Damiano & Abel, 1998). In this study, children with spastic cerebral palsy demonstrated strength gains in specific muscle groups, increased velocity of gait, and improvement in the ambulatory subtest of the Gross Motor Function Measure after a 6-week strengthening program.

How therapeutic exercises are carried out will vary depending on the age of the child and the severity of the brain injury. With an adolescent, the therapist may be able to complete a rote therapeutic exercise program with standard exercises and repetitions. Adolescents may also enjoy strengthening activities in a weight room with their peers. With a younger child, the therapist may need to choose appropriate developmental activities that will facilitate muscle strengthening in a given muscle group or pattern of movement. For example, if a 5-year-old child is demonstrating lower extremity weakness as a result of a traumatic brain injury, therapeutic activities could consist of climbing on equipment, squat to stand to retrieve game pieces, or step-stance activities while drawing on the wall. A pool is an excellent modality for this population. If a child is very weak with minimal active movements, the principles of buoyancy will assist with movement. For the stronger child, the principles of resistance of water will allow for increased strengthening. For the child who demonstrates ataxia, proximal strengthening will assist in the child's stability. For the pediatric physical therapist, therapeutic exercise is limited only by the imagination of the therapist (Fig. 22–3).

Contraindications to therapeutic exercise must be noted before initiating an exercise program. Limitations caused by fractures, skin involvement, or myocardial involvement must be noted. In the child who has a brain tumor, a specific set of guidelines should also be followed, because side effects of medical treatment may limit the child's performance. For example, the child who is fatigued after radiation therapy or who is nauseated after chemotherapy may be scheduled for physical therapy before radiation or chemotherapy. Because chemotherapy frequently affects blood parameters that are associated with clotting and tolerance of activity, blood cell counts should be considered when an exercise program is developed or modified. According to the hematology-oncology protocol at Egleston Children's Hospital, which was adapted from the work of Dietz (1980), exercise is recommended only for children whose hematocrit is greater than 25%,

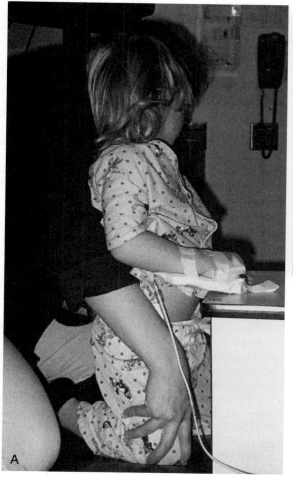

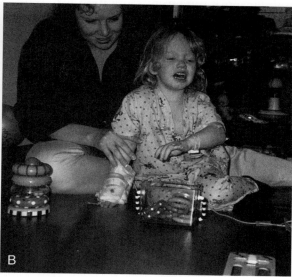

FIGURE 22–3. Three-year-old child with weakness and right hemiplegia after a traumatic brain injury. *A,* Strengthening for hip extensors in tall kneeling position. *B,* Right upper extremity weight bearing during play activity.

hemoglobin levels are greater than 10 mg/dl, platelet counts are greater than 50,000/mm^3, and white blood cell counts are greater than 500/mm^3.

Neuromuscular electrical stimulation (NMES) may be a useful adjunct to therapy in children with brain injury. NMES was found to increase ankle dorsiflexion at heel strike in children with cerebral palsy (Comeaux et al., 1997). Carmick (1997) published a guideline for clinical application of NMES for children with cerebral palsy that may also be useful for children with brain injury. Care must be taken to introduce electrical stimulus slowly to the child and to let the child initiate the movement during functional activities.

When impairments in ROM are present, the pediatric physical therapist has many options for intervention. For the child who demonstrates an increase in muscle tone and little active movement, passive ROM and positioning are the primary means of preventing contracture. Children who suffer severe submersion injury impairments may demonstrate severe spasticity and abnormal posturing, and as a result, adaptive equipment fabrication may constitute a significant component of intervention. Splinting or serial casting may also be used to maintain optimal ROM over time. For children who demonstrate active movement, ROM activities may be used in conjunction with strengthening and functional activities to maximize function and therapy time.

Joint mobilization or soft tissue massage in children with central nervous system disorders may help maintain ROM. Although much more research in the area of joint mobilization for children in general is needed, some basic precautions and contraindications should be noted. Absolute contraindications include malignancy involving the spinal cord, cauda equina lesions producing bowel and bladder dysfunction, bone disease of the spine, active inflammatory and infective arthritis, and rheumatoid collagen necrosis of vertebral ligaments (Harris, 1991). Aside from training in manual therapy techniques, the therapist should have knowledge in developmental biomechanics. Caution and care should be exhibited when using this method, particularly if the patient is unable to report pain or discomfort.

Changes in the child's cognitive status will also be an important consideration in the development of an exercise program that focuses on the improvement of balance and coordination skills, as well as other aspects of rehabilitation. Short-term memory deficits may make it difficult for a child to become independent in performing an exercise program. A lack of mastery at this task may be frustrating for both the child and the family. Variable levels of arousal within a session or from session to session will affect a child's ability to attend to instructions and to stay on task. A treatment plan for a given session may then need to be adjusted accordingly.

Intervention for Functional Limitations

Functional limitations are defined as a potentially remediable inability to perform a task as a result of an impairment. For example, a child who has lost ROM into dorsiflexion may be unable to ambulate because of poor ankle balance strategies. Intervention is used to help the child regain the transfer and mobility skills needed for independent or assisted ambulation in his or her immediate environment. In the functional limitations domain, increased independence in mobility skills, including bed mobility, transfer training, gait activities, and wheelchair mobility training, is emphasized.

Once again, the child's cognitive status must be considered. Difficulty learning new tasks and material or short-term memory problems may influence the method selected for instruction in transfer and mobility training. A child who demonstrates perseveration may have difficulty with reciprocal tasks or may become upset when asked to change from one activity to another. A child's short-term memory deficits or variable levels of arousal may necessitate frequent repetition of instructions and additional cueing while learning a task. These factors will also influence safety. For example, a child may be physically capable of performing a transfer but may not be able to attend to the task sufficiently to observe the necessary safety precautions, such as positioning a wheelchair or locking the brakes, to safely complete the task independently.

Children whose injuries are the result of a traumatic event may have other associated complications, such as fractures. This may change the management of mobility-related skills. For example, a child who demonstrates hemiplegia related to a brain injury but also has a fractured femur and humerus will be considerably more limited in mobility skills than the child who experiences neurologic or orthopedic injuries exclusively.

Functional training at home, at school, and in the community is important for children with brain injuries. Because brain injuries can lead to deficits in a broad range of skills, it is not appropriate to simply address impairments such as strengthening. A child with hemiplegia may be able to demonstrate adequate strength for independent ambulation but may be lacking visual-perceptual and cognitive skills that would allow him or her to do this functionally. The physical therapist must treat the whole child and treat the child in settings that will allow the child to practice functional skills. For a 1-year-old child with severe spasticity from a submersion injury, intervention involving functional training may involve work in sitting so that the child may be able to play in a functional sitting position. For an 11-year-old child with hemiplegia, a functional training session may involve work on bicycle riding so that the child may ride to school with friends.

Assessing for and fabricating assistive devices and equipment is an intervention that will lead to increased independence for the child with brain insult. Assessment is difficult in the early stages of recovery because of the difficulty in determining the amount of recovery a child may make. In this case, it may be best to create temporary devices before spending time and money on a permanent device. If a child is unable to ambulate initially after injury, a rental wheelchair may be more appropriate than purchase of a chair. Therapists can fabricate splints for the lower extremities initially to assess for later use of a foot orthosis in a child with poor motor control in the lower extremities. If complete neurologic recovery does not occur, custom orthoses and adaptive equipment may be purchased to facilitate independent functioning in the child's environment. Because of the potential for changes and growth in this population, equipment needs may change frequently.

Intervention for Disabilities

In the disability domain, a child's ability to function and be integrated into the community at large is a concern. Intervention is directed at assisting the child in the achievement of the highest possible levels of independent functioning in his or her home, school, and residential community. Intervention will be focused on the adaptive equipment, orthoses, and environmental modifications to allow the child to function as independently as possible in his or her natural environment.

Traumatic brain injury is a disability category under the Individuals with Disabilities Educational Act (IDEA). Therefore, any child who has a documented traumatic brain injury must be evaluated by school personnel for special services, including physical therapy, on reentry to schools. Although children who have sustained a submersion injury or a brain tumor do not fit specifically under this category, they should also be evaluated by school personnel on reentry because of the similar nature of their impairments, functional limitations, and disabilities.

The role of the school physical therapist in intervention with a child who has undergone treatment and rehabilitation for a brain tumor provides an illustration of treatment focused at preventing disability. Goals of treatment may include determination of the mode of mobility and required assistive devices to promote efficient functioning in the classroom and school building. An evaluation of the child's general endurance in relation to the demands of daily activity and the formulation of recommendations for modifications in the child's schedule will also be included.

Education of and support for parents as they adapt to changes in their child's transition to school and community living are appropriate goals to prevent disability and facilitate coping with inevitable societal barriers to full integration in society.

Intervention that focuses on helping the child become reintegrated into the community through the implementation of provisions in federal legislation such as the Americans with Disabilities Act (PL-101-336) may also be considered as an illustration of intervention to prevent disability. For example, working on improving the child's mobility in the community by securing public transportation mandated by federal legislation influences the child's ability to fully participate in the life of the community.

Referrals to support groups and community agencies can be valuable to the family, child, and siblings. In the case of the child with a brain tumor who experiences regrowth or for whom further treatment is not possible, physical therapists work with hospice organizations or home health agencies. In such cases, the physical therapist collaborates with the family and the child to help them cope with a progressively debilitating process in the child.

Outcomes

Outcomes in the pediatric population who have sustained brain injuries are variable. In children who suffer traumatic brain injuries, the prognosis is also variable with factors such as extent of primary injury, other injuries sustained, and amount of secondary damage. The severity of traumatic brain injury is the major factor associated with outcome. For children who have received traumatic brain injury, outcomes at discharge from the hospital in terms of neurologic sequelae were assessed in a study by Kraus and colleagues (1990). They found that at discharge, 3% of those who sustained a mild brain injury had neurologic sequelae, 94% of those who sustained a moderate brain injury had neurologic sequelae, and 100% of those who sustained a severe brain injury had neurologic sequelae. The effect of age at injury on neurologic outcome is complex, and the results of studies to date are inconsistent. Cerebral water content, extent of myelination, degree of brain development, stage of development of localization of cortical function, and neurochemical content vary in children of different ages, and each of these factors may affect brain plasticity and potential recovery of function (Michaud et al., 1993).

In the case of the child with a diagnosis of brain tumor, the amount of function that will be regained depends on whether the limitation is related to the lesion itself, to pressure effects, or to the effects of medical treatment such as surgery or radiation therapy. For example, if a child's hemiparesis is related to direct pressure of a tumor or associated edema, surgical excision of the tumor or treatment that shrinks it will probably be followed by recovery of function. If the hemiparesis is related to an exacerbation of symptoms that has been noted to occur with radiation therapy (Menkes & Till, 1990), recovery of some function may also be expected. If the hemiparesis is related to infiltration of the tumor into healthy tissue, function is less likely to be regained. Similarly, if healthy tissues have been surgically excised or damaged by radiation therapy, recovery is less likely to occur. Future recurrence of the tumor will also, of course, have an effect on the outcome of treatment.

Duration of the hypoxic-ischemic event is the primary determinant of prognosis of victims of submersion incidents. Studies vary, but most recently suggest that if patients do not die, or are not left in a persistive vegetative state, they are likely to have only minimal neurologic deficits (Fields, 1992). The prognosis of children with brain tumors will vary largely based on the type of tumor, the amount of healthy tissue damaged, and the rate of recurrence.

The therapist should consider outcomes at every level of care. Therapeutic outcomes should include minimization of functional limitation, optimization of health status, prevention of disability, and optimization of patient and family satisfaction. To minimize functional limitations and prevent further disability, the therapist must be proactive in all aspects of intervention. Aside from therapy services, the patient and family should be directed to community support groups.

Optimization of Health Status

In a recent study, adults who had sustained a traumatic brain injury were surveyed to determine what long-term health issues may be common in the traumatic brain injury population. The most frequently reported health issues were suggestive of ongoing neuroendocrine dysfunction, neurologic difficulties, and arthritic complaints (Hibbard et al., 1998). It is important to remember that our pediatric patients may have health issues that affect them for a lifetime, and therefore, our intervention should consider the possible long-term sequelae of brain injury.

Wellness is an area of rehabilitation for the child with a brain insult that is an integral but often overlooked part of the rehabilitation process. One way that a physical therapist can assist with wellness activities is to assist the child in maintaining activities that promote cardiovascular health and strength. A recent study found that adult patients with traumatic brain injury who exercised regularly had improved mood, less impairment, less disability, and perceptions of better health than those who did not exercise (Gordon et al., 1998).

For children with chronic neurologic sequelae, the therapist may need to help the child adapt an exercise program to maintain a level of cardiovascular fitness and strength. For example, a group of children with various mild motor impairments from traumatic head injuries may be seen weekly for a fitness group. Intervention could include strengthening and cardiovascular activities, as well as some general instruction about health and wellness. Children with more significant motor impairments may participate in a swimming program to address strength and cardiovascular endurance in a gravity-limited, buoyancy-assisted environment.

Prevention

A large part of the job of a physical therapist is education, and part of our educational efforts should be focused on prevention of brain injuries. Education of our patients should also extend to education of the general public. Brain injury prevention efforts have focused on use of helmets and appropriate motor vehicle restraints in children. There have also been educational efforts regarding safe-proofing houses and eliminating the use of baby walkers. It has been documented that after sustaining one traumatic brain injury, the risk of a further traumatic brain injury increases (Annegers et al., 1980). Some communities have local chapters of the Brain Injury Association that give free helmets and car seats to children who have suffered or are at risk for a traumatic brain injury.

Near-drowning prevention efforts have focused on general water safety. The U.S. Consumer Product Safety Commission has begun to look at regulations regarding pools in residential properties. Owners are being advised to have childproof barriers around their pool and have cardiopulmonary resuscitation training. Parent education about household dangers such as the bathtub and other dangerous water sources is also necessary.

Although brain tumors are largely unpreventable, physical therapists must be aware of early signs and symptoms. Children who are examined by a therapist for motor signs and symptoms of unknown etiology may benefit from a further workup by a neurologist to rule out tumor. This may allow for earlier identification and treatment of tumors.

Many local and national organizations have prevention efforts aimed at reducing injury in the pediatric population. The National SAFE Kids Coalition sponsors SAFE Kid Week nationally and other safety-related events throughout the year. Non-accidental injuries such as shaken baby syndrome are being targeted in national "Babies Are Fragile" campaigns.

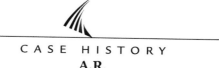

CASE HISTORY
A.R.

Examination

History. A.R. is a 51-month-old boy who experienced a traumatic brain injury. He was a pedestrian who was struck by a drunk driver. After initial impact, A.R. was dragged under the car and the upper part of his body became lodged in the wheel well of the car. A.R. was stabilized at the scene and transferred to the regional trauma center.

A computed tomography (CT) scan obtained in the emergency department showed a depressed skull fracture in the left frontotemporal area. He was taken to surgery immediately, where his skull fracture was elevated and an intracranial pressure bolt was placed. The neurosurgeon noted that although there was a good deal of gravel and dirt in the skull fracture, the dura remained intact. A CT scan obtained after surgery showed minimal swelling with no obvious damage to the brain. A.R. was intubated and remained on the ventilator for 11 days after the injury.

A.R. also suffered a degloving laceration starting at his left eyebrow and leading back past his left ear. He was also noted to have extensive wounds, down to the bone of both shoulders. He underwent extensive debridement and grafting for these wounds.

Rehabilitation services were initiated 4 days after the injury in the pediatric intensive care unit. He was evaluated and treated by a physical therapist, an occupational therapist, and a speech therapist during his acute care stay. Therapy in the acute care setting consisted of increasing level of alertness, endurance, feeding, cognitive assessment, and family education regarding brain injuries and the role of rehabilitation services. After 19 days in the acute care hospital, A.R. was transferred to the local rehabilitation hospital.

On admission to the rehabilitation hospital, A.R.'s history was reviewed, family contact was made, and the examination was completed. A.R.'s family consisted of two parents and five siblings. They expressed concerns regarding deficits and goals as follows:

1. A.R. will eat independently.
2. A.R. will walk again.
3. A.R. will talk with family members.

Systems review. On first meeting A.R. in the rehabilitation center, the following observations were made:

1. The child was still dependent on a wheelchair for mobility.
2. The child was demonstrating variable levels of alertness.
3. The child still had bandaging over both shoulders where grafting and debridement had been performed.
4. The child was demonstrating neglect of the left side of the body.
5. The child was dependent on nasogastric feeding.
6. The child had minimal verbal communication.

Through the review of systems, it was determined that the child would continue to receive physical, occupational, and speech therapy. It was also determined that physical therapy assessment would consist of administration of the Pediatric Evaluation of Disability Inventory (PEDI) and other tests and measures that would further examine the deficits noted in the systems review.

Tests and measures

Impairments. Range of motion was assessed, and A.R. was found to have full passive movement in both lower extremities and in the right upper extremity but limited shoulder flexion and abduction in the left upper extremity secondary to pain complaints noted over areas of wounds. He was unable to consistently move his extremities actively on request secondary to limitations in motor planning. He was, however, spontaneously moving all four extremities. Strength was not formally assessed because of difficulties with following instructions and motor planning. In functional movement, A.R. was able to support his weight through his lower extremities in supported standing. He was using his trunk to attempt to transition from supine to sit and using his upper extremities to pull himself to sit with assistance. He was able to lift his right arm above his head to reach for a toy but unable to lift his left arm above 90° flexion. When the integrity of A.R.'s sensory system was assessed, he demonstrated appropriate response on the right side of his body. He had a limited perception of sensory input in all forms on the left side of his body, frequently needing increased intensity or duration of stimulus on the left side to acknowledge the input. When A.R. was given minimal support, he was noted to be ataxic in his movements.

Functional limitations and disability. The PEDI was administered to determine the functional limitations of his injuries. Mobility scores are shown in Box 22-2. After administering the PEDI and tests for impairments, it was determined that A.R.'s primary disability was that he was unable to be integrated back into his home and family life at this time because of the extent of both his medical needs and his increased functional dependence.

Prognosis

Because of the moderate nature of his traumatic brain injury, the healing potential of orthopedic and skin wounds, and the progress made to date, it was determined that A.R. had an excellent prognosis for recovery of his physical skills. He was thought to be a good candidate for return to ambulation and some level of gross motor play. His prognosis for return of all prior cognitive skills was more guarded, however, based on the limited progress that he had demonstrated in this area to date.

Plan of care

It was determined at the first team conference that A.R. would benefit from 6 to 8 weeks of intensive rehabilitation within the rehabilitation center. It was also determined that he would most likely continue to demonstrate some deficits at discharge from rehabilitation and would benefit from both outpatient therapy services and school assessment and services. Physical therapy goals and outcomes were established as follows:

Goals:	*Outcomes:*
1. A.R. will have minimal scarring.	1. A.R. will ambulate independently in school environment.
2. A.R. will use both upper extremities for play.	2. A.R. will be able to participate in family activities.
3. A.R. will demonstrate full strength in lower extremities.	3. A.R. will climb six stairs independently.
4. A.R. will have full active ROM of all extremities.	4. A.R.'s family will demonstrate ability to interact and play to maximize his skills at home.

Intervention

Indirect physical therapy intervention was completed primarily in weekly team conferences and in communication in the patient chart. As discharge neared, communication expanded to include the school physical therapists who would be assessing A.R. after discharge from the rehabilitation center.

A.R. received direct physical therapy treatment

BOX 22-2. Admission PEDI Scores for A.R.

Domain	Raw Score	Normative Standard Score	Scaled Score
Mobility Functional skills	17	Below 10	39.3
Mobility Caregiver assistance	17	16.1	52.3

Modification Frequencies (7 items)

None	Child	Rehab	Extensive
3	4	0	0

twice daily during his stay at the rehabilitation center. He also received occupational and speech therapy services twice daily and therapeutic recreation daily. Physical therapy intervention addressed the goals in the plan of care. Therapy focused on increasing range of motion in the left upper extremity, wound management with fitting of pressure garments over the shoulders and face, proximal strengthening, and ambulation training. A variety of settings were used for these interventions. At first, because of A.R.'s agitation and poor attention, he was seen in a one-on-one setting. As his tolerance for activity and stimulation increased, so did the variety of his therapy sessions. Sessions progressed to include his mother, then his siblings, and finally therapy as part of a group of similar-age children.

Outcome

At discharge from the rehabilitation center, A.R. was demonstrating near age-appropriate gross motor skills as measured by the PEDI (Box 22-3) and the Peabody Developmental Motor Scales. His only limitation at discharge was a slight weakness noted in his left upper extremity. He continued to demonstrate some difficulties with cognitive skills involving executive functioning. Because of these two areas of difficulties, A.R. was followed twice weekly in the outpatient setting. Physical therapy intervention was divided between a weekly one-on-one visit in which issues relating to wound management, range of motion, and strengthening of the left upper extremity were addressed and a group session with similar-age peers in which general gross motor skills were taught and practiced. He also continued to receive occupational and speech therapy on an outpatient basis.

Because of A.R.'s near full recovery, when he was tested by the school district, his scores were too high to qualify him for services. However, because of the

BOX 22–3. Discharge PEDI Scores for A.R.

Domain	Raw Score	Normative Standard Score	Scaled Score
Mobility Functional skills	57	48.1	89.2
Mobility Caregiver assistance	35	60.7	100.0

Modification Frequencies (7 items)

None	Child	Rehab	Extensive
7	0	0	0

BOX 22–4. Admission PEDI Scores for L.L.

Domain	Raw Score	Normative Standard Score	Scaled Score
Mobility Functional skills	5	Below 10	20.9
Mobility Caregiver assistance	0	Below 10	0

Modification Frequencies (7 items)

None	Child	Rehab	Extensive
0	3	4	0

IDEA legislation qualifying all children who have sustained a traumatic brain injury, the school therapy team would reassess both cognitive and motor skills frequently.

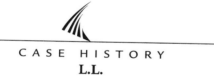

CASE HISTORY
L.L.

Examination

History. L.L. is an 18-month-old girl who was an unrestrained passenger in a motor vehicle accident. She sustained a small subdural hematoma, a subarachnoid hematoma, a skull fracture, an ischemic infarct, and bilateral retinal hemorrhages. She was in the intensive care unit for 2 weeks following her injury and had her intracranial pressures monitored while in intensive care. Other medical procedures included a period of assisted ventilation and placement of a nasogastric tube for nutrition. Physical therapy services were initiated immediately after removal of the intracranial pressure bolt in the pediatric intensive care unit.

The child was a daughter of a teenage mother who was living in a converted school bus on her parent's property in the mountains, 30 miles from the nearest town and 60 miles from the nearest pediatric rehabilitation center. The child had shown some mild delays early in her life and was being followed on a monthly basis by an educational development team before the injury. At the time of initial evaluation, L.L.'s mother was unable to specifically identify any deficits or goals other than to be able to take her child back home.

Review of systems. On initial examination of this child, the following were noted:

1. The child was not responding to any stimuli presented.
2. The child was unable to control secretions.
3. The child was positioned in a left-facing-only posture.
4. The child occasionally demonstrated random movement of the left side of her body.
5. The child was not vocalizing.

At this point, it was recommended that the child receive occupational and speech therapy in conjunction with physical therapy services to address feeding, cognition, and developmental skills.

Tests and measures

Impairments. Initially, L.L. was noted to have flaccid extremities on the right side. Her left extremities were demonstrating some movement and some resistance to passive movement. Her muscle tone in the left extremities was thought to be near normal. She demonstrated full passive range of motion of all extremities, but active range of motion was limited due to weakness in the extremities. She was unable to control her head in any upright position. Vital signs were stable during the examination activities. As noted in the review of systems, L.L. was not responding to tactile, visual, or auditory input. She did, however, show an increase in heart rate and respiratory rate with vestibular input.

Functional limitations and disability. The PEDI was administered to determine functional limitations. Scores for initial administration are shown in Box 22–4. L.L. was unable to demonstrate any active exploration of her environment, and her mother was unable to respond to her change in needs.

Diagnosis

Based on the examination information, the following diagnoses were determined: impaired vision, impaired arousal and attention, impaired motor function, and impaired sensory integration.

Prognosis

Because of the severity of both the physiologic changes and the resulting profound impairments and functional limitations, it was thought that L.L.'s prognosis was guarded as to the amount of motor function and skills that she would regain. However, because she was still very young and recently injured, it was thought that she had potential to regain some motor skills.

Plan of Care

Because of the distance of L.L.'s home from rehabilitation services and her continued medical and nutritional needs, it was determined that a stay in a rehabilitation center would provide the family and child with the best possible outcomes. For the rehabilitation stay, the following physical therapy goals and outcomes were established:

Goals:	*Outcomes:*
1. L.L. will tolerate change in positions without dramatic changes in vital signs.	1. L.L. will tolerate handling for routine care.
2. L.L. will hold her head independently in supported sitting.	2. L.L.'s mother will recognize deficits and strengths in the child's sensory motor system and respond accordingly.
3. L.L. will support weight through her lower extremities.	3. L.L. will explore environment with caregiver modification.
4. L.L. will actively use all extremities in play.	4. L.L. will sit independently and stand with assistance.
	5. L.L. will demonstrate two play skills.

Intervention

L.L. received extensive physical therapy services in the rehabilitation center over 2.5 months. Intervention involved weekly care conferences, staff training in developmental activities for nontherapy times, and extensive family training.

Direct physical therapy intervention was done twice daily. Emphasis was on sensorimotor stimulation, strengthening, postural stability, and establishing some forms of independent movement. Physical therapy sessions frequently coincided with speech therapy sessions. Multiple goals were accomplished during these sessions. First, L.L. was more active vocally with more active body postures. She also demonstrated

---

BOX 22–5. Discharge PEDI Scores for L.L.

Domain	Raw Score	Normative Standard Score	Scaled Score
Mobility Functional skills	7	Below 10	25.4
Mobility Caregiver assistance	9	54.4	40.9

Modification Frequencies (7 items)

None	Child	Rehab	Extensive
0	4	3	0

---

more active oral motor skills in terms of feeding in more dynamic positions. Also, because of the need for extensive handling, cotreatment with the speech therapist facilitated play.

Outcomes

L.L. was discharged from the rehabilitation center 3 months following her initial injury with discharge PEDI scores as shown in Box 22–5. At time of discharge she could roll from supine to prone independently, sit for brief periods of time independently with upper extremity propping, and take weight through her lower extremities. With assistance she was able to pull to sit, although still with a slight head lag. She demonstrated some purposeful movements in her left extremities. Movements of the right extremities were random and less frequent than movements of the left extremities. She responded intermittently to stimuli on the right side of her body. She appeared to track some toys and was able to reach for toys with variable accuracy with her left upper extremity. She continued to have significant deficits, and it was determined that L.L. would benefit from an intensive outpatient therapy program. Because of the rural area where she lived and the family's limited resources for transportation, she would be followed by a home health therapy team. No therapists on the home health team had pediatric experience, so a video demonstrating intervention techniques was made by the pediatric team on the day of discharge. L.L. was also scheduled to be followed every 3 months for reassessment by the pediatric therapy team at the rehabilitation center.

L.L.'s last follow-up visit was 3 years after her injury (Fig. 22–4). She was receiving therapy 4 days weekly in a developmental preschool. She was able to ambulate with a walker, using bilateral fixed ankle orthoses to assist with stability. She demonstrated an improved repertoire of play and had increased her vocabulary to include some two-word sentences. Her family contin-

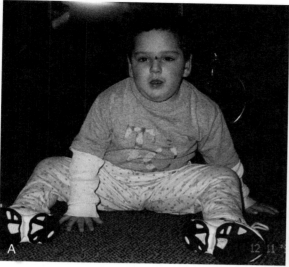
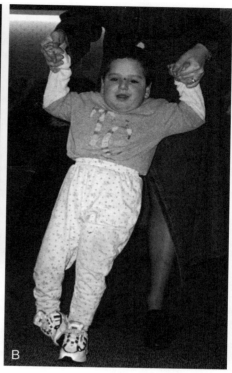

FIGURE 22–4. L.L. 3 years after injury at age 4.5. *A*, Preferred sitting posture; note continued low muscle tone and stabilizing patterns of upper extremity propping and wide base of support. *B*, Ambulation with caregiver assistance; note the posturing of the right foot with attempts to progress the right lower extremity forward.

ues to be thrilled with her progress and are very involved in her therapy activities.

Recommended Resources

Begali, V. Head Injury in Children and Adolescents: A Resource and Review for Allied Professionals. New York: Wiley, 1986.
Brain Injury Association. Alexandria, VA. Phone: 703-236-6000. Internet: www.biausa.org.
Sellers, CW, & Vegter, CH. Pediatric Brain Injury: A Practical Resource. Tucson, AZ: Communication Skill Builders, 1993.
Snow, JH. Pediatric Traumatic Brain Injury. Thousand Oaks, CA: Sage, 1994.
Ylvisaker, M: Head Injury Rehabilitation in Children and Adolescents. Boston: Butterworth-Heinemann, 1995.

References

American Physical Therapy Association. Guide to physical therapy practice. Physical Therapy, *77*:1163–1650, 1997.
Annegers, JF, Garbow, JD, Kurland, LT, & Laws, ER, Jr. The incidence, causes and secular trends of head trauma in Olmstead County Minnesota. Neurology, *30*:912–919, 1980.
Bastian, AJ. Mechanisms of ataxia. Physical Therapy, *77*:672–675, 1997.
Berry, MA. Radiation treatment for medulloblastoma: A 21-year review. Journal of Neurosurgery, *55*:43–50, 1981.
Beyda, DH. Pathophysiology of near-drowning and treatment of the child with a submersion incident. Critical Care Nursing Clinics of North America, *3*:273–280, 1991.

Blume, WT, Girvin, JP, & Kauffman, JCE. Childhood brain tumors presenting as chronic uncontrolled focal seizure disorders. Annals of Neurology, *12*:538–549, 1982.
Braun, SL, & Granger, CV. A practical approach to functional assessment in pediatrics. Occupational Therapy Practice, *2*:46–51, 1991.
Bray, PF, Carter, S, & Taveras, JM. Brainstem tumors in children. Neurology, *8*:1–9, 1958.
Bruininks, RH. Bruininks–Oseretsky Test of Motor Proficiency. Circle Pines, MN: American Guidance Service, 1978.
Campbell, SK. Measurement of motor performance in cerebral palsy. In Forrsberg, H, & Hirsch, H (Eds.), Movement Disorders in Children. Basel: Karger, 1992, pp. 264–271.
Carmick, J. Guidelines for the clinical application of neuromuscular electrical stimulation (NMES) for children with cerebral palsy. Pediatric Physical Therapy, *9*:128–136, 1997.
Castel, JC, & Caille, JM. Imaging of irradiated brain tumors: Value of magnetic resonance imaging. Journal of Neuroradiology, *16*:81–132, 1989.
Citta-Pietrolungo, TJ, Alexander, MA, & Steg, NL. Early detection of heterotopic ossification in young patients with traumatic brain injury. Archives of Physical Medicine and Rehabilitation, *73*:258–262, 1992.
Cochrane, DD, Gustavsson, B, Poskitt, KP, Steinbok, P, & Kestle, JR. The surgical and natural morbidity of aggressive resection for posterior fossa tumors in childhood. Pediatric Neurosurgery, *20*:19–29, 1994.
Cohen, AM, Parker, JA, Donahoe, K, Jansons, D, & Kolodny, GM. Three years experience with all-digital nuclear medicine department. Seminars in Nuclear Medicine, *20*:225–233, 1983.
Cohn, AW, Edmonds, JF, & Barker, GA. Near drowning in cold fresh water: Current treatment regimen. Canadian Anaesthetists Society Journal, *25*:259–265, 1980.

Comeaux, P, Patterson, N, Rubin, M, & Meiner, R. Effect of neuromuscular electrical stimulation during gait in children with cerebral palsy. Pediatric Physical Therapy, 9:103–109, 1997.

Damiano, DL, & Abel, MF. Functional outcomes of strength training in spastic cerebral palsy. Archives of Physical Medicine and Rehabilitation 79:119–125, 1998.

Dietz, JH. Adaptive rehabilitation in cancer: A program to improve quality of survival. Postgraduate Medicine, 68:145–153, 1980.

Epstein, F, & McCleary, EL. Intrinsic brain stem tumors of childhood: Surgical indications. Journal of Neurosurgery, 64:11–24, 1986.

Epstein, F, & Wisoff, JH. Intra-axial tumors of the cervico medullary junction. Journal of Neurosurgery, 67:483–487, 1987.

Epstein, F, & Wisoff, JH. Intrinsic brain stem tumors in childhood: Surgical indications. Journal of Neuro-oncology, 6:309–317, 1988.

Ewing-Cobbs, L, Lewin, HS, Fletcher, JM, Miner, ME, & Eisenberg, HM. Post-traumatic amnesia in children: Assessment and outcome. Paper presented at the meeting the International Neuropsychological Society. Vancouver, British Columbia, 1989.

Fields, AI. Near-drowning in the pediatric population. Progress in Pediatric Critical Care, 8:113–129, 1992.

Fisher, DH. Near-drowning. Pediatric Review, 14:148–151, 1993.

Gjerris, F. Clinical aspects and long-term prognosis in supratentorial tumors in infancy and childhood. Acta Neurologica Scandinavica, 57:445–456, 1978.

Gordon, WA, Sliwinski, M, Echo, J, McLoughlin, M, Sheerer, M, & Meili, T. The benefits of exercise in individuals with traumatic brain injury: A retrospective study. Journal of Head Trauma Rehabilitation, 13:58–67, 1998.

Gusnard, DA, & Zimmerman, RA. Computed tomography versus magnetic resonance imaging. Clinical Pediatrics, 29:136–157, 1990.

Hagen, C, Makmus, D, Durhham, P, & Bowman, K. Levels of cognitive functioning. In Rehabilitation of the Head-Injured Adult: Comprehensive Physical Management. Downey, CA: Professional Staff Association of Rancho Los Amigos Hospital, 1979, pp. 87–90.

Haley, SM, Coster, WJ, Ludlow, LH, Halliwanges, JT, & Andrellos, PJ. Pediatric Evaluation of Disability Inventory (PEDI), version 1.0. Boston: New England Medical Center, 1992.

Harris, SR, & Lundgren, BD. Joint mobilization for children with central nervous system disorders: Indications and precautions. Physical Therapy, 71:890–896, 1991.

Hibbard, MR, Uysal, S, Sliwinski, M, & Gordon, WA. Undiagnosed health issues in individuals with traumatic brain injury living in the community. Journal of Head Trauma Rehabilitation, 13:47–57, 1998.

Hurvitz, EA, Mandac, BR, Davidoff, G, Johnson, JH, & Nelson, VH. Risk factors for heterotopic ossification in children and adolescents with severe traumatic brain injury. Archives of Physical Medicine and Rehabilitation, 73:459–462, 1992.

Kosmidis, HV, Bouhoutsouu, DO, Varroutsi, MC, Papadatos, J, Stefanidis, CG, Vlachos, P, Scardoutsou, A, & Kostakis, A. Vincristine overdose experience with three patients. Pediatric Hematology and Oncology, 8:171–178, 1991.

Kraus, JF, Rock, A, & Hemyari, P. Brain injuries among infants, children, adolescents and young adults. American Journal of the Disabled Child, 144:684–691, 1990.

Lannering, B, Marky, I, & Nordborg, C. Brain tumors in childhood and adolescence in West Sweden, 1970–1984: Epidemiology and survival. Cancer, 66:604–609, 1990.

Lofgren, J, & Awetnow, NN. Cranial and spinal components of the cerebrospinal fluid pressure-volume curve. Acta Neurologica Scandinavica, 49:575–585, 1973.

Marcal, PV, & Nickell, RE. Assessment of coma and impaired consciousness: A practical scale. Lancet, 2:81–84, 1973.

McLean, DE, Kaitz, ES, Keenan, CJ, Dabney, K, Cawley, MF, & Alexander, MA. Medical and surgical complications of pediatric brain injury. Journal of Head Trauma and Rehabilitation, 10:1–12, 1995.

Menkes, JH, & Till, K. Tumors of the nervous sytem. In Menkes, JH (Ed.), Textbook of Child Neurology. Philadelphia: Lea & Febiger, 1990, pp. 526–582.

Michaud, LJ, Duhaime, AC, & Batshaw, ML. Traumatic brain injury in children. Pediatric Clinics of North America, 40:553–565, 1993.

Pang, D. Pathophysiologic correlates of neurobehavioral syndromes following closed head injury. In Ylviasaker, M (Ed.), Head Injury Rehabilitation. Austin, TX: Pro-Ed, 1985, pp. 3–70.

Safar, P. Resuscitation from clinical death: Pathophysiologic limits and therapeutic potentials. Critical Care Medicine, 16:923–941, 1988.

Shiminsky-Maher, T, Abbott, R, Ursoff, JH, & Epstein, FJ. Current trends in the management of brainstem tumors in childhood. Journal of Neuroscience Nursing, 23:356–362, 1991.

Shumway-Cook, A, & Horak, FB. Assessing the influence of sensory interaction on balance: Suggestions from the field. Physical Therapy, 66:1548–1550, 1986.

Stroink, AR. Diagnosis and management of pediatric brain stem gliomas. Journal of Neurosurgery, 19:745–754, 1986.

Teasdale, G, & Jennett, B. Assessment of coma and impaired consciousness: A practical scale. Lancet, 2:81–84, 1974.

CHAPTER
23

Myelodysplasia

KATHLEEN A. HINDERER, PT, MS, MPT
STEVEN R. HINDERER, PT, MD, MS
DAVID B. SHURTLEFF, MD

Children and adolescents with myelodysplasia, perhaps more than most diagnostic groups of children with disabilities, challenge pediatric physical therapists to use and integrate many facets of their knowledge and skills. The multiple body systems affected by this congenital malformation make intervention of these patients highly complex, more than the congenital spinal cord defect alone might imply. Awareness of the many possible manifestations of this condition, knowledge of methods to examine and detect their presence, and the ability to evaluate the relative contribution of each manifestation to current functional limitations are important. This knowledge, combined with the ability to anticipate future needs and potential problems, empowers the physical therapist to select interventions that will optimize function and prevent the development of secondary impairment. Conversely,

621

lack of awareness of these issues is not without consequences. As significant secondary permanent impairments can result when clinicians are not aware of or do not recognize early signs and symptoms of preventable complications related to myelodysplasia.

The objectives of this chapter are to familiarize the physical therapist with the numerous manifestations of myelodysplasia; describe its impact on body systems and functional skills; provide developmental expectations and prognosis based on the level of involvement; outline the roles of the various disciplines involved in team management; discuss methods of examination, evaluation, and diagnosis; and highlight intervention strategies for specific problems.

GENERAL OVERVIEW

Types of Myelodysplasia

Dorland's Medical Dictionary defines *myelodysplasia* as "defective development of any part (especially the lower segments) of the spinal cord." The various types of myelodysplasia are illustrated in Figure 23-1. *Spina bifida* is a commonly used term referring to various forms of myelodysplasia. Spina bifida is classified into *aperta* (visible or open) lesions and *occulta* (hidden or not visible) lesions (Lemire et al., 1975). The degree of motor and sensory loss from these lesions can range from no apparent loss to severe impairment. Regardless of initial level of neurologic impairment, individuals with *any* of these lesions are at risk for further loss of function over time. Paralysis may occur later in life as a complication of abnormal tissue growth (dysplasia) causing pressure on nerves (e.g., lipomatous or dermoid tissue). Lack of proper growth of associated connective tissues around the malformed spinal cord can also cause ischemia and progressive neurologic impairment by tethering of the cord.

Spina bifida aperta is commonly thought of as *myelomeningocele,* which is an open spinal cord defect that usually protrudes dorsally. Myelomeningoceles are not skin covered and are usually associated with spinal nerve paralysis (see Fig. 23-1A and 23-1B). Meninges and nerves can also protrude anteriorly or laterally, making them not visible externally but still associated with nerve paralysis. Some individuals with myelomeningocele do not have associated paralysis.

Meningoceles are also classified as spina bifida aperta. They are skin covered and are initially associated with no paralysis (see Fig. 23-1C). Meningoceles contain only membranes or nonfunctional nerves that end in the sac wall (Lemire et al., 1975). Other

skin-covered lesions, however, can be associated with paralysis.

The next most common form of myelodysplasia is a *lipoma* of the spinal cord. Lipomas are classified as spina bifida occulta, but most are visible. They may be large or small and manifest as distinct, subcutaneous masses of fat, frequently associated with abnormal pigmentation of the skin, hirsutism, skin appendages, and dimples above the gluteal cleft. A lipomatous or fibrous tract descends ventrally from the subcutaneous lipoma to varying extents into the subdural space adjacent to the spinal cord. Lipomas of the spinal cord are therefore classified based on the location of the tract. They can be (1) lipomyelomeningoceles with paralysis, (2) lipomeningoceles with no paralysis, (3) lipomas of the filum terminale usually with no paralysis, (4) lipomas of the cauda equina or conus medullaris either with or without paralysis, and (5) myelolipomas that are lipomas within the dural sheath associated with paralysis. Some lipomas involving the spinal cord are not associated with an extension to subcutaneous fat. Lipomas of the spinal cord may or may not be associated with bifid vertebrae (true spina bifida).

Diastematomyelia is a fibrous, cartilaginous, or bony band or spicule separating the spinal cord into hemicords, each surrounded by a dural sac. It can occur as an isolated defect along with vertebral anomalies or in conjunction with either myelomeningocele or lipomyelomeningocele. Depending on the associated involvement of the spinal cord and meninges, diastematomyelia may be associated with paralysis initially, or progressive weakness can develop later in occulta lesions as a result of cord tethering.

The least common of the myelodysplasias are separate or septated cysts. These *myelocystoceles* are separate from the central canal of the spinal cord and from the subarachnoid space. They occur in the low lumbar and sacral area and are skin covered. They may or may not be associated with nerve impairment or lipomas of the spinal cord. When a myelocystocele is associated with a primitive gut and an open abdomen, it is classified as an *exstrophy of the cloaca.* When the bony elements of the sacrum are missing or abnormal, such myelocystic lesions are termed *sacral agenesis.*

Pathoembryology

Embryologically, myelodysplastic lesions can be related to two different processes of nervous system formation: abnormal neurulation or canalization. *Neurulation* is the folding of ectoderm (primitive skin and associated structures) on each side of the noto-

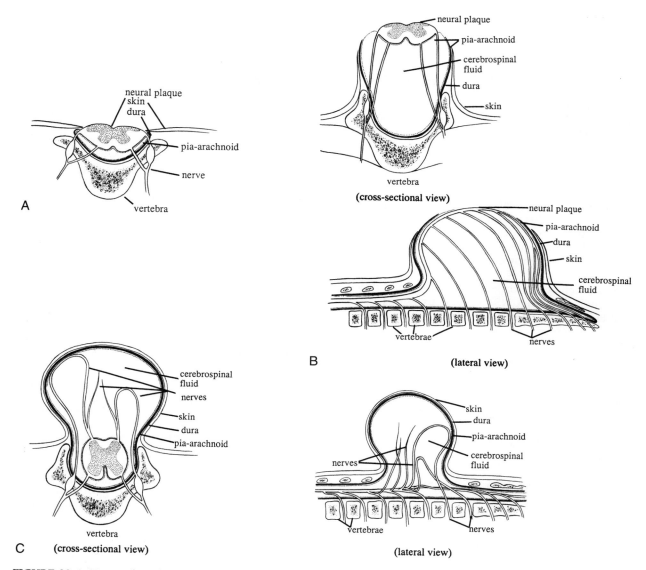

FIGURE 23–1. Types of myelodysplasia. *A*, An illustration of a *myelocele* with no cystic subarachnoid space anterior to the spinal cord as is observed with myelomeningocele. *B*, A *myelomeningocele* may barely protrude from the back or may be a large sessile lesion as pictured here. There is a covering membrane with nerves imbedded in the dome of the sac. These spinal nerves occasionally return to their appropriate neural foramina to exit from the spinal canal. *C*, This type of lesion may be incompletely covered or have a full-thickness skin covering as shown here. When such a lesion is completely skin covered and is associated with *no* paralysis, it is classified as a *meningocele*. Meningoceles have only a few or no nerves attached to the dome of the sac. (Adapted from Shurtleff, DB [Ed.]. Myelodysplasias and Exstrophies: Significance, Prevention, and Treatment. Orlando, FL: Grune & Stratton, 1986, pp. 44 and 45.)

chord (primitive spinal cord) to form a tube that extends from the hindbrain to the second sacral vertebra. Meningoceles can therefore occur both over the skull and along the spinal column. Encephaloceles (containing brain if along the midline of the skull) and myelomeningoceles, which can occur along the spinal canal from the C1 to S2 vertebrae, result from a failure of complete entubulation with associated abnormal mesodermal (primitive connective tissue, muscle, and nervous tissue) development. Abnormal mesodermal development produces epidermal sinus tracts, lipomas, and diastematomyelia, as well as unfused posterior vertebral laminae (i.e., true spina bifida) (Lemire et al., 1975). Neurulation occurs early in development, before day 28 of gestation.

The spinal cord distal to the S2 vertebra develops by *canalization*. Groups of cells in the dorsal, central midline of the mesoderm, distal to the S2 vertebra, become nerve cells. These cells clump together into masses, which develop cystic structures that join to form many canals. The canals ultimately fuse into one tubular structure that joins with the distal end of the spinal cord, which was developing from the neurulation process described previously. Failure of proper canalization, with subsequent retrogressive development of this region, embryologically explains the occurrence of skin-covered meningoceles, lipomas of the spinal cord, and myelocystoceles, all of which most frequently develop caudal to the L3 vertebra (Lemire et al., 1975).

The much better formed, essentially normal, central nervous system (CNS) observed in lesions associated with abnormal canalization and the frequency of CNS malformations (e.g., Arnold-Chiari type II, mental retardation, cranial nerve palsies, and hydrocephalus) associated with neurulation can be explained by the way that neurulation takes place. The neural crests first fuse at approximately the C1 vertebra, and closure of the neural tube progresses simultaneously in cephalad and caudal directions. The same embryologic neurulation processes are simultaneously forming the CNS from the tectal plate to the midlumbar area. It is therefore logical that an influence sufficient to interfere with neurulation along the spinal canal would also interfere with development of the cephalad end, producing CNS malformations above the spinal cord level, which are commonly exhibited in this population (Lemire et al., 1975). Because canalization occurs by different embryologic processes at a different time period than neurulation, any factor interfering with canalization will not necessarily affect neurulation, so the CNS forms normally above the midlumbar area.

Etiology

The cause of canalization disorders is unknown. This discussion therefore focuses on disorders of neurulation and, in particular, on myelomeningocele. These causes may also apply to other neural tube defects that can result from defective neurulation (anencephaly, encephalocele, meningocele, and lipomyelomeningocele, all with or without diastematomyelia). For brevity, we refer to all these lesions throughout this chapter as MM for *myelomeningocele* and its associated malformations (Shurtleff et al., 1986a).

Genetics

MM is often associated with genetic abnormalities, including chromosomal aberrations and other classic "syndromes." Each child born with MM, therefore, warrants a careful physical examination by a pediatrician because the "syndrome" is usually more important than the spinal lesion for defining prognosis. The recurrence risk for siblings in the United States is 2 to 3% (Shurtleff et al., 1986a).

The occurrence of MM varies among races and regions of the world. African blacks have the lowest incidence at 1 in 10,000. Celts (Eastern Irish, Western Scots, and all Welsh) had a birth incidence recorded as high as 1 in 80 in the recent past. The Spanish also have a high birth incidence; however, these patients have unusually good leg function and minimal CNS abnormalities considering their thoracic and high lumbar level lesions. Sikhs living in Vancouver, British Columbia, have another form of MM, with a higher frequency in birth incidence than many other genetically related groups. One can conclude from these data that either there are many different genetic causes for MM or that there are many different genetically determined responses to one or more teratogens (Shurtleff et al., 1986a).

Teratogens

Teratogens can cause MM. Excess maternal alcohol intake can produce a classic fetal alcohol syndrome with MM. Ingestion of valproic acid (an anticonvulsant medication) during pregnancy is also associated with an increased birth incidence of MM. Many other possible teratogens have been studied, but inadequate descriptions of the pathology of the lesions and the relative infrequency of their occurrence have resulted in inconclusive observations. The rachitic lesion illustrated by Jacobson and Berlin (1972) suggests that the MM they observed among progeny of street-drug abusers is a specific entity that is probably due to nutritional deprivation, teratogens, or a combination of these influences. More studies combining detailed family histories, pathologic anatomy, and detailed physical examinations must be conducted to determine the relative contribution of teratogens to MM formation (Shurtleff et al., 1986a).

Nutritional Deficiencies

Folic acid deficiency has been identified as a cause of MM in some populations. A significant decrease in the incidence of MM births and abortions was observed for MM diagnosed prenatally in the United Kingdom during a placebo-controlled trial of prenatal folic acid administration (CIBA, 1994; MRC

Vitamin Study Research Group, 1991). With the introduction of more foods containing folic acid in the Celtic regions of the United Kingdom, particularly during winter and early spring when potatoes are scarce (potatoes are high in folic acid and a staple of the diet in this region), there has been a decrease in the birth incidence of MM predating the research on folic acid supplementation (Elwood & Elwood, 1980). The decrease in birth incidence in the United Kingdom reflects a current worldwide trend. Conflicting reports raise the question of whether the European and United Kingdom studies regarding the benefit of supplementation of folic acid can be applied to the culturally and genetically more diverse population of the United States, where there are known racial and regional differences in the birth incidence of MM (Birth Defects and Genetic Diseases Branch of Birth Defects and Developmental Disabilities Office, 1991; Mills et al., 1989; Milunsky et al., 1989; Seller & Nevin, 1984). Regardless of the applicability of these studies to the population of the United States, we recommend advising women to take folic acid in an effort to reduce both the recurrence in families (MRC Vitamin Research Group, 1991) and the occurrence in families without a member with MM (Czeizel & Dudas, 1992). Women with a first-degree relative with MM or with history of having an open neural tube defect in a previous child or fetus should be advised to take 4 mg per day, and women without a positive history should be advised to take 0.4 mg per day. Both should begin the folic acid at least 3 months before conception. Folic acid is believed to be harmless in this age group because the only possible concern is the masking of pernicious anemia due to cobalamin deficiency allowing progression of the subacute combined degeneration of the spinal cord resulting from cobalamin deficiency. Cobalamin deficiency is rare in this age group, and awareness of the possibility of neurologic loss from spinal cord degeneration should lead to early detection before significant harm occurs. The only other precaution is to warn the women that taking folic acid reduces their risk by 70% but does not eliminate the occurrence of open neural tube defects and has no known effect on the occurrence of closed neural tube defects.

Incidence and Prevalence

Superimposed on a general worldwide decrease in the birth incidence of MM are a number of influences to cause both a reduction in birth incidence and increased prevalence. Better nutrition mentioned earlier for the Celtic region of the United Kingdom and Ireland applies to many areas of the industrialized world. Wider availability of maternal serum alpha-fetoprotein screening and more highly refined resolution of diagnostic ultrasonography for fetal examination have given parents an option to terminate pregnancies because their fetus has MM (Main & Mennuti, 1986; Nyberg et al., 1988). Conversely, prenatal diagnosis has allowed other parents to select prelabor caesarean section, avoiding trauma to the neural sac from vaginal delivery. The outcome of prelabor caesarean delivery has been children with less paralysis and with minimal risk for CNS infection, both of which were previously a cause for increased morbidity and early death (Luthy et al., 1991). Improved medical care has allowed for increased survival and, secondarily, an increased prevalence. Incidence at birth in the United States has been reported to range from 0.4 to 0.9 per 1000 births, depending on the reporting source (Shurtleff et al., 1986a).

Diagnostic Techniques

The past decade has altered the intervention of MM from a postnatal crisis of horrendous magnitude to a prenatal option of either pregnancy termination or improved pregnancy outcome by prelabor caesarean section birth. This advance has been made possible by widespread use of maternal serum alpha-fetoprotein screening and improved resolution of ultrasonography (Main & Mennuti, 1986). Unfortunately, this type of screening will not detect skin-covered neural defects such as meningoceles or canalization defects distal to the S2 vertebra.

Technical improvements are being made rapidly in ultrasonography so that minor variations in the frontal bones of the fetus and encapsulation of the midbrain by the cerebellum can be interpreted as the "lemon" and "banana" signs (Nyberg et al., 1988). These ultrasonographic signs are more accurate in defining the cranial malformations associated with MM than in detecting abnormalities of the spine. As discussed in the section on pathoembryology, these ultrasonographic signs are pertinent to neural tube defects cephalad to the S2 vertebra (i.e., neurulation defects) but not to canalization defects, which are usually not associated with cranial malformations responsible for the Arnold-Chiari type II malformation (Shurtleff, 1986e), the cause of the "lemon" and "banana" signs. Some spinal dysraphic states and dorsal lumbosacral masses consistent with canalization defects such as myelocystocele or lipomyelomeningocele can be identified with ultrasonography. Other anomalies consistent with syndromes or organ malformations that are incompatible with survival beyond intrauterine life (e.g., anencephaly) can also be detected.

A third modality for prenatal diagnosis, amniotic fluid analysis, is critical in the evaluation of a fetus with a neural tube defect. Up to 10% of fetuses with a neural tube defect, detected in the first half of the second trimester or before, have an associated chromosome error, usually trisomy 13 or 18 (Luthy et al., 1991). Chromosome analysis of amniotic cells is therefore essential to the parental decision-making process regarding abortion of the pregnancy. From the same amniotic fluid specimen obtained for chromosome analysis, the acetylcholinesterase level can be determined. This test is more accurate than determination of the amniotic fluid level of alpha-fetoprotein used previously because the former is positive only in a fetus with an open neural tube defect (Main & Mennuti, 1986). The presence of a dorsal spine lesion and a negative result of an acetylcholinesterase test suggest a skin-covered meningocele or other skin-covered MM, which is an indication for normal vaginal delivery. An MM lesion containing nerves protruding dorsal to the plane of the back, in the presence of fetal knee or ankle function observed on ultrasonography, warrants prelabor caesarean section, sterile delivery, and closure of the open-back lesion to preserve nerve function (Luthy et al., 1991).

IMPAIRMENTS

The discussions of pathoembryology and diagnosis describe the potential involvement of the brain and brainstem in addition to the spinal cord in individuals with MM. The multifocal involvement of the CNS results in several possible complex problems, making the care of these individuals more challenging than and substantially different from that of children with traumatic spinal cord injuries. The broad spectrum of problems encountered with MM requires a multidisciplinary team approach in a comprehensive care outpatient clinic setting. In this section the variety of impairments that can occur with MM are described. In addition, general examination and intervention issues related to each impairment are discussed. *Impairment,* for the purpose of this discussion, is defined as an abnormality of body system functions, whereas *functional limitation* is the inability to perform functional tasks as a consequence of impairments. Functional limitations and disabilities encountered at specific age levels, along with age-specific examination, evaluation, and intervention issues, are discussed in subsequent sections of this chapter.

Musculoskeletal Deformities

Spinal and lower limb deformities and joint contractures occur frequently in children with MM.

Orthopedic deformities and joint contractures negatively affect positioning, body image, weight bearing (both in sitting and standing), activities of daily living (ADL), energy expenditure, and mobility from infancy through adulthood. Several factors contribute to abnormal posture, limb deformity, and joint contractures, including muscle imbalance secondary to neurologic dysfunction, progressive neurologic dysfunction, intrauterine positioning, coexisting congenital malformations, arthrogryposis, habitually assumed postures after birth, reduced or absent active joint motion, and deformities after fractures (Mayfield, 1991; Shurtleff, 1986d). The upper limbs can also be involved as a result of spasticity or poor postural habits. The upper limb region most likely to have restricted motion is the shoulder girdle due to overuse of the arms for weight bearing and poor postural habits.

Postural stability is essential to effectively perform functional tasks. Symmetric alignment is important to minimize joint stress and deforming forces and to permit muscles to function at their optimal length. Uncorrected postural deficits can result in joint contractures and deformities, stretch weakness, and musculoskeletal pain. Deficits that may appear insignificant during childhood often become magnified once an individual has adult body proportions, resulting in functional limitations and discomfort (e.g., low back pain resulting from an increased lumbar lordosis and hip flexion contractures). Consequently, limb, neck, and trunk range of motion (ROM), muscle extensibility, and joint alignment should be monitored throughout the life span so that appropriate interventions can be implemented as indicated.

Typical postural problems include forward head, rounded shoulders, kyphosis, scoliosis, excessive lordosis, anterior pelvic tilt, rotational deformities of the hip or tibia (in-toeing, out-toeing, or windswept positions), flexed hips and knees, and pronated feet. It is important to observe posture and postural control after a given position has been maintained for a period of time to determine the effects of fatigue. Static and dynamic balance should be observed in sitting, four-point positioning, kneeling, half-kneeling, and standing, as well as during transitions between these positions. Symmetry and weight distribution should also be noted. In addition, typical sleeping and sitting positions should be identified to determine if habitual positioning is contributing to postural or joint deformities (e.g., "frog-leg" position in prone or supine, W-sitting, ring sitting, heel sitting, cross-legged sitting, and crouch standing). These habitual positions should be avoided because they may produce deforming forces and altered musculotendon length that result in the development of secondary impairments such as the progression of orthopedic deformities, joint contractures, and strength deficits. Photographs or videotapes of sitting and standing postures are often useful to document current status and to provide a visual baseline for future reference.

Postural deviations and contractures that are typical for individual lesion levels are summarized as follows. Individuals with high-level lesions (thoracic to L2) often have knee flexion, abduction, and external rotation contractures, knee flexion contractures, and ankle plantar flexion contractures. The lumbar spine is typically lordotic. Individuals with mid- to low-lumbar (L3–L5) lesion levels often have hip and knee flexion contractures, an increased lumbar lordosis, genu and calcaneal valgus malalignment, and a pronated position of the foot when bearing weight. They often walk with a pronounced crouched gait and bear weight primarily on their calcaneus. Individuals with sacral level lesions often have mild hip and knee flexion contractures and an increased lumbar lordosis, and the ankle and foot can either be in varus or valgus, combined with a pronated or supinated forefoot. They may walk with a mild crouch gait and may bear weight primarily on their calcaneus unless plantar flexor muscles are at least grade 3/5.

Crouch standing is a typical postural deviation that is observed across lesion levels and is characterized by persistent hip and knee flexion and an increased lumbar lordosis. The crouch posture often occurs because of muscle weakness (e.g., insufficient soleus strength to maintain the tibia vertical) and orthopedic deformities (e.g., calcaneal valgus, which results in obligatory tibial internal rotation and knee flexion). Hip and knee flexion contractures often occur secondarily, in response to adaptive shortening of muscles from prolonged positioning in the crouch-standing posture. Altered postures, such as crouch standing, may negatively affect both the task requirements (by increasing the muscle torque required to maintain the position) and the torque-generating capacity of the musculoskeletal system. It is important that appropriate intervention be implemented to ameliorate crouch standing so that the excessive physical demands and stress placed on the musculoskeletal system are reduced and the development of secondary impairments is prevented.

Scoliosis occurring with MM can be congenital or acquired; the congenital form is usually related to underlying vertebral anomalies and the curve is often inflexible, whereas the acquired type is usually caused by muscle imbalance and the curve is flexible until skeletal maturity is reached (Mayfield, 1991), at which point little further progression is usually observed (Shurtleff, 1986d). Scoliosis is more frequently observed in higher lesion level groups and

becomes more prevalent and increasingly severe with age in all groups (Mayfield, 1991).

Orthotic intervention, usually with a bivalved Silastic thoracolumbosacral body orthosis, is helpful in maintaining improved trunk position for functional activities but does not prevent progression of acquired spinal deformity (Mayfield, 1991). For children with progressive spinal deformities, orthotic intervention is continued until the child reaches a sufficient age to allow surgical fusion of the spine to prevent further progression of these deformities. Long spinal fusions before the skeletal age of 10 result in greater loss of trunk height because of ablation of the growth plates of vertebral bodies included in the fusion mass (Mayfield, 1991). In addition, surgery at too young a skeletal age is associated with an increased frequency of instrumentation failure as a result of fragile bones and skin breakdown over the bulky spinal instrumentation (Mayfield, 1991). The ideal minimum age for spinal fusion is 10 to 11 years old in girls and 12 to 13 years old in boys (Mayfield, 1991). In general, children with spina bifida reach puberty and their growth spurt earlier than their able-bodied peers, so only minimal truncal shortening occurs as a consequence of long spinal fusion when it is performed at the appropriate age.

Other spinal deformities that can occur in conjunction with, or separate from, scoliosis are kyphosis and lordosis deformities (Fig. 23–2). Kyphosis can occur in the lumbar spine with reversal of the lumbar lordosis, or the kyphosis can be more diffusely distributed over the entire spine. Hyperlordosis of the lumbar spine is another commonly observed deformity. Like scoliosis, both kyphosis and lordosis are more commonly observed in children with higher spinal lesions and the curves tend to progress with age (Mayfield, 1991). Severe kyphosis and scoliosis can limit chest wall expansion with consequent restriction of lung ventilation and frequent respiratory infections. This restrictive lung disease can limit exercise tolerance and can be life threatening in extreme cases (Mayfield, 1991).

Hip joints also are prone to deformity in children with MM. Children with high lumbar lesions (L1, L2) have unopposed flexion and adduction forces that gradually push the femoral head superiorly and posteriorly. The resulting contractures and secondary bony deformities of the proximal femur and acetabulum can lead to subluxation or dislocation (Fig. 23–3).

In children with hip subluxation or dislocation, long-term follow-up studies have indicated that reduction of the hips is not a prerequisite for ambulation. Mayfield (1991) states that a level pelvis and a good ROM are more important for function than hip reduction. Furthermore, he states that the

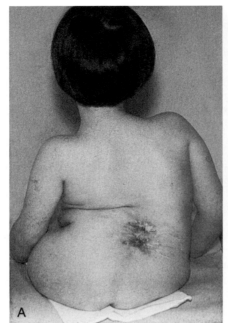
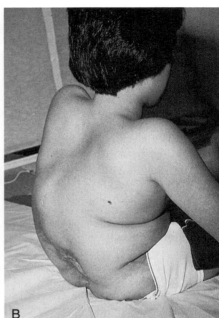

FIGURE 23–2. Spinal deformities. *A*, Collapsing type of lordoscoliosis. *B*, Kyphotic spinal deformity.

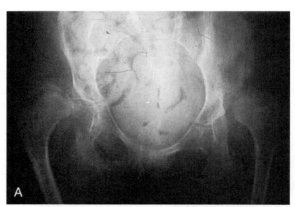
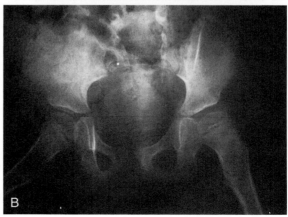

FIGURE 23–3. Lower limb deformities. *A*, Hip dislocation. *B*, Hip dysplasia and subluxation.

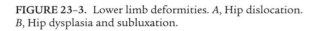

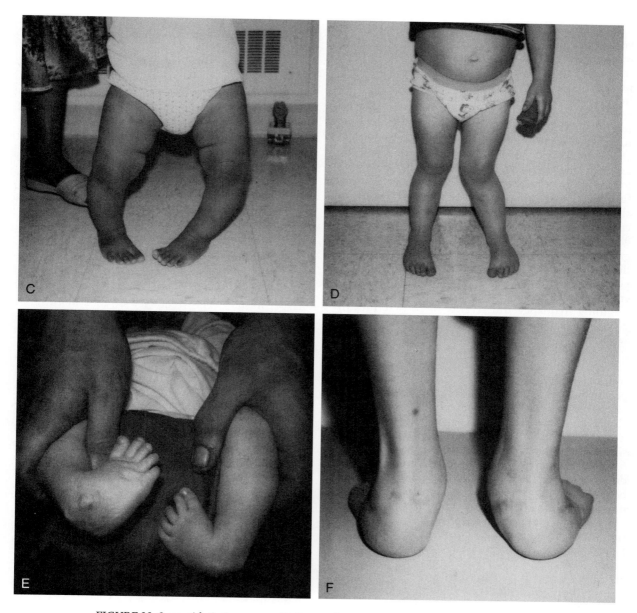

FIGURE 23–3, cont'd *C,* Genu varus. *D,* Genu valgus. *E,* Equinovarus. *F,* Calcaneal valgus.

presence of the femoral head in the acetabulum does not necessarily improve ROM at the hip or the ability to ambulate. In addition, unlike in children with cerebral palsy, it does not appear to affect the amount of orthotic support required, hip pain, or gait deviation (Ryan et al., 1991). The indications for hip surgery in children with MM continue to be controversial; however, a basic principle practiced at many centers is to operate only on children with a lesion level at or below L3, when quadriceps muscle function is present, because these children are more

likely to be functional ambulators into adulthood (Mayfield, 1991; Shurtleff, 1986d). An asymmetric pelvis caused by unilateral subluxation or dislocation, which interferes with sitting or standing posture and contributes to scoliosis, is another potential indication for surgical relocation of the hip, regardless of lesion level or ambulatory potential.

Shurtleff (1986d) evaluated the frequency of all types of hip contractures in large numbers of children with various spinal lesion level groups. He noted that contractures measured in infancy tended to decrease in severity until approximately age 3 to 4 years, then increased to much higher values by adolescence. The initial decrease in severity of hip contractures can potentially be explained as a normal physiologic phenomenon resulting from intrauterine positioning. The increase in severity of contractures by adolescence, however, is of special concern to physical therapists. Mild contractures of minimal functional significance in young children can increase dramatically during later childhood and adolescence, necessitating persistent intervention and follow-up by the therapist to prevent significant functional loss. Consequently, physical therapists should be proactive in preventing the progression of contractures. Thoracic and high lumbar (L1, L2) groups of children have a higher incidence and greater severity of contractures owing to unopposed iliopsoas function, regardless of whether they were participating in a standing program or not (Liptak et al., 1992). Shurtleff (1986d) reports progressively declining frequency and severity of contractures in groups of children with lesions at L3, L4 to L5, and sacral levels, respectively. An unexpected finding from Shurtleff's study was that only a certain percentage of children in each lesion level group had hip contractures, subluxation, or both. These relative percentages were not altered by surgical procedures on the hip and stayed constant across age groups. No clear reasons were discerned why certain individuals were susceptible to contractures while others with similar neurologic function were not.

The knee joints frequently have contractures or deformities in children with MM. These include both flexion and extension contractures; the former more commonly occur in children who primarily use a wheelchair for mobility (Liptak et al., 1992), and the latter often occur after periods of immobility from fractures, decubitus ulcers, or surgical procedures. Varus and valgus deformities (see Fig. 23–3) are also observed. As described earlier for the hip joints, Shurtleff (1986d) studied the frequency of knee contractures and deformities in children with different lesion levels. An initial decrease from the contractures measured in infants was also noted at the knees, with the lowest prevalence occurring at age 4 to 5 years for patients with L3 or higher lesions, and at age 2 to 3 years for children with lesions below L3. The frequency and severity of contractures increased in all groups from early childhood into adolescence. Knee joint contractures occurred in 65 to 70% of the thoracic and high lumbar groups by age 6 to 8, 20 to 25% of the L4 to L5 group by age 9 to 12, and sporadically among the children with sacral level lesions. Valgus and varus deformities were most frequently observed in the L3 and above groups, with a slight increase during adolescence.

Deformities of the ankles and feet can occur in both ambulatory and nonambulatory children and are most common in children with lesion levels at L5 and above (Shurtleff, 1986d). Partial innervation and consequent muscle imbalance determine the type of deformity that occurs. Even with surgical correction these deformities will recur unless the deforming forces are removed. Progressive ankle and foot deformities can also be observed in conjunction with the development of spasticity and motor strength loss associated with tethering of the spinal cord. Children with "skip" lesions (see section on motor paralysis) are particularly prone to progressive foot deformities (Shurtleff, 1986d).

A variety of foot and ankle deformities can occur (see Fig. 23–3), including ankle equinovarus (clubfeet), forefoot varus or valgus, forefoot supination or pronation, calcaneal varus or valgus, pes cavus and planus, and claw-toe deformities. The most frequent contracture observed is of the ankle plantar flexor muscles. The frequency of foot deformities varies from 20 to 50% between lesion level groups (Shurtleff, 1986d). Although some deformities are more frequently associated with certain neurosegmental levels (e.g., clubfeet in thoracic and high lumbar lesions, claw-toes in sacral lesions), all types of ankle and foot deformities are observed in children at every lesion level. The presence of ankle and foot deformities can greatly affect sitting and standing posture, balance, mobility, and shoe fit, regardless of lesion level. Weight-bearing forces often result in ankle and foot deformities. Even partial weight bearing on wheelchair footrests in poor alignment over time can result in deformities and even in decubiti. Consequently, achieving a plantigrade position of the feet is a priority, regardless of ambulatory status. Orthoses and assistive devices should be adjusted properly to maintain neutral subtalar alignment and a plantigrade foot position.

Torsional deformities are common. Excessive foot progression angles and windswept positions of the lower limbs are often present (Fig. 23–4) as a result of hip anteversion, hip retroversion, or tibial torsion. These torsional deformities negatively affect sitting and standing balance, weight distribution, and walking. See Cusick and Stuberg (1992) for factors that contribute to torsional deformities in individuals with developmental disabilities, examination procedures, normative values, and intervention suggestions.

Joint alignment and evidence of abnormal joint stress are often most apparent during dynamic activities, such as walking or wheelchair propulsion. Joint stresses are often magnified when walking on uneven surfaces, stairs, or curbs. Observing wear patterns on shoes and orthoses can provide additional clues to

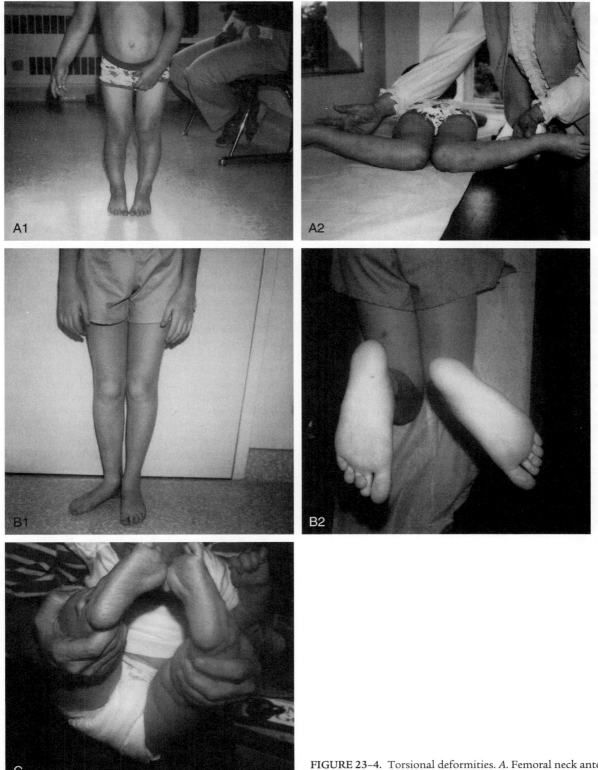

FIGURE 23–4. Torsional deformities. *A.* Femoral neck ante-version. *B.* External tibial torsion. *C,* Internal tibial torsion.

abnormal stress and malalignment. If joint deformities are supple, they may respond to stretching, combined with orthoses or positioning splints to maintain alignment. Fixed deformities may respond to serial casting (e.g., foot deformities) but will often require surgical intervention (e.g., scoliosis, unilateral hip dislocation, or tibial torsion). If muscle imbalance is severe and the deforming forces are not effectively counteracted by stretching, strengthening, or positioning, muscle transfers may be indicated (e.g., partial transfer of the anterior tibialis muscle to the calcaneus to achieve a plantigrade foot position by balancing the unopposed dorsiflexion force in a child with L5 motor function).

There are several reasons for maintaining joint ROM. Limited ROM can interfere with ADL, bed mobility, and transfers. Bed mobility is more efficient and self-care is easier for individuals who have maintained their flexibility (Hinderer & Hinderer, 1988). Restricted ROM, combined with muscle weakness, can result in poor postural habits and gait deviations. Adequate ROM must be maintained to perform ADL, such as bathing and toileting. Restricted joint motion can result in overlengthening of weak muscles, not permitting them to function in the optimal range of the length-tension curve. Limited ROM may result in discomfort, especially when lying down (e.g., tight hip flexors pulling on the lumbar spine). Severe contractures also can negatively affect body image. Contractures that may seem insignificant during childhood may become functionally limiting once the individual has adult-sized body proportions (e.g., knee extension contractures can interfere with the ability to maneuver in a wheelchair). In extreme cases, difficulty in managing paralyzed limbs because of joint contractures can put individuals at risk for skin breakdown and possibly amputations because of the increased incidence of injury (Hinderer et al., 1988). The impact of limited ROM on functional performance should be considered before deciding whether intervention is indicated.

ROM and positioning of paralytic limbs should be done carefully, without excessive force, to avoid fractures (Schneider, 1985). Caution should also be exercised when adducting the hips to avoid hip dislocation. The prone hip extension test (Staheli, 1977) for measuring hip extension is the method of choice in this population because of interference of spinal and pelvic deformities and lower limb spasticity with the traditional Thomas test method (Bartlett et al., 1985). Ankle ROM should always be measured with the ankle joint in subtalar neutral so that measurements are comparable.

There are several ways to minimize musculoskeletal stress and reduce the incidence of acquired orthopedic deformities. Improving traction of the hands by providing biking gloves for community wheelchair mobility reduces the grip forces required for wheelchair propulsion. Wheelchair seat positions influence propulsion effectiveness and the amount of stress on upper limb joints and muscles (Masse et al., 1992). For ambulators, shoes with nonskid soles improve foot traction. Symmetric neutral joint alignment should be maintained in both sitting and standing via appropriate orthotics or seating devices. It is important to avoid shifting weight to one leg when standing and to avoid crossing the legs when sitting. Extreme ROM should be avoided, especially when bearing weight. Crutch and walker handgrips should be angled to avoid hyperextension of the wrists, and weight should be distributed across a broad, cushioned area. Orthoses should provide total contact to minimize the risk of development of pressure areas. Excessive pressure on tendons and the palms of the hand should be avoided to reduce the risk of developing carpal tunnel syndrome. Overhead reaching and work activities should be minimized by adapting the home, school, and work environments. In addition, long-distance mobility options should be provided to reduce joint stresses. When sitting, weight bearing should be symmetric, pelvic tilt should be neutral with a slight lumbar lordosis, the hips and knees should be at 90°, and the feet should be flat on the floor. Good lumbar support should be provided. Inclining the seat backward 15° minimizes stress on the lumbar spine and helps keep the pelvis seated back in the chair (Chaffin, Andersson & Martin, 1999). Tilting the desk or table top upward improves the position of the upper trunk, head, and shoulders.

Osteoporosis

Decreased bone mineral density, thought to be secondary to hypotonic or flaccid musculature combined with decreased loading of long bones from altered mobility, is frequently observed in children with MM and often results in osteoporotic fractures. Stuberg (1992) suggests that standing programs are beneficial for children with developmental disabilities. He reports that the use of a standing program (60 minutes four or five times per week) appears to increase bone mineral density and enhance acetabular development in children with cerebral palsy. These issues must be studied further in the MM population, however. Bone responses in children with flaccid paralysis may be quite different. Rosenstein and associates (1987) examined this issue in the MM population and reported that bone mineral density was 38 to 44% higher in household or community ambulators compared with nonfunctional ambulators (exercise-only ambulators or nonambulators). Because the effects of lesion level were not controlled in this study, the potential contribution of muscle activity versus weight-bearing status to the differences in bone mineral density cannot be determined. In addition, neither study addressed the issue of reduction of the incidence of osteoporotic fractures.

Studying the frequency of fractures is a more direct and clinically significant method of examining the benefits of standing programs. Shurtleff (1986d) asked the question, "Are fractures less common among those patients in standing or ambulatory programs than among similarly paralyzed sedentary peers?" Asher and Olson (1983) showed no correlation between fractures and the use of wheelchairs. DeSouza and Carroll (1976) reported no fractures in 7 nonambulators and 38 fractures in 16 ambulators. Their data imply that exposure to forces that can produce fractures (i.e., upright mobility) is the important risk factor for fractures, rather than the level of flaccid paralysis, as would be expected. Liptak and associates (1992) found no difference in the frequency of fractures between a group of children who were wheelchair users and a comparable group of children who ambulated with orthoses. Clinically, the use of standing frames, parapodiums, or hip-knee-ankle-foot orthoses (HKAFOs) in children with high lumbar and thoracic lesions does not appear warranted for the purpose of fracture prevention. For children with lower lumbar and sacral lesion levels, for whom upright positioning and mobility is an important functional skill, undue restriction of physical activity for fear of a fracture is not indicated. The fact that passive weight bearing does not decrease the risk of fractures in these children makes sense if one considers that bone density is more likely maintained by torque generated from volitional muscle activity. Active muscle contraction generates forces through the long bones that are several times greater than the forces from passive weight bearing.

Motor Paralysis

The inherently obvious manifestation of MM is the paraplegia resulting from the spinal cord malformation. Upper limb weakness can also occur in this population, regardless of lesion level, and is often a sign of progressive neurologic dysfunction. Knowledge of the motor lesion level is useful for predicting associated abnormalities and for prognostication of functional outcome. A detailed discussion regarding developmental and functional expectations for each motor lesion level is provided later in the section on determinants of outcome and prognosis. Strategies for assessing strength and planning intervention programs to enhance motor function are provided in the section on age-specific examination and physical therapy intervention strategies.

The motor level is defined as the lowest intact, functional neuromuscular segment. For example, an L4 level indicates that the fourth lumbar nerve and the myotome it innervates are functioning, whereas segments below L4 are not intact. Table 23-1 provides the International Myelodysplasia Study Group (IMSG) criteria for assigning motor levels from manual muscle strength test results (IMSG, 1993). The IMSG criteria have been shown to best reflect the innervation patterns of individuals with MM as opposed to other spinal segment classification systems. MM spinal lesions can be asymmetric when motor or sensory function of the right and left sides of the body are compared. Consequently, motor function should be classified individually for the right and left sides.

Neuromuscular involvement of individuals with MM may manifest in one of three ways: (1) lesions resembling complete cord transection, (2) incomplete lesions, and (3) skip lesions (Shurtleff, 1986d). Lesions resembling complete cord transection manifest as normal function down to a particular level, below which there is flaccid paralysis, loss of sensation, and absent reflexes. Incomplete lesions have a mixed manifestation of spasticity and volitional control. Skip lesions are also observed, where more caudal segments are functioning despite the presence of one or more nonfunctional segments interposed between the intact more cephalad spinal segments. Individual skip motor lesions manifest either with isolated function of muscles noted below the last functional level of the lesion or with inadequate strength of muscle groups that have innervation higher than the lowest functioning group (Patient Data Management System, 1994). Consequently, it is important to evaluate muscles with lower innervation than the last functional level to determine whether a skip lesion exists. The presence of spasticity and reflexes should also be carefully documented.

McDonald and associates (1991b) demonstrated that muscle strength grades for the gluteus medius and medial hamstring muscles correlate more highly with strength grades of the hip adductors, hip flexors, and knee extensors than lower limb anterior compartment muscles that have been previously described as being innervated by the L4, L5, and sacral nerve roots. These data potentially explain the clinical observation that individuals with MM often have functional strength in the gluteus medius and medial hamstrings, despite having weak or nonactive lower limb anterior compartment muscles. It was concluded from this study that it is more useful clinically to group individuals with MM by the

TABLE 23–1. International Myelodysplasia Study Group Criteria for Assigning Motor Levels

Motor Level	Criteria for Assigning Motor Levels
T10 or above	Determined by sensory level and/or palpation of abdominal muscles.
T11	
T12	Some pelvic control is present in sitting or supine (this may come from the abdominals or paraspinal muscles). Hip hiking from the quadratus lumborum may also be present.
L1	Weak iliopsoas muscle function is present (grade 2).
L1–L2	Exceeds criteria for L1 but does not meet L2 criteria.*
L2	Iliopsoas, sartorius, and the hip adductors all must be grade 3 or better.
L3	Meets or exceeds the criteria for L2 *plus* the quadriceps are grade 3 or better.
L3–L4	Exceeds criteria for L3 but does not meet L4 criteria.
L4	Meets or exceeds the criteria for L3 and the medial hamstrings *or* the tibialis anterior is grade 3 or better. A weak peroneus tertius may also be seen.
L4–L5	Exceeds criteria for L4 but does not meet L5 criteria.
L5	Meets or exceeds the criteria for L4 and has lateral hamstring strength of grade 3 or better *plus one* of the following: gluteus medius grade 2 or better, peroneus tertius grade 4 or better, or tibialis posterior grade 3 or better.
L5–S1	Exceeds criteria for L5 but does not meet S1 criteria.
S1	Meets or exceeds the criteria for L5 *plus at least two* of the following: gastrocnemius/soleus grade 2 or better, gluteus medius grade 3 or better, or gluteus maximus grade 2 or better (can pucker the buttocks).
S1–2	Exceeds criteria for S1 but does not meet S2 criteria.
S2	Meets or exceeds the criteria for S1, the gastrocnemius/soleus must be grade 3 or better, *and* gluteus medius and maximus are grade 4 or better.
S2–3	All of the lower limb muscle groups are of normal strength (may be grade 4 in one or two groups). Also includes normal-appearing infants who are too young to be bowel and bladder trained (see "no loss").
"No loss"	Meets all of the criteria for S2–S3 *and* has no bowel or bladder dysfunction.

*When description states "meets criteria . . .," strength of muscles listed for preceding levels should be increasing respectively.

Adapted with permission from Patient Data Management System. Myelodysplasia Study Data Collection Criteria and Instructions, 1994. (Available from D.B. Shurtleff, MD, Professor, Dept. of Pediatrics, Univ. of Washington, Seattle, WA 98195.)

strength of specific muscle groups, as outlined in Table 23–1, rather than by traditional neurosegmental levels.

Sensory Deficits

Sensory deficits are often not clear-cut in this population, because sensory levels often do not correlate with motor levels and there may be skip areas that lack sensation. Because skip areas can occur within a given dermatome, it is important to test all dermatomes and multiple sites within a given dermatome to have an accurate baseline examination. Deficits should be recorded on a dermatome chart with areas of absent and decreased sensation color coded for the various sensory modalities (e.g., light touch, pinprick, vibration, and thermal). Proprioception and kinesthetic sense should also be evaluated in both the upper and lower extremities.

Based on the results of a study conducted on 30 adults with MM, testing with both light touch and pinprick stimuli is not necessary in this population because there is little discriminating value for detecting insensate areas (Hinderer & Hinderer, 1990). In contrast, vibratory stimuli could be felt one dermatome below light touch and pinprick sensation. Based on these results, vibration sensation should be

evaluated in addition to either light touch or pinprick sensation.

It is important for individuals with MM to be aware of their sensory deficits and to be taught techniques to compensate by substituting other sensory modalities (e.g., vision). The impact of decreased sensation on safety should be emphasized, especially when checking temperature (e.g., bath water or when sitting near a fireplace) and when barefoot. Skin inspection and pressure relief techniques should be taught early so that they are incorporated into the daily routine. The importance of pressure relief cushions and sitting push-ups for pressure relief should be emphasized. Proper intervention of lower limbs and joint protection techniques should be taught when learning how to perform ADL, such as transfers.

The impact of sensory deficits on functional performance should be kept in mind when teaching functional tasks. Individuals with MM may rely heavily on vision to compensate for sensory deficits (Shaffer et al., 1986). They may lack kinesthetic acuity that permits subconscious completion of many repetitive motor tasks. Consequently, visual attention may not be available to be directed at other factors in the environment (Andersen & Plewis, 1977). Adding small amounts of weight to the ankles

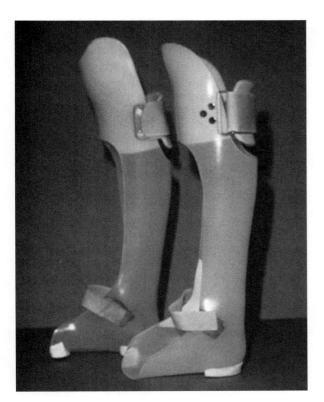

FIGURE 23–5. Ground-reaction ankle-foot orthosis. Polypropylene patellar tendon–bearing ground-reaction ankle-foot orthoses molded with the foot in a subtalar neutral position. Note the zero heel posts and posts under the first metatarsal heads.

or a walker may enhance proprioceptive awareness and facilitate gait training. Use of patellar tendon–bearing orthoses (Fig. 23–5) instead of traditional ankle-foot orthoses (AFOs) may also facilitate foot placement for individuals with innervation through L3 because the orthosis contacts the skin in an area of intact sensation.

Hydrocephalus

Hydrocephalus is excessive accumulation of cerebrospinal fluid (CSF) in the ventricles of the brain. Approximately 25% or more of children with MM are born with hydrocephalus. An additional 60% develop it after surgical closure of their back lesion (Reigel, 1993). If left untreated, the continued expansion of the ventricles can cause loss of cerebral cortex with additional cognitive and functional impairment. Cerebellar hypoplasia with caudal displacement of the hindbrain through the foramen magnum, known as the Arnold-Chiari type II malformation, is usually associated with hydrocephalus.

The hydrocephalus will occasionally arrest spon-

BOX 23–1. **Early Warning Signs and Symptoms of Shunt Dysfunction**
Changes in speech
Fever and malaise
Recurring headache
Decreased activity level
Decreased school performance
Onset of or increased strabismus
Changes in appetite and weight
Incontinence begins or worsens
Onset or worsening of scoliosis
Onset of or increased spasticity
Personality change (irritability)
Decreased or static grip strength
Difficult to arouse in the morning
Decreased visuomotor coordination
Decreased visual acuity or diplopia
Decreased visuoperceptual coordination
Onset or increased frequency of seizures

Adapted with permission from Shurtleff, DB, Stuntz, JT, & Hayden, P. Hydrocephalus. In Shurtleff, DB (Ed.), Myelodysplasias and Exstrophies: Significance, Prevention, and Treatment. Orlando, FL: Grune & Stratton, 1986, p. 142.

taneously; however, 80 to 90% of children with hydrocephalus will require a CSF shunt (Shurtleff et al., 1986b). A ventriculoperitoneal catheter shunts excess CSF from the lateral ventricles of the brain to the peritoneal space, where the CSF is resorbed. Because a shunt is a foreign body, it can be a nidus for infection or can become obstructed, requiring neurosurgical intervention. Repeated or prolonged shunt dysfunction and infections often lead to additional functional and cognitive decline of the child. Shunt dysfunction is often gradual, with subtle symptoms. Therapists should be familiar with these symptoms to facilitate early detection and appropriate referral to a physician for further evaluation. Box 23–1 provides a list of early symptoms and signs of shunt obstruction. Of particular interest are the findings of Kilburn and associates (1985), which suggest that static or declining grip strength measurements are potentially an early indicator of neurologic dysfunction such as shunt malfunction or symptomatic Arnold-Chiari malformation. Hydrocephalus persists throughout life with consequent need of ongoing follow-up by a physician who is familiar with the medical complications associated with MM.

Cognitive Dysfunction

Early closure of spinal lesions with antibiotic intervention to prevent meningitis and improved CSF shunt intervention have increased the expected cognitive function of children born with MM. The majority of children without hydrocephalus or with uncomplicated hydrocephalus (no infections or cerebral hemorrhage) will have intellect falling within the normal range on intelligence testing. The distribution of scores tends to be skewed toward the upper and lower ends of normal, however, with fewer children scoring in the middle of the curve and a greater proportion scoring at the lower end of the range (Shaffer et al., 1986). The intellectual performance of children who have had significant CNS infections is lower than those who have not had infection (Shurtleff et al., 1986b). Intelligence scores tend to be higher in lumbar and sacral lesion level groups than in thoracic lesion level groups (Shaffer et al., 1986). Verbal subtest scores usually exceed performance subtest scores (Shaffer et al., 1986). The poorer scores on performance subtests, however, may not represent true differences in verbal versus nonverbal reasoning skills. Instead, these differences can potentially be explained by upper limb dyscoordination (discussed later) and by memory deficits (Shaffer et al., 1986). Dyscoordination and memory deficits are manifested as distractibility on subtests assessing acquired knowledge (e.g., arithmetic), integrated right-left hemisphere function (e.g., picture arrangement, block design, and coding), speed of motor response (e.g., coding), and memory (e.g., digit span, coding, and arithmetic). Further controlled studies must be conducted to determine the source or sources of discrepant verbal versus performance intelligence scores observed in individuals with MM.

The "cocktail party personality" is a cognitively associated behavioral disorder that occurs in some individuals with hydrocephalus, regardless of age or intelligence level (Hurley, 1993). These individuals are articulate and verbose, superficially appearing to have high verbal skills. Close examination of the content of their speech, however, shows frequent and inappropriate use of clichés and jargon. Individual words are often misused. Despite the initial appearance of being capable, these individuals are often impaired, and their performance in daily life is below what they superficially appear able to do (Hurley, 1993). It is important for the physical therapist to directly observe skills that these children report that they can perform and to confirm regular performance of the task at home with parents and care providers to determine if information provided by the patient is accurate.

Language Dysfunction

Children with MM and hydrocephalus have been observed to have deficits in discourse, characterized by a high frequency of irrelevant utterances and poorer performance with abstract rather than con-

crete language. Culatta and Young (1992) administered the Preschool Language Assessment Instrument (PLAI) at four different levels of abstraction to children with MM and comparable language-age control children. Children with MM performed comparably to controls on concrete tasks of the PLAI, but they produced more "no response" and irrelevant responses than control participants on abstract tasks.

Upper Limb Dyscoordination

Upper limb dyscoordination is frequently observed in children with MM, especially those with hydrocephalus (Shaffer et al., 1986). The dyscoordination can potentially be explained by three possible causes: 1) cerebellar ataxia most likely related to the Arnold-Chiari type II malformation; 2) motor cortex or pyramidal tract damage secondary to hydrocephalus; or 3) motor learning deficits resulting from the use of upper limbs for balance and support rather than manipulation and exploration. These children perform poorly on timed fine motor skill tasks (Shaffer et al., 1986). Their movements can be described as halting and deliberate, rather than the expected smooth, continuous motion of able-bodied children. It often appears that there is a heavy reliance on visual feedback instead of kinesthetic sense. Consequently, even with extensive training, these children often have difficulty integrating frequently used fine motor movements at a subconscious level (Shaffer et al., 1986). Practicing fine motor tasks has been found to be beneficial, however, and often carries over into functional tasks (Fay et al., 1986). These coordination deficits have been described by some authors as apparent motor apraxias or motor learning deficits (Brunt, 1980; Land, 1977). Given the frequent occurrence of upper limb dyscoordination in these children, true apraxias are probably less common than these studies indicate.

An additional factor that may contribute to upper limb dyscoordination is delayed development of hand dominance (Shaffer et al., 1986). A large number of children with MM have mixed hand dominance or are left-handed, suggestive of possible left hemisphere damage (Shaffer et al., 1986). Brunt (1980) indicated that delayed hand dominance may contribute to deficits in bilateral upper limb function integration, resulting in further difficulty with fine motor tasks.

Visuoperceptual Deficits

Studies assessing visual perception have not clearly determined whether deficits in children with MM are common, as has been described in the literature (Miller & Sethi, 1971; Sand et al., 1973; Tew & Laurence, 1975). Tests that require good hand-eye coordination, such as the Frostig Developmental Test of Visual Perception, may artificially lower scores of children with MM as a result of the upper limb dyscoordination described earlier. When upper limb motor function has been removed as a factor in testing by using the Motor Free Visual Perception Test, children with MM have performed at age-appropriate levels (Shaffer et al., 1986). Consequently, results of visuoperceptual tests must be interpreted carefully, in conjunction with other examinations, before a diagnosis of a visuoperception deficit is made.

Cranial Nerve Palsies

The Arnold-Chiari malformation, along with hydrocephalus or dysplasia of the brainstem, may result in cranial nerve deficits. Ocular muscle palsies can occur (Shurtleff, 1986e), such as involvement of cranial nerve VI (oculomotor) with consequent lateral rectus eye muscle weakness and esotropia on the involved side. Correction with patching of the eye, prescription lenses, or minor outpatient surgery is necessary to prevent amblyopia and for cosmesis (Reigel, 1993). Gaston (1991) studied 322 children with MM for 6 years to monitor them for ophthalmic complications. Forty-two percent of these children had a manifest squint, 29% had an oculomotor nerve palsy or musculoparetic nystagmus, 14% had papilledema, and 17% had optic nerve atrophy. Only 27% of those surveyed had definite normal vision. Seventy percent of proven episodes of raised intracranial pressure (ICP) from CSF shunt malfunction had positive ophthalmologic evidence of the ICP. Shunt surgery is the first priority but may not restore normal ocular motility and visual function, requiring further compensatory interventions.

Cranial nerves IX (glossopharyngeal) and X (vagus) can also be affected with pharyngeal and laryngeal dysfunction (croupy, hoarse cry) and swallowing difficulties (Shurtleff, 1986e). Apneic episodes and bradycardia may occur with a severely symptomatic Arnold-Chiari type II malformation and can potentially be life threatening. These severe symptoms usually appear within the first few weeks of life but can occur at any time (Reigel, 1993). The survival rate is only about 40% in these severe cases (Shurtleff, 1986c). Those infants who do survive, however, have been noted to have gradual improvement in cranial nerve function. Neurosurgical posterior fossa decompression and high cervical laminectomies do not seem to substantially improve the outcome (Griebel et al., 1991; Shurtleff, 1986c). In contrast, surgical decompression of the Arnold-Chiari malformation has been shown to be beneficial for the intervention of progressive upper and lower limb spasticity (Griebel et al., 1991).

Spasticity

The muscle tone of infants and children with MM can range from flaccid to normal to spastic. Stack and Baber (1967) found that some upper motoneuron signs were present in approximately two thirds of children with MM whom they examined; however, only about 9% had true spastic paraparesis. The remainder of this group had predominantly a lower motoneuron presentation with scattered upper motoneuron signs (e.g., flexor withdrawal reflex). In the group of children without upper motoneuron signs, most had totally flaccid paralysis below the segmental level of their spinal lesion, but a small percentage had normal tone. As with other CNS conditions, spasticity and abnormal reflexes can affect function, positioning, or comfort in individuals with MM.

Progressive Neurologic Dysfunction

Minor improvements in strength or development of sensation, although rare, can occur even as late as the fourth decade of life. More important, however, is the deterioration from neurologic changes that are due to treatable complications. These changes include loss of sensation, loss of strength, pain at the site of the sac repair, pain radiating along a dermatome, initial onset or worsening of spasticity, development or rapid progression of scoliosis, development of a lower limb deformity not explained by previously documented muscle imbalance, or change in bowel or bladder sphincter control. Such changes can be due to cerebrospinal fluid shunt obstruction, hydromyelia (syringohydromyelia, syrinx), growth of a dermoid or lipoma at the site of repair, subarachnoid cysts of the cord, or spinal cord tethering. Cord tethering occurs from scarring of the neural placode or spinal cord to the overlying dura or skin with resultant traction on neural structures (Shurtleff et al., 1997). The tethered cord syndrome may also result from other congenital anomalies, including thickening of the filum terminale and diastematomyelia (Rekate, 1991). An acquired cause of progressive spinal cord dysfunction that has been reported is severe herniation of intervertebral discs into the spinal canal, causing compression of the cord (Shurtleff & Dunne, 1986).

Progressive deterioration of spinal cord function due to any of these causes can be arrested by neurosurgical interventions. Deterioration of the gait pattern is frequently the first complaint by patients or their parents. Because physical therapists see these patients more frequently than physicians or surgeons, the therapist often will be the first to observe these changes and should be alert to the need for immediate referral to a neurosurgeon. Owing to this risk of progressive loss of function, it is *essential* that individuals with MM be closely monitored throughout their life span.

Seizures

Seizures have been reported to occur in 10 to 30% of children and adolescents with MM (Shurtleff & Dunne, 1986). The etiologies of seizure activity include associated brain malformation, CSF shunt malfunction or infection, and residual brain damage from shunt infection or malfunction. Anticonvulsant medications, which are necessary for prophylaxis against seizures, unfortunately can also accentuate any cognitive deficits or dyscoordination already present (Gadow, 1986; Reynolds, 1983). Untreated seizures, however, can lead to permanent cognitive or neurologic functional loss, or even death.

Neurogenic Bowel

Fewer than 5% of children with MM develop voluntary control of their urinary or anal sphincter (Reigel, 1993). Abnormal or absent function of spinal segments S2 through S4, which provide the innervation to these organs, is the primary reason for the incontinence. The anal sphincter can be flaccid, hypotonic, or spastic, causing different manifestations of dysfunction during defecation. Anorectal sensation is also often impaired, preventing the individual from receiving sensory input of an imminent bowel movement so that he or she can take appropriate action. In addition to incontinence, constipation and impaction can also occur. Fortunately, conscientious attention to individually designed bowel programs can have effective results, minimizing problems of incontinence and constipation (King et al., 1994; Reigel, 1993; Wicks & Shurtleff, 1986a, 1986b). The presence of a bulbocavernosus or anal cutaneous reflex (indicating that lower motor neuron innervation of the sphincter is present) is highly predictive of success with a bowel training program (King et al., 1994). King and associates (1994) also report that instituting bowel training before age 7 years correlates with improved outcomes by means of better compliance. When stool incontinence is interfering with a child's school and social activities, the physical therapist may want to become involved to help address the problem. Incontinence often affects feelings of self-image and competence, which in turn can affect performance in other activities pertinent to the therapist's intervention program.

Neurogenic Bladder

Just as the nerves to control defecation are impaired, so are the nerves that produce bladder control. A variety of different types of dysfunctions can occur depending on the relative tonicity of the detrusor muscle in the bladder wall and the outlet sphincters of the bladder. Bladder intervention strategies are directed toward the point or points of dysfunction. The goal is infection-free social continence with preservation of renal function. Retrograde flow of urine from the bladder up the ureters to the kidneys, termed *vesicoureteral reflux,* can occur without symptoms or signs being evident until the later stages of irreversible renal failure. Inadequate emptying of the bladder with residual urine retention within the bladder provides an optimal culture medium for bacteria, causing recurrent urinary tract infections and possible generalized sepsis. Adequate bladder intervention is therefore an essential component of health maintenance and normal longevity of people with MM, in addition to being an important social issue.

For most individuals, effective bladder intervention is achieved with clean intermittent catheterization on a regularly timed schedule for voiding. A small catheter is inserted into the bladder through the urethra until urine begins to flow. After the bladder is empty or urine stops flowing, the catheter is withdrawn, cleansed with soap and water, and stored for future use. It has been shown that the clean method of catheterization, as opposed to sterile technique, is sufficient for prevention of urinary tract infections (Reigel, 1993). The risk of injury to the urethra or bladder from clean intermittent catheterization is sufficiently low to allow young children to be taught to catheterize themselves. Mastery of the technique is usually achieved by age 6 to 8 years depending on the severity of the involvement (Shurtleff & Mayo, 1986). Supplementation of clean intermittent catheterization with oral medication for spastic detrusor muscle function (e.g., oxybutynin [Ditropan] or propantheline [Pro-Banthine]), spastic sphincter function (phenoxybenzamine), or hypotonic sphincter function (ephedrine) is required in some children to achieve intervention goals. It is recommended that individuals with MM have regular follow-up with a urologist every 6 months until age 2 and yearly thereafter, throughout the life span (Kimura et al., 1986). The physical therapist must be aware of the method used for urine drainage as it relates to wheelchair positioning, transfer techniques, and orthoses so that assistive devices do not interfere with effective performance of urine drainage techniques. It is important to allow adequate time for patients with MM to attend to bowel and bladder needs before and after examination and therapy sessions so that they are comfortable and continent during physical activities. Discomfort from a distended bladder or rectum may impair performance. Patients are often not assertive in requesting necessary time for personal care, and therapists should encourage them to do so to avoid embarrassing accidents.

Skin Breakdown

Decubitus ulcers and other types of skin breakdown occur in 85 to 95% of all children with MM by the time they reach young adulthood (Shurtleff, 1986a). Okamoto and associates (1983) performed an extensive study of skin breakdown on 524 patients with MM who were 1 to 20 years old. Perineal decubiti and breakdown over the apex of the spinal kyphotic curve (gibbus) occurred in 82% of children with thoracic level lesions, 62% of those with high lumbar level lesions, and 50 to 53% of those with lower level lesions. Lower limb skin breakdown was approximately equivalent in all lesion level groups (30–46%). Although the sites and causes of skin breakdown varied among lesion level groups, the overall frequency was the same. The prevalence of skin breakdown at any one time was 20 to 25% for the population sampled. Several etiologies for skin breakdown were ascertained. In 42% of the children, tissue ischemia from excessive pressure was the cause. In 23% a cast or orthotic device produced the breakdown. In another 23% urine and stool soiling produced skin maceration. Friction and shear accounted for another 10%; burns accounted for 1%; and 1% of causes were not recorded or were unknown.

Other authors have described additional causes of skin breakdown (Shurtleff, 1986a). These include excessive weight bearing over bony prominences of the pelvis as a result of spinal deformity, obesity, lower limb autonomic dysfunction with vascular insufficiency or venous stasis, and tenuous tissue postoperatively over bony prominences.

Age is an important factor in the etiology of skin breakdown. Shurtleff (1986a) showed that young children who are not toilet trained have the greatest problem with breakdown from skin soiling (ammonia burns). Young active children with MM have the greatest frequency of friction burns on knees and feet from scooting along rugs, hot water scalds, and pressure ulcers from orthoses or casts. Older children, adolescents, and young adults develop skin breakdown over lower limb bony prominences (even if they did not have ulcers when they were younger) from the increased pressure of a larger body habitus, asymmetric weight bearing resulting from deformities, abrasions of the buttocks or lower limbs due to poor transfer skills, improperly fitted orthoses, and lower limb vascular problems. Strategies for prevention taught by the physical therapist therefore should be directed to the likely causes of skin breakdown for the age of the individual.

Obesity

Obesity is a common and difficult multifactorial problem occurring in children with MM. For children who are ambulatory, a greater expenditure of energy is required to participate in physical play activities, so it is likely that less time will be spent engaged in physical play and more sedentary activities (e.g., watching television) will be adopted. Children with mobility limitations, whether they are ambulatory or wheelchair mobile, may not be well accepted by able-bodied peers when they attempt to participate in physically challenging play, or they may feel conspicuous because of having difficulty keeping up. The likelihood of participation under these circumstances is diminished. As obesity develops, this further complicates participation and negatively affects self-image, creating an undesirable cycle perpetuating weight gain. In addition, children with MM probably are at a disadvantage physiologically. Studies evaluating the caloric intake required for children with MM (Shurtleff, 1986b) have shown that the intake should be lower than for able-bodied obese peers. This is probably not just a function of the decreased activity level of children with MM. Decreased muscle mass of large lower limb muscle groups diminishes the ability to burn calories (i.e., the basal metabolic rate of children with MM is probably lower than normal). This is consistent with the observation that children with high lumbar and thoracic lesions have greater problems with obesity. Weight control is therefore not just a function of decreased caloric intake for children with MM. The challenge of the physical therapist is to find age-appropriate physical activities for their clients that are fun and at which they can succeed; in this way, physical activity is positively reinforced and a lifelong pattern of engaging in such activities is developed.

The usual mechanism to screen for obesity in the general population is height-weight ratios; however, arm span–weight ratios are more appropriate for monitoring individuals with MM. Shurtleff (1986b) notes that height-weight ratios are not useful in children with MM because of their short stature, decreased linear length secondary to spine or lower limb deformities, and decreased growth of paretic limbs. He recommends monitoring individuals with MM by measuring serial subscapular skinfold thickness, linear length measured along the axis of long bones to take into consideration hip and knee joint contractures, arm span measured with a spanner, and weight measured on a platform scale (subtracting the weight of the wheelchair or adaptive aids). Results should be recorded on National Center for Health Statistics percentile charts (Hamill et al., 1979). Arm span measurements should be adjusted using correction factors to avoid underestimating body fat content: 0.9 arm span for children with no leg muscle mass (thoracic and high-lumbar levels), 0.95 arm span for those with partial loss of muscle mass (mid- and low-lumbar lesions), and 1.0 arm span for children with minimal or no muscle mass loss.

AGE-SPECIFIC EXAMINATION AND PHYSICAL THERAPY INTERVENTION

There are issues of particular importance for specific age groups with MM. Intervention should be provided to keep pace with the normal timing of development (Bleck & Nagel, 1982; Shurtleff, 1966). Throughout the life span, it is important to keep in mind the overall picture of the needs of the patient and family. The medical problems and the number of health care professionals involved in the care of individuals with MM can be overwhelming. Many members of other disciplines in addition to the physical therapist may also be making requests of the family's time. Each professional should prioritize his or her goals, relative to those of other disciplines, and coordinate planning so that the demands placed on the patient and the family are realistic. It is best to work as a team with the family and other disciplines to integrate appropriate intervention programs into the patient's daily routine. In addition, if conflicting information is provided to parents, they often become confused and may lack appropriate information to set realistic goals for their children and adolescents (e.g., goals for mobility, self-care, employment, and independent living). Consequently, multidisciplinary team collaboration with the family is important to establish appropriate goals and expectations.

The following sections focus on special considerations throughout the life span. Four age groups are discussed: infancy, preschool age, school age, and adolescence. Disabilities that are typically present, as well as the causes and impact of functional limitations on expected life roles, are discussed for each of the four age groups. Examination and evaluation of impairments, functional limitations, and disabilities, along with recommendations for ongoing monitoring, typical physical therapy goals, intervention, and strategies to prevent secondary impairments and functional limitations, are also discussed. In addi-

tion, typical secondary disabilities and functional limitations encountered during adolescence and their impact on the transition to adulthood are discussed in the section on adolescence and transition to adulthood. The information presented in this latter section has important implications for preventive intervention during childhood and adolescence to minimize the incidence of acquired impairments and functional limitations that often surface later in life.

It is important to keep in mind that the interaction of a multitude of impairments may affect an individual's functional performance, yet only a few key impairments are discussed for each age group. The reader is referred to the previous section on impairments for a more thorough discussion of other factors. Similarly, only key examination and intervention strategies that are specific to a given age category are discussed in each section.

Infancy

Typical Disabilities: Causes and Implications

The multiple impairments and overwhelming medical needs of a newborn with MM may interfere with parent-infant interaction. Parents are often afraid to handle their infant with MM, and the opportunities for handling and interacting with their child may be further limited by medical complications. Parents and extended family members may be cautious in handling the infant, resulting in decreased stimulation. Naturally occurring opportunities for early environmental stimulation, observation and exploration, and social interaction also may be limited as a result of somatosensory and motor deficits, hypotonia, and visual deficits. Family and infant interaction may be further impeded by the additional parental duties required (e.g., bowel and bladder intervention), frequent medical visits, and hospitalizations for complications.

The achievement of fine motor and gross motor developmental milestones is usually delayed during infancy because of multiple impairments, including joint contractures and deformities, motor and sensory deficits, hypotonia, upper limb dyscoordination, CNS dysfunction, visual and perceptual disorders, and cognitive deficits. The lack of normal infant movements, combined with impaired sensation, results in decreased kinesthetic awareness and inhibits perceptuomotor development. Independence with early ADL, such as holding a bottle or finger feeding, is also negatively affected by impairments resulting from MM, especially swallowing disorders, upper limb dyscoordination, and visuoperceptual deficits.

Examination of Impairments

As discussed in Chapter 4, therapists must be aware of normal physiologic flexion of the hips and knees when assessing newborns. Limitations of up to 35° are present in normal newborns. These contractures may be more pronounced at birth in the infant with MM after prolonged intrauterine positioning of the relatively inactive fetus. Physiologic flexion spontaneously reduces in able-bodied infants from the effects of gravity and spontaneous lower limb movements. Physiologic flexion of infants with MM typically does not spontaneously reduce, because of decreased or absent spontaneous lower limb activity secondary to muscle weakness. Consequently, contractures may develop even in children with sacral level function if they lack full strength of the gluteal muscles.

Two primary orthopedic concerns during this period are to identify and manage dislocated hips and foot deformities. Early orthopedic intervention of these deformities results in improved potential for standing balance and more timely achievement of motor milestones such as sitting and walking (Mayfield, 1991; Menelaus, 1976). Achieving a plantigrade foot position is important, regardless of ambulatory prognosis. Plantigrade alignment is optimal for shoe fit, positioning and weight distribution in sitting, and stability when bearing weight for standing pivot transfers or ambulation.

When assessing muscle tone in infants, the Movement Assessment of Infants (Chandler et al., 1980) is a useful tool. Hypotonia is typical in infants with MM, even if sacral level function is present (Wolf & McLaughlin, 1992). Poor head control, delayed neck and trunk righting, automatic reactions, and low trunk and lower limb muscle tone are typical. A mixture of hypotonia, hypertonia, and spastic movements may be present in the limbs. It is important to distinguish between voluntary and reflexive movements when assessing muscle function.

One of the key physical therapy considerations in managing the newborn with MM is to establish a reliable baseline of muscle function before and after back closure. This baseline is important for predicting future function and for monitoring status. In addition, it is important to identify muscle imbalance around joints and existing joint contractures that are unlikely to reduce spontaneously.

In the newborn, muscle function is assessed before and after surgical closure of the back to determine the extent of motor paralysis. Side lying is usually the position of choice for testing the newborn, to avoid injury to the exposed neural tissue (Schneider et al., 1995). The state of alertness must be considered and documented when testing newborns or infants. Repeated examinations may need to be conducted at different times of the day to observe the infant's muscle activity in various behavioral states. Optimal performance cannot be elicited if the infant is in a sleepy state. Muscle activity is best observed when the infant is alert, hungry, or crying. If the infant is drowsy, several techniques can be used to arouse the infant, including assessing limb ROM, rocking vertically to stimulate the vestibular system, and providing tactile and auditory stimulation (Hinderer & Hinderer, 1993; Schneider et al., 1995). Ideally, the infant's spontaneous activity should be observed in supine, prone, and side-lying positions before the examiner starts handling the infant. Handling the infant may suppress spontaneous activity. Movement can often be elicited through sounds, visual tracking, reaching for toys, tickling, placing limbs in antigravity positions to elicit holding responses, and moving limbs to end-range positions to see if the infant will move out of the position (Hinderer & Hinderer, 1993). For older infants, muscle activity can be observed, palpated, and resisted in developmental positions.

Therapists often do not record specific strength grades for infants and young children. Instead, either a dichotomous scale (present or absent) or a 3-point ordinal scale (apparently normal, weak, or absent) is often advocated (Murdoch, 1980; Pact et al., 1984; Schneider et al., 1995). This 3-point scale, however, lacks sensitivity and predictive validity (Murdoch, 1980). In contrast, specific manual muscle test strength scores (grades 0 to 5) have been found to provide useful information for infants and young children with MM and are predictive of later function (McDonald et al., 1986). Consequently, when strength is assessed manually, we recommend using the full manual muscle testing scale, regardless of age. The estimated quality of the examination should also be recorded, indicating the examiner's degree of confidence in the results, based on the child's level of cooperation. Neck and trunk musculature should be graded as "normal for age" if the child is able to perform developmentally appropriate activities (Kendall et al., 1999).

Testing sensation in infants and young children presents special challenges. Complete testing of multiple sensory modalities is not possible until the child has acquired sufficient cognitive and language abilities to accurately respond to testing (Schneider et al., 1995). Parents can often provide useful information to help focus on probable insensate areas. It is best to test the child in a quiet state. Testing with a pin or other sharp object should begin at the lowest level of sacral innervation and progress to more proximally innervated dermatomes until a noxious response is noted (e.g., crying or facial grimace).

Ongoing Monitoring

During the first year of life, it is important to monitor joint alignment, muscle imbalance, and the development of contractures. Typical lower limb contractures that develop are hip and knee flexion contractures, combined with external rotation at the hips. Children with weak or absent hip musculature often lie in a "frog-legged" position with the hips flexed and externally rotated and the knees flexed. Consequently, these muscle groups are typically in a shortened position. It is important to closely monitor ROM and muscle extensibility during periods of rapid growth. Soft tissue growth typically lags behind skeletal changes, resulting in decreased extensibility. Stretching exercises should be initiated early on, if indicated, when contractures are relatively flexible and respond well to intervention. If orthoses or night-positioning splints are used to correct orthopedic deformities, the fit of these devices should be monitored to prevent skin breakdown.

Changes in muscle tone and muscle function are observed with progressive neurologic dysfunction. Baseline measurements, therefore, are essential, and these parameters should be closely monitored. Therapists should also watch for behavioral changes, decreases in performance, and other subtle signs of shunt malfunction (see Box 23–1) or seizure disorders. Motor development must also be observed to determine whether an infant is keeping pace with normal developmental expectations. Abnormalities in any of these areas should be reported to the child's primary care physician.

Typical Physical Therapy Goals and Strategies

During the newborn period, physical therapists must be sensitive to the feelings and needs of parents and other extended family members who are learning to cope with the overwhelming problems of a child with MM. Parents go through a period of tremendous adjustment. They are required to meet the demands of a normal infant, plus deal with the extensive medical and surgical needs of their newborn and adjust to the long-term implications of their child's multiple impairments. Not all instructions may be assimilated at any one time given the large amount of information to which parents are asked to attend. Often instructions must be reviewed and reinforced during subsequent visits. Written instructions should be provided to augment verbal explanations.

If ROM is limited, parents should be instructed in positioning techniques. It is optimal to maintain ROM by means of positioning because little additional time is required of the family. If contractures do not resolve with positioning, or if contractures are not supple, parents should also be instructed in stretching exercises and soft tissue mobilization techniques. It is usually most efficient to perform stretching exercises and soft tissue mobilization techniques in conjunction with diaper changes.

For infants who exhibit hypotonia, parents should be instructed in handling techniques to facilitate head and trunk control. Techniques advocated for children with hypotonic cerebral palsy (e.g., Finnie, 1975) are often beneficial. Parents should be encouraged to provide sitting opportunities for the infant to facilitate the development of head and trunk control. Additional head and trunk support is often required in high chairs, strollers, and car seats. If motor development is significantly delayed and requires therapeutic intervention, a combination of neurodevelopmental intervention and proprioceptive neuromuscular facilitation techniques is beneficial. Therapeutic interventions and adaptive equipment should ideally be planned to keep pace with the normal timing of development so that the child is provided with typical developmental experiences. During the latter half of the first year, preparatory activities for mobility are indicated. Emphasis should be placed on balance, trunk control, and facilitating an upright posture as the child progresses through the developmental sequence.

Prevention of Secondary Impairments and Functional Limitations

Parents should be instructed in proper positioning, ROM, and handling techniques with the lower limbs in neutral alignment to prevent the development of contractures. If the hips are dislocated or subluxed, parents should be instructed in proper positioning, double diapering, and the use of a night-positioning orthosis, if indicated (Rowley-Kelly & Kunkle, 1993; Schafer & Dias, 1983). If surgery is indicated to relocate hip dislocations (see previous section on orthopedic deformities), it is generally performed after 6 months of age. Foot deformities are generally treated through serial casting or positioning splints.

Parents should also be instructed to inspect insensate skin areas during diaper changes and dressing for signs of pressure or injury. Parents need to understand the importance of skin inspection and that insensate areas should be inspected on a daily basis throughout the life span.

Toddler and Preschool Years

Typical Disabilities: Causes and Implications

The achievement of fine motor and gross motor developmental milestones continues to be delayed. Mobility is typically impaired in this population owing to orthopedic, motor, and sensory deficits. As the child nears the end of the first year of life, it is important to provide opportunities for environmental exploration. If the child does not have an efficient, effective mode of independent mobility by the end of the first year, provision of a mobility device is indicated.

Environmental exploration is essential for the development of initiative and independence. Limited early mobility may result in a lack of curiosity and initiative and may negatively affect other aspects of development (Becker, 1975; Butler et al., 1984; Shurtleff, 1986d). If a toddler does not have an effective means of independently exploring and interacting with the environment, he or she may learn to be passively dependent. The negative influence of limited early mobility on personality and behavior development can persist throughout life. Passive-dependent behavior is a commonly observed personality trait of adolescents and adults with MM.

Limited mobility also negatively affects socialization, especially interaction with other children. If a stroller is used as the primary mode of community mobility beyond the normal age of weaning a child from a stroller, other children will view the child with MM as a "baby." Play opportunities are also limited if a child does not have an effective means of mobility.

Independence with ADL is often impaired in this population because of fine and gross motor impairments, upper limb dyscoordination, and CNS dysfunction. Children who are not independent with ADL may miss out on normal childhood experiences (e.g., play time) while waiting for others to assist them with basic skills. Their self-esteem may also be negatively affected if other children tease them regarding their dependency.

It is important that parents, child care personnel, and preschool teachers be aware of other motor deficits that are often exhibited in this population, such as poor eye-hand coordination. The potential impact of these deficits on functional performance in handwriting and the acquisition of ADL skills such as feeding and dressing should be realized so that reasonable goals can be established and the use of appropriate adaptive equipment implemented.

Examination and Evaluation of Impairments and Functional Limitations

By the end of the first year, ROM is expected to be within normal limits. If limited ROM persists, it is important to distinguish between fixed and supple contractures, determine muscle extensibility, and evaluate orthopedic deformities to determine whether they are fixed or flexible.

To assess strength, functional muscle testing techniques are advocated for young children 2 to 5 years old because they may not cooperate with traditional test procedures (Hinderer & Hinderer, 1993; Pact et al., 1984). Functional activities that are helpful in determining the strength of key lower limb muscle groups include gait observations, heel- and toe-walking, climbing up and down a step, one-legged stand, toe touching, squat to stand, bridging, bicycling while supine, the Landau position, prone kicking, the wheelbarrow position, sit-ups, pull to sit, and sitting and standing push-ups. It is often possible for young children to cooperate with isolated muscle actions by having them push against a puppet to show how strong they are. To elicit the cooperation of older preschoolers (3- to 4-year-olds), it is often helpful to name the muscle and describe its "job" (the muscle action). The children think that the muscle names are humorous, maintaining their attention. Asking children to have the muscle do its "job" makes strength testing more understandable (Hinderer & Hinderer, 1993). We have found it possible to obtain objective, reliable measures of strength from children as young as 4 years of age using handheld myometry techniques (Hinderer & Hinderer, 1993). The degree of confidence regarding whether the child's optimal performance was elicited should be recorded.

Once the child is 2 years of age, light touch and position sense can usually be assessed by eliciting tickling responses or having the child respond to the touch of a puppet. Other sensory modalities can ordinarily be accurately tested once the child is 5 to 7 years old. The accuracy of responses often must be double-checked because of short attention span and response perseveration. Two sensory testing techniques help minimize perseveration of responses. The first is to randomly alternate between testing light touch and pinprick and have the child identify the type of sensation. The second is to have the child point to the spot that was touched and correctly state when no area was touched.

Fine and gross motor development should be assessed using appropriate standardized tests such as those discussed in Chapters 1 and 2. Examination of ADL should focus on what the individual actually does on a daily basis, in addition to what he or she is capable of doing. If independence with ADL is limited, appropriate adaptations and interventions should be implemented to foster independence. The Functional Activities Assessment (Okamoto et al., 1984; Sousa et al., 1976, 1983) is useful for this population (Fig. 23–6). Items may be scored by direct observation or by parent report. Assistive devices required to perform a given task are also documented. The "Can" and "Does" scoring format permits the examiner to record what the child can do versus what

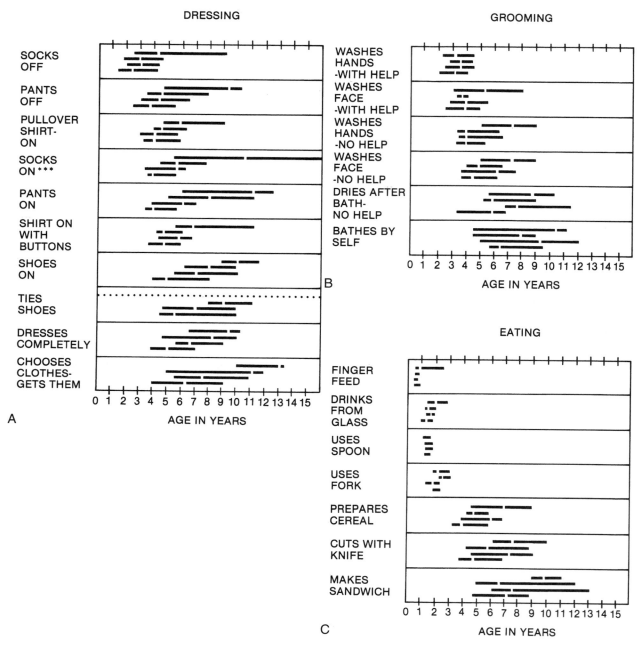

FIGURE 23–6. Functional Activities Assessment. The age at which 20%, 50%, and 80% of a group of 173 children learned (A) dressing, (B) grooming, and (C) eating skills is indicated by the beginning of, space between (*white space*), and end of the black bars, respectively. Triple asterisks indicate that this group never achieved an 80% learning proportion. Dotted line indicates activity was attempted with this group. The bars in each category represent, from top to bottom: 1) thoracic and L1–L2; 2) L3 and mixed lesions, L2–L4; 3) L4–L5; and 4) sacral-level groups. All data were recorded as the child achieved the skill during the 2.5-year period of the study, within 4 months of entering the study, or when the caretaker entered a specific date of achievement in the child's diary. These charts were created from data published by Okamoto and associates (1984) and Sousa and associates (1983). (From Shurtleff, DB [Ed.]. Myelodysplasias and Exstrophies: Significance, Prevention, and Treatment. Orlando, FL: Grune & Stratton, 1986, p. 376.)

the child actually does on a regular basis. In addition, if the child is directly observed performing the task, the degree of independence and the time to complete the task are recorded.

Ongoing Monitoring

Joint alignment, muscle imbalance, contractures, posture, and signs of progressive neurologic dysfunction should continue to be monitored. Contractures that seem insignificant during childhood may become functionally limiting once the individual has adult-sized body proportions. For example, knee extension contractures can interfere with the ability to maneuver in a wheelchair.

Typical Physical Therapy Goals and Strategies

Joint alignment, contractures, muscle strength, and postural alignment should continue to be treated, as necessary. Proper positioning in sleeping and sitting should continue. If stretching or strengthening exercises are indicated, it is often helpful to involve other family members in the exercise program so that the child does not feel singled out. For ambulatory candidates with weak hip and knee musculature, strengthening activities may be beneficial if the child is cooperative. In addition to traditional posture exercises (Kendall et al., 1999), many play activities promote strengthening and the development of good posture (Embrey et al., 1983). The use of therapy ball techniques to strengthen postural muscles is also beneficial. Muscle reeducation techniques, such as functional electrical stimulation and biofeedback, are useful to teach muscles to function in new ROM after stretching exercises. Electrical stimulation has also been found to be beneficial in increasing strength and enhancing functional performance in this population (Karmel-Ross et al., 1992).

During the preschool years, the focus is on improving the independence, efficiency, and effectiveness of ADL and mobility. Development of independence with dressing and feeding should be encouraged. Appropriate guidance should be provided so that parents have age-appropriate expectations. It is important for young children to actively participate in skin inspection, bowel and bladder intervention, donning and removing orthoses, wheelchair intervention, and other ADL tasks. Teaching these skills early on and actively involving the child facilitates independence and incorporation of these activities into the daily routine. As a result, these extra responsibilities required of the child with MM become as natural as other ADL, such as brushing teeth. Waiting to introduce tasks until the child

is older often is met with resistance, especially when the child observes that siblings do not have the same requirements.

By kindergarten age, children without disabilities are able to dress and toilet themselves (with the exception of some fasteners), eat independently, and be mobile (Fay et al., 1986). These skills must be emphasized at an early age in the MM populations so that independence is achieved by the time the child begins school. A wide range of age of achievement of independence with ADL is evident in this population when examining the normative data provided on the Functional Activities Assessment (see Fig. 23–6). This wide variability in age of achieving skills within a given motor level suggests that a significant percentage of children are delayed in ADL skill acquisition because of attitudes and expectations. Fay and associates (1986) suggest that these delays may be partially caused by low parental expectations and protective attitudes, perceptions that it is faster for the parent to perform the task, and parental difficulty accepting the reality of the child's functional impairments. Showing parents the ADL normative data for children with MM and promoting positive parental expectations of independence are beneficial. It is important for parents to positively reinforce the child's attempts to be independent so that he or she is motivated to achieve.

Skin inspection and pressure relief techniques should be taught early so that they are incorporated into the daily routine. Proper intervention of lower limbs and joint protection techniques should be taught to avoid injury of insensate areas when learning how to perform ADL, such as transfers. The impact of sensory deficits on functional performance should be kept in mind during gait training and when teaching other functional tasks.

Provision of an effective means of independent mobility is *essential* for young children. Consequently, if a child does not begin maneuvering effectively within the environment by 1 year of age, alternative means of mobility must be considered to achieve independent home and short-distance community mobility (Butler et al., 1984; Shurtleff, 1986d). Mobility options should be explored and implemented as frequently as is needed so that the child is able to actively participate in normal childhood activities. Various mobility options are available, from manual devices such as a caster cart to electric wheelchairs. Electric wheelchair use has been found to be feasible and beneficial for children as young as 24 months of age (Butler et al., 1984). If a wheelchair is indicated, it is important to present this option to the parents in a positive way. The use of a wheelchair does not preclude walking. In fact, children who use wheelchairs at an early age generally are more interested in mobility, independence, and environmental exploration. Consequently, they tend to be more independent in all forms of mobility later in life. Ryan and associates (1991) recommend introducing a wheelchair as early as 18 months to enable children to keep up with their peers, boost self-confidence, facilitate independence, and increase activity levels.

Preparatory activities for mobility are indicated for 1- to 2-year-olds. Emphasis should be placed on balance, trunk control, and facilitating an upright posture. For ambulatory candidates, once the child begins to pull to stand, the need for orthoses to improve weight-bearing alignment should be considered. It is important to anticipate future ambulatory needs when recommending orthoses to maximize their utility.

For children with high-level lesions (thoracic to L2), preparatory activities for wheelchair mobility should be emphasized (e.g., sitting balance, arm strengthening, transfer training, wheelchair propulsion, and electrical switch operation if indicated). The focus of wheelchair training for toddlers and preschoolers with high-level lesions should include mobility, environmental exploration, safety, and transfer skills. Household distance ambulation using a parapodium, HKAFO, knee-ankle-foot orthosis (KAFO), or reciprocating gait orthosis (RGO) may be attempted, but energy expenditure is very high. Consequently, wheelchairs are generally used for community mobility of children with thoracic to L2 motor function, particularly once body proportions increase.

Biped ambulation is feasible for toddlers and preschoolers with L3 and below motor function. It is essential to maintain adequate ROM and to emphasize an upright posture so that weight-bearing forces are properly distributed and muscles can function at their optimal length. Therapeutic activities that promote trunk control and balance are beneficial. Children with lumbar level lesions will require upper limb support for walking. In general, a reverse-facing walker is best when learning to walk because it allows the child to be upright and minimizes upper limb weight bearing. Reverse-facing walkers have been found to promote better postural alignment than anterior-facing walkers (Logan et al., 1990). Once an upright gait is established, the child can be advanced to forearm crutches.

If children with sacral level motor function require upper limb support to begin walking, a reverse-facing walker is also usually best to minimize upper limb weight bearing. Alternatively, forearm crutches can be used if the child is able to walk upright while manipulating the crutches. Children with L5 and S1 level lesions often abandon their upper limb aids when they are young and their center of mass is low

to the ground. Upper limb aids may still be indicated for endurance and to decrease trunk sway when walking long distances, for balance when walking on rough terrain, or to minimize the stress on weight-bearing lower limb joints. The need for upper limb aids should be reevaluated when the child is older and body proportions and environmental demands have changed.

The use of positive reinforcement is often recommended for this population to enhance cooperation with examination procedures and intervention programs. In general, food is not an appropriate form of reinforcement because obesity is often a concern. Verbal reinforcement is preferred at this age.

Prevention of Secondary Impairments and Functional Limitations

Individuals are at risk for joint contractures when there is muscle imbalance around joints, when a substantial portion of the day is spent sitting, when there is a prolonged period of immobilization or bed rest, following surgery, and during periods of rapid growth when soft tissue growth may lag behind skeletal changes. It is important to closely monitor individuals with MM during these periods so that intervention can be initiated early on, if needed, when contractures are still flexible and respond well to intervention. Early detection and intervention of contractures is important to prevent fixed deformities and stretch weakness of overlengthened muscles. Similarly, the importance of skin inspection of insensate areas, use of pressure relief cushions, and sitting push-ups for pressure relief should be emphasized at an early age so that these preventive measures become routine.

Habitual postural positions that contribute to deforming forces should be discouraged. It is essential to emphasize an upright posture when a child is learning to walk. If children are permitted to stand and walk in a crouched posture, habit patterns become established and it is difficult to teach a more upright posture because of the development of secondary impairments (e.g., joint contractures and stretch weakness of excessively lengthened muscles). Therapists should closely observe joint alignment and posture when a child is standing. Postural deviations that look insignificant when a child is young are often magnified once body proportions increase.

School Age

Typical Disabilities: Causes and Implications

Independence with ADL often continues to be impaired in this age group. Children who are not independent with ADL may miss out on normal childhood experiences (e.g., play time or recess) while waiting for parents or teachers to assist them with basic skills. Their self-esteem may continue to be negatively affected if other children tease them regarding their dependency.

Mobility limitations are magnified once a child begins school because of the increased community mobility distances and skills required. Advanced mobility skills are needed because of environmental barriers such as curbs, ramps, uneven terrain, and steps. Ineffective or inefficient community mobility can further reinforce dependent behaviors if other children carry his or her school books and lunch tray or push the wheelchair.

The negative effects of limited mobility and physical limitations on socialization become more apparent at this age. Play and recreational opportunities are restricted if a child does not have an effective method of mobility. Often children with MM are excluded from recess or physical education class. Consequently, they miss out on opportunities for social interaction. Even if they are included in these activities, often their involvement is peripheral (e.g., score keeper during physical education class). Mobility limitations, dependency with ADL, difficulties with toileting, and the difficulty of managing adaptive equipment often interfere with other aspects of peer interaction, such as going over to friends' houses to play or spending the night with friends.

Finally, it is important that parents and teachers be aware of perceptuomotor, visuoperceptual, and sensory deficits. The potential impact of these deficits on writing speed, legibility, and accuracy; the efficiency and effectiveness of performing ADL skills; problem solving; and cognitive abilities should be realized so that reasonable goals can be established and the use of appropriate adaptive equipment can be implemented. Multiple hospitalizations or medical complications can also negatively affect school performance.

Examination and Evaluation of Impairments and Functional Limitations

As with younger children, joint alignment, strength, muscle imbalance, contractures, muscle extensibility, and posture should continue to be monitored. Other parameters that should be assessed include sensation, coordination, fine motor skills, ADL, mobility, gait, body awareness, and functional skills.

Reliable, sensitive, objective measures of strength can be obtained in school-age children (Hinderer & Hinderer, 1993). We recommend that objective methods of strength examination, such as handheld myometry, be used to serially monitor strength of individuals with MM who are old enough to cooper-

ate (typically age 4 or older). Stationary isokinetic or strain gauge devices can also provide objective measures of strength, but these devices are not available in the typical clinic or school setting.

Independence with ADL should be assessed. In addition to the basic ADL skills evaluated in the Functional Activities Assessment, the school-age child's ability to carry items and assist with basic household chores should be evaluated. The adequacy of clearance, duration, frequency, and reliability of performance of wheelchair push-ups are also assessed by the physical therapist. Bowel and bladder function and the degree of continence are usually evaluated by a nurse. It is important that the physical therapist understand these functional impairments and degree of independence with bowel and bladder function, however, because positioning, adaptive equipment, and mobility issues can often restrict independence with bowel and bladder intervention programs.

The home, school, and community environments should be accessible so that individuals with MM can participate fully in all activities. The Americans with Disabilities Act of 1990 mandates access to all buildings, programs, and services used by the general public in the United States. Even partial exclusion from a school program can have lasting negative effects on a student's social and emotional development (Baker & Rogosky-Grassi, 1993). Providing accessibility to the entirety of school, home, and community activities lets individuals with MM know that they have the same opportunities and rights of access as everyone else. Limited access broadcasts a message of exclusion and estrangement. Both physical and social barriers to participation must be addressed. For a more thorough discussion of evaluating environmental accessibility in the school setting, see Baker and Rogosky-Grassi (1993). Community accessibility should also be evaluated. Ideally, the patient should have access to the community school, church, grocery and drug stores, post office, bank, cleaners, stores and shopping malls, library, restaurants, theaters, sports arenas, hospital, physician's office, work environment, and public transportation. Streets, sidewalks, crosswalks, and parking lots should also be accessible.

Ongoing Monitoring

Joint alignment, muscle imbalance, contractures, posture, and signs of progressive neurologic dysfunction should continue to be monitored. As school-age children mature, they should become more responsible for daily inspection of insensate skin areas when they are bathing and dressing. Appropriate performance of pressure relief strategies should also be monitored. Areas of skin breakdown should be noted so that appropriate adjustments in equipment and preventive behaviors can be implemented or reviewed.

School-age children should be observed closely during periods of rapid growth because they are at risk for loss of function as a result of cord tethering. Parents and teachers should be made aware of signs of progressive CNS complications so that they know when to refer the child to a primary care physician.

Typical Physical Therapy Goals and Strategies

The stretching and strengthening strategies discussed for the two previous age groups also apply to the school-age child. Improving the flexibility of low back extensor, hip flexor, hamstring, and shoulder girdle musculature should be emphasized. When possible, stretching and strengthening exercises should also be incorporated into the physical education program. It is important that children with MM participate in physical education classes and sports activities in a meaningful way.

Proper positioning while sleeping and sitting should continue. In the classroom, seating should provide stability and symmetric alignment. Feet should be flat on the floor or on wheelchair footrests. The seat and desk height should be adjusted to fit the child's body proportions. The desk top should be tilted up to improve neck and upper trunk alignment. Appropriate cushioning should be provided. The child's chair should be positioned in the room so that the teacher and blackboard can easily be viewed while maintaining neutral alignment, without having to turn in the chair.

If a child has not achieved independence with a given ADL task by the age at which 50% of the normative group achieved independence on the Functional Activities Assessment, the child's performance should be assessed to determine if adaptive equipment is required or if further interventions are indicated. Goals for ADL performance should include efficiency in addition to independence. If the child is not as efficient as the primary caretaker, the caretaker will most likely perform the task. The target goal, therefore, is for the child to be able to perform the task as efficiently as the primary caretaker. Showing parents the ADL normative data for children with MM and promoting positive parental expectations of independence are beneficial (see Fig. 23–6). It is important for parents to positively reinforce the child's attempts to be independent so that he or she is motivated to achieve. Pressure relief techniques should be incorporated into the daily routine. Joint protection measures should also be implemented early on to prevent the development of future degenerative changes.

Once children with MM begin school, it is important that they have an independent, efficient, and effective means of mobility for home and long community distances. Alternative means of mobility may need to be considered for long distances to ensure that children with MM are able to keep up with their peers and still have energy left to attend to classroom activities. Various mobility options should be evaluated according to the criteria outlined in Box 23–2 to determine the most effective means of mobility for a given environment. Community-level wheelchair and ambulation skills should be taught, emphasizing efficiency and safety. Community, home, and school environments should be assessed to determine if there are architectural barriers that interfere with daily activities. It is essential for normal social development to permit accessibility to all school, home, and community activities, including recess, physical education, and field trips (Baker & Rogosky-Grassi, 1993).

A functional environment should be created at home and school by removing obstacles and adapting the environment to facilitate efficient and independent function. Adaptive equipment and effective mobility devices should be provided to maximize function. Community mobility skills may need to be practiced to facilitate independent function. Endurance training may also be indicated to ensure that the individual has sufficient endurance and efficiency to function effectively in all activities.

Recreation and physical fitness are important for physical, psychologic, and social reasons. Psychosocial benefits of participation in recreational activities include enhancing confidence and self-esteem, increasing socialization, improving group participation skills, provision of a means of exercising in a more normal way, and increasing interest and motivation in maintaining flexibility, strengthening, and endurance. In contrast, perceived physical restrictions result in a sedentary lifestyle, potentially predisposing these individuals to problems with obesity and degenerative diseases. It is important to stimulate a lifelong interest in fitness and recreation. In addition, community resources, feasibility of transportation, and the family's lifestyle must be taken into account.

Recreation activities must be carefully selected to ensure that they are beneficial and feasible yet enjoyable so they will be continued on a regular basis. Ideally, recreation activities should incorporate forms of aerobic exercise, along with socialization. It is important for individuals with MM to be involved in regular aerobic exercise to maintain their physical fitness and effectively control their weight. Recreational and physical fitness goals include maintaining and improving flexibility, strength, endurance, aerobic capacity, cardiovascular fitness, and coordination and controlling weight. Low-impact aerobics are preferred to minimize stress on joints. Aerobic exercise videotapes have been developed for individuals with disabilities. Swimming is an ideal sport for this population, because they are often able to be competitive with their able-bodied peers and there is minimal stress on joints. Other low-impact activities include cycling, rowing, cross-country skiing, roller and ice skating, and aerobic dance.

Verbal reinforcement or implementation of a token economy system to earn special privileges is preferred at this age to enhance cooperation with examination procedures and intervention programs. As mentioned above, food is not an appropriate form of reinforcement.

Prevention of Secondary Impairments and Functional Limitations

Deficits that may appear insignificant during childhood often become magnified once an individual has adult body proportions, resulting in functional limitations and discomfort (e.g., low back pain resulting from an increased lumbar lordosis and hip flexion contractures).

Joint protection is also important, even at this early age. Joint trauma from excessive stress is cumulative over the life span. Children do not typically complain of pain, and children with MM may not be able to reliably detect pain in insensate areas. Consequently, sources of excess joint stress must be identified by carefully observing children while they perform ADL and transfers, walk, and propel their wheelchair.

Children and their parents should be involved as much as possible in the decision-making process and intervention of their disability. The rationale for assistive devices and therapeutic interventions should be explained so that they are in agreement with intervention plans and become knowledgeable regarding acquisition of medical care and services, rather than being passive recipients.

Adolescence and Transition to Adulthood

Typical Disabilities: Causes and Implications

Adolescence often brings expanded domains of travel for individuals with MM. School buildings become larger, with more environmental barriers for people with physical disabilities. To keep up with peers, community mobility must include mobility skills to travel long distances quickly and efficiently between classrooms, out to athletic fields as a participant or spectator, around shopping malls, and into

---

BOX 23–2. Feasibility of Wheelchair and Biped Ambulation: Criteria for Evaluation

Household Distances

Endurance
Adequate to go between rooms in house?
Adequate to get to yard and car?

Efficiency
Record heart rate and calculate energy expenditure.
Record normal and fast household walking speeds.
Is fast pace adequate for emergency situations?
Is normal pace practical for everyday activities?

Effectiveness
Independent with all transfers?
Able to carry, reach, lift, and climb?
Able to perform activities of daily living?
Able to go forward, backward, sideways, and turn?

Safety
Has good stability and balance?
Observes joint and skin protection?
Able to maneuver around obstacles?
Safe on smooth surfaces and rugs?
Safe when turning?

Accessibility
Maneuvers in and out of house independently?
Necessary household rooms accessible?
Emergency exit routes accessible?

Community Distances

Endurance
Sufficient at a functional speed for average community distances (e.g., going to school, store, medical appointments, and social activities)?
Adequate for play and recreational activities (e.g., playground, park, beach, theater, sports arenas, sports participation)?
Adequate for long-distance community distances (e.g., shopping mall, zoo, concert, sporting events, hiking)?

Efficiency
Record heart rate and calculate energy expenditure.
Record normal and fast walking paces.
Adequate speed to cross intersections?
Is typical pace practical for community distances?

Effectiveness
Independent with all transfers?
Able to maneuver in all directions?
Able to climb and step over obstacles?
Able to carry packages and groceries?
Able to reach and lift items from shelves?

Safety
Has good stability and balance?
Observes joint and skin protection?
Safe on wet or slippery surfaces?
Able to maneuver around obstacles?
Able to maneuver in congested areas?
Safe on uneven terrain, curbs, inclines, and steps?

Accessibility
Maneuvers in and out of car and bus independently?
Necessary community buildings accessible?

crowded movie theaters, dances, and night clubs. Independent adult living also requires mobility and balance skills that permit completion of advanced ADL tasks such as cooking, cleaning, clothes washing, shopping, yardwork, house and equipment maintenance, driving, riding on public transportation, and going to work. Children who have gotten by with slow, inefficient ambulation skills using cumbersome adaptive equipment or who have had basic wheelchair mobility on level surfaces but suddenly cannot handle ramps, hills, curbs, and uneven ground are "left in the dust." Nearly all of the adults in a study of 30 individuals with MM (Hinderer et al., 1988) required referral to a physical therapist to address advanced mobility or equipment issues. It has been the observation of the authors that many adolescents and young adults do not have sufficient mobility skills to succeed independently in the community and must play "catch-up" to achieve their functional potential. The price paid for this delayed development of functional community mobility and lack of independence is social incompetence, dependence for advanced living skills, and unemployability, all of which must subsequently be addressed once mobility skills are improved.

Changes in functional mobility skills often occur concurrently with the rapid changes of adolescence. Individuals who have previously been ambulatory often become more reliant on a wheelchair. Dudgeon and associates (1991) reported that adolescents with MM often exhibit changes in ambulation that are not explained by progressive complications. They suggest that these changes reflect adaptation of mobility to new environmental and social demands that require different speed, accessibility, and energy demands than those encountered in childhood. If orthotic stabilization of the hip, knee, or both is required, it is unlikely that adolescents with MM will maintain community ambulation; instead, most become nonambulators (Dudgeon et al., 1991). Wheelchair transfer skills are also observed to decline in some individuals. The study of 30 adults with MM (Hinderer et al., 1988) showed that 43% had declined in their mobility status from previous examinations performed during adolescence. Several potential factors can play a role in this decreased function.

Changes in body proportions and body composition occur throughout the growing years, but the rate of these changes is accelerated dramatically during adolescence (Hinderer & Hinderer, 1993). Increases in limb length affect the torque generated by muscles due to altered muscle length and resistance force moment arms. In addition, increases in height raise the location of the center of mass higher off the ground, making upright balance more difficult and

energy expenditure greater to perform mobility tasks. Changes in body composition also alter the biomechanics of movement and affect performance. The relative percentage of force-generating muscle to fat and bone tissue changes the ratio of force-producing tissue to the load of the limbs. The development of obesity often occurs during adolescence and can further accentuate these changes. In addition, it is known that during the adolescent growth spurt, the rate of skeletal growth exceeds the increase in muscle mass; the latter catches up after skeletal growth slows in late adolescence. Decreased flexibility of the trunk and two-joint limb muscles is often observed as part of this process. Normal adolescents frequently become clumsy during this period of adjustment while learning how to coordinate their longer limb lengths and increased muscle mass. Adolescents with MM already have a mechanical disadvantage and are consequently more susceptible to dyscoordination and decreased flexibility. It is likely that these developmental changes contribute to the decline in mobility that often occurs in adolescents with MM.

Progression of the neurologic deficit is another potential cause for decline in mobility function, and adolescents are particularly at risk during rapid periods of growth. Forty percent of the participants in our adult follow-up study (Hinderer et al., 1988) had lower limb strength loss compared with previous strength examinations as adolescents. Twenty-seven percent had a reduction in lower limb sensory perception. The greatest motor and sensory losses occurred in the group with lesions at L5 and below—the individuals with the most function to lose. In addition, 10% of study participants demonstrated upper limb strength loss. Progressive neurologic loss, therefore, appears to be an important factor in the changes in mobility status of many individuals during adolescence.

Immobilization for intervention of secondary complications of MM can also contribute to decreased mobility skills. The development of decubiti, fractures, and orthopedic surgeries such as spinal fusions often require extended periods of immobilization with consequent disuse weakness, decreased endurance, and contracture development, all of which can contribute to decreased performance of mobility and transfer tasks.

Prolonged periods of bed rest are often necessary to heal decubitus ulcers to avoid bearing weight on pressure areas. Adolescents often have an increased incidence of decubiti compared with younger children. This is due to their increased body mass causing greater pressure over bony prominences around the buttocks and because of the development of adult sweat patterns in these areas. Fifty-six percent of the adults evaluated in our study (Hinderer et al., 1988) had a history of skin breakdown since their last examination as adolescents; nearly 17% had breakdown present at the time of the examination. An alarming number of these people had little insight into the causes or methods for preventing skin breakdown despite their previous care in a large multidisciplinary pediatric clinic. Even more disturbing was the fact that three individuals (10%) had sustained lower limb amputations since adolescence (two bilateral, one unilateral) as a result of nonhealing ulcers that had progressed to osteomyelitis. Clearly, functional mobility is affected by decubitus ulcers and especially by limb loss.

Musculoskeletal problems can also affect the mobility of adolescents. Progression of spinal deformities often occurs during the growth spurt or in conjunction with one of the neurologic complications previously discussed. Sitting and standing balance can be affected by these spinal changes, leading to decreased mobility and transfer skills. Spinal orthoses prescribed to maintain optimal postural alignment also limit trunk ROM and hip flexion, interfering with wheelchair transfers and moving from sitting to standing. Surgical fusion of the spine to correct deformity and prevent its further progression can lead to immobilization with its consequent effects on mobility described earlier. Lower limb fractures secondary to osteoporosis can also necessitate immobilization with increased risk of functional loss.

Adolescents often begin to develop degenerative changes of weight-bearing joints and overuse syndromes as a result of the excessive loading of these joints necessitated by their neurologic deficit. Joint pain, ligamentous instability, or tendinitis can further limit mobility capabilities. Fifty percent of the adult study participants (Hinderer et al., 1988) complained of joint pain and 100% had joint or spinal deformities noted at the time of their examination.

Several other issues become important for the physical therapist to be cognizant of during adolescence. Independence with self-care and other daily activities is essential for normal socialization and for preparing individuals to lead normal adult lives. Bowel and bladder continence and independent intervention of bowel and bladder emptying are essential for social acceptance by peers and are even more critical at this stage because of the impact on dating, sexuality, higher education, employment, and independent living. Design and fit of wheelchair equipment, mobility aids, and orthoses affect independence with these tasks. Cosmesis is also a consideration with regard to equipment selection because body image and appearance become increasingly important issues during adolescence. Improper design

or fit of equipment can significantly limit normal development in these areas.

Examination and Evaluation of Impairments and Functional Limitation

Based on the discussion of disabilities and their causes, several impairments should be assessed by the physical therapist. Emphasis of specific impairments should be based on the known or suspected concurrent medical problems.

Joint ROM and muscle extensibility of two-joint muscles (especially hip and knee flexors) and trunk muscles should be assessed. Neck and low back motions are often restricted, particularly in adolescents and adults, because of muscle imbalance and poor postural habits. Joint swelling, ligamentous instability, crepitus, and pain with or without joint motion should be documented. If these conditions are progressive or severe enough to interfere with function, the patient should be referred to a physician for further evaluation and intervention. The distribution of degenerative joint changes should be noted with regard to performance of mobility tasks and obesity to determine the contribution of abnormal joint stresses to joint pain and dysfunction.

Muscle strength should continue to be monitored for all major upper and lower limb muscle groups. When progressive neurologic dysfunction is suspected, coordination testing and serial grip strength measurements can also be helpful. Posture and trunk balance in sitting and standing (for ambulators) should be assessed. Real or apparent leg length discrepancy may be present in individuals with foot and ankle deformities, lower limb contractures, unilateral or bilateral hip dislocation, or pelvic obliquity related to spinal curves.

Thorough examination of bed mobility, floor mobility, wheelchair mobility and transfers, and appropriateness and fit of wheelchair equipment is essential for wheelchair users. Endurance and effectiveness of mobility should be assessed to determine whether the individual's current mode of mobility is practical for community-level function. Box 23-2 provides further detail regarding important areas to assess. When orthoses are needed to maintain proper alignment or to facilitate efficient ambulation, the appropriateness and fit of the orthoses must be assessed by the physical therapist. Boxes 23-3 and 23-4 provide further information regarding lower limb orthoses used in this population.

Ongoing Monitoring

Given the multitude of potential problems that can occur during adolescence and adulthood,

---

BOX 23-3. Indicators for Lower Limb Orthoses

Foot Orthoses and Supramalleolar Orthoses

Advantages
Permits full active dorsiflexion and plantar flexion.
Maintains the subtalar joint in neutral alignment.
Provides medial and lateral ankle stability.

Motor function
S1 to "no loss."
Must have adequate toe clearance and sufficient gastrocnemius/soleus strength to provide adequate push-off and decelerate forward movement of tibia.

Indications
Unequal weight distribution, resulting in skin breakdown, foot deformities, or abnormal shoe wear.
Medial and lateral ankle instability, resulting in balance problems, especially difficulty traversing uneven terrain.
Poor alignment of the subtalar joint, forefoot, or rearfoot.

Ankle-Foot Orthoses (Standard AFOs and Ground-Reaction Force AFOs)

Advantages
In general, the ground-reaction force (see Fig. 23-5) is advantageous for this population. The proximal trim line can be extended medially to control genu valgus. The ground-reaction force AFO also facilitates push-off and knee extension during the stance phase and improves static standing balance. The ground-reaction force AFO has a patellar tendon–bearing design. This design distributes pressure across a broad area, preventing skin breakdown and lower leg deformities, which are common when traditional AFO anterior straps have been worn for an extended period of time. If traditional AFOs are used in this population, the anterior straps must be well padded.

Motor function
L4 to S1
Weak or absent ankle musculature
Knee extensors at least grade 4

Indications
Medial and lateral instability of knee or ankle
Insufficient knee extension moment (ground-reaction force AFO)
Lack of or ineffective push-off
Inadequate toe clearance
Crouched gait pattern

Knee-Ankle-Foot Orthoses

Advantages
If unable to maintain upright posture because of joint contractures or muscle weakness, or if the knee joints are unstable, KAFOs are indicated.

If the knee joint is primarily required for medial and lateral stability so the knee joint is unlocked, or if there is potential to progress to ambulation with the knee joints unlocked, it is best to incorporate the ground-reaction force AFO component into the KAFO design to provide the advantages listed earlier in the AFO section.

Motor function
L3 to L4
Weak knee musculature
Absent ankle musculature

Indications
Medial and lateral instability of knee
Weak quadriceps (grade 4– or less)

Reciprocating Gait Orthoses or Hip-Knee-Ankle-Foot Orthoses

Advantages
The reciprocating gait orthosis (RGO) cable system facilitates hip extension during stance phase and hip flexion during swing phase by coupling flexion of one hip with extension of the opposite hip.
Release of both cables permits hip flexion when sitting.
The RGO reduces the energy required for ambulation compared with walking with traditional KAFOs.

Motor function
L1 to L3 (some centers also advocate for thoracic level).
Weak hip flexion is required to effectively operate the cables.

Indications
Unable to maintain an upright posture with the hip joints extended.
RGO is indicated to facilitate hip extension and swing phase.

Thoracic-Hip-Knee-Ankle-Foot Orthoses, Parapodiums, or Verlos

Advantages
Upright positioning for high-level lesions
Generally for exercise walking only

Motor function
Thoracic to L2. Walking is usually nonfunctional for these high-level lesions because of the high energy expenditure required and the slow, cumbersome walking pace.

Indications
Limited distance mobility
Upright positioning
"Exercise" walking

---

comprehensive examinations should continue on at least a yearly basis, and potentially more frequently when problems are suspected or known to be present. Without regular reexamination, these individuals often "fall through the cracks" and endure permanent loss of function that was avoidable. An unfortunate example was one of the adult study participants with a diagnosis of lipomeningocele

BOX 23-4. Lower Limb Orthotic Specifications, Objectives, and Examination Criteria

Orthotic Specifications

Shoe heel height

A low heel (¼ to ½ inch) may improve balance by shifting the center of gravity forward in a person with a calcaneal weight-bearing position.

A low heel (¼ to ½ inch) may decrease knee hyperextension by shifting the center of gravity forward.

A high heel shifts the center of gravity too far forward and causes balance problems in a person with weak plantar flexors.

A high heel may result in increased hip and knee flexion, combined with an increased lordosis or swayback posture.

Ankle angle

Ideally molded or set in 5° *plantar flexion* with a rigid anterior and posterior stop to reduce energy requirements and to increase the knee extension moment (Lehmann et al., 1985), as long as toe clearance is adequate and the knee does not hyperextend. If foot clearance is a problem, set angle more acutely, no higher than neutral, at the minimum angle required to clear the foot during swing phase. Plastic orthoses must enclose the malleoli to effectively resist dorsiflexion and provide a rigid anterior stop (Lehmann et al., 1983).

Do not set ankle angle more acutely than a neutral angle unless trying to control a knee hyperextension problem, because the energy expenditure will increase.

Keel

Generally, keel should be rigid to the distal aspect of the metatarsal heads (to decrease energy expenditure by providing a longer lever). The plastic should extend to the end of the toes to maintain proper toe alignment, but it must be pulled thin distal to the metatarsal heads to provide a flexible toe break. If a flexible toe break is not provided, the knee extension moment may be excessive, resulting in knee hyperextension. The alternative is to trim the plastic at the metatarsal heads, but the toes are not adequately supported in this latter case.

Extending a rigid keel out to the end of the toes may be indicated to increase the extension moment at the knee. Do not extend the rigid lever arm to the end of the toes if it results in knee hyperextension or difficulty with balance (especially on stairs).

Plantar aspect

Posting may be required to accommodate the hindfoot and rearfoot position so that the subtalar joint is maintained in a neutral position, yet a plantigrade position is achieved (Weber & Agro, 1990).

Posting helps distribute the weight across the plantar aspect and prevents varus or valgus.

Straps

All straps should be well padded.

An instep strap angled at 45° helps hold the heel in place and prevents pistoning and friction.

KAFOs should have a three-point pressure distribution. A combined suprapatellar and infrapatellar strap distributes the pressure best. A spider knee cap pad can also be used but results in greater shear forces through the knee joint.

An infrapatellar strap often deforms the lower leg when worn for a prolonged period of time because the pressure is not well distributed. The patellar tendon–bearing orthotic trim line is preferred in this population because the pressure is better distributed.

Orthotic Fabrication Objectives

Increase medial and lateral stability

Mold in subtalar neutral position (Knutson & Clark, 1991; Weber & Agro, 1990).

Proximal trim line should be sufficiently proximal and anterior to provide adequate leverage to control the ankle and to distribute pressure evenly.

Increase base of support and equalize weight-bearing forces by means of external posting.

Valgus or pronated foot

Post medially under first metatarsal head and medial aspect of calcaneus.

Flare posting medially to increase the base of support and to prevent deviation into valgus.

Varus or supinated foot

Post medially under first metatarsal head to accommodate supinated position of forefoot and equalize pressure distribution.

Zero posting under calcaneus (with lateral flare if needed) to prevent deviation into supination at heel strike.

Orthoses must sit level in shoes, and the shoes should be fastened securely so they do not slide on orthoses.

Decrease energy expenditure

Ankle angle ideally molded or set at 5° plantar flexion with rigid anterior stop (see ankle angle, earlier)

Distal trim line at metatarsal heads to provide a long rigid lever arm

Provide adequate toe clearance and simulate push-off

Plantar flexion stop, ideally set at 5° of plantar flexion if able to adequately clear toe without increasing knee flexion during swing phase (see ankle angle, earlier).

Generally a rigid dorsiflexion stop is required, unless the patient has sufficient plantar flexor strength to control forward movement of tibia during stance phase.

Increase knee extension moment

Ground-reaction force, patellar tendon–bearing orthosis

Solid ankle, cushioned heel, or wedge heel anteriorly to move ground-reaction force forward at heel strike

Rigid dorsiflexion stop set in 5° plantar flexion (see ankle angle, earlier)

Continued

BOX 23–4. **Lower Limb Orthotic Specifications, Objectives, and Examination Criteria—cont'd**

Keel rigid to distal aspect of metatarsal heads to provide a long rigid lever and yet still permit a flexible toe break (see keel, earlier). An even greater extension moment can be provided by extending the rigid lever to the end of the toes. This is usually contraindicated, however, because it results in difficulties with balance (especially on stairs).

Prevent knee hyperextension

Prevent knee hyperextension by increasing knee flexion moment.

Flare heel posteriorly to move ground-reaction force behind knee joint axis at heel strike to produce a flexion moment.

Ankle set at neutral angle with rigid dorsiflexion and plantar flexion stop (if this does not adequately prevent knee hyperextension, the angle may need to be set more acutely, into dorsiflexion). The more acute the angle, however, the greater the energy expenditure (Lehmann et al., 1985).

A low heel (¼ to ½ inch) may decrease knee hyperextension by shifting the center of gravity forward.

Keel rigid to the distal aspect of the metatarsal heads to provide a long rigid lever to decrease energy expenditure. Plastic must be pulled thin beyond this point, however, to provide a flexible toe break (*do not* extend the rigid keel to the end of the toes because this will increase the knee extension moment at push-off).

If knee hyperextension cannot be adequately controlled with previously described modifications, use KAFOs with knee extension stops.

Improve pressure distribution

Use total contact orthoses.

All straps should be well padded.

Bony prominences should be padded (e.g., malleoli, prominent naviculi, patellar tendon region).

Posting to equalize pressure distribution on foot and minimize pressure on malleoli and naviculi.

Patellar tendon–bearing orthosis distributes pressure better than a proximal strap.

KAFOs: the combination of a suprapatellar and infrapatellar strap distributes pressure most effectively.

Improve balance

Adding a low heel (¼ to ½ inch) may improve balance by shifting the center of gravity forward in a person with a calcaneal weight-bearing position.

A high heel shifts the center of gravity too far forward and causes balance problems, particularly in a person with weak or absent plantar flexors.

Orthotic Examination Criteria

Check for pressure areas.

Heel must seat well in orthosis.

Check for rigid keel and flexible toe break.

Check knee alignment and congruency of knee joint axis.

All straps and bony prominences should be well padded.

Check medial and lateral alignment and make sure the orthosis is posted properly with subtalar joint in neutral.

Check angle at ankle (anterior/posterior and medial/lateral).

Check anterior and posterior stops to make sure they adequately control motion, facilitate push-off, and permit toe clearance during swing phase.

Insert orthosis in shoe to check alignment. If molded properly, the orthosis should be able to balance and stand without support on a flat surface.

---

and a neurosegmental classification of "no loss" as an adolescent. His lesion level was reclassified at an L5 level at the time of our study. His loss of neurologic function was caused by a recurrent lipoma on his spine that went undetected and was not surgically removed until permanent neurologic loss had occurred. This individual thought that because his original lesion was removed as an infant with preservation of his spinal cord function, he had no risk of future problems and therefore did not seek medical care until neurologic loss was irreversible. Early detection of progressive muscle strength loss, scoliosis, progression of spasticity, or contractures by the physical therapist with timely referral to a physician familiar with the potential complications associated with MM, along with aggressive physical therapy to reverse lost function (see section on prevention of secondary impairments and functional limitations), can prevent this scenario. This patient's story underscores the need for all individuals with MM to be followed *throughout life,* even if there are seemingly no current problems or their lesion has been classified as "no loss" after surgical closure.

Typical Physical Therapy Goals and Strategies

Functional goals for adolescents and adults are based on a number of factors that have been discussed in preceding sections of this chapter. The section on determinants of outcome and prognosis provides guidelines for outcome expectations based on neurologic system function. In general, the goal for all but the most severely involved patients is to achieve independent basic and community mobility skills. The physical therapist must, therefore, be aware of all environments, distances, and barriers the individual is required to negotiate to adequately prepare the patient for all eventualities. Instruction in advanced community skills, along with endurance training, is often indicated. Physical and occupational therapists often need to be involved with driver's education programs and with the provision of adaptive equipment required for driving.

Goodwyn (1990) expanded the Functional Activities Assessment format to include adolescent skills required for independent living. The items were selected from existing adult-oriented skill achievement tests, and normative data were studied in this population. The Kohlman Evaluation of Living Skills (McGourty, 1988) is also a useful screening tool for determining independence with adult living skills such as self-care, safety, health maintenance, money management, transportation, telephone use, and work and leisure activities. For adolescents and adults, the ability to lift and carry items such as a hot dish, grocery bags, a laundry basket, and heavy household items is also important to evaluate. It is particularly important to observe safety issues and the use of proper body mechanics for advanced living skills. In addition, the maximum carrying distance should be determined and contrasted with functional demands. If independence and effectiveness with ADL are limited, appropriate adaptations and interventions should be made to foster independence. Environmental adaptations or assistive devices required to perform functional tasks should be determined and specifically selected for application to social, educational, vocational, and work capacity requirements of the adolescent and adult. Vocational counseling and planning should begin early during the high school years. A social worker may need to be involved with the family to assist with the transition to independent living because a mutually dependent relationship is often fostered by the intense lifelong involvement of parents and siblings in assisting the individual with MM. Recreation therapy may be used to assist with shopping for and purchasing personal items, use of public transportation, and developing appropriate adult leisure activities. Occupational therapy may be useful to address advanced living skills such as cooking, cleaning, laundry, money management, and driver's training for appropriate candidates. A social worker can assist with locating accessible housing and obtaining appropriate support services for physical tasks that are too difficult for the patient. Depending on the practice setting, however, it may be necessary for the physical therapist to manage these areas. The expectation for individuals with MM who have intelligence in the normal range and sufficient motor function to care for themselves is the ability to thrive as an independent adult in our society.

Prevention of Secondary Impairments and Functional Limitations

The physical therapist plays an important role in anticipating the potential for functional loss when one of the medical complications of MM previously described increases the risk of secondary impairments. For example, when an adolescent undergoes a surgical procedure that requires extended bed rest, maintenance of muscle extensibility, joint ROM, and strength at the bedside followed by resumption of physical mobility tasks as soon as possible postoperatively can prevent long-term or permanent decline in mobility skills. Unfortunately, care providers are often not aware of these issues and intervention is not instituted until it is too late to recover lost function. The physical therapist must serve as an advocate for the patient under these circumstances.

Another mechanism for preventing secondary impairments is education of patients and their parents regarding the fit, specifications, condition, and maintenance of their adaptive equipment. They should know how to monitor skin tolerance and the fit of adaptive equipment. They should also understand the rationale for equipment and design features that are recommended. Knowledgeable consumers can detect and report potential problems before they result in complications such as decubiti. They need to be aware of the potential consequences of poorly fitted equipment so that they can advocate for the provision of quality equipment. The majority of adults in our follow-up study had improperly fitted equipment or lacked equipment that was essential for optimal function. These adults were also unaware of proper equipment maintenance techniques (Hinderer et al., 1988). As a result, many adults were functioning well below their capabilities and had skin breakdown, back pain, or joint pain as a result of poorly fitted orthoses or improper wheelchair design and seating.

DETERMINANTS OF OUTCOME AND PROGNOSIS

The motor function present is the most important factor for predicting outcome and prognosis. Common characteristics of each lesion level are described in this section. The functional motor level does not always correspond to the anatomic lesion level because of individual variations in nerve root innervation of muscles. The information presented here is intended to serve as general guidelines for expectations at a given level of motor function. Many factors besides muscle strength influence an individual's functional potential and result in variations of performance within a given lesion level group. These factors include age, body proportions, weight, sensation, orthopedic deformities, joint contractures, spasticity, upper limb function, and cognition. The relative contribution of these factors is highly individual, and a thorough examination and follow-up of each child is necessary to maximize potential capabilities.

Thoracic Level

Individuals with thoracic level muscle function have innervation of neck, upper limb, shoulder girdle, and trunk musculature, but no volitional lower limb movements are present. Neck, upper limb, and shoulder girdle muscle groups are innervated by the C1 to T4 spinal nerves; back extensors by the C2 to L4 spinal nerves; intercostals by the thoracic nerves; and abdominals by T5 to L1. Consequently, individuals with motor function at or above T10 have strong upper limbs and upper thoracic and neck motions, but their lower trunk musculature is weak. They have difficulty with unsupported sitting balance and may have decreased respiratory function. Sliding boards may be required to perform wheelchair transfers because of the combination of poor trunk control and upper limb dyscoordination.

Individuals with motor function at T12 have strong trunk musculature and good sitting balance and may have weak hip hiking by means of the quadratus lumborum (innervated by T12 to L3). Ambulation may be attempted for exercise at this level using a parapodium. A wheelchair, however, is required for functional household and community mobility.

Children with thoracic level lesions also tend to have greater involvement of other areas of the central nervous system, with corresponding cognitive deficits. Consequently, even though many of these people achieve independence with basic self-care skills and mobility by late childhood, they often require a supervised living situation throughout life. They are rarely competitively employed but often participate in sheltered workshop settings or perform volunteer work (Hinderer et al., 1988).

High Lumbar (L1–L2) Level

Individuals with high lumbar motor function have weak hip movements. The iliopsoas muscle is supplied by nerve roots L1 through L4, with its primary innervation at L2 and L3. The sartorius muscle is supplied by L2 and L3 and the adductors by L2 through L4. With L1 motor function, weak hip flex-

ion may be present, and with L2 motor function the hip flexors, adductors, and rotators are grade 3 or better. According to Schafer and Dias (1983), unopposed hip flexion and adduction contractures are often present at the L2 motor level, and this muscle imbalance often results in dislocated hips. Short-distance household ambulation is possible with high lumbar innervation (L1 and L2) when body proportions are small, using KAFOs or RGOs and upper limb support. These children generally use a wheelchair for community distances. By the second decade of life, a wheelchair is typically the sole means of mobility commensurate with increased energy requirements and enlarged body proportions (Hinderer et al., 1988; Shurtleff, 1986d).

The prognosis of children with high lumbar lesions for function and independent living as adults is similar to that of the thoracic group described earlier (Hinderer et al., 1988). More individuals in this group, however, achieve independent living status (approximately 50%), but they are rarely able to maintain competitive employment as adults.

L3 Level

Individuals with L3 muscle function have strong hip flexion and adduction, weak hip rotation, and at least antigravity knee extension. The quadriceps muscle group is innervated by nerve roots L2 through L4. Children with grade 3 quadriceps strength usually require KAFOs and forearm crutches to ambulate for household and short community distances and a wheelchair for long community distances. By adulthood, most individuals with L3 level lesions are primarily wheelchair mobile (Hinderer et al., 1988; Shurtleff & Lamers, 1978; Stillwell & Menelaus, 1983).

Approximately 60% of individuals with lesions at this level achieve independent living status as adults (Hinderer et al., 1988). Despite their higher level of independence, only a small percentage (about 20%) actively participate in full-time competitive employment (Hinderer et al., 1988).

L4 Level

At the L4 motor level, antigravity knee flexion and grade 4 ankle dorsiflexion with inversion may be present. The medial hamstrings are innervated by nerve roots L4 through S2, and the anterior tibialis is innervated primarily by L4 and L5, with some innervation from S1. An individual is considered to have L4 motor function if the medial hamstrings or anterior tibialis is at least grade 3. Calcaneal foot deformities are common at this motor level as a result of the unopposed action of the tibialis anterior muscle

(Schafer & Dias, 1983). Knee extension is usually strong, and these individuals are generally functional ambulators with AFOs and forearm crutches. When first learning to walk, however, KAFOs, a walker, or both may be required. A wheelchair is often needed for long distances.

In the adult follow-up study that we conducted, only 20% of individuals with L4 motor function continued to ambulate as adults (Hinderer et al., 1988). Many individuals stopped ambulation after their adolescent growth spurt. Others were unable to maintain ambulation because of ankle and knee valgus joint deformities and elbow and wrist pain resulting from years of weight bearing in poor alignment. To increase the likelihood of maintaining biped ambulation for individuals with L4 motor function throughout adulthood, upright posture should be emphasized when ambulating to minimize the weight-bearing stress on upper limb joints. Orthoses must be aligned properly and posted to support the ankle in a subtalar neutral position. If the ankle joint is malaligned, the knee joint position is adversely affected. It is essential to maintain the knee and ankle in neutral alignment when weight bearing. A flexed and valgus position should not be permitted. Often a patellar tendon–bearing, ground-reaction force orthotic design is optimal to protect the knee and increase the knee extension moment. The proximal medial trim line can be extended higher to provide additional medial knee support, if needed, to reduce a genu valgus deformity (see Fig. 23–5). Knee musculature should be strengthened to assist in maintaining the knee in neutral alignment when weight bearing. Every effort should be made to progress ambulation to using AFOs and forearm crutches to allow short-distance ambulation to easily be combined with long-distance wheelchair mobility. Crutches can be transported on the wheelchair, and AFOs are optimal because, unlike KAFOs, they do not interfere with dressing or toileting and do not cause skin breakdown when sitting. The prognosis for independent living and employment is similar to that for the group with L3 lesions.

L5 Level

According to the IMSG criteria, classification of an L5 motor level is based on the presence of lateral hamstring muscles with at least grade 3 strength, and either grade 2 gluteus minimus and medius muscles (L4–S1), grade 3 posterior tibialis muscles (L5–S1), or grade 4 peroneus tertius muscles (L4–S1). Therefore, an individual with an L5 motor level has at least antigravity knee flexion and weak hip extension using the hamstrings and may have weak hip abduction, as well as weak plantar flexion with inver-

sion, strong dorsiflexion with eversion, or both. Weak toe movements may also be present. Hindfoot valgus deformities or calcaneal foot deformities are common as a result of muscle imbalance. Individuals with motor function through L5 are able to ambulate without orthoses, yet require them to correct foot alignment and substitute for lack of push-off. A gluteal lurch is typically evident unless upper limb support is used. Bilateral upper limb support is usually recommended for community distances to decrease energy expenditure, decrease gluteal lurch and trunk sway, maintain symmetric alignment, protect lower limb joints, and improve safety. The need for upper limb support often becomes more apparent with increased height following growth spurts. Traversing uneven terrain is often difficult. A wheelchair may be required when there is a rapid change in body proportions (e.g., pregnancy) or for long distances on rough terrain. A bike is also useful for long community distances.

Approximately 80% of individuals with lesions at L5 and below achieve independent living status as adults (Hinderer et al., 1988). About 30% are employed full time and an additional 20% part time, well below the average employment rate of the general adult population.

S1 Level

With muscle function present through S1, at least two of the following additional muscle actions are present: gastrocnemius/soleus (grade 2), gluteus medius (grade 3), or gluteus maximus (grade 2). Individuals with S1 motor function have improved hip stability and can walk without orthoses or upper limb support. A weak push-off is evident when running or climbing stairs. A mild to moderate gluteal lurch is often present. Gait deviations and functional limitations are often more pronounced after the adolescent growth spurt. The toe musculature is generally strong. Foot deformities are less common at this level, but foot orthoses or AFOs may be required to improve lower limb alignment and permit muscle groups to function at a more optimal length. Medial and lateral stability at the ankle appears to be required for adequate function of the plantar flexor muscles during push-off (Lehmann et al., 1986).

S2, S2–S3, and "No Loss" Levels

Motor function is classified at the S2 level if the plantar flexor muscles are at least grade 3 and the gluteals grade 4. The only obvious gait abnormality present at this level is generally a decreased push-off and stride length when walking rapidly or running as a result of the decreased strength of the plantar flexor muscles. If all lower limb muscle groups have grade 5 strength except for one or two groups with grade 4 strength, the motor level is classified as S2–S3, according to the IMSG criteria. The term *no loss* is used if the bowel and bladder function normally and lower limb strength is judged to be normal through manual muscle testing. Functional deficits may be present, however, for individuals classified as having no loss. Foot orthoses are often beneficial to maintain the ankle in the subtalar neutral position and optimize ankle muscle function by maintaining optimal muscle length.

EXAMINATION, EVALUATION, AND DIRECT INTERVENTIONS FOR MUSCULOSKELETAL ISSUES, MOBILITY, AND FUNCTIONAL SKILLS

There are three primary reasons for evaluating the individual with MM: 1) to define an individual's current status so that appropriate program planning can occur, 2) to identify the potential for developing secondary impairments so that preventive measures can be implemented, and 3) to monitor changes in status that could indicate progressive neurologic dysfunction. Because of the complexity of problems associated with MM, numerous dimensions of disability must be assessed by various disciplines. The physical therapist provides essential information to other team members for program planning and to monitor status. Careful documentation is important for communication among team members and for serial comparisons over time. General examination and intervention strategies will be discussed in this section. Considerations that are specific to certain age categories are discussed in the section on age-specific examination and physical therapy interventions.

Examination Strategies

The dimensions typically assessed by physical therapists include ROM, muscle extensibility, joint alignment or orthopedic deformities, muscle tone, muscle strength and endurance, sensation, posture, motor development, ADL, mobility skills, equipment needs, and environmental accessibility. It is important to use standardized protocols, when available, that have good reliability and validity to permit comparison within and between individuals (Hinderer & Hinderer, 1998). If more than one measurement method exists (e.g., hip extension ROM), the specific method employed should be documented and used consistently. Comprehensive examinations should be conducted at regular intervals throughout the life span on all individuals with MM.

In addition, it is recommended that therapists remain blind to previous results of the more subjective measures (e.g., manual muscle testing scores or gait deviations) until the examination is complete to avoid potential biases from previous results. Videotapes and photographs are often a useful adjunct to clinical examination of gait, joint deformities, and posture. These visual records provide an excellent baseline for comparison purposes if deterioration in status is suspected. It is beneficial to conduct examination of activities that are influenced by environmental or endurance factors (e.g., wheelchair mobility, gait, or ADL) in more natural settings.

The IMSG recommends a comprehensive, multidisciplinary evaluation for *all* individuals with MM, regardless of functional level, because they all are at risk for progressive neurologic dysfunction, as discussed earlier. The following examination intervals are recommended: newborn preoperatively, newborn postoperatively, 6 months, 12 months, 18 months, 24 months, and annually thereafter, continuing through adulthood (Shurtleff, 1986c). Annual examinations are suggested to occur around an individual's birth date so that they are not forgotten. ROM, muscle extensibility, strength, endurance, coordination, and functional parameters should be monitored more closely during periods of rapid growth, when individuals with MM are at increased risk for loss of function. Preintervention and postintervention measurements should be obtained for individuals undergoing surgery or other therapeutic procedures. More frequent evaluation of specific goal attainment is indicated for individuals receiving ongoing therapeutic intervention. Mobility and independence with ADL should be reevaluated when body proportions or environmental demands change to determine if the individual has the strength, endurance, coordination, and adaptive equipment required to function effectively.

Shurtleff (1986c, 1991) advocates using the Patient Data Management System (PDMS) standardized protocol and recording format to serially monitor individuals with MM. The PDMS is composed of a comprehensive, interdisciplinary recording format, which consists of the dimensions typically assessed by each discipline. In addition, intervention data (e.g., surgery, medications, and therapy) are also documented. Scoring and recording criteria can be obtained by contacting the IMSG (IMSG, 1993). The PDMS computerized recording format is beneficial for monitoring this population because serial test results from birth to present can be efficiently scanned for each parameter to detect improvements or deterioration in status. In addition, an individual patient's status can be directly compared with that of other individuals with similar characteristics by using the interactive database. The standardized format facilitates communication between and within disciplines and intervention centers and promotes clinical research. Duplication of effort by the various health care professionals involved in the intervention of individuals with MM is minimized because each discipline is assigned specific PDMS areas to assess, yet all disciplines share the information in the combined database. The PDMS format has also been applied to several other pediatric populations, including those with cerebral palsy, cystic fibrosis, hemophilia, and traumatic brain injury (Shurtleff, 1991).

Individuals with MM should be evaluated on at least a yearly basis by multiple disciplines at a comprehensive care center. It is important, however, for comprehensive care centers and local school and intervention settings to coordinate their examinations, goals, and intervention programs to avoid duplication of effort and to ensure appropriate prioritization of intervention goals. The use of the PDMS facilitates communication. The School Needs Identification and Action Forms (Rowley-Kelly & Kunkle, 1993) also provide a useful format for identifying impairments, academic and functional limitations, and the remedial action recommended. The areas assessed by the school needs forms include health-related services required, physical intervention instructions, accessibility, safety and fire drills, preparation for school entry, educational rights and related services, academic difficulties, psychologic evaluation, perceptuomotor deficits, visuoperceptual deficits, self-help skills, social acceptance, social and emotional issues, parent and school relationships, transitional services, and other needs.

Intervention Strategies

Once primary and secondary impairments and disabilities are identified through a comprehensive evaluation, the functional significance must be determined to plan appropriate intervention strategies. Intervention of an impairment is indicated if it currently interferes with function or if the deficit can progress to a point where it may negatively affect future function. Intervention is also indicated if the efficiency, effectiveness, or safety of performance can be improved. Strength, endurance, and efficiency of performing tasks should be emphasized. Weight-bearing joints must be protected to prevent early onset of osteoarthritis and to prolong mobility. In addition, the most efficient and effective means of mobility for a given environment should be determined. Goal setting for intervention must consider the impact of the multiple impairments discussed earlier on functional performance expectations. The

cognitive, social, and behavioral issues discussed in the impairments section should also be considered.

Fay and associates (1986) recommend three specific intervention approaches for developmental delays in this population. The first is developmental programming in which children are encouraged by parents, teachers, and therapists with a "high dose" of normal developmental activities in "at-risk" areas. The philosophy behind this approach is that supplemental early emphasis and practice in potential problem areas will minimize later deficits. These early intervention programs are often initiated for children with MM before measurable delays are identified. The second approach, remediation, is implemented once problem areas are clearly identified. This approach consists of repetition of a set of graded tasks in the domain of concern. Improved performance through practice theoretically carries over into functional activities. The third approach is teaching compensatory skills. Compensation is often implemented when the other two approaches have not produced sufficient results or when the child is older or more severely inpaired. This intervention approach involves identifying functional impairments and developing strategies to help the child become as independent as possible or providing adaptive equipment to compensate for underlying problems and minimize disability in daily life.

Specific Examination and Intervention Strategies

Specific examination and intervention strategies as they pertain to strength, mobility, gait, and equipment issues are highlighted in this section because of the magnitude of the impact of these factors on function in this population, regardless of age or lesion level. Suggestions for impairment-specific parameters (e.g., ROM, orthopedic deformities, and sensation) were discussed in the section on impairments. Developmental issues were discussed in the section on age-specific examination and physical therapy interventions.

Strength

Upper limb, neck, and trunk musculature should be screened for weakness. If evidence of weakness exists, a more specific examination of strength should be conducted. For individuals with thoracic or high lumbar level involvement, it is important to palpate trunk musculature to determine which portions of muscle groups are functioning. Dynamometer values of grip and pinch strength should also be obtained. Kilburn and associates (1985) suggest that grip strength measurements can be a sensitive measure of progressive neurologic dysfunction. A standardized protocol for obtaining grip strength measurements and normative values for children has been provided by Level (1984).

Specific testing of isolated motions of lower limb muscles is essential to determine if individual muscles are functioning. Standardized test protocols should be used (e.g., Hislop & Montgomery, 1995; Janda, 1983; Kendall et al., 1999). It is *essential* to detect changes in strength in this population as soon as possible, because loss of strength can be a sign of progressive neurologic dysfunction. As a result, we recommend using quantitative strength measurements in conjunction with traditional manual muscle testing techniques. It is also important to distinguish between reflexive and voluntary movements. Reflexive movements should be documented, but they should not be considered when determining motor lesion levels.

Manual muscle testing is the most common method used to assess strength in this population because of its adaptability in a typical clinic setting. Manual muscle testing is the method of choice for screening muscle strength to determine the presence of volitional activity in specific muscles and to determine whether an individual muscle's function varies throughout the ROM. There are several limitations to relying only on manual muscle testing scores for serially monitoring strength, as discussed in Chapter 4.

Manual muscle testing has limited interrater and test-retest reliability (Hinderer & Hinderer, 1993). Manual muscle test scores must change more than one full grade to be confident that a true change in strength has occurred. In addition, manual muscle testing has poor concurrent validity compared with more quantitative measures. Several studies have demonstrated that deficits in strength exceeding 50% are *not* detected by manual muscle testing (Agre et al., 1987; Aitkens et al., 1989; Bohannon, 1986; Griffin et al., 1986; Miller et al., 1988). Agre and colleagues (1987) examined this issue in 33 adolescents with MM. Individuals who had been classified as having "no motor deficits" by means of manual muscle testing actually had strength deficits compared with normative data. These deficits were 40% for the hip extensor and 60% for the knee extensor muscles. The lack of concurrent validity of manual muscle testing compared with quantitative measurements demonstrates that the sensitivity of manual muscle testing in detecting weakness is very limited and is inadequate for detecting early strength loss in individuals with MM.

The *predictive validity* of manual muscle testing has been examined in two studies on children with MM. Murdoch (1980) examined the predictive validity of neonatal manual muscle testing examinations using a truncated 3-point scale. The correlation between muscle power of the newborn and subsequent mobility of the child at age 3 to 8 years was "very poor." In contrast, McDonald and associates (1986) examined the predictive validity of manual muscle testing for individual muscle groups on 825 children with MM using the complete 0- to 5-point grading scale. Predictive validity of manual muscle testing generally increased from birth to age 5. The probability that a given manual muscle test score precisely predicted future scores varied with age and the particular muscle group tested. These probabilities ranged from 23 to 68% for newborns and from 54 to 87% for older children. The probability that a single test score predicted future strength within ±1 manual muscle test grade, however, was considerably higher, ranging from 70 to 86% for newborns and from 87 to 97% for older children. These results indicate that manual muscle testing is useful for predicting future muscle function within one manual muscle test grade. Strength test results obtained in infancy using the complete manual muscle test scale, therefore, appear to provide useful information for prognosis and for planning the course of intervention.

The limited reliability and concurrent validity of manual muscle testing indicates that it is not the method of choice for monitoring changes in strength over time. In contrast, strength testing using handheld instruments has been found to be a reliable and sensitive method for assessing strength in children and adolescents with MM. Intraclass interrater and test-retest correlation coefficients using this technique ranged from .73 to .99 (Effgen & Brown, 1992; Hinderer, 1988). Other authors report good to high levels of reliability when testing the strength of other populations of children and adolescents with handheld instrumentation (Florence et al., 1988; Hinderer & Gutierrez, 1988; Hinderer & Hinderer, 1993; Hosking et al., 1976; Hyde et al., 1983; Mendell & Florence, 1990; Stuberg & Metcalf, 1988). Several portable, handheld instruments are available for use in conjunction with manual muscle testing (Hinderer & Hinderer, 1993). The advantages of these instruments over nonportable instruments are that they are easily applied in typical clinic settings and can be used with standard manual muscle testing techniques to obtain objective force readings from most muscle groups.

It is best to obtain three myometry trials and report the average score because the mean is more stable over time and between raters (Hack et al., 1981; Hinderer, 1988). Torque values should be reported (force times lever arm length) to permit comparison over time, regardless of changing body proportions, at least until skeletal maturity has been attained. Torque values also permit direct comparison of force production capabilities between individuals with different body proportions. Standardized testing techniques must be implemented when assessing strength with handheld instruments to ensure the consistency of measurements. Many factors influence test results and must be controlled for when testing, including test positions, instructions and commands provided, use of reinforcement and feedback, application of resistance, the type of contraction, and the examiner's body mechanics. For more information regarding techniques used in testing with handheld instruments, see Hinderer and Hinderer (1993).

Several factors should be considered when testing the muscle strength of children with MM, including age, developmental level, cognitive level, ability to follow directions, attention span, motivation, motor planning skills, sensation, and proprioception. The examiner must carefully watch for muscle substitutions. This is particularly challenging in the MM population because of altered angles of pull from orthopedic deformities. It is often difficult for multi-joint muscles such as the hamstrings to initiate motions. Any differences in function between end-range and midrange positions should be noted. Special considerations when testing infants and young children are discussed in the section on age-specific examination and physical therapy interventions.

As discussed in the impairments section, several CNS complications can account for loss of muscle function in this population, necessitating serial strength testing for early detection. There are many factors that can result in normal variations in strength, however, that should also be considered when interpreting test results. These factors include changes in body proportions, hormonal influences, motor learning, illness, injury, surgery, immobilization, physical or psychologic fatigue, the prior state of activity, seasonal variations, temporal factors, motivation, cooperation, and comprehension. Discussion of the specific influences of these factors is beyond the scope of this chapter. For further information regarding the impact of these factors on force production, see Hinderer and Hinderer (1993). Because of the multiple factors that can influence force production, it is important to repeat the testing at more frequent intervals, if strength loss is suspected, to determine whether consistent test results are obtained. Several variables should be considered when interpreting muscle test results, including the reliability and standard error of measurement of the testing method used, the concurrent and predictive validity of test results, and factors that can account for fluctuations in strength (Hinderer & Hinderer, 1993).

Static strength measurements should be correlated with functional measures to observe effects of fatigue and to determine the effect of reduced strength and limited endurance on function. Individuals with neurogenic muscle weakness may have a higher degree of variability in force production as a result of the lower threshold of fatigue and slower rate of recovery of weak musculature. Local muscle endurance appears to be deficient in some neuromuscular diseases (Bar-Or, 1986; Milner-Brown & Miller, 1989). Although this issue has not been specifically tested in the MM population, these results suggest that force production may be more variable in weak muscle groups of individuals with MM.

If function is present but weakness exists in muscle groups that are important for postural stability, ADL, mobility, or balance of muscle forces around joints, strengthening exercises are indicated. The specific muscle groups to emphasize vary depending on the lesion level and functional requirements. In general, strong upper limb muscle groups are required for performing transfers, for wheelchair propulsion, and when using assistive devices to walk. Increasing the strength of trunk musculature improves sitting balance and postural stability. Increasing the strength of key lower limb muscle groups that are critical for ambulation can improve gait and can possibly minimize the need for orthoses and assistive devices. For example, increasing the quadriceps and hamstrings strength in an individual with L4 motor function may enable progression of ambulation from using KAFOs to using AFOs (see the case history at the end of this chapter).

Muscle groups should be strengthened within functional ROM. In addition to traditional strengthening exercises, many play activities promote strengthening (Embry et al., 1983). Muscle reeducation techniques such as functional electrical stimulation and biofeedback are useful to teach muscles to function in new parts of the ROM. Electrical stimulation has also been found to be beneficial to increase strength and enhance functional performance in this population (Karmel-Ross et al., 1992). Strengthening programs should be implemented during periods when an individual is at risk for loss of muscle strength and endurance (e.g., after recent surgery, immobilization, illness, or bed rest) and during periods of rapid growth when individuals often lose function as a result of changes in body proportions.

Endurance activities are also important for weight control and to enhance aerobic capacity. Individuals with MM must have adequate endurance to meet the challenges of community mobility. Low-impact aerobic activities to minimize joint stress are preferable. In general, jumping activities should be avoided because joint stress is increased as a result of the inadequate deceleration provided by weak lower limb muscles. Indications for endurance training and instruction in energy conservation techniques include decreased aerobic capacity, high energy cost of mobility, and limited endurance.

Mobility

Ineffective mobility is a hallmark of MM. *Effective mobility* is defined as any efficient and effective means of moving about in space that enables the individual to easily traverse and explore the environment, grow and develop, and independently pursue an education, vocation, or avocation (Shurtleff, 1986d). Mobility options provided should meet these criteria for all environments encountered by the individual so that lifestyle is not limited by endurance and difficulty traversing uneven terrain.

Changes in body proportions can significantly affect mobility. Mobility options, orthoses, and assistive device requirements that are ideal at one time may not be effective once body proportions, environmental demands, or both change. Consequently, the appropriateness of adaptive equipment and mobility options must be reevaluated throughout the life span. Emphasis of this point to patients by their health care providers helps prevent the feeling of failure if alternative mobility options are required in the future. Too often, individuals with MM grow up being praised for walking instead of using a wheelchair or for walking without assistive devices, depending on their lesion level. This emphasis gives the impression that normal biped ambulation is the only socially acceptable form of mobility. Several of the adults in our follow-up study reported that it was difficult to accept the use of a wheelchair or other assistive devices as they grew up because they felt that they were a failure or that they would disappoint their parents and health care providers (Hinderer & Hinderer, 1988). It is important to emphasize that wheelchairs and other assistive devices are aids for effective mobility and that their use does not represent a failure of biped ambulation.

Bed mobility, floor mobility, wheelchair mobility, ambulation, and transfers should be assessed and compared with the requirements for independent function. Criteria for assessing mobility parameters are endurance, efficiency, effectiveness, safety, degree of independence, and accessibility. Objective information regarding these parameters is often helpful to convince patients and their parents that alternative methods of mobility should be considered. Efficiency can be estimated by measuring the time required to complete a task. Energy expenditure can be estimated by measuring heart rate. Regression equa-

tions have been determined for this population to equate heart rate with the energy expenditure required for a given task (Williams et al., 1983). The regression equations for energy expenditure and efficiency of this population are as follows:

Energy cost (ml O_2/kg min) = 0.073 (HR) + 6.119.

Energy efficiency (ml O_2/kg meter) = 0.006 (HR) − 0.313.

Criteria for determining the most practical and effective mode of mobility for household and community distances are provided in Box 23–2. Standardized tests that are useful for evaluating mobility in this population are discussed in Chapter 1. In addition, the Timed Test of Patient Mobility (Jebsen et al., 1970) is beneficial for assessing the efficiency of mobility because the time required to perform bed mobility, transfers, wheelchair mobility, and gait mobility tasks is documented. Normative data are available for comparison purposes. We suggest augmenting the efficiency time score of the Timed Test of Patient Mobility with a rating scale for the level of independence, safety, practicality, and assistive devices required for each task (Hinderer & Hinderer, 1988). Other evaluations that are specific to function in wheelchairs include the Functional Task Performance Wheelchair Assessment of positioning, reaching, and driving tasks (Deitz et al., 1991) and the Seated Postural Control Measure for sitting posture and functional movements (Fife et al., 1991).

Gait

Thorough examination and documentation of gait status are essential to monitor functional motor status and to watch for signs of progressive neurologic dysfunction. Patients or their parents typically notice changes in gait patterns and walking endurance before they notice increased muscle weakness. Careful gait observation is also needed to determine the most appropriate orthoses and assistive devices. Examination of orthoses and assistive devices for wear patterns helps determine if they are being used on a regular basis or just to perform in the clinic setting. Gait should be evaluated in a natural environment on a variety of walking surfaces. Patients should be observed walking for typical household and community distances to determine the effects of fatigue.

All too often decisions regarding gait problems and the need for orthoses and assistive devices are made by observing short-distance ambulation on a smooth clinic floor. Performance in the home or community environment may be vastly different than in a clinic situation, especially when walking around a number of obstacles, when in congested areas, when traversing uneven terrain, or with inclement weather. The impact of these factors must be considered when making recommendations.

Requirements for orthoses and ambulatory aids should be documented. Gait deviations should be closely observed and recorded. If possible, gait deviations and efficiency parameters should be observed both with and without orthoses and assistive devices. Typical gait parameters evaluated include arm swing, trunk position and sway, pelvic tilt and rotations, compensated or uncompensated Trendelenburg position, excessive hip flexion and rotation, excessive knee flexion or hyperextension, toe clearance, foot position, push-off effectiveness, and foot progression angle.

Observational gait analysis is the technique used most commonly to assess gait in clinical settings (Krebs et al., 1985). Video analysis augments clinical observations by allowing the evaluator to observe gait multiple times at slow speeds and by providing a permanent record that is invaluable for comparison purposes if deterioration of functional status is suspected. The interrater reliability of observational analysis through videotapes, however, has been reported to be low to moderate (Eastlack et al., 1991; Krebs et al., 1985). Footprint analysis is a low-cost method of obtaining objective information regarding velocity, cadence, foot progression angle, base of support, toe clearance, stride length, and step length (Shores, 1980). More sophisticated methods of objective gait analysis are described in Chapter 3.

Criteria for the effectiveness, efficiency, and safety of household and community ambulation are provided in Box 23–2. Efficiency and practicality of ambulation can be estimated by monitoring heart rate, normal and fast walking velocity, and maximum walking distance. Other time-distance variables (e.g., step and stride length, cadence, and cycle time) provide useful information regarding symmetry, stability, and function. These variables can be used for comparison purposes if they are normalized (adjusted) for stature (Rose et al., 1991).

Time-distance variables provide information about gait symmetry by comparing right-left differences in step lengths and stance–to–swing phase ratios. Examining cadence and the percentage of time spent in the stance phase versus the swing phase provides information regarding the stability of gait. For instance, a high cadence or an imbalance in the stance versus swing phase duration may indicate instability. Parameters such as walking velocity and cadence provide information regarding the functional practicality of gait. If the velocity is too low or step rate is too high, the individual may not be able to meet environmental demands.

It is essential to normalize time-distance variables for stature to compare these parameters serially over time for a given individual or to compare between individuals of different stature (e.g., comparing with normative data). These parameters are normalized by dividing by leg length. An alternative but less precise method of normalizing time-distance parameters is to divide by height because overall height is closely correlated to individual limb lengths. If these parameters are not normalized for stature, conclusions regarding differences in function may be confounded by changes in body proportions over time.

Indications for lower limb orthoses are provided in Box 23–3. Specifications and their effect on gait are outlined in Box 23–4. Indications for gait training include when a child is first learning to walk; when there is potential for progression to a new type of orthosis or upper limb aid; for progression to a more efficient gait pattern (e.g., from a four-point to a two-point alternative gait); when there is potential for improving gait (e.g., crouched gait pattern, excessive foot progression angle); to improve safety and confidence with advanced walking activities (e.g., walking on inclines, rough terrain, steps; learning to fall safely and stand up independently from floor; carrying and lifting objects); and to improve the efficiency and safety of gait, transfers, and intervention of aids.

Strength of the quadriceps muscles has been suggested by some authors to be the best predictor of ambulatory potential in children with MM (Schopler & Menelaus, 1987; Williams et al., 1983); others indicate that iliopsoas muscle strength is better (McDonald et al., 1991a). McDonald and associates (1991a) examined the relationship between the patterns of strength and mobility in 291 children with MM who had received at least three serial standardized strength examinations after age 5 and who were classified for their mobility status as community ambulators, partial (household) ambulators, and nonambulators. Iliopsoas muscle strength was found to be the best predictor of ambulation. The quadriceps, anterior tibialis, and gluteal muscles also were determined to have significant importance for ambulation in these children. Grade 0 to 3 iliopsoas strength was always associated with partial or complete reliance on a wheelchair. Patients with grade 4 to 5 iliopsoas and quadriceps muscle strength were almost all community ambulators, and no members of this group were completely wheelchair dependent. Children with grade 4 to 5 gluteal and anterior tibialis muscle strength were all classified as community ambulators and did not require the use of an assistive device or orthosis.

Key muscle groups for community ambulation, listed in order of importance, are the iliopsoas, gluteus medius and maximus, quadriceps, anterior tibialis, and hamstring muscles (McDonald et al., 1991a). Specific strength of these muscles accounted for 86% of the variance in mobility status. Gluteus medius muscle strength was found to be the best predictor of requirements for aids or orthoses. In individuals with gluteus medius strength grade 2 to 3, 72.2% required aids, orthoses, or both. If activity in this muscle was absent or trace, 95.7% required aids, orthoses, or both. In contrast, if gluteus medius strength was grade 4 to 5, only 11.2% required aids, orthoses, or both.

Agre and associates (1987) reported that maximum walking velocity was correlated with hip and knee extensor muscle strength. They compared the energy expenditure and efficiency of ambulation in children with MM versus able-bodied peers and found that children with MM exhibited 218% lower energy efficiency and a 41% lower ambulation velocity. They also reported that mobility in a wheelchair was considerably more efficient than walking, approximating normal gait in terms of energy requirements. In addition, individuals classified as having "no loss" by means of manual muscle testing had a decreased walking velocity and increased energy expenditure compared with able-bodied peers.

Equipment

A wide variety of adaptive equipment typically is required for individuals with MM. Equipment needs vary considerably with level of lesion and age. Therapists must be aware of the available options and be able to select the most appropriate type of equipment for a given situation. In addition, it is important to educate parents and patients regarding the fit and appropriateness of adaptive equipment so that they can be knowledgeable consumers. It is beyond the scope of this chapter to discuss specific equipment items. See Baker and Rogosky-Grassi (1993), Knutson and Clark (1991), and Pomatto (1991) for further information regarding adaptive equipment and orthoses for this population. In the following section the focus is on factors to consider when evaluating the appropriateness and fit of adaptive equipment. Indications for lower limb orthotics are provided in Box 23-3. Design specifications, objectives, and considerations when evaluating the components and fit of orthoses are included in Box 23-4.

Examinations of adaptive equipment and orthotics should be conducted on at least a yearly basis. Examinations should occur more often during periods of rapid growth; when environmental demands change (e.g., changing school or work settings); when there are changes in lifestyle, goals, or vocation; or when there is a change in status that may affect motor control or mobility.

SUMMARY

Few populations challenge the skill and knowledge domains of the physical therapist as extensively as individuals with MM. The previous discussion has highlighted the multitude and complexity of problems encountered by children and adolescents with MM. Each lesion level group has general functional expectations that help direct physical therapy goals from an early age. Although MM is a congenital-onset problem requiring intervention by the physical therapist during infancy and childhood, most of the impairments and functional deficits described in this chapter occur throughout the life span. Individuals with MM should be followed on a regular basis, even as adults, in multidisciplinary specialty clinics by care providers familiar with this population. Because the physical therapist has extended contact with these individuals from infancy through adolescence, the therapist plays an important role in screening and triaging for potential problems, in addition to more traditional physical therapy roles. The challenges and rewards of working with this population are therefore extraordinary. The following case history illustrates the principles of examination and intervention discussed in this chapter.

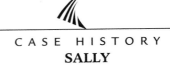

CASE HISTORY
SALLY

History

Sally is a 6-year-old girl with L4 level paraplegia resulting from a myelomeningocele. She was referred for physical therapy assessment to determine if her ambulation skills could be improved. She had a ventriculoperitoneal CSF shunt placed as an infant with one revision secondary to shunt infection. According to her mother Sally performs fine motor activities slowly. She is social, happy, and self-confident, however, and makes friends easily.

At 7 months Sally rolled from prone to supine position but could not sit independently. At 15 months she commando crawled and was able to get into quadruped position. She pulled to stand and had a modified quadruped crawl with little lower limb reciprocation at 2 years of age. She did not have an effective method of mobility until 3½ years of age when she was able to walk with AFOs and a wheeled anterior-facing walker. By 4 years of age, her gait with AFOs and the walker was crouched with little reciprocation and a wheelchair was her primary method of mobility. Her walking improved by switching to use of long leg braces (knees locked) at age 4½ years, and she began to walk with forearm crutches and KAFOs at age 5 years.

Systems review

Sally has frequent urinary tract infections that often cause her to miss school. Sally's mother performs intermittent catheterization every 4 hours, except when Sally is at school.

Tests and measures

Range of motion was within functional limits except for bilateral 15° hip flexion contractures and 20° knee flexion contractures. Her forefeet and hindfeet had a varus inclination when examined in a non–weight-bearing position with her subtalar joint positioned in neutral. This resulted in a valgus, everted position of her feet when bearing weight.

Motor level was L4 with weak quadriceps muscle strength (grade 4–), particularly in the shortened part of the range (from 40 to 20° of active knee extension), and grade 3 + hamstring muscle strength. Weakness in the terminal knee extension range had not been noted previously but was consistent with her history of knee flexion contractures and crouched gait. No volitional activity was present in the gluteal muscles or distal to the knee. Minimal spasticity was present in the hip adductor and hamstring muscles. Sensory level was intact through L3 but absent below this level.

Sally propelled independently in a lightweight wheelchair on level surfaces and on gradual inclines. She was independent for all transfers except to and from the floor because she was unable to independently operate the knee locks on her KAFOs. She walked with locked KAFOs and forearm crutches using a four-point gait pattern and was independent on level surfaces and gradual inclines. She had difficulty traversing uneven terrain and more severe inclines. When she attempted to walk without upper limb support, she had a severe gluteal lurch with lateral trunk sway and lost her balance after a few steps. She was a short-distance community ambulator (primarily walked at home and school and used a wheelchair for long distances). When bearing weight without orthoses or with the knees of her KAFOs unlocked, her hips and knees were severely flexed and her feet were dorsiflexed, everted, and pronated.

Her KAFOs were set in 5° of dorsiflexion and were aligned in valgus at the subtalar joint. The KAFO knee joint axis was not congruent with her anatomic knee joint axis. Only a narrow, infrapatellar anterior knee strap was present, and there was no padding on any of the KAFO straps. She was unable to independently manipulate the knee locks because of her knee flexion contractures. She had pressure marks from the infrapatellar straps and decubiti on her heels.

Evaluation

At the time of her initial assessment, Sally's orthoses did not fit properly and were causing pressure sores. Her parents requested that she progress to AFOs, if possible, so that she could be more independent with transfers. Her hip and knee flexion contractures prevented her from achieving the stable upright stance required for efficient ambulation with AFOs. Her weakness in terminal knee extension, in conjunction with the contractures, presented further difficulties for maintaining upright posture and ambulating with AFOs. Because this weakness had not been noted previously, and she exhibited mild lower limb spasticity, it was important to serially monitor her strength and muscle tone over the next several months to determine if she was experiencing progressive neurologic loss.

Despite the problems, in Sally's favor were the volitional quadriceps and hamstring muscle function present, a supportive family, and her personality with a willingness to try new and difficult tasks. Hip and knee flexion contracture reduction and healing of the heel decubitus ulcers were initial steps that had to be completed before AFOs could be fabricated. The unavailability of physical therapy at school provided an additional challenge. Her father worked full time and her mother had four other children to care for in addition to Sally, so frequent outpatient physical therapy sessions were not a practical alternative. Discontinuance of the improperly fitting KAFOs and good wound care healed the decubitus ulcers. In the meantime, an aggressive program of stretching and strengthening was implemented.

Direct interventions

An initial physical therapy session consisting of soft tissue mobilization followed by passive stretching resulted in 10° reductions in the hip and knee contractures. Sally's mother was instructed by the therapist in techniques for stretching the hip and knee flexors, which Sally performed daily. Strengthening exercises for the quadriceps and hamstring muscles were also implemented, including short arc quads, straight leg raises, knee flexion, and squat-to-stand exercises. Sally was seen biweekly by the therapist for reexamination and progression of her program. After 2 weeks of therapy, she continued to have difficulty with terminal knee extension and initiation of knee flexion. A home program of functional electrical stimulation was implemented to enhance volitional contractions of the quadriceps and hamstring muscles and to assist with muscle reeducation (Karmel-Ross et al., 1992). Strengthening exercises augmented with functional electrical stimulation resulted in significant increases in strength.

After 2 months of intervention, Sally had only 5° hip flexion contractures and her knees could fully extend. Quadriceps and hamstring muscle strength were grades 4 and 4–, respectively. Her decubiti were fully healed and she was anxious to resume bipedal ambulation. The child could stand and walk short distances with her knees and hips extended when she used a reverse-facing walker and concentrated on walking with an upright posture. She fatigued and was distracted easily, however, and still required support at the knees for community distances. The long-term goal remained progression to independent ambulation using AFOs and forearm crutches. Ground-reaction force AFOs (see Fig. 23–5) would most likely be the optimal design for advancing her to ambulation with AFOs, for the reasons outlined in Box 23-3. KAFOs were still currently indicated, however, to maintain an upright posture for community distances. If she regressed to a crouch gait pattern, contractures and stretch weakness could recur. After consultation with the orthotist, new KAFOs were fabricated that incorporated a ground-reaction force AFO component, along with removable metal knee joints, uprights, and thigh cuff sections. These orthoses enabled Sally to practice upright walking using a posture-control walker at home, with the knee joints either locked or unlocked. In therapy sessions, and under her mother's supervision, the thigh and knee components could be removed so that she could practice walking with the ground-reaction force AFOs.

Orthotic specifications included those listed in Box 23-4 for increasing medial and lateral stability, enhancing the knee extension moment, decreasing energy expenditure, providing adequate toe clearance, simulating push-off, distributing pressure evenly, and improving balance. The orthotist molded the feet in subtalar neutral, and the footplates of the AFOs were posted to accommodate forefoot and hindfoot varus and forefoot supination. The posting provided a wider base of plantigrade support to improve balance and prevented her feet from rolling over into pronation when weight bearing, thus maintaining good biomechanical alignment of the ankles and knees. The ankles were set in 5° of plantar flexion, providing an extensor moment at the knees to encourage more upright stance and gait.

Strengthening exercises and functional electrical stimulation were continued. Gait training began at home and in therapy sessions, initially using a posture-control walker and then progressing to forearm crutches. Gait training emphasized an upright posture and terminal knee extension with the KAFO knee joints

unlocked and removed. Functional electrical stimulation was used in conjunction with gait training for muscle reeducation (Kieklak & DeVahl, 1986; Packman & Ewaski, 1983). Videotaping of her gait pattern was used throughout the intervention process to provide visual feedback. Sally quickly progressed to ambulation with forearm crutches with the knee joints unlocked. Strength continued to increase; after 3 months of strengthening and gait training, quadriceps and hamstring muscle strength were grades 4+ and 4, respectively, and she was able to walk with ground-reaction force AFOs and forearm crutches for short community distances using a four-point gait pattern. She continued to use a wheelchair for long distances. Progression to a more efficient two-point gait was then emphasized. She mastered the two-point gait pattern following another month of gait training. Strengthening exercises and stretching have continued prophylactically three times a week. Her mother understood that it was essential to avoid regression to a crouched gait pattern and continued to monitor her ROM and posture closely, especially during periods of rapid growth. Sally continues to ambulate independently for short community distances with ground-reaction force AFOs and forearm crutches and uses a wheelchair for longer distances. She also has mastered wheelchair-to-floor transfers.

Sally was referred by the physical therapist for evaluation by a urologist because of her recurrent urinary tract infections. This physician started her on a daily suppressive dose of antibiotic medication and referred her to a nurse to learn self-catheterization. Owing to Sally's upper limb dyscoordination, it took her several months to master this skill, but the ability to catheterize herself, especially during school hours so that she no longer went 7 hours between catheterizations from before to after school, resulted in resolution of the recurrent infections.

Prognosis

It will be important to continue to teach her advanced wheelchair skills, including ramps and curbs, so that she is independent with the chair in the community; like many individuals with L4 level function, Sally will most likely continue to use the chair for long-distance community mobility as an adolescent and adult. Fortunately, neither Sally's lower limb weakness nor her spasticity progressed to suggest the presence of tethered cord syndrome; however, monitoring should continue at least annually throughout her life.

Recommended Resources

Patient Data Management System. Myelodysplasia Study Data Collection Criteria and Instructions, 1994. Available from D.B. Shurtleff, MD, Professor, Department of Pediatrics, University of Washington, Seattle, WA 98195.

References

Agre, JC, Findley, TW, McNally, MC, Habeck, R, Leon, AS, Stradel, L, Birkebak, R, & Schmalz, R. Physical activity capacity in children with myelomeningocele. Archives of Physical Medicine and Rehabilitation, 68:372–377, 1987.

Aitkins, S, Lord, J, Bernauer, E, Fowler, W, Lieberman, J, & Berck, P. Relationship of manual muscle testing to objective strength measurements. Muscle and Nerve, 12:173–177, 1989.

Andersen, EM, & Plewis, I. Impairment of motor skill in children with spina bifida cystica and hydrocephalus: An exploratory study. British Journal of Psychology, 68:61–70, 1977.

Asher, M, & Olson, J. Factors affecting the ambulatory status of patients with spina bifida cystica. Journal of Bone and Joint Surgery (American), 65:350–356, 1983.

Baker, SB, & Rogosky-Grassi, MA. Access to the school. In Rowley-Kelly, FL, & Reigel, DH (Eds.), Teaching the Student with Spina Bifida. Baltimore: Paul H. Brookes, 1993, pp. 31–70.

Bar-Or, O. Pathophysiological factors which limit the exercise capacity of the sick child. Medicine and Science in Sports and Exercise, 18:276–282, 1986.

Bartlett, MD, Wolf, LS, Shurtleff, DB, & Staheli, LT. Hip flexion contractures: A comparison of measurement methods. Archives of Physical Medicine and Rehabilitation, 66:620–625, 1985.

Becker, RD. Recent developments in child psychiatry: I. The restrictive emotional and cognitive environment reconsidered: A redefinition of the concept of therapeutic restraint. Israeli Journal of Psychiatry and Related Sciences, 12:239–258, 1975.

Birth Defects and Genetic Diseases Branch of Birth Defects and Developmental Disabilities Office, National Center for Environmental Disease and Injury. Use of folic acid prevention of spina bifida and other neural tube defects, 1983–1991. Morbidity and Mortality Weekly Report, 40:1–4, 1991.

Bleck, EE, & Nagel, DA. Physically Handicapped Children—A Medical Atlas for Teachers. Orlando, FL: Grune & Stratton, 1982.

Bohannon, RW. Manual muscle test scores and dynamometer test scores of knee extension strength. Archives of Physical Medicine and Rehabilitation, 67:390–392, 1986.

Brunt, D. Characteristics of upper limb movements in a sample of meningomyelocele children. Perceptual Motor Skills, 51:431–437, 1980.

Butler, C, Okamoto, GA, & McKay, TM. Motorized wheelchair driving by disabled children. Archives of Physical Medicine and Rehabilitation, 65:95–97, 1984.

Chaffin, DB, Andersson, GBJ, & Martin, BJ. Occupational Biomechanics, 3rd ed. New York: John Wiley & Sons, 1999.

Chandler, LS, Andrews, MS, & Swanson, MW. Movement Assessment of Infants: A Manual. Rolling Bay, WA: Authors, 1980.

CIBA. CIBA Symposium No. 191: Neural Tube Defects. London: CIBA Foundation, 1994.

Culatta, B, & Young, C. Linguistic performance as a function of abstract task demands in children with spina bifida. Developmental Medicine and Child Neurology, 34(5):434–440, 1992.

Cusick, BD, & Stuberg, WA. Assessment of lower extremity alignment in the transverse plane: Implications for management of children with neuromotor dysfunction. Physical Therapy, 72:3–15, 1992.

Czeizel, AE, & Dudas, I. Prevention of first occurrence of neural tube defects by periconceptual vitamin supplementation. New England Journal of Medicine, 327:131–137, 1992.

Deitz, JC, Jaffe, KM, Wolf, LS, Massagli, TL, & Anson, DK. Pediatric power wheelchairs: Evaluation of function in the home and school environments. Assistive Technology, 3:24–31, 1991.

DeSouza, L, & Carroll, N. Ambulation of the braced myelomeningocele patient. Journal of Bone and Joint Surgery (American), 58: 1112–1118, 1976.

Dudgeon, BJ, Jaffe, KM, & Shurtleff, DB. Variations in midlumbar myelomeningocele: Implications for ambulation. Pediatric Physical Therapy, 3:57–62, 1991.

Eastlack, ME, Arvidson, J, Snyder-Mackler, L, Danoff, JV, & McGarvey, CL. Interrater reliability of videotaped observational gait-analysis assessments. Physical Therapy, 71:465–472, 1991.

Effgen, SK, & Brown, DA. Long-term stability of hand-held dynamometric measurements in children who have myelomeningocele. Physical Therapy, 72:458–465, 1992.

Elwood, JM, & Elwood, JH. Epidemiology of Anencephalus and Spina Bifida. Cambridge: Oxford University Press, 1980.

Embrey, D, Endicott, J, Glenn, T, & Jaeger, DL. Developing better postural tone in grade school children. Clinical Management in Physical Therapy, 3:6–10, 1983.

Fay, G, Shurtleff, DB, Shurtleff, H, & Wolf, L. Approaches to facilitate independent self-care and academic success. In Shurtleff, DB (Ed.), Myelodysplasias and Exstrophies: Significance, Prevention, and Treatment. Orlando, FL: Grune & Stratton, 1986, pp. 373–398.

Fife, SE, Roxborough, LA, Armstrong, RW, Harris, SR, Gregson, JL, & Field, D. Development of a clinical measure of postural control for assessment of adaptive seating in children with neuromotor disabilities. Physical Therapy, 71:981–993, 1991.

Finnie, NR. Handling the Young Cerebral Palsied Child at Home, 2nd ed. New York: EP Dutton, 1975.

Florence, JM, Pandya, S, King, W, Schierbecker, J, Robison, JD, Signore, LC, Mandel, S, & Arfken, C. Strength assessment: Comparison of methods in children with Duchenne muscular dystrophy (Abstract). Physical Therapy, 68:866, 1988.

Gadow, K. Children on Medication. San Diego: College Hill Press, 1986.

Gaston, H. Ophthalmic complications of spina bifida and hydrocephalus. Eye, 5:279–290, 1991.

Goodwyn, MA. Biomedical Psychological Factors Predicting Success with Activities of Daily Living and Academic Pursuits. Unpublished doctoral dissertation. Seattle: University of Washington, 1990.

Griebel, ML, Oakes, WJ, & Worley, G. The Chiari malformation associated with myelomeningocele. In Rekate, HL (Ed.), Comprehensive Management of Spina Bifida. Boca Raton, FL: CRC Press, 1991, pp. 67–92.

Griffin, JW, McClure, MH, & Bertorini, TE. Sequential isokinetic and manual muscle testing in patients with neuromuscular disease: Pilot study. Physical Therapy, 66:32–35, 1986.

Hack, SN, Norton, BJ, & Zahalak, GI. A quantitative muscle tester for clinical use (Abstract). Physical Therapy, 61:673, 1981.

Hamill, PV, Drizd, TA, Johnson, CL, Reed, RB, Roche, AF, & Moore, WM. Physical growth: National Center for Health Statistics percentiles. American Journal of Clinical Nutrition, 32:607–629, 1979.

Hinderer, KA. Reliability of the Myometer in Muscle Testing Children and Adolescents with Myelodysplasia. Unpublished master's thesis. Seattle: University of Washington, 1988.

Hinderer, KA, & Gutierrez, T. Myometry measurements of children using isometric and eccentric methods of muscle testing (Abstract). Physical Therapy, 68:817, 1988.

Hinderer, KA, & Hinderer, SR. Mobility and transfer efficiency of adults with myelodysplasia (Abstract). Archives of Physical Medicine and Rehabilitation, 69:712, 1988.

Hinderer, KA, & Hinderer, SR. Muscle strength development and assessment in children and adolescents. In Harms-Ringdahl, K (Ed.), International Perspectives in Physical Therapy, Vol. 8, Muscle Strength. London: Churchill Livingstone, 1993, pp. 93–140.

Hinderer, SR, & Hinderer, KA. Sensory examination of individuals with myelodysplasia (Abstract). Archives of Physical Medicine and Rehabilitation, 71:769–770, 1990.

Hinderer, SR, & Hinderer, KA. Quantitative methods of evaluation. In DeLisa, JA, & Gans, BM (Eds.), Rehabilitation Medicine: Principles and Practices, 3rd ed. Philadelphia: Lippincott-Raven, 1998, pp. 109–136.

Hinderer, SR, Hinderer, KA, Dunne, K, & Shurtleff, DB. Medical and functional status of adults with spina bifida (Abstract). Developmental Medicine and Child Neurology, 30(suppl 57):28, 1988.

Hislop, HJ, & Montgomery, J. Daniels and Worthingham's Muscle Testing, 6th ed. Philadelphia: WB Saunders, 1995.

Hosking, GP, Bhat, US, Dubowitz, V, & Edwards, RHT. Measurements of muscle strength and performance in children with normal and diseased muscle. Archives of Disease in Childhood, 51:957–963, 1976.

Hurley, AD. Conducting psychological assessments. In Rowley-Kelly, FL, & Reigel, DH (Eds.), Teaching the Student with Spina Bifida. Baltimore: Paul H. Brookes, 1993, pp. 107–124.

Hyde, S, Goddard, C, & Scott, O: The myometer: The development of a clinical tool. Physiotherapy, 69:424–427, 1983.

IMSG. International Myelodysplasia Study Group Database Coordination. David B. Shurtleff, MD, Department of Pediatrics, University of Washington. Seattle, WA: 1993.

Jacobson, CB, & Berlin, CM. Possible reproductive determent in LSD users. Journal of the American Medical Association, 222:1367–1373, 1972.

Janda, V. Muscle Function Testing. Boston: Butterworths, 1983.

Jebsen, RH, Trieschman, RB, Mikulic, MA, Hartley, RB, McMillan, JA, & Snook, ME. Measurement of time in a standardized test of patient mobility. Archives of Physical Medicine and Rehabilitation, 51:170–175, 1970.

Karmel-Ross, K, Cooperman, DR, & Van Doren, CL. The effect of electrical stimulation on quadriceps femoris muscle torque in children with spina bifida. Physical Therapy, 72:723–731, 1992.

Kendall, FP, McCreary, EK, & Provance, PG. Muscles: Testing and Function, 4th ed. Baltimore: Williams & Wilkins, 1999.

Kieklak, H, & DeVahl, J. Respond II: Protocol for Pediatric Applications. Minneapolis, MN: Medtronics, Inc., 1986.

Kilburn, J, Saffer, A, Barnes, L, Kling, T, & Venes, J. The Vigorimeter as an early predictor of central neurologic malformation in myelodysplastic children. Paper presented at the meeting of the American Academy for Cerebral Palsy and Developmental Medicine, Seattle, 1985.

Kimura, DK, Mayo, M, & Shurtleff, DB. Urinary tract management. In Shurtleff, DB (Ed.), Myelodysplasias and Exstrophies: Significance, Prevention, and Treatment. Orlando, FL: Grune & Stratton, 1986, pp. 243–266.

King, JC, Currie, DM, & Wright, E. Bowel training in spina bifida: Importance of education, patient compliance, age, and anal reflexes. Archives of Physical Medicine and Rehabilitation, 75:243–247, 1994.

Knutson, LM, & Clark, DE. Orthotic devices for ambulation in children with cerebral palsy and myelomeningocele. Physical Therapy, 71:947–960, 1991.

Krebs, DE, Edelstein, JE, & Fishman, S. Reliability of observational kinematic gait analysis. Physical Therapy, 65:1027–1033, 1985.

Land, LC. Study of the sensory integration of children with myelomeningocele. In McLaurin, RL (Ed.), Myelomeningocele. Orlando, FL: Grune & Stratton, 1977, pp. 115–140.

Lehmann, JF, Condon, SM, de Lateur, BJ, & Price, R. Gait abnormalities in peroneal nerve paralysis and their corrections by orthoses: A biomechanical study. Archives of Physical Medicine and Rehabilitation, 67:380–386, 1986.

Lehmann, JF, Condon, SM, de Lateur, BJ, & Smith, C. Ankle-foot orthoses: Effect on gait abnormalities in tibial nerve paralysis. Archives of Physical Medicine and Rehabilitation, 66:212–218, 1985.

Lehmann, JF, Esselman, PC, Ko, MJ, de Lateur, BJ, & Dralle, AJ. Plastic ankle-foot orthoses: Evaluation of function. Archives of Physical Medicine and Rehabilitation, 64:402–404, 1983.

Lemire, RJ, Loeser, JD, Leech, RW, & Alvord, ED (Eds.). Normal and Abnormal Development of the Human Nervous System. Hagerstown, MD: Harper & Row, 1975.

Level, MB. Spherical Grip Strength of Children. Unpublished master's thesis. Seattle: University of Washington, 1984.

Liptak, GS, Shurtleff, DB, Bloss, JW, Baitus-Hebert, E, & Manitta, P. Mobility aids for children with high-level myelomeningocele: Parapodium versus wheelchair. Developmental Medicine and Child Neurology, 34:787–796, 1992.

Logan, L, Byers-Hinkley, K, & Ciccone, CD. Anterior versus posterior walkers: A gait analysis study. Developmental Medicine and Child Neurology, 32:1044–1048, 1990.

Luthy, DA, Wardinsky, T, Shurtleff, DB, Hollenbach, KA, Hickok, DE, Nyberg, DA, & Benedetti, TJ. Cesarean section before the onset of labor and subsequent motor function in infants with myelomeningocele diagnosed antenatally. New England Journal of Medicine, 324:662–666, 1991.

Main, DM, & Mennuti, MT. Neural tube defects: Issues in prenatal diagnosis and counseling. Journal of the American College of Obstetrics and Gynecology, 67:1–16, 1986.

Masse, LC, Lamontagne, M, & O'Riain, MD. Biomedical analysis of wheelchair propulsion for various seating positions. Journal of Rehabilitation Research and Development, 29:12–28, 1992.

Mayfield, JK. Comprehensive orthopedic management in myelomeningocele. In Rekate, HL (Ed.), Comprehensive Management of Spina Bifida. Boca Raton, FL: CRC Press, 1991, pp. 113–164.

McDonald, CM, Jaffe, KM, Mosca, VS, & Shurtleff, DB. Ambulatory outcome of children with myelomeningocele: Effect of lower-extremity muscle strength. Developmental Medicine and Child Neurology, 33:482–490, 1991a.

McDonald, CM, Jaffe, K, & Shurtleff, DB. Assessment of muscle strength in children with meningomyelocele: Accuracy and stability of measurements over time. Archives of Physical Medicine and Rehabilitation, 67:855–861, 1986.

McDonald, CM, Jaffe, KM, Shurtleff, DB, & Menelaus, MB. Modifications to the traditional description of neurosegmental innervation in myelomeningocele. Developmental Medicine and Child Neurology, 33:473–481, 1991b.

McGourty, LK. Kohlman Evaluation of Living Skills (KELS). In Hemphill, BJ (Ed.), Mental Health Assessment in Occupational Therapy. Thorofare, NJ: Black, 1988, pp. 131–146.

Mendell, JR, & Florence, J. Manual muscle testing. Muscle and Nerve, 13(suppl):16–20, 1990.

Menelaus, MB. Orthopedic management of children with myelomeningocele: A plea for realistic goals. Developmental Medicine and Child Neurology, 18(suppl 37):3–11, 1976.

Miller, E, & Sethi, L. The effect of hydrocephalus on perception. Developmental Medicine and Child Neurology, 13(suppl 25):77–81, 1971.

Miller, LC, Michael, AF, Baxter, TL, & Kim, Y. Quantitative muscle testing in childhood dermatomyositis. Archives of Physical Medicine and Rehabilitation, 69:610–613, 1988.

Mills, JL, Rhoads, GG, Simpson, JL, Cunningham, GC, Conley, MR, Lassman, MR, Walden, ME, Depp, R, & Hoffman, HJ. The absence of a relation between the periconceptual use of vitamins and neural tube defects. New England Journal of Medicine, 321:430–435, 1989.

Milner-Brown, HS, & Miller, RG. Increased muscular fatigue in patients with neurogenic muscle weakness: Quantification and pathophysiology. Archives of Physical Medicine and Rehabilitation, 70:361–366, 1989.

Milunsky, A, Jick, H, Jick, SS, Bruell, CL, MacLaughlin, DS, Rothman, KJ, & Willett, W. Multivitamin/folic acid supplementation in early pregnancy reduces the prevalence of neural tube defects. Journal of the American Medical Association, 262:2847–2852, 1989.

MRC Vitamin Study Research Group. Prevention of neural tube defects: Results of the Medical Research Council vitamin study. Lancet, 338:131–137, 1991.

Murdoch, A. How valuable is muscle charting? A study of the relationship between neonatal assessment of muscle power and later mobility in children with spina bifida defects. Physiotherapy, 66:221–223, 1980.

Nyberg, DA, Mack, LA, Hirsch, J, & Mahoney, BS. Abnormalities of fetal cranial contour in sonographic detection of spina bifida: Evaluation of the "lemon" sign. Radiology, 167:387–392, 1988.

Okamoto, GA, Lamers, JV, & Shurtleff, DB. Skin breakdown in patients with myelomeningocele. Archives of Physical Medicine and Rehabilitation, 64:20–23, 1983.

Okamoto, GA, Sousa, J, Telzrow, RW, Holm, RA, McCartin, R, & Shurtleff, DB. Toileting skills in children with myelomeningocele: Rates of learning. Archives of Physical Medicine and Rehabilitation, 65(4):182–185, 1984.

Packman, RA, & Ewaski, B. Respond II: Gait Training Protocol. Minneapolis, MN: Medtronics, 1983.

Pact, V, Sirotkin-Roses, M, & Beatus, J. The Muscle Testing Handbook. Boston: Little, Brown & Co., 1984.

Patient Data Management System. Myelodysplasia Study Data Collection Criteria and Instructions, 1994.

Pomatto, RC. The use of orthotics in the treatment of myelomeningocele. In Rekate, HL (Ed.), Comprehensive Management of Spina Bifida. Boca Raton, FL: CRC Press, 1991, pp. 165–183.

Reigel, DH. Spina bifida from infancy through the school years. In Rowley-Kelly, FL, & Reigel, DH (Eds.), Teaching the Students with Spina Bifida. Baltimore: Paul H. Brookes, 1993, pp. 3–30.

Rekate, HL. Neurosurgical management of the newborn with spina bifida. In Rekate, HL (Ed.), Comprehensive Management of Spina Bifida. Boca Raton, FL: CRC Press, 1991, pp. 1–28.

Reynolds, EH. Mental effects of antiepileptic medication: A review. Epilepsia, 24(suppl 2):S85–S95, 1983.

Rose, SA, Ounpuu, S, & DeLuca, PA. Strategies for the assessment of pediatric gait in the clinical setting. Physical Therapy, 71:961–980, 1991.

Rosenstein, BD, Greene, WB, Herrington, RT, & Blum, AS. Bone density in myelomeningocele: The effects of ambulatory status and other factors. Developmental Medicine and Child Neurology, 29:486–494, 1987.

Rowley-Kelly, FL, & Kunkle, PM. Developing a school outreach program. In Rowley-Kelly, FL, & Reigel, DH (Eds.), Teaching the Student with Spina Bifida. Baltimore: Paul H. Brookes, 1993, pp. 395–436.

Ryan, KD, Pioski, C, & Emans, JB. Myelodysplasia—The musculoskeletal problem: Habilitation from infancy to adulthood. Physical Therapy, 71:935–946, 1991.

Sand, PL, Taylor, N, Rawlings, M, & Chitnis, S. Performance of children with spina bifida manifesta on the Frostig Developmental Test of Visual Perception. Perceptual Motor Skills, 37:539–546, 1973.

Schafer, MF, & Dias, LS. Myelomeningocele: Orthopaedic Treatment. Baltimore: Williams & Wilkins, 1983.

Schneider, JW, Krosschell, K, & Gabriel, KL. Congenital spinal cord injury. In Umphred, DA (Ed.), Neurological Rehabilitation, 3rd ed. St. Louis: Mosby, 1995, pp. 454–483.

Schopler, SA, & Menelaus, MB. Significance of strength of the quadriceps muscles in children with myelomeningocele. Journal of Pediatric Orthopaedics, 7:507–512, 1987.

Seller, MJ, & Nevin, NC. Periconceptual vitamin supplementation and the prevention of neural tube defects in south-east England and northern Ireland. Journal of Medical Genetics, 21:325–330, 1984.

Shaffer, J, Wolfe, L, Friedrich, W, Shurtleff, H, Shurtleff, D, & Fay, G. Developmental expectations: Intelligence and fine motor skills. In Shurtleff, DB (Ed.), Myelodysplasias and Exstrophies: Significance, Prevention, and Treatment. Orlando, FL: Grune & Stratton, 1986, pp. 359–372.

Shores, M. Footprint analysis in gait documentation. Physical Therapy, 60:1163–1167, 1980.

Shurtleff, DB. Timing of learning in the myelomeningocele patient. Journal of the American Physical Therapy Association, 46(2):136–148, 1966.

Shurtleff, DB. Decubitus formation and skin breakdown. In Shurtleff, DB (Ed.), Myelodysplasias and Exstrophies: Significance, Prevention, and Treatment. Orlando, FL: Grune & Stratton, 1986a, pp. 299–312.

Shurtleff, DB. Dietary management. In Shurtleff, DB (Ed.), Myelodysplasias and Exstrophies: Significance, Prevention, and Treatment. Orlando, FL: Grune & Stratton, 1986b, pp. 285–298.

Shurtleff, DB. Health care delivery. In Shurtleff, DB (Ed.), Myelodysplasias and Exstrophies: Significance, Prevention, and Treatment. Orlando, FL: Grune & Stratton, 1986c, pp. 449–514.

Shurtleff, DB. Mobility. In Shurtleff, DB (Ed.), Myelodysplasias and Exstrophies: Significance, Prevention, and Treatment. Orlando, FL: Grune & Stratton, 1986d, pp. 313–356.

Shurtleff, DB. Selection process for the care of congenitally malformed infants. In Shurtleff, DB (Ed.), Myelodysplasias and Exstrophies: Significance, Prevention, and Treatment. Orlando, FL: Grune & Stratton, 1986e, pp. 89–116.

Shurtleff, DB. Computer data bases for pediatric disability: Clinical and research applications. In Jaffe, KM (Ed.), Physical Medicine and Rehabilitation Clinics of North America: Pediatric Rehabilitation. Philadelphia: WB Saunders, 1991, pp. 665–688.

Shurtleff, DB, Duguay, S, Duguay, G, Moskowitz, D, Weinberger, E, Roberts, T, & Loesre, J. Epidemiology of tethered cord with meningomyelocele. European Journal of Paediatric Surgery, 7(suppl 1):7–11, 1997.

Shurtleff, DB, & Dunne, K. Adults and adolescents with myelomeningocele. In Shurtleff, DB (Ed.), Myelodysplasias and Exstrophies: Significance, Prevention, and Treatment. Orlando, FL: Grune & Stratton, 1986, pp. 433–448.

Shurtleff, DB, & Lamers, J. Clinical considerations in the treatment of myelodysplasia. In Crandal, DB, & Brazier, MAB (Eds.), Prevention of Neural Tube Defects: The Role of Alpha-fetoprotein. New York: Academic Press, 1978, pp. 103–122.

Shurtleff, DB, Lemire, RJ, & Warkany, J: Embryology, etiology and epidemiology. In Shurtleff, DB (Ed.), Myelodysplasias and Exstrophies: Significance, Prevention, and Treatment. Orlando, FL: Grune & Stratton, 1986a, pp. 39–64.

Shurtleff, DB, & Mayo, M. Toilet training: The Seattle experience and conclusions. In Shurtleff, DB (Ed.), Myelodysplasias and Exstrophies: Significance, Prevention, and Treatment. Orlando, FL: Grune & Stratton, 1986, pp. 267–284.

Shurtleff, DB, Stuntz, JT, & Hayden, PW. Hydrocephalus. In Shurtleff, DB (Ed.), Myelodysplasias and Exstrophies: Significance, Prevention, and Treatment. Orlando, FL: Grune & Stratton, 1986b, pp. 139–180.

Sousa, JC, Gordon, LH, & Shurtleff, DB. Assessing the development of daily living skills in patients with spina bifida. Developmental Medicine and Child Neurology, 18(suppl 37):134–142, 1976.

Sousa, JC, Telzrow, RW, Holm, RA, McCartin, R, & Shurtleff, DB. Developmental guidelines for children with myelodysplasia. Journal of the American Physical Therapy Association, 63:21–29, 1983.

Stack, GD, & Baber, GC. The neurological involvement of the lower limbs in myelomeningocele. Developmental Medicine and Child Neurology, 9:732, 1967.

Staheli, LT. Prone hip extension test: Method of measuring hip flexion deformity. Clinical Orthopedics, 123:12–15, 1977.

Stillwell, A, & Menelaus, MB. Walking ability in mature patients with spina bifida. Journal of Pediatric Orthopedics, 3:184–190, 1983.

Stuberg, WA. Considerations related to weight-bearing program in children with developmental disabilities. Physical Therapy, 72:35–40, 1992.

Stuberg, WA, & Metcalf, WK. Reliability of quantitative muscle testing in healthy children and in children with Duchenne muscular dystrophy using a hand-held dynamometer. Physical Therapy, 68:977–982, 1988.

Tew, B, & Laurence, KM. The effects of hydrocephalus on intelligence, visual perception, and school attainments. Developmental Medicine and Child Neurology, *17*(suppl 35):129–134, 1975.

Weber, D, & Agro, M. Clinical Aspects of Lower Extremity Orthotics. Winnipeg, Manitoba: Canadian Cataloguing in Publication Data/Canadian Association of Prosthetists and Orthotists, 1990.

Wicks, K, & Shurtleff, DB. An introduction to toilet training. In Shurtleff, DB (Ed.), Myelodysplasias and Exstrophies: Significance, Prevention, and Treatment. Orlando, FL: Grune & Stratton, 1986a, pp. 203–219.

Wicks, K, & Shurtleff, DB. Stool management. In Shurtleff, DB (Ed.), Myelodysplasias and Exstrophies: Significance, Prevention, and Treatment. Orlando, FL: Grune & Stratton, 1986b, pp. 221–242.

Williams, LV, Anderson, AD, Campbell, J, Thomas, L, Feiwell, E, & Walker, JM. Energy cost of walking and of wheelchair propulsion by children with myelodysplasia: Comparison with normal children. Developmental Medicine and Child Neurology, *25*:617–624, 1983.

Wolf, LS, & McLaughlin, JF. Early motor development in infants with myelomeningocele. Pediatric Physical Therapy, *4*:12–17, 1992.

CHAPTER
24

Assistive Technology

SHIRLEY J. CARLSON, PT, PCS, MS
CAROLE RAMSEY, OTR/L, ATP

Physical therapists have long been involved in the practice of providing individuals with physical impairments with devices or pieces of equipment that are designed to help achieve or improve independent function. Attempts to increase carryover of therapy goals in the home and classroom settings often included homemade adaptive equipment for positioning, mobility, and communication. The application of technologic advances to health care, rehabilitation, and special education settings began slowly several decades ago and has rapidly accelerated. Assistive, or rehabilitation, technology now encompasses a vast range of materials, designs, and applications. It is used to promote the development and acquisition of skills that a client lacks as a result of disease or injury. It can also provide compromises or adaptations in motor function when the attainment of certain skills is unrealistic or impossible. Also referred to as enabling technology, assistive technology can often generate new opportunities and open new doors for individuals with physical impairments.

In the past 25 years there has been a virtual explosion in the number and type of assistive devices. The creation of several federally funded rehabilitation engineering centers in 1972 focused efforts on research and development of new products, as well as on the delivery of services to the consumer (Hedman, 1990). This process brought together professionals from many fields, such as biomedical and rehabilitation engineering, physical therapy, occupational therapy, speech and language pathology, and special education. RESNA, the Rehabilitation Engineering and Assistive Technology Society of North America, an outgrowth of this shared interest, is an interdisciplinary association of professionals who bring applied technology to persons with disability.

Since 1975, many laws have been enacted to ensure the rights of people with disabilities to be included in natural education and work environments.

These laws have helped to focus attention on, and create a growing market for, new technologies and products. Consumer demands for increased durability and performance have induced manufacturers to apply technologies created by the aerospace, medical, and information industries. The field of assistive technology is now well established as a cross-disciplinary specialty.

The Technology-Related Assistance for Individuals with Disabilities Act of 1988 (Tech Act) was the first piece of federal legislation to define assistive technology devices and services and to recognize the importance of technology in the lives of individuals with disability. States and territories were granted moneys to develop comprehensive Assistive Technology Projects to ensure access to the technology needed for integration and inclusion within the community and the workforce. Services vary from state to state and may include information and referral services (databases, 800 numbers, and web sites), centers for trying out devices and equipment, equipment exchange and recycling programs, funding resource guides, financial loan programs, mobile van outreach services, protection and advocacy services, and training programs on funding and self-advocacy. The Assistive Technology Act of 1998 has extended funding to develop permanent comprehensive technology-related programs. All states and territories are eligible for 10 years, and states that have completed 10 years are eligible for an additional 3 years of federal funding.

The purpose of this chapter is to discuss five major elements of assistive technology frequently employed in pediatric physical therapy, focusing on the role physical therapists play in selecting and obtaining appropriate pieces of equipment for their clients. The elements include postural support systems (adaptive seating), wheeled mobility, augmentative and alternative communication (AAC), computers, and electronic aids to daily living (EADLs). Emphasis is on application of these devices to individuals with severe physical impairments.

ASSISTIVE TECHNOLOGY TEAMS

Despite the diversity of technologic devices, most still require modification or customization in design, implementation, or attachment (Hedman, 1990). The complexity and expense of most of the devices required by individuals with severe physical impairments demand a thorough and careful process of selection and construction. Many professionals and lay people may need to be involved, each contributing a particular area of knowledge and expertise. All individuals who interact with the client and the equipment on a regular basis need to be considered part of the team and contribute important information.

The configuration of the team (Fig. 24–1) varies depending on the types of assistive technology needed and on the setting in which the evaluation and prescription are being conducted. Central to the team are the child and family. Family-centered intervention stresses the need to involve the client and primary caregivers in the goal-setting and decision-making process to ensure realistic and meaningful solutions. The professional component of the core should include experts with thorough training and experience in the areas being examined (mobility, seating, AAC, computers, and EADLs) and usually includes some or all of the following: physical therapist, occupational therapist, speech and language pathologist, rehabilitation engineer, and rehabilitation technology supplier.

Surrounding this core are several groups who share important roles and information. In the client's school or work setting, classroom teachers and aides, administrative personnel, psychologists, vocational counselors, and work supervisors may all need to be consulted. The client may have primary physical, occupational, and speech and language therapists in these settings with whom the development of goals and strategies must be coordinated. Within the medical setting, the client's family physician, as well as other medical specialists and nurses, may need to be involved. Problems requiring collaboration with medical personnel may include management of deformity and contracture, pressure ulcerations, incontinence, self-injury and safety, and visual and other sensory deficits. The issue of funding establishes a third group of contributors, including third-party payers, state-sponsored medical equipment programs, civic organizations, and other outside funding agencies. Many clinics and centers employ a funding specialist (often a social worker) whose role is to identify and obtain funding for prescribed technology. A final group within the team includes other community and family members who engage in day-to-day interactions or who provide special support services such as transportation or revision of architectural barriers.

The makeup of the team and the setting in which it functions can vary. For example, in many hospitals and rehabilitation centers with comprehensive technology service delivery programs, physicians (especially physiatrists and orthopedic surgeons) may be an integral part of the core team. In schools and residential centers, one or more of the client's primary therapists, along with an equipment vendor, may function as the core team.

A successful team will recognize that each of these members, even a minor player, has important information and perspective. Equally important is that communication must be bidirectional. The core team must impart information regarding proper

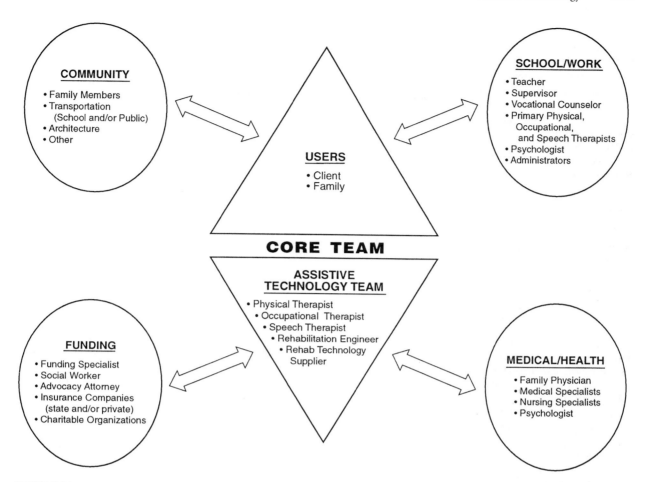

FIGURE 24–1. Core team interactions important in selecting and procuring assistive technology. Members and roles of each component may fluctuate depending on specific client problems and settings.

use, training, maintenance, responsibility, and safety relative to the prescribed devices to appropriate individuals.

Through a survey of 227 adults with various disabilities, Phillips and Zhao (1993) studied factors that predict abandonment of assistive technology devices. Nearly 30% of all devices were completely abandoned, with mobility devices abandoned most often. Devices were most frequently abandoned in the first year or after the fifth year. Four factors were significantly related to abandonment. The first was lack of consideration of the user's opinion during the selection process. Ease of procurement was a second factor, with easily obtained items purchased directly from a vendor (without team consultation) the most likely to be abandoned. A third factor was poor device performance, which reflected the user's perception of the device's ability to enhance his or her own performance in an easy, reliable, and comfortable manner. The fourth factor was the change in

users' needs and priorities over time, including functional changes, as well as changes in lifestyle and activities.

Credentialing of professionals in assistive technology was established in 1995 by RESNA for the purposes of ensuring consumer safeguards and increasing consumer satisfaction. Two types of credentialing examinations are offered:

- Assistive Technology Practitioner (ATP) Certificate: for service providers involved in analysis of a consumer's needs and training in use of a particular device
- Assistive Technology Supplier (ATS) Certificate: for service providers involved in the sale and service of commercial devices

A Rehabilitation Technology Supplier (RTS) is an individual who provides enabling technology in areas of wheeled mobility, seating and alternative positioning, ambulation assistance, environmental controls, and activities of daily living (note that

AACs and computers are not included). A National Registry of Rehabilitation Technology Suppliers (NRRTS) identifies qualified suppliers by confirming, through a review process, an individual's work experience, references from professional associates, adherence to the Code of Ethics and Standards of Practice and Protocol, and commitment to ongoing continuing education. A Certified RTS (CRTS) is an NRRTS member in good standing who has successfully completed the RESNA Assistive Technology Supplier examination.

LEVELS OF INTERVENTION

Several chapters in this book refer to the use of assistive technology to achieve the goals of physical therapy for children with particular disorders. The benefits of assistive technology can be discussed according to the National Center for Medical Rehabilitation Research (NCMRR) model of the disabling process, beginning at the level of impairment. Correctly prescribed and used, assistive technology, especially therapeutic positioning (adaptive seating), may help prevent secondary impairments such as skin breakdown, cardiopulmonary compromise due to scoliosis or slouched posture, and contractures or deformity due to inadequately supported body segments. Other potential benefits at this level are the reduction of tone or excessive muscle activity and a decrease in pathologic movements.

Assistive technology devices are essentially functional devices, and the most common reason for their use is to provide alternatives to functional limitations imposed by the client's disorder, thereby preventing or minimizing disability in activities of daily life. The inability to sit unsupported; the inability to walk or move from one place to another; the inability to use the hands well as the result of a weak, unstable trunk; or the inability to produce speech are often primary reasons for prescribing a seating system, a power wheelchair, or an electronic communication device.

Assistive devices intervene in the disability dimension of the NCMRR model by improving the ability to perform socially appropriate activities. A power wheelchair may allow independent access to school or work. An AAC system may facilitate interactions with peers or promote social skills. An EADL may make the difference between less restricted living in a supervised apartment or living in a nursing home or intermediate care facility. On the other hand, if careful thought is not given to the selection of appropriate devices, we may potentially add to the disability by limiting transportation options or increasing the client's reliance on others during repairs or maintenance.

Regarding societal impact, we must consider whether the use of technology can decrease medical or care costs, such as hospitalizations for decubitus healing or the need for live-in personal attendants. Social policies and attitudes have an impact on the success of clients in obtaining and using their assistive devices productively. Technology also has the potential to alter those attitudes and policies as clients' appearance and visibility improve and their capabilities become recognized.

Documentation of these benefits is often based empirically on clinical experience and observation. The literature is replete with descriptions of creative solutions for individual client problems. More difficult to find are carefully controlled studies of the effectiveness of assistive technology intervention on any of these dimensions of the disabling process. In this chapter we examine some of the literature within the framework of the NCMRR model.

LIFE-SPAN TECHNOLOGY

Assistive technology can be applied across the life span, and, indeed, the individual's needs change with growth and development. Intervention at each stage must be carefully planned to achieve maximum benefits. For example, positioning the infant is essential to promote social interaction and development of early concepts such as cause and effect and object permanence. Switch-activated toys and power-driven mobility toys can help the preschooler learn how to self-initiate movement and control the organization of his or her environment. The school-age child needs the postural support and comfort to enable learning and to help reinforce functional goals of therapy. He or she needs a reliable way to indicate needs and make choices. The adolescent needs to keep up with peers and be accepted socially. He or she should be included in decision making regarding choice of mobility, seating, or communication options whenever possible. The young adult needs to be able to get to and from a job or day setting and rely as little as possible on others to achieve basic functions, such as position changes, communicating, eating, and toileting. Because these individuals tend to spend many more hours at a time in one position, hygiene and skin care become especially important.

THE SELECTION PROCESS

An environment is a person's surroundings or a setting in which he or she spends a great deal of time. Children function in a series of environments throughout the day. Selection of assistive technologies must consider all of those environments in which they are to be used. In addition, the wheelchair itself, with its adaptive seating and communication systems, becomes a primary microenvironment for many severely impaired clients (Bergen, 1992). The ultimate responsibility of the assistive technology team must be to solve the client's identified problem without creating new problems, in an affordable manner with obtainable and durable equipment that can and will be serviced as needed and will meet the client's needs for the foreseeable future until a new device is appropriate (Hedman, 1990). Once a referral has been made, the steps followed by the assistive technology team resemble the HOAC decision-making model discussed in Chapter 7.

Step 1. *Collect initial data* regarding the client and her or his environments. *Client information* includes diagnosis, age, developmental levels, recent assessments of performance and skills, and current equipment and its shortcomings. *Environment information* identifies the context in which the client functions, that is, where and when potential devices will be used and for what tasks. Support and caretaking individuals and their responsibilities are identified.

Step 2. *Generate a problem statement* by identifying the client's overall needs and specific problems. Client and family input is vital to prioritize problems and assist with establishing goals. Thorough needs identification will ensure that the right team members are assembled and the required equipment is on hand for examination and simulation.

Step 3. *Establish realistic goals and outcomes* that reflect the desired functional gains, as well as any possible remediation of physical impairment. Resource constraints, such as funding and availability of devices, influence this process.

Step 4. *Perform the physical examination,* consisting of tests and measures particular to each type of assistive technology. Body dimensions, range of motion, functional strength and endurance, postural control, functional skills, and communication skills are typical examples. Simulation with trial devices is especially helpful at this point and may require more than one session.

Step 5. *Generate a working hypothesis,* or a clinical impression, regarding the impact of impairment on functional limitations and disability. This step can be particularly useful, because it provides the justification for choosing different components or configurations. For example, you may chose a forward-slanted seat to address tight hamstrings and allow the pelvis to be vertical, which in turn allows the client to sit more erect, increasing his or her reaching range.

Step 6. *Plan the intervention strategy.* Formulate a global concept of the assistive technology package while considering the relationships among the various components. The key to this step is to match the products and their features to the client's problems and capabilities. Particular attention is paid to the ability to interface components and to growth capabilities. The rehabilitation technology supplier is instrumental in identifying appropriate equipment choices, and a rehabilitation engineer is invaluable in creating unique solutions to difficult problems. Refer to other specialists if necessary for remediation or treatment of certain problems, such as surgery to correct severe deformity. Determine training needs of all involved with the new equipment. Assign responsibilities for each task in step 7 and a time line for completion.

Step 7. *Implement the intervention strategy,* including the following specific tasks:

a) *Select components and interfaces.* Generate a list of equipment items specifying the correct size, style, and model for each component. Carefully select mounting hardware such as brackets, extension arms, and locking pins to provide correct alignment, as well as strong and durable interfaces between components. This will ensure safety, easy detachment when taking apart a system for cleaning or transportation, and adjustability and growth of the system.

b) *Secure funding.* Submit the equipment justification and itemized price list to the funding agency. Customarily, equipment and devices that are considered to be "medically necessary" (wheelchairs, walkers, braces) will be approved before devices that might be considered "recreational," such as EADLs, computer equipment, switches, and, sometimes, communication devices. Be prepared to justify a more expensive choice, if indicated by the client's needs, when a less costly alternative exists.

c) *Assemble or construct the assistive technology package.* Order commercial equipment and fabricate customized pieces, such as molded seats and backs. The latter items may need to be delayed until the former are received to avoid errors due to growth and structural or functional changes. Perform frequent fittings with the client and be prepared to revise the original plan if necessary.

d) *Deliver the system.* Perform final fittings, programming of electronic devices, testing, and adjustments. Instruct primary users (the client and family or caregivers) in proper use of all parts. Share warranty, safety, and maintenance information with the client and family.

  e) *Provide training.* Extended training is often required for devices such as power wheelchairs, electronic speech devices, and EADLs, and this may occur in a different setting such as the home or school. Therefore, the team may need to train family members or the child's primary therapists or teachers both in the use of the device and in the best way to train the child.

Step 8. *Follow-up and reassessment.* For the child who is physically challenged, the previous process is usually only one of many repetitions of a cycle. Mechanical and electronic equipment wears out and breaks down, making repairs and fine-tuning necessary. The child's problems and needs change with age, development of new skills, and change of environments. As technologies continue to improve or be introduced, new solutions become available.

Effects of Managed Care on Acquisition of Assistive Technology

State-funded Medicaid programs, traditionally a major source of funding for the pediatric disabled population, have contracted much of their coverage to private managed care insurance organizations, which in many cases has affected accessibility to durable medical equipment and specialized devices (Whitney, personal communication, 1998). Denials for requested items may be increased, either because a narrower interpretation of the state's terminology is used in determining medical necessity, or because nonstandard or customized items do not fit the billing codes. The time between the initial request and approval may be prolonged if the reviewers are less experienced in this specialized population and need more explanation, making repeated requests and justification necessary. Choice of products may be restricted because allowables (amount that will be paid for a given item) are often based on simpler adult equipment designs and do not cover the full cost of more expensive or more customized pediatric designs, or because the capitated rate paid to medical equipment suppliers is inadequate to cover actual expenses, cutting their profit margins and making it difficult to provide and service sophisticated or customized equipment. In addition, many private insurance companies, as well as state-funded programs, have contracted with specific manufacturers to provide bulk orders of wheelchairs or other durable medical equipment, further restricting choice. Medical and equipment needs of the disabled population are much higher than what many private companies anticipate. Some managed care companies have dropped contracts for state Medicaid patients, leaving those individuals with little or no choice of coverage, and often requiring a change of provider.

In the next decade we will face the dilemma of reconciling the huge variety of devices that can be designed and tailored for achieving independent function with the increasing restrictions in funding, choice, and accessibility to those devices. Health care management and health care reform are issues that will continue to change in unpredictable ways in the foreseeable future.

POSTURAL SUPPORT SYSTEMS

The purpose of the seating system is to provide external postural support for the child with functional limitations in sitting as a result of impairments in musculoskeletal alignment, postural control, muscle tone, or strength. The goal is to enable the child to compensate for functional limitations and thereby prevent or minimize disability. Letts (1991) stated that to achieve stable sitting, biomechanical forces and moments in all planes must be balanced. "Good positioning" usually consists of an upright midline orientation of the entire body with a near-vertical alignment of the trunk and head. The "90-90-90 rule" (degrees of flexion at the hips, knees, and ankles) was deemed best practice until recently, when therapists recognized that to preserve the trunk stability necessary for head and upper extremity control, pelvic and lower extremity alignment may need to be altered to accommodate contracture or deformity (Bergen, 1992). Kangas (1991) has seriously challenged the idea of static positioning, stating that it is unnatural and impedes function. In this section, studies that have examined the effectiveness of postural support systems are reviewed using the NCMRR model as outlined earlier. Considerations in the prescription of postural support systems are then discussed.

Research on Effects of Therapeutic Seating

Major concerns in the seating management of individuals with cerebral palsy (CP) or head injuries are normalization of muscle tone and improvement of upper body postural control to enhance functional skills of the head and hands. Much of the research on therapeutic seating for this group has examined the effects of variables such as hip flexion angles (or seat-to-back angles) and orientation of the trunk and head (or angle-in-space). The former is achieved by independently changing the seat back angle; the latter is achieved by tilting the entire system. There has been considerable interest in the anteriorly tipped (or forward-inclined) seat, in which the front edge of the seat is rotated downward, thus increasing the seat-to-back angle while maintaining a near-vertical back. Most clients with myelodysplasia or spinal cord injuries tolerate and function well in a typical upright position; however, sitting pressures and the prevention of skin ulcerations are of concern. Various types of sitting surfaces and adjustments to postural alignment have been studied in the attempt to reduce pressure and decrease the incidence of decubiti. In children with muscular dystrophy, prevention of spinal collapse, preservation of upper extremity function, and comfort are major goals of positioning.

Impairment

NEUROMUSCULAR FUNCTION AND PATHOLOGIC MOVEMENT PATTERNS

A long-standing principle of therapeutic seating is that increased muscle tone, here defined as muscle activity at rest, can be reduced by altering seating angles. Seats are oriented either horizontally, wedged (front edge raised), or anteriorly tipped (front edge lowered). Backs are placed vertically, reclined (opening the hip angle to less flexion), or forward inclined (closing the hip angle to more flexion). The seat-back combinations and the degree to which they can be varied are therefore numerous. Several studies have examined the effect of altered seating angles on electromyographic (EMG) activity in children with CP. In a study that varied the hip angle by reclining the back or wedging the seat, lumbar EMG was lowest in vertical sitting, with a horizontal seat and a 90° hip angle (Nwaobi et al., 1983). Lumbar EMG was higher the more reclined the position regardless of the hip angle. Hip adductor activity was decreased when the back was vertical and the seat was wedged 15° (Nwaobi & Cusick, 1980). When the hip angle was kept constant at 90° and the entire system was tilted 30° posteriorly, EMG of both paraspinal and hip adductor muscle groups was significantly higher (Nwaobi, 1986).

The reclined position also resulted in the highest EMG in leg muscles (rectus femoris, adductor longus, biceps femoris, and gastrocnemius) in subjects with CP, as well as in normal control subjects (Myhr & von Wendt, 1993), and the addition of an abduction orthosis decreased leg muscle EMG in all positions. For subjects with the most severe impairments, EMG responses of back extensors and medial hamstrings to position changes were much more individualized (Fife et al., 1988).

Children with CP who sat on anteriorly tipped seats without back support showed a decrease in midthoracic EMG and an increase in lumbar EMG (Bablich et al., 1986). Myhr and von Wendt (1993) also advocated use of an anteriorly tipped chair, but they added an abduction orthosis and a cutout table for upper extremity support of forward leaning. EMG of leg muscles was lowest in the forward-leaning position with the abduction orthosis compared with vertical or reclined sitting. The frequency of pathologic movements (a single spastic or tonic reflex pattern defined for each subject) was significantly reduced in the experimental sitting position when compared with the subjects' own traditional systems (Myhr & von Wendt, 1991).

PHYSIOLOGIC FUNCTIONS

Most studies in this category have measured how pulmonary function is affected by variation of seating parameters. Supportive seating in a modular seating system with adjustable support components was superior to seating in a nonadapted wheelchair with standard sling seat and back for children with spastic CP in the three pulmonary functions measured (Nwaobi & Smith, 1986). The differences were attributed to changes in the shape, structure, and capacity of the thorax and abdomen and to improved control of the respiratory muscles in the supported, upright position.

In a group of children with muscle weakness due to neuromuscular disease who were ambulatory and without scoliosis, forced vital capacity (FVC) was slightly decreased in supine position compared with sitting (Noble-Jamieson et al., 1986). In a second group of nonambulatory children with scoliosis, however, the decrease in FVC while supine compared with sitting was much greater. When tested again in sitting position with their spinal brace on, FVC was further reduced. The more severe the scoliosis, and the greater the reduction of the spinal curve by the brace, the greater the decrease in FVC.

Anteriorly tilted sitting may have some potential to improve respiratory function in children with moderate CP. Tidal volume and minute ventilation in subjects with CP were increased compared with controls when seated on a 10° anteriorly tipped bench without back support (Reid & Sochaniwskyj, 1991).

SKELETAL DEFORMITY, CONTRACTURE, AND PASSIVE RANGE OF MOTION

Studies that pertained to these types of impairments examined the management of scoliosis in patients with Duchenne muscular dystrophy. Carlson and Payette (1985) used a combination of molded seating systems with soft spinal corsets and found a reduction of curves on radiography. Seeger and associates (1984b), however, found no significant difference in spinal curves when modular seats, custom-molded seats, unmodified wheelchair seats, and spinal jackets were compared.

The principle that postural support systems can maintain or increase range of motion (ROM) or prevent and control contracture and deformity, particularly for clients with increased postural tone, has not been studied. In theory, maintaining normalized skeletal alignment of the trunk and lower extremities should help prevent structural changes such as scoliosis and hip dislocation by achieving the balance of forces advocated by Letts (1991). This may be particularly true for the young child without contractures but with preferred postures, where gravity has a significant effect over time. It can be argued, however, that for those with severely increased tone, strong deforming muscle forces, especially asymmetric ones, cannot be overcome through seating.

POSTURAL STABILITY AND CONTROL

This research has mostly hypothesized that anteriorly tilted seats will improve upright posture or stability. Measurement methods generally include instrumented systems or clinical rating scales. Two typical designs of anterior seats are 1) a flat bench with no trunk support, with feet flat on the floor, and 2) a forward-leaning system with an anterior trunk or upper extremity surface for support. Using the first type of bench seat, Bablich and colleagues (1986) measured postural stability with a three-dimensional tracking system that monitored a point on the top of the head. The anteriorly tipped seat resulted in a more upright and stable posture compared with a flat seat by increasing trunk extension and decreasing deviation from the midline in subjects with CP.

The position of the C7 spinous process was tracked to yield a *radius of stability,* with a smaller radius indicating reduced postural sway and thus increased postural stability (Reid et al., 1991). During quiet sitting on a flat bench, children with CP and with head injury showed no significant difference in the amount of postural sway when compared with age-matched controls, although they did show more variability. On a 10° anteriorly tilted seat, half of the children with CP (described as having spasticity with tight hamstrings) had a decrease in sway and a more upright posture (vertical measurement of C7 height) on the anterior seat. The other half of the children with CP (described as having low trunk tone and tight hamstrings) had an increase in sway on the anterior seat but also a more upright posture.

Video-digitized displacements of the head, shoulder, hip, knee, and ankle and seat reaction forces were studied as indicators of postural stability when the seating surface was varied between horizontal, 5° anterior tilt, and 5° posterior tilt (McClenaghan et al., 1992). Significant differences were found between children with and without motor impairment, as well as between quiet and active sitting for both groups, but this small degree of seat inclination did not affect postural stability.

Active control of trunk extension was rated using a four-point scale, and trunk extension was measured as the linear distance between defined marks on the spine (Miedaner, 1990). Young subjects with various motor impairments and delays sat on the floor, a level bench, a bench tipped anteriorly 20°, a bench tipped anteriorly 30°, and a commercial TherAdapt Posture Chair (TherAdapt Products, Bensonville, IL), an anteriorly tipped seat with a leg support to provide weight bearing through the knees and shins rather than the feet. Back extension was greatest in the TherAdapt Posture Chair, perhaps because of the levering action provided by the leg supports.

Head and postural control were clinically measured in Myhr and von Wendt's (1991) study of the forward-leaning seating system. The mean duration of head control during a 5-minute test period and postural control of the head, trunk, and feet, as scored on a four-point sitting assessment scale developed by the authors, all improved in the anterior position. The critical features of the Seating and Mobility (SAM) system (Pope et al., 1994) are a saddle seat, a solid anterior chest support, and a tray to support forward leaning. Qualitative changes in independent sitting ability, improved or maintained trunk posture in sitting, and power driving ability were observed in 10 children after 3 years of using the system.

The Sitting Assessment for Children with Neuromotor Dysfunction (SACND) is a standardized, observational rating scale, designed to assess the quality of sitting at rest and during upper extremity movements of children older than age 2 years (Reid, 1995, 1997). The scale rates postural tone, proximal stability, postural alignment, and balance, using four descriptors for each item. In young children with CP, the total rest score of the SACND was better on a saddle seat with 15° anterior tilt, foot support, and no trunk support, compared with sitting on a flat bench. Postural tone and postural alignment items showed the most change, indicating a more upright head and trunk and better alignment between body segments, and correlated with improved spinal extension measured by motion analysis (Reid, 1996).

PRESSURE AND PREVENTION OF DECUBITI

Several factors contribute to the development of pressure sores (Crenshaw & Vistnes, 1989), including skin temperature, moisture, and shear and compressive forces. Pressure (compressive force) has been the most-studied variable, because it has a clear relationship to the development of decubiti and is relatively easy to measure and manipulate during wheelchair seating. The risk of a pressure sore is directly related to the length of time soft tissue is compressed and inversely related to the area being compressed. Serious pressure sores are a common impairment in children with spinal cord injury and myelodysplasia in which immobility and insensate tissue compound the problem of prolonged sitting. Clients who are immobilized by severe CP or other neuromuscular impairment also need special considerations for pressure relief in sitting. Skeletal asymmetries such as pelvic obliquity, hip dislocation, and scoliosis predispose children who sit in wheelchairs to pressure problems.

Pressure mapping devices have become highly sophisticated and are commonly used to study differences in pressure distribution in subjects with and without motor impairment, reduction of seat interface pressure using various seat surfaces, and prevention of decubiti. Normal adult subjects displayed an even pressure distribution from side to side and a biphasic pattern of pressure concentration with a posterior concentration on the ischial tuberosities and a second, but lesser, concentration on the distal thighs (Drummond et al., 1982). A similar biphasic pattern was found in normal adolescent boys; however, over a 3-hour period, pressure tended to be skewed slightly to one side or the other (Pate, 1988). Patients with "unbalanced sitting" due to pelvic obliquity or scoliosis showed a pronounced shift of pressure laterally and often posteriorly, thereby severely loading one of the ischial tuberosities (Drummond et al., 1982).

For subjects without impairment, return to upright after a short period of recline in a wheelchair resulted in higher pressures and shear forces than in the original upright position (Gilsdorf et al., 1990). Leaning forward off the backrest returned the forces to initial values. Also, when the footrests were elevated, pressure under the ischial tuberosities was increased. There was no difference in pressure under the ischial tuberosities between upright sitting and 10° of recline in adults without impairment, but there was reduction of pressure in both positions when a lumbar support was added (Shields & Cook, 1988). The reclined position with lumbar support was recommended for patients with spinal cord injury because they slide or rotate off the lumbar support in upright position due to tight hamstrings or weak trunk musculature.

Magnetic resonance imaging can be used to evaluate soft tissue contours of the buttocks during loading. In a subject with paraplegia, less sitting pressure was required before soft tissue became compressed by a bony prominence, and there was increased stiffness and lateral shifting of the gluteal muscle mass (Reger et al., 1986). Foam cushions that were contoured to match the shape of the buttocks, as opposed to flat foam, improved the load transfer from buttocks to cushion because the total contact surface area was greater (Sprigle et al., 1990a). Foam stiffness was also important in determining the seat contours, with a stiffer foam having less deflection under the load. When clients with spinal cord injury were seated on flat versus contoured foam cushions of various stiffness, pressures were lower on the contoured cushions than on the flat cushions, and on the more compliant foam than on the stiffer foam (Sprigle et al., 1990b). The buttocks were encompassed more on the contoured and softer cushion with less tissue distortion. The authors cautioned that too soft a foam would deform too much and "bottom out" quickly. In contrast, when subjects with paraplegia sat with their trunks bent laterally, the mean pressure difference between the left and right ischial tuberosities was greater on a foam cushion than on a commercial air-bladder cushion (Koo et al., 1996).

Several studies have compared sitting pressures, skin temperature, and relative humidity in subjects seated on a number of commercially available cushions (Garber & Dyerly, 1991; Palmieri et al., 1980; Seymour & Lacefield, 1985; Stewart et al., 1980). The findings indicate that no one type of cushion is universally effective for all clients and that a variety of cushion options are needed to meet a variety of needs. The subjects in most of these pressure studies were adults with spinal cord injury; the unique needs of children, particularly those with severe pelvic and spinal deformity, as in myelodysplasia and CP, have not been studied.

Functional Limitations

UPPER EXTREMITY CONTROL AND HAND FUNCTION

Several authors have investigated the effect of varying seating configurations on upper body control and function. Wedging the seat did not improve hand function on a joystick-controlled targeting task in subjects with marked extensor spasticity (Seeger et al., 1984a), nor did it increase movement time of shoulder horizontal adduction to trigger a switch in subjects with CP (Nwaobi et al., 1986). Movement time was faster with the hips in a 90° position than in a wedged position, and slowest at a hip angle of 50°. When the hips were maintained at 90° of flexion but the entire system tilted posteriorly to 15 or 30°, or anteriorly to 5°, performance on the same shoulder adduction task was best in the vertical position and worst in the anterior position (Nwaobi, 1987).

Arm and hand function scores on a four-point rating scale were higher in the anteriorly tipped, forward-leaning position described by Myhr and von Wendt (1991). Performance on six upper extremity tasks did not change appreciably for subjects with or without CP at seat angles of 0°, 5° anterior tilt, or 5° posterior tilt (McClenaghan et al., 1992), possibly, as noted earlier, because of the very small change in seat angle. Reid's study (1996) using the saddle seat found that more than half of the subjects demonstrated faster and more accurate reaching movements.

Typing speed and accuracy of an 8-year-old boy with spastic athetoid CP was not measurably different when he sat in his typical position of posterior pelvic rotation (sacral sitting), compared with sitting in a therapeutic alignment with neutral pelvic rotation (McCormack, 1990). Perhaps seating adjustments have a less immediate or measurable effect on such a well-learned or long-practiced task as typing than on a more novel or spontaneous task.

ORAL-MOTOR, SPEECH, AND COMMUNICATION FUNCTIONS

Very young children with multiple handicaps demonstrated improvements in observed oral-motor skills associated with eating and drinking when seated in individually selected therapeutic seating devices over a period of many weeks (Hulme et al., 1987). No significant improvements were seen in self-feeding or independent drinking. Larnert and Ekberg (1995) used videofluoroscopy to examine swallowing in young children with severe CP who had feeding difficulties since birth. At 30° of recline, with the neck flexed, aspiration decreased in all five children, oral leak diminished in two children, and retention improved in one child compared with their typical upright eating position.

Spontaneous vocalizations in very young children with spasticity or hypotonia were sampled from 3 months before to 6 months after delivery of an adaptive seating system (Hulme et al., 1988). Increased frequency of speech sounds was found in seven children, and increased types of sounds were found in six. Bay (1991) studied a woman with spastic athetoid CP who activated her electronic communication device with a head-mounted light sensor. Her rate of head-controlled typing increased, but her accuracy decreased when she was seated in her power wheelchair with lateral trunk supports and properly adjusted foot support, compared with seating in her manual wheelchair with no foot or trunk support and excessive seat height.

MOBILITY

Several researchers have examined the effect of seating position on efficiency of manual wheelchair propulsion in adults (Hughes et al., 1992; van der Woude et al., 1989). Altering seat height, seat inclination, or anterior-posterior orientation for individual subjects affected upper extremity patterns of joint motion and wheeling efficiency. Wheeling performance can be optimized by adjusting seating configurations in relation to the propulsion mechanism (hand-rims or lever), based on the functional characteristics of each user. The effect that standard wheelchair configurations and the addition of seating systems has on the ability of young children with disabilities to learn self-wheeling has not been addressed. Pope and colleagues (1994) included a description of improved power driving ability over a period of 3 years in their subjects, who used the forward-leaning SAM system, although their results were based on subjective assessment and lacked controls.

Disability

The assumption is often made that individuals who experience an increase in functional skills also decrease their level of disability and improve their ability to fill societal roles. The families of 41 individuals who were nonambulatory and developmentally disabled, and who ranged in age from 1 to 67 years, were surveyed after receipt of adaptive seating equipment that included wheelchairs, travel chairs, and strollers, with custom adaptations as needed (Hulme et al., 1983). Changes in motor behavior included increased ability to sit upright without leaning, more time spent in sitting and less time lying down, increased ability to grasp an object, and improved ability to eat with a spoon. Social behavior changes included an increased number of community places visited, more time during the day spent with someone else, and less time spent in the bedroom. Although there was no change in frequency of leaving the home, caregivers reported improved ease of taking the clients on outings.

School-age children with profound multiple disabilities were positioned in a wheelchair, a sidelyer, and a freestyle position on a mat on the floor, and social-communicative interactions with classroom staff were measured (McEwen, 1992). Adults initiated interactions more often when the students were in the wheelchair, whereas there was no difference in student initiations between the positions. For the lower-functioning group, the average duration of interaction during the structured session was higher in the freestyle position than in either of the other two positions, but there was no difference for the higher-functioning group.

Summary

When the relevant studies are summarized, the gaps in information and the number of questions that remain to be answered regarding best options in seating become evident. There is supporting evidence in the literature that therapeutic seating systems that provide external postural support may improve pulmonary function in subjects with CP; reduce scoliosis when combined with a soft orthosis in subjects with muscular dystrophy; possibly have effects on upper extremity function in some subjects with CP; and potentially improve oral-motor skills, vocalizations, and social interaction behaviors in subjects with multiple disabilities. More specifically, an upright orientation appears to correlate with decreased myoelectric activity of extensor muscles at rest in cerebral palsy, improve pulmonary function in subjects with muscle weakness compared with supine positioning, improve an upper extremity (shoulder adduction) task in subjects with CP, and increase the number of adult-initiated interactions with subjects who have profound involvement compared with floor-lying positions. Hip flexion greater than 90° did not reduce myoelectric activity in extensors, nor did it improve upper extremity function. For clients with the most severe involvement, effects of orientation in space and seat-to-back angles are more variable and individualized than for clients with mild-to-moderate involvement. This must be considered when assessing clients with severe impairments and supports the use of postural support system simulation. The purpose in providing postural support for these clients often is focused more on improving comfort and alignment, which in turn allows greater participation in daily activities.

The effects of anteriorly tipping the seat are more controversial. Although anteriorly tipped seats appear to increase back extension and improve spinal alignment, it is unclear whether they improve stability or upper extremity function. Clinically, anteriorly tipped seats are used to encourage more "active sitting," with the goal of improving pelvic and spinal alignment in the presence of tight lower extremity musculature. The more vertical orientation of the pelvis that is possible with an anteriorly tipped seat may place the lumbar extensors at a better biomechanical advantage and reduce the need for the thoracic extensors to be excessively active to compensate for upper body flexion. As an active sitting position, the effects of long-term seating on performance and fatigue must be studied.

There is evidence that use of contoured cushions improves pressure distribution in subjects with spinal cord injury. Lumbar rolls tend to decrease pressure under the ischial tuberosities. The results with commercially available pressure relief cushions are variable, but of interest is the number of manufacturers of these cushions that are adding blocks and foam pieces to provide custom-contouring of their products.

Much work remains to be done in defining the features and components of postural support systems that reduce impairment, improve function, and increase social access for individuals with severe physical impairments. Identifying the specific disorders and severity of involvement and consistently reporting this information in all research reports are also necessary. Even in studies with relatively homogeneous subjects, results tend to be highly variable, indicating individualized responses. Objective clinical tools for identifying functional levels and measuring change as a result of intervention with a postural support system, such as the SACND and seat interface pressure monitors and shape sensors, must be developed and refined in terms of validity, reliability, and ease of clinical use.

The societal impact of use of adaptive seating, as well as of assistive technology clinics and programs, must be studied in detail. Potentially, these can reduce costs of hospitalizations due to decubiti and corrective surgery. Comprehensive regional centers may be the most cost-effective way to deliver advanced technology to the greatest number of people; however, rural mobile vans may promote a broader range of access. In some cases, receipt of expensive assistive technology and vocational training may increase a client's employability but reduce his or her eligibility for Medicaid or other supplemental assistance.

Principal Concepts in the Prescription of Postural Support Systems

Standardization of Terminology

Assistive seating technology has been evolving rapidly in many different regions of North America, creating a confusion of locally adopted language and terminology. RESNA has published a list of standardized seating terminology that is helpful in improving communication among research and service centers, clients, and funding sources (Medhat & Hobson, 1992).

Matching the Intervention to the Client's Level of Need

Classification schemes have been developed by many authors and are based on different dimensions

TABLE 24–1. **Classification of Sitting Needs**

Trefler (1984)	Tredwell & Roxborough (1991)

Group I
  Good head control
  Good to fair trunk control
  Good to fair fine motor skills
  Symmetric posture readily attainable
  Joint range of motion within normal limits
	Hand-Free Sitter
	  Sits for long periods without using hands for support

Group II
  Good to fair head control
  Fair to poor trunk control
  Fair to poor fine motor skills
  Up to and including moderate deformities
	Hand-Dependent Sitter
	  Needs one or both hands to maintain sitting
	  Needs some form of trunk or pelvic support to be able
	    to use hands for activities of daily living

Group III
  Fair to poor head control
  Poor trunk control
  Poor fine motor skills
  Deformities at the severe end of the scale, with limitation
    in range of motion due to contractures
	Propped Sitter
	  Unable to sit without major modification for pelvis
	    and trunk
	  Often requires head support
	  Severe structural and functional deformity

of the NCMRR model. Two methods of classification are compared in Table 24–1. Trefler (1984) described three classifications of seating clients based on the level of impairment of neuromotor control and deformity, whereas Tredwell and Roxborough (1991) used functional criteria to describe three similar categories.

The levels of intervention achieved with postural support systems have also been classified in many ways, but most investigators agree on three basic categories based on the amount of support the systems provide (Bergen et al., 1990). The first level of intervention is the *planar system* and consists of a flat seat and back. Good postural stability and sitting balance, with a minimum of deformity, are required, and this type of system is most appropriate for clients at the first level of the classification schemes. The seat and back consist of a solid base (plywood or plastic), covered by foam, and upholstered with vinyl or knit fabric. Flat trunk or pelvic supports may be added laterally. Many commercial variations are available, or they can be easily constructed in the clinic.

The second level of intervention is the *contoured system*, which provides external postural control by increasing the points of contact, especially laterally. The seat and back surfaces are rounded by shaping layers of firm foam to correspond to the curves of the body. Contours also help distribute pressures more evenly. Contouring can range from simple to aggressive. Although contoured systems are most typically used for clients at the second classification level, simple contouring can improve comfort and stability for many clients at the first level, and aggressive contouring may provide enough support for some

clients at the third level. Many varieties are fabricated in the clinic of a solid base with varying densities and configurations of foam, or there are a number of standardized modules commercially available.

The third level of intervention is the *custom-molded system*. It provides an intimate fit by closely conforming to the shape of the client's body, thereby giving the most postural support. When carefully molded it also provides the greatest amount of pressure relief. The time and expense involved in the fabrication of these systems is considerable, and the molding process requires a great deal of skill. Production of the mold usually involves either a vacuum consolidation method or a chemical reaction of liquid foams injected into a special bag. Several varieties of custom-molded systems are available, including those that can be completed on site and those that are sent to a central fabrication center. Computer-aided design technology allows the clinician to bypass the making of molds by mapping and digitizing body shape data directly using an instrumented simulator. The information is then transferred via computer disc, fax, or modem to a computer-driven carving machine that produces the cushion.

Examination and Simulation

Physical examination of the client for prescription of postural support systems is a pivotal role of the physical therapist on the technology team. The physical therapist applies knowledge of anatomy, kinesiology, biomechanics, and principles of neuromuscular control of posture and function when examining the child. Early strategies for seating intervention used by therapists often focused on con-

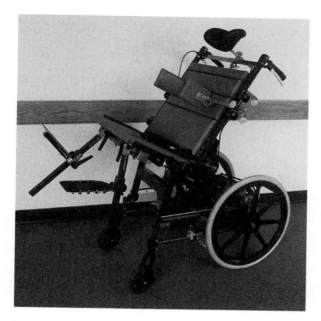

FIGURE 24–2. Commercially available seating simulator with multiadjustable components and angles. Shown mounted on a power mobility base that also allows assessment of driving ability and appropriate controls and switches.

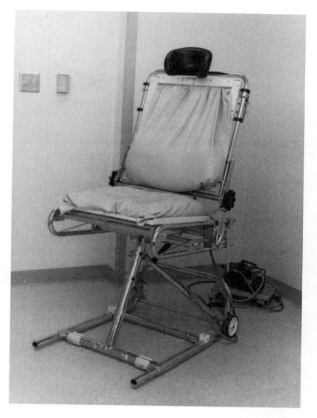

FIGURE 24–3. Commercially available seating simulator with adjustable angles. Shown with Contour-U (Invacare, Elyria, OH) vacuum-molding units for custom-contoured seat and back inserts.

trolling tone and reflexes according to Bobath-based principles. Letts (1991) and Myhr and von Wendt (1993) stressed the critical need to thoroughly understand and apply the principles of biomechanics to seating intervention as well.

Bergen has provided the most current and complete discussion of the examination process (Bergen, 1992; Bergen et al., 1990). The client should be examined both supine and sitting. A simulator chair works especially well for measuring linear dimensions, determining seating angles, and determining the amount of contouring needed, particularly for the more severely involved client who requires a very individualized solution. Two seating simulators that are commercially available are shown in Figures 24–2 and 24–3; however, many centers have made their own using modular components.

The assessment of posture in a wheelchair begins with the pelvis and its relationship to its adjacent segments. The orientation and range of mobility of the pelvis in all three planes will in turn determine the alignment and support needed at the trunk, head, and extremities. The measurements taken with the client supine and sitting are summarized in Figures 24–4 through 24–7. The effect of hip flexion and knee extension range of motion on the vertical orientation of the pelvis is among the most critical

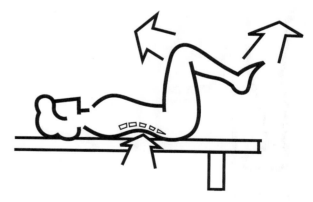

FIGURE 24–4. The examiner must monitor the lumbar curve as the hips are flexed and the knees extended. (Redrawn with permission from Bergen, AF, Presperin, J, & Tallman, T. Positioning for Function: Wheelchairs and Other Assistive Technologies. Valhalla, NY: Valhalla Rehabilitation Publications, 1990.)

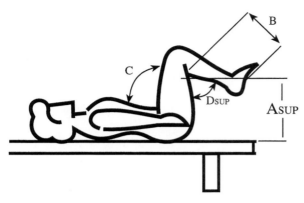

FIGURE 24–5. Hip (C) and knee (Dsup) angles, thigh/hip length (Asup), and calf length (B) are measured first in supine position. (Redrawn with permission from Bergen, AF, Presperin, J, & Tallman, T. Positioning for Function: Wheelchairs and Other Assistive Technologies. Valhalla, NY: Valhalla Rehabilitation Publications, 1990.)

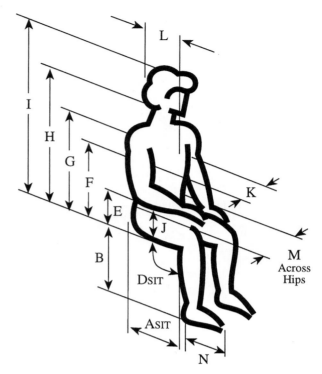

FIGURE 24–7. The following measurements are added to those taken with the client supine: Asit (R & L), behind hips to popliteal fossa; B (R & L), popliteal fossa to heel; Dsit, knee flexion angle; E, sitting surface to pelvic crest; F, sitting surface to axilla; G, sitting surface to shoulder; H, sitting surface to occiput; I, sitting surface to crown of head; J, sitting surface to hanging elbow; K, width across trunk; L, depth of trunk; M, width across hips; N, heel to toe. (Redrawn with permission from Bergen, AF, Presperin, J, & Tallman, T. Positioning for Function: Wheelchairs and Other Assistive Technologies. Valhalla, NY: Valhalla Rehabilitation Publications, 1990.)

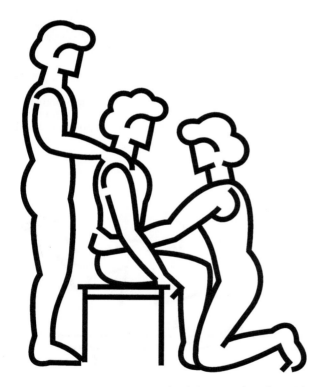

FIGURE 24–6. Measurements in sitting must be taken with the client sitting on a surface with a thin top. This will allow the knees to flex as needed. (Redrawn with permission from Bergen, AF, Presperin, J, & Tallman, T. Positioning for Function: Wheelchairs and Other Assistive Technologies. Valhalla, NY: Valhalla Rehabilitation Publications, 1990.)

factors in selecting seating angles and components. If there are minimal contractures of the hamstrings, hip extensors, and hip flexors, the pelvis should retain a considerable amount of mobility, and vertical orientation of the pelvis with a well-aligned trunk above will be possible. If any or all of these muscles are tight, the pelvis may be locked in either an anterior or a posterior tilt and the client will require a much more individualized solution.

Identification of the severity and type of deformities during examination and simulation will influence the type of system and components chosen. A *flexible deformity*—one that can be manually corrected and maintained with a reasonable amount of force—can often be maintained in optimal alignment with the appropriate and balanced use of support components. Postural support systems, however, are not intended to stretch tight musculature or correct bony deformity. Stretching invariably results in sacrifice of the optimum posture because the child will attempt to move and avoid the uncomfortable forces. *Fixed deformities*—those that are not correctable without an undue amount of force—and severe muscle contractures must be accommodated in the postural support system, and reduction must be addressed through other interventions. Letts (1991) strongly advocates surgical intervention to achieve a balance of sitting forces in much the same way that a goal of surgery is to improve symmetry of gait for individuals who are ambulatory.

Although the primary focus of the assessment is the pelvis, the primary goal of intervention is to provide a stabilized trunk for upright posture and for function (Bergen et al., 1990). With many individuals, the trunk alignment is achieved by first establishing the optimum pelvic positioning. For clients with severe scoliosis and pelvic obliquity, however, neutral alignment of the pelvis is not always possible and does not result in acceptable trunk and head alignment. In such cases, it is better to start with a relatively vertical head and level shoulders and allow the pelvis to be tilted and rotated.

In clients at risk for skin breakdown due to pressure problems, measurement of seat and back interface pressures should be included in the assessment process. Devices such as the Xsensor Pressure Mapping System (Crown Therapeutics, Belleview, IL) are increasingly common in the clinic for comparing pressures while seated on various cushions. Shortcomings of such devices are that accuracy of the monitor decreases with an increasingly contoured cushion and the monitor itself can interfere with the cushion's ability to conform to the bony prominence. In addition, pressure in deep tissues, especially near bone, can be higher than a reading of seat interface pressures might indicate (Crenshaw & Vistnes, 1989). Variable-tilt and variable-recline features of manual and power wheelchairs can provide another source of pressure relief throughout a long day of sitting for some clients.

Prescription and Application of Postural Support Systems

The scope of this chapter and the rapidly evolving nature of technology preclude a thorough discussion of all options and features of postural support systems. Many excellent resources exist describing these in more detail and provide problem-solving lists and charts (Bergen et al., 1990; Letts, 1991; Trefler, 1984; Trefler et al., 1993). In this section attention is

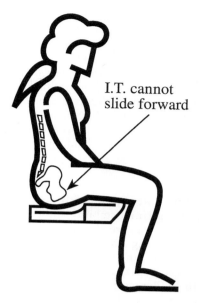

FIGURE 24–8. An antithrust seat can help hold the pelvis back on the seat by blocking forward sliding of the ischial tuberosities (I.T.). (Redrawn with permission from Bergen, AF, Presperin, J, & Tallman, T. Positioning for Function: Wheelchairs and Other Assistive Technologies. Valhalla, NY: Valhalla Rehabilitation Publications, 1990.)

focused on some of the most salient points in the decision-making process.

SEATS

In most cases, the seat is the most critical element of the postural support system. The use of true planar seats is becoming rare because most clinicians have found that a small amount of lateral contouring for even the highest-level sitter adds comfort and stability (Bergen, 1992; Bergen et al., 1990). The benefit of adding contours to help relieve pressure problems is evidenced by the number of commercially available air and gel pressure cushions that have foam blocks and wedges to allow customization of cushion shape. On the other hand, strategically placing commercial gel pads in a custom-made, contoured foam cushion can also supply that extra, critical amount of pressure relief needed by some clients. Antithrust seats (Fig. 24–8) have a block of high-density foam placed just anterior to the ischial tuberosities that keeps the pelvis from sliding forward and equalizes pressure distribution along the thighs (Siekman & Flanagan, 1983). Antithrust seats can be added to planar as well as contoured systems, but they are thought to work best with deep lateral contours of the pelvis and lateral thigh supports (adductor pads).

Seat placement within the wheelchair frame is another important consideration. A thick cushion or inappropriate mounting hardware can place the seat too high, causing loss of independent transfers or wheeling, or can change the center of gravity to an unsafe position. Forward or backward placement, especially in very small children, can affect the knee angle required for foot placement on the footrests and can change the ease of wheeling by affecting access to the wheel rims or loading or unloading the front casters.

BACKS

A back support with a gently curved surface can improve lateral trunk stability and comfort. Simple contouring for a prominent rib hump can be achieved by cutting a hole in the plywood or plastic to allow the overlying foam some give. More aggressive contouring can be achieved using blocks of high-density foam (Bergen et al., 1990). A custom-molded back should be used for clients with severe fixed spinal deformity.

Sagittal plane alignment of the spine has traditionally been adjusted using lumbar rolls; however, control of sagittal curves begins with the pelvis and sacrum rather than the lumbar spine (Margolis, 1992; Margolis et al., 1988). A "biangular back" has a vertical section behind the pelvis, with the section above the pelvis angled back a few degrees to encourage lumbar extension, or sacral disks or pads can be added to the back surface. The client must have sufficient range of motion and flexibility for these items to work.

PELVIC STABILIZATION

A seat belt placed at a 45° angle at the seat-back junction is the most typical form of pelvic stabilization. For highly functional individuals, placement of the belt across the anterior thighs, just in front of the hips, allows more natural active trunk and pelvic mobility (Bergen et al., 1990).

The subASIS bar is a form of rigid pelvic stabilization consisting of a padded bar attached to plates lateral to the pelvis (Margolis et al., 1988). The pelvis must be maintained in a vertical orientation or the client will slide under the bar. A less rigid variation is the semirigid pelvic stabilizer (SRPS) (Carlson, 1987; Carlson & Grey, 1988) (Fig. 24–9). Constructed of high-density foam mounted on a reinforcing strip of thermoplastic splinting material, it incorporates wedges that fit under the anterior superior iliac spine while providing relief across the lower abdomen. Like the subASIS bar, the SRPS provides direct control of the pelvis for stabilization, yet the angle of placement can be varied, as with a seat belt, making it an option for clients with a mild fixed posterior

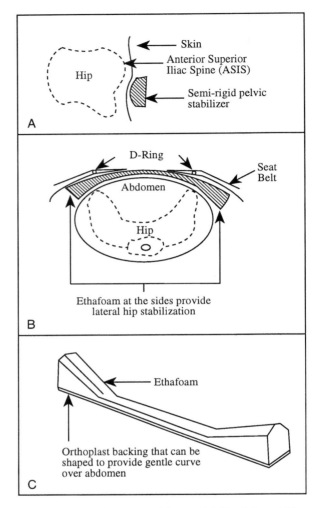

FIGURE 24–9. Placement of the semirigid pelvic stabilizer from a side view *(A)* and from a top view *(B)*. *C*, Detail of the stabilizer shape. (Redrawn with permission from Carlson, SJ. The semi-rigid pelvic stabilizer for seating control. Assistive Devices Information Network Newsletter [University of Iowa, Iowa City, IA], *1*[1]:2–3, 1987.)

pelvic tilt. The flexibility of the SRPS may result in fewer pressure problems than the subASIS bar, and it works especially well for clients who demonstrate a strong asymmetric thrusting pattern.

A promising new form of dynamic pelvic stabilization uses individually contoured pads that fit around the pelvis, with a pivot mechanism allowing anterior-posterior tilting of the pelvis without loss of stability (Noon et al., 1998). Adjustments allow accommodation of deformity, control of direction and amount of tilting, and a dynamic force to return the pelvis to a neutral position. Anterior knee blocks, another form of pelvic stabilization

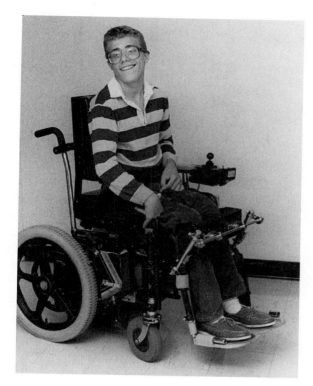

FIGURE 24–10. Knee blocks used to stabilize pelvis and prevent sliding on an anteriorly tipped seat. (From Carlson, SJ. Knee gate for control of forward sliding in wheelchair. Assistive Devices Information Network Newsletter [University of Iowa, Iowa City, IA], *2*[3]:2–3, 1988.)

(Fig. 24–10), direct a force up the length of the femurs to counter sliding of the pelvis (Bergen et al., 1990; Carlson, 1988).

ANGLES

There is no consensus as to the effects of seat and spatial angles on alignment and function. Factors that must be considered in determining fixed angles include severity and nature of postural tone abnormalities, contractures, and deformities; level of motor control for sitting; and design and purpose of the mobility base. Although the concept of upright 90-90-90 sitting is theoretically sound, it is neither a natural functional sitting position (Kangas, 1991) nor a logistically possible option for many clients. Slight wedging of the seat or posterior tilt may improve head alignment or keep very young children from sliding. Opening the hip angle may be necessary when hip extension contractures are present. By allowing the knees to flex, thus bringing the feet back under the seat, the rotatory force on the pelvis may be reduced in the presence of tight hamstrings.

The anteriorly tipped seat has potential for clients with hypoextensible lower extremity musculature but fair to good upper body control who "sacral sit" on a flat surface. It is also used for the more severely involved child in a forward-lean position with a solid anterior chest support. Good pelvic stabilization must be achieved to prevent sliding. Unfortunately, when anteriorly tipped seating is used in wheelchairs, the client often lacks enough knee extension to keep the heels from interfering with caster movement. Figure 24–11 shows one solution for a young man with severe spastic athetoid CP in which one legrest arrangement was used for functional tasks in the stationary chair and the other, although not an ideal position, was used for wheeling.

Variable angles allow adjustments of tilt and recline throughout the day. Tilt is useful for relief of pressure or relief of trunk or neck fatigue, and it provides a combination of active sitting and rest positions. Recline is useful for relief of fatigue, for hip or back pain, and if catheterizations or other hygiene procedures must be performed in the chair.

Some clinics have been engineering dynamic or compliant seating systems for clients with severe and abrupt extensor spasms (Evans & Nelson, 1996; Orpwood, 1996). Often the severity of tone or spasms is exacerbated by the rigidity of a conventional system. The new devices use hinges, pivot points, and springs to allow movement of the seat or back with the child and provide a gentle returning force. Clients who used these systems exhibited a decrease in the severity of spasms or fluctuating tone over a period of weeks. Comfort and ease of transfers were improved.

UPHOLSTERY

Synthetic knit fabrics with waterproof backing have for the most part replaced vinyl upholstery. They are less slippery, thus decreasing shear, and can be removable for easy cleaning. Contoured cushions are easier to cover with knit fabric, but fabric that is pulled too tightly will interfere with deep contours. Vacuum methods allow even aggressively contoured cushions to be covered with durable, fabric-backed vinyl that is easy to clean and protects the cushions from urine and food spills.

LEG SUPPORTS

Leg supports, usually a component of the mobility base, are discussed here because of their direct influence on the entire seating system. Elevated legrests are offset forward of the seat more than fixed legrests and can contribute to forward sliding on the seat or poor positioning of the feet for weight bearing. They should never be ordered unless they are specifically required. Choice of footrests on small, pediatric chairs can be especially difficult because they frequently interfere with caster action.

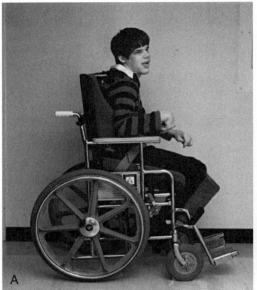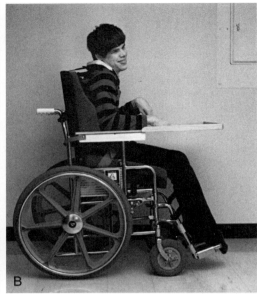

FIGURE 24–11. Anteriorly tipped seat mounted in a manual wheelchair. *A,* An anterior knee and shin support was used to decrease stretch on the hamstrings and improve pelvic and trunk alignment; this support is used for stationary sitting only, because the feet interfere with caster motion. *B,* An alternative foot position on the footrests allowed wheeling but contributed to sliding and slouching.

Footplates that extend backward under the seat are helpful when clients have tight hamstrings. Foot straps hold the feet in the desired location to assist with lower body stability and weight bearing. For clients with deformity or limited joint movement, forcing the foot into neutral alignment on the footrest may impose undesirable stresses at the knees or hips (Bergen et al., 1990). Other clients exhibit natural postural adjustments and placement of the feet during weight shifting and active movement, and their feet should be left free.

LATERAL AND MEDIAL SUPPORTS

Lateral trunk supports (or scoliosis pads) range from simple, flat, padded blocks to contoured, wraparound supports. Swivel or swing-away mounting hardware is usually needed for wraparound supports. Contoured seats usually provide the most effective lateral thigh and pelvic support, as well as the best pressure relief. Square or rectangular pads used as lateral thigh supports are still sometimes used for mildly impaired clients. Medial thigh supports (abductor wedges or pommels) are intended to maintain hip alignment in neutral or slight abduction and not to stretch tight adductors or prevent sliding of the pelvis. Removable or swing-away supports facilitate transfers and urinal or catheter use (Bergen et al., 1990).

ANTERIOR SUPPORTS

Anterior trunk supports keep the spine erect over the pelvis. Butterfly-shaped straps apply more direct control at the sternum and shoulders than single horizontal belts or H- or Y-straps; however, the lower end of one strap must be permanently attached to the backrest or to the seat behind the pelvis so that it cannot ride up and choke the client. Rigid shoulder retractors that project over the top of the backrest provide even more anterior shoulder control, but may be poorly tolerated. Padded axillary straps are becoming much more popular. They attach to the underside of the lateral thoracic support, are directed superiorly and medially over the front of the axilla, and attach at the top of the backrest, controlling shoulder protraction without crossing the chest.

HEADREST

Facilitating good head position can be one of the most difficult tasks. In an otherwise totally immobile client, the head is the one part that is likely to move. Poor head positioning can make an otherwise effective postural support system look awful. On the other hand, our own observations of barium swallow studies suggest that some clients with the most severe physical and mental impairments may need to adopt a forward-hanging head position to cope with increased oral secretions or reflux. Correcting these clients' heads to a position that "looks good" may increase their risk of aspiration or choking.

Support under the occiput is better than a flat contact on the back of the head. Neck rings, two-step (with an occipital ledge), and contoured head supports are several options. Halos encircle the forehead and should always be used with caution, particularly during vehicular transport, because of the potential for neck injury. Static and dynamic forehead straps are newer options. Collars with soft anterior chin support, that are not attached to the wheelchair, may be effective for the client who has constant neck flexion regardless of seating angles.

UPPER EXTREMITY SUPPORTS

Cutout trays are the most typical form of upper extremity support and can be designed for a multitude of special purposes. Posterior elbow blocks and scapular pads are used to reduce the tendency to retract the arms; however, if these are needed, it may be necessary to reassess whether the seating angles are appropriate. Clients with severe dystonia often prefer wrist or arm cuffs to reduce unwanted movement of one or both arms.

WHEELED MOBILITY

The purpose of the mobility base is dependent on the child's level of function. For some, the primary purpose will be independent mobility, and the therapist must determine how best to achieve this. For others, the purpose of the base is to provide a means of being transported by a companion, and this must be accomplished in a comfortable and efficient manner. In either case, the base serves the additional role of supporting the seating system. Selection of a mobility base requires consideration of the client's lifestyle, the seating system it will support, and the environments in which it will function. Assessment for a new mobility base should ideally be done at the same time as assessment and simulation for the postural support system, because much of the same information regarding the client and the environment must be gathered.

Research on Mobility

Excessive energy expenditure during locomotion is a common impairment of people with movement dysfunction. Persons with disability decrease their walking speed so that energy expenditure approaches a normal range, and assistive devices that increase effort will be abandoned (Fisher & Gullickson, 1978). Children with CP walked at nearly half the velocity of children without disability and consumed more oxygen per kilogram of body weight per minute doing so (Campbell & Ball, 1978).

Fifty percent of children with myelomeningocele who were ambulatory with braces stopped walking between ages 10 and 20 years (DeSouza & Carroll, 1976). In children with myelomeningocele, ambulation was 218% less energy efficient than for children without disability, energy expenditure was significantly lower during wheelchair propulsion than during walking, and wheelchair propulsion was as fast and as energy efficient as normal walking (Williams et al., 1983). Children with a higher lesion (L2 or above) expended energy equal to their maximal aerobic capacity when walking at slow speed, whereas those with lower lesions (L3–L4) used 85% of their maximal aerobic capacity (Agre et al., 1987). Wheelchair propulsion required 42% less energy than crutch walking at the same speed. When the wheelchair was propelled at typical walking speed of children without disability, oxygen consumption was only 9% greater than for the nondisabled children during walking.

Future studies of wheelchair ergometrics in children with other disabilities would be useful. For example, energy expenditure is likely to be excessive during wheeling a manual wheelchair in children with CP with upper extremity involvement, and power wheelchair driving would allow a reduction of energy expenditure.

Excessive energy expenditure during locomotion leads to functional limitation, such as fatigue, and to disability, such as poor academic performance. Academic performance measures (reading fluency, visuomotor accuracy, and manual dexterity) were taken at the end of each school day, after subjects either propelled their wheelchair or walked with assistive devices (Franks et al., 1991). Visuomotor accuracy was significantly decreased for all three subjects during the ambulation phase compared with the wheelchair phase. Manual dexterity decreased for only one subject, and reading fluency did not change for any of the subjects.

Lepage and colleagues (1998) conducted a study of 98 children with all types of CP to determine the association between type of locomotion and the accomplishment of life habits, which included six activities of daily living and six social roles. The greatest disruption of life habits was found in children who used manual wheelchairs; children who used power wheelchairs showed somewhat less disruption in five of the life habit categories. More manual wheelchair users showed associated problems such as visual and auditory impairments, epilepsy, and comprehension difficulties. Ambulatory children showed fewer disruptions of life habits than those using wheelchairs, with children who walked without technical aids showing the least disruption in four categories.

Many factors affect performance and mobility in users of manual wheelchairs, including human physiologic capacities, such as strength and endurance, which are dependent on the user's diagnosis, age, sex, lifestyle, and build (Brubaker, 1986, 1988). The position of the individual within the wheelchair, particularly in relation to the handrims or other propulsion method, determines the mechanical advantage of the user to act on the chair. Wheelchair factors that affect mobility are rolling resistance, control, maneuverability, stability, and dynamic behavior. These are dependent on the quality and construction of the wheelchair, such as weight, rigidity of the frame, wheel alignment, mass distribution, and suspension. Wheelchair propulsion in children with spinal cord injury was similar to that in a neurologically matched group of adults (Bednarczyk & Sanderson, 1994). The adults wheeled faster, but the children spent a similar proportion of the wheeling cycle in propulsion, and the angular changes in the kinematics of the elbow and shoulder over time were the same for both groups. Therefore, applications intended to improve wheeling efficiency in adults may be appropriate for children as well.

The developmental consequences of impaired movement is another area of functional limitation and disability. The nondisabled infant's experience with independent forward progression has a profound impact on perceptual, cognitive, emotional, and social processes (Kermoian, 1997). For the immobile child, early provision of artificial forms of locomotion has the potential to minimize the deficits in spatial, cognitive, affective, and social functions. Prone scooters, caster carts, and walkers are alternatives for some young children with functional upper extremities. For the child with more severe involvement, however, early power mobility offers the best choice.

Traditionally, prescription of power wheelchairs was put off until children reached their teens, when all attempts at effective ambulation were exhausted. Power wheelchairs were considered too expensive and too difficult for young children to learn to drive, and walking was too important a goal to give up. Studies indicate that children as young as 24 months can successfully learn independent power mobility within a few weeks (Butler, 1986; Butler et al., 1983). Benefits attributed to the use of power mobility include increases in self-initiated behaviors, including change in location, rate of interaction with objects, and frequency of communication (Butler, 1986). Other benefits reported are increased peer interaction; increased interest in other forms of locomo-

tion, including walking; increased family integration such as inclusion in outings; and decreased perception of helplessness by family members (Butler et al., 1983; Paulsson & Christoffersen, 1984; Schiaffino & Laux, 1986; Verburg et al., 1984).

Performance characteristics of various power bases is another important area of study. Deitz and colleagues (1991) studied the performance of children without disability on functional tasks while using four different power wheelchairs representing different designs, including a standard chair, a modular (all-terrain) base, a three-wheeled scooter, and the Turbo, a unique pediatric base with a power elevating seat (now called the GoBot by Permobil). Functional positioning tasks required the subjects to position themselves at a standard table, at a classroom desk, and at the blackboard. Access to environment tasks had the children opening a door, retrieving books from shelves, retrieving a book from the floor, turning on a water faucet, and turning on a light switch. Wheelchair maneuvering skills included U-turns, making left and right turns on a pathway, and speed and accuracy in straight driving. No chair was superior in all the tasks, although certain designs were advantageous for some tasks. The scooter and Turbo allowed positioning at the table and desk, respectively, whereas the other two bases did not. The Turbo offered the widest range of reaching; however, maneuverability was least for the Turbo and greatest for the conventional chair.

When performance characteristics of conventional power chairs, all-terrain bases, three-wheelers, and children's all-terrain devices from six manufacturers were evaluated, results showed each chair to have advantages and disadvantages in straight driving speed, speed on a graded run with a 90° turn, curb jumps of varying thickness, and load pulling (Jones, 1988). Performance characteristics must be matched with the client's intended use, lifestyle, and comfort during the selection process.

An interdisciplinary U.S. Wheelchair Standards Committee, administered through RESNA and approved by the American National Standards Institute, has completed a document on wheelchair standards. The standards represent a comprehensive approach to testing and disclosing information about wheelchairs (Bryant, 1991). Manufacturers, suppliers, and consumers can use this information to improve their products, select chairs with the best performance for the cost, and identify chairs that meet specific performance needs. Thacker and colleagues (1994) have written a useful manual detailing the engineering and technical features of each component on the wheelchair, from frame construction, to caster bearings, to drive trains and batteries.

Selection of a Mobility Base

The goal in selecting a mobility base is to provide an appropriate means of getting from one location to another efficiently. It is inappropriate to require someone to rely on his or her everyday mobility for exercise. Prohibiting the use of a manual wheelchair for a child with marginal ambulation, or that of a power wheelchair for a child with marginal manual wheelchair skills, places their functional and academic performance at risk due to excessive energy expenditure. A creative and structured fitness program is a more appropriate way of addressing strength and cardiovascular endurance goals.

It is generally agreed that positioning needs take precedence over the issuance of a mobility device. At the same time, the design of the postural support system should maximize potential for independent function in the wheelchair whenever possible. This, in turn, influences chair modifications and the interface hardware needed. For example, if a 3-inch, modular composite foam cushion is necessary for pressure relief, yet the client has short extremities as in myelodysplasia, both independent transfers and wheeling will be more difficult. A possible solution is to order a chair frame with a lower seat height and without upholstery so that drop brackets can be used to lower the cushion between the seat rails.

To assess driving skills and controller placement once the desired seating position has been obtained, some seating simulators can be mounted on a power base. A remote, attendant-held control can override the user's control, ensuring safety and appropriate feedback during assessment and training. The client should be offered test drives in a variety of bases with as appropriately simulated postural support as possible.

The first step in selecting a mobility base is to determine what type of functional mobility is desired. Three general types of mobility bases are companion chairs for dependent wheeling, standard manual wheelchairs, and power wheelchairs. Ideally, the selection should be based on the potential level of independent mobility, but other factors often come into play, including methods of transportation, availability of training or supervision, and availability of funding.

The second consideration is choice of style of the base. Within each type, there are several styles with different features and performance characteristics. Factors that influence this choice are the level and type of postural support system required, the level of independence in other skills such as transfers and activities of daily living, the specific environments in which the chair will be used, the method of transportation, and the needs of caregivers.

Selection of size may influence both the style and type chosen and is based on client size, expected growth rate, growth capabilities of the chair itself, and the size and style of the postural support system. Mobility bases designed specifically for pediatrics are available in a variety of sizes and designs. Growth capabilities have been greatly improved as funding sources have demanded longer life from purchased items.

The final consideration is the model and manufacturer of the chair. Often the finer details of construction are important at this stage, such as the proportions of the chair, angles, orientations, adjustability of parts such as footrests and armrests, and swing-away, detachment, or folding mechanisms. Other important influencing factors are performance characteristics, styling, comfort, rate of breakdown, availability of parts, service record, and cost. Regional preferences for various models and manufacturers are evident across North America.

Companion Wheelchairs

Companion wheelchairs, transporter chairs, and dependent mobility bases (Fig. 24–12) are intended for individuals who will not need to access the wheels for independent mobility, including those with the most severe impairments and very young children. In other cases, this type of chair may be used as backup transportation for a child who ambulates or uses a power wheelchair. Manual wheelchairs are frequently used as dependent bases, but there are many other styles as well. They often include firm seats and backs and have a wide variety of positioning components as options. Alternatively, contoured or custom-molded postural support systems can be fabricated and mounted on the frames. Some of these chairs can be used as vehicular transport seats and comply with federal safety standards. Others are designed for very young children and look and perform like a stroller.

When choosing a dependent mobility base, the primary caregiver must be considered a user as well. Attention should be given to his or her comfort and ease of use, including push handle height, rolling resistance, maneuverability, and ease of disassembly and transport. Parents of young children who are receiving their first mobility base and seating system may be very sensitive to the need for a wheelchair. Stroller bases that look least like a wheelchair are popular and are often much less threatening. Some funding sources deny stroller bases because of their limitations in growth and ability to be adapted if the child's independent capabilities progress.

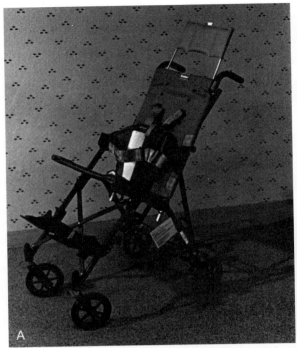

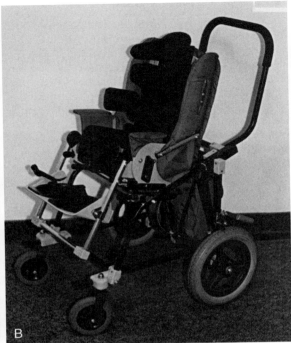

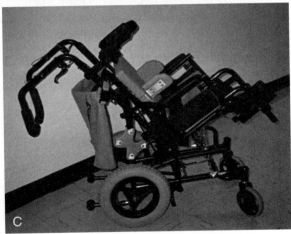

FIGURE 24–12. Companion or transporter chairs. *A,* Collapsible stroller base. *B,* Stroller base with removable modular seating system. *C,* Manual wheelchair-style base with smaller rear wheels, stroller handles, and tilt mechanism.

Manual tilt and recline features are incorporated into many companion chairs. A fixed angle of tilt or recline can be useful when designing the postural support system for some clients. For others, the ability to vary the amount of tilt or recline throughout the day is critical for prevention of pressure sores, fatigue, and discomfort.

Manual Wheelchairs

The standard manual wheelchair has two large wheels, usually in back, for independent propul-sion, and two small swiveling casters in front. Manual wheelchairs are often chosen as dependent mobility bases as well because of their ability to accept custom-designed postural support systems, their ease of use, and their tilt and recline options (Fig. 24–13). For independent wheelers, the 1980s was the "new age" of manual wheelchairs when lightweight chairs and chairs designed for recreational use and athletic competition became widely available. Lightweight and durable metals and fabrics, alternative wheel placement, improved frame proportions and designs, adjustability, and adaptability

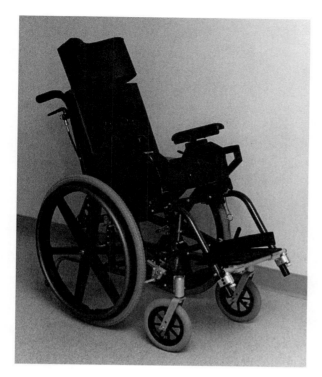

FIGURE 24–13. Standard lightweight manual wheelchair with manual tilt mechanism, shown with a contoured seating system.

to custom seating have all helped streamline the manual wheelchair to improve efficiency and control, ease of transfers, portability, and appearance. Lightweight chairs with the large wheels in front are much easier for young children to propel for short distances indoors. For the very active person, ultra-lightweight, high-performance chairs incorporate rigid frames and high-quality bearings for the best chair responses. The serious athlete can find specialized designs dedicated to specific performance needs and that sometimes barely resemble the traditional concept of a wheelchair.

One-arm–drive wheelchairs are designed for individuals with significant asymmetry of upper extremity strength and function that prevents bimanual propulsion. The classic style is the double-handrim on one side, with a linkage system to the other wheel. Styles that use a pumping action with a lever and ratchet system, although rarely used now, are generally easier and more efficient for both wheeling and steering but create more problems in dependent wheeling by caregivers. Operation of a one-arm–drive chair may exacerbate existing asymmetry in clients with tonal disorders such as CP. However, it may be the best option for the child or teen with severe cognitive impairment who does not have the where-withal to operate a power chair, but who can get around in her or his familiar environment with a one-arm drive.

Power Mobility

Hays (1988) described four functional categories of children for whom power mobility is indicated. The first group includes children who will never ambulate and who experience no independent mobility without the use of a power device. The second group includes children with inefficient mobility, that is, they ambulate or use a manual wheelchair but with unacceptable speed or endurance. The third group consists of children who have lost independent mobility through disease, brain injury, or spinal cord trauma. For this group, the developmental implications of independent mobility may be less important, but the acceptance of assisted mobility is a more significant issue. The fourth group includes children who require assisted mobility temporarily, either because they gain new ambulation skills through surgery or maturation or they recover lost function.

Advances in technology have brought independent power mobility to a greater number of individuals with severe disabilities than ever before. If the 1980s was the decade of the lightweight wheelchair, the 1990s is the decade of electronic control development. Today a variety of power bases and options are available, with more reliable and precise controls than ever before possible. The three main types of power wheelchairs are the conventional design with integral seat and chassis (evolved from the traditional, tubular manual wheelchair frame), the power-base or modular design with separate seat and chassis (often called an all-terrain wheelchair), and scooters with either three- or four-wheeled platforms (Fig. 24–14). Power chairs may be ordered with seats that tilt, backs that recline, units that recline and tilt, legrests that elevate, and headrests that adjust, all with the touch of a switch. Manufacturers have responded to an increased demand for pediatric-sized power wheelchairs by producing wheelchairs that are lighter in weight, are correctly proportioned for children, and have growth capabilities. Major advances in electronics have produced a greater variety of controls that are easier to access, more durable, and easier to adjust and customize.

The style of power base chosen will depend in part on the client's upper body control. Scooters are steered using a tiller that requires a significant amount of upper extremity active range of motion and sitting balance. The control functions are usually mounted on the tiller and require a grip-type action of the thumb or fingers. Jones (1990)

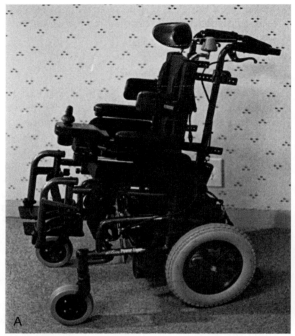

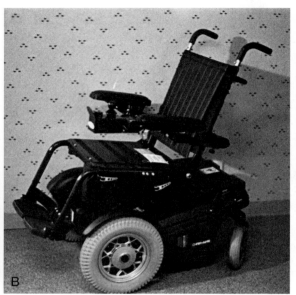

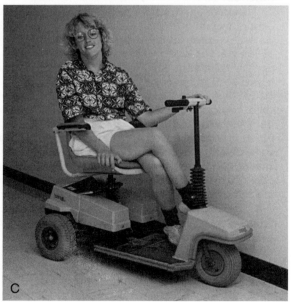

FIGURE 24–14. Power wheelchairs. *A,* Typical, pediatric-sized, rear wheel, direct-drive model, shown with standard armrest-mounted proportional control. *B,* Modular, front wheel, direct-drive model. *C,* Three-wheeled power chair, or "scooter."

described a range of scooters from "light duty mall crawlers to heavy duty barnyard rut jumpers." Scooters are easier to dismantle and transport in the trunk of a car and look least like a wheelchair. Although they remain popular among adults, funding is often denied based on their limited indoor mobility and poor vehicle tie-down capabilities. Manufacturers

have responded by making them more rugged and suited to outdoor use.

The conventional and powerbase designs offer the greatest range of seating and control options. The entire seating unit can be removed from the pedestal mount of the modular base. The traditional belt-driven chair is obsolete; the direct-drive motors of the powerbase improve power, as well as control in turning. Drive systems have recently expanded to include choices between front-, mid-, and rear-wheel drive. Each offers different advantages and disadvantages in stability while driving and stopping, stability during recline or tilt, maneuverability in tight spaces, and ability to climb curbs. The type of drive system chosen for any given client must be as carefully considered as any other component of the wheelchair and seating system.

Power recline and power tilt wheelchairs offer excellent alternatives to individuals who need position changes throughout a long day of sitting to perform different functions or because of pain, fatigue, or pressure concerns associated with sitting too long (Fig. 24–15). The act of reclining, however, causes shearing of tissues due to the disproportionate movement between the client and the postural support system. On returning to the upright position, most clients will have shifted position in the system, and the more complex the seating system, the more significant the effects. Power recliners are available in low-shear and zero-shear models to help address these problems. Power tilt models work well for the client with severe hypertonia or contractures who cannot tolerate having the seat-to-back angle opened up or who, once having done so, cannot return to an upright position without significant sliding.

Controls for power wheelchairs are available in two basic types: proportional and microswitch. The former has a proportional relationship between movement of the joystick and speed of the chair or sharpness of turning, whereas the latter has an on/off relationship to chair movement. The proportional control is the standard joystick found on most power wheelchairs. It is customarily mounted on either armrest and will move in a 360° arc. The movement of the joystick controls the speed and the direction of the wheelchair. An alternative to the standard joystick is a remote proportional joystick that is smaller and more compact. This feature allows a great deal of flexibility for joystick placement, provided sturdy mounting hardware is used. Proportional joysticks are also available in short-throw models that require less movement and force for activation and in heavy-duty models that can withstand a great deal of force. Head control joysticks are also available for some wheelchairs.

A microswitch control consists of four separate switches, with each switch controlling one direction—forward, reverse, left, and right. All four switches might be in one control box (resembling a standard proportional control) or assembled into a smaller, more compact, remote control. Microswitches are also available in heavy-duty and short-

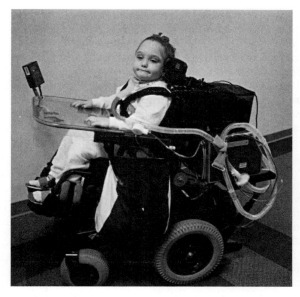

FIGURE 24–15. This child with a C4 spinal cord injury is learning to drive her power wheelchair with a proximity switch head array. The chair is equipped with power tilt for frequent pressure relief, low-shear power recline to allow catheterization procedures without a transfer, and a swivel-mounted ventilator and suction machine tray that remains horizontal during tilt and recline. She is able to activate all driving and position functions, as well as access her computer, through the head array. The monitor to the right of her tray indicates which function mode she has chosen with the head switch.

throw models, as are the proportional controls. Microswitches are somewhat more flexible for assessment purposes. For example, they may be separated and set up in arrays to evaluate head control, or each of the four switches may be positioned at different body sites. The wafer board and arm-slot control are examples of microswitch technology. Microswitch-driven chairs tend to be less precise and smooth while turning and changing directions because each direction is controlled by a separate switch.

With the recognition that age is no longer the determining factor in successful use of power mobility has come the need to define appropriate selection criteria. Schiaffino and Laux (1986) reported that children needed a cognitive level of at least 2 years of age, although these children would take longer to train than children with cognitive skills at the 3-year level or above. More recently, transitional mobility programs are being developed for children as young as 12 to 14 months (Wright-Ott, 1997). Barnes (1991) described a "motoric language" needed to learn to drive a powered chair that includes relational vocabulary (in, on, under), substantive vocabulary (nouns), directionality (forward, backward, right, left), perceptual concepts (visual and auditory feedback with switch activation), spatial concepts (depth perception, location of self in an environment, and problem solving to avoid obstacles), and serial or sequential concepts (first, second; before, after).

It is possible that many of these concepts could actually be taught through training in a power device. Kangas (1997) provides a compelling argument for an experiential power mobility assessment for very young children that is based not on "readiness for driving" skills, but on the need for assistive mobility in any or all environments. She suggests that the child be allowed to explore movement in the device over a period of many sessions, by first being restricted to a single turning direction in a small, safe environment. Only after the child has experienced going, and stopping for the sake of being able to go again, has she experienced mobility, without regard for direction or purpose. This parallels the development of independent walking in toddlers. The child is never praised for "good driving" because this is meaningless to her. As the child's control over mobility expands, and the verbal labels for what she is doing are provided, the concepts described previously will develop. Power toys that are available at local toy stores make an excellent inexpensive alternative for power training of young children when the devices can be suitably adapted for seating and control.

Galka and Lombard (1992) described functional criteria for safe driving, including the ability to turn the chair on and off, follow a straight course, turn both left and right, back the chair up, maneuver around objects and persons, and stop quickly. The "marginal driver" is one of any age who may show borderline cognitive or physical skills or whose visuoperceptual problems significantly interfere with driving ability. With supervision, these children may do well driving in a very specific setting, such as their school, but are not successful in novel or unpredictable community settings. The value of a power chair in increasing self-esteem and promoting independence in specific skills must be carefully weighed against the expense and amount of training and supervision required.

Besides the client criteria, there are several practical considerations that are unique to selection of power mobility. Building accessibility and space will affect where and how the device is used. Often it is kept and maintained at school and a manual base is used at home. Care and maintenance of the power

chair are more complex, and the batteries must be recharged on a daily basis. Transportation is also a more complicated issue. Some school districts refuse to transport certain types of power wheelchairs, such as scooters. The family may need a van for transporting the chair, and a ramp or a lift may be required for loading and unloading. Funding options for more expensive power wheelchairs may be more restrictive. Usually, a backup manual chair is also required, especially during maintenance or repair of the power base. Responsibility for supervision, training, and routine wheelchair care must be assigned for all environments.

The evaluation process is also more complicated than for other types of wheelchairs. First, a variety of power bases should be available for trial and preferably with capabilities to adjust speed, acceleration, deceleration, turning speed, sensitivity, and tremor-dampening of the joystick. Children generally perform better in a pediatric-sized wheelchair rather than an adult-sized wheelchair, so options should be available. Because proper support is critical to performance in a power wheelchair, the therapist needs access to a variety of seating components, supports, and straps to provide stability to the client that will, in turn, enhance best functional movement patterns for operating the controls. A variety of controls and mounting options should also be available for trial. Evaluation should take place over a period of several days to weeks, and ideally in a variety of settings, especially for young and inexperienced drivers, who require much practice with different options before reaching a final decision.

A standard proportional control mounted on the armrest should be the first option the therapist evaluates if a child is found to have reasonable upper extremity control because this is the simplest and least expensive. If a more midline position of the joystick is desired, placement of the control bracket on the inside of the wheelchair armrest is relatively easy.

Site options for the control increase with the use of a remote joystick and the proper hardware. Some possibilities include center mounting of the joystick close to the user to compensate for decreased range of motion or strength, mounting the joystick at arm's length on top of a lap tray to provide support and increased stability when dyskinetic movements or fluctuating muscle tone is present, or mounting the joystick for chin or foot operation. For clients with limited functional movements and site options, an integrated control permits operation not only of the wheelchair but also of other equipment such as a communication aid, electronic aid to daily living, or computer equipment.

Transportation Safety

Safety in transportation of clients in wheeled mobility devices is an important issue. More and more testing is being done of various wheelchairs and restraint systems (Shaw, 1987) in both private and public transportation vehicles (Shaw, 1998). Many issues have yet to be addressed, including whether the use of standard tie-downs and belts is effective or safe with customized wheelchair users, such as one who is ventilator dependent in a power recline chair. In general, wheelchairs in vans or buses should never be in a side-facing position. There should be two sets of restraints, one for the chair and one for the occupant, and only tie-downs that meet federal safety standards should be used. Letts (1991) provides a list of restraint options for children with special needs such as premature infants, children with poor head and trunk control, children dependent on ventilators, and children in hip spica casts. Concern for transportation safety must also extend to the components of postural support systems, especially to stress tolerances of straps, buckles, D-rings, and mounting hardware (Arnold, 1988).

EXAMINATION AND EVALUATION FOR ASSISTIVE TECHNOLOGY

Assistive technologies offer children with motor or cognitive impairments an opportunity to participate more fully and become more independent in their daily lives. In addition to manual or powered mobility and specialized seating, these technologies include specialized switches, communication devices, computers, and electronic aids to daily living. Often the term *assistive technology* is used specifically to designate these latter four types of electric or electronic devices, although the Tech Act and RESNA include all forms of mobility, positioning, and related devices in the definition of assistive technology. The assessment and selection process for each of these types of assistive technology tends to be similar.

Before evaluation for use of assistive technology, a child who is nonambulatory should have a mobility device and be well positioned to minimize the effects of abnormal muscle tone, weakness, and pathologic movement patterns that interfere with controlled movement and function. The physical therapist, as a member of the assistive technology team, is responsible for completing the physical skills examination for technology use. A comprehensive physical examination includes range of motion, muscle strength, muscle tone, endurance, and gross and fine motor abilities. The therapist also examines righting and equilibrium reactions and notes the presence of primitive reflexes. These data provide the team with information concerning a child's functional motor abilities such as head and trunk control, the variety and quality of active movements, and the ability to isolate one movement from another. For successful technology use, these functional movements must be voluntary, reliable, repeatable, and in some cases sustainable. The movement patterns should not contribute to fatigue or pain, nor should they elicit pathologic reflexes or increase postural tone (Cook & Hussey, 1995; Dickey & Shealy, 1987; Stowers et al., 1987).

Given the influences of managed care, collaboration among health professionals and agencies is vital to avoid duplication of services and unnecessary expense to families and third-party payers. Recent physical therapy examinations performed in the child's primary care setting can be shared with a consulting assistive technology team from another facility in several ways. A detailed written report, a videotape or still pictures, a telemedicine videoconference, and the physical presence of the examining therapist are different ways in which findings, preferred positioning, planning, and recommendations can be shared.

The physical therapist, along with the other team members, also contributes information regarding the child's sensory, perceptuomotor, and cognitive abilities. Sensory skills needed for successful use include visual and auditory discrimination and responses to tactile, kinesthetic, and proprioceptive input. Visual acuity allows a youngster to focus sharply on an image such as a switch, joystick, or computer screen, and visual accommodation allows the eyes to adjust to near and far objects. Limitations in visual field necessitate placement of controls or displays within the functional visual range of the child. Tracking is the ability to follow a moving object with the eyes, and scanning is when the eyes move to find an object, necessary skills for successful computer use. Hearing impairments compromise a child's ability to receive auditory information, as well as to produce and monitor speech output (Cook & Hussey, 1995). When the assistive technology team members know how a child processes sensory information, they are able to select devices that are highly motivating and ensure success. Children tend to learn to use devices that provide a variety of sensory cues more quickly than devices that do not. Auditory clicks or beeps, visual light displays, and tactile and proprioceptive cues such as textured or vibrating switches can be highly motivating teaching techniques.

The team also needs prior knowledge of a child's level of cognitive functioning, as well as his or her learning style as a basis for selection of appropriate access, feedback, application, and training with the various devices. During the evaluation, the team will be able to directly observe a child's understanding of cause and effect, attention span, and short-term memory; ability to follow directions, sequence, and problem solve; and intention and motivation for technology use (Swinth, 1996).

SWITCHES, CONTROLS, AND ACCESS SITES

Children with motor impairments may require special switches or controls to operate communication aids, computers, power wheelchairs, or EADLs. Switches are also called *control interfaces* and *input devices*, and practitioners who specialize in this area are referred to as *interface specialists*. Switch technology can help teach cause and effect, encourage independent play, promote group participation, and give a child control over a part of his or her environment. A child who does not have to depend on others to interact for her or him may be less likely to develop learned helplessness or disruptive behaviors (Angelo, 1997).

Typically an access site (a body part that can produce a consistent movement) is selected first and then the switch or control to operate a device is chosen. If a child is capable of any purposeful, controlled movement of any body part, the team can identify a suitable switch. A variety of switches and controls are available from manufacturers who specialize in technologic aids for people with special needs. They vary in size, shape, cost, performance capabilities, and ways in which they are activated. Switches may be single (perform an on/off function), dual (perform on/off and a select function), or mul-

tiple (perform on/off and several functions). Examples of multiple-switch configurations are joysticks, wafer boards, slot controls, head arrays, and keyboards. Methods for activating switches include air pressure, light, magnetic fields, sound waves, and physical contact (Mann & Lane, 1995).

A child as young as 6 months is capable of using hand or head switches for computer access (Swinth et al., 1993). Using the hands to activate switches is the typical mode for most children; however, switches can be operated by other body parts such as the head, chin, tongue, eyebrows, elbows, or lower extremities. At times, children will require additional support or extension devices to use a switch or control such as a head or chin pointer, a mouth stick, finger or hand splints, styluses, mobile arm supports, or overhead slings (Fig. 24–16).

Some switches have been especially designed to use with a certain body part, such as an eyebrow switch, an eye blink switch, or a tongue touch keypad. Proximity switches will activate when a user gets near the switch, but actual physical contact is not required. A practical application of this technology is to imbed four proximity switches (one each for forward, reverse, right, and left) in an acrylic tray to operate a power wheelchair. Heavy-duty contact switches may be the most suitable choice for children with fluctuating muscle tone who have difficulty controlling the force of their movements, and tiny fiber-optic switches may be suitable for the user with very limited range and strength. At one spinal cord treatment facility, switch evaluations are performed at bedside as soon as the patient is stable. Functional movements are examined, including use of tongue, lips, eyes, eyelids, eyebrows, and jaw (Mitchell, 1995). Users with high-level spinal cord injuries often use pneumatic breath control switches

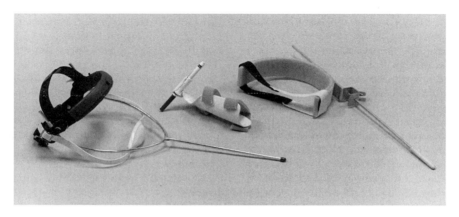

FIGURE 24–16. Devices for pointing or indicating that may be used with communication aids or electronic aids to daily living. *From left to right:* Chin pointer, thermoplastic hand splint with stylus, headstick.

to operate their assistive technology devices, and many find that integrated controls provide them with access to several types of technology.

An integrated control is one that controls several devices and may be the best choice for individuals who use a variety of assistive technology devices. For example, a power wheelchair joystick can be designed as an integrated control that will also operate a communication device, computer equipment, or environmental controls. Guidelines to determine when an integrated control is the optimal choice include the following: when a user has a single reliable access site; if the access method is the same for all devices used; when speed, accuracy, or endurance is improved; or when it is the user's or family's personal preference (Guerette & Sumi, 1994). There are also disadvantages to using integrated controls, including the higher cost of more sophisticated electronics required to perform several functions. Because the user is able to operate only one device at a time with the control, he or she will lose all functions if the controller breaks down and repairs are needed.

AUGMENTATIVE AND ALTERNATIVE COMMUNICATION

In addition to spoken or verbal output, communication includes body language, gestures, facial expressions, and written output. Speech impairments in children may occur as a result of congenital or acquired dysarthria, developmental apraxia, developmental aphasia, congenital anomalies, mental retardation, autism, or deafness (Cohen, 1985). When the ability to communicate and interact is not functional, some form of augmentative or alternative communication (AAC) should be explored. *Augmentative communication* is the use of aids or techniques to supplement a child's existing vocal or verbal communication. *Alternative communication* refers to the communication method used by a person without vocal ability (Reichle et al., 1991). In earlier years, AAC users were primarily those with adequate cognition but limited speaking ability. Users now include those with cognitive limitations, those needing written augmentation, and those with a temporary limitation in expression due to illness or injury (Guerette & Sumi, 1994).

The speech and language pathologist, along with the child and family members, assume the lead roles in identifying the best choice for an AAC system. In addition to contributing to the team evaluation, the physical therapist plays an important ongoing role in the classroom in determining optimal positions and equipment needed for communicating. Many classrooms contain a variety of chairs, corner chairs, prone or supine standers, and sidelyers, which typically require adjustment or adaptation for a particular child. The physical therapist should train the speech and language pathologist, the teacher and associates, and family members in proper use of selected positioning devices that enhance a child's communication abilities. Early intervention therapists are in a unique position to influence development of effective communication skills in infants and young children. Attermeier (1987) encourages therapists to establish treatment goals that include developing head control, developing the ability to separate head and neck movements from eye movements, allowing the child to make choices, developing a method of indication, and encouraging family members to talk to and read to their youngsters.

A number of techniques and devices for augmenting communication are available and may or may not employ electronics. Supplementation techniques are referred to as either unaided or aided communication (Mann & Lane, 1995; Stowers et al., 1987). Unaided techniques such as eye gaze, signing, or gesturing do not require external devices or equipment but rely on the user's ability to physically respond in some consistent manner. Aided techniques include the use of an external device, which may or may not be electronic. A communication sheet or notebook (with pictures, symbols, or words) is an example of a nonelectronic aided device.

Electronic communication aids offer a much greater range of capabilities and options for users, and as the capabilities of the devices increase, so do the costs. Simple devices may run less than $100; high-end devices cost several thousand dollars. One inexpensive aid is a tape recorder equipped with a loop tape message that repeats each time the switch is activated. This device may be a good starting place when assessing young children for augmentative communication because it is inexpensive and can be readily adapted with different switches mounted at various access sites. Some low-cost durable devices play a single message or series of messages, whereas others offer four, eight, or more messages. Generally, the messages can be quickly changed as desired.

At the other end of the spectrum are sophisticated, computer-driven AAC devices that allow a variety of input methods (direct, scanning, or coded), high-quality voice output, storage capability for vocabulary and phrases, printouts, and the capability to run a computer or EADL through the communication device (Fig. 24–17). Laptop computers with speech capabilities have multiple functions in addition to the ability to augment communication. Third-party payers may deny funding for laptops if they are viewed as educational equipment that should be provided by the student's local education agency. New devices are continually evolving that are

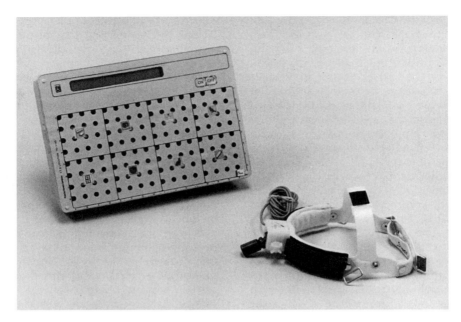

FIGURE 24–17. This electronic communication device may be directly operated with an optical headpointer. Many other selection techniques are also possible, including row and column scanning, two-switch scanning, and joystick use.

more compact, durable, lighter in weight, and easier to transport than many earlier models. More important, operation and programming of newer AAC devices have been simplified. Given the ever-expanding variety of AAC devices available, the assistive technology team should be able to identify a device that meets the motor and cognitive abilities of each child.

The input, or selection, method for AAC devices and computers includes three choices: direct, scanning, and encoding. Children with mild to moderate involvement often have sufficient motor control to use direct selection, which is preferred over scanning to operate a communication device because it is faster. The child simply makes a choice from the options presented. For example, when a child touches a location on a communication device with a picture of a glass, the spoken response might be, "May I have a drink please?"

Children with severe motor impairment may need to rely on scanning to operate their AAC or computer. The device runs through a sequence of choices (usually rows, then columns), repeating the sequence until the user makes a selection. The scanning rate is adjustable, which allows beginners ample time to become familiar with the new equipment and to build confidence and accuracy before increasing the speed. In most cases the selection is made by using a special switch positioned to allow independent access. Examples include a pressure switch mounted on a laptray and activated with the touch of the

hand, a lever switch positioned near the child's temporal region and operated with lateral head movements, and a chin switch mounted on a collar and operated by flexion and extension movements of the head. Scanning can be both motorically and cognitively demanding for some users because they must be able to wait for the appropriate selection, activate the switch at the right moment, release the switch, and repeat these steps for the next selection.

Encoding is the third access option and uses symbols (such as the dots and dashes used in Morse code) to represent words. The cognitive demands are higher with this method because the user must be able to remember the code, where messages are stored, and how to sequence stored messages. In some cases, the user must also learn how to program the device independently if a knowledgeable assistant is not available. Encoding may be used with either direct or scanning modes.

COMPUTER TECHNOLOGY

Computers are typically used for word processing to compose and edit the written word, data collection and storage, graphics for drawing and publishing, communication via E-mail and the Internet, and various educational and recreational activities. A computer is operated through a keyboard, the mouse, or both. Computers, as well as many computer-based devices such as communication

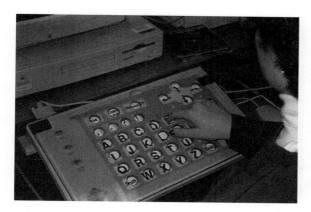

FIGURE 24–18. A keyshield or keyguard placed over a modified keyboard can eliminate unwanted keystrokes for individuals with poor fine motor control or accuracy.

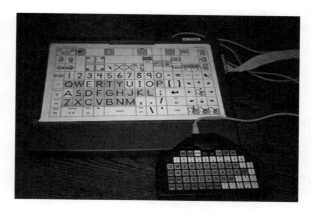

FIGURE 24–19. An expanded keyboard and a mini-keyboard are examples of alternative keyboards.

aids, environmental controls, and power wheelchair controllers, are readily adaptable and can be customized as needed. More than 500 products are commercially available to adapt a computer for an individual with special needs (Anson, 1997), an important feature for users whose needs may change due to improvement in motor or cognitive responses, or due to loss of skill if a progressive condition is present. Input to computers, as with communication devices, can be direct or indirect (scanning or Morse code), with direct access being faster and generally more intuitive.

Keyboard Adaptations and Alternatives

A keyguard attached over a keyboard is used to prevent unwanted keystrokes when fine motor control or finger isolation is impaired (Fig. 24–18). Ergonomic keyboards or wrist-arm supports may be beneficial to a child requiring distal support or if tremor, pain, fatigue, or lack of endurance interferes with typing. Mobile arm supports and overhead slings also benefit users with muscle weakness. Software is available to decrease additional keystrokes, minimize repetition of the same key, and allow activation of more than one key at a time.

Alternatives to the standard keyboard include mini-keyboards, expanded keyboards, chord keyboards, and one-handed keyboards (Fig. 24–19). Mini-keyboards are beneficial to children such as those with muscular dystrophy who have accurate fine motor abilities but limited range of motion, decreased strength, or low endurance. Expanded or enlarged keyboards are helpful for children with poor coordination and difficulty isolating a finger. These keyboards have up to 128 pressure-sensitive

areas referred to as keys, and because the number, size, shape, and location of these keys can be redefined, the possibilities for customization are numerous. For example, this type of keyboard could be set up to offer four choices with large contact areas, rather than 128 choices. A chord keyboard consists of an array of keys (typically 5 to 10 depending on the model) that is operated by pressing a predetermined combination of keys to type a character. Court reporters use this type of technology. Chord keyboards are available in one-handed and two-handed models. Standard keyboards, mini-keyboards, and enlarged keyboards may be set up in the typical *qwerty* pattern, in an *alphabetic* layout, or in a *frequency of use* layout. Dvorak keyboard patterns place frequently used keys near the home row and are available in one-handed or two-handed models (Anson, 1997; Cook & Hussey, 1995).

Touch screens may be attached to the computer monitor or used on a table top or wheelchair laptray. A touch screen is one example of a *concept keyboard,* which replaces the letters and numbers of a typical keyboard with pictures or symbols of the subject matter being taught. Because touch screens use direct selection, they tend to be less cognitively demanding, which may be important to children being introduced to computer technology (Cook & Hussey, 1995).

Children with visual impairments require technology specifically developed to meet their needs, such as software or hardware adaptations to enhance auditory feedback, tactile keyboards, screen readers that translate text to the spoken word, screen magnifiers, or software that will enlarge the text on the screen up to 16 times.

Mouse Alternatives

Mouse functions include moving the cursor to a specific location on the screen, dragging a selected item to a different location on the screen, and clicking or double clicking to select items and functions (Anson, 1997). Modifications to the cursor such as enlarging it, changing its color, slowing it down, or giving it tails may make it easier for a child to locate the cursor on the computer screen. Keyboard functions using the arrow keys or the numeric keypad may assist a child who is unable to use a mouse effectively. Alternative mouse options are available, both on the general market and through manufacturers of special equipment, and include joysticks, trackballs, mousepads, keypad mice, and head-controlled mice (Fig. 24–20). Practitioners are encouraged to become familiar with commercially available mice, as well as those developed for users with special needs, because they are often less expensive.

Virtual or on-screen keyboards display an image of a keyboard on the monitor, and the user moves the cursor to the desired key with a mouse, joystick, trackball, head-controlled mouse, or switch array. A selection is then made using a second switch or by dwelling on the key for a predetermined amount of time. On-screen keyboards with scanning programs are commonly used by children who rely on a single or dual switch to access assistive technology devices. Keyboard and mouse functions can also be achieved using light beams, infrared, ultrasonic, and speech recognition technology.

Rate Enhancement

Practitioners are encouraged not only to become familiar with different access and input methods, but to personally try them, because each access and input method requires different motor responses and cognitive processes. Consider that a trained typist without a disability is capable of transcribing text at an average of 100 words per minute. The same person typing, while composing text, averages 50 words per minute. Court reporters, using special chord keyboards, enter text at 150 words per minute. Contrast that with an average of 10 to 12 words per minute for a person typing with just one finger. The person using scanning usually averages 3 to 5 words per minute (Cook & Hussey, 1995). Overall speed of production, although not an issue for all users, can become an issue for students in regular education who are expected to produce a similar amount of written output as nondisabled peers. Productivity also becomes an issue during transition planning if prospective employment opportunities require a certain degree of proficiency in computer use.

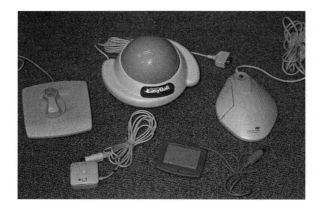

FIGURE 24–20. Examples of mouse alternatives.

When use of a computer or communication device is effortful and time consuming, use of macros, abbreviation expansion, or word prediction to enhance productivity should be investigated. Macro programs allow users to combine and automate tasks. Abbreviation expansion automatically types out an entire word or phrase when two or three letters have been typed. For example, a user can command the computer to type out "Physical Therapy" each time the user inputs the letters "PT." With word prediction software, the computer tries to predict what word is being typed after only two or three characters are entered. A numbered list of likely choices appears on the screen and the correct number is selected.

ELECTRONIC AIDS TO DAILY LIVING

An electronic aid to daily living (EADL), previously known as an environmental control unit (ECU), is a device or system of devices that allows the operation of electrical appliances or equipment in a variety of ways and places. Each of us encounters this technology on a daily basis in the form of energy- and time-saving devices such as electronic garage door openers, portable telephones, and remote controls for television and audio equipment. Many of these affordable, commercially available products require precise fine motor control, which precludes their use for those with motor dysfunction; however, a range of environmental control devices is available from manufacturers of equipment for children and adults with special needs. The purpose of an EADL is to apply technology to facilitate the user's control over the environment, to promote independent access to items required for daily living, and to improve the quality of life (MacNeil, 1998).

Control of the environment for a preschooler might include operating a blender with a head-

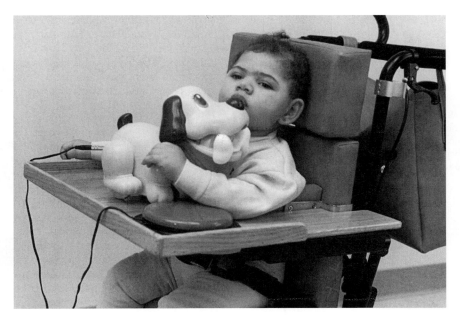

FIGURE 24-21. A large pressure switch can be used to activate a battery-operated toy placed on a laptray.

activated switch to prepare treats at school or activating a pressure switch with the hand to operate a battery toy during free time (Fig. 24-21). An older child may use a headstick to operate the television's remote control to select a channel, control the volume, and turn off the set when done. Adapted phone equipment that can be programmed to store several numbers, automatically dial a number, and answer calls with the touch of a switch can allow a teenager access to important, age-appropriate socialization. These independent, functional activities help instill a sense of responsibility and independence from caregivers.

Benefits of EADLs for adults include increased personal satisfaction, increased participation in life activities, possible return to work, and possible reduction in cost for personal care attendants (Dickey & Shealy, 1987). The use of EADLs in one residential facility to operate televisions, radios, lights, tape recorders, and stereos reduced the amount of nursing care required by about 2 hours per day per participant (Symington et al., 1986). Both residents and nursing staff reported reduced frustration following introduction of EADLs. Persons with spinal cord injuries who used EADLs participated more often in telephone use, were more inclined to travel, and spent more time in educational pursuits than nonusers (Efthimiou et al., 1981). Radio use by elderly nursing home residents with mobility and fine motor impairments increased threefold compared with a control group once the participants were equipped

with and trained in the use of remote devices to turn radios on and off (Mann, 1992).

An EADL generally includes three parts: the main control unit (central processing unit), the switch (transducer), and any devices (peripherals) to be controlled or activated. Most EADLs emit some type of tactile, visual, or auditory feedback that immediately indicates which function has been selected before the function is activated. Feedback can be an essential feature to the user with memory impairments and is helpful in initial assessment and training sessions with systems capable of multiple functions.

There are two basic types of EADLs: direct and remote. In a direct system, the devices to be controlled are plugged directly into the main control unit. In a remote system, the control unit acts as a transmitter, sending radio waves, ultrasonic signals, or infrared light beams to remote receivers, which, in turn, are connected to the devices to be activated. The remote system has the advantages of operating a number of devices or appliances from one location such as a wheelchair or bed and the absence of wires running from the unit to the device (Cook & Hussey, 1995).

Capabilities of systems vary from simply turning one device on and off to operating whole-house configurations and integrated computer workstations. Common functions include operation of a small electrical appliance, stereo, television, videocassette recorder, light fixture, door lock, intercom or call signal, electric bed, and telephone and computer

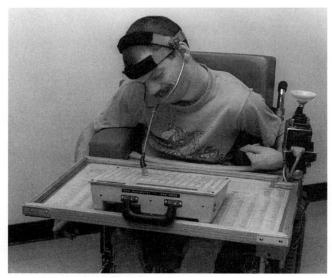

FIGURE 24–22. Scott, sitting in his custom-molded seating system, mounted in his power wheelchair with swing-away chin control joystick. He is using his custom headstick to activate a Light Talker. His communication sheet, sealed in the frame on his laptray, is also visible.

equipment. EADLs can be activated through the wide variety of switches and controls described previously, through voice activation, or through the user's power wheelchair controller, electronic communication aid, or computer. Lange has produced a chart to assist practitioners in comparing the various features of popular EADLs on the market (MacNeil, 1998). The chart includes input options; what type of equipment can be controlled; what devices the EADL will interface with, such as a computer or communication aid; whether battery backup is included; cost; and comments.

CASE HISTORY
SCOTT

Scott was born in 1963 with spastic athetoid CP (Fig. 24–22). Scott is dependent on others for all personal care, including feeding, dressing, grooming, hygiene, toileting, transfers, and mobility, unless he is in his power wheelchair. Functional arm and hand usage is limited, with purposeful movement dominated by reflexive patterns and fluctuating tone. His speech is dysarthric, but his ability to communicate is excellent. Scott agreed to be featured in this chapter to provide a consumer's viewpoint of assistive technology. His words and thoughts (in italics) reflect many of the points made in this chapter regarding the need for team consultation, communication, respect for the

client's opinion, customization of equipment and devices, and the revisions to equipment required over a lifetime.

Before passage of Public Law 94-142 in 1975, few local school districts were able or inclined to provide educational services for children with severe physical disabilities. Scott's early education (from preschool in 1967 to junior high in 1975) was at a residential program at the University of Iowa. After he returned to his home school district, he continued to receive assistive technology services at the same facility, which was converted to a regional evaluation and consultation center.

In addition to classes, his early years were filled with individual therapy sessions, including speech, occupational, and physical therapy. A variety of assistive devices (called adaptive equipment at the time) were used over the years in Scott's therapeutic management, including Pope night splints; short leg braces; long leg braces with pelvic band; stand-up boxes; bilateral upper arm restraints; pelvic restraints; chest restraints; wooden armchairs; footboards with footstraps; cutout tables; various bowls, spoons, cups, and straws for feeding; communication boards; headsticks; electric typewriters with keyshield; and last, but not least, wheelchairs.

"Manual wheelchairs . . . at first these required little or no adapting. As I got older, we tried one fancy chair I remember well. The back was in sections and could adjust to different positions. I remember about five people in the P.T. room working all day to adapt it to fit me." Wheelchairs were generally not adapted in the 1960s, and children relied on seat belts and pelvic or chest restraints; in some

cases, their long leg braces locked in flexion at the hips and knees kept them safely in their chairs.

Records indicate that Scott was evaluated for his first seating system in 1973 and was provided with *"a wedged seat with 15° angle, a wedge between thighs, and a high back."* His long leg braces were discontinued because the seating inserts were believed to provide adequate postural support for sitting. Over the next 20 years, Scott's seating systems changed from simple linear wood and foam inserts, to wood and foam with contouring, to orthotic molded inserts, to his currently used, custom-molded Contour-U (PinDot Products, Chicago, IL) seat and back cushions. Changes in his seating requirements closely paralleled changes in his musculoskeletal status over the years, which included slowly progressing kyphoscoliosis, hip flexion and adduction contractures, and knee flexion contractures.

Scott began using a headstick between 3 and 4 years of age for pointing and to manipulate objects in his environment. He soon developed proficiency with his head stick and eventually switched to a custom-made chin pointer style that he has had for over 15 years. *"I'm careful picking equipment out. I want the least amount of equipment on me as possible. This is so no more extra attention, looks, or glares come my way. However, I wear my headstick because it's my life. People see it before they see my face. But I think of it as a part of me. Once people get to know me, the headstick becomes less noticeable and everyone's happy."*

While Scott was learning headstick skills, he was introduced to picture and word boards for communication. The combination of headstick skill plus his ability to spell and write to communicate progressed over the years, as did his selection and use of technology. *"Language boards/Touch Talkers . . . This has been a very 'lucky' area for me. I've had a word board ever since age 3. As I grew, so did my boards. My first try at a voice [electronic device with voice output] was a bomb! Other people were telling ME what I wanted! Finally, I took a stand and said 'No' to that device, and most people took that as my not wanting a 'voice.' That wasn't so, it was just too much work with a poor voice. I was saying, 'Let's wait.' My word board did fine back then. But as my life got busier, I had a greater need to communicate. I knew that was when I needed a voice output. The 1989 Touch Talker had a pretty good voice to it and so I fell in love with it. Now, with the Liberator [a highly sophisticated AAC device from Prentke Romich Co., Shreve, OH, with voice or print output, ability to operate computers and EADLs, and ability to perform math and calculator functions], I'm in heaven."*

"Power wheelchairs . . . I still remember my first electric chair. I had a big say in the driving method. Everyone was thinking 'headstick,' and I said, 'No, try my chin!' I was shocked at how well I could drive power chairs once the right method was found. Now better controls are coming out so who

knows what will be next." Scott received his first power wheelchair in 1981 and his second chair in 1988. *"My power wheelchair. It is my legs, my little home. I have everything in my backpack, it holds as much as a small house."* After fabrication and assembly of seating components, a custom swing-away mounting arm to hold the chin control was designed and fabricated by a rehabilitation engineer who worked closely with Scott to meet his needs. With this custom device, Scott is able to move the chin control into position for driving or swing it out of the way with his arm to access his communication equipment independently. Most important, the mounting hardware is sturdy, is durable, and does not slip out of alignment. The capability to customize cannot be overemphasized when providing technology for individuals with severe physical disabilities. One-of-a-kind designs and devices often provide the best solutions to technology puzzles. *"My chin control arm. It has no wires or batteries, it works off my power. Being homemade, it's made to last. My headstick is another good example."*

In the early years, much of Scott's therapeutic management and adaptive equipment reflected an attempt to intervene at the impairment level, such as by preventing contractures and increasing weight bearing with braces and standing boxes. Functional limitations were also addressed by providing alternatives to speech and walking, such as headsticks, communication boards, and wheelchairs. As Scott became older, it was evident that many of his impairments (scoliosis and contractures) needed to be accommodated, rather than corrected, to maximize function.

Now, as a young adult, Scott's priorities lie with minimizing his disabilities and increasing acceptance of his role in society. In 1995, he found a data entry position two mornings a week at a local law firm. About this time he also experienced weight loss secondary to lifelong oral-pharyngeal dysfunction with dysphagia. He subsequently developed a pressure sore over his right ischial tuberosity. A custom Silhouette seat was molded for Scott, which decreased sitting pressures, provided comfort, and promoted quick healing of the sore. He was then able to gradually increase his working hours to about 6 hours a day. Scott must carefully monitor how much income he earns to avoid reduction of his Medicaid entitlement. He continues to live in a group home with four other young men with physical disabilities and manages his personal life and affairs with the assistance of care attendants.

Technology has made a definite impact on Scott's life over the years. *"In general, special devices have changed my life in a good way. I'm doing more and more for myself. However, rapid changes in equipment design makes knowing what to buy very hard."* Future plans include working toward getting his own apartment with one or two hired personal care attendants and perhaps taking classes at the university or community college.

Resources

PROFESSIONAL ORGANIZATIONS AND CONFERENCES

Communication Aids Manufacturers (CAMA)
612 Davis Street, Suite 211
Evanston, IL 60202-4644
Phone: 800-441-2262
Distributes free packet of materials and list of member manufacturers; holds workshops that feature AAC devices.

Closing The Gap (CTG)
P.O. Box 68
Henderson, MN 56044
Phone: 612-248-3294; Internet: www.closingthegap.com
Publishes a bimonthly newspaper; holds annual conference, thought by many to be the premier computer access conference in the country.

Rehabilitation Engineering and Assistive Technology Society of North America (RESNA)
1700 Moore Street, Suite 150
Arlington, VA 22209-1903
Phone: 703-524-6686; Internet: www.resna.org

Foundation for Technology Access
2173 E. Francisco Boulevard, Suite L
San Rafael, CA 94901
Provides a list of Alliance for Technology Access centers in the United States and distributes a newsletter.

International Society for Augmentative and Alternative Communication (ISAAC)
P.O. Box 1762, Suite R
Toronto, Ontario, Canada M40 4A3
Phone: 416-737-9308
Information on AAC; publishes a journal and newsletters; holds an annual conference.

Rehab Report
P.O. Box 8987
Malibu, CA 90265-8987
Phone: 800-543-4116; Internet: www.teamrehab.com
A monthly publication on rehabilitation technology and services; covers up-to-date legislative, product, and practice issues.

Trace Research and Development Center
Room S-151, Waisman Center
1500 Highland Ave.
University of Wisconsin
Madison, WI 53707
Phone: 608-262-6966
Information on communication and microcomputer technology.

References

Agre, JC, Findley, TW, McNally, MC, Habeck, R, Leon, AS, Stradel, L, Birkebak, R, & Schmalz, R. Physical activity capacity in children with myelomeningocele. Archives of Physical Medicine and Rehabilitation, 68:372–377, 1987.

Angelo, J. Assistive Technology for Rehabilitation Therapists. Philadelphia: FA Davis, 1997.

Anson, DK. Alternative Computer Access: A Guide to Selection. Philadelphia: FA Davis, 1997.

Arnold, RL. Safe transportation for persons with disabilities. Assistive Devices Information Network Newsletter (University of Iowa, Iowa City, IA), 2(1):1–2, 1988.

Attermeier, SM. Augmentative communication: An interdisciplinary challenge. Physical and Occupational Therapy in Pediatrics, 7(2): 3–11, 1987.

Bablich, K, Sochaniwskyj, A, & Koheil, R. Positional and electromyographic investigation of sitting posture of children with cerebral palsy (Abstract). Developmental Medicine and Child Neurology, 28(suppl 53):25, 1986.

Barnes, KH. Training young children for powered mobility. Developmental Disabilities Special Interest Section Newsletter (American Occupational Therapy Association, Rockville, MD), 14(2):1–2, 1991.

Bay, JL. Positioning for head control to access an augmentative communication machine. American Journal of Occupational Therapy, 45:544–549, 1991.

Bednarczyk, JH, & Sanderson, DJ. Kinematics of wheelchair propulsion in adults and children with spinal cord injury. Archives of Physical Medicine and Rehabilitation, 75:1327–1334, 1994.

Bergen, AF. Seating and positioning principles for the neurologically involved client. Presented at the American Physical Therapy Association Combined Sections Meeting, San Francisco, February 1992.

Bergen, AF, Presperin, J, & Tallman, T. Positioning for Function: Wheelchairs and Other Assistive Technologies. Valhalla, NY: Valhalla Rehabilitation Publications, 1990.

Brubaker, CE. Wheelchair prescription: An analysis of factors that affect mobility and performance. Journal of Rehabilitation Research and Development, 23(4):19–26, 1986.

Brubaker, CE. Manual mobility. Presented at the Fourth International Seating Symposium, Vancouver, BC, February 1988.

Bryant, L. Wheelchair standards ready to roll. TeamRehab Report, May-June 1991, pp. 44–45.

Butler, C. Effects of powered mobility on self-initiated behaviors of very young children with locomotor disability. Developmental Medicine and Child Neurology, 28:325–332, 1986.

Butler, C, Okamoto, GA, & McKay, TM. Powered mobility for very young disabled children. Developmental Medicine and Child Neurology, 25:472–474, 1983.

Campbell, J, & Ball, J. Energetics of walking in cerebral palsy. Orthopedic Clinics of North America, 9:374–377, 1978.

Carlson, JM, & Payette, M. Seating and spine support for boys with Duchenne muscular dystrophy. In Proceedings of the 8th Annual Conference on Rehabilitation Technology. Washington, DC: RESNA Press, 1985, pp. 36–38.

Carlson, SJ. The semi-rigid pelvic stabilizer for seating control. Assistive Devices Information Network Newsletter (University of Iowa, Iowa City, IA), 1(1):2–3, 1987.

Carlson, SJ. Knee gate for control of forward sliding in wheelchair. Assistive Devices Information Network Newsletter (University of Iowa, Iowa City, IA), 2(3):2–3, 1988.

Carlson, SJ, & Grey, TL. The semi-rigid pelvic stabilizer for seating control. Presented at the Fourth International Seating Symposium, Vancouver, BC, February 1988.

Cohen, C. Augmentative communication: A perspective for pediatricians. Pediatric Annals, 14:3, 1985.

Cook, A, & Hussey, SM. Assistive Technologies: Principles and Practice. St. Louis: Mosby, 1995.

Crenshaw, RP, & Vistnes, LM. A decade of pressure sore research: 1977–1987. Journal of Rehabilitation Research and Development, 26:63–74, 1989.

Deitz, J, Jaffe, KM, Wolf, LS, Massagli, TL, & Anson, D. Pediatric power wheelchairs: Evaluation of function in the home and school environments. Assistive Technology, 3:24–31, 1991.

DeSouza, LJ, & Carroll, N. Ambulation of the braced myelomeningocele patient. Journal of Bone and Joint Surgery (American), 58:1112–1118, 1976.

Dickey, R, & Shealy, SH. Using technology to control the environment. American Journal of Occupational Therapy, 41: 717–721, 1987.

Drummond, DS, Narechania, RG, Rosenthal, AN, Breed, AL, Lange, TA, & Drummond, DK. A study of pressure distributions measured during balanced and unbalanced sitting. Journal of Bone and Joint Surgery (American), 64:1034–1039, 1982.

Efthimiou, MA, Gordon, WA, Sell, GH, & Stratford, C. Electronic assistive devices: Their impact on the quality of life of high-level quadriplegic persons. Archives of Physical Medicine and Rehabilitation, 62:131–134, 1981.

Evans, MA, & Nelson, WB. A dynamic solution to seating clients with fluctuating tone. In Proceedings of the 19th Annual Conference on Rehabilitation Technology. Arlington, VA: RESNA Press, 1996, pp. 189–190.

Fife, S, Roxborough, L, Cooper, D, & Steinke, T. Tonic electromyographic activity in seated subjects with spastic quadriplegia: A pilot study. Presented at the Fourth International Seating Symposium, Vancouver, BC, February 1988.

Fisher, SV, & Gullickson, G. Energy cost of ambulation in health and disability: A literature review. Archives of Physical Medicine and Rehabilitation, 59:124–133, 1978.

Franks, CA, Palisano, RJ, & Darbee, JC. The effect of walking with an assistive device and using a wheelchair on school performance in students with myelomeningocele. Physical Therapy, 71:570–579, 1991.

Galka, G, & Lombard, T. So . . . You're Considering Power Mobility. Iowa City, IA: Occupational Therapy Department, Division of Developmental Disabilities, University Hospital School, University of Iowa, 1992.

Garber, SL, & Dyerly, LR. Wheelchair cushions for persons with spinal cord injury: An update. American Journal of Occupational Therapy, 45:550–554, 1991.

Gilsdorf, P, Patterson, R, Fisher, S, & Appel, N. Sitting forces and wheelchair mechanics. Journal of Rehabilitation Research and Development, 27:239–246, 1990.

Guerette, P, & Sumi, E. Integrating control of multiple assistive devices: A retrospective review. Assistive Technology, 6(1):67–76, 1994.

Hays, RM. Childhood motor impairments: Clinical overview and scope of the problem. Presented at the Fourth International Seating Symposium, Vancouver, BC, February 1988.

Hedman, G. Overview of rehabilitation technology. Physical and Occupational Therapy in Pediatrics, 10(2):1–10, 1990.

Hughes, CJ, Weimar, WH, Sheth, PN, & Brubaker, CE. Biomechanics of wheelchair propulsion as a function of seat position and user-to-chair interface. Archives of Physical Medicine and Rehabilitation, 73:263–269, 1992.

Hulme, JB, Bain, B, & Hardin, MA. The influence of adaptive seating devices on vocalization (Abstract). Developmental Medicine and Child Neurology, 30(suppl 57):35, 1988.

Hulme, JB, Poor, R, Schulein, M, & Pezzino, J. Perceived behavioral changes observed with adaptive seating devices and training programs for multihandicapped, developmentally disabled individuals. Physical Therapy, 63:204–208, 1983.

Hulme, JB, Shaver, J, Acher, S, Mullette, L, & Eggert, C. Effects of adaptive seating devices on the eating and drinking of children with multiple handicaps. American Journal of Occupational Therapy, 41:81–89, 1987.

Jones, CK. A sampler of available powered mobility bases: Hard facts and a little opinion. Presented at the Fourth International Seating Symposium, Vancouver, BC, February 1988.

Jones, CK. In search of power for the pediatric client. Physical and Occupational Therapy in Pediatrics, 10(2):47–68, 1990.

Kangas, KM. Seating, positioning, and physical access. Developmental Disabilities Special Interest Section Newsletter (American Occupational Therapy Association, Rockville, MD), 14(2):4, 1991.

Kangas, KM. Clinical assessment and training strategies for the child's mastery of independent powered mobility. In Furumasu, J (Ed.), Pediatric Powered Mobility: Developmental Perspectives, Technical Issues, Clinical Approaches. Arlington, VA: RESNA Press, 1997.

Kermoian, R. Locomotion experience and psychological development in infancy. In Furumasu, J (Ed.), Pediatric Powered Mobility: Developmental Perspectives, Technical Issues, Clinical Approaches. Arlington, VA: RESNA Press, 1997.

Koo, TK, Mak, AF, & Lee, YL. Posture effect on seating interface biomechanics: Comparison between two seating cushions. Archives of Physical Medicine and Rehabilitation, 77:40–47, 1996.

Larnert, G, & Ekberg, O. Positioning improves the oral and pharyngeal swallowing function in children with cerebral palsy. Acta Paediatrica, 84:689–692, 1995.

Lepage, C, Noreau, L, & Bernard, PM. Association between characteristics of locomotion and accomplishment of life habits in children with cerebral palsy. Physical Therapy, 78:458–469, 1998.

Letts, RM (Ed.). Principles of Seating the Disabled. Boca Raton, FL: CRC Press, 1991.

MacNeil, V. Electronic aids to daily living: A change for the better. TeamRehab Report, 9(11):53–56, 1998.

Mann, WC. Use of environmental control devices by elderly nursing home patients. Assistive Technology, 4(2):60–65, 1992.

Mann, WC, & Lane, JP. Assistive Technology for Persons with Disabilities, 2nd ed. Bethesda, MD: American Occupational Therapy Association, 1995.

Margolis, S. Lumbar support issues. Presented at the Eighth International Seating Symposium, Vancouver, BC, February 1992.

Margolis, SA, Wengert, ME, & Kolar, KA. The subASIS bar: No component is an island: A five-year retrospective. Presented at the Fourth International Seating Symposium, Vancouver, BC, February 1988.

McClenaghan, BA, Thombs, L, & Milner, M. Effects of seat-surface inclination on postural stability and function of the upper extremities of children with cerebral palsy. Developmental Medicine and Child Neurology, 34:40–48, 1992.

McCormack, DJ. The effects of keyguard use and pelvic positioning on typing speed and accuracy in a boy with cerebral palsy. American Journal of Occupational Therapy, 44:312–315, 1990.

McEwen, IR. Assistive positioning as a control parameter of social-communicative interactions between students with profound multiple disabilities and classroom staff. Physical Therapy, 72:634–647, 1992.

Medhat, MA, & Hobson, DA. Standardization of Terminology and Descriptive Methods for Specialized Seating: A Reference Manual. Arlington, VA: RESNA Press, 1992.

Miedaner, JA. The effects of sitting positions on trunk extension for children with motor impairment. Pediatric Physical Therapy, 2:11–14, 1990.

Mitchell, CL. Switch access, environmental control and computer access: The evaluation process. Technology Special Interest Section Newsletter (American Occupational Therapy Association, Bethesda, MD), 5(1):3–4, 1995.

Myhr, U, & von Wendt, L. Improvement of functional sitting position for children with cerebral palsy. Developmental Medicine and Child Neurology, 33:246–256, 1991.

Myhr, U, & von Wendt, L. Influence of different sitting positions and abduction orthoses on leg muscle activity in children with cerebral palsy. Developmental Medicine and Child Neurology, 35:870–880, 1993.

Noble-Jamieson, CM, Heckmatt, JZ, Dubowitz, V, & Silverman, M. Effects of posture and spinal bracing on respiratory function in neuromuscular disease. Archives of Disease in Childhood, 61:178–181, 1986.

Noon, JH, Chesney, DA, & Axelson, PW. Development of a dynamic pelvic stabilization system. In Proceedings of the 21st Annual Conference on Rehabilitation Engineering. Arlington, VA: RESNA Press, 1998, pp. 209–211.

Nwaobi, OM. Effects of body orientation in space on tonic muscle activity of patients with cerebral palsy. Developmental Medicine and Child Neurology, 28:41–44, 1986.

Nwaobi, OM. Seating orientations and upper extremity function in children with cerebral palsy. Physical Therapy, 67:1209–1212, 1987.

Nwaobi, OM, Brubaker, CE, Cusick, B, & Sussman, MD. Electromyographic investigation of extensor activity in cerebral-palsied children in different seating positions. Developmental Medicine and Child Neurology, 25:175–183, 1983.

Nwaobi, OM, & Cusick, B. The effect of hip flexion angle on the electrical activity of the hip adductors in cerebral palsied children. Unpublished report, 1980.

Nwaobi, OM, Hobson, DA, & Trefler, E. Hip angle and upper-extremity movement time of children with cerebral palsy (Abstract). Developmental Medicine and Child Neurology, 28(suppl 53):24, 1986.

Nwaobi, OM, & Smith, PD. Effect of adaptive seating on pulmonary function of children with cerebral palsy. Developmental Medicine and Child Neurology, 28:351–354, 1986.

Orpwood, R. A compliant seating system for a child with extensor spasms. In Proceedings of the 19th Annual Conference of Rehabilitation Engineering. Arlington, VA: RESNA Press, 1996, pp. 261–262.

Palmieri, VR, Haelen, GT, & Cochran, GV. Comparison of sitting pressures on wheelchair cushions as measured by air cell transducers and miniature electronic transducers. Bulletin of Prosthetic Research, 17(1):5–8, 1980.

Pate, G. Patterns of pressure during normal sitting. Presented at the Fourth International Seating Symposium, Vancouver, BC, February 1988.

Paulsson, K, & Christoffersen, M. Psychological aspects of technical aids: How does independent mobility affect the psychosocial and intellectual development of children with physical disabilities? In Proceedings of the 2nd International Conference on Rehabilitation Engineering. Washington, DC: RESNA Press, 1984.

Phillips, B, & Zhao, H. Predictors of assistive technology abandonment. Assistive Technology, 5:36–45, 1993.

Pope, PM, Bowes, CE, & Booth, E. Postural control in sitting the SAM system: Evaluation of use over three years. Developmental Medicine and Child Neurology, 36:241–252, 1994.

Reger, SI, Chung, KC, & Paling, M. Weightbearing tissue contour and deformation by magnetic resonance imaging. In Proceedings of the 9th Annual Conference on Rehabilitation Technology. Washington, DC: RESNA Press, 1986, pp. 387–389.

Reichle, J, York, J, & Sigafoos, J. Implementing Augmentative and Alternative Communication: Strategies for Learners with Severe Disabilities. Baltimore: Paul H. Brookes, 1991.

Reid, DT. Development and preliminary validation of an instrument to assess quality of sitting of children with neuromotor dysfunction. Physical and Occupational Therapy in Pediatrics, 15(1):53–81, 1995.

Reid, DT. The effects of the saddle seat on seated postural control and upper extremity movement in children with cerebral palsy. Developmental Medicine and Child Neurology, 38:805–815, 1996.

Reid, DT. Sitting Assessment for Children with Neuromotor Dysfunction: A Standardized Protocol for Describing Postural Control. San Antonio, TX: Therapy Skill Builders, 1997.

Reid, DT, & Sochaniwskyj, A. Effects of anterior-tipped seating on respiratory function of normal children and children with cerebral palsy. International Journal of Rehabilitation Research, 14:203–212, 1991.

Reid, DT, Sochaniwskyj, A, & Milner, M. An investigation of postural sway in sitting of normal children and children with neurological disorders. Physical and Occupational Therapy in Pediatrics, 11(1):19–35, 1991.

Schiaffino, S, & Laux, J. Prerequisite skills for the psychosocial impact of powered wheelchair mobility on young children with severe handicaps. Developmental Disabilities Special Interest Section Newsletter (American Occupational Therapy Association, Rockville, MD), 9(2):1, 3, 8, 1986.

Seeger, BR, Caudrey, DJ, & O'Mara, NA. Hand function in cerebral palsy: The effect of hip-flexion angle. Developmental Medicine and Child Neurology, 26:601–606, 1984a.

Seeger, BR, Sutherland, AD, & Clark, MS. Orthotic management of scoliosis in Duchenne muscular dystrophy. Archives of Physical Medicine and Rehabilitation, 65:83–86, 1984b.

Seymour, RJ, & Lacefield, WE. Wheelchair cushion effect on pressure and skin temperature. Archives of Physical Medicine and Rehabilitation, 66:103–108, 1985.

Shaw, G. Vehicular transport safety for the child with disabilities. American Journal of Occupational Therapy, 41:35–42, 1987.

Shaw, G. Travel hazards. TeamRehab Report, 9(10): 23–24, 1998.

Shields, RK, & Cook, TM. Effect of seat angle and lumbar support on seated buttock pressure. Physical Therapy, 68:1682–1686, 1988.

Siekman, AR, & Flanagan, K. The anti-thrust seat: A wheelchair insert for individuals with abnormal reflex patterns or other specialized problems. In Proceedings of the 8th Annual Conference on Rehabilitation Engineering. Washington, DC: RESNA Press, 1983, pp. 203–205.

Sprigle, S, Chung, KC, & Brubaker, CE. Factors affecting seat contour characteristics. Journal of Rehabilitation Research and Development, 27:127–134, 1990a.

Sprigle, S, Chung, KC, & Brubaker, CE. Reduction of sitting pressures with custom contoured cushions. Journal of Rehabilitation Research and Development, 27:135–140, 1990b.

Stewart, SFC, Palmieri, V, & Cochran, GVB. Wheelchair cushion effect on skin temperature, heat flux, and relative humidity. Archives of Physical Medicine and Rehabilitation, 61:229–233, 1980.

Stowers, S, Altheide, MR, & Shea, V. Motor assessment for unaided and aided augmentative communication. Physical and Occupational Therapy in Pediatrics, 7(2):61–77, 1987.

Swinth, Y. Evaluating toddlers for assistive technology. Occupational Therapy Practice, 1(3):32–41, 1996.

Swinth, Y, Anson, D, & Dietz, J. Single switch computer access for infants and toddlers. American Journal of Occupational Therapy, 47:1031–1038, 1993.

Symington, DC, Lywood, DW, Lawson, JS, & Maclean, J. Environmental control systems in chronic care hospitals and nursing homes. Archives of Physical Medicine and Rehabilitation, 67:322–325, 1986.

Thacker, JG, Sprigle, SH, & Morris, BO. Understanding the Technology When Selecting Wheelchairs. Arlington, VA: RESNA Press, 1994.

Tredwell, S, & Roxborough, L. Cerebral palsy seating. In Letts, RM (Ed.), Principles of Seating the Disabled. Boca Raton, FL: CRC Press, 1991.

Trefler, E (Ed.). Seating for Children with Cerebral Palsy. Memphis: University of Tennessee, 1984.

Trefler, E, Hobson, DA, Taylor, SJ, Monahan, LC, & Shaw, CG. Seating and Mobility for Persons with Physical Disabilities. Tucson, AZ: Therapy Skill Builders, 1993.

van der Woude, LHV, Veeger, DJ, Rozendal, RH, & Sargeant, TJ. Seat height in handrim wheelchair propulsion. Journal of Rehabilitation Research and Development, 26:31–50, 1989.

Verburg, G, Snell, E, Pilkington, M, & Milner, M. Effects of powered mobility on young handicapped children and their families. In Proceedings of the 2nd International Conference on Rehabilitation Engineering. Washington, DC: RESNA Press, 1984.

Williams, LO, Anderson, AD, Campbell, J, Thomas, L, Feiwell, E, & Walker, JM. Energy cost of walking and of wheelchair propulsion by children with myelodysplasia: Comparison with normal children. Developmental Medicine and Child Neurology, 25:617–624, 1983.

Wright-Ott, C. The transitional powered mobility aid: A new concept and tool for early mobility. In Furumasu, J (Ed.), Pediatric Powered Mobility: Developmental Perspectives, Technical Issues, Clinical Approaches. Arlington, VA: RESNA Press, 1997.

SECTION
IV

MANAGEMENT OF CARDIOPULMONARY CONDITIONS

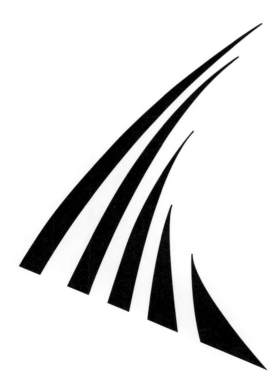

SUZANN K. CAMPBELL, PT, PhD, FAPTA

Section Editor

CHAPTER
25

Children with Ventilator Dependence

M. KATHLEEN KELLY, MS, PT

Case History submitted by HELENE DUMAS, MS, PT, PCS

OVERVIEW AND INCIDENCE

The U.S. Government Office of Technology Assessment (OTA) (1987) defines the technology-dependent child as "one who needs both a medical device to compensate for the loss of a vital body function, and substantial and ongoing nursing care to avert death or further disability." This technology may range from apnea monitors and intravenous medications to dialysis and mechanical ventilators. Because of recent advances in medical care and in the use of aggressive respiratory management for critically ill infants and children, the number of children who are dependent on mechanical ventilation is estimated to be between 680 and 2000 per year (Criner et al., 1994; OTA, 1987). Significant improvements in the technical aspects of ventilation have also reduced the incidence of barotrauma and oxygen toxicity, often associated with chronic lung disease in infants (Leonard et al., 1989; Mallory & Stillwell, 1991; OTA, 1987; Raulin & Shannon, 1986). Geographic differences with respect to the incidence

of children with ventilator dependence also exist largely as a result of differing parental attitudes and differing medical practices (Mallory & Stillwell, 1991; OTA, 1987).

A distinctive aspect of this group of children is that they are united by a dependence on technology, not on a common diagnosis. Rather, a wide variety of diagnoses exist that can result in the underlying respiratory failure. Although the degree of care and support varies from child to child, all of these children require expensive care that demands sophisticated equipment and round-the-clock vigilance and monitoring. The child with ventilator dependence represents a unique challenge for all health care professionals as we have moved beyond the goal of increasing their survival; rather, we are now in the era of defining best practices as those that result in optimal quality-of-life outcomes. For pediatric patients, this includes optimizing their developmental potential and reducing the incidence of functional limitations and disabilities. The role of the pediatric

711

physical therapist is an obvious and important one in addressing the latter issue. This chapter attempts to move beyond the individual diagnostic categories to which the children belong to suggest a framework for the examination, diagnosis, and intervention strategies for these children based on their ventilator dependence. The pathophysiologic processes that are commonly seen in pediatric practice are discussed, as well as the common modes of ventilatory support. The reader will be referred to several sources for a more in-depth discussion of ventilatory strategies and clinical management.

PATHOPHYSIOLOGY OF CHRONIC RESPIRATORY FAILURE

Adequate respiratory function requires effective pulmonary exchange of oxygen and carbon dioxide. Respiration requires an organ of gas exchange, the lungs, and a "pump" mechanism consisting of the rib cage and respiratory muscles and the neural control centers (Watchko et al., 1991). Under normal conditions, this pump mechanism can adapt to satisfy the changing metabolic needs that may occur during exercise, hyperthermia, or other demands (Bureau & Begin, 1983), but when these systems are unable to deliver oxygen and remove carbon dioxide from the pulmonary circulation, respiratory failure ensues and gas exchange is impaired (Pagtakhan & Chernick, 1983).

Chronic respiratory failure is not a specific disease entity but a pathophysiologic state defined by treatment with mechanical ventilation for more than 28 days, usually as a result of abnormal gas exchange caused by either primary lung failure or failure of the respiratory pump (Roussos, 1985). Primary lung failure is typically associated with acute respiratory disease such as bronchopulmonary dysplasia (BPD). In this case, primary lung or airway disease compromises pulmonary gas exchange. On the other hand, failure of the respiratory pump mechanism may be caused by impaired neural control of respiration or by inadequate force generation of the respiratory muscles as the result of primary muscle disease, spinal cord injury, chest wall defects, or muscle fatigue.

A number of conditions may predispose children to chronic respiratory failure, but the most common pathophysiologic process is respiratory distress leading to respiratory failure (Box 25-1). Some of the more common diagnoses requiring long-term ventilation in the pediatric population include BPD, neuromuscular disease, traumatic or congenital spinal cord injuries, congenital anomalies such as congenital heart disease and various airway abnormalities, and congenital central hypoventilation syndrome (CCHS; also called Ondine's curse). The mechanisms

---

BOX 25-1. Clinical Signs of Respiratory Failure

Respiratory
Tachypnea
Altered depth and pattern of respiration (deep, shallow, apnea, irregular)
Chest wall retractions
Nasal flaring
Cyanosis
Decreased or absent breath sounds
Expiratory grunting
Wheezing or prolonged expiration

General
Fatigue
Excessive sweating

Cardiac
Tachycardia
Hypertension
Bradycardia
Hypotension
Cardiac arrest

Cerebral
Restlessness
Irritability
Headache
Mental confusion
Papilledema
Seizures
Coma

Laboratory Findings
Hypoxemia (acute or chronic)
Hypercapnia (acute or chronic)
Acidosis (metabolic or respiratory)

From Pagtakhan, RD, & Chernick, V. Intensive care for respiratory disorders. In Kendig, EL, & Chernick, V (Eds.), Disorders of the Respiratory Tract in Children. Philadelphia: WB Saunders, 1983, p. 148.

---

that can lead to respiratory failure can be broadly categorized into four major groups: central nervous system (CNS) disease; muscle disease and musculoskeletal abnormalities; intrinsic pulmonary disease; and airway abnormalities (Box 25-2).

CNS disease is characterized by disorders affecting the central respiratory centers (i.e., the brainstem or cervical spinal cord) (Fig. 25-1). CCHS is a rare disorder that manifests shortly after birth or early in infancy. It is characterized by the failure of the autonomic control of ventilation in the absence of primary pulmonary or neuromuscular disease. The anatomic and biochemical mechanisms of central dysfunction are not completely known, but are postulated to be due to abnormalities of the chemoreceptors (Cutz et al., 1997; Woo et al., 1992). This

---

BOX 25–2. Common Pathophysiologic Mechanisms Leading to Chronic Respiratory Failure

Central Nervous System	Intrinsic Muscle Disease	Intrinsic Pulmonary Disease	Congenital Airway Abnormalities
Congenital hypoventilation syndrome	Congenital abnormalities of thoracic rib cage	Congenital heart disease	Tracheoesophageal fistula
Viral encephalitis	Congenital myopathies	Respiratory distress syndrome or bronchopulmonary dysplasia	Subglottic stenosis
Brain tumors	Duchenne muscular dystrophy		Laryngomalacia
Arnold-Chiari malformation	Phrenic nerve trauma	Tumors	Choanal atresia
Traumatic spinal cord injuries	Diaphragmatic dysfunction	Aspiration syndromes	Various syndromes
Anterior horn cell disease	Myasthenia gravis	Pneumothorax	
Apnea of prematurity	Botulism		
Intracranial hemorrhage			
Hypoxic encephalopathy			

Data from Mallory, GB, & Stillwell, PC. The ventilator-dependent child: Issues in diagnosis and management. Archives of Physical Medicine and Rehabilitation, *72*:43–55, 1991; Goldsmith, JP, & Karotkin, EH. Introduction to assisted ventilation. In Goldsmith, JP, & Karotkin, EH (Eds.), Assisted Ventilation of the Neonate, 2nd ed. Philadelphia: WB Saunders, pp. 1–21; 1988; and Pagtakhan, RD, & Chernick, V. Intensive care for respiratory disorders. In Kendig, EL, & Chernick, V (Eds.), Disorders of the Respiratory Tract, 4th ed. Philadelphia: WB Saunders, 1983, pp. 205–224.

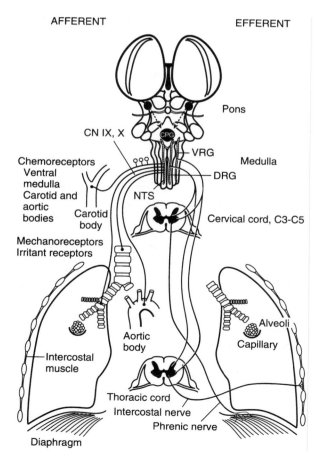

FIGURE 25–1. Schema outlining the various contributions to the neural control of respiration. *NTS,* Nucleus tractus solitarius; *VRG,* ventral respiratory group; *DRG,* dorsal respiratory group; *CPG,* central pattern generator. (From Brazy, JE, Kinney, HC, & Oakes, WJ. CNS structural lesions causing apnea at birth. Journal of Pediatrics, *111*:163–175, 1987.)

disorder is generally diagnosed in the neonatal period when the infant experiences apneic episodes during sleep or while awake. CCHS is known to be associated with other systemic or oncologic conditions such as Hirschsprung disease or neuroblastoma (Woo et al., 1992).

Although the incidence of CCHS is low, these patients face a lifelong dependence on mechanical ventilation. The severity of CCHS varies, as does the degree of dependence on a mechanical ventilator. Because these children have absent or negligible ventilatory sensitivity to hypercapnia and variable sensitivity to hypoxemia during sleep, they are dependent on a ventilator during the night or during sleep (Weese-Mayer et al., 1992; Woo et al., 1992). Artificial ventilation in these patients is done almost exclusively with positive-pressure ventilators or diaphragmatic pacemakers. For children who require 24-hour-a-day ventilation, these options seem to be the most reasonable and the least invasive.

Children with CCHS usually have otherwise unremarkable medical histories. The most vulnerable period is before the diagnosis is made when the infant may experience hypoxic episodes resulting in permanent neurologic damage. With early diagnosis and aggressive management of respiratory failure, the adverse sequelae of hypoxia should be minimized and most of these children can enjoy a relatively "normal" and productive life.

Acquired disorders of the brainstem that affect respiration typically result from either infectious disease processes, brainstem tumors, or complications of Arnold-Chiari malformations. In these instances chronic respiratory failure may be transient or long term. Spinal cord injury or disease can also result in chronic respiratory failure, leading to dependence on mechanical ventilation. The rate of recovery of breathing and motor function after the injury separates those infants and children with satisfactory outcomes from those with poor outcomes (i.e., complete dependence on mechanical ventilation). The level of spinal cord injury dictates the degree of respiratory compromise. Typically, with injuries involving the upper cervical or cervicothoracic area, respiration is compromised because of phrenic and intercostal nerve root damage affecting the function of the diaphragmatic and accessory muscles of respiration. Patients with cervical-level injuries usually require mechanical ventilation either throughout the entire day or only at night. The prognosis for dependence on mechanical ventilation depends on the level of the lesion, the extent of nerve damage, and the nature of the lesion (MacKinnon et al., 1993).

Anterior horn cell disease represents another group of disorders affecting the spinal cord. Spinal muscular atrophy is one of the most common anterior horn cell diseases seen in children since the polio era (Mallory & Stillwell, 1991). There are different types of spinal muscular atrophy, the most common being type I (Werdnig-Hoffman disease). Werdnig-Hoffman disease is a hereditary and progressive disease that typically leads to respiratory failure within a few months after birth. The infant with Werdnig-Hoffman disease typically has generalized hypotonia and paralysis of the limb and trunk musculature with facial sparing. The presence of bulbar weakness results in difficulty with swallowing and sucking, putting these infants at great risk of aspiration, which complicates their already compromised respiratory status. If respiratory involvement is present and noted in the early postnatal period, it is usually severe, leading to respirator dependence very early in the child's life (see Chapter 14).

Intrinsic muscle disease is another common cause of chronic respiratory failure in children. Those with congenital myopathies typically manifest symptoms of respiratory failure early in the course of the disease, whereas those with muscular dystrophies typically do not develop respiratory compromise until late childhood or early adolescence. In either case, mechanical ventilation may be warranted to compensate for the significantly reduced respiratory muscle function (Bureau & Begin, 1983).

Congenital anomalies of the thorax may also predispose the infant to respiratory failure. Thoracic abnormalities are associated with a variety of syndromes (e.g., asphyxiating thoracic dystrophy and dwarfism), as well as scoliosis. In all cases, the rib cage abnormalities result in pulmonary hypoplasia and significantly decreased lung volumes. Treatment of these various impairments will vary; however, in some cases the child may require mechanical ventilation.

Respiratory failure associated with preterm birth probably represents the most common category of pediatric patients who are ventilator dependent. Although the advent of mechanical ventilation has decreased the mortality and morbidity rates of neonates with respiratory distress syndrome (RDS), respiratory failure continues to be a major cause of neonatal mortality. RDS accounts for approximately 30% of all neonatal deaths and 50 to 70% of preterm infant deaths. Because of anatomic and physiologic immaturities, the infant is predisposed to respiratory dysfunction such as atelectasis, airway obstruction, increased pulmonary vascular resistance, and pulmonary edema. They are also predisposed to diaphragmatic fatigue and instability in the neural control of breathing (Make et al., 1998). Ventilatory management of acute RDS often results in damage to lung tissue because of the high inspiratory pressures needed to adequately ventilate. Unfortunately, many infants with RDS go on to develop the chronic lung disease, BPD.

BPD, first described by Northway in 1967, is the most common chronic lung disease in infants (Bregman & Farrell, 1992). BPD is associated with low birth weight, prematurity, and severe initial lung disease, but it has also been described in full-term infants treated with extracorporeal membrane oxygenation (ECMO) (Gannon et al., 1998; Kornhauser et al., 1998). It is thought that structural changes in the lung parenchyma occur as a result of both increased ventilatory pressures over a period of time and prolonged exposure to high levels of oxygen tension. Only after the acute disease has subsided can BPD be accurately distinguished from complications of other acute lung injury (Northway, 1979). BPD was originally defined as oxygen dependence greater than 30% beyond 28 to 30 days with accompanying radiographic changes in the lungs. The infants described in Northway's original work were over 31 weeks of gestational age, and only one weighed less than 1500 g; thus the criteria that he used may no longer be applicable. In fact, the more recent definition of BPD has been modified to include infants who have oxygen requirements at 36 weeks of postconceptional age (Gregoire et al., 1998).

The treatment of BPD, as well as of other forms of chronic lung disease, includes nutritional support, respiratory support, and pharmacologic management, in addition to addressing the child's psychosocial and developmental needs. Commonly used pharmacologic approaches include bronchodilators and diuretics to improve airway conductance, decrease edema, and increase gas exchange; sedatives for persistent agitation; and high-dose corticosteroids to decrease inflammation of the respiratory tract. All of these have adverse side effects that may alter the child's developmental and medical course. The respiratory management may range from supplemental oxygen given by nasal cannula to a tracheostomy with mechanical ventilatory support and oxygen. Nevertheless, these infants and children require ongoing monitoring of their physiologic status to ensure physiologic stability.

Although there have been no major breakthroughs in the prevention of BPD, the long-term outcomes have improved and the disease severity is reduced as a result of medical and pharmacologic improvements (Bancalari & Sosenko, 1990). Two of the most recent additions to the armamentarium for treatment of neonatal respiratory distress are the use of high-frequency ventilators and surfactant replacement in the early neonatal period. The goals of high-frequency ventilation are to adequately ventilate at lower intrapulmonary pressures and smaller tidal volumes, thereby reducing the degree of barotrauma and volutrauma to the immature airways, and to reduce the risks of pulmonary air leaks.

The use of surfactant therapy is now standard practice for the treatment of RDS. A wide variety of surfactant types exist, including both artificial surfactant and surfactant derived from animal sources. A recent review of several clinical trials assessing the efficacy of synthetic surfactant replacement concluded that there were improved clinical outcomes (Soll, 1998).

Because lung tissue continues to grow postnatally, most infants will recover from BPD and eventually function independent of assisted ventilation and supplemental oxygen if conditions for growth are optimized (Farrell & Fost, 1989). Nevertheless, a relatively small proportion of the infants who develop BPD go on to require prolonged ventilation.

Thus far, it appears that the best prevention of BPD is the ability to avoid prematurity, barotrauma, overuse of the ventilator, and the release of free oxygen radicals (possibly with the use of antioxidants) associated with the inflammatory process.

MECHANICAL VENTILATION

Mechanical ventilators have played and continue to play an important role in critical care medicine for both adults and children. Although the underlying disease processes and severity of respiratory failure differ considerably among individuals, mechanical ventilation is the final common treatment approach for individuals with chronic respiratory failure (Table 25-1) (Pilmer, 1994). Mechanical ventilation and the artificial airways used to facilitate it are designed to either assist or substitute for a person's respiratory efforts (i.e., moving air into and out of the lungs) (Luce, 1996; Pagtakhan & Chernick, 1983). In addition to the major goal of restoring adequate gas exchange, it is also essential that complications be avoided or at least minimized (Dick & Sassoon, 1996).

The decision to institute long-term mechanical ventilation is increasingly being made electively to preserve physiologic function and to improve quality of life. In many instances, the clinical decision is made to take advantage of the growth and developmental potential of the lungs (Make et al., 1998). Thus, the desired outcome for many patients is medical stability with adequate growth and healing of the lungs, and eventual withdrawal of the assisted ventilation.

Since the beginning of the modern era of mechanical ventilation in the 1950s, ventilators have undergone, and continue to undergo, significant technologic advances (Goldsmith & Karotkin, 1988; Perel & Stock, 1992). Since the 1950s, 300 to 400 different

TABLE 25-1. Selection Criteria for Mechanical Ventilation

Parameter	Findings
Clinical	
Respiratory*	Apnea; decreased breath sounds; rigorous chest wall movement; weakening ventilatory effort
Cardiac	Asystole; peripheral collapse; severe bradycardia or tachycardia
Cerebral	Coma; lack of response to physical stimuli; uncontrolled restlessness; anxious facial expression
General	Limpness; loss of ability to cry
Laboratory†	
Pa_{CO_2}	Newborn: >60–65 mm Hg Older child: >55–60 mm Hg Rapidly rising >5 mm Hg
Pa_{O_2}	Newborn: <40–50 mm Hg Older child: <50–60 mm Hg

From Pagtakhan, RD, & Chernick, V. Intensive care for respiratory disorders. In Kendig, EL, & Chernick, V (Eds.), Disorders of the Respiratory Tract in Children. Philadelphia: WB Saunders, 1984, p. 160.

*More than one episode of apnea with bradycardia or an episode of cardiac arrest is an adequate indication for initiating mechanical ventilation even in the absence of blood gas data.

†Laboratory values less extreme than those indicated must be supplemented by clinical evidence of severity to warrant initiating mechanical ventilation.

types of ventilators have been on the market at one time or another (Perel & Stock, 1992; Tremolieres, 1991). Specifically, pediatric mechanical ventilation has undergone continual changes that reflect an increased knowledge and understanding of, and appreciation for, the developing cardiorespiratory system. Currently, ventilation strategies use a "lung protective" approach. This strategy minimizes the potential for lung injury through the use of maximal alveolar pressures, minimal positive end-expiratory pressure, and permissive hypercapnia (Elixson et al., 1997; Gannon, 1998). Contemporary knowledge of respiratory physiology and a more detailed understanding of the pathophysiologic mechanisms underlying diseases of the respiratory system continue to drive research and development in this area. Although it is beyond the scope and intent of this chapter—and of physical therapy practice—to detail the technical information that exists on mechanical ventilation, brief descriptions of the major ventilator types are provided.

There are various classifications of assisted ventilation, ranging from noninvasive ventilation to conventional mechanical ventilation with a tracheostomy. This chapter focuses on the use of conventional ventilation with a tracheostomy, which is the most common mode of long-term ventilation in children. Ventilators can be simply classified into positive- and negative-pressure ventilators. With negative-pressure ventilation (NPV), a pressure gradient is established by creating a negative pressure around the person's entire body from the neck down during inspiration, causing air to enter the lungs. The interface used with this type of ventilatory strategy is a chest shell, wrap or poncho, or tank. The major advantages of NPV are that an artificial airway is not needed, thereby reducing the risks of infection, and there is no need to interrupt ventilation for suctioning (Dougherty, 1990; Make et al., 1998). NPV has been used most successfully for patients with neuromuscular diseases and patients with pulmonary disease who require periodic or nocturnal ventilatory support (McPherson, 1995). It has also been successfully used to avoid or delay the need for a tracheostomy. The limitations of NPV are that it can cause airway occlusion in infants and young children during sleep, and the chest shell or wrap is not effective for children who require high respiratory rates, tidal volumes, or distending pressures. Overall, negative-pressure ventilators tend to be less powerful and less versatile than positive-pressure ventilators.

Positive-pressure ventilation (PPV) is the more commonly used ventilation strategy and is the preferred type used in portable ventilators for children who are at home (Table 25–2). With PPV, pressurized gas is delivered into the vent circuit and airways during inspiration; it can be administered via a tracheostomy or a nasal mask. Because there is not a secure airway with nasal mask ventilation, nasal mask ventilation is usually reserved for an intensive care unit (ICU) or acute care setting. This type of ventilation strategy is not used routinely with pediatric patients and is still considered to be experimental for use with small children. PPV can be further classified according to degree and timing of ventilatory support and the type of cycling used to end the inspiratory phase (Box 25–3).

Because many combinations of ventilatory attributes can obtain desirable results, practices are far from uniform (Froese, 1991) and often cannot be supported by scientific research (Rasanen & Downs, 1990). The optimal settings for each patient vary and are determined by the patient's metabolic requirements, respiratory drive, and pulmonary mechanics (Shneerson, 1996). The type of mechanical ventilation and the various parameters chosen depend on a number of considerations. These include an understanding of the underlying disease process that precipitated ventilatory failure, available equipment, knowledge of the current literature, previous experience with specific types of machines, and whether

TABLE 25–2. Common Classification of Positive Pressure Ventilation

Type of Ventilation	Description
Controlled mechanical ventilation (CMV)	Delivers a preselected ventilatory rate, tidal volume, and inspiratory flow rate independent of spontaneous effort by the patient.
Continuous positive-pressure ventilation (CPPV)	Similar to CMV except the airway pressure never returns to 0.
Assisted mechanical ventilation	Also known as "patient-triggered" positive-pressure ventilation; the ventilator will not deliver a breath unless the patient initiates a spontaneous breathing effort.
Assist-control ventilation	Combines assisted mechanical ventilation and CMV, whereby the ventilator may be triggered by the patient's spontaneous efforts or by a timing device, whichever comes first. There is a minimal preselected rate determined, so CMV acts as a backup in the event of apnea or an attempt to breathe at a rate lower than that preselected.
Intermittent mandatory ventilation (IMV)	Allows the patient to breathe spontaneously with a mechanical inflation provided at preset intervals; the ventilatory rate cannot be influenced by the patient. In addition to the spontaneous breaths from the patient, IMV should be titrated to deliver only the support needed to maintain normal alveolar ventilation and $Paco_2$.
Synchronized intermittent mandatory ventilation (SIMV)	Similar to IMV; however, at regular intervals the mandatory breath is synchronized to begin with the next spontaneous inhalation. (This technique was introduced to avoid the phenomenon of "breath stacking.")
Mandatory minute ventilation	Patient is guaranteed a preselected minute volume either through spontaneous ventilation or as a positive-pressure breath from the ventilator. (If the desired minute volume is achieved by the patient's spontaneous breaths, no mandatory breaths are delivered by the ventilator.)
Continuous positive airway pressure (CPAP) ventilation	Positive-pressure modes are used in conjunction with spontaneous breaths; can be used individually or with mechanical ventilation.
Expiratory positive-pressure ventilation	Similar to CPAP except that the airway pressure is 0 or negative during inhalation but increases at the end of exhalation to a predetermined positive pressure.

From Perel, A, & Stock, MC (Eds.). Handbook of Mechanical Ventilatory Support. Baltimore: Williams & Wilkins, 1992, pp. 7–30. Copyright 1992, the Williams & Wilkins Co., Baltimore.

the patient will be cared for outside of an ICU environment (Perel & Stock, 1992). Numerous complications can occur with mechanical ventilation (Box 25–4), and it is essential that individuals who work with these children have a knowledge of normal and pathologic respiratory physiology, as well as an intimate knowledge and understanding of how the machine interfaces with the patient's physiology (Kirby et al., 1990; Perel & Stock, 1992).

A number of complex decisions are made before choosing the appropriate method and type of ventilation. For the infant or child who is facing long-term ventilator dependence, the possibilities and options of going home should weigh heavily in the decision making. Advances in design, efficiency, and portability have all contributed to an increased use of mechanical ventilators outside the acute care environment. In the past 5 to 10 years there has been a

---

BOX 25–3. Cycling Mechanisms on Positive Pressure Ventilators

Time-cycled ventilation: Mechanical ventilation terminates after a preselected inspiratory time (T_1) elapses.

Volume-cycled ventilation: Mechanical inhalation terminates after a preselected volume (V_T) has been ejected from the ventilator irrespective of changes in pulmonary mechanics.

Pressure-cycled ventilation: Mechanical ventilation terminates when a preselected peak inspiratory pressure is achieved within the breathing circuit tubing.

Flow-cycled ventilation: Mechanical ventilation is terminated when the inspiratory flow rate delivered by the ventilator decreases to a critical value, independent of inspiratory time or tidal volume.

From Perel, A, & Stock, MC (Eds.). Handbook of Mechanical Ventilatory Support. Baltimore: Williams & Wilkins, 1992, pp. 7–30. Copyright 1992, the Williams & Wilkins Co., Baltimore.

BOX 25-4. Complications Associated with Mechanical Ventilation

Respiratory

Tracheal lesions (erosion, edema, stenosis, granuloma, obstruction, perforation)

Accidental endotracheal tube displacement or actual extubation

Air leaks (pneumothorax, pneumomediastinum, interstitial emphysema)

Infection (tracheitis, pneumonitis)

Trapping of gas (hyperinflation)

Excessive secretions (atelectasis)

Oxygen hazards (depression of ventilation, bronchopulmonary dysplasia)

Pulmonary hemorrhage

Circulatory

Impairment of venous return (decreased cardiac output and systemic hypotension)

Oxygen hazard (retrolental fibroplasia, cerebral vasoconstriction)

Septicemia

Intracranial hemorrhage

Hyperventilation (decreased cerebral blood flow)

Metabolic

Increased work of breathing ("fighting the ventilator")

Alkalosis (potassium depletion, excessive bicarbonate therapy)

Renal and Fluid Balance

Antidiuresis

Excess water in inspired gas

Equipment Malfunction

Power source failure

Improper humidification (overheating of inspired gas, inspiratory line condensation)

Improper tubing connections (kinked line, disconnection)

Ventilation malfunction (leaks, valve dysfunction)

Adapted from Pagtakhan, RD, & Chernick, V. Intensive care for respiratory disorders. In Kendig, EL, & Chernick, V (Eds.), Disorders of the Respiratory Tract in Children. Philadelphia: WB Saunders, 1983, p. 162.

shift in the emphasis on home care, and it is now standard practice for ventilator-dependent children who are medically stable to be cared for outside the hospital. A number of studies have demonstrated that appropriately selected infants and children can be safely cared for at home (for review, see Make et al., 1998).

WEANING

The transition to unassisted breathing is a complex issue. Weaning the patient from the support of a mechanical ventilator is highly individualized, but it should be the ultimate goal for most patients. The primary assessment of weaning capability is to determine at what point the patient is capable of maintaining adequate alveolar ventilation while breathing spontaneously. This requires the ventilatory pump to support the work required for breathing (Hodgkin et al., 1984). Various determinants of physiologic and medical stability such as pulmonary function, gas exchange, neuromuscular function, respiratory muscle strength, and ventilatory pattern are used to determine weaning capabilities. Knisely and co-workers (1988) found an association between prolonged ventilatory dependence in infants and diaphragmatic muscle atrophy. These investigators suggested that these changes could certainly affect the weaning process because the diaphragm would be predisposed to fatigue. The process of weaning tends to be done by trial and error where the time off the ventilator is variable, dependent on when hypercapnia and hypoxia develop (Gozal et al., 1993). Numerous weaning strategies may be used. Some use an all-or-none strategy whereby the vent is removed for periods of time during the day; the time off is dictated by the patient's physiologic responses. Another strategy is to combine continuous positive airway pressure (CPAP) with time off the vent so that the transition is less drastic.

Weaning can be an arduous task both physiologically and psychologically, and it should be done with caution (Hodgkin et al., 1984). During this time, the child's schedule of activities may need to be altered. It is imperative that the physical therapist coordinate and communicate with the medical team as to the amount of physical exertion that can be tolerated safely. At all costs, both muscular and respiratory fatigue must be avoided.

DISABILITIES ASSOCIATED WITH MECHANICAL VENTILATOR DEPENDENCE

In addition to a new category of patients being "created," chronic dependence on assisted ventilation has created a new category of developmental disabilities. As elucidated previously, a wide range of pathophysiologic mechanisms underlie dependence on mechanical ventilation. Hence, this "medical" diagnosis represents a diverse and heterogeneous group of children with varying impairments and developmental capabilities. Despite differences, however, these children are all medically fragile and vulnerable. It has been known for a number of years that medically fragile infants and children are at risk for physical, mental, and social disabilities. Although the predictive value of any one risk factor is not well established, it appears that long-term outcome depends on a number of risk factors and their interac-

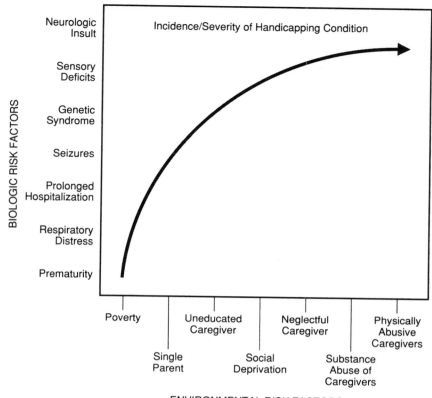

FIGURE 25–2. Relationship between multiple risk factors. This example illustrates how various biologic risk factors in combination with multiple environmental risks can magnify the incidence of disabilities associated with the given pathophysiologic process. (From Schaaf, RC, & Davis, WS. Promoting health and wellness in the pediatric disabled and "at risk" population. In Rothman, J, & Levine, R [Eds.], Prevention Practice: Strategies for Physical Therapy and Occupational Therapy. Philadelphia: WB Saunders, 1992, p. 273.)

tions (Fig. 25–2). Schaaf and Davis (1992) suggest that environmental factors become increasingly more important to the child's eventual outcome, a concept that is receiving much attention in the literature on the outcome of children with disabilities (Escalona, 1982; Hunt et al., 1988; Schafer et al., 1987; Slater et al., 1987).

Few studies have specifically examined the developmental outcome of children who are ventilator dependent. One group that has probably been studied most extensively are infants and children with BPD. The morbidity associated with BPD includes not only the associated chronic respiratory problems, but other growth- and development-related factors. For example, linear and anthropometric growth are often adversely affected by BPD (Bregman & Farrell, 1992; Kurzner et al., 1988; Meisels et al., 1986). Although optimal nutrition is an important goal in the care of infants with respiratory distress, it is often difficult to achieve because of the increased energy expenditure, increased work

of breathing, and limited fluid intake (Bregman & Farrell, 1992; Kurzner et al., 1988). Weinstein and Oh (1981) reported a 25% increase in resting oxygen consumption of preterm infants with BPD compared with normal infants. In addition, the caloric requirements of infants with BPD are 25 to 50% greater than those of normal infants. Kao and colleagues (1988) found that when pulmonary mechanics were improved and work of breathing decreased, oxygen consumption did not decrease. These results suggest that other factors such as inflammation, repair processes of the lung, and pulmonary tension might account for the increased metabolic rate, and hence the increased oxygen consumption (Weinstein & Oh, 1981). These children may also experience a failure to thrive because of an intolerance for feeding secondary to oral motor sensitivity, a poor suck, or decreased physical stamina to sustain the demands of feeding (Bregman & Farrell, 1992; Yu et al., 1983).

Because a small percentage of the preterm infant's birth weight is fat, those specific nutrients supply little caloric reserve and decrease the antioxidant functions that play a role in lung repair and protection from lung injury. Thus, the inadequate nutrition may adversely affect lung growth and development, increasing the infant's susceptibility to hyperoxia and barotrauma.

In general, a paucity of literature exists on the long-term developmental outcomes of chronically ventilated infants with BPD or other diagnoses requiring prolonged mechanical ventilation. Discrepancies exist regarding the impact of chronic lung disease on developmental outcomes beyond infancy. Bozynski and colleagues (1987) assessed the relationship between mechanical ventilation and developmental outcome. They found prolonged ventilator dependence to be the best predictor of poor developmental progress during the first 18 months. Even when the effects of intracranial hemorrhage were controlled, chronic lung disease was associated with lower scores on the Bayley scales. Bregman and Farrell (1992) suggest that length of mechanical ventilation does not necessarily correlate with developmental outcome. More recently, O'Shea and colleagues (1996) found that chronic lung disease was associated with long-term effects on cognitive development. In this study, IQ tests were administered to 4- to 5-year-old children who were very low birth weight infants, had similar medical outcomes, and were without evidence of major abnormalities on cranial ultrasound. Those children who had recovered from severe chronic lung disease had significantly lower full-scale and performance IQ scores. Singer and colleagues (1997) found that infants with BPD who were followed longitudinally to 3 years of age performed poorly on developmental indices. Regression analyses revealed that BPD predicted a poor motor outcome. Gregoire and colleagues (1998) discuss these discrepancies in terms of the definitions of BPD being used and whether there were associated neurologic lesions that coexisted with the chronic lung disease. In their study, the developmental outcomes of two groups were compared: one with traditionally defined BPD (O_2 dependence at 28 days) and the other with the "revised" definition of O_2 dependence at 36 weeks of postconceptional age. In their cohort, those with O_2 dependence at 36 weeks had a greater incidence of developmental delay, but not greater neurologic impairments, at 18 months. The presence of chronic lung disease (and ventilator dependence) alone puts a child at the same risk of neurodevelopmental impairments as the child with only a neurologic insult such as an intraventricular or periventricular hemorrhage or periventricular leukomalacia. Thus, the presence of both, as is commonly seen, would place the child at an even higher risk for chronic developmental disabilities.

Even in the presence of an otherwise unremarkable medical history, the child on a ventilator is at risk for functional limitations related to communication, mobility, and fatigue related to poor cardiorespiratory endurance. This is not surprising when one considers the extent of the child's "world" when the child is ventilator dependent. The context for motor learning is highly limiting for the child who is hospitalized for prolonged periods or who is constrained by lifesaving equipment. The lack of practice and of variable practice opportunities makes skill acquisition difficult, so the repertoire of skills in a variety of developmental domains is limited. (See Chapter 6 for further details on motor learning concepts.) As a point of illustration, the acquisition of independent mobility in typically developing children allows them to acquire information about their world and develop perceptions on which they can act. Thus, development of cognitive skills such as object permanence are facilitated through motoric competencies (Bai & Bertenthal, 1992). This interleaving of developmental domains and their interdependence is a well-known phenomenon, so the impact of atypical circumstances and a lack of environmental affordances can be substantial. It is easy to see why these children often have global developmental delays, despite having no history of neurologic insults.

In addition to the aforementioned developmental risks, the additive effects of secondary complications such as recurrent hypoxic episodes, recurrent infections, poor weight gain, and poor physical growth can directly result in a number of impairments (Bos et al., 1998; Singer et al., 1997). For example, because of the often prolonged periods of immobility or restricted activity early in the course of their disease, these children may demonstrate such problems as sensory defensiveness, generalized weakness, and soft tissue or muscular tightness. Likewise, if the child has had some type of hypoxic or ischemic episode, there may be neurologic damage that limits normal motor skill acquisition and execution. However, if these children have been spared the associated problems (most commonly the frequent hypoxic episodes), there is a good chance that they can grow and develop normally. For example, children with CCHS have a favorable prognosis and the capacity for normal or near-normal intelligence if they are diagnosed early and managed aggressively (Weese-Mayer et al., 1992). Similarly, infants with BPD who have not had major neurologic insults also have an excellent chance of being weaned from oxygen dependence and the ventilator, as well as functioning independently in their school years (Mallory & Stillwell, 1991).

Regardless of the reason for being dependent on

assisted ventilation, appreciation of the fact that the child is at a disadvantage in terms of developmental risks is a compelling reason to begin early intervention as soon as the infant or child is medically stable. Because of the risks for abnormal neurodevelopmental sequelae in children who are ventilator dependent, physical therapists should be involved with providing developmental intervention early in the course of an infant's hospitalization. Delays in the initiation of rehabilitation or habilitation can place the child at risk for developing secondary impairments and functional limitations that could otherwise be prevented.

ELEMENTS OF PATIENT MANAGEMENT

The physical therapy examination and evaluation of the infant or child who is mechanically ventilated must encompass a wide range of skills and observations. In addition to an understanding of typical and atypical motor skill development, one must have knowledge of cardiorespiratory physiology and the implications of a compromise to that system in the developing infant or child. The complexity of the technical environment also makes this a challenging population. First, the physical therapist must be familiar with the equipment, both the ventilator and its attachments, as well as the physiologic monitoring devices (Table 25-3). Although the infant or child may be medically stable, the presence of an artificial airway creates a critical situation because of the potential for its being dislodged or occluded. Because the infant or young child may not yet communicate well, it is up to the therapist to interpret any signs of impending or actual distress. The essence of the intervention is to ensure that no harm be done in the delivery of services and to optimize the child's developmental potential.

Before any examination or treatment session, the therapist should confer with the child's primary nurse or caregiver to determine the child's most recent medical status, in addition to the child's baseline physiologic parameters. Depending on the nature and severity of the predisposing condition, the cardiorespiratory parameters may vary from what is considered to be normal for the child's age (Table 25-4). It is always prudent to establish the "safe" physiologic parameters within which to work. Typically, heart rate, respiratory rate, and oxygen saturation are monitored while the child is on the ventilator. In the home or outpatient setting, one may choose to monitor these parameters periodically; however, *there is no substitute for the keen visual observation of signs of distress.*

TABLE 25-3. Commonly Encountered Noninvasive Monitoring Devices*

Equipment	Physiologic Parameters Monitored
Cardiorespiratory monitors	Heart rate and respiratory rate
Pulse oximeter†	Transcutaneous arterial oxygen saturation to monitor hypoxemia
Ventilator alarms	Various modes chosen for the individual case, as well as airway pressures, gas concentrations, and expiratory tidal volumes
Transcutaneous Po_2 and Pco_2	Partial pressure of oxygen and carbon dioxide in the arterial blood
Oxygen analyzers on the ventilator	Oxygen supply in the ventilator circuit
Sphygmomanometer	Blood pressure

*These are some noninvasive devices that one may use to monitor response to activity and general status. Before any examination or treatment session the therapist should be familiar with *all* of the equipment used for the child.

†Pulse oximeters are not useful for discriminating hyperoxia because the blood is fully saturated at Pao_2 of 150 mm Hg.

TABLE 25-4. Approximate Normal Physiologic Values*

Parameter	Newborn	Older Infant and Child
Respiratory rate	40–60	20–30 (≤6 years) 15–20 (>6 years)
Heart rate	120–200	100–180 (≤3 years) 70–150 (>3 years)
Po_2 (mm Hg)	60–90	80–100
Pco_2 (mm Hg)	30–35	30–35 (≤2 years) 20–24 (>2 years)
Blood pressure (mm Hg)		
Systolic	60–90	75–130 (≤3 years) 90–140 (>3 years)
Diastolic	30–60	45–90 (≤3 years) 50–80 (>3 years)
Arterial oxygen saturation (%)	87–89 (low) 94–95 (high) 90–95 (preterm infant)	95–100

Data from Comer, DM. Pulse oximetry: Implications for practice. Journal of Obstetric, Gynecologic and Neonatal Nursing, 21:35–41, 1992; and Pagtakhan, RD, & Chernick, V. Intensive care for respiratory disorders. In Kendig, EL, & Chernick, V (Eds.), Disorders of the Respiratory Tract in Children, 4th ed. Philadelphia: WB Saunders, 1983, pp. 145–168.

*These values represent "normal" physiologic values; in the case of infants and children with varying pathophysiologic processes, the "normal" values may be different.

Physical Therapy Examination

Although the most obvious impairment in patients on ventilators is their cardiopulmonary system, it is essential that the approach to patient management be multidimensional. These patients probably have coexisting impairments, functional limitations, and disabilities in various areas. Thus, once the necessary history and systems review is completed, the appropriate tests and measures are chosen to adequately examine aerobic capacity and endurance, adequacy of respiration, motor function, musculoskeletal performance, and general adaptive behaviors that are age appropriate.

In terms of the respiratory examination, at a minimum the therapist should be comfortable observing the patient for signs of respiratory distress, skin color changes indicative of hypoxia, changes in respiratory rate, breathing pattern, symmetry of chest expansion, posture, and general comfort (DeCesare & Graybill, 1990). (In neonates, visual inspection for hypoxia is not effective because neonates generally do not appear cyanotic until the Pao_2 is dangerously low, below 40 mm Hg [Null et al., 1990].) Signs of respiratory distress such as retractions, nasal flaring, expiratory grunting, and stridor may not be evident when a child is on a mechanical ventilator (Crane, 1990). For more information specific to the assessment of the cardiorespiratory system, the reader is referred elsewhere (DeCesare & Graybill, 1990; Gould, 1991; Waring, 1983).

The neuromuscular examination should provide information about the infant's or child's general musculoskeletal status and includes strength, sensation, posture, and general movement competencies. The examination procedures vary depending on the age and cognitive level of the child, and the areas of emphasis may be different depending on the diagnosis. Last, the measurement of neuromotor development and motor control is an important aspect of the examination for these children because they are at great risk for global developmental delays that may or may not have a pathophysiologic component.

The physical therapy examination alone does not begin to represent the wide range of competencies that must be monitored. Ideally, all aspects of the child's development will be assessed periodically by members of the health care team. It cannot be emphasized enough that a multidisciplinary team approach is necessary in the management of these children and should be the standard of practice, regardless of the physical therapist's practice setting.

The child needs to be functional within the context of his or her environment; therefore, an examination of the child's functional level is as important as the respiratory and neuromotor assessments that the physical therapist would typically perform. The functional examination should include age-appropriate basic and instrumental activities of daily living, general mobility skills, communication skills, and an evaluation of the child's role within the family and within the relevant environment. At the very least, the functional assessment provides an indication of how well the child is integrated into the family and community lifestyle.

The importance of the disablement framework (see Chapter 7) relative to the examination of motor function is nicely elucidated by Haley and colleagues (1993). These authors stress the significance of assessing motor skills during spontaneous activity and of obtaining parental impressions of function. Their emphasis on functional considerations is translated into the recommendation that the environment and social context be an essential part of any examination to determine the nature of the child's functional limitations and disabilities. The child requiring assisted ventilation exemplifies this concept because it would be impossible to isolate the effects of the restrictive environment in an examination of the child's sensorimotor development. The types of formal developmental tests used will vary with the age of the child (see Chapter 1). Although useful to some degree with this population, most developmental tests are inadequate because they fail to take into account the effects of medical and physiologic instability; long-term hospitalization; decreased mobility; and separation from "normal" social, emotional, and physical life experiences. As a result, the use of any standardized test requires that the therapist be familiar with the purpose of the test, its limitations, and its relevance to the outcome measures of interest. Specifically, the user must understand the generalizability of the test results because many assessments are normed on children without disabilities. Supplementing any standardized examination should be the therapist's individualized assessment of the infant's or child's developmental competencies. Haley and colleagues (1993) caution that standardized and criterion-referenced testing of neuromotor behaviors and movement analyses do not always give information at all levels of the disablement spectrum. They recommend sampling motor outcomes across the entire disablement framework and suggest the use of judgment-based assessments, which can provide additional information that is a useful adjunct to that obtained from standardized or criterion-based tests. Judgment-based assessments do not require observation of the actual performance of the motor task; however, the respondent is asked to make a judgment about the ability of the child to perform a task based on prior observations and a knowledge of how the child would typically perform.

This allows one to distinguish between what the child is capable of and how the child actually performs during day-to-day functional tasks. Parent or caregiver participation should be encouraged in the examination, as well as in the formulation of therapy goals (see Chapter 31).

Evaluation and Diagnosis

Considering the complexity of impairments in many children who are ventilator dependent, the evaluation is especially important. Ideally, a multidimensional approach to the use of tests and measures should be employed and the results correlated to the relevant functional limitations and disabilities interfering with the child's quality of life. This important step in the process will be used to define the physical therapy diagnosis and to describe the specific plan of care for the child (American Physical Therapy Association, 1997). For the child with ventilator dependence, the range of diagnoses can be broad. For example, the child with chronic lung disease and mechanical ventilator dependence secondary to chronic lung disease (e.g., BPD) may have coexisting neurologic impairments, gastrointestinal abnormalities, and growth disturbance. The physical therapy diagnosis might therefore include developmental delay, aerobic capacity and endurance limitations, and decreased repertoire of movement patterns. On the other hand, a child with the medical diagnosis of congenital central hypoventilation syndrome may be otherwise medically stable and is at risk for developmental delay only if the child is hospitalized for a prolonged period of time. With appropriate attention to ensuring adequate and appropriate developmental intervention, these children can lead fairly normal lives. Thus, at this stage of clinical decision making, the diagnostic and prognostic determinations used for developing a physical therapy plan of care will vary depending on the age of the child, the severity and chronicity of the lung disease, and the coexisting diagnoses.

Intervention Considerations

Regardless of the cause for requiring chronic mechanical ventilation, once a child is diagnosed with chronic respiratory failure and the decision is made to begin artificial ventilation, prevention and treatment of the associated complications must be a primary goal of medical and rehabilitative management. These children require early and aggressive developmental intervention. Although the degree and intensity may vary, the intervention strategy should maximize the child's developmental and functional potential. After the acute medical condition of any of these patient groups is stabilized, considerable efforts should be aimed at promoting growth and development. In many centers, specialized units exist that exclusively serve the medical and developmental needs of infants and children who are ventilator dependent (Mallory & Stillwell, 1991; Schreiner et al., 1991). These units often attempt to provide individualized care and management while trying to maintain as normal an environment as possible.

No one intervention strategy is unanimously embraced by physical therapists for any diagnostic group. Similarly, in the case of children with ventilator dependence, physical therapy varies widely because of differing philosophies of management and the wide range of problem areas that might be identified. Thus, the intent of this section is not to prescribe specific treatment but to present a conceptual framework from which one can organize an appropriate plan of care and to emphasize considerations unique to this group of children.

Typically developing infants and children are capable of using a variable repertoire of motor skills to explore and learn (see Chapter 1). This normal acquisition of skills presumes an interaction of the cardiopulmonary and musculoskeletal systems, as well as the presence of the necessary cognitive requirements. Inactivity in children is never normal, and they usually require minimal encouragement to be active and spontaneous. In the case of a child with chronic respiratory insufficiency, however, compromised physiologic stability alone may limit the seemingly endless exploration and practice in which children typically engage. In children with a chronic illness, a reduced capacity for activity or exercise can be a direct or an indirect result of their underlying pathophysiologic process (Bar-Or, 1986). Regardless of the cause, a vicious cycle of inactivity → reluctance to move and explore → decreased endurance and "fitness" → inactivity ensues. Another consideration is that these children may associate movement with negative experiences such as fatigue, hypoxia, and pain, which limits their "motivation" to be as active as their peers. It is not always easy to distinguish among the various factors that lead to a paucity of movement, especially in the absence of neurologic deficits.

A major goal of the physical therapist in the management of children who are dependent on ventilators should be secondary prevention (i.e., prevent deprivation of sensory and motor experiences and all of the various sequelae that result from that deprivation). Regardless of the child's medical diagnosis, treatment should be aimed at providing a variety of opportunities for movement challenges and for exploration, as well as increasing the child's capacity for exercise. Depending on whether the child has a specific motor impairment, these goals may be accomplished with or without the use of assistive devices. For example, in the case of a child with BPD who also had an intraventricular hemorrhage, assistive devices may be needed for positioning because of poor antigravity trunk control, or for ambulation because of lower extremity weakness and spasticity. In contrast, the child with CCHS and no neurologic injuries leading to motor impairments may be completely independent in all motor skills. In the context of functional limitations, exercise intolerance is a problem in this group of children. Any activity in which these infants or children engage should be viewed as "exercise" and seen as a means of improving their tolerance for movement. A paucity of literature exists on the role developmental intervention plays in improving cardiopulmonary status and exercise tolerance, *in addition* to achieving developmental goals.

Simply stated, the "normal" response to exercise is an increase in heart rate, followed by a return to baseline. Ventilation also increases linearly with the metabolic rate until approximately 60% of the oxygen consumption, at which time it increases more rapidly. (See Chapter 5 for a summary of the cardiorespiratory and musculoskeletal components of exercise and fitness.) These relationships, as well as the other physiologic processes that support adequate ventilation and perfusion during exercise, are altered in conditions of lung disease. Whereas exercise is normally cardiac limited, in those with chronic lung disease exercise may be ventilatory limited as a result of deficient exercise capacity, deficient gas exchange, or poor pulmonary mechanics (Darbee & Cerny, 1990). Each child's specific pathophysiologic process determines the response to exercise and the capacity for improvement.

The beneficial effects of exercise have been well documented in certain populations such as individuals with cystic fibrosis and asthma (Darbee & Cerny, 1990), but less information exists that objectively documents the effects of any type of structured exercise program on either short- or long-term outcomes of children who are dependent on ventilators. Bader and colleagues (1987) examined the long-term pulmonary sequelae and exercise tolerance of 10 children with BPD at a mean of 10 years of age. All children in the study had required either mechanical ventilation or oxygen therapy for at least 30 days. Half of the group had exercise-induced bronchospasms, but no significant differences from normal values were found in maximal oxygen consumption, suggesting that their aerobic fitness was comparable to that of the "normal" group.

Despite similar cardiovascular function to normal children, those with BPD demonstrated pulmonary limitations to exercise evidenced by a decrease in arterial oxygen saturation and an increased $Paco_2$. Although some of the children were mechanically ventilated for a very short time during their acute disease course, it would be erroneous to extrapolate the findings to the population of children who remain chronically dependent on mechanical ventilation. More long-term studies are needed to determine the effectiveness of exercise programs in this group.

One of the ultimate goals for pediatric physical therapists should be to promote the concept of lifelong fitness. Regardless of the underlying medical diagnosis there is usually no reason not to encourage some type of physical activity in children who are dependent on a ventilator. The long-term benefits of physical activity and lifelong fitness include not only physiologic and health-related ones, but also mental health benefits such as improved self-esteem and confidence.

In all circumstances the physical therapist must recognize the potential for physiologic jeopardy when implementing any intervention program with these infants and children. The amount and type of motor activities must be individualized and graded to the child's level of tolerance so that the risks associated with the physiologically immature or unstable systems are not magnified. Decisions regarding the mode, intensity, and frequency of activity should be made in conjunction with the other members of the child's medical team and modified as the disease process changes.

Coordination and Communication

Although physical therapists play an important role in direct treatment, consultation, parent teaching, and discharge planning, they represent only one aspect of the care that children dependent on ventilators require. The lives of these children are complex, so it is imperative that they be managed by a multidisciplinary team rather than by fragmented individual service providers. Typically, the multidisciplinary team might consist of physician and nurse specialists, therapists, nutritionists, and other professionals who address the psychosocial aspects of the child and family in their community. Communication and collaboration among team members are essential to the child's and family's well-being and to an understanding of the disability. Short- and long-term goals developed by the team should be formulated in conjunction with the family, keeping in mind the ultimate goal of maximizing function from a physical, cognitive, social-emotional, and family dynamics perspective. It is not uncommon for parents to be naive to the disease process and the implications for future function. As a protective mechanism, many parents are often overprotective of a "sick" child and actually contribute to sustaining the child's fear of movement challenges or lack of activity. Especially in relation to functional mobility and fitness, the physical therapist has an important role to play in educating the family toward maximizing the child's *abilities* rather than imposing limitations because of the child's *disabilities*. In the case of the child who is at home, this role may extend to community therapists and school personnel as well. The most effective outcomes occur when the focus of the team is on the integration of the child into the family and then, at the right time, into the community (Raulin & Shannon, 1986; Schaaf & Davis, 1992). In fact, it is the integration of the child into the community—schools, play groups, structured social activities, and so forth—that represents optimal outcomes when considering quality-of-life measures. This is a challenge that requires and deserves the attention of numerous professionals and the child's family (Make et al., 1998; Sevick & Bradham, 1997).

Family-centered intervention is mandated by law, representing a departure from the traditional child-focused programs of the past (Kolobe, 1992). For reasons other than legal ones, however, the involvement of the parents and family in the life of the child with a disability is essential for optimal child development and family dynamics. Probably no situation better demonstrates the need for inclusion of the family in the child's entire care plan more than in the case of the child who is dependent on mechanical ventilation. The role of the family in shaping the child's environment to be the most conducive to learning and optimal development is crucial. More important, from a practical point of view, the child's life depends on the parents' knowledge about the intensive care needed to maintain the child's fragile life.

HOME CARE OF THE CHILD WITH VENTILATOR DEPENDENCE

Once the decision has been made to mechanically ventilate an infant or a child for an extended length of time, the long-term impact of a prolonged hospitalization should be considered. It is unfortunate that despite the well-known benefits of being in one's natural environment, far too many children with ventilator dependence stay in an ICU setting long past the point of clinical stability and readiness for discharge (DeWitt et al., 1993). Although most would agree that it is beneficial to have a child who is dependent on a ventilator remain at home, the impact of caring for a child with chronic medical needs and disabilities causes varying degrees of stress on families (American Thoracic Society, 1990; Bach et al., 1990; Fields et al., 1991; Frates et al., 1985; Make et al., 1998). The dilemma of whether a child with ventilator dependence can be cared for at home is not made solely on the basis of medical stability. Rather, family and social supports, as well as financial resources, are as important as the medical and technical management skills that are required. The parents of a child who is dependent on mechanical ventilation also have the added burden of needing highly qualified child care resources, making leisure time or needed respite care difficult to arrange. As the degree and complexity of impairment and disabilities increase, the quality of life usually decreases—especially if financial, psychosocial, and emotional supports dwindle. Keeping this in mind, one of the most important roles of the various disciplines is to work closely with family members as the child is being considered for discharge. Parents should expect the health care professionals to give them as much information as needed to make an informed decision about their abilities to care for their child at home, as well as the risks and benefits. The family's coping skills and lifestyle needs should always be at the forefront of any parent-professional relationship and a major consideration of any rehabilitation program that might be recommended. It is essential that the child's therapy program be integrated into the family's daily routine and not be the sole focus of the family's daily schedule (Kolobe, 1992).

It is imperative that the family or designated caregivers be involved in, and capable of learning, all aspects of the child's care (American Thoracic Society, 1990; Frates et al., 1985; Make et al., 1998; Mallory & Stillwell, 1991). This care includes not only managing the ventilator and other monitoring equipment, but also being able to provide emergency medical procedures if the child experiences distress, and most important, the ability to recognize signs of distress. The high degree of medical and technologic expertise required by parents or caregivers can be a tremendous drain on a family, and it "strains the traditional conceptions of parental responsibilities" (Mallory & Stillwell, 1991). The critical nature of this type of family teaching goes beyond our normal expectations of the family unit, and caregivers need extensive support from the various team members. Parents who decide *not* to have their child cared for at home on a ventilator, or those who do not have a choice, will also need ongoing support as they continue to be "parents from a distance" and without the luxury of the home environment. The reality is that home care is possible and feasible only when the financial costs and caregiver needs are adequately met (Campbell & Pierce, 1998). Unfortunately, in many instances the rate-limiting factor for discharge is the excessive amount of time it takes to process the paper trail associated with applying for home care funding (DeWitt, 1993).

In recent years there has been a rapid growth in high-tech pediatric home care and increasing support for managing children with chronic illnesses at home (Andrews & Nielson, 1988; Lantos & Korman, 1992; Quint et al., 1990). Changes in health care financing also reflect a greater acceptance of home care as an alternative to hospitalization. Since 1981, U.S. legislative efforts in the area of financial assistance have made it economically more feasible for families to care for children at home. The Omnibus Reconciliation Act of 1981 (OBRA) resulted in an expansion of Medicaid benefits for U.S. children by financing medical and nonmedical support services and allowing the purchase of equipment to be used in the home. It also expanded Medicaid eligibility by considering only the child's income and essentially disregarding parental income when calculating the allotment of funds. Originally, these waivers were individually approved through the Health Care Financing Administration (HCFA), but in 1982 the Medicaid Home and Community Based waiver program (also known as the Katie Beckett waiver) was developed, allowing each state to establish its own program under the waiver (Burr et al., 1983).

Provided the home is safe and nurturing, children with chronic illnesses or disabilities have a much better chance of optimal development when cared for at home. The cost of home care, although thought to be less than that of hospital care, is still high because many of the children are expected to survive well beyond early childhood. In many cases an often overlooked indirect cost is that the primary caregiver has to leave the workforce to care for the child (Billeaud et al., 1992; Burr et al., 1983; Fields et al., 1991; OTA, 1987; Sevick et al., 1996). Even in the best of situations, the burden on the family continues to be great not only because the family is expected to bear some portion of the financial cost, but also because the psychologic, social, and personal resources necessary to keep a child who is dependent on technology at home are great. As a result, the cost savings often associated with home care can be attributed to the family's willingness to assume the major responsibilities for the day-to-day care of the patient (Sevick & Bradham, 1997; Sevick et al., 1996). Despite this burden, the majority of caregivers report that caring for

their child at home is less stressful than the separation of the child being hospitalized and that they feel that they provide better care than the hospital personnel (Make et al., 1998).

CASE HISTORY

This case illustrates the physical therapy management of a child with ventilator dependence and several comorbidities and uses the *Guide to Physical Therapist Practice* (American Physical Therapy Association, 1997) as a framework for the presentation.

Practice Patterns

Neonate (0 to 5 months): Cardiopulmonary Pattern J: Impaired Ventilation, Respiration and Aerobic Capacity and Endurance Secondary to Respiratory Failure in the Neonate

5 months to 2 years 9 months (age of discharge): **Cardiopulmonary Pattern I:** Impaired Ventilation and Respiration with Mechanical Ventilation Secondary to Respiratory Failure *and* **Neuromuscular Pattern A:** Impaired Motor Function and Sensory Integrity Associated with Congenital or Acquired Disorders of the Central Nervous System in Infancy, Childhood, and Adolescence

---

Initial data collection: Peter was born prematurely at 28 weeks of gestation by cesarean section following onset of preterm labor due to preeclampsia and breech presentation; birth weight was 970 g and Apgar scores were 4^1 and 7^5. Peter's medical history was significant for congenital heart defects, a diaphragmatic hernia, G-tube, grade III intraventricular hemorrhage (IVH), BPD, tracheomalacia, and ventilator dependence with tracheostomy tube placement at 3 months of age.

Peter was hospitalized for the first 5 months of life in the neonatal intensive care unit (NICU). At 5 months chronologic age, Peter was transferred to a pediatric rehabilitation hospital for admission to a pulmonary rehabilitation program. The projected outcomes were determined before his initial admission to justify the transfer to his payer (state Medicaid program) and to assist his parents in their decision making and expectations of the rehabilitation stay. The anticipated outcomes for Peter's hospitalization were as follows: elimination or reduction of impairment (Peter's lung disease); elimination or reduction of functional limitations (developmental delay); elimination or reduction of disability (ability to participate in age-appropriate family and social roles); health promotion for Peter, education for Peter's family, and the prevention of life-limiting illness. Peter's projected discharge disposition was home to the care of his parents with appropriate medical and educational services in place. Peter's team at the rehabilitation hospital included Peter's family, an attending pediatrician, a pediatric pulmonologist, a primary nurse, a physical therapist, an occupational therapist, a speech-language pathologist, a respiratory therapist, a social worker, a dietitian, a case manager, a pastoral care associate, and a child-life specialist. Peter was on multiple medications and had several transfers back to the acute care hospital with readmissions to the rehabilitation facility after acute medical management and stabilization.

Generation of problem statement and functional, time-referenced goals: The problem list and goals were developed from the projected hospitalization outcomes and confirmed based on the results of Peter's physical therapy examination and evaluation. Peter's problem list included ventilator dependence; moderate hypotonia with potential for musculoskeletal deformity due to hypermobility and postural instability, poor endurance and strength, and presence of abnormal movement patterns; delay in acquisition of gross motor skills; and limited opportunity and endurance for sensory, social, and cognitive development.

Physical therapy examination: Peter's age, diagnosis, and medical history, as well as the service delivery setting and reason for referral, were considered with respect to which tests and measures to use (based on the *Guide*). Initial examination findings for Peter included the following:

Arousal, attention, and cognition. Peter did not interact with the therapist or family members (e.g., no eye contact, no smiling) and did not respond to any auditory or visual stimuli by tracking or focusing or attempting to locate sounds; positive startle reaction was noted, and Peter often closed his eyes and cried during interaction.

Aerobic capacity and endurance. Peter's aerobic capacity and endurance were guided by his ventilator settings and monitored by cardiac and apnea monitors, pulse oximetry, and clinical observation and assessment. With physical handling for more than 5 to 10 minutes, Peter became bradycardic and desaturated to 60 to 70% oxygen level; Peter was able to tolerate prone positioning for no more than 15 to 30 seconds before becoming bradycardic and desaturating. With nonphysical interaction, Peter was able to maintain his oxygen saturation level and heart rate but would close his eyes and cry after more than 1 to 2 minutes.

Ventilation, respiration, and circulation. Peter's ventilation, respiration, and circulation were externally con-

trolled and monitored by his ventilator. Peter used a Sechrist ventilator with a synchronized intermittent mandatory ventilation (SIMV) of 40 breaths per minute, a peak inspiratory pressure (PIP) of 25 cm H_2O, a positive end-expiratory pressure (PEEP) of +7 cm H_2O, and an FIo_2 of 0.35 to 0.40%.

Range of motion/joint integrity and mobility. Peter's passive range of motion (ROM) measured within normal limits; noted clonus with tightness at the end range of bilateral ankle dorsiflexion; no pain in response to movement; no limitations or abnormalities in anatomic structures or biomechanical functions.

Muscle performance. Axial and appendicular hypotonia noted; minimal antigravity movement of extremities, no antigravity movement of trunk, and decreased head control in prone and supported sitting positions relative to age-appropriate expectations.

Posture. Symmetric alignment noted in supine position, with exception of preferred head rotation due to position of ventilator tubing; decreased antigravity head and trunk control in supported sitting position (flexible kyphosis).

Reflex integrity. The reflexes emerging or present on initial examination included rooting, sucking, Galant, flexor withdrawal, tonic labyrinthine in prone position, and the positive and negative supporting reactions.

Sensory integrity. Responded to tactile stimulation, movement, and cold temperatures with crying, eye closing, and desaturation.

Integumentary integrity. Noted skin trauma around tracheostomy site due to moisture and friction from tracheostomy ties.

Motor function/neuromotor development and sensory integration. Observed active head turning to the left (approximately 30°) in prone and supine position; unsuccessful attempts at maintaining antigravity head control in supported sitting position; lower extremity extension and weight bearing in supported standing position. On the Peabody Developmental Motor Scales (PDMS) Gross Motor section (Folio & Fewell, 1983), Peter's basal age level was 0 to 1 month and ceiling age level was 2 to 3 months, with an age equivalent of 0 to 1 month at 2 months adjusted age.

Environmental, home, and work (job/school/play) barriers. The physical space in the crib and hospital room revealed limited positioning options due to short ventilator tubing, the position of the tubing on the left side, and excessive lighting and noise in the room.

Evaluation of clinical data/generation of the clinical impression: Peter's motor dysfunction was hypothesized to be the result of neurologic and cardiopulmonary impairments, as well as cognitive, perceptual, social, and environmental factors, including premature birth and extended hospitalization. A physical therapy diagnosis of developmental delay and neuromotor movement dysfunction was made, and the goals for intervention were developed. Peter's physical therapy plan of care included the following major goals during his 2-year stay at the rehabilitation hospital:

Goals	Time frame
1. Tolerance of physical inter-action without desaturation	First 6 months
2. Antigravity head and trunk control in all positions (acqui-sition and maintenance of anti-gravity control) (Fig. 25–3)*	First 6 months
3. Maintenance of joint ROM and mobility	Throughout stay
4. Independent floor mobility for exploration and play	6–12 months
5. Independent acquisition and maintenance of sitting (Fig. 25–4)	6–12 months
6. Independence in transitional skills in all positions from floor through standing	12–18 months
7. Independent standing and ambulation	16–24 months
8. Increased repertoire of move-ment skills	Throughout stay
9. Enhanced opportunities for movement and exploration in the hospital surroundings	6–24 months

---

*Although the child shown in Figures 25–3 through 25–6 is not Peter, his skills and goals are representative of the child in the case.

Intervention

The three components of physical therapy inter-vention—coordination, communication, and docu-mentation; patient-related instruction; and direct in-terventions (American Physical Therapy Association, 1997)—were used throughout Peter's care to encour-age functional independence and for health promo-tion. Interventions focused on these goals with specific activities were geared toward the impairment and functional limitation levels. Throughout Peter's stay, the specific treatment activities were selected and modified based on Peter's level of medical and behav-ioral stability. Treatment frequency was three to five times per week during his rehabilitation stay. Gradually over time, Peter was able to tolerate sessions that lasted up to 45 minutes.

- **Direct Interventions (from the *Guide*)**

Therapeutic exercise: Using age-appropriate develop-mental activities, focused on muscle strengthening and ROM (including soft tissue massage), joint mobility, cardiorespiratory endurance, and balance/coordina-tion in all positions.

Functional training in self-care and home manage-ment: Focused on transitional skills in all positions up through standing.

Functional training in community and work (job/school/ play) integration or reintegration; prescription, application, and fabrication of devices and equipment: Keeping in mind that play is the work of children, assistive devices were used to optimize positioning/mobility and leisure task adaptation (activities promoting motor skill acquisi-tion). Accommodation of the ventilator was a major consideration in the choice of wheeled mobility op-tions (Fig. 25–5).

Airway clearance techniques: Chest percussion, vibra-tion, postural drainage, and suctioning were used by nursing and respiratory therapy to manage Peter's airway.

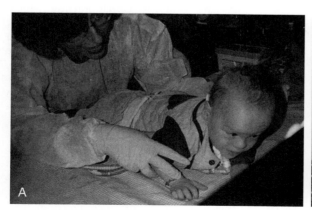 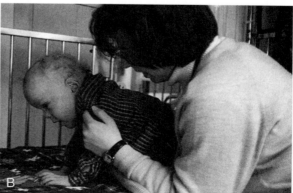

FIGURE 25–3. Goals for the first 6 months of Peter's rehab stay included acquisition and maintenance of antigravity head control *(A)*. Peter struggled with this task but eventually was able to independently achieve and maintain a stable head and neck position *(B)*.

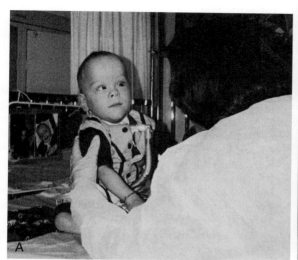

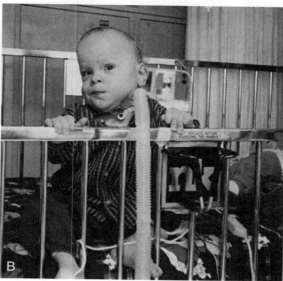

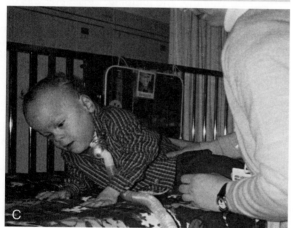

FIGURE 25–4. As Peter's physiologic status stabilized, he was able to tolerate upright sitting without compromise *(A)*. It was several months (after admission) before this task was possible without significant desaturation. Eventually, Peter acquired the ability to sit independently *(B)* and was able to push up to sitting through side lying with assistance *(C)*.

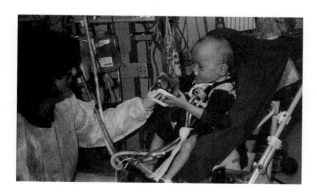

FIGURE 25–5. Until Peter was able to be independently mobile, he used a Graco (commercially available) stroller to increase his independence and to allow him to freely explore his environment. The stroller had to be fitted for transporting a portable ventilator.

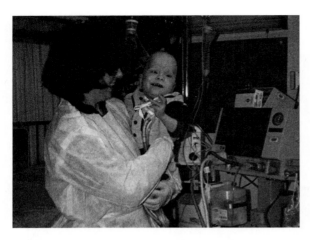

FIGURE 25–6. This was Peter's "world" for the first 2 years of his life. Fortunately, he was able to go home to a less intensive "high-tech environment." Peter was ultimately discharged on supplemental oxygen via his tracheostomy.

- **Coordination, Communication, and Documentation; Patient-Related Instruction**

Beginning at admission, the team worked together to prepare both Peter and his family for his eventual discharge from the rehabilitation center (Fig. 25-6). The patient/family-related instruction for Peter's family was done both formally and informally. Formally, teaching was done through family/team meetings and during his physical therapy sessions. Peter's parents were instructed in the role and rationale of physical therapy services throughout his hospitalization, and ongoing teaching was focused at a functional limitation level, a meaningful level for Peter and his family. The expectations for the family were expressed in terms of their becoming "experts" in his medical care, as well as promoting his developmental (all domains) and fitness goals. Physical therapy teaching concentrated on developmental activities that would facilitate play, motor function, and interaction, as well as addressing equipment needs and use. Carryover of treatment goals by the family and caregivers was emphasized throughout Peter's rehabilitation.

Evaluation of treatment goals: Monthly examinations assessed progress toward established goals and were used to determine the appropriate ongoing treatment frequency. The use of the Peabody Developmental Motor Scales was discontinued after the initial assessment, and the Gross Motor Function Measure (GMFM) (Russell et al., 1993) was then used every 3 to 6 months to assess qualitative and functional changes in neuromotor function.

Ventilatory status: Before discharge, Peter was eventually weaned from the ventilator using CPAP during the transition. Once off CPAP, Peter was weaned to a 30% supplemental oxygen requirement via his tracheostomy tube. Throughout his hospitalization, changes in Peter's cardiopulmonary status and progress in his ventilator weaning affected his ability to participate in activities requiring physical exertion. Events such as a change in ventilatory settings, a tracheostomy change, a bronchoscopy, or the need for frequent suctioning often resulted in a deferred physical therapy session or a change in the intensity of the activities to avoid undue distress.

Discharge status: Peter was discharged home to the care of his family 2 years and 3 months after admission. He required home nursing services because of his tracheostomy tube and the 30% supplementary oxygen requirement. Peter was enrolled in an early intervention program and received physical therapy, occupational therapy, and speech-language therapy. Peter still demonstrated the need for further physical therapy because he continued to demonstrate motor delays and deviances. Peter's GMFM scores at discharge were as follows: lying and rolling, 100%; sitting, 95%; crawling and kneeling, 76%; standing, 76%; and walking, running, and jumping, 29%. Peter was using a Passey-Muir valve to allow for early vocalization in combination with early sign language. After entering school the following September, therapy services were delivered as part of his school programs outlined in an individualized education plan.

SUMMARY

Because of improved medical and technologic management, a large number of children who are mechanically ventilated are likely to survive and eventually be discharged from the intensive care environment. More than likely, the rate of medical and technologic progress will continue to exceed the strides made in rehabilitation and prevention of disabilities and in policies that support an uncomplicated transition into the home and community.

Although physical therapists can do little to prevent chronic respiratory failure and ventilator dependence, they have an important role to play in fostering the child's development and endurance for physical activity. Uncertainty regarding the prognosis for weaning from the ventilator or a child's prognosis for a productive and independent life may persist for an extended period of time. For the family there is the additional stress relating to the child's fragile medical status and the constant possibility of sudden death if the mechanical equipment should fail. When children go home on mechanical ventilation, normal family routines are replaced with highly structured schedules with little room for spontaneity. It is essential that health care professionals present the parents with a realistic picture of the benefits, cost, and burden of caring for a child at home and help them realize that advanced technologic capacity does not necessarily ensure or equate to a benefit for the patient or the family (Mallory & Stillwell, 1991).

From early on in the neonatal intensive care unit through school age, physical therapists are in a unique position to be involved with these children and families. Some aspects of care may be specific medically related interventions, such as percussion and postural drainage; however, the majority of time is spent addressing various aspects of the child's development. In dealing with any population at risk for disability, one of the major roles of physical therapists is to integrate treatment goals into everyday activities and help the caregivers or parents appreciate the relevance of their involvement. The ecologic validity of the treatment goals increases if those goals are made a part of functionally relevant tasks.

The care of this group of children will continue to be a challenge to physical therapists and other health care professionals because they possess a wide range of impairments, functional limitations, and disabilities. One should not expect uniformity in the examination and treatment of these children. This should not be discouraging, but should force physical therapists to organize clinical judgments according to the "disabling" dimension that most clearly affects the child's ultimate functional outcome.

Recommended Resources

Bregman, J, & Farrell, EE. Neurodevelopmental outcome in infants with bronchopulmonary dysplasia. Clinics in Perinatology, 19: 673–694, 1992.

Capen, CL, & Dedlow, ER. Discharging ventilator-dependent children: A continuing challenge. Journal of Pediatric Nursing, 13(3):175–184, 1998.

Gould, A. Cardiopulmonary evaluation of the infant, toddler, child, and adolescent. Pediatric Physical Therapy, 3:9–13, 1991.

Make, BJ, Hill, NS, Goldberg, AI, Bach, JR, Criner, GJ, Dunne, PE, Gilmartin, ME, Heffner, JE, Kacmarek, R, Keen, TG, Oppenheimer, EA, & Dominique, R. Mechanical ventilation beyond the intensive care unit: Report of a Consensus Conference of the American College of Chest Physicians. Chest, 113(5):289S–344S, 1998.

Mallory, GB, & Stillwell, PC. The ventilator-dependent child: Issues in diagnosis and management. Archives of Physical Medicine and Rehabilitation, 72:43–55, 1991.

McKibben, AW, & Ravenscraft, SA. Pressure-controlled and volume-cycled mechanical ventilation. Clinics in Chest Medicine, 17(3): 395–410, 1996.

Pilmer, SL. Prolonged mechanical ventilation in children. Pediatric Clinics of North America, 41(3):473–512, 1994.

Parents and professionals might be interested in the International Ventilator Users Network (IVUN), 5100 Oakland Ave, #206, St. Louis, MO 63110-1406. The IVUN is a worldwide network of ventilator users and health professionals. This group is a strong advocate for home care and long-term ventilation and provides numerous resources for professionals, patients, and families of children with ventilator dependence.

References

American Physical Therapy Association. Guide to physical therapist practice. Physical Therapy, 77(11):1371–1382, 1536–1555, 1997.

American Thoracic Society. Home mechanical ventilation of pediatric patients. American Review of Respiratory Disease, 141:258–259, 1990.

Andrews, MM, & Nielson, DW. Technology-dependent children in the home. Pediatric Nursing, 14:111–151, 1988.

Bach JR, Intinola, P, Alba, AS, & Holland, IE. The ventilator-assisted individual: Cost analysis of institutionalization vs rehabilitation and in-home management. Chest, 101:26–30, 1990.

Bader, D, Ramos, AD, Lew, CD, Platzker, ACG, Stabile, MW, & Keens, TG. Childhood sequelae of infant lung disease: Exercise and pulmonary function abnormalities after bronchopulmonary dysplasia. Journal of Pediatrics, 110:693–699, 1987.

Bai, DL, & Bertenthal, BI. Locomotor status and the development of spatial search skills. Child Development, 63:215–226, 1992.

Bancalari, E, & Sosenko, I. Pathogenesis and prevention of neonatal chronic lung disease: Recent developments. Pediatric Pulmonology, 8:109–116, 1990.

Bar-Or, O. Pathophysiological factors which limit the exercise capacity of the sick child. Medicine and Science in Sports and Exercise, 18:276–282, 1986.

Billeaud, C, Piedboeuf, B, & Chessex, P. Energy expenditure and severity of respiratory disease in very low birth weight infants receiving long-term ventilatory support. Journal of Pediatrics, 120:461–464, 1992.

Bos, AF, Martijn, A, van Asperen, RM, Hadders-Algra, M, Okken, A, & Prechtl, HFR. Qualitative assessment of general movements in high-risk preterm infants with chronic lung disease requiring dexamethasone therapy. Journal of Pediatrics, 132:300–306, 1998.

Bozynski, MEA, Nelson, MN, Matalon, TAS, O'Donnell, KJ, Naughton, PM, Vasan, U, Meier, WA, & Ploughman, L. Prolonged mechanical ventilation and intracranial hemorrhage: Impact on developmental progress through 18 months in infants weighing 1,200 grams or less at birth. Pediatrics, 79:670–676, 1987.

Brazy, JE, Kinney, HC, & Oakes, WJ. CNS structural lesions causing apnea at birth. Journal of Pediatrics, 111:163–175, 1987.

Bregman, J, & Farrell, EE. Neurodevelopmental outcome in infants with bronchopulmonary dysplasia. Clinics in Perinatology, 19: 673–694, 1992.

Bureau, MA, & Begin, R. Chest wall diseases and dysfunction in children. In Kendig, EL, & Chernick, V (Eds.), Disorders of the Respiratory Tract in Children. Philadelphia: WB Saunders, 1983, pp. 601–616.

Burr, BH, Guyer, B, Todres, ID, Abrahams, B, & Chiodo, T. Home care for children on respirators. New England Journal of Medicine, 21:1319–1323, 1983.

Campbell, DA, & Pierce, RJ. Long-term ventilatory support at home: Any progress? Medical Journal of Australia, 168:7–8, 1998.

Comer, DM. Pulse oximetry: Implications for practice. Journal of Obstetric, Gynecologic, and Neonatal Nursing, 21:35–41, 1992.

Crane, LD. Physical therapy for the neonate with respiratory disease. In Irwin, S, & Tecklin, JS (Eds.), Cardiopulmonary Physical Therapy. St. Louis: Mosby, 1990, pp. 389–416.

Criner, GJ, Tzouanakis, A, & Kreimer, DT. Overview of improving tolerance of long-term mechanical ventilation. Critical Care Clinics, 10(4):845–865, 1994.

Cutz, E, Ma, TKF, Perrin, DG, Moore, AM, & Becker, LE. Peripheral chemoreceptors in congenital central hypoventilation syndrome. American Journal of Respiratory and Critical Care Medicine, 155: 358–363, 1997.

Darbee, J, & Cerny, F. Exercise testing and exercise conditioning for children with lung dysfunction. In Irwin, S, & Tecklin, JS (Eds.), Cardiopulmonary Physical Therapy. St. Louis: Mosby, 1990, pp. 461–476.

DeCesare, JA, & Graybill, CA. Physical therapy for the child with respiratory dysfunction. In Irwin, S, & Tecklin, JS (Eds.), Cardiopulmonary Physical Therapy. St. Louis: Mosby, 1990, pp. 417–460.

DeWitt, PK, Jansen, MT, Davidson Ward, SL, & Keens, TG. Obstacles to discharge of ventilator-assisted children from the hospital to home. Chest, 103:1560–1565, 1993.

Dick, CR, & Sassoon, CSH. Patient-ventilator interactions. Clinics in Chest Medicine, 17(3):423–438, 1996.

Dougherty, JM. Negative pressure devices in pediatric practice. Pediatric Nursing, 16(2):135–138, 1990. pp. 328–341.

Elixson, EM, Myrer, ML, & Horn, MH. Current trends in ventilation of the pediatric patient. Critical Care Nursing Quarterly, 20(1):1–13, 1997.

Escalona, SK. Babies at double hazard: Early development of infants at biologic and social risk. Pediatrics, 70:670–676, 1982.

Farrell, PM, & Fost, NC. Long-term mechanical ventilation in pediatric respiratory failure: Medical and ethical considerations. American Review of Respiratory Disease, 140:S36–S40, 1989.

Fields, AI, Rosenblatt, A, Pollack, MM, & Kaufman, J. Home care cost-effectiveness for respiratory technology-dependent children. American Journal of Diseases in Children, 145:729–733, 1991.

Folio, MR, & Fewell, RR. Peabody Developmental Motor Scales and Activity Cards. Allen, TX: DLM Teaching Resources, 1983.

Frates, RC, Splaingard, ML, Smith, EO, & Harrison, GM. Outcome of home mechanical ventilation in children. Journal of Pediatrics, 106:850–856, 1985.

Froese, AB. Mechanical ventilation. In Chernick, V, & Mellins, RB (Eds.), Basic Mechanisms of Pediatric Respiratory Disease: Cellular and Integrative. Philadelphia: BC Decker, 1991, pp. 418–431.

Gannon, CM, Wiswell, TE, & Spitzer, AR. Volutrauma, Paco$_2$ levels, and neurodevelopmental sequelae following assisted ventilation. Clinics in Perinatology, 25(1):159–175, 1998.

Goldsmith, JP, & Karotkin, EH. Assisted Ventilation of the Neonate, 2nd ed. Philadelphia: WB Saunders, 1988.

Gould, A. Cardiopulmonary evaluation of the infant, toddler, child, and adolescent. Pediatric Physical Therapy, 3:9–13, 1991.

Gozal, D, Shoseyev, D, & Keens, TG. Inspiratory pressures with CO$_2$ stimulation and weaning from mechanical ventilation in children. American Review of Respiratory Diseases, 147:256–261, 1993.

Gregoire, MC, Lefebvre, F, & Glorieux, J. Health and developmental outcomes at 18 months in very preterm infants with bronchopulmonary dysplasia. Pediatrics, 101:856–860, 1998.

Haley, SM, Baryza, MJ, & Blanchard, Y. Functional and naturalistic frameworks in assessing physical and motor disablement. In Wilhelm, IJ (Ed.), Physical Therapy Assessment in Early Infancy. New York: Churchill Livingstone, 1993, pp. 225–256.

Hodgkin, JE, Gray, LS, & Burton, GG. Techniques of ventilatory weaning. In Burton, GG, & Hodgkin, JE (Eds.), Respiratory Care: A Guide to Clinical Practice. Philadelphia: JB Lippincott, 1984, pp. 648–655.

Hunt, J, Cooper, B, & Tooley, W. Very low birthweight infants at 8 and 11 years of age: Role of neonatal illness and family status. Pediatrics, 82:596–603, 1988.

Kao, LC, Durand, DJ, & Nickerson, BG. Improving pulmonary function does not decrease oxygen consumption in infants with bronchopulmonary dysplasia. Journal of Pediatrics, 112:616–621, 1988.

Kirby, RR, Banner, MJ, & Downs, JB (Eds.). Clinical Applications of Ventilatory Support. New York: Churchill Livingstone, 1990, pp. 173–198.

Knisely, AS, Leal, SM, & Singer, DB. Abnormalities of diaphragmatic muscle in neonates with ventilated lungs. Journal of Pediatrics, 113:1074–1077, 1988.

Kolobe, THA. Working with families of children with disabilities. Pediatric Physical Therapy, 4:57–62, 1992.

Kornhauser, MS, Baumgart, S, Desai, SA, Stanley, CW, Culbane, J, Cullen, JA, Wiswell, TE, Graziani, LJ, & Spitzer, AR. Adverse neurodevelopmental outcome after extracorporeal membrane oxygenation among neonates with bronchopulmonary dysplasia. Journal of Pediatrics, 132:307–311, 1998.

Kurzner, SI, Garg, M, Bautista, DB, Sargent, CW, Bowman, M, & Keen, TG. Growth failure in bronchopulmonary dysplasia: Elevated metabolic rates and pulmonary mechanics. Journal of Pediatrics, 112:73–80, 1988.

Lantos, JD, & Kohrman, AF. Ethical aspects of pediatric home care. Pediatrics, 89:920–924, 1992.

Leonard, BJ, Brus, JD, & Choi, T. Medicaid model waiver program. Public Health Reports, 104:465–472, 1989.

Luce, JM. Reducing the use of mechanical ventilation. The New England Journal of Medicine, 335:1916–1917, 1996.

MacKinnon, JA, Perlman, M, Kirpalani, H, Rehan, V, Sauve, R, & Kovacs, L. Spinal cord injury at birth: Diagnostic and prognostic data in twenty-two patients. Journal of Pediatrics, 122:431–437, 1993.

Make, BJ, Hill, NS, Goldberg, AI, Bach, JR, Criner, GJ, Dunne, PE, Gilmartin, ME, Heffner, JE, Kacmarek, R, Keen, TG, Oppenheimer, EA, & Dominique, R. Mechanical ventilation beyond the intensive care unit: Report of a Consensus Conference of the American College of Chest Physicians. Chest, 113(5):289S–344S, 1998.

Mallory, GB, & Stillwell, PC. The ventilator-dependent child: Issues in diagnosis and management. Archives of Physical Medicine and Rehabilitation, 72:43–55, 1991.

McPherson, SP. Respiratory Care Equipment. St. Louis: Mosby, 1995.

Meisels, SJ, Plunkett, JW, Roloff, DW, Pasick, PL, & Steifel, GS. Growth and development of preterm infants with respiratory distress syndrome and bronchopulmonary dysplasia. Pediatrics, 77:345–352, 1986.

Northway, WH. Observations on bronchopulmonary dysplasia. Journal of Pediatrics, 95:815–817, 1979.

Null, D, Berman, LS, & Clark, R. Neonatal and pediatric ventilatory support. In Kirby, RR, Banner, MJ, & Downs, JB (Eds.), Clinical Applications of Ventilatory Support. New York: Churchill Livingstone, 1990, pp. 199–238.

Office of Technology Assessment. Technology-Dependent Children: Home vs Hospital Care. A Technical Memorandum. Washington, DC: U.S. Government Printing Office, 1987.

O'Shea, TM, Goldstein, DJ, de Regnier, RA, Sheaffer, CI, Roberts, DD, & Dillard, RG. Outcome at 4 to 5 years of age in children recovered from neonatal chronic lung disease. Developmental Medicine & Child Neurology, 38:830–839, 1996.

Pagtakhan, RD, & Chernick, V. Intensive care for respiratory disorders. In Kendig, EL, & Chernick, V (Eds.), Disorders of the Respiratory Tract in Children, 4th ed. Philadelphia: WB Saunders, 1983, pp. 145–168.

Perel, A, & Stock, MC. Introduction to ventilatory support. In Perel, A, & Stock, MC (Eds.), Handbook of Mechanical Ventilatory Support. Baltimore: Williams & Wilkins, 1992, pp. 3–6.

Pilmer, SL. Prolonged mechanical ventilation in children. Pediatric Clinics of North America, 41(3):473–512, 1994.

Quint, RD, Chesterman, E, Crain, LS, Winkleby, M, & Boyce, WT. Home care for ventilator-dependent children: Psychosocial impact on the family. American Journal of Diseases in Children, 144:1238–1241, 1990.

Rasanen, J, & Downs, JB. Modes of mechanical ventilatory support. In Kirby, RR, Banner, MJ, & Downs, JB (Eds.), Clinical Applications of Ventilatory Support. New York: Churchill Livingstone, 1990, pp. 173–198.

Raulin, AM, & Shannon, KA. PNPs: Case managers for technology-dependent children. Pediatric Nursing, 12:338–340, 1986.

Roussos, C. Ventilatory failure and respiratory muscles. Lung Biology in Health and Disease, 29:1253–1279, 1985.

Russell, DJ, Rosenbaum, PL, Gowland, C, Hardy, S, Lane, M, Plews, N, McGavin, H, Cadman, D, & Jarvis, S. Gross Motor Function Measure Manual, 2nd ed. Owen Sound, Ontario, Canada: Gross Motor Measures Group, 1993.

Schaaf, RC, & Davis, WS. Promoting health and wellness in the pediatric disabled and "at risk" population. In Rothman, J, & Levine, R (Eds.), Prevention Practice: Strategies for Physical Therapy and Occupational Therapy. Philadelphia: WB Saunders, 1992, pp. 270-283.

Schafer, DS, Spalding, JB, & Bell, AP. Potential predictors of child progress as measured by the Early Intervention Developmental Profile. Journal of the Division for Early Childhood, 11(2):106-117, 1987.

Schreiner, MS, Donar, ME, & Kettrick, RG. Pediatric home ventilation. Pediatric Clinics of North America, 34:47-60, 1987.

Sevick, MA, & Bradham, DD. Economic value of caregiver effort in maintaining long-term ventilator-assisted individuals at home. Heart and Lung, 26:148-157, 1997.

Sevick, MA, Kamlet, MS, Hoffman, LA, & Rawson, I. Economic cost of home-based care for ventilator-assisted individuals. Chest, 109:1597-1606, 1996.

Shneerson, JM. Techniques in mechanical ventilation: Principles and practice. Thorax, 51:756-761, 1996.

Singer, L, Yamashita, T, Lilien, L, Collin, M, & Baley, J. A longitudinal study of developmental outcome of infants with bronchopulmonary dysplasia and very low birth weight. Pediatrics, 100:987-993, 1997.

Slater, MA, Naqvi, M, Andrew, L, & Haynes, K. Neurodevelopment of monitored vs nonmonitored very low birth weight infants: The importance of family influences. Developmental and Behavioral Pediatrics, 8:278-285, 1987.

Soll, RF. Synthetic surfactant treatment for preterm infants with respiratory distress syndrome (Cochrane Review). In The Cochrane Library, Issue 4, 1998. Oxford: Update Software.

Tremolieres, F. Description of a ventilator. In Lemaire, F (Ed.), Mechanical Ventilation. New York: Springer-Verlag, 1991, pp. 3-18.

Waring, WW. The history and physical examination. In Kendig, EL, & Chernick, V (Eds.), Disorders of the Respiratory Tract in Children. Philadelphia: WB Saunders, 1983, pp. 57-78.

Watchko, JF, Mayock, DE, Standaert, TA, & Woodrum, DE. The ventilatory pump: Neonatal and developmental issues. Advances in Pediatrics, 38:109-134, 1991.

Weese-Mayer, DE, Silvestri, JM, Menzies, LJ, Morrow-Kenny, AS, Hunt, CE, & Hauptman, SA. Congenital central hypoventilation syndrome: Diagnosis, management, and long-term outcome in thirty-two children. Journal of Pediatrics, 120:381-387, 1992.

Weinstein, MR, & Oh, W. Oxygen consumption in infants with BPD. Journal of Pediatrics, 99:958-961, 1981.

Woo, MS, Woo, MA, Gozal, D, Jansen, MT, Keens, TG, & Harper, RM. Heart rate variability in congenital central hypoventilation syndrome. Pediatric Research, 31:291-296, 1992.

Yu, VYH, Orgill, AA, Lim, SB, Bajuk, B, & Astbury, J. Growth and development of very low birthweight infants recovering from bronchopulmonary dysplasia. Archives of Disease in Childhood, 58:791-794, 1983.

CHAPTER

26

Cystic Fibrosis

JO A. ASHWELL, BScPT
JENNIFER L. AGNEW-COUGHLIN, BScPT, BHK

Cystic fibrosis (CF) was first defined as a clinical entity 60 years ago when Andersen published a paper describing the clinical course of a number of children who had died of pulmonary and digestive problems. She labeled the disorder "cystic fibrosis of the pancreas" (Andersen, 1938). This disease was thereafter classified as a disorder of exocrine gland function, influencing the respiratory system, pancreas, reproductive organs, and sweat glands. At times the first presenting sign has been the subjective report "my child tastes salty to kiss"; the "sweat test" has confirmed the diagnosis. Subsequent study and interest led to clearer understanding of the disease and a coordinated approach to treating the associated impairments. Over time the disorder that had so intrigued Andersen has come to be known as cystic fibrosis, and research has continued, yielding a vast knowledge base about this chronic illness. In 1989 a major scientific breakthrough occurred with discovery of the precise locus on chromosome 7 of the gene responsible for CF (Riordan et al., 1989). Investigations and research have followed to define the pathologic basis of the physical manifestations of CF.

Although at present the time-honored definition of this disease as the most commonly inherited life-shortening illness in the white population remains appropriate, our present growing understanding of CF may prove to temper its impact. More research must be done before treatment may allow people with CF to lead lives free of the complications currently implicit in this diagnosis. Current management of the manifestations of CF has, however, promoted improved quality of life and a better prognosis for life expectancy for people with CF (MacLusky & Levison, 1990).

Classified as a hereditary disease, CF has long been understood to be inherited in an autosomal recessive pattern (MacLusky & Levison, 1990). Two copies of the gene responsible for CF are inherited by an affected individual. Both parents of a child diagnosed with CF are, therefore, known to be carriers of at least one copy of a mutation at the gene locus responsible for CF. Those persons with one copy of the CF gene are termed *heterozygote carriers* and are not diagnostically positive for CF.

CF is diagnosed in 1 in 2000 children born to white parents, and statistical analysis of this incidence yields a best estimate of the rate of heterozygote carriers as about 5% of the population in areas of the world where significant white populations have settled (MacLusky et al., 1987). The incidence of CF in African, African-American, and Asian peoples is considerably lower than that in whites—approximately 1 in 17,000 births in the African-American population and an estimated 1 in 90,000 births in Asian societies (MacLusky et al., 1987). Recent research and new possibilities for carrier screening are producing more precise statistical estimates of the actual incidence of individuals who are heterozygote CF carriers, suggesting that previous rates were underestimated (Witt et al., 1992). Prenatal diagnosis of CF is now sometimes possible, as is screening for carrier status, which is discussed in detail later in this chapter.

The identification in 1989 of the site of the gene responsible for CF by an international team of researchers, led by Drs. Tsui, Collins, and Riordan, was an extraordinary achievement in molecular genetics (Kerem et al., 1989). Subsequent research advances in numerous laboratories worldwide have yielded an unprecedented quantity of data on the genetic and pathologic components of CF. Well over 600 distinct mutations within the CF gene have been identified. A specific trinucleotide deletion (delta-F508, resulting in the loss of phenylalanine from the product protein) is the most common mutation associated with clinical CF, identified in 70% of patients. Various degrees of disease expression are associated with the different mutations, and significant variability exists in the incidence of the different mutations in ethnic populations (MacLusky & Levison, 1998).

The nature of the disease, its multisystemic involvement, and the variety of needs of affected individuals and their families dictate that professional intervention in the management of CF is generally concentrated in regional CF clinics. Comprehensive treatment programs for CF were established about 35 years ago (Doershuk et al., 1964) and are now the primary mode of delivery of associated health care needs. CF centers can offer their clients the services of respirologists, gastroenterologists, physical therapists, dietitians, psychologic and genetic counselors, social workers, and specialty care nursing personnel. These multidisciplinary teams are dedicated to the delivery of the most effective and palatable treatments available in promoting the optimal level of well-being for their patients with CF. The team can offer crucial support to affected families. Worldwide, CF centers are also dedicated to the collaborative process, as clinical expertise and the knowledge base expand to suggest new possibilities in the treatment of this disease and new hopes for an ultimate cure.

In this chapter considerations for choosing appropriate intervention for patients with CF are outlined. An increasing number of people with CF are reaching the third and even fourth decades of life (Orenstein, 1997), and surgical advances in lung transplantation offer hope of prolonging life for people with chronic pulmonary disabilities. Physical therapists are serving an expanded role in management programs for people with CF. It is of crucial importance that clinical decisions be directed by careful consideration of the available scientific evidence and that therapists continue to seek out the means to scientifically evaluate empiric experiences. A clear understanding of the pathophysiology, etiology, diagnostic indicators, methods of examination, and medical management is essential for the physical therapist working with the CF population to ensure a comprehensive incorporation of the issues in developing management strategies and goals. The reader is also urged to consult the appropriate sections of the *Guide to Physical Therapist Practice* (section 6H 1-5 is particularly helpful) (American Physical Therapy Association, 1997) whenever designing or reevaluating the management or process of examining clients with CF. A discussion of the evolution of self-management through infancy, for preschool and school-age children, and during adolescence and adulthood is included. Improving adherence to a plan of care through the promotion of self-efficacy may prove to enhance the effectiveness of treatment and help prevent or delay the onset of functional impairments characteristic of this disorder. As a result, well-being and improved quality of life will be promoted.

PATHOPHYSIOLOGY

The primary pathologic feature of CF is obstruction of mucus-secreting exocrine glands by hyperviscous secretions (MacLusky et al., 1987). Blockage of exocrine gland products prevents their delivery to target tissues and organs and creates clinical abnormalities in these body systems. The most impaired organs are the lungs and pancreas, with significant involvement of the reproductive system, sinuses, and sweat glands. An elevated level of sodium chloride in the sweat has been the principal diagnostic indicator for CF for almost 40 years (Gibson & Cooke, 1959).

The pulmonary impairments of CF are characterized by accumulation of hyperviscous secretions leading to progressive airway obstruction, secondary infection by opportunistic bacteria, inflammation, and subsequent bronchiectasis and irreversible airway damage. Airways may be further obstructed by bronchoconstriction. Impaired respiratory muscle function under conditions of malnutrition and weakness or deconditioning also has an impact on progression of the functional limitations of the respiratory system in patients with CF, as does the mechanical disadvantage that results from chronic lung hyperinflation.

The obstruction of the small airways in CF and subsequent air trapping and atelectasis result in ventilation and perfusion mismatching, which leads to hypoxemia. Long-standing hypoxemia may result in pulmonary artery hypertension and cor pulmonale or right ventricular failure. Large airway bronchiectasis combined with small airway obstruction reduces vital capacity and tidal volume and results in decreased volumes of air flow at the alveolar level and a progressively increasing arterial carbon dioxide tension ($Paco_2$), which may lead to hypercapnic respiratory failure (Yankaskas, 1992). Respiratory failure accounts for 95% of the mortality rate in CF (Orenstein, 1997).

Viscous secretions begin to obstruct the pancreatic duct in utero, and periductal inflammation and fibrosis cause the loss of the pancreatic exocrine function. The resulting maldigestion of fats and protein leaves the pancreatic-insufficient patient with clinical steatorrhea (Durie et al., 1984); the stools are described as bulky, frequent, and "greasy" and, perhaps most noticeably, as having a strongly offensive odor. In infancy, patients with CF can display evidence of protein-calorie malnutrition with a protruding abdomen, muscle wasting, and initial diagnosis of failure to thrive despite the reports from parents of these children's hearty appetites (MacLusky & Levison, 1990). Compensating for loss of pancreatic function remains a critical feature of management throughout these children's lives.

Another pathologic finding that presents in 10 to 15% of diagnosed cases of CF, is meconium ileus which is demonstrated in neonates (Park & Grand, 1981). The combination of abnormal pancreatic function and hyperviscous secretions of the intestinal glands creates an altered viscosity of the meconium causing an obstruction at the distal ileum, thus preventing passage of meconium in the first neonatal days (MacLusky & Levison, 1990). Distal intestinal obstruction is seen in some older patients, associated with abnormal intestinal secretions and increased adherence of mucus in the intestines (Durie, 1988).

Abnormal secretions may cause hepatobiliary involvement, recurrent pancreatitis, and, for about 7% of patients with CF, diabetes mellitus (MacLusky & Levison, 1990). Obstruction of the vas deferens causes infertility in 98% of males with CF (Taussig et al., 1972). The fertility rate in females with CF is estimated as 20 to 30% of normal (Matson & Capen, 1982).

In the upper respiratory tract, sinusitis may cause persistent headache, and nasal polyps occur in 7 to 26% of patients with CF and often necessitate surgical resection. There is a 50 to 80% recurrence rate of nasal polyps once polypectomy is performed (MacLusky et al., 1987). Hypertrophic pulmonary osteoarthropathy is often associated with advanced severity of pulmonary disease and is most noticeable in the clinical finding of "clubbing," which is rounded hypertrophic changes in the terminal phalanges of the fingers and toes (MacLusky & Levison, 1990).

ETIOLOGY

The etiology of CF is traced to the abnormal gene product, the cystic fibrosis transmembrane conductance regulator (CFTR) protein, which seems to be most abundantly expressed in the apical membrane surface of epithelial cells of the respiratory, gastrointestinal, reproductive, and sweat glands (Collins, 1992). Normal epithelial cells secrete fluid by allowing chloride (a negatively charged ion) to pass through the luminal membrane of the cell. Because this membrane is permeable to sodium (positively charged), it passively follows; increased levels of sodium chloride then stimulate fluid secretion. Fluid levels in the airways must be maintained at a sufficient level to provide for normal mucociliary transport. Structural defects in the CFTR protein lead to abnormalities in cell membrane function. The resulting electrolyte abnormality (chloride impermeability and sodium hyperpermeability) results in abnormal amounts of fluid being removed from the airway lumen, which results in thick, dry mucus (MacLusky & Levison, 1998). Abnormal expression of the CFTR protein in airway epithelial cells is the primary cause of the respiratory manifestations of CF.

A main focus of current research in CF is aimed at normalizing the defective electrolyte transport of the epithelium. This may be achieved in various ways, either by transferring normally functioning genes into the CFTR gene locus or by mediating the chloride channel by other means (Orenstein, 1997). Research on various gene transfer techniques will be further discussed in this chapter.

DIAGNOSIS AND MEDICAL MANAGEMENT

Early diagnosis, including prenatal determination of the presence of CF gene mutation, has enabled researchers to follow the expression and progression of the disease from birth in many patients. Impairment of the respiratory system does not manifest immediately, and at birth the lungs appear normal on radiologic examination. In the most distal small airways, however, dilation and hypertrophy of mucus-secreting goblet cells begins early in life and subsequent impaired mucociliary clearance can cause obstructive mucus plugs and associated air trapping and atelectasis. Signs of hyperinflation may be present on radiography. The presentation of infants with failure to thrive and nutritional losses through steatorrhea accounts for up to 85% of the cases of CF diagnosed in infancy. A history of respiratory illness such as repeated respiratory tract infections, recurrent bronchiolitis, or even pneumonia is often reported, but in 80% of newly diagnosed cases, there is no known family history of CF (MacLusky & Levison, 1998).

A quantitative pilocarpine iontophoresis sweat test, an analysis of chloride levels in the sweat, is the accepted test to confirm the diagnosis of CF. Because of the quantity of sweat required to provide an accurate analysis and the difficulty in inducing adequate amounts when testing infants in the first few months of life, positive diagnosis may be delayed until a valid test can be performed. Values greater than 60 mEq/L of sweat chloride are considered positive for CF (MacLusky & Levison, 1998).

In the few centers with the capacity (the specialized laboratory and the trained personnel), another diagnostic test, nasal potential difference (PD), is possible. This test measures the electrical charge (potential difference) across the epithelial surface (mucous membrane) of the nose. In normal subjects a small charge of −5 to −30 mV is present, whereas subjects with CF demonstrate values between −40 and −80 mV (Orenstein, 1997).

Screening tests for prospective parents who are known carriers (with prior offspring with CF or with CF themselves) are now possible and raise a number of ethical issues when CF is suggested prenatally. Genetic counseling is therefore available at CF centers. Analysis of the blood of known heterozygote parents and tissue from the fetus obtained through amniocentesis or chorionic villi sampling can determine the presence of the CF gene mutation common to the family history. With identity of the same pattern of inherited genetic material in the fetus as in an affected sibling, there is a 98% probability the fetus is also affected (Dean et al., 1987). Mass carrier screening in prenatal populations of up to 4000 women has been undertaken in both the United States and England to investigate the value and feasibility of population screening for CF heterozygotes. In California, where 6 to 12 of the most common mutations were sought, this type of screening identified more than 90 female heterozygotes. Screening of their partners revealed five male heterozygotes and therefore five high-risk pregnancies (Witt et al.,

1992). Among adults with CF and parents of affected children, attitudes and debate about prenatal diagnosis and heterozygote screening reflect a variety of concerns. Although up to 74% of questioned adults with CF in one study reported supporting carrier testing of their siblings (Lemke et al., 1992) and 93% supported screening for carriers in the general population, only a minority saw prenatal diagnosis as an absolute indication for termination of pregnancy (Conway & Allenby, 1992). The future of carrier screening and any possible effects prenatal diagnosis may have on the incidence rate of CF remain to be seen.

Medical management of pulmonary disability in CF generally focuses on attempts to limit the effects of impairments in the disease, namely, the airway obstruction due to chronic bronchorrhea (abnormal mucus secretions) and the progressive inflammation that is secondary to chronic bacterial colonization (MacLusky et al., 1987). Nutritional management is also vitally important because most patients with CF will have some pancreatic insufficiency and therefore require enzyme supplementation to compensate for losses of enzymes crucial to fat and protein digestion. Patients are followed periodically, and quantitative sputum cultures are regularly performed. (Clinics vary as to frequency of assessment; generally, appointments are made every 3 months.) Radiologic assessment, pulmonary function testing (PFT), nutritional status, and any pattern of weight loss combined with subjective reports of treatment adherence assist the CF clinical team to gauge the ever-changing therapeutic needs of patients with CF and to initiate treatment regimens with the aim of preventing or slowing development of the functional limitations of CF.

Throughout their lives, most people with CF battle the tendency toward malnutrition that comes from protein and calorie deficits. Special attention to a properly balanced, high-calorie diet with supplementary pancreatic enzymes requires acceptance and compliance in patients of all ages with CF but may aid in slowing the rate of deterioration of lung function. During acute episodes of respiratory exacerbations, the anorexia that accompanies the frequent racking cough, increase in mucus production, and increased work of breathing poses a challenge to provide adequate nutritional intake. Levels of resting energy expenditure are reportedly higher in patients with CF with more progressive pulmonary disease (Fried et al., 1991; Spicher et al., 1991), and this has implications for the degree of caloric input necessary for patients with advanced pulmonary dysfunction. Caloric supplementation may be necessary in the form of feedings given nasogastrically or intravenously. Nutritional management for patients with intractable weight loss can be provided by nocturnal feedings through indwelling gastrostomy or jejunostomy tubes (MacLusky & Levison, 1990).

Most of the morbidity seen in CF is associated with deteriorating pulmonary status; medical intervention is, therefore, focused on attempts to influence the rate of progression of the pathogenesis of pulmonary dysfunction in CF. Antibiotic therapy appears to have significantly influenced the effects of the chronic endobronchial colonization that typifies CF and has been a mainstay of treatment regimens for 30 years (MacLusky & Levison, 1990). Sputum cultures show colonization by a number of organisms in a common pattern that changes with severity of disease and age of the patient. *Staphylococcus aureus, Pseudomonas aeruginosa, Burkholderia cepacia, Haemophilus influenzae,* and *Klebsiella* are the organisms most commonly seen. Combinations of colonizing organisms are common, particularly when disease severity and age of the patient advance. Prophylactic antibiotics are advocated by some but remain controversial. Inhaled antibiotics, such as the aminoglycosides tobramycin and gentamicin, which have shown some effect on *Pseudomonas* species, have not shown universal therapeutic value (MacLusky et al., 1989). Ceftazidime and aminoglycosides are used intravenously to target *Pseudomonas* infections in the hospitalized patient, but eradication of this organism is rare. *Pseudomonas aeruginosa* is now the most common pathogen in CF, with reported clinic rates as high as 70% of patients affected (Corey et al., 1984a). Pharmacologic therapies are needed to inhibit the adherence of the initiating bacteria in *P. aeruginosa* colonization because this pathogen has demonstrated an extraordinary affinity for the airways of patients with CF (Prince, 1992).

Burkholderia cepacia is an opportunistic pathogen in hospitalized patients and other compromised hosts. Although normally nonpathogenic in healthy immunocompetent individuals, patients with CF are at significant risk of colonization (MacLusky & Levison, 1998). *Burkholderia cepacia* is recognized as a particularly virulent pathogen because of its high level of intrinsic antibiotic resistance, its tenacity to persist in the lungs, and its association with more advanced pulmonary disease. Synergy studies combining antibiotics may help identify a more effective antimicrobial therapy for these colonized patients (Burns, 1997). Evidence that transmission of this organism may occur through interpatient mechanisms (Pegues et al., 1994; Tablan et al., 1985) has initiated segregation practices and attempts to control cross-contamination of equipment in many centers.

Several of the virulent products of bacterial colonization cause airway inflammation and pro-gressive epithelial destruction and therefore contribute significantly to the severity of the pulmonary impairment in CF (MacLusky & Levison, 1990). Anti-inflammatory corticosteroids may slow the progressive pulmonary deterioration (Auerbach et al., 1985) but are associated with numerous side effects when used on a long-term basis and require careful consideration before use (MacLusky & Levison, 1998).

Although 25 to 50% of patients with CF have evidence of increased airway hyperactivity, the mechanism for bronchoconstriction in CF appears to differ from that of asthma (MacLusky & Levison, 1990). When assessed by methacholine challenge, higher doses are necessary to produce a response, and the bronchodilation achieved through albuterol therapy is both slower and less dramatic than in patients with asthma (Skorecki et al., 1976). Evaluation by exercise challenge, using a bicycle ergometer or treadmill and using the change in peak expiratory flow rate as a measure of lung function, indicates that a majority of children with CF demonstrate bronchial hyperreactivity with the increased respiratory effort of exercise (Day & Mearns, 1973). Inhaled sympathomimetic agents do demonstrate the effect of bronchodilation in many patients and may also improve mucociliary function and therefore serve to complement airway clearance techniques (Ormerod et al., 1980) (Fig. 26–1). When used immediately before exercise or pulmonary physical therapy, bronchodilators may help prevent induced bronchospasm and are therefore often prescribed as an important adjunct to physical therapy (MacLusky & Levison, 1990). Anticholinergics, such as ipratropium bromide (Atrovent), have also been shown to be effective bronchodilators in patients with CF (Wiebicke et al., 1990).

Many medications employed in the treatment of CF require nebulization. As a result, the performance characteristics of the nebulizer must be considered when selecting a method of delivery for inhaled medications. Studies comparing the efficiency of different aerosol delivery systems found that there was a significant difference among systems in particle size, total delivery of fluid, and time taken to deliver the medication (Coates et al., 1998; Loffert et al., 1994). Less drug wastage, reduced treatment time, and a more specific match of the delivery system to the breathing pattern of the individual is therefore possible (Coates et al., 1998).

Providing effective pulmonary hygiene by promoting improved clearance of mucus-obstructed airways benefits the pulmonary environment, allowing for improvements in gas exchange and limiting the tissue damage associated with infection. Physical therapy techniques to promote airway clearance in-

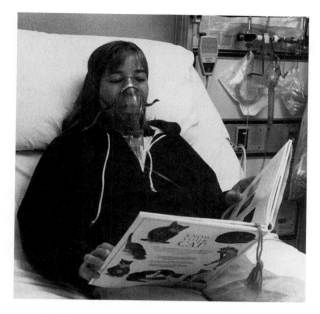

FIGURE 26–1. Receiving inhalation therapy in hospital.

clude postural drainage and manual or mechanical percussion of segmental lobes, vibratory facilitation of ciliary function, directed breathing techniques such as the active cycle of breathing technique (ACBT) (formerly known as FET, for forced expiratory technique) and autogenic drainage, use of positive expiratory pressures (PEP) through valve-equipped facial masks and oscillating PEP (Flutter), and high-frequency chest wall oscillations, as well as exercise prescription, assisted coughing, and postural realignment exercises.

More research is needed to scientifically support the efficacy of the use of pulmonary physical therapy modalities in CF. A comparative study of the literature demonstrated a need for more adequate controls, randomized design and sampling, larger sample sizes, and use of valid outcome measures (Boyd et al., 1994). The studies reviewed were evaluated and classified according to the level of evidence supported by the research design as proposed by Sackett (1986). Our analysis suggested support for exercise, "conventional" physical therapy (postural drainage, percussion, and vibration), and PEP mask therapies in treatment of children with CF in chronic stages of the disease when PFT results were used as an outcome measure. In acute exacerbations of respiratory status, both PEP mask therapy and conventional physical therapy (CPT) showed some evidence of improving pulmonary function scores. A moderate cycling program used to replace two of the three daily CPT sessions produced equivalent improvement in

PFT results (Boyd, et al., 1994). A 2-year study of 66 subjects found that PEP therapy is a valid alternative to CPT (Gaskin et al., 1998). In another long-term study, pulmonary function scores improved in subjects using PEP versus CPT and indicated that PEP was preferred by subjects, thereby increasing adherence (McIlwaine et al., 1997). Oscillating PEP (Flutter) has gained popularity as an airway clearance mechanism, and short-term studies indicate its usefulness as an alternative modality to CPT (Konstan et al., 1994). A more long-term comparison of Flutter versus PEP found that Flutter was not as effective as PEP in maintaining pulmonary function over a 1-year period (McIlwaine et al., 1997).

New strategies for treating CF by pharmacologic means (gene therapy) continue to show promise (Collins, 1996). Research has demonstrated that to successfully treat the respiratory dysfunction of CF, 5 to 10% of the airway epithelial cells must be corrected with normal CFTR expression. To achieve this, a method of delivering the normal gene to the airways is needed. Three different vector delivery systems—modified adenovirus, adeno-associated virus, and liposomes—are being extensively investigated worldwide (Crystal, 1997). An undesirable immune response that targets and destroys corrected epithelial cells remains problematic. Reducing or eliminating this unwanted immune response is a primary focus of current research (Wilson, 1996).

Studies with high-dose preservative-free aerosolized tobramycin have demonstrated improved pulmonary function, decreased sputum bacterial densities, and decreased risk for hospitalization (Ramsey, 1997). Other drugs under investigation include ibuprofen (to decrease airway inflammation), recombinant human DNase (to improve mucous surface properties and transportability) (Galabert et al., 1996), and other mucolytic agents such as hypertonic saline.

The unprecedented volume of current research and the emergence of new, successful therapies for CF dictate a need for conscientious practitioners to remain educated and receptive to adjusting their management plans and critical pathways for care of patients with CF.

LUNG TRANSPLANTATION

Organ transplantation is now a treatment option in many different terminal illnesses, including CF. In the past decade advances in surgical technique and postoperative care with improved immunosuppressive therapies have given some patients with CF a new lease on life. (See Chapter 28 for a more detailed discussion of the involvement of physical therapy in postsurgical care.)

In North America, both heart-lung and double-lung transplants have been performed on patients with CF with end-stage pulmonary disease. The Toronto Lung Transplant Group were pioneers in this field and performed the world's first successful double-lung transplant in 1987 (Pizer, 1991). Through April 1996, the St. Louis International Lung Transplant Registry reported that 746 lung transplants had been performed on patients with CF worldwide. Survival rates continue to improve as the current estimate for 3-year survival is 56% for CF patients with transplants since 1992, and the current 5-year survival rate is 48% (Yankaskas et al., 1998). Living-donor lobar lung transplantation has been performed since 1993, but because it involves recruitment of two donors and the surgical procedure carries inherent risks to the donors, it is not without its problems. This technique's impact on survival statistics appears comparable to that of other approaches, but long-term analysis is needed (Yankaskas et al., 1998). Most complications arise from infections or development of graft rejection. The development of obliterative bronchiolitis may be evidence of chronic rejection (Paradowski, 1992) and is a significant cause of posttransplant death (Egan, 1992). The problem with malabsorption that patients with CF have dictates difficulties with the therapeutic regimen for adequate immunosuppression after transplantation. Individual transplant centers should direct and monitor the immunosuppressive regimen because close monitoring of serum levels and adjustment of doses are vital to successful posttransplant management (Yankaskas et al., 1998).

Criteria for acceptance on a waiting list for lung transplantation include severe pulmonary disease with marked hypoxemia, increased frequency and duration of hospitalizations for pulmonary exacerbations, increasing antibiotic resistance of colonizing bacteria, no significant dysfunction or disease of other vital organs, a history of compliance with medical treatment, and an acceptable psychosocial profile (Yankaskas et al., 1998). A referral for transplant (and acceptance onto the waiting list) must be made early enough to allow for a substantial wait for a suitable donor and creates a need for the development of a preoperative program of conditioning for these patients, which is a component of the lung transplantation program in many centers. These conditioning programs are designed to optimize the patient's functional ability and exercise tolerance, as well as help maintain emotional well-being during the long wait for a transplant (Craven et al., 1990). Physical therapists play a primary role in development and implementation of both preoperative and postoperative exercise programs, which are described later in this chapter.

Double-lung transplantation is now most often performed by bilateral anterolateral thoracotomies using bilateral submammary incisions as first described in 1990 (Pasque et al., 1990). The lungs are transplanted as sequential single-lung grafts. The lung with the worst pulmonary function is replaced first while oxygenation and ventilation are maintained by the native lung. Replacement of the second lung can then proceed with the newly implanted lung supporting the patient (Winton, 1992). Use of this technique has reduced to 30 to 35% the number of patients requiring anticoagulation and cardiopulmonary bypass during surgery (Winton, 1992). This surgical innovation has also reduced the degree of complication from perioperative bleeding, which can be a significant problem for patients with CF because of the presence of inflammatory adhesions within the pleural space (Winton, 1992).

Single-lung transplants are not performed on patients with CF because the remaining native lung continues to be ventilated after transplantation and its overexpansion will compress the transplanted lung (MacLusky & Levison, 1990). Contamination of the native lung could also spread infection to the transplanted lung (Egan, 1992).

IMPAIRMENTS

Examination and Implications

The primary physiologic abnormalities in CF include (1) a dysfunctional chloride channel in transepithelial electrolyte transport, creating abnormal increases in the concentrations of sodium and chloride in serous gland secretions; (2) blocked exocrine gland function due to obstruction by hyperviscous secretions; and (3) an extraordinary susceptibility to chronic endobronchial colonization by specific groups of bacteria, apparently compounded by impaired or deficient ciliary clearance. Although patients with CF show significant differences in levels of clinical impairment, all patients with CF have these three abnormalities (MacLusky & Levison, 1990).

The degree of functional limitation that these impairments impose varies greatly among people with CF. Proper measurement of these limitations is crucial to determining the proper interventions. Examination techniques to quantify the impairments seen in CF measure the functioning of the respiratory and gastrointestinal systems and the limitations in exercise tolerance. Quality-of-life questionnaires and other subjective reports provide information on the patient's perceived level of disability.

A number of clinical scoring systems have been proposed in an attempt to standardize measurement of CF severity. The most commonly used is the Shwachman score (Shwachman & Kulczycki, 1958). Points are awarded under four categories: (1) chest radiography, (2) growth and nutrition, (3) pulmonary (physical findings and cough), and (4) case history, which includes subjective reports of activity tolerance. Findings that reflect no impairment or limitation ("normal" findings) are awarded 25 points; therefore a "perfect" Shwachman score is 100. The lower the score, the worse the clinical condition of the patient. A patient scoring 40 points may have an increased anterior-posterior diameter on chest radiography with atelectatic patches and noticeable hyperinflation, subnormal weight and height, poor muscle strength, marked reduction of fat on skinfold testing, chronic productive cough, rapid respiration and pulse, moderate to severe overexpansion of the lungs, rattles and wheezes on auscultation, breathlessness on exertion, listlessness or lethargy, poor school attendance, limited exercise tolerance, postural abnormalities of protracted shoulders and extended neck, clubbing of the phalanges, and poor appetite or anorexia (Shwachman & Kulczycki, 1958) (Fig. 26–2). This scoring system has good interobserver reliability and correlates well with PFT scoring systems (Lewiston & Moss, 1987), permitting use in clinical comparisons of disease morbidity.

Measuring Pulmonary Impairment

PFT scores provide incremental knowledge of the extent of bronchial obstruction and a means of tracing the degree of restriction of lung function. PFTs include measurement of static and dynamic lung volumes and airflow. Evidence of reactive airway disease can be quantified. Spirometry can be used to record acute deterioration of pulmonary function and to monitor recovery. Vital capacity (VC), total lung capacity (TLC), inspiratory reserve volume (IRV), and expiratory reserve volume (ERV) are directly measured by spirometry. Spirometry can measure airflow rates during different phases of expiration, yielding an indication of the amount of bronchial obstruction. The measure of forced expiratory volume in 1 second (FEV_1) chronicles the early portion of expiration, whereas FEV_3 reflects the terminal stages of a maximal expiratory effort. FEV_1 is often reported as a ratio to forced vital capacity (FVC). In a healthy individual, FEV_1/FVC is 0.70 to 0.80, indicating that 70 to 80% of the FVC is expired in the first second of a forced exhalation (Miller, 1987). Changes in this ratio can reflect an obstructed expiratory airflow.

Analysis of spirometric flow-volume curves enables the early detection of abnormalities in the

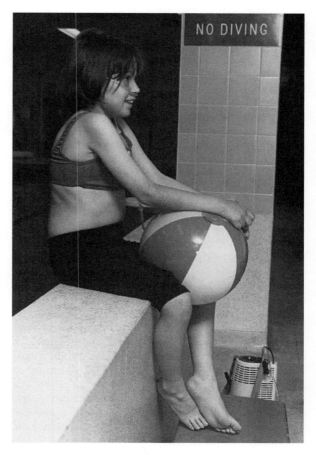

FIGURE 26–2. An example of postural changes in one individual: elevation of the shoulders and an increased anterior-posterior diameter of the chest. Note intercostal indrawing.

smaller airways (Orenstein, 1997). Convexity of the curve in relation to the volume axis is one of the most sensitive indicators of early obstruction of the peripheral airways (Mellins, 1969). Forced expiratory flow between 25 and 75% ($FEF_{25-75\%}$) is the measurement of flow between 25 and 75% of vital capacity and reflects airflow at high lung volumes. Miller (1987) suggests that $FEF_{25-75\%}$ is more sensitive than FEV_1 or FEV_1/FVC in detecting changes in small airway obstruction and provides an important indication of early pulmonary disease in individuals with CF because initial abnormalities involve the small airways (Mellins et al., 1968). Timed volumes at high lung volumes (e.g., FEV_1) may remain within normal limits because the contribution of the small airways to overall resistance is low (Kattan, 1987). FEV_1 is therefore not a sensitive test in early lung disease but indicates obstruction of the central bronchi and becomes markedly abnormal as disease progresses (MacLusky & Levison, 1990).

With more severe pulmonary dysfunction, air trapping results in increases in residual volume (RV) and functional reserve capacity (FRC) (both are measured by a more complicated PFT than spirometry) and an increase in RV/TLC. Restrictive disease can be reflected in decreases in TLC and VC (Altose, 1979). The presence of both restrictive and obstructive components of pulmonary dysfunction may compensate for each other in some measurements (Miller et al., 1987). For example, restrictive disease (in the absence of an obstructive component) results in a normal RV/TLC and obstructive disease (in the absence of a restrictive component) results in an increase in this ratio. When both components coexist, RV/TLC "may not reflect the anatomic changes" (Miller et al., 1987).

Spirometry is the simplest type of PFT performed in the hospital or clinic. Spirometric measurements are all generated by "effort-dependent" means, however, and cannot be used as a test for young children. Children younger than age 6 cannot perform the necessary forced expirations in a reliable way. Modifications to the classic methods of measuring ventilatory parameters in infants and young children are described in the literature (Buist et al., 1980; Doershuk et al., 1970; England, 1988; Sammut & Morgan, 1987; Taussig, 1977; Tepper et al., 1988).

In older children and adults, many other factors, such as sputum retention, poor nutrition, and fatigue, can influence the individual's performance on spirometric PFTs. Notably, many children with CF show performance scores on repeat tests that have a significantly greater range of variability than that of scores of normal test subjects (Cooper et al., 1990). Interpretation of the pulmonary function of an individual with CF therefore also must include other PFTs, such as the closed-circuit helium dilution method, the open-circuit nitrogen washout technique, or a method colloquially known as the "body box"—total-body plethysmography. Ruppel (1991) provides detailed descriptions of these tests. In the plethysmograph, the volume of air is a constant; the test measures the changes in air pressure within the sealed chamber as the patient breathes through a mouthpiece. These measures yield an accurate calculation of the patient's lung volumes, the FRC and RV (Altose, 1979). Some claustrophobia may be experienced by subjects undergoing testing in the "body box," and plethysmography may not be appropriate for all young children.

The U.S. National Institutes of Health's comparative review of 307 cases of CF reported that PFT scores showed a common pattern: progressive declines in flow rates and VC and an increase in the RV/TLC ratio, correlating with clinically gauged worsening of disease (di Sant'Agnese & Davis, 1979).

As pulmonary disease becomes progressively more severe, deteriorating PFT scores can be used to help predict life expectancy. In one study patients with poor arterial gases and an FEV_1 of less than 30% of predicted value had 2-year mortality rates of greater than 50% (Kerem et al., 1992). Individuals with CF demonstrate a characteristic decline in midexpiratory flow rate ($FEF_{25-75\%}$); noting the rate of this decline becomes an important prognostic indicator (Gurwitz et al., 1979). Steadily worsening PFT scores reliably correlate with declining clinical condition and are used as an indicator in assessment for lung transplantation (Khaghani et al., 1991).

Progressive hypoxemia is one of the earliest signs of increasing pulmonary disease and can occur before any other detectable abnormality in lung function (Lamarre et al., 1972). Mucous plugging and bronchiolitis in the patient's airways cause ventilation-perfusion abnormalities, and the subsequent hypoxemia worsens as severity of the obstruction increases (MacLusky & Levison, 1990). Further declines in arterial oxygenation can occur during sleep, so blood gases may have to be monitored throughout the night to assess the need for nocturnal supplementation of oxygen (Muller et al., 1980). Increased oxygen demands during exercise can be a contributing factor to hypoxemia in the patient with CF. Although arterial blood gas measures are considered the "gold standard" in blood gas analysis (Zadai, 1992), they are not commonly used in patients with CF because of their invasive nature. Other noninvasive techniques such as pulse oximetry are preferred. Pulse oximetry to gauge the level of oxygen saturation in the blood as the patient performs exercise contributes to assessment of the suitability of supplemental oxygen during exercise.

Other changes in blood gas readings forewarn of serious disability. Hypercapnia in CF indicates advanced pulmonary disease and carries a poor prognosis. In a study of survival patterns of patients with CF who demonstrated hypercapnia, it was found that death usually occurred within 1 year of the development of chronic hypercapnia (Wagener et al., 1980).

Chest radiographs can provide detailed evidence of the progressive nature of pulmonary disease in CF. In the initial stages of pulmonary involvement, the chest radiograph may reveal signs of hyperinflation and peribronchial thickening. As the disease progresses, bronchiectasis can become apparent, particularly in the upper lobes, and pulmonary infiltrates appear as nodular shadows on radiographs. With severe pulmonary disease the hyperexpanded lungs can precipitate flattening of the diaphragm, thoracic kyphosis, and bowing of the sternum, all detectable on radiography (MacLusky & Levison,

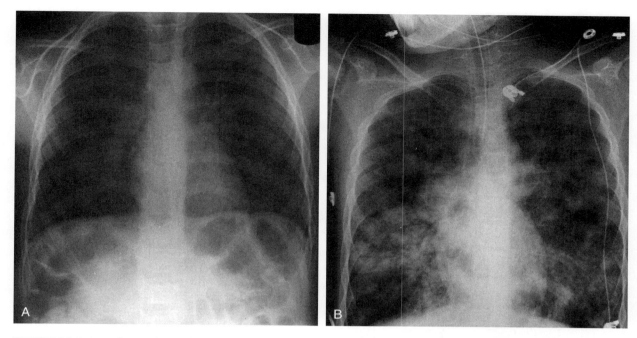

FIGURE 26–3. Two chest radiographs of same individual showing marked deterioration over course of 8 years. *A*, On diagnosis there is evidence of bronchial wall thickening and slight prominence of pulmonary arteries. *B*, At the preterminal stage there is diffuse bilateral bronchiectasis and fibrosis, with severe hyperinflation and bilateral areas of consolidation.

1990) (Fig. 26–3). Confirmation of the development of a pneumothorax can also be provided by examining the chest radiographs. When pulmonary disease is advanced, pulmonary artery hypertrophy may be noticed on radiography as a sign of the pulmonary hypertension associated with cor pulmonale (MacLusky & Levison, 1990).

Cultures from sputum of a patient with CF identify the variety of bacteria that has infected the lower respiratory tract (Gilljam et al., 1986). Sensitivity studies can then be performed to identify effective antibiotic therapies (Orenstein, 1997). CF centers perform regular sputum bacteriology tests to ensure adequate antibiotic coverage for their patients and to help monitor the state of bacterial colonization (MacLusky et al., 1987).

Physical examination of the patient also gathers valuable information. Chest assessment includes inspection, palpation, percussion, and auscultation. Inspection can reveal postural abnormalities, modifications of breathing pattern (Fig. 26–4), or signs of respiratory distress. Evidence of a chronic productive cough may be apparent. Examination of the comparative dimensions of the chest in the anterior-posterior and transverse planes may reveal the barrel chest deformity common to obstructive lung diseases (Humberstone, 1990). Palpation and accurate evaluation of the findings of tactile fremitus will

reveal atelectasis, pneumothorax, or large airway secretions (Humberstone, 1990). Examination of the resonance pattern of the chest, as demonstrated by audible changes on percussion, can provide an indication of abnormally dense areas of the lungs (Humberstone, 1990).

Age of the patient may highly influence the reliability and clinical usefulness of different components of the physical examination. In an infant, measurement of chest wall expansion may be difficult and percussion may not be appropriate (Crane, 1990).

Careful auscultation of the chest can contribute information on the quality of airflow and evidence of obstruction in different areas of the lungs. Reduced ventilation is suggested by decreased breath sounds or presence of inspiratory crackles (also called rales). If crackles are heard throughout the ventilatory cycle, it suggests impaired secretion clearance. Diffuse airway obstruction may cause polyphonic wheezing (Humberstone, 1990).

The examiner must be aware that chronically hyperinflated lungs tend to mask or make it difficult to hear adventitious sounds on auscultation (Humberstone, 1990). It is also important to note that use of a stethoscope, described as the "most frequently used tool in medicine" (Loudon, 1987), is not consistent or reliable among health care provid-

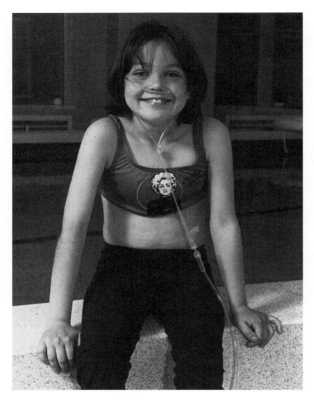

FIGURE 26–4. Use of accessory muscles of respiration is apparent on physical inspection.

ers (Pasterkamp et al., 1987). Validity and reliability of auscultation may be affected by a disparity in nomenclature, the quality of the stethoscope used, and a lack of correlation between pathologic findings and lung sounds (Aweida & Kelsey, 1989). When various health care workers were compared, significant differences were noted in the terminology used to describe tape-recorded adventitious sounds (Pasterkamp et al., 1987). Despite auscultation's limitations in interobserver reliability, it continues to serve as a valuable element of clinical examination. Familiarization with the usual pattern of a patient's lung sounds can be a critical component of evaluation of examination results because an alteration of the typical pattern may signal a pulmonary change that might otherwise have gone undetected.

The long-term prognosis of CF patients with significant pulmonary disease worsens when there is also evidence of protein-calorie malnutrition (Park & Grand, 1981). Patients who are pancreatic insufficient need oral supplementary enzymes to enable them to absorb adequate nutrients from their diet and prevent the devastating effects of malnutrition. Identifying the need for enzyme supplementation is, therefore, a critical component in the treatment of CF. Pancreatic function may be determined by a number of testing methods, including fecal fat assessment, pancreatic substrate assays, and direct collection of pancreatic secretions by duodenal intubation (MacLusky & Levison, 1990). Individuals with CF who have significant preservation of pancreatic function and therefore can maintain normal fat absorption have less pulmonary dysfunction and a better prognosis than those individuals who have pancreatic insufficiency (Corey et al., 1984b).

A number of clinicians and researchers have examined various prognostic indicators in CF. Sustaining adequate nutritional requirements to ensure the maintenance of appropriate growth percentiles is one such indicator (Corey et al., 1984b). Other factors that are associated with a preferred prognosis include single organ involvement at diagnosis, absent or single-organism sputum colonization, and a normal chest radiograph 1 year after diagnosis. Multiple organ involvement, abnormal chest radiographs at diagnosis, colonization of multiple organisms in the sputum, a falloff from typical growth curves, and recurrent hemoptysis are all factors associated with a poor prognosis. There also appears to be a gender bias in severity of disease expression, with male patients possessing a better prognosis than their female counterparts (MacLusky et al., 1987).

PHYSICAL THERAPY: EXAMINATION AND INTERVENTION

Infancy

A diagnosis of CF for their child can mean many things to parents. At the most basic level, it means they have a child with "special needs," and those needs can be seen to influence the family dynamics (Lloyd-Still & Lloyd-Still, 1983). The child's family members are forced to familiarize themselves with CF and both the psychologic and practical demands implicit with this diagnosis. Education of the family is a crucial goal, and this seems best achieved by regional CF centers because a number of different specialty services can be provided in one place. A physical therapist at a CF center is part of a cohesive team of interested investigators and caregivers. Educating the patients and their families while measuring and treating the myriad complications in this disease is the ongoing goal of a CF center's staff.

Preventing Disability: Parental Education

Intervention often must be implemented immediately on diagnosis, and the family needs assistance in making the necessary adjustments and provisions to ensure adherence with any suggested therapeutic regimen. Physical therapists evaluate which essential elements of the child's care must be addressed by them and then provide instruction for the family in the proper administration of the physical therapy modalities that appear appropriate. The therapist should demonstrate sensitivity and equanimity while interacting with these children and their families, remembering that this is a very stressful time for those involved and that what the family may "hear" can differ from what is actually said to them (Bush, 1997).

What families seem to need most is information that acknowledges the seriousness of the disease while still emphasizing the likelihood of a happy and fulfilling family life. Developing the types of strategies that permit some flexibility in intervention regimens promotes a better integration of the child's treatment needs into the family's routines (Maxwell, 1991). Parents may have many concerns and a host of questions and can be especially confused by all the uncertainty that typifies the disease. Because the progression of CF is so variable from case to case, an ongoing examination of the child's status is the only way to ensure meeting the child's individual requirements. This means that the family members must have continued association with the CF center and need to appreciate their role as integral members of the caregiving team.

Children with a chronic condition have been shown to have increased risk of psychosocial dysfunction, particularly when parental anxiety is overwhelming (Cappelli et al., 1989; Green & Solnit, 1964). Because excessive parental overprotection is strongly linked to the existence of psychosocial maladjustment in children, the parents of a child with CF must be alerted to the dangers of unnecessarily shielding their child from aspects of normal life. In infancy, this may take the form of overdressing the child to guard against drafts or neglecting to allow the child to participate in normal exploratory play. Physical therapists should reassure parents that infants with CF have the same requirements as other infants with respect to physical and emotional development. Excellent reference materials are available in most CF centers. Teaching manuals, designed to supplement the information imparted by the CF center staff, are often distributed to families and can be made available to other interested caregivers such as child care workers or school teachers. Orenstein's book *Cystic Fibrosis: A Guide for Patient and Family* (Orenstein, 1997) is highly recommended.

Management of Impairment

In the neonate, the most frequently seen symptoms of CF are meconium ileus, malabsorption of nutrients, and failure to thrive, all of which are associated with the gastrointestinal tract (Rosenstein & Langbaum, 1984). Overt pulmonary involvement is not apparent in the neonatal period because the lungs are morphologically normal at birth (Hardy et al., 1989; MacLusky & Levison, 1990). Within a few months, however, some infants with CF develop signs of impaired respiratory function, manifesting symptoms suggesting bronchiolitis. Pronounced wheeze, an indication of hyperactive airways, is sometimes apparent, and chest radiographs can reveal evidence of hyperinflation (Phillips & David, 1987). Obstruction of airflow in these infants may be related to airway inflammation, mucosal edema, copious mucus secretions, and increased airway tone (Tepper, 1992). The bronchioles are considered the main site of airflow obstruction in infancy (Taussig et al., 1984). Studies using bronchoalveolar lavage revealed that every infant with CF—whether symptomatic or not—has evidence of small airway obstruction in the form of bronchial mucous casts (Wood, 1993).

Measurements to assess possible limitation of pulmonary function cannot be taken in the conventional way (e.g., spirometry) in infants; therefore researchers have had to modify standard methods to accommodate testing in this age group. Infants with CF demonstrate low values of pulmonary compliance (Phelan et al., 1969), decreased lung compliance, and a less homogeneous distribution of ventilation when compared with normal controls (Tepper et al., 1988). Tepper and colleagues (1987) found these changes in both symptomatic and asymptomatic infants. Abnormalities in flow-volume curves (Godfrey et al., 1983) and low values of maximal expiratory flow (Hiatt et al., 1988) indicate that the limitations to airflow in infancy are associated with bronchoconstriction (Hardy et al., 1989). Infants with CF have indeed displayed altered bronchial tone after the administration of a bronchodilator, as revealed by the fact that airflow rates showed significant increases not seen in a control group (Hiatt et al., 1988). Methacholine challenge testing also revealed heightened airway responsiveness (Ackerman et al., 1991).

These research studies have yielded valuable insight into the early pulmonary manifestations of CF in infancy. The formal PFTs used in these studies, however, are not feasible or practical for the infant population of most clinics or CF centers. Examination of pulmonary involvement in infancy is usually limited to physical findings, history of respiratory symptoms, and chest radiographs. Carefully observing for signs of respiratory distress, such as nasal flaring, expiratory grunting, retractions of the chest wall, tachypnea, pallor, or cyanosis, produces an indication of respiratory status. Auscultation of an infant or young child is less than ideal owing to the deceptively easy transmission of sounds from the close structures underlying the thin chest wall (Crane, 1990), but careful auscultation is necessary to ascertain if there is any evidence of wheezing. Changes visible on radiography are the most reliable indication of early pulmonary involvement, because it has been demonstrated that airflow obstruction may precede the presence of overt respiratory symptoms and because lack of cooperation in this population diminishes the reliability of the physical examination. Historical accounts of respiratory illness must also be carefully considered.

It has been suggested that the rate of deterioration of pulmonary function in individuals with CF might be slowed by early initiation of treatment (Taussig et al., 1984). Because research has shown changes in respiratory patterns and mechanics in asymptomatic infants newly diagnosed with CF (Tepper et al., 1988) and evidence of small airway obstruction in the form of bronchial mucous casts (Wood, 1993), early therapeutic intervention might actually delay the onset of overt symptoms of respiratory impairment. The value of initiating pulmonary treatment before development of symptoms remains controversial, but various theoretic arguments for initiating therapy as soon as possible can be presented. Adherence to a therapy routine may be improved if it is accepted as a routine part of life, and prevention of respiratory impairment is an easily supported goal (Wood, 1993).

A study was conducted to evaluate the combined effect of a bronchodilator and chest physical therapy on infants newly diagnosed with CF, addressing the controversy surrounding treatment for asymptomatic children (Hardy et al., 1989). Baseline, preintervention measurements of the mechanics and energetics of breathing were obtained for all subjects. Twenty minutes after the inhalation of a bronchodilator, chest physical therapy was given to the subjects, consisting of 20 minutes of chest percussions and vibrations applied in five different postural drainage positions. Immediately after the physical therapy session, repeat pulmonary function measurements were taken. Most of the infants (10 of 13) demonstrated decreases from baseline values in pulmonary resistance, with subsequent decreases in the work of breathing, after the administration of the bronchodilator and chest physical therapy (Hardy et al., 1989). The researchers postulated that the bronchodilator relieved subclinical bronchospasm and aided the reduction of mucosal edema, and that chest physical therapy, assisting the immature mucociliary system, was effective in mobilizing secretions, thereby improving the patency of the airways (Hardy et al., 1989). When serial PFTs are possible, objective measures of the progression of impairment

and the effects of specific treatments may provide future evidence of the efficacy of early intervention (Hardy et al., 1989).

Prevention of obstructive mucous plugging is the initial goal of pulmonary physical therapy in this population. The primary modalities used for promotion of clearance of secretions for infants with CF are postural drainage, percussion, and vibrations. The physiologic rationale and precise methodology of these modalities are well described in most comprehensive texts on physical therapy (e.g., Frownfelter, 1987; Irwin & Tecklin, 1990; Mackenzie, 1989), but important modifications to the proper use of these modalities for infants will be discussed.

In obstructive airway diseases such as CF, the effectiveness of the antireflux mechanism at the esophagogastric junction is reduced (Orenstein & Orenstein, 1988). The increases in intra-abdominal pressure that can be associated with coughing also promote gastroesophageal reflux (Scott et al., 1985). Of newly diagnosed infants with CF, 35% had symptomatic gastroesophageal reflux in one study (Vinocur et al., 1985), and 24-hour esophageal monitoring revealed abnormalities in 10 successive infants newly diagnosed with CF in another (Dab & Malfroot, 1988). Because gastroesophageal reflux can result in aspiration of gastric contents, head-down positions for postural drainage may have to be modified. A 12-month comparison of standard (tipped position) versus modified (no tip) found both techniques equally effective for this population (younger than 12 months of age) (Button et al., 1997). Timing the physical therapy around feeding schedules may also be necessary to reduce the risk of gastroesophageal reflux. Postural drainage positions are easily achieved by arranging the infant in the required manner on the caregiver's lap. Holding the small child in this way also seems to offer the child an extra measure of security. Adapting hand position (by "tenting" of the middle finger) suits the application of percussion on a tiny chest wall. The applied force of percussion should vary with size and condition of the infant, and conscientious monitoring of the infant's response to treatment should guide the amount of vigor used in percussion. Timing of manual vibrations to coincide with the expirations of an infant is difficult owing to the infant's rapid respiratory rate, and this technique may be very difficult to teach to parents.

Education for the family in the application of prescribed physical therapy modalities should be ongoing. Periodically asking the parent or caregiver to demonstrate treatment positions and manual technique allows the therapist to identify possible problems with proper application. In some CF centers the physical therapist is also responsible for ordering, demonstrating, and arranging for the maintenance of the equipment necessary for the aerosol delivery of medications. Instruction in the care and use of these nebulizers is vitally important to ensure correct delivery of prescribed medications.

Adherence with any suggested therapeutic regimen requires commitment on the part of the caregiver. The demands of caring for a child with CF can seem extreme when considering the extra attention to nutritional issues, medications, and physical therapy that this diagnosis entails. Signs of excessive stress or evidence that the family is having difficulty in coping with the caregiving requirements may become obvious. Referral to a social worker or a psychologist might help identify the family in crisis and aid the family in developing strategies to enable adjustment to the various challenges that lie ahead of them as they nurture their child with CF.

Preschool and School-Age Period

Prevention of Disability

Approximately 75% of children with CF are now diagnosed before their third birthday (Lloyd-Still & Lloyd-Still, 1983). When there is a positive family history of CF, parents are familiar with the disease, but in many cases there is no prior knowledge of the disorder and the diagnosis can be startling. Initial shock may be followed by disbelief, anger, or grief (Lloyd-Still & Lloyd-Still, 1983). The age of the child when diagnosed affects parental reaction to some extent. The longer the prediagnostic stage (the older the child), the greater the likelihood of the parents experiencing extreme shock at the time of diagnosis (Burton, 1975). Sensitivity for the anguish experienced by the family must be shown.

The clinical status of children with CF is highly variable. Some toddlers may have already experienced pulmonary complications and been hospitalized repeatedly, whereas others exhibit little or no detrimental impact on their respiratory status. The effects of protein-calorie deficits due to malabsorption may be manifest in stunted development such as small stature or a lower than average weight-to-height ratio; therefore, a difference in appearance from their healthy siblings or friends may already be perceptible.

Young children need to develop the ability to function socially outside the family circle. Demands of school and new friendships dictate a lessening of parental attachments and a capacity for some measure of independence (Lloyd-Still & Lloyd-Still, 1983). This type of autonomy may be difficult to achieve for the child with CF. If parents perceive that their child is fragile with exceptionally vulnerable health, they may become overprotective. McCollum

and Gibson (1970) examined issues of family adaptation to CF and found that 47% of parents in the study admitted granting less independence to their child with CF than to their healthy children. Cappelli and colleagues (1989) found a strong correlation between parental overprotection and psychologic maladjustment in the child; the attempt to shield her or him from harm can negatively affect a child's ability to adapt to social pressures. Behavior problems such as restlessness, excessive daydreaming, and inattentiveness are found more often in children with medical conditions such as CF than in their healthy peers (McCollum & Gibson, 1970). Encouraging children with CF to participate in a variety of social and physical activities could prove beneficial to both their physical and emotional health. The physical therapist should stress the importance of incorporating an active lifestyle into the family dynamic.

Assisting children to gain a sense of self-efficacy is an important goal at this time. A key factor of lifelong adherence to necessary treatment is incorporating a sense of self-efficacy (the confidence that one has the ability to perform a behavior). This results from exposure to a credible role model, the encouragement to perform the tasks of self-management, and developing competency (Bartholomew et al, 1993). Annual self-management workshops at the Hospital for Sick Children in Toronto, Canada, have been initiated to increase the knowledge and commitment to treatment for children and their families by teaching age-appropriate tasks in a multisensory, multidisciplinary setting. Individual care plans are developed with each child, and a self-care manual is provided to the families to act as a guide. By initiating this education when the child is young, it is hoped that it may influence the negative correlation between adherence and aging identified by Passero (Passero et al., 1981).

The CF Family Education Project at Baylor College of Medicine and Texas Children's Hospital developed an educational program that emphasized self-management by providing individual learning packages for parents and patients in early childhood, middle childhood, and adolescence. The curriculums were developed based on social cognitive theory and target behavioral capability, self-efficacy, and outcome expectations. The program was designed to be implemented as an integral component of the health care of these families, facilitating learning by the reciprocity between the clients and the health care environment (Bartholomew et al., 1996).

Measurement of Functional Limitations

Measurement of impairment and functional limitations in the young child includes history, physical examination, chest radiographs, blood gases, oximetry, and sputum bacteriology. The pulmonary function of children who are able to execute the necessary voluntary maneuver (usually by age 6) can now be assessed by spirometry.

Examination by the physical therapist should include thorough history taking, a physical examination including posture, and, when applicable, some type of exercise tolerance testing. Young children with CF may have a chronic cough, hypoxemia, and decreased compliance of the lungs (Tepper et al., 1988), leading to restrictions in maximal oxygen consumption, an increase in work of breathing, and an increase in resting energy expenditure (Shepherd et al., 1988). These factors will all compromise exercise tolerance.

Exercise testing is an objective method in which the physical therapist can quantify the subject's pulmonary deterioration, as well as determine the subject's response to physical therapy. Individuals with CF will often not be aware of the extent of their physical limitations owing to the slow progression of their disease (Cerny & Darbee, 1990). An exercise test can detect mild pulmonary dysfunction, which may go undetected during investigations at rest, and will also help reveal how the individual copes with work despite his or her disability (Godfrey, 1974).

When choosing an exercise test protocol, the purpose for the test and the age and disease severity of the subject should be carefully considered. To evaluate functional limitations, the exercise test should be progressive and stress the subject's cardiorespiratory system to a symptom-limited maximum. The test should also be reproducible and capable of providing meaningful results (Singh, 1992).

Cycle ergometers are often used for testing exercise capacity in children with pulmonary disease (Cerny et al., 1982; Nixon et al., 1992). An accurate prediction of oxygen consumption can be obtained because the mechanical efficiency for pedaling a cycle is independent of body weight and therefore is almost identical for all individuals (Cerny & Darbee, 1990). Although the treadmill test generally yields higher oxygen consumption values, the cycle ergometer has the advantages of being relatively inexpensive, portable, and safe. Because cycling is also a familiar exercise for many people, it is less likely to cause apprehension. As with the treadmill test, cycle ergometry is reproducible (Fox & Mathews, 1981). In addition, the subject is relatively stationary and therefore vital signs are easily monitored. Most ergometers have adjustable seat heights suitable for children, and it is important to be able to adjust handlebars and pedal crank length.

Several progressive exercise protocols are used on the cycle ergometer to determine maximum oxygen consumption or individual peak work capacity (see Chapter 5). Cerny and colleagues (1982) examined subjects with CF matched to a normal control sample to monitor cardiopulmonary response to incrementally increased workloads with cycle ergometry. Workloads were increased every 2 minutes until the subject could not continue. The study demonstrated that normal subjects needed an increased workload of 0.32 W/kg on average to effect an increase in heart rate of 10 beats per minute. Subjects with CF required workload increases ranging from 0.15 to 0.35 W/kg, depending on the severity of their disease, to demonstrate the same change in heart rate. Cerny and colleagues concluded that the limiting factor in exercise tolerance was severity of pulmonary involvement and not cardiovascular limitation (Cerny et al., 1982).

If the child is too small to successfully use a cycle ergometer, a treadmill can be used because only the ability to walk is required (Fig. 26-5). The child should be monitored closely to maintain a sense of confidence during the test. The elevation and speed are adjusted according to the size and skill of the subject and should be selected to allow even the subject with severe dysfunction to exercise at two to three levels of difficulty (Cerny & Darbee, 1990).

For individuals with severe lung disease, field walking tests such as 6- or 12-minute walks (Butland et al., 1982) or the shuttle walking test (Scott et al., 1990) may be preferred. The reliability and validity of the 6-minute walk test with children with CF has been demonstrated (Gulmans et al., 1996). Walking tests are simple, are inexpensive, and can be performed by individuals of all ages and abilities with little risk of injury (Porcari et al., 1989). Because they are highly reproducible, walking tests correspond closely to the demands of everyday activity (Guyatt et al., 1985). Another quick and portable test that may prove useful in a clinical setting is the 3-minute step test, which illustrated similar results as the 6-minute walk test when outcome measures were arterial oxygen saturation, maximum pulse rate, and the Modified Borg Dyspnea Scale (Balfour-Lynn et al., 1998).

Subjects performing an exercise test must be closely monitored and special notice must be given to signs of increased work of breathing, disproportionate to what is expected (Cerny & Darbee, 1990). Subjective measures of the perceived level of respiratory labor with a dyspnea scale such as Borg's Scale of Ratings of Perceived Exertion (Borg, 1982) can be taken before, during, and after the exercise test. Borg's scale is a good indicator of both physiologic and psychologic strain and allows individuals to

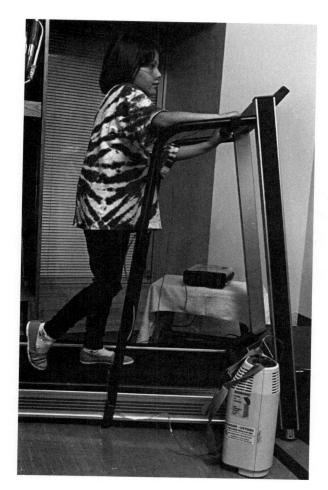

FIGURE 26–5. Treadmill testing with a young patient on oxygen.

interpret the intensity of their exercise according to subjective impressions (Paley, 1997).

Maximal work capacity is limited by ventilation in individuals with pulmonary disease (Cerny & Darbee, 1990). Deficiencies in gas exchange and poor pulmonary mechanics compound the effects of decreased exercise capacity (Cerny et al., 1982; Henke & Orenstein, 1984). That limitation to exercise is due to pulmonary restrictions is further evidenced by the failure to reach predicted peak heart rates in exercise test subjects with CF, suggesting that exercise capacity is not limited by cardiovascular factors (Canny & Levison, 1987).

A complete physical examination should assist in revealing the individual's level of fitness, thus aiding the physical therapist in choosing the most appropriate exercise testing protocol. Individual exercise

programs can then be designed to improve exercise capacity and fitness level.

Management of Pulmonary Impairment

People with CF demonstrate a wide variance in the severity of illness, because the disease progresses in individuals at different rates, but some amount of chronic airflow obstruction is often already present in childhood. The small peripheral airways are the site of most of these early pulmonary changes, and patchy atelectasis and ventilation-perfusion abnormalities lead to increases in functional dead space and discernible hypoxemia (MacLusky & Levison, 1990).

The goals of a physical therapy program for the young child should encompass the improvement of exercise tolerance with continued attention to secretion clearance techniques. Correction and maintenance of proper postural alignment are also stressed. Goals of treatment should be designed with the child and her or his family and account for the developmental stage of the child and the uniqueness of the family's circumstances. The learning environment must accommodate the child's learning style and avoid prescriptive tasks that are beyond the child's capabilities in order to promote self-efficacy and adherence. Education of the caregivers must incorporate similar strategies because their full cooperation and participation is essential.

Postural drainage, percussion, and vibration (conventional physical therapy) are common modalities for secretion mobilization in this population. Once children have grown too large to be positioned in the caregiver's lap for postural drainage, equipment such as a drainage board will have to be introduced. Mechanical percussors may be used to ease the work involved with manual percussion and to provide the child with an aid for self-treatment (Fig. 26–6). Children with a chronic illness should be encouraged to assume a degree of responsibility for their own treatment. Feeling some level of control over one's own health fosters self-esteem and helps subdue anxiety (Kellerman et al., 1980). Children with CF may find it difficult to sustain the performance of manual percussion, even on easily accessible lung segments, and mechanical percussors can therefore help alleviate this problem.

Although CPT has long been used in the treatment of CF, it has been criticized as being too time-consuming and difficult to perform independently. Compliance with a daily physical therapy regimen is reported as lower than with all other aspects of treatment (Passero et al., 1981). Proof of efficacy might promote compliance, but research studies to

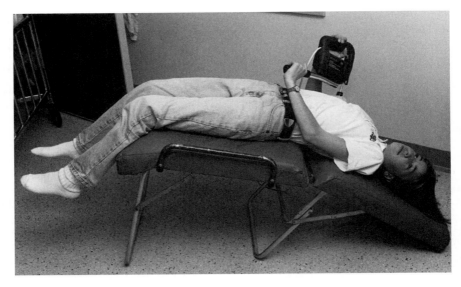

FIGURE 26–6. Self-administered postural drainage and percussion using a mechanical percussor.

examine the effectiveness of CPT are difficult to evaluate because they use a wide variety of outcome measures, including different PFTs, volume of secretions produced, and participants' subjective impressions (Starr, 1992). It is also problematic to compare studies done in different stages of the disease or with differences in study populations. Identifying the independent variable is sometimes troublesome because of the diverse combinations of techniques used; for example, percussion is rarely performed independently of postural drainage and coughing, making it difficult to definitively state which aspect of the treatment investigated has proven effective.

In a study by Lorin and Denning (1971), the short-term effect of CPT for patients with CF, compared with cough alone, was production of more sputum. Other studies support the effectiveness of CPT in increasing amounts of sputum expectorated by subjects when excess secretion production is already a feature of the patient's condition (Bateman et al., 1979; Mazzacco et al., 1985). The amount of sputum produced may be quantified by volume or weight, but caution must be used when interpreting the findings from this type of measurement. Because many individuals may swallow a portion of their sputum, the output can underestimate the true volume produced. The amount of saliva that contaminates the product is difficult to determine, and this has resulted in the measurement of the dry weight of sputum in some studies. Measurement of dry weight is not practical in most clinical settings. In addition, the amount of sputum produced does not indicate where it originated.

Alternative methods for mobilizing secretions and stimulating cough have been suggested, usually involving directed breathing techniques. These include huffing, PEP, oscillating PEP (Flutter), autogenic drainage, and active cycle of breathing (formerly known as FET).

The rationale for use of huffing, a type of forced expiration with a similar mechanism to coughing, was suggested by a study that bronchoscopically demonstrated that maintenance of an open glottis throughout the maneuver stabilized the collapsible airway walls of subjects with chronic airflow obstruction (Hietpas et al., 1979). The glottis normally closes in the compression phase of a cough, translating high compressive pressures on the tracheobronchial tree that may cause bronchiolar collapse (Starr, 1992). Uncontrolled coughing is often nonproductive and exhausting. To perform huffing, the subject is asked to take a deep inspiration and then, without allowing the glottis to close, to render a strong contraction of the abdominal muscles to aid in forceful expiration. Maintaining an open glottis can be compared to vocalizing "ha" (Starr, 1992). Huffing is an uncomplicated breathing technique that can be easily taught to young children, and performing huffs can introduce the child to the concept of controlled or directed breathing techniques.

Descriptions of the forced expiratory technique vary in the literature. Generally, it employs forceful expirations combined with an open glottis as in huffing, interspersed with controlled breathing at mid to low lung volumes. A 3-year study was conducted by Reisman and associates (1988) to compare the treat-

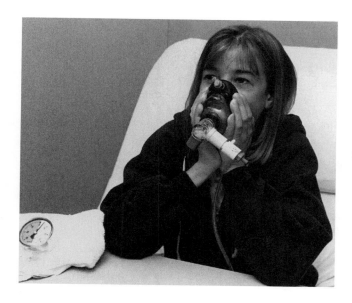

FIGURE 26-7. Use of a PEP mask.

ment effects of FETs in isolation (without postural drainage) versus CPT in subjects with mild to moderate pulmonary involvement. The study assessed the rates of deterioration in PFT scores, exercise challenge tests, and Shwachman clinical scores for all study subjects. The subjects who performed only FETs had significantly greater rates of decline in measures of FEV_1, midexpiratory flow rates ($FEF_{25-75\%}$), and Shwachman score than the group performing CPT.

Other studies support the use of FET when used as an adjunct to postural drainage for secretion clearance (Pryor et al., 1979; Sutton et al., 1983; Sutton et al., 1985; Van Hengstrum et al., 1988). These studies describe FETs differently than Reisman and associates did, use dissimilar outcome measures (sputum yield and clearance of radioaerosol particles), and combine the maneuver with postural drainage, so the results are not easily compared with those of Reisman and associates.

Clarification of the use of FET that always includes finer breathing control techniques and thoracic expansion exercises required that FET be reclassified as active cycle of breathing techniques by Pryor and associates (Pryor, 1991). The three components are combined in a set cycle: relaxation and breathing control and three to four thoracic expansion exercises repeated twice, then relaxation and breathing control followed by one or two forced expirations. When secretions reach the larger, proximal airways they may be cleared by a huff or a cough at high lung volume. Postural drainage positions may augment the effect, but the sitting position may be used if a gravity-assisted position is contraindicated (Pryor & Webber, 1993).

Use of PEP (Fig. 26-7) as a means of secretion mobilization for individuals with CF has been proposed. Introduced for use in this population in the 1980s in Denmark, PEP has been shown to be as effective as CPT in both chronic (baseline) stages of CF (Gaskin et al., 1998; McIlwaine et al., 1997b; Oberwaldner et al., 1986) and during an acute exacerbation of pulmonary complications (Oberwaldner et al., 1991). The transmural pressure generated by maintaining resistant pressure throughout the expiration phase is thought to allow airflow to reach some obstructed alveoli through use of collateral airway channels. Airways are "splinted open" through the maintenance of PEP, thereby facilitating movement of peripheral secretions toward central airways (Lannefors, 1992). The reader is urged to refer to the studies mentioned earlier to gain a better understanding of PEP as an airway clearance modality for CF.

Oscillating PEP (Flutter therapy) was developed to generate a controlled oscillating positive pressure and interruptions to the airflow during expiration through a handheld device. The only long-term study reported to date found that using Flutter in isolation from other airway clearance techniques did not prove as effective as PEP, when outcome measures were pulmonary function scores and frequency of hospitalizations (McIlwaine et al., 1997a). Flutter may be useful as an adjunct to other airway clearance techniques, however, because ease of use and portability of the device makes it attractive to some individuals.

An inflatable fitted vest attached to a pump that generates high-frequency oscillations applied to the external chest wall has been developed and is currently used in some CF centers. The high-frequency chest wall compression that the Vest delivers helps mobilize secretions and can be used simultaneously with other airway clearance techniques. The device is costly, however, and long-term studies of efficacy are necessary (Hardy, l994).

Exercise has also been shown to be a useful therapeutic modality for secretion clearance, as evidenced by improved expiratory flow rates in subjects with stable CF with mild pulmonary disease (Zach et al., 1981). A 30-month study of the effects of discontinuing other airway clearance modalities in favor of participation in aerobic exercise activities demonstrated no significant declines in clinical status (Shwachman score), radiographic results, or PFT outcomes (Andreasson et al., 1987). In an acute exacerbation, exercise proved as effective as CPT for the study subjects when pulmonary function was reviewed. The group assigned to "exercise" continued to receive one bronchial hygiene treatment session by a physical therapist daily, whereas the CPT group received three of these sessions per day. Cerny concluded that hospitalized patients could substitute exercise for part of the standard in-hospital care (Cerny, 1989).

Salt and fluid requirements need special attention in the individual with CF who is participating in exercise, especially in hot weather. The higher sodium and chloride concentrations in the perspiration of people with CF impose an elevated demand for salt and fluid replacement while exercising, which may not always be apparent to the individual (Orenstein et al., 1983).

Benefits of an exercise program extend beyond increases in peak oxygen consumption, increased maximal work capacity, improved mucus expectoration, and improved expiratory flow rates (Heijerman et al., 1991; Orenstein et al., 1981; Zach et al., 1981). Participation in a prescribed exercise program has also been shown to improve self-concept (Folkins, 1972) and may provide increased social interaction.

Fitness level has implications as a prognostic indicator. An improved survival rate is found in individuals with CF who demonstrate higher levels of aerobic fitness. Although this may simply reflect less severe illness, the ability to maintain aerobic fitness appears to have value in improving longevity (Nixon et al., 1992). Further research is necessary to determine what precise role prescriptive exercise programs play in improving survival.

Young children with CF should be encouraged to use those treatment modalities that best suit their requirements for adequate secretion clearance and prevention of deterioration of clinical status. Attitudes toward adherence with treatment can greatly influence the effectiveness of any therapeutic regimen, and the challenge for the physical therapist is to design a treatment strategy for these children that is useful both for efficacy and practicality. Factors that must be considered in designing a therapy program include disease presentation and severity; patient's age; documented effectiveness; motivation and ability to concentrate; physician, caregiver, and patient goals; training considerations; work required; need for assistance or equipment; and costs (Hardy, 1994). Children who learn to adopt their physical therapy as an aspect of daily living, as opposed to a burden or punishment, will be more likely to comply with treatment plans.

Adolescence

Adolescence is a time of rapid transformation in many areas of development. Sexual maturation comes about as a result of the major changes in circulating hormones occurring around the time of maturity of the skeletal system, normally when the child is about 11 or 12 years old. These hormonal secretions cause a "growth spurt" in the adolescent (Green, 1983). "Delay of maturity" occurs when there has been slowed or prolonged skeletal maturation. This is often the cause of delayed puberty in adolescents with CF (di Sant'Agnese & Davis, 1979; Mitchell-Heggs et al., 1976). Arrested sexual development, combined with a smaller than average physical build, can intensify feelings of isolation from healthy peers (McCollum & Gibson, 1970). Osteopenia (low bone mass) is a possible complication of CF and may be linked to nutritional factors and delayed puberty (Bhudhikanok et al., 1996). The risk of fractures in these patients must be considered when developing a therapy program.

A need for increasing independence can conflict with the demands of daily medical care, making compliance with the routine seem arduous. The adolescent with CF who looks and feels disparate from the perceived "norm" may rebel against the continuation of time-consuming treatments that reinforce his or her sense of being dissimilar or abnormal (Boyle et al., 1976).

Management of Impairment

Adherance with the "conventional" physical therapy routine of daily postural drainage and percussion sessions is poor in the adolescent population (McCollum & Gibson, 1970; Passero et al., 1981). One challenge with this population is to promote self-efficacy with alternative methods of treatment. The use of PEP, active cycle of breathing technique, or a program of regular exercise may help promote independence and has already been discussed. Autogenic drainage (AD) is another treatment modality involving self-controlled breathing techniques.

AD requires no equipment or special environment to execute and relies on the user's ability to control both inspiratory and expiratory airflow to generate maximum airflow within the different generations of bronchi (Chevaillier, 1984). Three separate phases of the technique are believed to "unstick" mucus in the peripheral airways, "collect" the mucus in the middle airways, and "evacuate" it from the central airways according to the volume level of the controlled breaths (McIlwaine et al., 1992). Mobilization of airway secretions by AD does not rely on the gravity assistance needed for postural drainage and can be performed in a sitting position.

There is a scarcity of research studies validating the long-term efficacy of AD. A study was published comparing AD with CPT and PEP in patients with CF (McIlwaine et al., 1988), and a 2-year comparison trial of AD and CPT has also been reported and showed no significant differences between treatment groups when clinical status and PFT scores were used as outcome measures (Davidson et al., 1992).

Learning the technique of AD poses difficulties for both the subject and the trainer. It requires concentration and the ability to use proprioceptive and sensory cues to localize the secretions in the various levels of bronchi. A hands-on approach is essential, with a minimum of environmental distractions. Frequent training sessions and reviews are necessary. This type of concentrated self-directed activity is usually not achievable by children younger than age 12. The mechanism for collateral ventilation through the channels of Lambert and pores of Kahn is not fully developed in young children (DeCesare & Graybill, 1990), providing another limitation to the use of AD.

Maintenance of proper posture is important for individuals with CF to provide efficient breathing mechanics. The changes in the length-tension relationships of the respiratory musculature that may occur with increases in FRC create a mechanical disadvantage and contribute to increased work of breathing and muscle fatigue (Cerny & Darbee, 1990). Several postural changes are found in CF to varying degrees, associated with chronically hyperinflated lungs, including increased anterior-posterior diameter of the chest, shoulder elevation, and forward protraction and abdominal flexion (Rose & Jay, 1986). The incidence of thoracic kyphosis in CF is approximately 15% (Denton et al., 1981), which predisposes affected individuals to chronic back pain. Estimates of the rate of back pain among people with CF are as high as 80% (Rose & Jay, 1986).

The physical therapist must examine the patient for postural abnormalities and determine which changes may be reversible or amenable to treatment. Exercises to promote improved posture include a strengthening program for the supporting muscles of the back and spine, stretching of contracted musculature, and training the subject to develop a keener sense of his or her postural alignment. Projecting a good appearance is usually very important to adolescents, and informing the teenager with CF of the benefits of a good postural maintenance program may provide the incentive necessary to ensure adherence to recommendations for exercises.

Secondary effects of strength training with weights may be an improvement in self-confidence in the adolescent because training has been shown to be beneficial in promoting weight gain (Strauss et al., 1987). As pulmonary impairment worsens, nutritional status is a consideration that requires a great deal of focus. Individuals who are malnourished have reduced exercise capacity; therefore, the ability to maintain adequate weight gain is essential to the goal of improving exercise tolerance (Canny & Levison, 1987). The dietitian serving the population with CF contributes considerable expertise in identifying situations in which intervention is necessary and may be a valuable ally to reinforce the message that exercise can promote weight gain when appropriately managed. A liaison with the dietitian can ensure coordination of dietary and physical therapy recommendations.

Transition to Adulthood

When CF was first described in 1938, fewer than half of the patients survived their first year (Davis, 1983), but CF is no longer a purely pediatric disease. With contemporary methods of management, almost 80% of patients should reach adulthood (MacLusky & Levison, 1990), and it is currently estimated that the life expectancy of children born with CF in 1990 is 40 years (Elborn et al., 1992). Although many of the issues physical therapists are concerned with in the pediatric patient are similar for adults, some special differences should be considered.

The psychosocial issues in adulthood are distinct because the normal progression of psychologic maturation brings new concerns with each developmental stage (Davis, 1983). Greater clinical awareness, early treatment, and more effective management of CF have all contributed to the improvement of prognosis (Pinkerton et al., 1985). Choices regarding education, employment, marriage, and family will have to be made. These choices are more complex than usual for the adult with CF, who has to consider not only present health status but also must attempt to predict future health status.

Physically demanding occupations may not be appropriate for the adult with CF with pulmonary limitations; therefore, a careful consideration of the physical demands of any task must be undertaken. Jobs involving constant exposure to dust, chemical fumes, or smoke should be avoided (Davis, 1983; Orenstein, 1997). Many adults with CF will be socially and vocationally fully functioning members of society, however, and their physical therapy plan of care must accommodate their busy lifestyles. Physical therapists should help the adult incorporate strategies for fitting treatment into work schedules. Methods that are more convenient and promote independence, such as the PEP mask, Flutter, or AD, may be more agreeable to the adult at work or school.

Because many adults with CF witness mortality among their peers, deterioration of their own health may have heightened significance for them. The adult who as an adolescent chose to be noncompliant with a physical therapy regimen may decide to initiate one again. Generally, individuals with CF have a strong positive outlook and are able to fully enjoy many of the normal pleasures of adulthood despite having to contend with unusual difficulties (Orenstein, 1997). Patients' attitudes and outlook on life can have a tremendous influence on the medical progression of CF and are considered in prognostic scores (Davis, 1983).

Because of the progressive nature of CF, many adults will have more symptoms and functional limitations than they had as children (Orenstein, 1997). Minor hemoptysis occurs in up to 60% of adults with CF (di Sant'Agnese & Davis, 1979), and, in most cases, the cause is an increase in bronchial infection that has irritated a blood vessel (Orenstein, 1997). *Massive hemoptysis,* which is also strongly related to advancing age (Davis, 1983), is defined as a rupture of a bronchial blood vessel into the airways producing greater than 300 ml of blood in 24 hours (Cohen, 1992). It is reported to occur in 5 to 7% of adults with CF (Porter et al., 1983) and warrants hospitalization and possible blood transfusion (Lloyd-Still, 1983).

Pneumothorax, which is one of the most common respiratory complications in adulthood, occurs in approximately 19% of individuals older than 13 years of age (MacLusky & Levison, 1990). A common cause of pneumothorax is the spontaneous rupture of apical bullae, which develop due to increased air trapping and microabscess formation in the diseased lung (MacLusky & Levison, 1990).

Episodes of hypertrophic pulmonary osteoarthropathy also increase in prevalence with advancing age (Davis, 1983). Digital clubbing can become more noticeable in people whose pulmonary disease is severe (Orenstein, 1997).

In general, cardiac status is related to severity of pulmonary involvement: the more severe the pulmonary adaptation to hypoxemia, the worse the pulmonary hypertension and right-sided heart strain. With comparable degrees of pulmonary disease, adults, especially those with mild lung disease, have more severe echocardiographic abnormalities than children. This may reflect the accumulative effects of episodes of mild hypoxemia and nocturnal oxygen desaturation that occur in even minimally affected individuals (Davis, 1983).

Management of Impairment

Because the incidence of respiratory complications increases with age, physical therapists must work with the individual to adapt the treatment program accordingly. For the individual experiencing hemoptysis, physical therapy may have to be altered, although there are conflicting opinions in the literature as to the extent of the modification necessary. MacLusky and Levison (1990) report that CPT is usually discontinued until there is no longer blood in the sputum. Lloyd-Still (1983) is also in favor of temporarily discontinuing CPT. Orenstein (1997), however, believes that if the cause of minor hemoptysis is an increase in bronchial infection irritating a blood vessel, treatment should be the same as for other types of increased infection. He believes that bleeding within the lungs can worsen infection by providing a more hospitable environment for bacteria. He does caution that if a particular treatment position aggravates the bleeding, that position should be avoided.

Other reports in the literature on hemoptysis include the opinion that chest physical therapy should not be withheld for all individuals who produce blood in their sputum (Mackenzie, 1989). The use of postural drainage, percussion, and shaking, along with huffing or FETs, may be less likely to increase the amount of bleeding than the frequent uncontrolled coughing that may occur with abandonment of the manual techniques (Starr, 1992). DeCesare and Graybill (1990) conclude that decisions should be based on individual situations and stress the importance of modified but continued physical therapy. In summary, it would seem logical that if a particular technique, such as percussion, makes the individual's situation worse, it should be discontinued. Other modalities using breathing techniques may be beneficial at this time.

Chest physical therapy is contraindicated in the presence of an untreated, progressing, or tension pneumothorax (DeCesare & Graybill, 1990); however, treatment can continue with a small, stable pneumothorax (DeCesare & Graybill, 1990;

Mackenzie, 1989) and with a pneumothorax that has resolved through treatment with a thoracotomy and insertion of a chest tube for vacuum drainage of air (DeCesare & Graybill, 1990). Percussion must not be performed directly over the chest tube site owing to the danger of displacement, but percussion may be safely performed elsewhere on the thorax as tolerated. The PEP mask would not be the treatment of choice, because theoretically it could make the pneumothorax worse as a result of increased pressures generated in the airways.

Standard anti-inflammatory agents are used to treat the joint pain associated with hypertrophic pulmonary osteoarthropathy (Phillips & David, 1986). Physical therapists have a role in helping to relieve pain while maintaining joint range of motion. A home treatment program consisting of stretching, muscle strengthening, and range-of-motion exercises for the specific joints involved can be easily added to the individual's existing exercise program.

When pulmonary disease becomes so disabling that the individual is having difficulty performing activities of daily living, physical therapy goals should encompass these needs. The patient may have to be instructed in energy conservation techniques such as diaphragmatic pursed-lip breathing and assuming positions that relieve breathlessness. These positions should promote comfort and relaxation and should encourage mobility of the thorax and support of the spinal column. They should also include hip flexion to relax the abdominal musculature and aid in increasing intra-abdominal pressure for coughing (DeCesare & Graybill, 1990). Examples of energy conservation positions are shown in Figure 26–8. Retraining of the respiratory pattern using pursed-lip breathing in conjunction with diaphragmatic excursion has shown temporary benefits in increased tidal volume, decreased respiratory rate, reduction in $Paco_2$ levels, and improved Pao_2 levels, as well as subjective benefits reported by patients (Ciesla, 1989). It may be that pursed-lip breathing improves confidence and decreases anxiety by providing some temporary control over oxygenation (Ciesla, 1989).

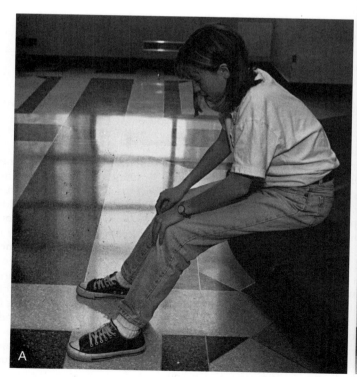
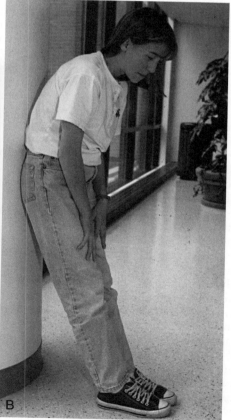

FIGURE 26–8. *A* and *B*, Positioning for energy conservation, promoting relaxation and ease of breathing.

Oxygen needs with exercise may have to be assessed at this time. Continuation of an active lifestyle should be promoted for all individuals with CF to optimize physical condition and maintain an optimistic outlook. If the individual is considering lung transplantation as an option, physical therapists must involve the individual in a formalized exercise program.

The Toronto Lung Transplant Program at the Toronto Hospital has a well-established rehabilitation program. Exercise capacity is determined by using a 6-minute walk test and ear oximetry, or the Modified Bruce Protocol on the treadmill (Craven et al., 1990). For a 6-minute walk test, the subject is instructed to walk as quickly and comfortably as possible on a level, measured distance for 6 minutes. If the patient becomes short of breath or too exhausted to continue, he or she is allowed to rest but then must continue the test as soon as symptoms subside. The distance travelled and the rest periods the subject takes are recorded. Subjects' pulse and respiratory rates and oxygen saturation are measured and recorded before, during, and at the conclusion of the test. The purpose of performing a test of exercise capacity is to help determine if severity of disability warrants consideration for transplant. A 6-minute walk test result of less than 400 meters was found to be a significant indicator for a patient to be listed for transplantation (Kadikar et al., 1997).

Individuals can also be monitored at regular intervals with these tests to gauge potential deterioration in their functional status. Once accepted into the lung transplantation program, most centers require attendance at a formal rehabilitation program (Grossman, 1988) featuring aerobics, muscle strengthening, stretching, and light calisthenics.

Expected physical therapy outcomes for the adult with CF include optimizing functional ability, physical exercise tolerance, and emotional well-being. For the individual awaiting a lung transplant, improvement in overall function should enable him or her to handle the actual surgery and immediate postoperative period with less difficulty (Craven et al., 1990). Arnold and associates (1991) found that 13 patients with end-stage CF showed improvement in their functional exercise capacity by participation in pulmonary rehabilitation while awaiting double-lung transplantation. Pulmonary rehabilitation entailed treadmill walking and lower extremity ergometry 3 to 5 times per week, initiated at the time of listing for double-lung transplant. Six-minute walks were performed biweekly to assess changes in functional exercise capacity, and workload on the treadmill and bicycle ergometer was recorded. Six-minute walk distances and treadmill and bicycle workloads all increased significantly. The conclusions from this data confirm the possibility of improving functional exercise capacity in patients with end-stage CF awaiting double-lung transplantation, despite severe limitations in pulmonary function. There is a role for aerobic exercise in improving physical conditioning, exercise tolerance, and quality of life for all patients with CF.

The physical therapist's contact with those individuals in the terminal stages of their disease should not be discontinued. Intervention at this stage must include the provision of comfort measures and be directed by the patient's wishes. Treatment sessions may have to decrease in duration and be offered with increased frequency throughout the day. Adaptations to postural drainage positions may have to be adopted so treatment can be tolerated. As the work of coughing becomes too tiring or painful, other modalities such as splinting and huffing can be reviewed. Pain control measures and relaxation and anxiety-reducing techniques, such as massage, may be the primary need of the dying patient. Simply listening to the concerns of these patients can be therapeutic. The value of a compassionate ear should not be underestimated. Physical therapists treating terminally ill patients should be careful to incorporate the families' needs, respecting the fact that this is an emotionally volatile time for all involved.

CASE HISTORY
SUZETTE

This section of the chapter presents a case history of a child with CF. Parenthetical comments provide reflection on how practice might be improved based on current knowledge.

Suzette was diagnosed with CF at age 5 months after an admission to hospital with failure to thrive. The diagnosis of CF was based on her presenting symptomatology of poor appetite, vomiting following feedings, bulky and foul-smelling stools, chronic cough, a recurrent rectal prolapse and laboratory investigations that demonstrated right lower lobe pneumonia and partial atelectasis of the right middle lobe on a chest radiograph, presence of *Staphylococcus aureus* in nasopharyngeal aspirate, and elevated sweat chloride level. Suzette was discharged with prescriptions for enzyme supplements, multivitamins, cloxacillin, and a bronchodilator. Goals for physical therapy were to improve ventilation and promote secretion clearance, so a CPT regimen was taught consisting of postural drainage and manual percussions concentrating on the right middle and lower lobes.

Suzette was next admitted to hospital at 1 year of age with recurrent vomiting. During this admission, her sputum culture showed colonization by *Pseudomonas aeruginosa*. Three years later she was again admitted to hospital for treatment of acute bronchitis. Her chest radiographs showed patchy atelectasis and peribronchial thickening of the right middle lobe and a partial collapse of the right lower lobe. She was treated with a 10-day course of intravenously administered antibiotics and postural drainage, percussion, and vibration three times per day. Her CPT techniques were reviewed with her parents before discharge. Suzette remained on the same medications as before except for the change of her oral antibiotic to cephalexin. She remained stable for the next few years.

When Suzette was 6, she participated in a standardized series of exercise challenge tests administered in the school system based on the Canada Fitness Awards Test (Canadian Association for Health, Physical Education and Recreation, 1980) and scored in the top third percentile for her age category. The exercise assessment included an endurance run, speed sit-ups, flexed arm hang, standing broad jump, sit and reach, and flexibility measures. She also underwent her first PFT. Her FVC was 1.05 liters, 72% of the predicted value of 1.45 liters, and her FEV_1 was 0.82 liter, 78% of predicted value. She was classified as having "mild obstruction."

Soon after she turned 7, Suzette was admitted to hospital with an exacerbation of respiratory symptoms. Immediately after discharge she was tested at school with the same series of exercise challenge tests as before and was awarded a gold medal for consistently excellent results. Two weeks later she was readmitted to hospital for acute bronchitis. At this time, because of her chronic chest radiographic findings of bronchiectasis of the right middle lobe and collapsed right lower lobe, the possibility of lobectomy was considered. A bronchoscopy revealed mild bronchiectasis and secretions in both right-stem and left-stem bronchi. After consulting with Suzette's parents and considering her clinical presentation with the maintenance of good fitness levels, the decision was made to defer performing a lobectomy. Suzette was not judged to have severe enough impairment to justify this course of action.

On a routine clinic appointment 6 months later, Suzette and her parents reported that her recurrent vomiting was interfering with completion of physical therapy. She was also experiencing mild, streaky hemoptysis with severe coughing. On questioning, the family related that physical therapy was regularly given 30 minutes after meals to accommodate parental work schedules. The physical therapist aided the family in devising a schedule that allowed treatment sessions to be completed before meals. A recommendation was also made to modify treatment with the use of active cycle of breathing techniques if Suzette continued to experience vomiting. The family was instructed in this technique, and Suzette was able to mobilize secretions with this method. The family was requested to keep a record of when episodes of hemoptysis occurred.

During the following year, a subjective record of continued frequent hemoptysis was reported, correlating with severe bouts of uncontrolled coughing. Suzette was admitted to hospital twice with hemoptysis. The bleeding typically persisted for 2 to 7 days and occurred about every 2 weeks.

Physical examination revealed no cyanosis, moderate clubbing, decreased breath sounds in the right lower lobe, and diffuse coarse inspiratory crepitations heard throughout both lower lobes posteriorly. The parents were again consulted and asked to consider a right middle lobe lobectomy because this was the presumed causative site of Suzette's recurrent hemoptysis. Her parents were resistant to this course and asked to defer the decision until the following spring with the hopes that the frequency of episodes of hemoptysis would decrease. They vowed to continue with the treatment plan of attempting to control coughing with the previously learned ACBT combined with relaxed diaphragmatic pursed-lip breathing. When she was followed up in clinic the following spring, she showed marked clinical improvement with no further episodes of hemoptysis. In view of this, along with the previous bronchoscopic evidence of involvement in more than one lobe, a lobectomy was not indicated.

When she performed spirometric PFTs at age 9, her FVC was 83% of predicted, FEV_1 was 79% of predicted, and $FEF_{25-75\%}$ was 60% of predicted. Obstruction was still considered to be mild. Suzette told the physical therapist on this occasion that she was "sad," and mentioned the recent separation of her parents as being the source of her mood, so a referral to the social worker was initiated.

Three months later, Suzette looked drawn and pale at her clinic visit. She complained of frequent nocturnal wakings caused by a racking cough that was productive of a large amount of thick yellowish sputum. She reported that she had no appetite and had lost 2.5 kg (5.5 lb) since the last clinic visit. She admitted to reduced compliance with physical therapy as a result of severe epigastric pain when in a head-down position. Evidence of gastroesophageal reflux was subsequently found. Suzette was admitted to hospital for 2 weeks. She received intravenous antibiotic therapy and physical therapy 3 times per day, modified to tolerance. (Today a 9-year-old patient with this history would be taught PEP therapy in an attempt to reduce reflux symptoms.) During a physical therapy session Suzette began to relate a number of fears surrounding her attendance at a new school. She had recently moved with her mother into a home with her mother's boyfriend, and Suzette had concerns about fitting in with her new classmates. She had to leave the classroom once a day for inhalation therapy and physical therapy, making her feel different from the other students. She was afraid they would ask her many questions about CF, and she did not feel comfortable answering these types of questions. All of the concerns were related to the social worker responsible for Suzette's case.

The social worker arranged for one of the nurses from the CF clinic to travel to the school and give a talk on CF to Suzette's class. This reassured Suzette greatly, and she started to look forward to returning to school. With the social worker's help, Suzette also began to confront some of her feelings about her parents' separation. Ongoing counseling was made available to the entire family. (Self-management workshops and programs such as the Baylor CF Family Education Program might have assisted Suzette and her family at this time.)

Suzette remained clinically stable for the next year until she was again admitted to hospital with a respiratory exacerbation. She was discharged after 10 days but reported never feeling "right" for the next few months and was readmitted to hospital. Suzette's performance on spirometric PFTs at the time of admission revealed an FVC of 60%, an FEV_1 of 52%, and an $FEF_{25-75\%}$ of 23% of expected values. A decision was made to add an inhaled antibiotic (tobramycin) to Suzette's usual medications to be continued after discharge. The physical therapist reviewed proper inhalation technique and use of the aerosol delivery system, as well as her airway clearance techniques. During her next clinic visits, Suzette relayed a positive subjective response to the new medication and showed steady clinical improvement. The following year, the results of her PFTs demonstrated significant improvement: her FVC was 85%, FEV_1 was 85%, and $FEF_{25-75\%}$ was 72% of predicted values. Suzette continued on the inhaled tobramycin for the next year and remained clinically stable.

Almost 3 years later, when Suzette was 13, the clinic physical therapist discovered that she was not complying with her physical therapy regimen. Suzette did not feel that she wanted to do daily treatments because they interfered with the time she wanted to spend with her friends. Suzette's mother admitted to being frustrated with the "continual struggle" against compliance and sought alternatives to Suzette's treatment plan. The physical therapist suggested a cycle ergometer test to establish a baseline measure of Suzette's exercise tolerance. Suzette completed only 2 minutes on the ergometer before being overcome with a prolonged spell of coughing, necessitating discontinuation of the test. A discussion of the benefits of regular

exercise followed. Suzette admitted to being fearful of exertion as a result of her embarrassment over the severe, productive coughing that usually ensued. An exercise program was proposed by the physical therapist that featured a walking program of very gradually increasing difficulty, and Suzette agreed to try the program for 2 months. Suzette then underwent a 6-minute walk test, and although she complained of severe dyspnea, she completed 460 meters. (The Borg's Scale of Perceived Exertion, The Dyspnea Index, or the San Diego Shortness of Breath Questionnaire [Eakin et al., 1998] could have provided objective measures of the patient's perceived exercise tolerance, if introduced at this time.)

Over the next three clinic appointments, Suzette remained clinically stable and reported steady improvement with her exercise program but continued to have difficulty with adherence to daily physical therapy. The physical therapist undertook an in-depth educational review with emphasis on self-management skills with Suzette.

At 16, Suzette came to clinic complaining of a prolonged malaise; her weight had dropped 2 kg (4.4 lb). She suffered from intermittent fevers and had a frequent cough, productive of large amounts of thick, green sputum that was occasionally tinged with blood. Chest radiography revealed new extensive infiltrates in her right middle lobe and a complete right lower lobe collapse. Results of her PFTs were FVC of 59%, FEV_1 of 52%, and $FEF_{25-75\%}$ of 31% of predicted values. She required an intravenous course of antibiotics and extensive physical therapy and was therefore hospitalized.

Suzette had two more hospital admissions during the next 5 months, both for respiratory exacerbations. During this time, Suzette was instructed in the use of a PEP mask. She quickly demonstrated the proper application of the mask and reported that she "liked" using it. The physical therapist proposed that she attempt to use the mask three times daily and Suzette agreed to try this regimen.

Three months later, Suzette came to her clinic appointment in obvious distress. She was now 17 and was complaining of "almost continuous" shortness of breath, daily fevers, a severely decreased tolerance for exercise, and frequent episodes of hemoptysis. Chest radiography revealed a lobar consolidation. She reported feeling "very sick" for about 10 days but had not come in earlier because she was reluctant to submit to another hospitalization. However, Suzette did need to be hospitalized. The social worker became involved as Suzette became withdrawn during this admission and was found to be severely depressed. The frequency of Suzette's hospital admissions and declining clinical status over the past few years had exacted an emotional toll. With psychologic counseling and emotional support from all members of the multidisciplinary team, Suzette gradually came to embody a more optimistic demeanor. On discharge, Suzette thanked various members of the team who had cared for her and vowed to "keep fighting." She proposed a "new beginning" and resolved to comply with her entire therapeutic regimen, "even physical therapy." Just before discharge Suzette performed a 6-minute walk test and finished 700 meters. She maintained a broad smile throughout the distance.

CONCLUSION

The management of CF poses many challenges for physical therapists. The multisystemic involvement and chronicity of the disorder compel physical therapists to continually interact with a team of professionals to shape appropriate treatment plans. Collaboration with this type of multidisciplinary health care team is always stimulating and fosters creative and fulfilling practice of physical therapy. New advances suggest exciting possibilities for the future care of people with CF, and physical therapists serving this population are required to continually adapt their management approach in light of new research. The aspiration to discover a cure seems to be approaching fulfillment. Meanwhile, the challenge for all those involved is in finding effective means to slow (or prevent) the disabling effects of this disease.

Recommended Resources

Baylor College of Medicine and Texas Children's Hospital. CF Family Education Program. Baylor College of Medicine, 1994.
Hardy, KA. A review of airway clearance: New techniques, indications, and recommendations. Respiratory Care, 39(5):440–452, 1994.
International Physiotherapy Group for Cystic Fibrosis. Physiotherapy in the treatment of cystic fibrosis (CF). IPG/CF, 1995. Contact person: Maggie McIlwain, Physiotherapy Department, B.C.'s Children's Hospital, Vancouver, BC, Canada (phone: 604-875-2123).
Irwin, S, & Tecklin, JS (Eds.). Cardiopulmonary Physical Therapy. St. Louis: Mosby, 1990.
MacLusky, IB, & Levison, H. Cystic fibrosis. In Cherniak, V (Ed.), Kendig's Disorders of the Respiratory Tract in Children, Vol. 5. Philadelphia: WB Saunders, 1990, pp. 692–730.
Orenstein, DM. Cystic Fibrosis: A Guide for Patient and Family, 2nd ed. New York: Lippincott & Raven, 1997.

References

Ackerman, V, Montgomery, G, Eigen, H, & Tepper, R. Assessment of airway responsiveness in infants with cystic fibrosis. American Review of Respiratory Disease, 144:344–346, 1991.
Altose, MD. The physiological basis of pulmonary function testing. Clinical Symposia, 31(2):1–39, 1979.
American Physical Therapy Association. Guide to Physical Therapist Practice. Physical Therapy, 77(11): 1997.
Andersen, DH. Cystic fibrosis of the pancreas and its relation to celiac disease: A clinical and pathologic study. American Journal of Diseases of Children, 56:344–395, 1938.

Andreasson, B, Jonson, B, Kornfalt, R, Nordmar, E, & Sandstrom, S. Long-term effects of physical exercise on working capacity and pulmonary function in cystic fibrosis. Acta Paediatrica Scandinavica, 76:70–75, 1987.
Arnold, CD, Westerman, JH, Downs, AM, & Egan, TM. Benefits of an aerobic exercise program in C.F. patients waiting for double lung transplant. Pediatric Pulmonology Supplement, 6:287, 1991.
Auerbach, HS, Williams, M, Kirkpatrick, JA, & Colten, HR. Alternate-day prednisone reduces morbidity and improves pulmonary function in cystic fibrosis. Lancet, 2:686–688, 1985.
Aweida, D, & Kelsey, CJ. Accuracy and reliability of physical therapists in auscultating tape-recorded breath sounds. Physiotherapy in Canada, 42(6):279–282, 1989.
Balfour-Lynn, IM, Prasad, SA, Laverty, A, Whitehead, BF, & Dinwiddie, R. A step in the right direction: Assessing exercise tolerance in cystic fibrosis. Pediatric Pulmonology, 25(4):223–225, 1998.
Bartholomew, LK, Czyzewski, DI, & Swank, PR. Short-term outcomes of the CF Family Education Program (CF FEP): What we know and what we don't know. Pediatric Pulmonology Supplement, 13:154–155, 1996.
Bartholomew, LK, Parcel, GS, Swank, PR, & Czyzewski, DI. Measuring self-efficacy expectations for the self-management of cystic fibrosis. Chest, 103:1524–1530, 1993.
Bateman, JRM, Newton, SP, Daunt, KM, Pavia, D, & Clarke, SW. Regional lung clearance of excessive bronchial secretions during chest physiotherapy in patients with stable chronic airway obstruction. Lancet, 1:294–297, 1979.
Bhudhikanok, GS, Lim, J, Marcus, R, Harkins, A, Moss, RB, & Bachrach, LK. Correlates of osteopenia in patients with cystic fibrosis. Pediatrics, 97:103–111, 1996.
Borg, GAV. Psychophysical bases of perceived exertion. Medicine and Science in Sports and Exercise, 14:377–381, 1982.
Boyd, S, Brooks, D, Agnew-Coughlin, J, & Ashwell, J. Evaluation of the literature on the effectiveness of physical therapy modalities in the management of children with cystic fibrosis. Pediatric Physical Therapy, 6(2):70–74, 1994.
Boyle, IR, di Sant'Agnese, PA, & Sack, S. Emotional adjustment of adolescents and young adults with cystic fibrosis. Journal of Pediatrics, 88:318–326, 1976.
Buist, AS, Adams, BE, Sexton, GJ, & Azzam, AH. Reference values for functional residual capacity and maximal expiratory flow in young children. American Review of Respiratory Disease, 122:938–988, 1980.
Burns, JL. Treatment of cepacia: In search of the magic bullet. Pediatric Pulmonology Supplement, 14:90–91, 1997.
Burton, L. The Family Life of Sick Children: A Study of Families Coping with Chronic Childhood Disease. London: Routledge & Kegan Paul, 1975.
Bush, A. Giving the bad news—Your child has cystic fibrosis. Pediatric Pulmonology Supplement, 14:206–208, 1997.
Butland, RJA, Pang, J, Gross, ER, Woodcock, AA, & Geddes, DM. Two, six and 12-minute walking test in respiratory disease. British Medical Journal, 284:1607–1608, 1982.
Button, BM, Heine, R, Catto-Smith, A, Olinsky, A, Phelan, PD, & Story, I. A 12 month comparison of standard vs. modified chest physiotherapy in 20 infants with cystic fibrosis. Pediatric Pulmonology Supplement, 14:299a, 1997.
Canadian Association for Health, Physical Education and Recreation. Fitness Performance: Second Test Manual—Canadian Youths, Ages 6–17. Ottawa: CAHPER, 1980.
Canny, GJ, & Levison, H. Exercise response and rehabilitation in cystic fibrosis. Sports Medicine, 4:143–152, 1987.
Cappelli, M, McGrath, PJ, MacDonald, NE, Katsanis, J, & Lascelles, M. Parental care and overprotection of children with cystic fibrosis. British Journal of Medical Psychology, 62:281–289, 1989.

Cerny, FJ. Relative effects of bronchial drainage and exercise for in-hospital care of patients with cystic fibrosis. Physical Therapy, 69:633–639, 1989.

Cerny, FJ, & Darbee, J. Exercise testing and exercise conditioning for children with lung dysfunction. In Irwin, S, & Tecklin, JS (Eds.), Cardiopulmonary Physical Therapy. St. Louis: Mosby, 1990, pp. 461–475.

Cerny, FJ, Pullano, TP, & Cropp, GJA. Cardiorespiratory adaptations to exercise in cystic fibrosis. American Review of Respiratory Disease, 126:217–220, 1982.

Chevaillier, J. Autogenic drainage. In Lawson, D (Ed.), Cystic Fibrosis: Horizons. New York: Wiley, 1984, p. 235.

Ciesla, N. Postural drainage, positioning and breathing exercises. In Mackenzie, CF (Ed.), Chest Physiotherapy in the Intensive Care Unit. Baltimore: Williams & Wilkins, 1989, pp. 93–133.

Coates, AL, MacNeish, CF, Lands, LC, Meisner, D, Kelemen, S, & Vadas, EB. A comparison of the availability of tobramycin for inhalation from vented vs. unvented nebulizers. Chest, 113(4):951–956, 1998.

Cohen, AM. Hemoptysis: Role of angiography and embolization. Pediatric Pulmonology Supplement, 8:85–86, 1992.

Collins, FS. The C.F. gene: Perceptions, puzzles and promises. Pediatric Pulmonology Supplement, 8:63–64, 1992.

Collins, FS. CF Research: Highlights of 1996. Pediatric Pulmonology Supplement, 13:74, 1996.

Conway, SP, & Allenby, K. Parental and patient attitudes in an adult CF clinic to prenatal screening programmes. Pediatric Pulmonology Supplement, 8:238, 1992.

Cooper, PJ, Robertson, CF, Hudson, IL, & Phelan, PD. Variability of pulmonary function tests in cystic fibrosis. Pediatric Pulmonology, 8:16–22, 1990.

Corey, M, Allison, L, Prober, C, & Levison, H. Sputum bacteriology in patients with cystic fibrosis in a Toronto hospital during 1970–1981. Journal of Infectious Diseases, 149:283, 1984a.

Corey, M, Gaskin, K, Durie, P, Levison, H, & Forstner, G. Improved prognosis in C.F. patients with normal fat absorption. Journal of Pediatric Gastroenterology and Nutrition, 3(suppl 1):99–105, 1984b.

Crane, L. Physical therapy for the neonate with respiratory disease. In Irwin, S, & Tecklin, JS (Eds.), Cardiopulmonary Physical Therapy. St. Louis: Mosby, 1990, pp. 389–416.

Craven, JL, Bright, J, & Dear, CL. Psychiatric, psychosocial, and rehabilitative aspects of lung transplantation. Clinics in Chest Medicine, 11:247–257, 1990.

Crystal, RG. Gene therapy for cystic fibrosis: Where have we been and where are we going? Pediatric Pulmonology Supplement, 14:73, 1997.

Dab, I, & Malfroot, A. Gastroesophageal reflux: A primary defect in cystic fibrosis. Scandinavian Journal of Gastroenterology Supplement, 143:125–131, 1988.

Davidson, AGF, McIlwaine, PM, Wong, LTK, & Pirie, GE. Long-term comparative trial of conventional percussion and drainage physiotherapy versus autogenic drainage in cystic fibrosis. Pediatric Pulmonology Supplement, 8:a298, 1992.

Davis, PB. Cystic fibrosis in adults. In Lloyd-Still, JD (Ed.), Textbook of Cystic Fibrosis. Stoneham, MA: Wright, 1983, pp. 351–370.

Day, G, & Mearns, M. Bronchial lability in cystic fibrosis. Archives of Disease in Childhood, 48:355–359, 1973.

Dean, M, O'Connell, P, Leppert, M, Park, M, Amos, JA, Phillips, DG, White, R, & Vande Woude, GF. Three additional DNA polymorphisms in the met gene and D7S8 locus: Use in prenatal diagnosis of cystic fibrosis. Journal of Pediatrics, 111:490–495, 1987.

DeCesare, JA, & Graybill, CA. Physical therapy for the child with respiratory dysfunction. In Irwin, S, & Tecklin, JS (Eds.), Cardiopulmonary Physical Therapy. St. Louis: Mosby, 1990, pp. 417–460.

Denton, JR, Tietjen, R, & Gaerlan, PF. Thoracic kyphosis in cystic fibrosis. Clinical Orthopaedics and Related Research, 155:71–74, 1981.

di Sant'Agnese, PA, & Davis, PB. Cystic fibrosis in adults: 75 cases and a review of 232 cases in the literature. American Journal of Medicine, 66:121–132, 1979.

Doershuk, CF, Downs, TD, Matthews, LW, & Lough, MD. A method for ventilatory measurements in subjects one month to five years of age: Normal results and observations in disease. Pediatric Research, 4:165–174, 1970.

Doershuk, CF, Matthews, LW, & Tucker, AS. A five-year clinical evaluation of a therapeutic program for patients with cystic fibrosis. Journal of Pediatrics, 65:1112–1113, 1964.

Durie, PR. Gastrointestinal motility disorders in cystic fibrosis. In Willa, JP (Ed.), Disorders of Gastrointestinal Motility in Childhood. New York: Wiley, 1988, pp. 91–99.

Durie, PR, Gaskin, KJ, Corey, M, Kopelman, H, Weizman, Z, & Forstner, GG. Pancreatic function testing in cystic fibrosis. Journal of Pediatric Gastroenterology and Nutrition, 3:89–98, 1984.

Eakin, EG, Resnikoff, PM, Prewitt, LM, Ries, AL, Kaplan, RM. Validation of a new dyspnea measure: the VCSD Shortness of Breath Questionnaire, University of California, San Diego. Chest, 113(3):619–24, Mar 1998.

Egan, TM. Overview of lung transplantation for cystic fibrosis. Pediatric Pulmonology Supplement, 8:204–205, 1992.

Elborn, JS, Shale, DJ, & Britton, JR. Cystic fibrosis: Current survival and population estimates to the year 2000. Thorax, 45:783a, 1992.

England, SJ. Current techniques for assessing pulmonary function in the newborn and infant: Advantages and limitations. Pediatric Pulmonology, 4:48–53, 1988.

Folkins, C. The effects of physical training on mood. Journal of Clinical Psychology, 32:583–588, 1972.

Fox, EL, & Mathews, DK. The Physiological Basis of Physical Education and Athletics, 3rd ed. Philadelphia: Saunders College, 1981.

Fried, MD, Durie, PR, Tsui, LC, Corey, M, Levison, H, & Pencharz, PB. The cystic fibrosis gene and resting energy expenditure. Journal of Pediatrics, 119:913–916, 1991.

Frownfelter, DL (Ed.). Chest Physical Therapy and Pulmonary Rehabilitation. Chicago: Year Book Medical, 1987.

Galabert, C, Zahm, JM, Chaffin, C, de Bentzmann, S, Grosskopf, C, Chazalette, JP, Puchelle, E. Improvement by rhDNASE of cystic fibrosis mucus transport capacity is related to the release of surface active molecules. Pediatric Pulmonology Supplement, 13:283a, 1996.

Gaskin, L, Shin, J, Reisman, JJ, Thomas, J, Tullis, E. Long term trial of conventional postural drainage and percussion vs. positive expiratory pressure. Pediatric Pulmonology Supplement, 15:345a, 1998.

Gibson, LE, & Cooke, RE. A test for the concentration of electrolytes in sweat in cystic fibrosis of the pancreas utilizing pilocarpine by iontophoresis. Pediatrics, 23:545–549, 1959.

Gilljam, H, Malmborg, A, & Strandvik, B. Conformity of bacterial growth in sputum and contamination free endobronchial samples in patients with cystic fibrosis. Thorax, 41:641–645, 1986.

Godfrey, S. Exercise Testing in Children. Philadelphia: WB Saunders, 1974.

Godfrey, S, Bar-Yishay, E, Arad, I, Landau, LI, & Taussig, LM. Flow-volume curves in infants with lung disease. Pediatrics, 72:517–522, 1983.

Green, M, & Solnit, AJ. Reactions to the threatened loss of a child: A vulnerable child syndrome. Pediatrics, 34:58–66, 1964.

Green, OC. Endocrinological complications associated with cystic fibrosis. In Lloyd-Still, JD (Ed.), Textbook of Cystic Fibrosis. Stoneham, MA: Wright, 1983, pp. 329–349.

Grossman, RF. Lung transplantation. Medical Clinics of North America, 24:4572–4579, 1988.

Gulmans, VAM, van Veldhoven, NHMJ, de Meer, K, & Helders, PJM. The six-minute walking test in children with cystic fibrosis: Reliability and validity. Pediatric Pulmonology, 22:85–89, 1996.

Gurwitz, D, Corey, M, Francis, PJ, Crozier, D, & Levison, H. Perspectives in cystic fibrosis. Pediatric Clinics of North America, 26(3):603–615, 1979.

Hardy, KA. A review of airway clearance: New techniques, indications, and recommendations. Respiratory Care, 39(5):440–452, 1994.

Hardy, KA, Wolfson, MR, Schidlow, DV, & Shaffer, TH. Mechanics and energetics of breathing in newly diagnosed infants with cystic fibrosis: Effect of combined bronchodilator and chest physical therapy. Pediatric Pulmonology, 6:103–108, 1989.

Heijerman, HGM, Bakker, W, Sterk, P, & Dijkman, JH. Oxygen-assisted exercise training in adult cystic fibrosis patients with pulmonary limitation to exercise. International Journal of Rehabilitation Research, 14:101–115, 1991.

Henke, KG, & Orenstein, DM. Oxygen saturation during exercise in cystic fibrosis. American Review of Respiratory Disease, 129:708–711, 1984.

Hiatt, P, Eigen, H, Yu, P, & Tepper, RS. Bronchodilator response in infants and young children with cystic fibrosis. American Review of Respiratory Disease, 137:119–122, 1988.

Hietpas, B, Roth, R, & Jensen, W. Huff coughing and airway patency. Respiratory Care, 24:710, 1979.

Humberstone, N. Respiratory assessment and treatment. In Irwin, S, & Tecklin, JS (Eds.), Cardiopulmonary Physical Therapy. St. Louis: Mosby, 1990, pp. 283–322.

Kadikar, A, Maurer, J, & Kesten, S. The six-minute walk test: A guide to assessment for lung transplantation. Journal of Heart and Lung Transplantation, 16(3):313–319, 1997.

Kattan, M. Pediatric pulmonary function testing. In Miller, A (Ed.), Pulmonary Function Tests: A Guide for the Student and House Officer. Philadelphia: WB Saunders, 1987, pp. 199–212.

Kellerman, J, Zeltzer, L, & Ellenberg, L. Psychological effects of illness in adolescence: Anxiety, self-esteem and perception of control. Journal of Pediatrics, 97:126–131, 1980.

Kerem, BS, Rommens, JR, Buchanan, JA, Markiewicz, D, Cox, TK, Chakravarti, A, Buchwald, M, & Tsui, LC. Identification of the cystic fibrosis gene: Gene analysis. Science, 245:1073–1080, 1989.

Kerem, E, Reisman, J, Corey, M, Canny, GJ, & Levison, H. Prediction of mortality in patients with cystic fibrosis. New England Journal of Medicine, 326:1187–1191, 1992.

Khaghani, A, Madden, B, Hodson, M, & Yacoub, M. Heart-lung transplantation for cystic fibrosis. Pediatric Pulmonology Supplement, 6:128–129, 1991.

Konstan, MW, Stern, RC, & Doershuk, CF. Efficacy of the Flutter VRPI in airway mucus clearance in cystic fibrosis. Pediatrics, 124:689–693, 1994.

Lamarre, A, Reilly, BJ, & Bryan, AC. Early detection of pulmonary function abnormalities in cystic fibrosis. Pediatrics, 50:291–298, 1972.

Lannefors, L. Different ways of using positive expiratory pressure to loosen and mobilize secretions. Pediatric Pulmonology Supplement, 8:136–137, 1992.

Lemke, A, Lester, L, Lloyd-Still, J, & Powers, C. Attitudes toward genetic testing among adults with cystic fibrosis. Pediatric Pulmonology Supplement, 8:238, 1992.

Lewiston, N, & Moss, R. Interobserver variance in clinical scoring for cystic fibrosis. Chest, 91:878–882, 1987.

Lloyd-Still, DM, & Lloyd-Still, JD. The patient, the family and the community. In Lloyd-Still, JD (Ed.), Textbook of Cystic Fibrosis. Stoneham, MA: Wright, 1983, pp. 443–446.

Lloyd-Still, JD. Pulmonary manifestations. In Lloyd-Still, JD (Ed.): Textbook of Cystic Fibrosis. Stoneham, MA: Wright, 1983, pp. 165–198.

Loffert, DT, Ikle, D, & Nelson, HS. A comparison of commercial jet nebulizers. Chest, 106:1788–1792, 1994.

Lorin, MI, & Denning, CR. Evaluation of postural draight by measurement of sputum volume and consistency. American Journal of Physical Medicine and Rehabilitation, 50:215–219, 1971.

Loudon, RG. The lung exam. Clinics in Chest Medicine, 8:265, 1987.

Mackenzie, CF. Undesirable effects, precautions, and contraindications of chest physiotherapy. In Mackenzie, CF (Ed.), Chest Physiotherapy in the Intensive Care Unit. Baltimore: Williams & Wilkins, 1989, pp. 321–344.

MacLusky, IB, Canny, GJ, & Levison, H. Cystic fibrosis: An update. Paediatric Reviews and Communications, 1:343–384, 1987.

MacLusky, IB, Gold, R, Corey, M, & Levison, H. Long-term effects of inhaled tobramycin in patients with cystic fibrosis colonised with Pseudomonas aeruginosa. Pediatric Pulmonology, 7:42–48, 1989.

MacLusky, IB, & Levison, H. Cystic fibrosis. In Chernick, V (Ed.), Kendig's Disorders of the Respiratory Tract in Children, Vol. 5. Philadelphia: WB Saunders, 1990, pp. 692–730.

MacLusky, IB, & Levison, H. Cystic fibrosis. In Chernick, VI (Ed.), Kendig's Disorders of the Respiratory Tract in Children, Vol. 6. Philadelphia: WB Saunders, 1998, pp. 838–882.

Matson, JA, & Capen, CV. Pregnancy in the cystic fibrosis patient. Journal of Reproductive Medicine, 26:373, 1982.

Maxwell, B. Nursing aspects of C.F. care. Pediatric Pulmonology Supplement, 6:85–86, 1991.

Mazzacco, MC, Owens, GR, Kirilloff, LH, & Rogers, RM. Chest percussion and postural drainage in patients with chronic bronchiectasis. Chest, 88:360–363, 1985.

McCollum, AT, & Gibson, LE. Family adaptation to the child with cystic fibrosis. Journal of Pediatrics, 77:571–578, 1970.

McIlwaine, PM, Davidson, AGF, Wong, LTK, & Pirie, GE. Autogenic drainage. Pediatric Pulmonology Supplement, 8:134–135, 1992.

McIlwaine, PM, Davidson, AGF, Wong, LTK, Pirie, GE, & Nakielna, EM. Comparison of positive expiratory pressure and autogenic drainage with conventional percussion and drainage therapy in the treatment of cystic fibrosis. Pediatric Pulmonology, 4(suppl 2):132a, 1988.

McIlwaine, PM, Wong, LT, Peacock, D, & Davidson, GF. "Flutter versus pep": A long-term comparative trial of positive expiratory pressure (PEP) versus oscillating positive expiratory pressure (Flutter) physiotherapy techniques. Pediatric Pulmonology Supplement, 14:299, 1997a.

McIlwaine, PM, Wong, LT, Peacock, D, & Davidson, GF. Long-term comparative trial of conventional postural drainage and percussion versus positive expiratory pressure physiotherapy in the treatment of cystic fibrosis. Pediatrics, 131(4):570–574, 1997b.

Mellins, R. The site of airway obstruction in cystic fibrosis. Pediatrics, 44:315–318, 1969.

Mellins, R, Levine, OR, Ingram, RH, Jr, & Fishman, AP. Obstructive disease of the airways in cystic fibrosis. Pediatrics, 41:560–573, 1968.

Miller, A. Spirometry and maximum expiratory flow-volume curves. In Miller, A (Ed.), Pulmonary Function Tests: A Guide for the Student and House Officer. Philadelphia: WB Saunders, 1987, pp. 15–32.

Miller, WF, Scacci, R, & Gast, LR. Laboratory Evaluation of Pulmonary Function. Philadelphia: JB Lippincott, 1987, pp. 105–176.

Mitchell-Heggs, P, Mearns, M, & Batten, JC. Cystic fibrosis in adolescents and adults. Quarterly Journal of Medicine, 45:479–504, 1976.

Muller, N, Frances, P, Gurwitz, D, Levison, H, & Bryan, AC. Mechanisms of hemoglobin desaturation during rapid-eye movement sleep in normal subjects and in patients with cystic fibrosis. American Review of Respiratory Disease, 119:338, 1980.

Nixon, PA, Orenstein, DM, Kelsey, SF, & Doershuk, CF. The prognostic value of exercise testing in patients with cystic fibrosis. New England Journal of Medicine, 327:1785–1788, 1992.

Oberwaldner, B, Evans, JC, & Zach, MS. Forced expirations against a variable resistance: A new chest physiotherapy method in cystic fibrosis. Pediatric Pulmonology, 2:358–367, 1986.

Oberwaldner, B, Theissl, B, Rucker, A, & Zach, MS. Chest physiotherapy in hospitalized patients with cystic fibrosis: A study of lung function effects and sputum production. European Respiratory Journal, 4:152–158, 1991.

Orenstein, DM. Cystic Fibrosis: A Guide for Patient and Family, 2nd ed. New York: Lippincott-Raven, 1997.

Orenstein, DM, Franklin, BA, Doershuk, CF, Hellerstein, HK, Germann, KJ, Horowitz, JG, & Stern, RC. Exercise conditioning and cardiopulmonary fitness in cystic fibrosis. Chest, 80:292–298, 1981.

Orenstein, DM, Franklin, BA, Doershuk, CF, Hellerstein, HK, Germann, KJ, Horowitz, JG, & Stern, RC. Exercise conditioning and cardiopulmonary fitness in cystic fibrosis. Chest, 80:292–298, 1981.

Orenstein, DM, Henke, KG, & Cerny, FJ. Exercise and cystic fibrosis. Physician and Sports Medicine, 2:57–63, 1983.

Orenstein, SR, & Orenstein, DM. Gastroesophageal reflux and respiratory disease in children. Journal of Pediatrics, 112:847–858, 1988.

Ormerod, LP, Thompson, RA, & Anderson, CM. Reversibility of airways obstruction in cystic fibrosis. Thorax, 35:768–772, 1980.

Paley, CA. A way forward for determining optimal aerobic exercise intensity? Physiotherapy, 83(12):620-624, 1997.

Paradowski, LJ. The CF patient post lung transplant: The UNC experience. Pediatric Pulmonology Supplement, 8:210–212, 1992.

Park, RW, & Grand, RJ. Gastrointestinal manifestations of cystic fibrosis: A review. Gastroenterology, 81:1143–1161, 1981.

Pasque, MK, Cooper, JD, Kaiser, LR, Haydock, DA, Triantafilloy, A, & Trulock, EP. Improved technique for bilateral lung transplantation: Rationale and initial clinical experience. Annals of Thoracic Surgery, 49:785–791, 1990.

Passero, MA, Remor, B, & Solomon, J. Patient-reported compliance with cystic fibrosis therapy. Clinical Pediatrics, 20:264–268, 1981.

Pasterkamp, H, Montgomery, M, & Wiebicke, W. Nomenclature used by health care professionals to describe breath sounds in asthma. Chest, 92:346–352, 1987.

Pegues, DA, Carson, LA, Tablan, OC, FitzSimmons, SC, Roman, SB, Miller, JM, Jarvis, WR, and the Summer Camp Group. Acquisition of *Pseudomonas cepacia* at summer camps for patients with cystic fibrosis. Summer camp study group. Pediatrics, 124:694–702, 1994.

Phelan, PD, Gracey, M, Williams, HE, & Anderson, CM. Ventilatory function in infants with cystic fibrosis. Archives of Disease in Childhood, 44:393–400, 1969.

Phillips, BM, & David, TJ. Pathogenesis and management of arthropathy in cystic fibrosis. Journal of the Royal Society of Medicine, 79(suppl 12):44–49, 1986.

Phillips, BM, & David, TJ. Management of the chest in cystic fibrosis. Journal of the Royal Society of Medicine, 80(suppl 15):30–37, 1987.

Physiotherapy in the Treatment of Cystic Fibrosis (CF). International Physiotherapy Group for Cystic Fibrosis Mucoviscidosis Association 1995. (Available by the secretary of IPG/CF, www.ipg-cf.fw.hu).

Pinkerton, P, Trauer, T, Duncan, F, Hodson, M, & Batten, J. Cystic fibrosis in adult life: A study of coping patterns. Lancet, 2:761–763, 1985.

Pizer, HF. Organ Transplants: A Patient's Guide. Cambridge, MA: Harvard University Press, 1991.

Porcari, JP, Ebbeling, CB, Ward, A, Freedson, PS, & Rippe, JM. Walking for exercise testing and training. Sports Medicine, 8:189–200, 1989.

Porter, DK, Van Every, MJ, Anthracite, RF, & Mack, JW, Jr. Massive hemoptysis in cystic fibrosis. Archives of Internal Medicine, 143:287–290, 1983.

Prince, A. *Pseudomonas aeruginosa* gene products associated with epithelial colonization. Pediatric Pulmonology Supplement, 8:75–76, 1992.

Pryor, JA, Webber, BA, Hodson, ME, & Batten, JC. Evaluation of the forced expiration technique as an adjunct to postural drainage in treatment of cystic fibrosis. British Medical Journal, 2:417–418, 1979.

Pryor, JA. The forced expiratory technique. In: Pryor J. ed. Respiratory Care. London: Churchill Livingstone. 1991:79–100.

Ramsey, BW. New clinical developments: From the test tube to the bedside. Pediatric Pulmonology Supplement, 14:137–138, 1997.

Reisman, JJ, Rivington-Law, B, Corey, M, Marcotte, J, Wannamaker, E, Harcourt, D, & Levison, H. Role of conventional physiotherapy in cystic fibrosis. Journal of Pediatrics, 113:632–636, 1988.

Riordan, JR, Rommens, JM, Kerem, BS, Alon, N, Rozmahel, R, Grzelczak, Z, Zielensky, J, Lok, S, Plavsic, N, Drumm, ML, Iannuzzi, MC, Collins, FS, & Tsui, LC. Identification of the cystic fibrosis gene: Cloning and characterization of complementary DNA. Science, 245:1066–1073, 1989.

Rose, J, & Jay, S. A comprehensive exercise program for persons with cystic fibrosis. Journal of Pediatric Nursing, 1:323–334, 1986.

Rosenstein, B, & Langbaum, T. Diagnosis. In Taussig, LM (Ed.), Cystic Fibrosis. New York: Thieme-Stratton, 1984, pp. 85–115.

Ruppel, G. Manual of Pulmonary Function Testing. St. Louis: Mosby, 1991.

Sackett, DL. Rules of evidence and clinical recommendations on the use of antithrombotic agents. Chest, 89(suppl):25–35, 1986.

Sammut, P, & Morgan, WJ. Volume-independent assessment of forced expiratory flow in young children. American Review of Respiratory Disease, 135:A238, 1987.

Scott, RB, O'Loughlin, EV, & Gall, DG. Gastroesophageal reflux in patients with cystic fibrosis. Journal of Pediatrics, 106:223–227, 1985.

Scott, SM, Walters, DA, Singh, SJ, Morgan, MDL, & Hardman, AE. A progressive shuttle walking test of functional capacity in patients with chronic airflow limitation. Thorax, 45:781a, 1990.

Shepherd, R, Vasques-Velasquez, L, Prentice, A, Holt, TL, Coward, W, & Lucas, A. Increased energy expenditure in young children with cystic fibrosis. Lancet, 2:1300–1303, 1988.

Shwachman, H, & Kulczycki, LL. Long-term study of 105 patients with cystic fibrosis. American Journal of Diseases of Children, 96:6–15, 1958.

Singh, S. The use of field walking test for assessment of functional capacity in patients with chronic airways obstruction. Physiotherapy, 78:102–104, 1992.

Skorecki, K, Levison, H, & Crozier, DN. Bronchial lability in cystic fibrosis. Acta Paediatrica Scandinavica, 65:39–44, 1976.

Spicher, V, Roulet, M, & Schultz, Y. Assessment of total energy expenditure in free-living patients with cystic fibrosis. Journal of Pediatrics, 118:865–972, 1991.

Starr, JA. Manual techniques of chest physical therapy and airway clearance techniques. In Zadai, CC (Ed.), Pulmonary Management in Physical Therapy. New York: Churchill Livingstone, 1992, pp. 99–133.

Strauss, GD, Osher, A, Wang, CI, Goodrich, E, Gold, F, Colman, W, Stabile, M, Dobrenchuk, A, & Keens, T. Variable weight training in cystic fibrosis. Chest, 92:273–276, 1987.

Sutton, PP, Lopez-Vidriero, MT, Pavia, D, Newman, SP, & Clay, MM. Assessment of percussion, vibratory-shaking and breathing exercises in chest physiotherapy. American Review of Respiratory Disease, 66:147–152, 1985.

Sutton, PP, Parker, RA, Webber, BA, Newman, SP, & Garland, N. Assessment of the forced expiration technique, postural drainage and directed coughing in chest physiotherapy. European Journal of Respiratory Disease, 64:62–68, 1983.

Tablan, OC, Chorba, TL, Schidlow, DV, White, JW, Hardy, KA, Gilligan, PH, Morgan, WM, Carson, MS, Martone, WJ, Jason, JM, & Jarvis, WR. *Pseudomonas cepacia* colonization in patients with cystic fibrosis: Risk factors and clinical outcome. Pediatrics, 107:382–387, 1985.

Taussig, LM. Maximal expiratory flows at functional residual capacity: A test of lung function for young children. American Review of Respiratory Disease, 116:1031–1038, 1977.

Taussig, LM, Landau, LI, & Marks, MI. Respiratory system. In Taussig, LM (Ed.), Cystic Fibrosis. New York: Thieme-Stratton, 1984, pp. 115–174.

Taussig, LM, Lobeck, CC, di Sant'Agnese, PA, Ackerman, DR, & Kattwinkel, J. Fertility in males with cystic fibrosis. New England Journal of Medicine, 287:587–589, 1972.

Tepper, RS. Assessment of pulmonary function in infants with cystic fibrosis. Pediatric Pulmonology Supplement, 8:165–166, 1992.

Tepper, RS, Hiatt, P, Eigen, H, Scott, P, Grosfeld, J, & Cohen, M. Infants with cystic fibrosis: Pulmonary function at diagnosis. Pediatric Pulmonology, 5:15–18, 1988.

Tepper, RS, Hiatt, PW, Eigen, H, & Smith, J. Total respiratory compliance in asymptomatic infants with cystic fibrosis. American Review of Respiratory Disease, 135:1075–1079, 1987.

Van Hengstrum, M, Festen, J, & Beurskens, C. Conventional physiotherapy and forced expiration technique maneuvers have similar effects on tracheobronchial clearance. European Respiratory Journal, 1:758, 1988.

Vinocur, CD, Marmon, L, Schidlow, DV, & Weintraub, WH. Gastroesophageal reflux in the infant with cystic fibrosis. American Journal of Surgery, 149:182–186, 1985.

Wagener, JS, Taussig, LM, Burrows, B, Hernried, L, & Boat, T. Comparison of lung function survival patterns between cystic fibrosis and emphysema or chronic bronchitis patients. In Sturgess, JM (Ed.), Perspectives in Cystic Fibrosis. Mississauga, Canada: Imperial Press, 1980, pp. 236–245.

Webber, BA, Pryor JA. Physiotherapy for Respiratory and Cardiac Problems. New York: Churchill and Livingstone, 1993.

Wiebicke, W, Pownter, A, Montgomery, M, & Pagtakhan, R. The effect of dipratropium bromide on lung function in patients with cystic fibrosis. Pneumonologie, 44(suppl 1):277–278, 1990.

Wilson, CB. The immune system: The devil within or the good guy. Pediatric Pulmonology Supplement, 13:75, 1996.

Winton, T. Double lung transplantation for cystic fibrosis: Operative technique and early post-operative care. Pediatric Pulmonology Supplement, 8:208–209, 1992.

Witt, DR, Blumberg, B, Schaefer, C, Fitzgerald, P, Fishbach, A, Holtzman, J, Kornfeld, S, Lee, R, Nemzer, L, Palmer, R, Sato, M, & Jenkins, L. Cystic fibrosis carrier screening in a prenatal population. Pediatric Pulmonology Supplement, 8:235, 1992.

Wood, RE. Why commence conventional chest physiotherapy for CF at diagnosis? Pediatric Pulmonology Supplement, 9:89–90, 1993.

Yankaskas, JR. Respiratory failure in CF: Pathophysiology and treatment, including the role of mechanical ventilation. Pediatric Pulmonology Supplement, 8:87–88, 1992.

Yankaskas, JR, Mallory, GB, and the Consensus Committee. Lung transplantation in cystic fibrosis: Consensus conference statement. Chest, 113(1):217–226, 1998.

Zach, MS, Purrer, B, & Oberwaldner, B. Effect of swimming on forced expiration and sputum clearance in cystic fibrosis. Lancet, 2:1201–1203, 1981.

Zadai, CC. Comprehensive physical therapy evaluation: Identifying potential pulmonary limitations. In Zadai, CC (Ed.), Pulmonary Management in Physical Therapy. New York: Churchill Livingstone, 1992, pp. 55–78.

CHAPTER
27

Asthma

CYNTHIA L. MAGEE, PT, MS

Bronchial asthma is a chronic inflammatory disorder of the respiratory system. Complex interactions occur between various cells and cellular elements resulting in recurrent episodes of shortness of breath, chest tightness, and coughing. There is usually an associated obstruction of airflow that may reverse spontaneously or with pharmacologic treatment. Bronchial hypersensitivity to a variety of stimuli is also increased (National Heart, Lung, and Blood Institute [NHLBI], 1997). These stimuli are classified as extrinsic or intrinsic. Extrinsic, or allergic, stimuli include pollen, mold, animal dander, cigarette smoke, foods, drugs, and dust. Intrinsic, or nonallergic, stimuli include viral infections, inhalation of irritating substances, exercise, emotional stress, and environmental factors such as the weather or climate changes. An individual may be sensitive to either type of stimuli or to both types. A study of 298 children with asthma, ages 5 months to 14 years 11 months, revealed that the most common triggers included upper respiratory tract infections (virtually all children), exercise (60% of children), changes in the weather (63%), grass pollen (63%), animal danders (cats 55%, dogs 36%, and feathers

21%), and even strong odors (about 50%) (Mercer & Van Niekerk, 1991).

The prevalence of asthma is increased in the extended families of persons who demonstrate asthma or allergic rhinitis. Mercer and Van Niekerk (1991) reported that 76.8% of 298 children with asthma had allergic rhinitis, 17.1% had eczema, and 91% had a family history of allergy in first- or second-degree relatives.

The prevalence of reported asthma in children younger than age 17 is 8 to 10%, making asthma the most common lung disease in children (Evans et al., 1987). A study conducted in Great Britain (Burney et al., 1990) demonstrated an increasing prevalence of asthma in children 5 to 12 years of age over the period from 1973 to 1986. Although the prevalence of bronchitis decreased over this same time period (down 4.7% for boys and 5.8% for girls), the prevalence of asthma increased by 6.9% for boys and 12.8% for girls. The increase in asthma, therefore, cannot be explained solely by a change in diagnosis.

A survey conducted by the Centers for Disease Control and Prevention (CDC) in the United States (CDC, 1998) reported an increase in asthma incidence, morbidity, and mortality between 1979 and 1995. In 1995, more than 13 million people were affected by asthma and over 4 million of these were children under age 15. The incidence increased between 1980 and 1993–1994 by 160% for children ages 0 to 4 years and by 74% for children ages 5 to 14 years. Average office visits with asthma as the first-listed diagnosis increased between 1985 and 1993–1995 by 63% for children ages 0 to 4 years and by 20% for children ages 5 to 14 years. Average death rates with asthma as the underlying cause increased between 1979–1980 and 1993–1995 by 12% for children ages 0 to 4 years and 146% for children ages 5 to 14 years.

Genetic research continues to isolate the locations of the genes responsible for asthma. Different genes have been found for different races, as summarized in Table 27–1 (Collaborative Study on the Genetics of Asthma, 1997). An autosomal dominant pattern of inheritance with variable patterns of expression has been demonstrated. Cookson and colleagues (1989) reported that 85% of those who carry the gene displayed some symptoms, 60% had wheezing, and 20% had been diagnosed with asthma. Although it is not possible to predict which individuals who carry the gene will be more severely affected, a child who has two parents with asthma has a greater chance of having severe symptoms.

This chapter will present an overview of the pathophysiology of asthma; the current diagnosis criteria and recommended medical management; and the secondary impairments, functional limitations, and disabilities that may occur throughout childhood. Physical therapy examination and intervention from infancy to adulthood will be discussed. A case history following a child with asthma from infancy to adulthood with a retrospective look at how his medical treatment would have been changed based on current knowledge concludes the chapter.

PATHOPHYSIOLOGY

The physical, neurogenic, chemical, or pharmacologic factors that are associated with asthma are specific to each individual. They stimulate or trigger the immune system to release chemical mediators, which in turn cause constriction of the bronchial muscles, increased mucus production, and swelling of the mucous membranes. These effects result in increased resistance to airflow, increasing the work of breathing and decreasing pulmonary ventilation. Mucus accumulation may cause blockage of the airways, resulting in further air trapping, hyperinflation, and, eventually, atelectasis. In some patients, there is hypertrophy of the smooth muscles of the airways with new vessel formation, an increase in the number of goblet cells, and deposition of interstitial collagen, which may not be reversible and results in fibrosis of the basement membrane (NHLBI, 1997). In the acute stage, the early recruitment of cells results in inflammation. In the subacute stage, the recruited and activated resident cells result in a more persistent inflammation. Persistent cell damage and ongoing repair result in chronic inflammation.

The pathophysiology of asthma is one of five types of hypersensitivity reactions mediated by the immune system (Male, 1986). Asthma is considered a type 1 or immediate-type hypersensitivity reaction. Subsequent to exposure to a bronchial challenge, serum molecules and cells of the immune system migrate to the site of inflammation where they stimulate increased blood supply, increased capillary permeability, migration of cells out of the blood vessels into the tissues, smooth muscle contraction, increased mucus secretion, inhibition of mucociliary clearance, and activation of neurons (NHLBI, 1997; Stempel, 1998). These inflammatory cells and mediators, which include T lymphocytes, mast cells, macrophages, eosinophils, neutrophils, histamine, prostaglandins, leukotrienes, platelet activating factor (PAF), bradykinin, adenosine, anaphylatoxins, substance P, thromboxane, serotonin, oxygen radicals, complement fragments, and neurokin A, may also produce a secondary late reaction 6 to 8 hours later (Stempel, 1998).

The release of chemical mediators of the allergic response depends on the relative intracellular concentrations of cyclic adenosine monophosphate (cAMP) and cyclic guanosine monophosphate (cGMP) (Crofton & Douglas, 1981). A higher concentration of cAMP will inhibit the release of mediators, resulting in bronchodilation, decreased mucus production, and decreased histamine production. A higher concentration of cGMP will enhance the release of mediators, resulting in bronchoconstriction, increased mucus production, and increased histamine production. cAMP can be increased by stimulation of the sympathetic nervous system through the beta-adrenergic receptors. cGMP can be increased by stimulation of the sympathetic nervous system

TABLE 27–1. **Identified Gene Locations**

Race	Chromosome Location
African-American	5p15, 17p11.1-q11.2
Caucasian	5q23-31, 6p21.3-23, 11p15, 12q14-24.2, 13q21.3-qter, 14q11.2-13, 19q13
Hispanic	2q33, 12q14-24.2, 21q21

Compiled from The Collaborative Study on the Genetics of Asthma. A genome-wide search for asthma susceptibility loci in ethnically diverse populations. Nature Genetics, 15:389–392, 1997.

through the alpha-adrenergic receptors or by stimulation of the parasympathetic nervous system. Knowledge of the pathophysiology of immune system hypersensitivity reactions has been used to develop effective pharmacologic control of asthma.

Mucociliary transport in patients with asthma has been investigated and found to be abnormal (Kurashima et al., 1992; Mezey et al., 1978). Six patients with ragweed hypersensitivity, ages 18 to 48 years, and seven controls, ages 19 to 29 years, participated in one study (Mezey et al., 1978). Tracheal mucus velocity (TMV) was measured before and after antigen challenge. Forced expiratory volume during the first second of exhalation (FEV_1) was measured by spirometry and used to determine lung function. Mean baseline TMV was 54% of normal ($p < .01$) even though FEV_1 was normal or only slightly abnormal. After the antigen challenge when FEV_1 had reached maximal decrease ($p < .01$), the mean TMV had decreased to 72% of baseline ($p < .05$). TMV continued to decrease to 47% of baseline ($p < .05$) even though FEV_1 had returned to baseline values.

PRIMARY IMPAIRMENT

Diagnosis

The diagnosis of asthma is made on the basis of history, physical examination, auscultation and palpation, and pulmonary function tests (PFTs). Wheezing and rhonchi may be detected and may even be present when the child demonstrates no breathing difficulty. Coughing, wheezing, difficulty breathing, and chest tightness may be reported as being worse at night or early in the morning. Hyperexpansion of the thorax, decreased use of the diaphragm with increased use of accessory muscles, postural changes, increased nasal secretions, mucosal swelling, nasal polyps, "allergic shiners" (darkened areas under the eyes), and evidence of an allergic skin condition may be noted on physical examination.

The severity of asthma is classified as mild intermittent, mild persistent, moderate persistent, or severe persistent (Table 27–2) (NHLBI, 1997). During an acute asthma attack, the child may evidence an increased respiratory rate, expiratory grunting, intercostal muscle retractions and nasal flaring, an alteration in the inspiration-expiration ratio, and coughing. In severe cases, a bluish color of the lips and nails may be noted.

Pulmonary Function Tests

PFTs are performed to determine the degree of respiratory impairment and the reversibility of bronchoconstriction following administration of a bronchodilator. A variety of PFT equipment is available to obtain specific PFT parameters. The Wright Peak Flow Meter (Armstrong Medical Industries, Northbrook, IL) is the most commonly used device because of the relative ease of use, availability, and cost of the unit (Fig. 27–1). Spirometry can be used to obtain several PFT measurements during one test. Plethysmography, or the "body box," is the least used and is found in pulmonary clinics. Obtained test values are compared with predicted values based on age, sex, height, race, and air temperature. Many computer programs are available that provide actual values, predicted values, and percentage of predicted values. An unofficial interpretation of the results may also be given. The degree of impairment may be classified on four or five levels (normal to severe or very severe) based on results of percentage of predicted values. Different laboratories may use different values for determining degree of impairment. An example is given in Table 27–3.

Asthma is a disease of both the large and the small airways. The predominant site of flow limitation varies with the individual. Various PFT parameters are sensitive to different areas of obstruction (Buckley & Souhrada, 1975; Ruppel, 1982). The airway obstruction in asthma typically results in difficulties during expiration. PFT measurements may reveal decreases in forced vital capacity (FVC), forced expiration during the first second of FVC (FEV_1), forced expiratory volume compared with forced vital capacity (FEV/FVC), and peak expiratory flow rate (PEFR) due to airway obstruction in large or small airways; decreases in forced expiratory flow during 25 to 75% of FVC ($FEF_{25-75\%}$) due to airway obstruction specifically in small airways; and increases in residual volume (RV) and functional residual capacity (FRC) due to air trapping. Decreases in $FEF_{25-75\%}$ are common in early stages of obstructive disease before other measurements are abnormal (Ruppel, 1982).

Even when the child is free of symptoms, some impairment may be noted (Crofton & Douglas, 1981). Table 27–3 shows the PFT results of a 14-year-old boy who had no symptoms at the time of the test. Values within the normal range are noted for FVC, FEV_1, and PEFR; however, a moderate degree of impairment in $FEF_{25-75\%}$ was found.

The most commonly reported PFT measurements are PEFR and FEV_1. Many investigators, however, recommend using more than one PFT parameter to detect individual differences in the predominant site of airway obstruction (Buckley & Souhrada, 1975; Cropp, 1979; Kattan et al., 1978). From the PFT results in Table 27–3, it is clear that if only PEFR

TABLE 27–2. **Classification of Asthma Severity**

	Clinical Features Before Treatment*		
	Symptoms†	Nighttime Symptoms	Lung Function
Step 4—Severe persistent	Continual symptoms Limited physical activity Frequent exacerbations	Frequent	FEV_1 or PEF ≤60% predicted PEF variability >30%
Step 3—Moderate persistent	Daily symptoms Daily use of inhaled short-acting β_2 agonist Exacerbations affect activity Exacerbations ≥2 times a week; may last days	>1 time a week	FEV_1 or PEF >60%–<80% predicted PEF variability >30%
Step 2—Mild persistent	Symptoms >2 times a week but <1 time a day Exacerbations may affect activity	>2 times a month	FEV_1 or PEF ≥80% predicted PEF variability 20–30%
Step 1—Mild intermittent	Symptoms ≤2 times a week Asymptomatic and normal PEF between exacerbations Exacerbations brief (from a few hours to a few days); intensity may vary	≤2 times a month	FEV_1 or PEF ≥80% predicted PEF variability <20%

From The National Heart, Lung, and Blood Institute. Expert Panel Report 2: Guidelines for the Diagnosis and Management of Asthma. Pub no. 97-4051. Bethesda, MD: National Institutes of Health, 1997.

*The presence of one of the features of severity is sufficient to place a patient in that category. An individual should be assigned to the most severe grade in which any feature occurs. The characteristics noted in this figure are general and may overlap because asthma is highly variable. Furthermore, an individual's classification may change over time.

†Patients at any level of severity can have mild, moderate, or severe exacerbations. Some patients with intermittent asthma experience severe and life-threatening exacerbations separated by long periods of normal lung function and no symptoms.

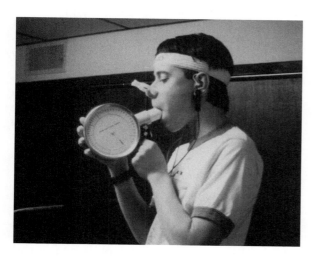

FIGURE 27–1. Boy with asthma using a Wright peak flow meter. The nose clip prevents him from exhaling air through his nose.

or FEV_1 was used to determine airway obstruction, no impairment would have been reported. By including $FEF_{25-75\%}$, a moderate degree of impairment would be reported and proper treatment could be initiated.

TABLE 27–3. **Results of Spirometry in 14-Year-Old Boy with Asthma***

Test	Actual	Predicted	% Predicted
FVC	2.57	2.51	102
FEV_1	2.17	2.16	100
PEFR	5.36	3.62	148
$FEF_{27-75\%}$	2.22	2.94	76
FEV_1/FVC	84	86	

*Results show normal values for FVC, FEV_1, and PEFR and moderate impairment for $FEF_{25-75\%}$. This boy was free of symptoms at the time of testing.

Primary Impairment in Infancy and Early Childhood

During infancy and early childhood, asthma attacks are often triggered by viral infections, in particular by respiratory syncytial virus. A diagnosis of wheezy bronchitis, recurrent upper respiratory tract infections, chronic bronchitis, or recurrent pneumonia may be made, rather than a diagnosis of asthma (NHLBI, 1997).

Although the majority of children with asthma experience their first episode before age 3, it is difficult to obtain objective measurements for diagnosis in toddlers. PFTs are not usually used with this age group. Asthma severity scales using parameters other than PFTs have been investigated. One study (Kerem et al., 1991) compared clinical signs (accessory muscle use, heart rate, respiratory rate, pulsus paradoxus, dyspnea, and wheezing) to spirometric values (FEV_1) and transcutaneous arterial oxygen saturation ($tcSao_2$) in 71 children, ages 5 to 17 years, during an acute asthmatic attack. Significant correlations were found between FEV_1 and accessory muscle use ($p < .001$), dyspnea ($p < .001$), and wheezing ($p < .001$). Significant correlations were also found between $tcSao_2$ and FEV_1 ($p < .001$) and accessory muscle use ($p < .001$); however, a low FEV_1 was not always associated with a low $tcSao_2$ or a high clinical score. Kerem and colleagues (1991) emphasize the need to use both subjective and objective measures in evaluating the severity of an asthma attack.

Another study (Bishop et al., 1992) investigated the ability of a clinical asthma severity scale, clinical judgment rating, and oxygen saturation level to predict the severity of an acute asthma attack for 60 children, ages 6 months to 17 years. The asthma severity scale score was obtained by pediatricians' ratings of accessory muscle use, wheeze, and heart rate, each on a four-point scale. The clinical judgment rating was obtained by the pediatricians' clinical judgment of the severity of the asthma attack, also on a four-point scale (mild, moderate, severe, or very severe). Severity of oxygen desaturation, obtained by pulse oximetry, was rated on a three-point scale (mild, moderate, severe). The severity of the asthma attack was determined by admission, length of inpatient stay, frequency and duration of inhalation therapy, and parental assessment of subsequent days unwell. Wheezing and accessory muscle use were found to be the most valuable in predicting the severity of the asthma attack.

In a study by Wennergren and co-workers (1986), a clinical symptom grading system based on respiratory rate; rhonchi; wheezing; retractions; fatigue; anxiety; cyanosis, pallor, and cold sweat; and breath sounds and degree of consciousness was compared with transcutaneous oxygen pressure ($tcPo_2$) and transcutaneous carbon dioxide pressure ($tcPco_2$) in children younger than 2 years of age during an acute asthmatic attack. At very slight signs of obstruction, $tcPo_2$ was decreased and continued to decrease with severity of signs and symptoms. The $tcPco_2$ remained almost unchanged until moderate obstruction was evident.

These studies demonstrate that objective measurements can be obtained for children who are too young or in too much distress to adequately perform PFTs. The acute asthmatic attack can be monitored

with standardized protocols for documentation of signs and symptoms.

Physicians are often hesitant to make the diagnosis of asthma. Wheezy bronchitis and acute bronchiolitis are considered temporary diseases, whereas asthma is a chronic and recurring condition. Unfortunately, if a diagnosis of asthma is not made, the child will receive inappropriate treatment and will not benefit from prophylactic treatment of asthma. Unnecessary or inappropriate medication may be prescribed, and the child may continue to have undiagnosed respiratory problems.

A retrospective study in an "asthma aware" medical practice examined the medical records of 52 children with diagnosed asthma ages 18 months to 11 years (Levy & Bell, 1984). Eight of these children were diagnosed in the hospital, and 44 were diagnosed by general practitioners. An average of 16 to 20 (range, 1–48) consultations for respiratory problems was required before the diagnosis of asthma was recorded. Thirty-five of the 52 children had their first consultation for respiratory problems before age 1, another 10 (total 45) between 1 and 2 years of age, another 6 (total 51) by age 4, and all 52 by age 5. In 31 patients, an objective diagnosis was made based on a change in PEFR of at least 20%. In 21 patients, a subjective diagnosis was made based on a history suggestive of asthma combined with a positive response to bronchodilators or asthma prophylaxis. Symptoms recorded during consultations included cough (96% of children), wheeze (75%), difficulty sleeping (31%), and difficulty breathing (25%). A preoccupation with infection as the primary cause of recurrent respiratory problems in the children was revealed by physicians' treatments. Before the diagnosis of asthma was made and recorded, 43% of prescriptions were for antibiotics, 38% were for cough suppressors, and 17% were for bronchodilators.

Impairment in Childhood

An increased prevalence of asthma during childhood has been reported in children who have a history during infancy of wheezy bronchitis, croup, respiratory syncytial virus infection, bronchopulmonary dysplasia, and viral bronchiolitis, and in children with extremely low birth weight (500–999 g) (Crofton & Douglas, 1981; Gold et al., 1989; Li & O'Connell, 1987; McConnochie & Roghmann, 1984; Pullan & Hey, 1982; Rickards et al., 1987; Smyth et al., 1981). An increased prevalence of chronic or recurrent otitis media with effusion has been reported in children with upper respiratory tract allergy (Fireman, 1988). Otitis media with effusion has been related to an abnormal function of the eustachian tube and has been associated with allergy, infection, and enlarged adenoids. It may be an intrinsic trigger for asthma.

During childhood, PFT measures become an easy and effective diagnostic tool. Overt wheezing is the major presenting sign. Some children may exhibit respiratory difficulty only after exercise, at night, or in cold air (de Benedictis et al., 1990). Some children may have trouble keeping up with peers or with strenuous exercise. Routine PFT results may be normal; however, the history may indicate that an allergen or exercise challenge test should be performed. The prevalence of exercise-induced bronchospasm (EIB) is 70 to 90% in individuals with documented asthma who have performed an exercise challenge test; however, a positive history of EIB is not always given (Schroeckenstein & Busse, 1988; Sly, 1986; Voy, 1986).

The exercise challenge test requires the child to run on a treadmill for 6 to 8 minutes at the slope and speed needed to attain a heart rate of 75 to 90% of the predicted maximum heart rate for the child's age. PFT measures are then taken at 5-minute intervals for 20 to 30 minutes after the run. The test is positive if PFT measures drop by more than 15% from pre-exercise baseline measures or if the child develops a cough or wheeze (Burr et al., 1974; Cropp, 1979; Taussig et al., 1980). If bronchospasm is elicited, the diagnosis is made if signs and symptoms are reversed by administration of bronchodilator medications (de Benedictis et al., 1990). Table 27-4 shows the results of an exercise challenge test for a 17-year-old girl who did not have positive results for EIB. In fact, the exercise resulted in some bronchodilation. Table 27-5 shows the positive test results of an exercise challenge test for a 14-year-old boy and the reversal of bronchoconstriction 15 minutes after the administration of bronchodilator medication by nebulizer. After the 6-minute exercise challenge, this boy demonstrated severe impairment in $FEF_{25-75\%}$, mild impairment in FEV_1, and normal values for PEFR. His PFT measures, however, dropped by more than 15% from pre-exercise baseline values for each parameter. The time at which the lowest value is reached may vary among individuals and between parameters for one individual. Even though this boy had severe bronchoconstriction, his oxygen saturation remained at or above 98%.

Impairment in Adolescence

By adolescence, symptoms often decrease. Even when free of symptoms, however, the adolescent may have significant impairment revealed by PFT measures. Continued decrease in severity and frequency of asthma attacks during adolescence results in the belief that children "outgrow" asthma. Research has not demonstrated this to be true. In a study of 286 subjects at age 28, first studied at age 7 and again at ages 10, 14, and 21, it was found that asthma severity at age 28 was similar to that at age 14 (Kelly et al., 1988). Asthma that had worsened during adolescence continued to worsen in early adulthood. In another study, 331 children with asthma and 77 controls were examined at ages 7, 14, and 21 (Martin et al., 1980). Although in some subjects there was amelioration of symptoms, they did continue to wheeze.

TABLE 27-4. Negative Exercise Challenge Test Results*

Time (min)	PEFR	FEV_1	$FEF_{25-75\%}$	RPE	Heart Rate	%O_2 Saturation
0	5.08/112%	2.36/84%	2.82/75%	7	105	94
1				14	165	94
3				15	177	94
5				14	175	94
6/0				14	175	94
/3	5.42/119%	2.46†/89%	2.98/79%			94
/5	5.42/119%	2.49/89%	2.98/79%			94
/10	5.34/118%	2.62/93%	2.90†/77%			94
/15	4.83†/106%	2.49/89%	3.19/85%			94
/20	4.91/108%	2.49/8%	3.02/80%			94
		Change from baseline				
	4.9% drop	5.5% rise	2.8% rise			

RPE, Rating of perceived exertion.

*Results of an exercise challenge test for a 17-year-old girl with asthma. Test consisted of a 6-minute run on a treadmill followed by 20 minutes of monitoring. Results are negative for exercise-induced asthma.

†Lowest value after exercise.

TABLE 27–5. **Positive Exercise Challenge Test Results***

Time (min)	PEFR	FEV$_1$	FEF$_{25-75\%}$	RPE	Heart Rate	%O$_2$ Saturation
0	6.01/166%	2.53/117%	2.42/82%	6	96	98
1	—	—	—	11	160	100
3	—	—	—	12	166	99
5	—	—	—	13	167	98
6/0	—	—	—	14	167	98
/3	3.98/110%	1.69/78%	1.10/37%	—	—	100
/5	3.98/110%	1.77/82%	1.02†/35%	—	—	99
/10	3.39†/94%	1.60†/74%	1.03/35%	—	—	100
/15	3.81/105%	1.65/76%	1.35/46%	—	—	100
/20	4.83/133%	1.90/88%	1.49/51%	—	—	100
		Change from baseline				
	43.5% drop	36.8% drop 15 minutes after nebulizer	57.3% drop			
	5.42/150%	**2.66/125%**	**3.02/103%**			

RPE, Rating of perceived exertion.

*Results of an exercise challenge test for a 14-year-old boy with asthma. Test consisted of a 6-minute run on a treadmill followed by 20 minutes of monitoring. Results are positive for exercise-induced asthma. Reversal of bronchoconstriction 15 minutes after nebulizer treatment with albuterol is indicated in **bold type.**

†Lowest value after exercise.

Medical Management

Episodes of asthma attacks are usually reversible and can be prevented or modified to some degree when the individual-specific triggers have been identified. The frequency, duration, and severity of attacks are highly variable even for the same individual.

Acute treatment is aimed at reversing the bronchoconstriction. Bronchodilator medications are administered by inhalation or injection. If the asthma attack is severe and does not respond to bronchodilator medications, the diagnosis of status asthmaticus may be made and is considered a life-threatening medical emergency. Hospitalization will be required to administer medications intravenously, to monitor blood gases, and to administer oxygen.

The goals of long-term management are to prevent chronic and troublesome symptoms, to maintain pulmonary function and physical activity level, to prevent recurrent exacerbations, to minimize the need for emergency room visits or hospitalizations, to provide optimal pharmacotherapy, and to meet the patient's and family's expectations of and satisfaction with asthma care (NHLBI, 1997). This is accomplished through periodic examination, ongoing monitoring, and education. The patient should be taught to self-monitor asthma symptoms and patterns, response to medications, quality of life, and functional status and to perform and record peak flow readings. A written action plan should be developed and reviewed and revised periodically. This action plan should be shared with school and other personnel who are involved with the child. Some allergens such as cigarette smoke, animal dander, or dust can be handled by environmental control. Desensitization ("allergy shots") may be used for triggers such as pollen or mold. Triggers such as emotional stress may be handled by relaxation exercises and education.

Medications

Many individuals with asthma require daily medication. These medications may be administered by inhalation (metered-dose inhaler [Fig. 27–2], breath-activated inhaler, dry powder inhaler, space-holding chamber, face mask, nebulizer [Fig. 27–3]) or systemically (oral, subcutaneous, intravenous) and have their effect at points A, B, or C in Figure 27–4. Inhaled medications deliver a concentrated dose most effectively with fewer systemic side effects and a shorter onset of action than other routes of administration. The primary medications in current use are anti-inflammatory agents (corticosteroids, cromolyn sodium, nedocromil), bronchodilators (β$_2$ agonists), leukotriene inhibitors, and theophylline. These medications are classified as either quick relief or long-term control medications. The quick relief or rescue medications are used as needed to provide quick relief of bronchospasm or to inhibit EIB. Long-term control or maintenance medications are taken daily and target the underlying pathology. The type of medication prescribed depends on the asthma severity. A step-wise approach is recommended

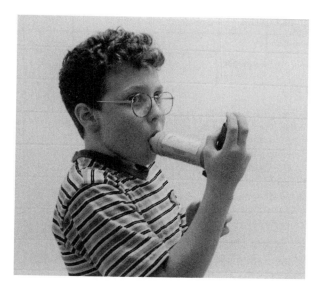

FIGURE 27–2. Boy using metered-dose inhaler with spacing chamber. This boy is using his accessory muscles and decreased diaphragmatic movement as evidenced by his raised shoulders.

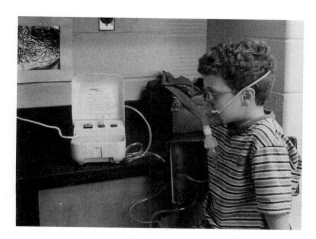

FIGURE 27–3. Boy using a nebulizer with face mask. This boy is receiving a nebulizer treatment at school 3 days after an asthma episode. His shoulders are elevated and he is using his accessory muscles and decreased diaphragmatic movement.

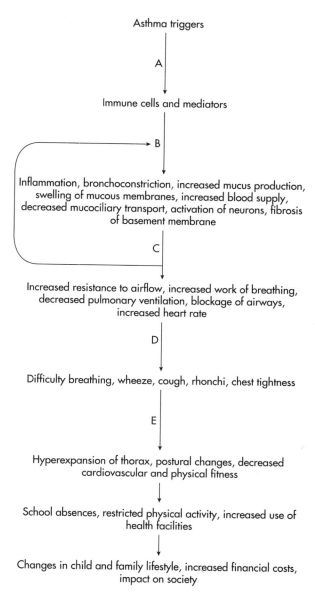

Asthma triggers

A

Immune cells and mediators

B

Inflammation, bronchoconstriction, increased mucus production, swelling of mucous membranes, increased blood supply, decreased mucociliary transport, activation of neurons, fibrosis of basement membrane

C

Increased resistance to airflow, increased work of breathing, decreased pulmonary ventilation, blockage of airways, increased heart rate

D

Difficulty breathing, wheeze, cough, rhonchi, chest tightness

E

Hyperexpansion of thorax, postural changes, decreased cardiovascular and physical fitness

School absences, restricted physical activity, increased use of health facilities

Changes in child and family lifestyle, increased financial costs, impact on society

Medical intervention occurs at points A, B, and C. Physical therapy intervention occurs at points C, D, and E.

FIGURE 27–4. Progression of asthma to secondary impairments, functional limitations, disabilities, and impact on family and society.

(Table 27–6) with the patient's treatment moving up or down the steps in relation to the present state of the asthma severity (NHLBI, 1997).

Corticosteroids (Beclovent, Azmacort, budesonide, prednisone) are the most potent and effective anti-inflammatory agents and can be given by inhalation or systemically. They decrease inflammation and may inhibit the production of cytokines, recruitment of eosinophils, and release of inflammatory mediators. Research in the area of corticosteroids is directed toward inhaled agents with higher topical potency but without the systemic side effects; corticosteroids that are targeted for specific inflammatory cells, such as macrophages; and the use of

TABLE 27-6. **Recommended Medical Intervention for Age 5 and Older**

Step	Quick Relief	Long-Term Control	Education
4—Severe persistent	Inhaled short-acting β_2 agonist as needed	*Increase* anti-inflammatory (inhaled corticosteroid) to high dose AND *Add* long-acting bronchodilator (long-acting inhaled β_2 agonist, sustained-release theophylline, or long-acting oral β_2 agonist) or systemic corticosteroid	Steps 2 and 3 PLUS Refer to individual education/counseling
3—Moderate persistent	Inhaled short-acting β_2 agonist as needed	*Increase* anti-inflammatory (inhaled corticosteroid) to medium dose OR *Add* long-acting bronchodilator (long-acting inhaled β_2 agonist, sustained-release theophylline, or long-acting oral β_2 agonist)	Step 1 PLUS Teach self-monitoring Refer to group education Review and update self-management and action plans
2—Mild persistent	Inhaled short-acting β_2 agonist as needed	*Add* daily anti-inflammatory (inhaled corticosteroid low dose, cromolyn, or nedocromil)	Step 1 PLUS Teach self-monitoring Refer to group education Review and update self-management and action plans
1—Mild intermittent	Inhaled short-acting β_2 agonist as needed	None	Teach basic facts about asthma and inhaler technique Discuss medications and environmental control Develop self-management and action plans

Adapted from The National Heart, Lung, and Blood Institute. Expert Panel Report 2: Guidelines for the Diagnosis and Management of Asthma. Pub no. 97-4051. Bethesda, MD: National Institutes of Health, 1997.

liposomes to deliver corticosteroids to specific sites (Barnes, 1991). Another important goal of research is to develop nonsteroidal drugs that mimic the benefits of corticosteroids but without the side effects.

Cromolyn sodium and nedocromil work by inhibiting the release of the immune system mediators. They also have anti-inflammatory properties, inhibit both immediate and late hypersensitivity reactions, and inhibit the response to exercise and cold, dry air. Cromolyn has been shown to improve mucociliary transport in patients whose transport is abnormal and to offer partial protection from antigen-induced bronchospasm (Mezey et al., 1978). It is one of the safest medications, but it is inconvenient in that dosage is required 4 times a day. The administration of 20 mg of cromolyn 3 times per day over 3 years has been shown to decrease histamine sensitivity and overall asthma severity (Wantanabe, 1992).

Although 4 times daily is the recommended dosage, nedocromil has been shown to be effective when used twice daily. Newer cromolyn-like drugs are being studied (Spector, 1989).

Bronchodilators reverse the contraction of the smooth muscles. The most widely used and most effective are the β_2 agonists, which are given by inhalation or orally. They stimulate β_2 receptors, thus increasing cAMP. They are equally effective on the large and small airways and inhibit mast cells and mediator release, decrease vascular permeability, and increase mucociliary clearance. Short-acting inhaled β_2 agonists (Ventolin, Proventil) work in 15 to 30 minutes and are effective for a few hours. Long-acting β_2 agonists (salmeterol, sustained-release albuterol) take longer to work but are effective for 12 hours or more.

A newer class of medication is the leukotriene

inhibitors (Accolate, Singulair). They are given orally once or twice per day in patients older than age 12 who have mild persistent asthma. These drugs can cause drug-drug interactions, and liver function must be monitored.

Theophyllines (Slo-Bid, Slo-Phyllin) have been important in the treatment of asthma for more than 50 years. Theophylline is administered once or twice per day orally in a sustained-release tablet or capsule. Theophyllines inhibit phosphodiestrase and possibly adenosine, resulting in smooth muscle relaxation, and they may affect eosinophil infiltration, T lymphocyte numbers, diaphragmatic contactility, and mucociliary clearance.

The goal of present research is to find drugs that will stop the inflammatory process at an earlier point (Vogel, 1997). Drugs that target specific cytokines are under investigation. T lymphocyte T_H1 protects the body against bacteria and tumor cells. T lymphocyte T_H2 is involved with allergies and is a factor in asthmatic reactions. The activity of one of these suppresses the activity of the other. Certain bacteria that induce T_H1 responses are being investigated, and their DNA is being used to desensitize individuals to their allergies. Because viruses would induce a T_H1 response, but are known to be an asthma trigger, it is possible that they may attack the lining of the lung, which then becomes susceptible to T_H2.

Other mechanisms to induce bronchodilation are under investigation (Barnes, 1991). Drugs that stimulate production of cAMP or inhibit the breakdown of cAMP have been investigated, but their use is limited by cardiovascular side effects, nausea, and vomiting. Anticholinergics, calcium antagonists, and potassium channel activators have demonstrated some potential for benefit, but selectivity and side effects continue to need research. The use of immunomodulators such as methotrexate, cyclosporine, and gold is also under investigation (Barnes, 1991; Spector, 1989).

Another problem area of asthma under investigation is decreased mucociliary clearance. Nineteen adults with asthma, ages 28 to 75 years, and 30 control subjects participated in a study to investigate the drug thromboxane A_2 synthetase inhibitor (OXY-046) (Kurashima et al., 1992). Before the treatment period, the mean velocity of mucociliary transport for the group with asthma was 25% of the mean for the control group. OXY-046 was administered orally twice daily for 4 weeks. Following the treatment period, the frequency of asthma attacks decreased. Mean sputum volume decreased by 28.3% ($p < .01$) at 2 weeks and by 44.5% ($p < .001$) at 4 weeks. The mean score for difficulty of sputum expectoration decreased by 64% ($p < .001$) at 2 weeks and by 60% ($p < .01$) at 4 weeks. Mean velocity of mucociliary

transport improved by 119.7% ($p < .01$) from baseline, but remained significantly ($p < .01$) decreased from the control group. No significant changes were found in the velocity of mucociliary transport in the control subjects who received OXY-046.

In the study by Mezey and co-workers (1978), after administration of cromolyn sodium, mean TMV increased to 132% of baseline in patients with asthma. Following antigen challenge when FEV_1 had significantly ($p < .05$) decreased, mean TMV was 162% of baseline. After 1 hour, mean TMV continued to be increased to 134% of baseline. No change in TMV was reported in the control group.

The future holds many possibilities for new drugs. As the understanding of the pathophysiology and genetics of asthma increases, new medications with more specific but fewer side effects will be developed. Future research must consider disease severity, disease volatility, concurrent medications and comorbidity, age, and gender as factors in drug responsivity. The exciting field of genetic research should aid in the development of drugs that can specifically turn off asthma genes.

SECONDARY CONDITIONS

Recurrent asthma attacks may result in secondary impairments, functional limitations, and disabilities beginning in early childhood and continuing throughout life. Restricted physical activity, school absences, school difficulties, changes in family lifestyle, and increased use of health care facilities are examples of some disabilities that may begin in early childhood. As the child approaches adolescence, self-esteem concerns become prominent. As adulthood is reached, concerns such as choice of vocation and living location become increasingly more important to consider.

Restrictions in Daily Life

Asthma is a condition that may alter or interfere with the daily life of the individual and his or her family. In a study of 420 children with asthma, ages 7 to 16 years, 13% had school absences of more than 5 days as a result of asthmatic symptoms (Braback & Kalvesten, 1988). The results of a study (Anderson et al., 1983) of 284 children with asthma and 92 control subjects are presented in Table 27–7. Fortunately, little effect on social activities was reported. Belonging to clubs, swimming, and special lessons, such as music lessons, were reported as equally frequent among the children with asthma and the controls.

A study of 1083 children in first through sixth grade (Hessel et al., 1996) found that 70.5% of the

TABLE 27-7. **Effects of Asthma on Daily Life**

Activity Affected by Asthma	Percent of Children Affected
School absence due to wheezing	58%
School absences of more than 30 days	12%
At least one day of bed rest required	34%
Wheezing severe enough to interfere with speaking	13%
Nocturnal wheezing interrupting sleep	40%
Activities around the house	29%
Mother's activities affected	42%
Activities affected a lot	7%
Special household arrangements required	13%
Special arrangements of child's bedroom	29%
Special allowances made for child	29%
Family pet removed	20%
Family choice of holiday activities	11%

Data compiled from a study of 284 children with asthma: Anderson, HR, Bailey, PA, & Cooper, JS. Morbidity and school absence caused by asthma and wheezing illness. Archives of Disease in Childhood, 58:777–784, 1983.

children with asthma had limited their activities for a health reason compared with 6.6% of the children without asthma, and 32.7% of the children with asthma had missed 2 or more days of school in the preceding month compared with 14.8% of the children without asthma.

Townsend and associates (1991) investigated the impact of asthma on the lives of 100 children ages 7 to 18 years who were diagnosed with mild-to-moderate asthma and on the lives of their parents. The children and their parents were asked if each item on their respective questionnaires was a problem for them and then to rate those items on a 5-point scale (1 = does not bother you much; 5 = bothers you very, very much). The children's questionnaire consisted of 77 items, which included 29 items dealing with respiratory symptoms and fatigue, 21 items dealing with emotional function, and 16 items dealing with limitations in physical activities. A separate medication side effects category and a wishes category were included for each child. The children reported that respiratory symptoms such as wheezing, asthma attacks, shortness of breath, and feeling out of breath were the most bothersome. Emotional items such as fear, frustration, and anger were identified by more than 45%. Feeling frightened by an asthma attack was reported by 49%. In the limitations in physical activity category, running was reported by 85%. In the medication side effects category, 32% reported difficulty in falling asleep, and 22% reported not being able to sit still and feeling restless. Seventy-six percent reported at least one problem, including inability to concentrate in school. The wishes focused mostly on being able to perform a current activity better or longer. Thirty-

nine percent wished they could own a pet. For the parents, the questionnaire consisted of 69 items: 13 dealing with interference of the disease in day-to-day activities, and 56 dealing with the emotional impact on parents, which included basic health concerns, as well as financial concerns. The emotional items scored higher than interference with daily life items. Major areas were concern about drug side effects and long-term effects, permanent lung damage, and feeling helpless during an attack.

The effect of asthma on the daily life of 150 adults, ages 18 to 70 years, was investigated by Juniper and colleagues (1992). A questionnaire consisting of 32 items assessed asthma symptoms, emotional problems caused by asthma, activities restricted by asthma, and troublesome environmental stimuli. The subjects were asked to rate each item on a 5-point scale (not very important to extremely important). Major asthma symptoms reported included shortness of breath, chest tightness, and wheezing. Emotional problems were not rated very highly. Major restrictions in physical activities included jogging and running. Major environmental triggers included cigarette smoke, dust, and air pollution. Exposure to and avoidance of environmental stimuli were classified as two different types of limitations. Choosing not to go to a party because of cigarette smoke was a different problem than choosing to go and then dealing with the consequent symptoms. Limitations were reported to be greater for younger than for older adults and greater for women than for men.

Restrictions in Physical Activity

In 70 to 90% of individuals with diagnosed asthma, exercise has been identified as a trigger (Sly, 1986). The degree of bronchial spasm caused by exercise is variable among individuals and may vary on a daily basis depending on other triggers to which the child has been exposed. Asthma caused by exercise can be inhibited or modified by proper medication, proper warm-up and cool-down, or both.

Children with asthma may restrict their physical activity on their own. Teachers or parents may discourage the child from participation because of fear of an asthma attack. Regular physical education may be modified, and the child may avoid sports activities to prevent an asthma attack. In a study of 420 children with asthma, ages 7 to 16 years, 40% reported restricted physical activity of more than 10 days per year because of asthmatic symptoms; an additional 24% reported occasional restriction (Braback & Kalveston, 1988). This hypoactivity may lead to decreased cardiovascular fitness. A pattern of hypoactivity, isolation from peers, and focus on disability may then become established.

TABLE 27–8. **Reported Cardiopulmonary Responses in Children with Asthma at Rest, During Exercise, After Exercise, and During Bronchospasm**

Response	Rest	During Exercise	After Exercise	During Bronchospasm
Cardiac output	N	N	N	I
Blood pressure	N	N		I
Blood volume	N			I
Heart volume	N			
Stroke volume	N			N/I
Total hemoglobin	N			
Alveolar-arterial O$_2$ gradient	N/I		N/I	I
Pao_2 tcPo_2	N	N/I/D	D	I/D
Paco_2 tcPco_2	N	N/I		N/I
Ventilation-perfusion	N/Abn		Abn	Abn
Minute ventilation	N	I	I/N	
Physiologic dead space	N/I			I
Arterial blood lactate		I		

Data from Anderson and colleagues (1972), Bevegard and co-workers (1976), Chryssanthopoulos and colleagues (1984), Freyschus and co-workers (1984), Hedlin and others (1984, 1986), & Wennergren and colleagues (1986).
Reported results do not include pulmonary function test measurements.
N, Normal; *Abn*, abnormal; *I*, increased from normal; *D*, decreased from normal.

The need for physical activity and the normal effects of conditioning and training on the cardiovascular and pulmonary systems are discussed in Chapter 5. The need for fitness in children with asthma is no less important than in children without asthma.

Cardiopulmonary responses other than PFT measures before, during, and after exercise and during bronchoconstriction have been studied in children with asthma. These responses as reported by various researchers are summarized in Table 27–8. In children with severe asthma, obstructive changes and disturbed pulmonary gas exchange have been reported even at rest when asymptomatic (Bevegard et al., 1976; Hedlin et al., 1986).

Repeated asthma attacks with increased production and accumulation of mucus combined with the abnormal mucociliary clearance associated with asthma may result in an altered breathing pattern, poor posture, and decreased cardiovascular fitness. Expiration may become an active rather than a passive process. Continued use of the accessory muscles of inspiration rather than the diaphragm may result in decreased thoracic mobility, hypoextensibility of pectoral muscles, elevated and adducted shoulders, winging scapulae, kyphosis, hypertrophied neck muscles, forward-head posture, and hypoextensibility of the hip and knee flexor muscles. Chronic lung hyperinflation may result in chest deformities.

Medication Side Effects

Although the medications used in the management of asthma are necessary, the side effects of these medications also may have an impact on daily life. Side effects of oral corticosteroids in the typical doses used for treatment of asthma include increased appetite and weight gain, fluid retention, increased bruising, and mild elevation of blood pressure. In corticosteroid-dependent individuals, increased body fat composition, myopathy of type II (fast-twitch) fibers, decreased proximal muscle strength, acne exacerbation, hirsutism, linear growth suppression, and osteoporosis have been reported (Hollister & Bowyer, 1987). A study by Picado and associates (1990) investigated respiratory and skeletal muscle strength and endurance time, examined biopsy specimens of deltoid muscles for type I and type II fibers, and assessed nutritional status of oral corticosteroid–dependent subjects and of controls. No difference was found in respiratory or skeletal muscle strength or endurance time. Atrophy of type II muscle fibers was found to be associated with decreased nutritional status rather than with corticosteroid use. Another study evaluating fitness in children with moderately severe to severe asthma found increased skinfold thickness (body fat) present more often than normally (Strunk et al., 1988). The investigators, however, did not believe it to be likely that corticosteroids played a primary role in this finding. Side effects of beta-sympathomimetics include nervousness, headache, trembling, heart palpitations, dizziness or light-headedness, dryness or irritation of the mouth and throat, heartburn, and bad taste in the mouth. Side effects of cromolyn include bad taste in the mouth and cough. Side effects of theophylline include nausea and heartburn, headaches, restlessness, insomnia, muscle spasms, anxiety, irritability, tremulousness, muscle incoordination, speech disturbances, heart palpitations, excessive perspiration, and frequent urination.

The side effects and dosage schedule of medication may call attention to the child. During the school day, the child may need to leave the classroom to receive medication. Theophylline has side effects that may interfere with schoolwork. Increased attention, concentration, and memory ability were noted by psychologic testing of children with asthma after 2 weeks off theophylline and on cromolyn (Furukawa et al., 1984). Parents reported decreased restlessness, distractibility, and irritability; increased manageability; and better sleeping during the time off theophylline. In a second study comparing theophylline and cromolyn therapy over 4 weeks, psychologic tests revealed abnormal visuospatial planning in children with an intelligence quotient (IQ) of 87 to 105 compared with children with IQs of 111 to 134 when on theophylline (Springer et al., 1985).

Another study of children 6 to 12 years of age with mild asthma who had not been on any long-term oral medications for at least 6 months evaluated the effect of short-term (4 weeks) use of theophylline (Rachelefsky et al., 1986). Assessments were made by psychologic tests, a parent questionnaire and daily diary, and a teacher checklist. Psychologic tests were used to measure memory and learning, attention span, spatial visualization, and IQ. The parent questionnaire was designed to evaluate the child's behavior and consisted of 26 associated behaviors and 21 activity-attention behaviors. The daily diary was used to record medications and signs and symptoms. The teacher checklist was designed to characterize the child's ability to control activity and attention. Thirty-three associated behaviors and 20 activity-attention behaviors were rated comparing the child with other students. Significant ($p < .001$) negative effects were reported during theophylline use. Specific areas noted by teachers were "trouble finishing task," "seems to do things fast without thinking," "easily distracted from work," "gets into fights," and "gets angry easily."

Attention should be given to asthma-related behaviors used to get attention or to avoid demanding situations. Conditioned fear and anxiety may occur owing to repeated breathlessness and unpleasant treatments (Dahl et al., 1990). Vividly remembered incidents of intense fear and anger have been shown to significantly ($p < .05$) decrease FEV_1 (Tal & Micklich, 1976).

Growth and Development

Another effect of asthma that is particularly important for self-esteem in adolescence is delayed growth and development. Both sexual and skeletal maturation are frequently delayed. Bone age has been correlated to height rather than to age (Snyder et al., 1967). In infancy, no delay is evident, but a small consistent delay has been recorded in childhood (Hauspie et al., 1977). By adolescence, growth delay is marked. The adolescent growth spurt is delayed by approximately 1.3 years. The total length of the growth period is extended, however, and children with asthma eventually reach normal height and weight. The more severe the asthma, the greater the delay. This delay has not been found to be related to allergies or to short-term use of corticosteroids, and the explanation is still unknown (Shohat et al., 1987).

Impact on Family and Society

Asthma is thought to be a mild chronic disorder, but increases in morbidity and mortality have been reported over the past few decades (CDC, 1998). Between the years 1975 and 1993–1995, there was a 123% increase in office visits with asthma as the first-listed diagnosis. Between the years 1992 and 1995 there was a 27% increase in emergency department visits. Between the years 1979–1980 and 1993–1994, there was a 21% increase in hospitalizations. The increases were greater for females than for males and for nonwhites than for whites.

A study of 71,818 children ages 1 to 17 years who were enrolled in a health maintenance organization (Lozano et al., 1997) was conducted to measure the impact of asthma on the use and cost of health care. Children with asthma incurred 88% more costs than children without asthma. Of the total health care received by the children with asthma, 37% was for asthma care, with two thirds of this care being for nonurgent care and prescriptions. Children with asthma received 65% more nonurgent visits and filled 2.77 times as many prescriptions as children without asthma.

Asthma also has a major impact on the national economy. Direct and indirect costs for the family and society multiply if more than one child in a family is affected by asthma. Direct costs would include health insurance premiums, copayments for doctor visits and prescriptions, deductibles, and nonreimbursed expenses. Durable medical equipment such as a home nebulizer may not be covered by medical insurance and becomes an additional out-of-pocket expense for the family. Indirect costs would include days missed from school or work, caregiver expenses, travel expenses, and travel and waiting times. An impact on society is also generated by the increased cost of health care and decreases in worker productivity. The cost related to asthma was estimated to be $6.2 billion in 1990 (Weiss et al., 1992). Hospitalizations were the largest single direct expense, accounting for $1.6 billion. Forty-three percent of the economic impact of asthma was associated with emergency department use, hospitalizations, and death.

Asthma may cause changes in the family's lifestyle. Opportunities may be lost or plans may have to be changed depending on the current status of the child with asthma. There is an emotional toll on the family when the child is having difficulty breathing and especially when hospitalization is required, but working with the child on relaxation and breathing exercises, performing percussions, and reviewing the action plan benefits both the child and the parents.

PHYSICAL THERAPY: EXAMINATION AND INTERVENTION

The purpose of physical therapy is to prevent secondary difficulties resulting from recurrent asthma attacks. In Figure 27–4 this occurs specifically at points C, D, and E. The physical therapist conducts an examination, including history, systems review, and tests and measures to identify impairments, functional limitations, and disabilities. Goals and expected outcomes are established, and intervention is initiated. Asthma does not fit into one preferred practice pattern in the American Physical Therapy Association's *Guide to Physical Therapist Practice* (1997). Depending on the impairments and functional limitations identified in the individual child, several of the preferred practice patterns may be useful. Under the Musculoskeletal section of the *Guide,* these include the following: 4B Impaired Posture; 4C Impaired Muscle Performance; and 4E Impaired Joint Mobility, Muscle Performance, and Range of Motion Associated with Ligament or Other Connective Tissue Disorders. Under the Cardiopulmonary section, these include 6B Impaired Aerobic Capacity and Endurance Secondary to Deconditioning Associated with Systemic Disorders; 6C Impaired Ventilation, Respiration, and Aerobic Capacity Associated with Airway Clearance Dysfunction; 6F Impaired Ventilation, Respiration, and Aerobic Capacity and Endurance Associated with Ventilatory Pump Dysfunction; and 6H Impaired Ventilation and Respiration with Potential for Respiratory Failure. Education, relaxation, increasing or maintaining range of motion and muscle strength, improving thoracic mobility and posture, improving breathing pattern and bronchial hygiene, and improving cardiovascular and physical fitness would be applicable goals for all ages, although different goals and outcomes may be stressed at different points in the life cycle.

Infancy and Preschool Period

For the infant or preschool child, parent education and involvement are most important. The parent can learn to recognize signs of an impending asthma attack. Administering medication and calming the child can prevent the attack from progressing. The parent can be sure that the child drinks plenty of liquids to help thin any secretions. Research has demonstrated that postural drainage with percussion will help clear the lungs when mucus accumulations occur (Huber et al., 1974). Twenty-one children with mild-to-moderate airway obstruction were divided into treatment and control groups. The treatment group received chest physical therapy with vibration and percussion. Thirty minutes after treatment, the treatment group demonstrated up to 40% increases in FEV_1. Many children also find percussion to be calming.

School-Age and Adolescence Period

The older child can and should become more actively involved in independently managing his or her asthma. The child can receive education on identifying specific triggers, signs and symptoms of an impending attack, and proper medication technique. Exercises to improve or maintain range of motion, muscle strength, posture, and fitness can be taught. Relaxed diaphragmatic breathing and effective coughing techniques should be practiced often and in settings that cause difficulties. Relaxed diaphragmatic breathing may be performed to prevent or lessen the severity of an attack. Deep inspirations, however, should be avoided because they have been shown to induce bronchoconstriction (Gayrard et al., 1975). Relaxed diaphragmatic breathing exercises and pursed-lip exhalations can slow the respiratory rate and give the child a sense of control (King et al., 1984). Pursed-lip exhalation helps maintain the intra-airway pressure and prevent collapse of the airways. The forced expiration technique or "huffing" combined with relaxed diaphragmatic breathing does not increase airway obstruction and is effective in clearing airway secretions (Pryor & Webber, 1979).

In a study by Girodo and co-workers (1992), 92 adults participated in an exercise program using abdominal, dorsal, and oblique muscles to decrease their respiratory rate. Pretest to posttest results showed significant ($p < .01$) decreases in medication use and asthma severity, and a significant ($p < .01$) increase in physical activity. These changes were not maintained at an 8-week follow-up, which emphasizes the need for continued practice.

Exercise-Induced Bronchospasm

Because EIB is so common, any breathing difficulties associated with exercise should be assessed by means of a standardized exercise challenge test conducted by qualified laboratory personnel. If a

TABLE 27–9. **Exercise Challenge Test Results Following Pre-exercise Inhalation of a Bronchodilator***

Time (min)	PEFR	FEV$_1$	FEF$_{25-75\%}$	RPE	Heart Rate	%O$_2$ Saturation
0	3.52/97%	2.50/116%	2.08/71%	6	83	98
1	—	—	—	8	159	99
3	—	—	—	11	161	98
5	—	—	—	12	163	97
6/0	—	—	—	13	168	98
/3	3.43†/95%	2.29/106%	1.86/63%	—	—	100
/5	6.18/187%	2.25/104%	2.73/83%	—	—	98
/10	5.44/150%	1.92†/89%	1.80†/61%	—	—	98
/15	3.43/95%	2.34/108%	2.05/70%	—	—	98
/20	3.94/109%	2.42/112%	1.98/67%	—	—	99
		Change from baseline				
	2.1% drop	23.3% drop	14.1% drop			

RPE, Rating of perceived exertion.

*Results of an exercise challenge test 15 minutes after proper inhalation of a bronchodilator for a 14-year-old boy with asthma. Test consisted of a 6-minute run on a treadmill followed by 20 minutes of monitoring. Results indicate a positive exercise-induced asthma response.

†Lowest value after exercise.

positive test is obtained, the child may be given medication to be used before exercising. In some children, however, medication does not totally prevent bronchoconstriction following exercise. Table 27–9 shows the results of an exercise challenge test performed 15 minutes following the proper administration of a bronchodilator inhaler for the 14-year-old previously presented in Table 27–5. Although the bronchodilator provided some protection against the exercise-induced bronchoconstriction, a positive test for EIB was still obtained. For these children, enjoyable physical activities and sports activities may need to be specifically selected to encourage exercising for fitness. Frequency, duration, and intensity should then be gradually increased.

An interesting aspect of EIB is that the degree of bronchoconstriction experienced is affected by type, duration, and intensity of exercise; air temperature and humidity; and time since the previous exercise (Sly, 1982). Short exercise periods (less than 2 minutes) are less likely to cause difficulty than prolonged exercise of 5 minutes or more. Exercise at a lower heart rate is also less problematic. Exercising in cold, dry air will cause heat loss from the respiratory mucosa and result in more problems than exercising in warm, humid air (Ben-Dov et al., 1982; Strauss et al., 1978). For example, baseball would cause fewer difficulties than basketball. Swimming is less likely to cause difficulty than running. Hyperventilation at rest under conditions that simulate the hyperpnea of exercise (same minute ventilation) has been shown to induce bronchoconstriction equivalent to that during exercise (Deal et al., 1979). The bronchoconstriction was increased when dry, cold air was breathed and inhibited when warm, humid air was breathed. It has been concluded, therefore, that the

major stimulus for EIB may be heat loss caused by the hyperpnea of exercise rather than by the exercise itself.

Previous strenuous exercise can result in a refractory period during which there is a decreased bronchoconstriction response to exercise. This refractory period can last up to 2 hours and has been related to the intensity of the first exercise period (Edmunds et al., 1978). Exercising in warm, humid air, however, can inhibit EIB and also result in a refractory period to a second exercise period (Ben-Dov et al., 1982). A prolonged submaximal warm-up lasting 30 minutes and completed 21 minutes before a standard EIB test has also been shown to inhibit EIB (Reiff et al., 1989). Seven repeated 30-second short sprints with a 2½-minute rest between them completed 20 minutes before a standard exercise test have also been shown to inhibit EIB (Schnall & Landau, 1980). Refractoriness, therefore, is not dependent on the degree of bronchoconstriction occurring during previous exercise.

Conditioning Programs and Physical Fitness

Conditioning programs can improve the response of the cardiovascular and respiratory systems to exercise. An increase in cardiac output results from an increase in cardiac stroke volume. A similar oxygen requirement can then be met by a lower heart rate. Ventilation improves with lower frequency and higher tidal volume. Improved oxygen utilization can result from an increase in the size and number of muscle mitochondria (Orenstein, 1988; Sharkey, 1979). An increase in fitness will result in an improved minute ventilation with a consequent decreased stimulus for EIB. Children with asthma have been shown to be able to attain normal maximum oxygen consumption (Vo_2max) levels (Bevegard et al., 1976; Chryssanthopoulos et al., 1984; Hedlin et al., 1986). Fit adults with asthma have been shown to be able to exercise significantly ($p < .001$) longer than unfit adults with asthma even though both groups were able to attain the same heart rate (Haas et al., 1985).

Children with asthma have participated safely in various exercise programs to improve their physical fitness when receiving preventive medication. Three types of programs will be described. In the first study (Henrickson & Nielson, 1983), 42 children with EIB and generally poor physical fitness were divided into a training group of 28 and a control group of 14. The training group participated in a 6-week endurance training program consisting of 15 minutes of warm-up, 15 minutes of ball games, 10 minutes of running, 20 minutes of gymnastic exercises, 20 minutes of circuit training, and 10 minutes of team games. The training sessions lasted 90 minutes and were scheduled twice per week. Following the 6-week program, the training group demonstrated a significantly increased aerobic capacity ($p < .05$) and a significantly decreased resting heart rate ($p < .05$). The second study (Fitch et al., 1976) examined the effects of a swimming program. Forty-six children participated in a 5-month program. The program began with three sessions per week and increased in intensity, duration, and frequency up to five 1-hour sessions per week. At the conclusion of the program, improved posture and fitness, decreased fat folds measures, and enhanced swimming ability were reported, although no statistical analysis was reported. The third study (Nickerson et al., 1983) examined the effect of a running program. Fifteen children ran 4 days per week for 6 weeks. The daily distance was gradually increased over 2 weeks to 3.2 km. Fitness was assessed by measuring the distance run in 12 minutes. At the conclusion of the program, the average distance the children could run in 12 minutes was significantly increased above baseline measures ($p < .005$).

Varray and associates (1991) have emphasized the need to individualize physical fitness or aerobic training. Fourteen children with asthma, ages 9 to 13 years, were divided into a training group and a control group. The training group participated in two types of swimming training: aerobic training and high-intensity training, each conducted two times per week for 3 months. During the aerobic training the individual's ventilatory threshold (VTh, the point at which a nonlinear increase in ventilation occurs) was used to determine the training swimming speed (VTh velocity, the speed required to maintain the heart rate at VTh). During each session,

the children swam three times for 10 minutes at their individual VTh velocity. The high-intensity training sessions were conducted during the second 3 months and consisted of two series of 6- to 25-meter laps at maximum speed with a 1-minute rest between laps at each session. After aerobic training, Vo_2max was significantly ($p < .001$) higher for the training group than for the controls. Mean VTh increased in the training group by 20% from baseline ($p < .001$). A significant ($p < .001$) increase in O_2 pulse max (Vo_2/HRmax) in the training group was also found, indicating improved cardiac adaptation and oxygen extraction. After high-intensity training, Vo_2max did not change. VTh and O_2 pulse max decreased after the high-intensity training sessions and were not significantly different from baseline. The use of VTh to determine exercise intensity decreases the hyperventilation stimulus for EIB during training and individualizes the aerobic training protocol.

The effect on EIB itself of programs to improve fitness has been reported, but results are contradictory. On closer examination, it can be observed that programs that reported a decrease in EIB (e.g., Henricksen & Nielsen, 1983) retested the children at the same heart rate, whereas the programs that reported no change in EIB (e.g., Fitch et al., 1976; Nickerson et al., 1983) altered the exercise stress level on retesting to compensate for the improved fitness and to ensure the same EIB stimulus. As mentioned, one of the benefits of improved fitness is a lower respiratory rate, which has been shown to decrease the stimulus for EIB. This is an interesting and important observation demonstrating the value of improving and maintaining cardiovascular fitness in children with asthma.

Other areas of fitness have been evaluated by Strunk and associates (1988). Seventy-six children, ages 9 to 17 years, with moderately severe to severe asthma were tested for fitness by a timed 9-minute run, skinfold thickness, number of sit-ups completed in 60 seconds, and flexibility determined by reaching toward the toes while sitting on the floor with outstretched legs. The primary area of difficulty was found to be endurance: 91% of the children scored at or below the 50th percentile, 74% at or below the 25th percentile, and 51% at or below the 10th percentile. An increase in skinfold thickness was also present more frequently than normal: 21% at or below the 10th percentile. The results were not well explained by the severity of the disease.

Some children with EIB may reach Olympic levels of physical fitness. In the 1984 summer Olympics, 67 of 597 U.S. Olympic athletes had EIB. These athletes participated in 29 different events and won 41 medals (Voy, 1986).

The psychologic adjustment to asthma has been found to be at least as important as the severity in determining fitness (Strunk et al., 1989). Ninety children, ages 9 to 17 years, with moderate-to-severe asthma, were tested by bicycle ergometry to determine cardiovascular fitness. Forty-eight percent were found to be more than 2 standard deviations below the mean, with an additional 5% 1 to 2 standard deviations below the mean. Medical variables (recent exacerbation of disease, FEV_1, and specific airway conductance) and the psychologic adjustment in terms of the child's relationship to family and peers, overall school adaptation, and the presence of psychiatric symptoms then were correlated with fitness separately and jointly. Medical variables as predictors of fitness resulted in an $R^2 = 0.08$ ($p < .19$). When psychologic variables were added to the equation, the variance explained increased to 0.18 ($p < .003$). Psychologic variables alone resulted in an R^2 of 0.12 ($p < .001$). Psychologic variables were, therefore, more important in predicting fitness than medical factors.

Education

The proper use of medications must be discussed as part of an educational program. Many teenagers may underdose or overdose to "belong." With the present stress on drug education, some teenagers may be hesitant to take their medications for fear of being teased about "being on drugs." Other teenagers may have such a strong desire to participate in activities that they take extra doses, especially of metered-dose inhalers, at the slightest feeling of tightness. Still others may deny the symptoms and not take their medication when it is appropriate (Dahl et al., 1990).

The proper use of metered-dose inhalers has been taught to children as young as preschoolers. The majority of children, however, do not use a correct technique (see Fig. 27-2). An increased number of errors has been demonstrated by children younger than 6 years of age (Pedersen et al., 1986). Lee (1983) found that when time was taken to ensure that the child performed the maneuver correctly, use of proper technique was retained on retesting 6 months later.

Another area in which physical therapists in the educational environment may be helpful is in teacher education. In many classrooms, a child may be exposed to a variety of triggers. Classroom pets, plants, chalk dust, laboratory chemicals, and carpeting are a few examples. School performance may be affected by some asthma medications. School personnel should be instructed in the signs and symptoms of asthma and in relaxation and breathing exercises. They should know what to do to assist a child who is experiencing an asthma attack. Advanced notification of planned class experiences that might trigger attacks should be given to parents so that proper medications can be used if necessary. Occasionally, it may be necessary to alter the planned experience.

Children with asthma and EIB do not always feel that they receive sufficient support from instructors at school. In a study of 420 children with asthma, ages 7 to 16 years, 29% of those who had occasional restrictions and 62% of those who had frequent restrictions stated that they had insufficient support from the instructor (Braback & Kalvesten, 1988). Physical education teachers may not have an adequate knowledge of asthma and, in particular, of EIB. The child who experiences EIB may be accused of being out of shape or lazy and pushed too much. Conversely, the instructor may not encourage the child to participate to his or her ability.

Behavioral management programs have proven helpful in increasing the child's participation in his or her own monitoring of asthma. Easily available specific programs include "Superstuff" (Superstuff [Item 0317], American Lung Association, New York), "Open Airways" (Open Airways/Respiro Abierto: Asthma Self Management Program, National Heart, Lung, and Blood Institute, Bethesda, MD), and "Asthma Care Training" (Asthma Care Training for Kids, Asthma and Allergy Foundation of America, Washington, DC). These programs are aimed at increasing self-management skills, helping families adjust to the demands that asthma imposes on family life, changing the use of health care services (e.g., decreased use of emergency departments), and improving school attendance and performance. Learning to discriminate early asthma symptoms is important for the proper use of relaxation and breathing exercises and of medication. A significant ($p < .05$) positive correlation has been found between subjectively experienced asthma and experienced panic in connection with asthma and school absenteeism (Dahl et al., 1990). A significant ($p < .05$) positive correlation has also been found between the perception of panic in asthmatic situations and the number of "as needed" doses of medication.

Education programs have been found to assist the child and family in developing coping skills. In one study, changes in compliance behavior and reductions in emergency department visits and days in the hospital were noted after education sessions (Lewis et al., 1984). The children demonstrated increased self-care and increased use of relaxation exercises. The parents demonstrated improved communication with their children and changes in smoking behavior and played a more active role during an attack. Another study (Dahl et al., 1990) examined the effect of behavioral intervention on children with severe asthma who were on oral β_2 agonists and used inhalers on an as-needed basis. The behavioral intervention consisted of symptom discrimination, self-management techniques for breathlessness and to decrease the psychologic dependence on spray medications, and modification of asthma-related behaviors (e.g., using asthma as a way to gain an advantage or to avoid a demanding situation). Relaxation and breathing exercises were taught to decrease anxiety and panic, to allow more appropriate use of the spray medication, and to aid in symptom discrimination. The intervention group demonstrated a significantly ($p < .05$) decreased use of as-needed β_2 agonist sprays and a significantly ($p < .05$) decreased number of school absences when compared with a control group.

Physical therapy can assist the child with asthma and his or her family in prevention of secondary impairments that can lead to functional limitations and disabilities. Maintenance of a good breathing pattern and bronchial hygiene for elimination of secretions will minimize poor posture and thoracic deformities. Improving or maintaining range of motion, muscle strength, and cardiovascular endurance will result in good physical fitness. Education will help the family learn to accept some lifestyle changes that will be necessary and to deal with the asthma attacks that do occur. Consultation with school personnel, scout leaders, camp counselors, and coaches will allow the child to participate in activities to his or her maximum ability.

Transition to Adulthood

During transition to adulthood, the individual-specific triggers may need to be considered when selecting future living and employment. When selecting a college roommate, for example, whether or not the person is a smoker may need to be considered. Reserve Officers' Training Corps and the military academies will not accept a candidate who has a history of asthma, and the military services will not enlist a person with a history of asthma. Employment may be limited by allergens or asthma. Continued physical fitness should be stressed. Although it is believed that children outgrow asthma owing to a decrease in the number and severity of asthma attacks, adults who had asthma as children often demonstrate a positive bronchoconstriction response when sufficiently challenged (de Benedictis et al., 1990).

CASE HISTORY
TERRY

Terry was born in December 1974. He had signs and symptoms as an infant suggestive of allergies to cow's milk and eggs. These foods were avoided and Terry drank a soy formula. During his infancy and toddler years, he also experienced several episodes of croup. At age 19 months, he had a severe reaction to baby aspirin. Urticarial lesions appeared on his legs and arms, and the pediatrician was concerned about the reaction spreading to his lungs.

At age 2 years 6 months, Terry experienced his first asthma attack. It occurred after midnight, and therefore he was seen in the emergency department of the local hospital. Wheezing, nasal flaring, expiratory grunting, intercostal retractions, and abdominal respirations were noted. Terry was treated with injections of epinephrine and released when his breathing difficulties abated. He was examined the following morning by his pediatrician and, continuing with medication, recovered within 1 week. Of significance to his asthmatic attack is that he had been treated by the pediatrician 5 days earlier for upper respiratory tract infection, gastroenteritis, and otitis media.

At this time, Terry was referred to an allergist for evaluation. Skin prick allergen testing was positive for nearly every allergen tested. Very strong reactions to chicken, turkey, cow's milk, and eggs, as well as to mold, cat, and tobacco, were found. A familial history of asthma was strong on the father's side and minimal on the mother's side. The allergist recommended placing Terry on theophylline, eliminating as many of the reactive foods as possible, and then gradually reintroducing them to obtain a more definite picture of the response to allergens. The parents were instructed in environmental control and to encourage liquids.

Terry experienced strong nervous system and gastrointestinal system side effects to the theophylline, and the medication was changed to metaproterenol (Alupent), a beta sympathomimetic. Although the side effects decreased, they did not disappear and affected his ability to eat and sleep.

During the 15 months (age 2 years 6 months to 3 years 9 months) after Terry's first episodes of otitis media and asthma, he experienced four more episodes of otitis media and five episodes of respiratory congestion, wheezing, and bronchioasthmatic-type attacks that required examination and treatment by the pediatrician. A myringotomy with tubes was performed at age 2 years 11 months. Other mild asthma attacks were handled by medication at home. Terry's mother performed chest physical therapy as needed, along with calming, encouraging fluids, and administering medications.

At age 3 years 9 months, Terry was hospitalized for status asthmaticus. He was in significant respiratory distress with intercostal and substernal retractions, nasal flaring, expiratory stridor, and wheezing. He received intravenous aminophylline and was placed in a humidified oxygen tent. Terry recovered quickly and was discharged after 4 days. He was kept on Robitussin with ephedrine and a tapering dose of oral prednisone for a few days. While Terry was hospitalized, his parents were questioned about a family history of cystic fibrosis. After the hospitalization, the allergist recommended desensitization (allergy shots). Terry received an injection once per week for 6 weeks, and, interestingly, he would grind his teeth throughout that night.

After the myringotomy tubes fell out, Terry began to experience otitis media again. A second myringotomy with tubes and an adenoidectomy were performed when Terry was 4 years old.

During the next 2 years (age 4 to 6), Terry was followed by a different allergist, who recommended discontinuing the desensitization series and continuing with the daily medications and encouraging fluids. Subsequent wheezing episodes were milder and were handled with medications, fluids, and chest physical therapy. Between acute asthmatic attacks, signs and symptoms were negative and peak flow rates were greater than 100% of predicted values. Relaxed diaphragmatic breathing was practiced, and Terry would request chest physical therapy when he began to feel congestion. Terry was aware of the foods and situations that would cause difficulty and would try to avoid them if possible. If at a friend's house for lunch, for example, he would inform the friend's mother that he was allergic to milk and refuse to drink it even though often the mother was skeptical.

From age 6 to adulthood, Terry required treatment in the doctor's office for an acute asthma attack only once. Terry and his parents became aware of signs and symptoms that would indicate the beginning of an asthma attack. These were often associated with a cold. A home stethoscope was used to detect wheezing or decreased airflow. Using relaxation techniques, breathing exercises, and chest physical therapy, as well as medication, Terry was able to lessen or inhibit asthma attacks. Oral Alupent was not used daily but only as needed.

At age 13, Terry's mother learned that while playing with friends, Terry often had to stop to rest and catch his breath or to recover from coughing. He had not been interested in playing organized team sports but had enjoyed playing games with his friends just for fun. Unfortunately, the possibility of EIB had never been examined. After a consultation with the doctor, Terry was prescribed and instructed in the use of an albuterol (Ventolin) inhaler to use before physical education or other physical activity. A cromolyn (Intal) inhaler was also prescribed. At age 14, Terry participated in a research project on EIB. Until that time, the severity of his EIB had never been documented. The results in Tables 27–5 and 27–9 are for Terry. His physical education teachers were informed of his condition and worked with Terry in improving his physical fitness. At age 13, Terry was tested in physical education class using the test from the American Alliance for Health, Physical Education, Recreation, and Dance (Reston, VA). Results are presented in Table 27–10. At the time of the testing, Terry had not yet started using the Ventolin inhaler before physical activity. It can be seen that Terry was at or below the 30th percentile in all tests but shuttle run and that his major difficulty was in the 600-yard run. Results from testing at age 17 are reported in Table 27–11. Although the high school physical education teachers were very strict in assessing quality of performance, the improvement in his physical fitness can be seen. The testing was completed

TABLE 27–10. Results of Standardized Physical Education Fitness Testing for 13-Year-Old Boy with Asthma

Test	Score	Percentile Rank
Sit-ups in 60 seconds	33	30th
Pull-ups	0	<20th
Long jump	5 feet 2 inches	25th
Shuttle run	10.2 seconds	60th
50-yard dash	7.8 seconds	30th
60-yard run	3 minutes 5 seconds	<5th*

Data from Hunsicker, P., & Reiff G. AAHPER Youth Fitness Test Manual, Rev. ed. Reston, VA: AAHPER Publications (American Alliance for Health, Physical Education, and Recreation), 1976, pp. 38–53.

*Major difficulty was found on prolonged running.

TABLE 27–11. Results of Standardized Physical Education Fitness Testing for 17-Year-Old Boy with Asthma

Test	Score	Attainment Standard* (45th Percentile)	Outstanding Achievement* (80th Percentile)
Sit-ups	53	46	55
Sit and reach	20	17	20
Pull-ups	7	8	11

*Standards are from the Chrysler Fund–Amateur Athletic Union Physical Program, Poplars Building, Bloomington, IN 47405.

during the fall when the pollen was high, and, therefore, Terry did not complete the 1-mile test as per physician recommendation.

This history exemplifies the need to question and test any child who seems to demonstrate the possibility of having EIB. Terry had reasoned that he had asthma; just as he could not eat turkey on Thanksgiving, he had difficulty with running. He had never known any different and so had never mentioned it.

Terry and his parents learned to recognize signs and symptoms of an impending asthma attack and how to inhibit or minimize the attack, as well as allergens that needed to be avoided. This awareness resulted in decreased visits to the doctor and decreased absences from school. Family life and vacations and teenage social life always took potential asthma attacks into account. Medication was carried by Terry for use as needed.

Unfortunately, not all asthma attacks could be prevented. Occasionally, a decision was made to try a potentially asthma-inducing situation after preventive medication. A hay ride resulted in bronchoconstriction. An overnight school camping experience resulted in a severe reaction to the mold and pollen. A Boy Scout backpack hike and sleep out was canceled at the last minute when asthma symptoms were noted; however, a 12-mile bike ride was accomplished without difficulties and a skiing trip was experienced with minimal problems. Terry participated in school dances and sporting activities with friends. He occasionally had problems in his school science laboratories when strong chemicals were used, but a second dose from his inhaler and relaxed breathing usually inhibited the bronchoconstriction.

Terry was always short for his age, usually at or below the 5th percentile. Decreased height was not a problem that needed to be discussed, however, because he was one of the oldest students in his class due to the cutoff date for starting school and consequently was within the 10th to 25th percentile for the class. He had his adolescent growth spurt around ages 15 to 16½ and is now at about the 25th percentile for adult height and weight.

Fortunately, Terry did not develop many of the secondary problems associated with asthma. He benefited from having a mother who was able to work with him on breathing and relaxation exercises and postural drainage with percussion. Unfortunately, any decreases in physical activity and fitness were attributed to the asthma and not investigated further. Terry's physical education teachers were aware that he had asthma and allowed him to participate in physical education classes according to his own assessment of his daily asthma status.

Terry has now graduated from college and has assumed an adult role in society. He continues to use his inhalers as needed. Under the new classification, Terry's asthma would be classified as mild intermittent. In the future, any children that Terry may have will benefit from the expanding knowledge of asthma control and prevention.

Based on the present knowledge of the pathophysiology of asthma and the new medications, Terry's medical treatment would have included cromolyn or nedocromil and β_2 agonists while still a preschooler. The decreased side effects and increased effectiveness of these medications compared with the ones available when Terry was young would have improved his ability to eat, sleep, and participate in physical activities. Testing for EIB at an earlier age with consequent prescriptions for Intal and Ventolin would have allowed Terry to more fully participate in physical education classes and other physical activities throughout elementary and middle school.

CONCLUSION

Asthma is a common childhood condition that may produce functional limitations and interfere with daily life. It is a lifelong condition and, therefore, the main objective is to accept the condition and learn how to best prevent or minimize primary and secondary impairments that limit function and lead to disability. New developments in genetic research, however, hold promise for major advances in prevention and management of asthma. Much is available to assist the child and family in dealing with asthma. The physical therapist has much to offer the child, family, and others and is a wonderful resource in the educational system.

Recommended Resources

American Lung Association.
Internet: http://www.lungusa.org.
National Heart, Lung, and Blood Institute. Expert Panel Report 2: Guidelines for the Diagnosis and Management of Asthma. Pub. no. 97-4051. Bethesda, MD: National Institutes of Health, 1997.

References

American Physical Therapy Association. Guide to Physical Therapist Practice. Physical Therapy, *77*(11):1240–1263, 1276–1288, 1461–1482, 1505–1514, 1526–1535, 1997.

Anderson, HR, Bailey, PA, Cooper, JS, Palmer, JC, & West, S. Morbidity and school absence caused by asthma and wheezing illness. Archives of Disease in Childhood, *58*:777–784, 1983.

Anderson, SD, Silverman, M, & Walker, SR. Metabolic and ventilatory changes in asthmatic patients during and after exercise. Thorax, *27*:718–725, 1972.

Barnes, PJ. New therapeutic approaches. British Medical Bulletin, *48*: 231–247, 1991.

Ben-Dov, I, Bar-Yishay, E, & Godfrey, S. Refractory period after exercise-induced asthma unexplained by respiratory heat loss. American Review of Respiratory Disease, *125*:530–534, 1982.

Bevegard, S, Eriksson, BO, Graff-Lonnevig, V, Kraepelien, S, & Saltin, B. Respiratory function, cardiovascular dimensions and work capacity in boys with bronchial asthma. Acta Paediatrica Scandinavica, 65:289-296, 1976.

Bishop, J, Carlin, J, & Nolan, T. Evaluation of the properties and reliability of a clinical severity scale for acute asthma in children. Journal of Clinical Epidemiology, 45:71-76, 1992.

Braback, L, & Kalvesten, L. Asthma in schoolchildren: Factors influencing morbidity in a Swedish survey. Acta Paediatrica Scandinavica, 77:826-830, 1988.

Buckley, JM, & Souhrada, JF. A comparison of pulmonary function tests in detecting exercise-induced bronchoconstriction. Pediatrics, 56(suppl):883-889, 1975.

Burney, PGJ, Chinn, S, & Rona, R. Has the prevalence of asthma increased in children? Evidence from the national study of health and growth 1973-86. British Medical Journal, 300:1306-1310, 1990.

Burr, ML, Eldridge, BA, & Borysiewicz, LK. Peak expiratory flow rates before and after exercise in schoolchildren. Archives of Disease in Childhood, 49:923-926, 1974.

Centers for Disease Control and Prevention. Surveillance for asthma—United States 1960-1995. Morbidity and Mortality Weekly Report, 47(SS-1):12-17, 1998.

Chryssanthopoulos, C, Maksud, MG, Gallen, WG, & Hause, LL. Cardiopulmonary responses of asthmatic children to strenuous exercise. Clinical Pediatrics, 23:384-388, 1984.

Collaborative Study on the Genetics of Asthma. A genome-wide search for asthma susceptibility loci in ethnically diverse populations. Nature Genetics, 15:389-392, 1997.

Cookson, WO, Sharp, PA, Faux, JA, & Hopkin, JM. Linkage between immunoglobulin E response underlying asthma and rhinitis and chromosome 11q. Lancet, 1:1292-1295, 1989.

Crofton, J, & Douglas, A (Eds.). Bronchial asthma. In Respiratory Diseases, 3rd ed. Boston: Blackwell Scientific, 1981, pp. 478-515.

Cropp, GJA. The exercise bronchoprovocation test: Standardization of procedures and evaluation of response. Journal of Allergy and Clinical Immunology, 64:627-633, 1979.

Dahl, J, Gustafsson, D, & Melin, L. Effects of a behavioral treatment program on children with asthma. Journal of Asthma, 27:41-46, 1990.

Deal, EC, McFadden, ER, Ingram, RH, & Jaeger, JJ. Hyperpnea and heat flux: Initial reaction sequence in exercise-induced asthma. Journal of Applied Physiology, 46:476-483, 1979.

de Benedictis, FM, Canny, GJ, & Levison, H. The progressive nature of childhood asthma. Lung, 168:278-285, 1990.

Edmunds, AT, Tooley, M, & Godfrey, S. The refractory period after exercise-induced asthma: Its duration and relation to the severity of exercise. American Review of Respiratory Diseases, 117:247-254, 1978.

Evans, R, Mullally, DI, Wilson, RW, Gergen, PJ, Rosenberg, HM, Grauman, JS, Chevarley, FM, & Feinleib, M. National trends in the morbidity and mortality of asthma in the US: Prevalence, hospitalization and death from asthma over two decades: 1965-1984. Chest, 91(suppl):65S-74S, 1987.

Fireman, P. Otitis media and its relationship to allergy. Pediatric Clinics of North America, 35:1075-1090, 1988.

Fitch, KD, Morton, FR, & Blanksby, BA. Effects of swimming training on children with asthma. Archives of Disease in Childhood, 51:190-194, 1976.

Freyschus, U, Hedlin, G, & Hedenstierna, G. Ventilation-perfusion relationships during exercise-induced asthma in children. American Review of Respiratory Disease, 130:888-894, 1984.

Furukawa, CT, Shapiro, GG, DuHamel, T, Weimer, L, Pierson, WE, & Bierman, CW. Learning and behaviour problems associated with theophylline therapy. Lancet, 1:621, 1984.

Gayrard, P, Orehek, J, Grimaud, C, & Charpin, J. Bronchoconstrictor effect of a deep inspiration in patients with asthma. American Review of Respiratory Disease, 111:433-439, 1975.

Girodo, M, Ekstrand, KA, & Metevier, CG. Deep diaphragmatic breathing: Rehabilitation exercises for the asthmatic patient. Archives of Physical Medicine and Rehabilitation, 73:717-720, 1992.

Gold, DR, Trager, IB, Weiss, ST, Tosteson, TD, & Speizer, FE. Acute lower respiratory illness in childhood as a predictor of lung function and chronic respiratory symptoms. American Review of Respiratory Disease, 140:877-884, 1989.

Haas, F, Pineda, H, Axen, K, Gaudino, D, & Haas, A. Effects of physical fitness on expiratory airflow in exercising asthmatic people. Medicine and Science in Sports and Exercise, 17:585-592, 1984.

Hauspie, R, Susanne, C, & Alexander, F. Maturational delay and temporal growth retardation in asthmatic boys. Journal of Allergy and Clinical Immunology, 59:200-206, 1977.

Hedlin, G, & Freyschuss, U. Cardiac output and blood pressure in asthmatic children before and during induced asthma. Acta Paediatrica Scandinavica, 73:441-447, 1984.

Hedlin, G, Graff-Lonnevig, V, & Freyschuss, U. Working capacity and pulmonary gas exchange in children with exercise-induced asthma. Acta Paediatrica Scandinavica, 75:947-954, 1986.

Henricksen, JM, & Nielson, TT. Effect of physical training on exercise-induced bronchoconstriction. Acta Paediatrica Scandinavica, 72:31-36, 1983.

Hessel, PA, Sliwkanich, T, Michaelchuk, D, White, H, & Nguyen, TH. Asthma and limitation of activities in Fort Saskatchewan, Alberta. Canadian Journal of Health, 87:397-400, 1996.

Hollister, JR, & Bowyer, SL. Adverse side effects of corticosteroids. Seminars in Respiratory Medicine, 8:400-405, 1987.

Huber, AL, Eggleston, PA, & Morgan, J. Effect of physiotherapy on asthmatic children (Abstract). Journal of Allergy and Clinical Immunology, 53:109, 1974.

Juniper, EF, Guyatt, GH, Epstein, RS, Ferrie, PJ, Jaeschke, R, & Hiller, TK. Evaluation of impairment of health related quality of life in asthma: Development of a questionnaire for use in clinical trials. Thorax, 47:76-83, 1992.

Kattan, M, Keens, TG, Mellis, CM, & Levinson, H. The response to exercise in normal and asthmatic children. The Journal of Pediatrics, 92:718-721, 1978.

Kelly, WJ, Hudson, I, Raven, J, Phelan, PD, Pain, MC, & Olinsky, A. Childhood asthma and adult lung function. American Review of Respiratory Disease, 138:26-30, 1988.

Kerem, E, Canny, G, Tibshirani, R, Reisman, J, Bentur, L, Schuh, S, & Levison, H. Clinical-physiological correlations in acute asthma of childhood. Pediatrics, 87:481-486, 1991.

King, JT, Bye, MB, & Demopoulos, JJ. Exercise programs for asthmatic children. Comprehensive Therapy, 10:67-71, 1984.

Kurashima, K, Ogawa, H, Ohka, T, Fujimura, M, & Matsuda, T. Thromboxane A_2 synthetase inhibitor (OXY-046) improves abnormal mucociliary transport in asthmatic patients. Annals of Allergy, 68:53-56, 1992.

Lee, HS. Proper aerosol inhalation technique for delivery of asthma medications. Clinical Pediatrics, 22:440-443, 1983.

Levy, M, & Bell, L. General practice audit of asthma in childhood. British Medical Journal, 289:1115-1116, 1984.

Lewis, CE, Rachelefsky, F, Lewis, MA, de la Suta, A, & Kaplan, M. A randomized trial of ACT. Pediatrics, 74:478-486, 1984.

Li, JT, & O'Connell, EJ. Viral infections and asthma. Annals of Allergy, 59:321-328, 1987.

Lozano, P, Fishman, P, VonKorff, M, and Hecht, J. Health care utilization and cost among children with asthma who were enrolled in a health maintenance organization. Pediatrics, 99:757-764, 1997.

Male, D. Immunology: An Illustrated Outline. St Louis: Mosby, 1986.

Martin, AJ, McLennan, LA, Landau, LI, & Phelan, PD. The natural history of childhood asthma to adult life. British Medical Journal, 280:1397-1400, 1980.

McConnochie, KM, & Roghmann, KJ. Bronchiolitis as a possible cause of wheezing in childhood: New evidence. Pediatrics, 74:1-10, 1984.

Mercer, MJ, & Van Niekerk, CH. Clinical characteristics of childhood asthma. South African Medical Journal, 79:77-79, 1991.

Mezey, RJ, Cohn, MA, Fernandez, RJ, Januszkiewicz, AJ, & Wanner, A. Mucociliary transport in allergic patients with antigen-induced bronchospasm. American Review of Respiratory Disease, 118:677–684, 1978.

National Heart, Lung, and Blood Institute. Expert Panel Report 2: Guidelines for the Diagnosis and Management of Asthma. Pub. no. 97-4051. Bethesda, MD: National Institutes of Health, 1997.

Nickerson, BG, Bautista, DB, Namey, MA, Richards, W, & Keens, TG. Distance running improves fitness in asthmatic children without pulmonary complications or changes in exercise-induced bronchospasm. Pediatrics, 71:147–152, 1983.

Orenstein, DM. Exercise tolerance and exercise conditioning in children with chronic lung disease. Journal of Pediatrics, 112:1043–1047, 1988.

Pederson, S, Frost, L, & Arnfred, T. Errors in inhalation technique and efficiency in inhaler use in asthmatic children. Allergy, 41:118–124, 1986.

Picado, C, Fiz, JA, Montserrat, JM, Grau, JM, Fernandez-Sola, J, Luengo, MT, Casademont, J, & Agusti-Vidal, A. Respiratory and skeletal muscle function in steroid-dependent bronchial asthma. American Review of Respiratory Disease, 141:14–20, 1990.

Pryor, JA, & Webber, BA. An evaluation of the forced expiration technique as an adjunct to postural drainage. Physiotherapy, 66:304–307, 1979.

Pullan, CR, & Hey, EN. Wheezing, asthma, and pulmonary function dysfunction ten years after infection with respiratory syncytial virus in infancy. British Medical Journal, 284:1665–1669, 1982.

Rachelefsky, GS, Wo, J, Adelson, J, Mickey, MR, Spector, SL, Katz, RM, Siegel, SC, & Rohr, AS. Behavior abnormalities and poor school performance due to oral theophylline use. Pediatrics, 78:1133–1138, 1986.

Reiff, DB, Choudry, NB, Pride, NB, & Ind, PW. The effect of submaximal warm-up exercise on exercise-induced asthma. American Review of Respiratory Disease, 139:479–484, 1989.

Rickards, AL, Ford, GW, Kitchen, WH, Doyle, LW, Lissenden, JV, & Keith, CG. Extremely low-birthweight infants: Neurological, psychological, growth, and health status beyond five years of age. Medical Journal of Australia, 147:476–481, 1987.

Ruppel, G. Manual of Pulmonary Function Testing. St. Louis: Mosby, 1982.

Schnall, RP, & Landau, LI. Protective effects of repeated short sprints in exercise-induced asthma. Thorax, 35:828–832, 1980.

Schroeckenstein, DC, & Busse, W. Exercise and asthma: Not incompatible. Journal of Respiratory Diseases, 9:29–45, 1988.

Sharkey, BJ. Physiology of Fitness. Champaign, IL: Human Kinetics, 1979.

Shohat, M, Shohat, T, Kadeem, R, Mimouni, M, & Danon, YL. Childhood asthma and growth outcome. Archives of Disease in Childhood, 62:63–65, 1987.

Sly, RM. Management of exercise-induced asthma. Drug Therapy, 12(March):95–100, 1982.

Sly, RM. History of exercise-induced asthma. Medicine and Science in Sports and Exercise, 18:314–317, 1986.

Smyth, JA, Tabachnik, FE, Duncan, JW, Reilly, BJ, & Levison, H. Pulmonary function and bronchial reactivity in long-term survivors of bronchopulmonary dysplasia. Pediatrics, 68:336–340, 1981.

Snyder, RD, Collip, PJ, & Greene, JS: Growth and ultimate height of children with asthma. Clinical Pediatrics, 6:389–392, 1967.

Spector, SL. Outpatient treatment of asthma. Annals of Allergy, 63:591–597, 1989.

Springer, C, Goldenberg, B, Ben-Dov, I, & Godfrey, S. Clinical, physiologic, and psychologic comparison of treatment by cromolyn or theophylline in childhood asthma. Journal of Clinical Immunology, 76:64–69, 1985.

Stempel, DA. Leukotriene modifiers in the treatment of asthma. Respiratory Care, 43:481–489, 1998.

Strauss, RH, McFadden, ER, & Ingram, RH. Influence of heat and humidity on the airway obstruction induced by exercise in asthma. Journal of Clinical Investigation, 61:433–440, 1978.

Strunk, RC, Mrazek, DA, Fukuhara, JT, Masterson, J, Ludwick, SK, & LaBrecque, JF. Cardiovascular fitness in children with asthma correlates with psychological functioning of the child. Pediatrics, 84:460–464, 1989.

Strunk, RC, Rubin, D, Kelly, L, Sherman, B, & Fukuhara, J. Determination of fitness in children with asthma: Use of standardized tests for functional endurance, body fat composition, flexibility, and abdominal strength. American Journal of Disease in Childhood, 142:940–944, 1988.

Tal, A, & Miklich, DR. Emotionally induced decreases in pulmonary flow rates in asthmatic children. Psychosomatic Medicine, 38:190–199, 1976.

Taussig, LM, Chernick, V, Wood, R, Farrell, P, Mellins, RB, & Members of the Conference Committee. Standardization of lung testing in children. Journal of Pediatrics, 97:668–676, 1980.

Townsend, M, Feeny, DH, Guyatt, Furlong, W, Seip, AE, & Dolovich J. Evaluation of the burden of illness for pediatric asthmatic patients and their parents. Annals of Allergy, 67:403–408, 1991.

Varray, AL, Mercier, JG, Terral, CM, & Prefaut, CG. Individualized aerobic and high intensity training for asthmatic children in an exercise readaptation program: Is training always helpful for better adaptation to exercise? Chest, 99:579–586, 1991.

Vogel, G. New clues to asthma therapies. Science, 276:1643–1646, 1997.

Voy, RO. The U.S. Olympic Committee experience with exercise-induced bronchospasm, 1984. Medicine and Science in Sports and Exercise, 18:328–330, 1986.

Wantanabe, H. The effect of disodium cromoglycate against bronchial hyperresponsiveness in asthmatic children. Journal of Asthma, 29:117–120, 1992.

Weiss, KB, Gergen, PJ, & Hodgson, TA. An economic evaluation of asthma in the United States. New England Journal of Medicine, 326:862–866, 1992.

Wennergren, G, Engstrom, I, & Bjure, J. Transcutaneous oxygen and carbon dioxide levels and a clinical symptom scale for monitoring the acute asthmatic state of infants and children. Acta Paediatrica Scandinavica, 75:465–469, 1986.

CHAPTER 28

Thoracic Surgery

BETSY A. HOWELL, PT, MS

Approximately 8 to 10 in 1000 children born each year have congenital heart defects (Callow, 1989). The impact a congenital heart defect has on a child varies greatly depending on the type of defect, as well as the individual child. For example, two children, each diagnosed with a ventricular septal defect, may have entirely different histories. One child may go undiagnosed for several years, whereas the other child may require surgery in infancy. Formerly, most congenital heart defects were repaired when the child was at least 1 year old, often older. More of these surgeries are now being performed during infancy, which is likely to affect how children with congenital heart defects grow and develop. The likelihood of treating a child who has previously had open-heart surgery is greater with more children surviving open-heart surgery. Physical therapists examining this population should closely monitor and document the nature and extent of developmental differences that may result from earlier surgical repair, as well as potential neurologic deficits possibly secondary to deep hypothermic circulatory arrest. To prepare therapists for this task, this chapter describes congenital heart defects; surgical repairs, including heart and heart-lung transplantation; acute and chronic physical impairments secondary to heart defects and surgery; profound cyanosis or neurologic complications; and physical therapy intervention for the population of children with cardiac defects.

CONGENITAL HEART DEFECTS

The cause of congenital heart defects is unknown; however, the occasional presence of more than one child with congenital heart disease in the same family suggests a possible genetic component. Approximately 10% of children with congenital heart defects also have other physical malformations (Noonan, 1981). Heart defects may be associated with Down syndrome, Turner syndrome, Williams syndrome, Marfan syndrome, Costello syndrome, DiGeorge syndrome, and the Vater association. Infants of diabetic mothers also have an increased incidence of congenital heart disease (Clarke et al., 1991).

Diagnosis of cardiac problems may occur at birth and be followed by further evaluation at that time. Some infants with severe cyanotic disease are not diagnosed before they are discharged to home, but several weeks later they may be diagnosed with a heart defect when they develop symptoms of septic shock. Other cardiac defects may not be diagnosed until much later, even as late as adolescence. For example, coarctation of the aorta is occasionally diagnosed during a sports physical examination when a large difference between upper and lower extremity blood pressure or an abnormally high upper extremity blood pressure is observed.

The infant with a congenital heart defect often has abnormal respiratory signs, including a labored breathing pattern and an increased respiratory rate. The infant may be diaphoretic and tachycardic. Edema around the eyes and decreased urine output (evidenced by dry diapers) may also be observed. Eating problems result from difficulty in coordinating sucking and swallowing with breathing at an increased rate. Irritability that is difficult to assuage may be noted. These symptoms of congestive heart failure can lead to the diagnosis of a cardiac defect or provide evidence of the worsening of a known defect.

Congenital heart defects are usually classified as acyanotic or cyanotic. In acyanotic lesions, the child is pink and has normal oxygen saturation. If there is mixing or shunting of blood within the heart, the blood shunts from the left side of the heart to the right side, so oxygenated blood goes to the lungs as well as to the body. Common acyanotic lesions include atrial septal defects, ventricular septal defects, patent ductus arteriosus, coarctation of the aorta, pulmonary stenosis, and aortic stenosis.

In cyanotic defects, blood is typically shunted from the right side of the heart to the left side. Unoxygenated blood is then returned to the body, resulting in arterial oxygen saturation levels 15 to 30% below normal values. Common cyanotic lesions include tetralogy of Fallot, transposition of the great arteries, tricuspid atresia, pulmonary atresia, truncus arteriosus, total anomalous pulmonary venous return, and hypoplastic left-heart syndrome.

Type and timing of intervention depends on the defect and the child's age. Some defects are repaired immediately, whereas others require a staged procedure, with the first several surgeries being palliative rather than corrective. Some acyanotic defects are not repaired until the child is several years old. Less impairment of growth and weight gain, however, occurs when surgery is performed in the first 2 years of life (Rosenthal, 1983; Suoninen, 1971). However, there has been some recent concern about neurologic complications in the newborn after heart surgery (duPlessis, 1997). Low-flow cardiopulmonary bypass (Zimmerman et al., 1997) and neurophysiologic monitoring during surgery help minimize the possibility of neurologic complications (Austin et al., 1997). Acyanotic and cyanotic defects are described in the next two sections and may be compared with normal anatomy of the heart (Fig. 28-1).

ACYANOTIC DEFECTS

Atrial Septal Defect

Atrial septal defect, one of the most common congenital heart defects, is an abnormal communication between the left and right atria (Fig. 28-2).

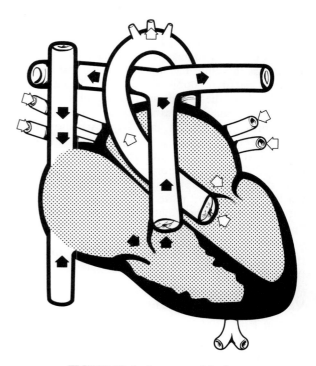

FIGURE 28-1. Anatomy of the heart.

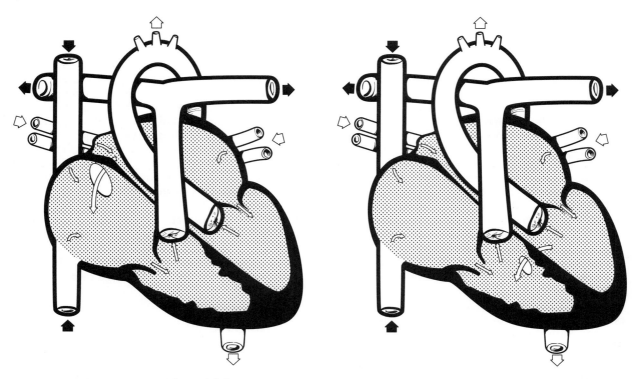

FIGURE 28–2. Atrial septal defect.   **FIGURE 28–3.** Ventricular septal defect.

The defect is classified by its location on the septum. Blood is generally shunted from the left atrium to the right atrium. This defect has traditionally been repaired when a child is between 4 and 6 years old because of slow progression of damage to the heart and lungs. If a child has more severe symptoms, the defect is repaired sooner (Mee, 1991). Some adults with signs of heart failure are found to have a previously undiagnosed atrial septal defect. As medical technology advances, late diagnoses should become rare.

Surgical repair has traditionally been made through a median sternotomy incision; however, a right thoracotomy approach has also been used primarily for cosmetic reasons. The defect is usually sutured together, or a patch closure is used when necessary (Kopf & Laks, 1991). The timing of surgery depends on the age of the child, when the diagnosis is confirmed, and how symptomatic the child is, but it typically occurs during the first 5 years of life.

Ventricular Septal Defect

Ventricular septal defect is the most common congenital heart defect (20–30% of all children with congenital defects) (Graham et al., 1989). It can be present alone or in association with other defects such as the tetralogy of Fallot and transposition of the great arteries. Ventricular septal defect alone is discussed here. A ventricular septal defect is a communication between the ventricles that allows blood to be shunted between them, generally from left to right (Fig. 28–3). The increase in blood flow through the right ventricle to the lungs may lead to pulmonary hypertension. In severe cases, in which pulmonary pressures exceed systemic pressures, shunting switches from right to left, which is often termed *Eisenmenger syndrome* (Graham et al., 1989). A large defect may lead to early left ventricular failure. An infant with a large ventricular septal defect has signs of severe respiratory distress, diaphoresis, and fatigability, especially during feeding, when the infant's endurance is stressed (Giboney, 1983). The infant's weight is dramatically affected in this situation. A child this severely affected has a much earlier surgical repair than a child who is asymptomatic.

Small defects may close spontaneously. Defects that compromise the clinical status of the patient must be surgically closed. The timing of surgery varies, depending on the child's tolerance of the defect. A child with a larger defect undergoes surgery earlier to diminish the negative effects on growth and the pulmonary system. Surgical intervention is through a mediastinal approach and usually requires a syn-

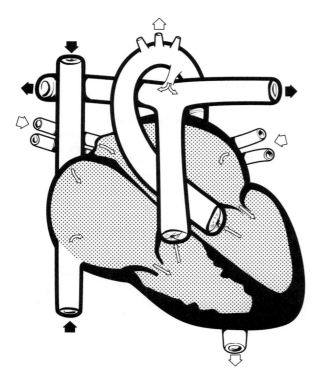

FIGURE 28–4. Patent ductus arteriosus.

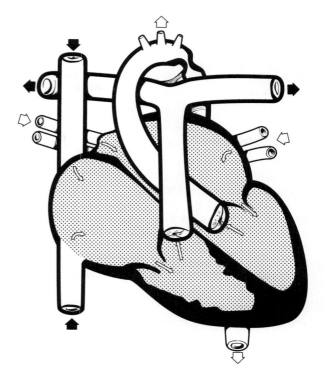

FIGURE 28–5. Coarctation of the aorta.

thetic patch closure (Arciniegas, 1991). The mortality rate for surgical closure of a ventricular septal defect without other associated defects is very low (1%) (Arciniegas, 1991).

Patent Ductus Arteriosus

The ductus arteriosus is a large vessel that connects the main pulmonary artery to the descending aorta (Fig. 28–4). It usually closes soon after birth but dilates (remains patent) in response to hypoxia or prostaglandins E_1 and E_2 (Levitsky & del Nido, 1991). The ability to maintain patency of the ductus arteriosus becomes important in certain cyanotic heart defects to be discussed later. The spontaneous closing of the ductus arteriosus can create a critical situation in the infant with an undiagnosed heart defect. A high incidence of patency is found in premature infants because of respiratory distress syndrome and the resulting hypoxia. Surgical repair is generally performed by a left thoracotomy incision. The ductus is ligated and sutured.

Coarctation of the Aorta

Coarctation of the aorta is defined as a narrowing or closing of a section of the aorta (Fig. 28–5). Patent

ductus arteriosus was observed in approximately 23% of diagnosed cases of coarctation of the aorta (Waldhausen et al., 1991). Infants with a severe narrowing may develop left ventricular failure (Girlando et al., 1988). Early repair is necessary when a child is severely symptomatic. The child or adult without symptoms may go undiagnosed until a routine physical examination reveals an abnormally high upper extremity blood pressure.

Surgical intervention is the primary method of treating coarctation of the aorta. Access to the aorta is through a left thoracotomy, after which the aorta is repaired with an end-to-end anastomosis, a subclavian flap, or a patch aortoplasty (Waldhausen et al., 1991). The operative mortality rate for surgical repair is low (3%) (Waldhausen et al., 1991).

Pulmonary Stenosis

Pulmonary stenosis is a narrowing of the right ventricular outflow tract and is classified by the location of the narrowing relative to the pulmonary valve. It often occurs in association with other heart defects. Timing of surgery depends on the severity of the narrowing and the degree of functional compromise.

Surgery is performed through a median sternotomy; the type of surgical procedure depends on the site of narrowing. A valvotomy may be performed, or in severe cases, the valve may need to be replaced (Moulton & Malm, 1991). Mortality rate varies with the age of the child at the time of repair. Children older than 2 years have a low mortality rate (0.5%), whereas the rate for those younger than 1 year increases to 10% (Moulton & Malm, 1991).

Aortic Stenosis

Aortic stenosis is a narrowing of the left ventricular outflow tract and is classified by its relation to the aortic valve (supravalvular, valvular, or subvalvular) (Fig. 28–6). An aortic valvotomy is performed through a median sternotomy in infants and children with severe stenosis. In severe cases, a valve replacement may be necessary if a valvotomy cannot be performed (Weldon et al., 1991). Mortality rate around the time of surgery is 6% (Weldon et al., 1991).

CYANOTIC DEFECTS

Tetralogy of Fallot

The tetralogy of Fallot is the most common cyanotic cardiac defect, accounting for almost 50% of all cyanotic lesions. The primary abnormalities that oc-

cur in the tetralogy of Fallot are a ventricular septal defect, right ventricular outflow tract obstruction, an aorta that overrides the right ventricle, and hypertrophy of the right ventricle (Laks & Breda, 1991a) (Fig. 28–7). Clinical manifestations of the defect depend on severity of the obstruction of the right ventricular outflow tract. With increasing severity, an increase in cyanosis is observed that becomes more marked when the child is overexerted or upset. Clubbing of the nailbeds occurs and becomes more apparent after the first 6 to 8 months. The child's height and weight are often affected. Cyanotic or blue episodes occur, which are thought to be caused by an abrupt decrease in pulmonary blood flow and are characterized by dyspnea, syncope, and deepening cyanosis (Laks & Breda, 1991a; Page, 1986). The cyanotic episodes are typically relieved by squatting or by bringing the knees to the chest. These maneuvers are believed to increase systemic vascular resistance and ultimately to increase pulmonary blood flow. Oxygen or morphine or both may also need to be administered (Laks & Breda, 1991a).

Surgical intervention depends on the patient's symptoms and overall clinical picture. Early palliation may be necessary if an infant is severely involved and would probably not survive corrective surgery. The palliative procedure used most often is a Blalock-Taussig (BT) shunt performed through a

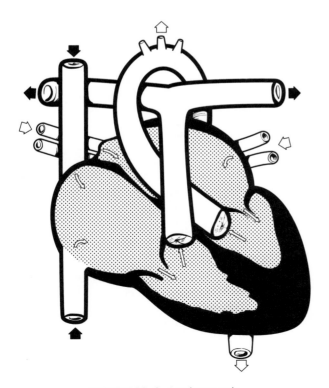

FIGURE 28–6. Aortic stenosis.

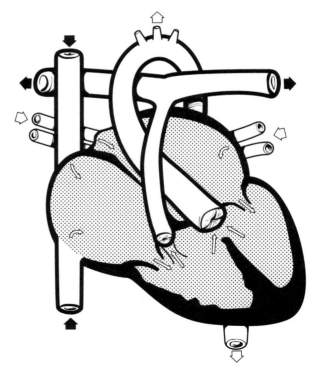

FIGURE 28–7. Tetrology of fallot.

thoracotomy. The BT shunt involves an anastomosis of the subclavian artery to the pulmonary artery, providing increased pulmonary blood flow while the infant gains more time to grow before undergoing corrective surgery. Mild growth retardation may occur in the upper extremity on the side of the shunt, but it has not been viewed as a major problem (Page, 1986). Another important consequence of early palliation is continued cyanosis until complete repair is performed.

Corrective surgery involves closing the ventricular septal defect and relieving the right outflow tract obstruction. After surgical repair, an exercise stress test is warranted before the initiation of an exercise program because of a 14% incidence of ventricular arrhythmias at rest and a 30% incidence during exercise (Garson et al., 1980). With advances in surgical technique, mortality rates for surgical repair (5%) have been drastically reduced (Laks & Breda, 1991a).

Transposition of the Great Arteries

In transposition of the great arteries, the pulmonary artery arises from the morphologic left ventricle, and the aorta arises from the right ventricle (Callow, 1989) (Fig. 28–8). In the absence of other defects, the systemic blood returns to the body unoxygenated and pulmonary blood returns to the lungs

fully oxygenated. This situation is obviously not compatible with life unless the ductus arteriosus remains patent. Immediate intervention, usually with the infusion of prostaglandin E_1, is necessary to keep the ductus arteriosus open. An atrial septostomy is performed by a cardiac catheterization to keep the child alive until surgical intervention occurs.

The type of surgical intervention used for correction of transposition of the great arteries depends largely on the surgeon's preference. In some institutions, a Mustard or Senning technique is used to redirect the venous return to the atria, either by baffles or flaps of atrial wall, respectively (de Leval, 1991; Trusler, 1991). These techniques leave the right ventricle as the pumping chamber for the systemic system.

The Rastelli procedure is a surgical technique used when a severe left ventricular outflow tract obstruction and a ventricular septal defect coexist. Repair usually occurs when the child is between 4 and 6 years old. A conduit diverts blood from the left ventricle through the ventricular septal defect and right ventricle to the aorta, a right ventricle to pulmonary artery conduit is formed, and any previous shunts are eliminated (Williams, 1991). Reoperation for conduit enlargement is not uncommon. Depression of right ventricular function over time has been reported in some patients whose defects were corrected with these procedures (Jarmakani & Canent, 1974; Nakazawa et al., 1986).

The preferred technique, when anatomically possible, is the arterial switch procedure. Surgery during the first 2 to 4 weeks of life is preferred so that the left ventricle meets the systemic demands. Surgical repair occurs through a median sternotomy and involves transecting the aorta and pulmonary artery. The coronary arteries are excised with a wide button of aortic tissue and reimplanted in the old pulmonary arterial vessel; the great vessels are then switched and anastomosed so that the aorta connects to the left ventricle and the pulmonary artery connects to the right ventricle. The arterial switch procedure produces results that are free of the dysrhythmias and right ventricular failure associated with the techniques described previously (Callow, 1989). Survival rates at major centers in which this technique is performed have been good (greater than 90%) (Castaneda & Mayer, 1991).

Tricuspid Atresia

Tricuspid atresia is the failure of development of the tricuspid valve, resulting in a lack of communication between the right atrium and right ventricle. Usually, an atrial septal defect or a ventricular septal defect or both exists to allow pulmonary blood flow (Fig. 28–9). The right-to-left shunt allows mixing of

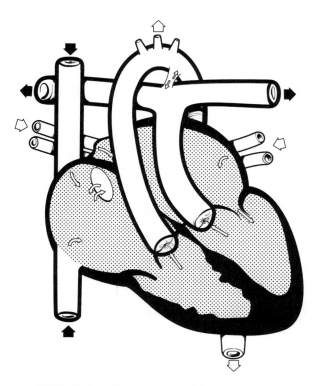

FIGURE 28–8. Transposition of the great arteries.

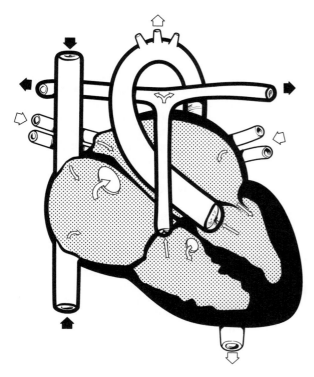

FIGURE 28-9. Tricuspid atresia.

unoxygenated and oxygenated blood, causing the child to be cyanotic. The right ventricle is frequently underdeveloped.

Surgical repair is staged, with the initial operation shunting blood from the body to the lungs with a BT shunt through a thoracotomy. However, if the ventricular septal defect is large and too much blood is going to the lungs, a band may be placed around the pulmonary artery to decrease blood flow to the lungs. The child remains cyanotic for several years.

The next stage of surgical repair is often the Fontan procedure (or a modification thereof) performed through a median sternotomy in which the right atrium is attached to the pulmonary artery or directly to the right ventricle, using a conduit or baffle. The ventricular septal defect may be surgically closed (Laks & Breda, 1991b). It is not uncommon to have significant chest tube drainage for weeks after the Fontan surgery, thereby increasing the length of hospital stay.

In some institutions, a bidirectional Glenn procedure performed before the Fontan procedure leads to an improved outcome. In the Glenn procedure, the superior vena cava is anastomosed to the right pulmonary artery. The child remains cyanotic but gains time for growth before undergoing the Fontan operation. Operative mortality rates have decreased from 15 to 30% to less than 5% with improved surgical technique and patient selection (Laks & Breda, 1991b).

Pulmonary Atresia

Pulmonary atresia occurs when the pulmonary valve fails to develop, resulting in obstruction of blood flow from the right side of the heart to the lungs. Blood flow to the lungs is initially maintained by a patent ductus arteriosus. An atrial septal defect or a ventricular septal defect may also be present, allowing shunting of blood from the right to the left side of the heart and ultimately back to the body. The size of the right ventricle may vary, affecting later surgical decisions. Early intervention involves maintaining patency of the ductus arteriosus to increase blood flow to the lungs until surgery can be performed. An atrial septostomy is usually performed during the initial cardiac catheterization. A BT shunt is often performed as soon as possible.

Later surgery involves ligating the previous shunt, closing the atrial septal defect, and opening the pulmonary valve by a valvulotomy, an infundibular graft, or a right ventricle–to–pulmonary artery conduit. If the ventricle is poorly developed, the Fontan procedure may be performed to provide communication through a conduit between the right atrium and pulmonary artery (Puga, 1991). Children remain cyanotic during their early developmental years until the Fontan operation is performed. Surgical mortality rates approach 10% (Puga, 1991).

Truncus Arteriosus

Truncus arteriosus occurs when the aorta and pulmonary artery fail to separate in utero and form a common trunk arising from both ventricles (Fig. 28-10). Four grades of the condition are differentiated, depending on the location of the pulmonary arteries. Early surgical intervention is necessary. Surgical repair is through a median sternotomy and involves removing the pulmonary arteries from the truncus, closing the ventricular septal defect, and connecting the pulmonary arteries to the right ventricle by an extracardiac baffle. Mortality rates are lower in patients operated on in the first 6 months of life (9% vs. 18% for later repair) (Milgalter & Laks, 1991; Peetz et al., 1982).

Total Anomalous Pulmonary Venous Return

Total anomalous pulmonary venous return occurs when the pulmonary veins fail to communicate with the left atrium and instead connect to the coro-

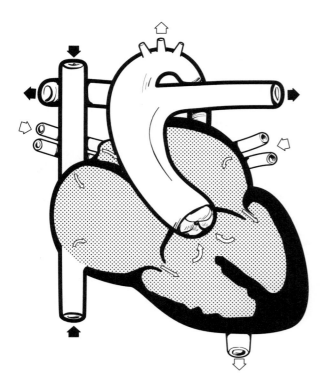

FIGURE 28–10. Truncus arteriosus.

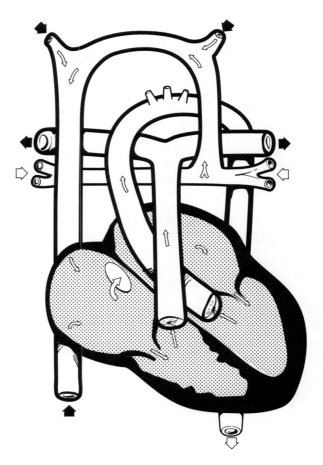

FIGURE 28–11. Total anomalous pulmonary venous return.

nary sinus of the right atrium or to one of the systemic veins. The ductus arteriosus often remains patent (Fig. 28–11). The increase in flow through the right side of the heart and into the lungs may lead to congestive heart failure. Anastomosis of the pulmonary veins to the left atrium through a median sternotomy is usually performed as soon as possible. Postoperative ventilation may be difficult because of stiffness and wetness of the lungs from the previous excessive blood flow (Byrum et al., 1982; Hammon & Bender, 1991). Mortality rates continue to improve but remain nearly 30% for infants (Hammon & Bender, 1991).

Hypoplastic Left-Sided Heart Syndrome

Hypoplasia (incomplete development or underdevelopment) or absence of the left ventricle and hypoplasia of the ascending aorta mark hypoplastic left-sided heart syndrome, the most common form of a univentricular heart, often coexisting with severe aortic valve hypoplasia. A patent ductus arteriosus provides systemic circulation until surgical intervention. Without surgical intervention, death is certain; however, the surgical mortality rate at 24% is still higher than other congenital heart surgeries (Lloyd, 1996). Lloyd (1996) reported that the sur-

vival rate after the second-stage palliation is now 97%, and the survival rate is 81% after the Fontan operation. However, Lloyd also reported that some of the survivors of the Fontan operation were observed to have neurologic conditions (6%) and respiratory conditions (11%).

Three options are available to parents of infants diagnosed as having hypoplastic left-sided heart syndrome. One option is no surgical intervention. As a second option, the child's name may be placed on a waiting list for a heart transplant, or as a third, the child may undergo a series of palliative procedures. The initial surgical procedure (Norwood I) involves enlarging the atrial septal defect, transecting the main pulmonary artery and anastomosing it to the aorta, and reconstructing the aortic root. A BT or central shunt is placed to allow pulmonary blood flow. The second stage is a bidirectional Glenn procedure anastomosing the superior vena cava to the pulmonary arteries and ligating the BT shunt. The Fontan procedure may be performed several months to a few years later. This procedure provides continuity between the right atrium and pulmonary artery, and the pulmonary venous return is separated from the systemic system. As a result, the right ventricle pumps fully oxygenated blood to the body (Johnson & Davis, 1991; Norwood, 1991a, 1991b). Heart transplantation is also offered as a second-stage possibility. The postoperative stay is usually lengthy, and children often have difficulty in being weaned from the ventilator. Although infants who survive the first stage may die (10%) before reaching the second stage, surgical interventions continue to lower the mortality rate (Bailey & Gundry, 1990). Table 28–1 summarizes the common types of congenital heart defects, their typical surgical repair, and associated impairments and functional limitations.

Heart Transplantation

Cardiac transplantation is a viable option for children with end-stage heart failure secondary to congenital malformations or for children with cardiomyopathy. Introduction of cyclosporine to control rejection has increased survival rates to 65% after 5 years, and 92% survival in infants has been reported (Bauer et al., 1998). The previous indication for

TABLE 28–1. **Summary of Congenital Heart Defects, Surgical Repair, and Associated Issues**

Type of Defect	Surgical Repair	Associated Issues	Physical Therapy Issues
Atrial septal defect (ASD)	Suture or patch closure		Early mobility
Ventricular septal defect (VSD)	Dacron patch closure	Failure to thrive; pulmonary hypertension	Failure to thrive
Atrial ventricular septal defect/endocardial cushion defect	Pericardial patch	Down syndrome; failure to thrive	Developmental delay
Coarctation of the aorta	Subclavian patch/end-to-end anastomosis	Hypertension	Upper extremity range of motion
Pulmonary stenosis	Valvotomy		
Aortic stenosis	Valvotomy; aortic valve replacement; conduit		
Tetralogy of Fallot	VSD closed; right ventricular outflow tract resected	"Tet" spells	
Transposition of the great arteries (dextro)	Arterial switch operation	Edema; poor left ventricle function	
Pulmonary atresia (PA) with a VSD	Blalock-Taussig shunt (BT); VSD closed; right ventricle–to–pulmonary artery conduit	Developmental delay; poor oral intake	Developmental delay; feeding issues
Pulmonary atresia without a VSD	Valvotomy/BT shunt; right ventricular outflow tract patch, ASD closed, Fontan procedure	Very sick postoperatively, low oxygen saturations	Developmental delay
Total anomalous pulmonary venous return	Anomalous veins connected to left atrium; ASD closed	Failure to thrive	Failure to thrive
Tricuspid atresia	1. Atrial septostomy, BT shunt 2. Bidirectional Glenn or hemi-Fontan procedure 3. Fontan procedure	Low oxygen saturations	Failure to thrive
Truncus arteriosus	VSD closure, right ventricle–to–pulmonary artery conduit	Pulmonary hypertensive crisis	Developmental delay; failure to thrive
Hypoplastic left-sided heart syndrome	1. Division of the main pulmonary artery; suture PA to the aorta; BT shunt and patent ductus arteriosus ligation 2. Bidirectional Glenn or hemi-Fontan procedure 3. Fenestrated Fontan procedure	Low oxygen saturations	Poor oral feeders; developmental delay; may not crawl

transplantation in children was largely cardiomyopathy (62%). Since 1988, however, the number of transplants for congenital heart defects has surpassed that of cardiomyopathy (Kriett & Kaye, 1991; Pennington et al., 1991). The increase is at least partly related to the fact that cardiac transplantation is being offered more frequently as an option for children with hypoplastic left-sided heart syndrome. As a result, a greatly increased number of children under 1 year of age have received a cardiac transplant (Bailey et al., 1988; Bove, 1991; Pennington et al., 1991; Starnes et al., 1992). Razzouk and associates (1996) have observed an 84% 1-year and 72% 7-year survival rate in infants under 1 year of age undergoing cardiac transplantation.

Surgery is performed through a median sternotomy and involves removal of the recipient heart with residual atrial cuffs remaining. The atria are reanastomosed with the donor heart, and then the great arteries are connected (Haas et al., 1991). Severing of the vagus nerve and the cervical and thoracic sympathetic cardiac nerves leaves the heart denervated (Clough, 1990; Kent & Cooper, 1974). An intrinsic control system exists within the heart, so it is not dependent on innervation for function. Cardiac impulse formation occurs because of spontaneous depolarization of the sinoatrial node (Kent & Cooper, 1974). The sinus node firing rate is faster than the usual heart rate in resting humans, so the heart rate of an individual after transplantation is faster than normal (Uretsky, 1990).

Several other influences on myocardial contractility remain, including the Frank-Starling effect, the Anrep effect, and the Bowditch effect. The Frank-Starling effect is the increase in cardiac output by an increase in stroke volume after an increased input or venous return (Kent & Cooper, 1974). This is an important effect that helps the body meet its early oxygen needs for exercise after transplantation. With the Anrep effect retained, the cardiac muscle increases its contractile force when the aortic pressure rises (afterload). The Bowditch effect describes an augmented contractile force of the heart with an increase in heart rate (Clough, 1990; Kent & Cooper, 1974). The transplanted heart has an increased sensitivity to circulating catecholamines (epinephrine and norepinephrine). Epinephrine increases the heart rate and the force of myocardial contraction, and norepinephrine increases the peripheral vascular resistance (Clough, 1990). The hormonal release takes several minutes to have an effect on the heart's rate and contractility, so it is generally advised that patients perform several minutes of warm-up exercises before vigorous exercise. It also takes several minutes for the body to reduce the hormones to normal levels, so a cool-down period at the end of

exercise is also advised. The resting heart rate is higher than usual in transplant recipients, and the peak heart rate is lower; both should be taken into account when transplant patients are exercising (Uretsky, 1990).

Antirejection treatment begins with triple therapy of cyclosporine, azathioprine (Imuran), and prednisone. The use of steroids is discontinued as soon as possible and reinstituted only if rejection occurs (Bailey et al., 1988; Pennington et al., 1991). The use of steroids should be taken into consideration when the weight and height percentiles of transplant recipients are reviewed. The majority of children increase their weight dramatically without a concomitant increase in height (Fricker et al., 1990; Pennington et al., 1991). Cyclosporine has been noted to cause hypertension, hyperplasia of the gastrointestinal mucosa, hirsutism, and gingival hyperplasia (Haas et al., 1991). The immunosuppressive medications also accelerate atherosclerosis, even in children, as well as decrease the body's ability to fight infections.

Rejection is an ongoing issue in all transplant patients. Signs and symptoms of rejection range from fever, malaise, poor appetite, weight gain, tachycardia, tachypnea, and low urine output to poor perfusion, complete heart block, pulmonary edema, and shock (Haas et al., 1991). Severe rejection has been observed in several adolescent transplant recipients after missing just one dose of cyclosporine.

Several complications are common in the pediatric heart transplant population. Hypertension and seizures have been observed in a number of patients. Seizures are believed to be caused by high cyclosporine levels; however, they do not generally recur once the patient is on a therapeutic dose of anticonvulsants (Fricker et al., 1990; Pennington et al., 1991). Other central nervous system disturbances have been observed in children, ranging from lethargy and confusion to localized neurologic defects and behavioral disturbances. Central nervous system dysfunction occurs more commonly in children than in adults; fortunately, the impairment is usually transient (Haas et al., 1991).

Conditions Requiring Lung and Heart-Lung Transplantation

More than 200 heart-lung transplantations take place each year, with a small proportion of those being in children. In 1990, 214 single-lung and 60 double-lung transplants were reported (Kriett & Kaye, 1991). Primary pulmonary hypertension and Eisenmenger syndrome are the indications for over 50% of the heart-lung transplants being done, with a small percentage performed for congenital heart disease and about 30% performed for cystic fibrosis. Primary pulmonary disease is the usual diagnosis of lung transplant recipients; however, some transplants are necessary secondary to lung failure caused by congenital heart defects. Lung transplants in these cases are usually associated with cardiac repair. Previous thoracotomy is no longer considered a contraindication for heart-lung or lung transplantation; however, it does increase the risk of perioperative bleeding (Whitehead et al., 1990). The mortality rate for children has been reported at nearly 30% in the first year after transplant and less than 10% later (Wilkinson, 1989).

The surgical procedure for a heart-lung transplantation is performed through a median sternotomy. The recipient heart and then lungs are removed. The donor organs are placed inside the chest cavity with the trachea anastomosed several rings above the carina. The right atrial anastomosis is performed and followed by anastomosis of the aorta (Bonser & Jamieson, 1990). Because of the risk of tracheal dehiscence, an omentum wrap around the suture line is typically used (Griffith et al., 1987).

The surgical procedure for a single-lung transplantation is performed through a thoracotomy incision. The removal of diseased lung is followed by the placement of the donor lung. The bronchial anastomosis is completed with an omentum wrap and followed by anastomosis of the pulmonary artery (Bolman et al., 1991).

When both lungs are transplanted, pulmonary innervation is lost (Jamieson et al., 1984). An early study observed bronchial hyperresponsiveness to inhaled methacholine, which was thought to be caused by denervation hypersensitivity (Glanville et al., 1989). Since that time, however, the postganglionic cholinergic nerve responses have been observed to be intact, as demonstrated by a normal bronchoconstrictor response to a stimulant. Therefore airway hypersensitivity is most likely a result of intact postganglionic cholinergic nerve response instead of denervation hypersensitivity (Stretton et al., 1990). Hypersensitivity was not observed during exercise (Glanville et al., 1989).

Because secretions below the tracheal anastomosis in the denervated lung do not excite the cough reflex, percussion, postural drainage, and breathing exercises are required to aid expectoration (Bonser & Jamieson, 1990). A certain amount of atelectasis is observed in all patients, especially when the transplanted lungs must be compressed to fit into the thoracic cage (Jamieson et al., 1984). Pulmonary edema is also commonly observed in the early postoperative period. Positive end-expiratory pressure is often used with mechanical ventilation to reduce atelectasis and pulmonary edema (Whitehead et al., 1990).

The diagnosis of rejection is made based on clinical signs and symptoms suggesting a deterioration in function. Chest radiographic findings and pulmonary function test results are noninvasive indicators. If necessary, a transbronchial biopsy is performed when patients are breathless and febrile and have rales and wheezes on auscultation (Hutter et al., 1988).

Pulmonary infection occurs in most transplant recipients, usually repeatedly. Obliterative bronchiolitis is also a common posttransplant complication that has been reported to affect 71% of long-term survivors (Glanville et al., 1990; Starnes et al., 1991). The acute phase of obliterative bronchiolitis is characterized by varying degrees of bronchiolar obstruction by plugs of granulation tissue; in the chronic phase, the bronchioles are partially to completely occluded (Aziz & Jamieson, 1991). Severe damage may necessitate retransplantation. With improvements in immunosuppression, obliterative bronchiolitis is becoming less common in adults; the same progress is anticipated in children.

The education of parents and children about the implications and ramifications of a heart, heart-lung, or lung transplantation must be thorough and frank, including discussion of the implications of being on a waiting list and the extent of the postoperative care after transplantation. Geographic and social dislocation may occur during assessment and during the wait for a transplant (Warner, 1991). Warner (1991) stresses that families must be aware that, although transplantation is a last resort, it still may not be the answer. Many centers require transplant candidates to participate in a formal exercise rehabilitation program before receiving the transplant to minimize postoperative complications, maximize the transplant, and assess compliance. Compliance before transplantation may be an indicator of posttransplant compliance. Noncompliance is a contraindication for transplantation because rigid adherence to the immunosuppressive regimen is imperative. Missed doses of cyclosporine can result in death.

Technologic Support

Mechanical ventilation is common after open-heart surgery in the pediatric patient but should not deter the physical therapist from beginning treatment. Recent improvements in cardiopulmonary bypass, decreased operating time, and improved postoperative fluid management have allowed early extubation, often within 8 hours of surgery (Prakanrattana et al., 1997). This has led to decreased costs, early patient mobility, and fewer respiratory complications. However, some patients may require the use of high-frequency jet ventilation in the period after open-heart surgery in pediatric patients, which will prevent initiation of early physical therapy. High-frequency jet ventilation introduces a small tidal volume at a very rapid rate. Its use allows delivery of oxygen and removal of carbon dioxide at reduced mean airway and peak inspiratory pressures, and it is often used in unstable patients for whom physical therapy is contraindicated (Norwood & Civette, 1991). The three main advantages of high-frequency ventilation over conventional approaches to ventilation are improvement in the ventilation/perfusion ratio, less reduction of cardiac output, and minimized barotrauma (McWilliams, 1987).

Nasal intermittent positive pressure ventilation has been used for short periods in the pediatric surgical patient who has had difficulty in remaining extubated. This type of ventilation provides respiratory support through a preset tidal volume or inspiratory time, resulting in improved arterial blood gas tensions, improved alveolar ventilation, and decreased work of breathing (Bott et al., 1992). Nitric oxide is now being used successfully with patients who have pulmonary hypertension postoperatively (Russell et al., 1998).

Extracorporeal membrane oxygenation may be used for cardiovascular support in children after open-heart surgery. Indications for biventricular support by extracorporeal membrane oxygenation in the early postoperative period include progressive hypotension, increased ventricular filling pressures, poor peripheral perfusion, decreased urine output, and decreased mixed venous oxygen saturation (Weinhaus et al., 1989). Extracorporeal membrane oxygenation is especially effective in treating conditions with right-sided heart failure and has also been used as a support while waiting for a heart, heart-lung, or lung transplantation (Weinhaus et al., 1989). The extracorporeal membrane oxygenation pump takes over oxygenation and perfusion of the child's body while the heart and lungs are "rested."

MANAGEMENT OF ACUTE IMPAIRMENT

Education

The majority of acute impairments after thoracic surgical procedures occur in the immediate or early postoperative period. Rockwell and Campbell (1976) described a preoperative program to assist in minimizing postoperative complications and to educate the parents of children 3 to 12 years of age. Educa-

tion is facilitated through an audiotape and a puppet show, as well as by a coloring book that shows the child what will happen after surgery. Preoperative programs probably benefit the parents as much as the child in alleviating some anxiety about the surgery. Preoperative education for the child younger than 5 years is also described by Page (1986). The program lists concepts that may be helpful in teaching and preparing the child and family for surgery. A doll is used to educate the child about placement of tubes and incisions; pictures are used for parents. Preparing children before the surgery should assist in obtaining their cooperation after surgery, as well as minimize their fears.

Pulmonary Management

The primary area to be addressed after heart repair is the pulmonary status of the patient. Numerous articles describe pulmonary complications and physical therapy in the postoperative pediatric patient (Ali et al., 1974; Bartlett, 1980, 1984; Bartlett et al., 1973a, 1973b; Gamsu et al., 1976; Krastins et al., 1982; Thoren, 1954; Van De Water et al., 1972; Vraciu & Vraciu, 1977). Although intervention varies with the age of the child, the primary goals are to mobilize secretions, increase aeration, and increase general mobility (Fig. 28–12).

Mucus transport is slowed after surgery and can lead to atelectasis (Gamsu et al., 1976). Atelectasis also occurs secondary to an altered breathing pattern, prolonged positioning in supine, and possible diaphragmatic dysfunction in the early postoperative period (Bartlett, 1984). In early studies by Bartlett and co-workers (Bartlett, 1980; Bartlett et al., 1973a) lack of deep breaths was observed as a causative factor in atelectasis. The yawn maneuver or

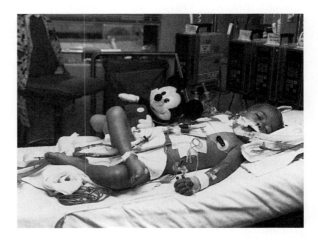

FIGURE 28–12. Two-year-old boy 24 hours after open-heart surgery.

prolonged inspiration with normal or increased inflation prevented atelectasis (Bartlett et al., 1973b). Bartlett (1984) observed that a collapsed lung expands only after the normal lung is fully inflated. This is achieved with prolonged inspiration. The restriction in ventilation has also been attributed to incoordination and reduction of rib expansion after sternotomy (Locke et al., 1990).

Incentive spirometry is an effective tool for reducing the occurrence of atelectasis in the pediatric population (Krastins et al., 1982). The primary emphasis with incentive spirometry or any other respiratory intervention should be on prolonged inspiration. When the inspiration is held for at least 3 seconds, arterial oxygen tension improves (Ward et al., 1966). Huckabay and Daderian (1990) observed an increase in compliance with breathing exercises after surgery when children were given a choice and some control regarding breathing exercises. With young children, tools such as bubble blowing or blowing on a windmill can be used (Rockwell & Campbell, 1976) (Fig. 28–13). Although these are expiratory maneuvers, a child often takes in a large inspiration before exhaling. Other respiratory techniques can also be performed to mobilize secretions and increase aeration, such as percussion and postural drainage, vibration, segmental expansion, and assisted cough techniques (Hussey, 1992) (Fig. 28–14).

Segmental expansion techniques may be performed to reduce postoperative complications and increase segmental aeration (Vraciu & Vraciu, 1977). This technique is performed by placing a hand over a particular segment and allowing it to move with the ventilator or respiratory cycle. Gentle pressure may be applied to the chest wall during exhalation at the end of the expiratory phase just before the inspiratory phase. This facilitates airflow to the specific segment (Massery, 1987). When a specific lobe or segment has decreased aeration, this technique, used in conjunction with gentle sustained pressure on the opposite upper lobe, may increase aeration to the affected area. When the patient is in a side-lying position, gentle rocking may also stimulate segmental expansion and relax the patient (Massery, 1987). This technique is particularly effective when the child is upset or does not tolerate percussion or other treatment techniques. It may also decrease the respiratory rate and is especially useful with infants who cannot respond to verbal relaxation instructions. Segmental expansion techniques are also beneficial when the patient is having excessive bleeding after surgery and use of more vigorous techniques is contraindicated (Johnson, 1991). The author has used this technique with lung transplant recipients who have been unable to cooperate or follow commands for deep breathing and coughing and found

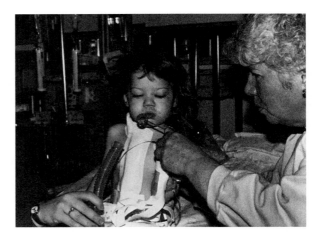

FIGURE 28–13. Child blowing bubbles 24 hours after open-heart surgery.

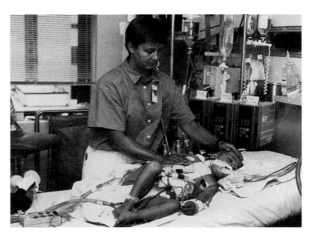

FIGURE 28–14. Child receiving percussion after open-heart surgery.

it to work well in decreasing atelectasis and increasing oxygen saturation. Segmental expansion techniques performed before other respiratory techniques may further enhance their benefit.

Percussion may need to be performed to assist in removal of excess secretions. *Percussion* is defined as a rhythmic clapping with cupped hands over the involved lung segment performed throughout the respiratory cycle, with the goal of mechanically dislodging pulmonary secretions (Imle, 1981). Vibration also assists in mobilization of secretions. It is performed by creating a fine oscillating movement of the hand on the chest wall just before expiration and continuing until the beginning of inspiration (Imle, 1981).

Both percussion and vibration techniques can be performed in conjunction with postural drainage.

Optimal positions are described and pictured in Frownfelter's text on chest physical therapy (Crane, 1987). Positioning must be used with caution in the postoperative patient; use of the Trendelenburg position, for example, is often contraindicated after open-heart surgery. It is important to confirm with the nurse or the physician whether it is even suitable for the child to be flat in bed. Despite limitations, percussion and vibration can be performed in the positions available. It has been the author's experience that children respond well to both percussion and vibration, even on the first postoperative day. Encouraging the child to tell you if the treatment hurts—because it should not be painful—often facilitates cooperation. It may also be helpful to coordinate the treatment with administration of pain medications. Percussion may be contraindicated when platelets are low, pulmonary artery pressures are too high, or the child becomes too agitated with treatment. Vibration can generally be safely used instead. Blood pressure and intracardiac pressures should be closely monitored throughout the treatment because they are indicators of intolerance to treatment. The physician usually establishes parameters, set on an individual basis.

Massery (1987) described a counterrotation technique for altering respiratory rate in the neurologically impaired patient that has also been safely used in the pediatric patient after open-heart surgery through a median sternotomy only. The technique has been used by the author to slow the respiratory rate and increase expansion of the lateral segment. It generally relaxes patients and increases their tidal volume. When the technique is used in the postoperative cardiac patient, extreme caution must be exercised to avoid disturbing chest tubes and other intravenous lines. This treatment is recommended only after intracardiac lines have been removed. The sternal incision has not been a problem; because it is stable, it does not undergo any mobilization during application of this technique. The counterrotation technique is performed with the therapist standing behind the side-lying patient near the patient's buttocks. One hand is placed on the anterior iliac spine and the other hand is placed on the patient's posterior shoulder. On inspiration the hand on the buttocks pulls down and posteriorly while the hand on the shoulder gently pushes up and anteriorly. On expiration the therapist's hands and the patient's body return to neutral. This is repeated several times in cycle with the patient's breathing. It should be very relaxing and comfortable for the patient.

The techniques just described not only facilitate increased lung expansion but also mobilize secretions. Once mobilized, secretions act as an irritant in the airway when the child takes a deep breath and a spontaneous cough usually occurs (Bartlett, 1984). The child may need some assistance in removing excess secretions, owing either to lack of cooperation or to inability to cooperate secondary to age. This may be accomplished by coughing or airway suctioning.

If the child is intubated, suctioning is done to clear secretions and maintain patency of the tube. Children who have cyanotic heart defects, such as hypoplastic left-sided heart syndrome, tend to desaturate during suctioning. It is extremely important to hyperventilate these patients with oxygen and a resuscitation bag before and after suctioning and to monitor their oxygen saturation and other hemodynamic parameters (Boutros, 1970; Fox et al., 1978; Hussey, 1992; Rosen, 1962). It is also important to monitor how far the suction catheter is inserted so that it only goes approximately 0.5 to 1 cm past the end of the endotracheal tube and does not touch the patient's carina. During suctioning, normal sterile saline may be instilled through the endotracheal tube to thin the thickened secretions. If the child is not intubated and is unwilling to cough, nasal pharyngeal suctioning may be performed to stimulate a cough and clear secretions. If the child is able to drink, a small sip of water or juice may also stimulate a cough. During coughing, a blanket or soft stuffed animal may be used to help splint the incision and minimize discomfort (Johnson, 1991).

Pain

Postoperative pain can be detrimental to the child's recovery. Pain medications must be given regularly, not only to reduce anxiety (which further increases pain from splinting) but also to encourage deeper breathing. A child in pain does not take deep breaths, even spontaneously. Morphine, a commonly used postoperative narcotic, depresses spontaneous sighing; patients receiving morphine should be encouraged to voluntarily take deep breaths (Egbert & Bendixon, 1964).

Other techniques now being used to manage postoperative pain include epidural morphine administration and patient-controlled analgesia (Asantila et al., 1986; Wilson, 1991). Both have proved effective in management of postoperative pain, especially in thoracotomy patients. Proper pain management is also extremely important in mobilizing the patient.

Early Mobilization

Postoperative immobility can lead to a variety of problems, including reduced ventilation and perfusion distribution (Peters, 1979), shallow breathing

(Risser, 1980; Scheidegger et al., 1976), fever (Chulay et al., 1982), retention of secretions (Pairolero & Payne, 1991), fluid shifts (Rubin, 1988), and generalized discomfort from immobility. The child should be mobilized as soon as possible to minimize these deleterious effects.

Range-of-motion exercises should be initiated as soon as possible. It may not be possible to attain normal range of motion immediately because of discomfort or intravenous or arterial lines, but any movement helps to mobilize the patient. Range-of-motion exercises are extremely important for the child with a thoracotomy incision because this incision tends to produce more guarding than does a median sternotomy. Passive to active-assisted range of shoulder motion to 90 degrees of flexion is usually tolerable. Discomfort often occurs when the arm is returned to a neutral position. The therapist may apply gentle resistance to the arm as the child attempts to return the arm to a neutral position because contraction of the arm muscles tends to minimize discomfort (Johnson, 1991).

The child's position should be changed regularly to avoid retention of secretions in the dependent portion of the lung (Pairolero & Payne, 1991). Regular turning has been observed to decrease postoperative fevers (Chulay et al., 1982). It also assists in decreasing postoperative chest wall immobilization, which is thought to decrease ventilation (Peters, 1979). The supine position alone contributes to airway closure (Dean, 1985; Risser, 1980) and a shift in blood volume to the dependent side (Rubin, 1988).

Arterial oxygen saturation is also affected by body position because of ventilation and perfusion matching (Dean, 1985). The supine position tends to decrease ventilation, which affects ventilation and perfusion matching and may ultimately decrease oxygen saturation. Positioning the patient effectively can reduce the pulmonary dysfunction that occurs most commonly when perfusion is greater than ventilation (Dean, 1985). The prone position has been observed to be associated with a significantly higher arterial oxygen tension than the supine position (Fox & Molesky, 1990), as well as an increased tidal volume and improved lung compliance (Dean, 1985). This position can be especially beneficial in preventing respiratory difficulty in a child who is extubated.

The side-lying position has been observed to be a better position than the supine position for improving oxygenation (Banasik et al., 1987; Dean, 1985). In studies, adult patients became better oxygenated when the "good" lung was in the dependent position (Banasik et al., 1987; Todd, 1990). In children, however, the opposite was observed, namely, improved gas exchange with the good lung uppermost (Davies et al., 1985). It has been observed in lung transplant recipients that regional differences in blood flow distribution produced by position changes may lead to significant changes in oxygenation. Positioning the patient in a side-lying position, with the best lung dependent, may improve ventilation and perfusion matching (Todd, 1990). The best lung may or may not be the transplanted lung in the early postoperative period; thus tolerance to having the transplanted lung dependent should be confirmed with the surgeons before placing the patient in this position.

Early ambulation after surgery reduces both pulmonary and circulatory complications (Webber, 1991). It has been observed to be as effective as deep-breathing exercises in minimizing complications in adults (Dull & Dull, 1983). Ambulation was observed to be beneficial in returning respiratory function toward normal by inducing more frequent and deeper sigh respirations (Scheidegger et al., 1976). Activity and mobility have been clinically observed to minimize chest tube output. At our center, children ambulate as soon as atrial lines and groin lines are removed and the child is extubated. Children often ambulate for the first time with any or all of the following: central venous pressure line, peripheral intravenous line, arterial line, chest tubes, temporary pacemakers, and oxygen (Fig. 28–15). The first walk is often only for 5 to 10 feet and may be difficult for the patient. Anxiety often plays as great a role in the perceived difficulty as does the discomfort. It may be beneficial for the patient to receive some pain medication before the first walk. Parents are also anxious, so the benefits of early ambulation should be explained to them ahead of time, with emphasis on the problems that can occur by remaining in bed. This is also a good time to review with parents the importance of picking their child up under the bottom and

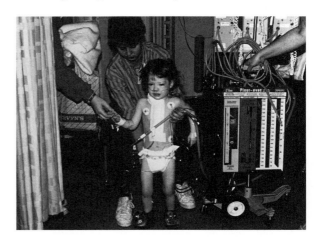

FIGURE 28–15. A child walking 1 day after open-heart surgery.

back as they did when the child was an infant. They should avoid picking up the child under the child's arms for 4 to 6 weeks after surgery to allow the sternum time to heal.

Medical Complications

Several medical complications can affect postoperative function. Secondary to phrenic nerve palsy, some children may have a paralyzed diaphragm after surgery that affects their early postoperative course, as well as their long-term respiratory status and endurance. The paralyzed diaphragm may persist but is seldom permanent (Markland et al., 1985; Morriss & McNamara, 1975). Infants have horizontal ribs and lack the normal bucket handle movement, relying primarily on use of the diaphragm for respiration. Paralysis of the diaphragm by unilateral or bilateral phrenic nerve palsy can cause further respiratory problems, including difficulty in weaning from the ventilator (Hussey, 1992).

Peroneal nerve palsy is another complication of surgery, usually caused by improper positioning of the lower extremity during surgery. The resultant drastic alteration in the child's gait must be addressed as soon as possible. An ankle-foot orthosis can improve gait and should be necessary for only a short time.

Postoperative neurologic impairments can occur subsequent to prolonged surgical time, usually related to length of hypothermic arrest, low cardiac output, or arrhythmias after surgery (Ferry, 1990; Wells et al., 1983). Hemodynamic instability and coagulation disturbances are risk factors for postoperative neurologic problems in infants (duPlessis, 1997). Thirty-five percent of premature infants weighing less than 2 kg who had open-heart surgery developed neurologic complications (Rossi et al., 1998). Neurologic consequences can also be the result of an air embolus, a prolonged hypotensive period (van Breda, 1985), or complications of long-term cyanosis (Amitia et al., 1984). Choreoathetosis has been observed in some children after they have been on cardiopulmonary bypass. When a basal ganglia lesion is also seen the prognosis is poor (Holden et al., 1998). It is encouraging to note that of almost 700 children who underwent a Fontan operation, less than 3% suffered a stroke (duPlessis et al., 1995). The child who has suffered a neurologic insult requires both early intervention and long-term physical therapy. A child with severe extensor tone may benefit from inhibitive casts on the lower extremities and hand splints to decrease the effects of increased tone and maintain range of motion. Parent education concerning the impact of a neurologic insult should begin as soon as the diagnosis is confirmed,

including information on handling and positioning the child with increased tone, appropriate stimulation, use of adaptive equipment, and long-term follow-up.

The following case history describes a typical course of surgeries, with complications that resolved, in a child with cyanotic heart disease.

CASE HISTORY
DAVID

David was born with severe cyanotic congenital heart disease. He was diagnosed with total anomalous pulmonary venous return, transposition of the great arteries, hypoplastic left ventricle syndrome, atrial-ventricular septal defect, and pulmonary atresia. He had two surgeries performed within the first month of life. At 10 days of age, he had ligation of the ductus arteriosus and a modified BT shunt. At 4 weeks of age, he required repair of his right pulmonary artery. Then, at 4 months of age, he underwent surgery to repair his total anomalous pulmonary venous return. After this surgery, it took approximately 4 weeks to wean him from the ventilator, owing to a left phrenic nerve palsy. He was discharged to home on nasogastric feedings, which continued until he was 1 year old. He advanced from nasogastric feedings to baby food and liquid from a "tippy" cup.

David experienced some delay in achieving developmental milestones. He sat independently at 9 months of age. At 16 months of age, David had a bidirectional Glenn procedure and his BT shunt taken down. He did well after this surgery and was discharged to home within 1 week of his surgery date. He developed well over the next 18 months, with marked improvement in his activity level. For instance, David crawled at 17 months of age and then walked at 19 months.

At 3 years of age, David had a Fontan procedure performed, which he tolerated well until seizures occurred on the third postoperative day. A computed tomography scan revealed a right frontal lobe infarct, and increased tone and briskness of reflexes were noted on his left side. He was irritable and difficult to console. Initially, David demonstrated left-sided neglect and a decrease in his protective reactions to the left. Within 1 week, his tone was only minimally increased and he was able to use his left extremities with cueing. Within 2 weeks, his protective reactions were symmetric, and he was shifting his weight and using either extremity readily. His ambulation was typical of a child after surgery, with slight balance problems and the use of a wide base of support. He did have difficulty coming to a standing position from sitting without support, which resolved within 4 weeks.

David's parents are attentive and recognize tasks that are difficult for him. They have continued home exercises to encourage use of his left extremities and have had better cooperation from him than have the therapists. He continued to be followed for reexamination several times a year to monitor his progress and update his home program.

Four years later, David goes to school every day and does well. His overall endurance and risk taking are less than his peers, but generally he gets along well.

Age-Specific Disabilities in the Immediate Postoperative Period

The infant who undergoes surgery within the first few days of life suffers immediate disruption of all aspects of normal newborn life. The infant is often sedated, restrained, and intubated, all of which interfere with being held, bundled, and fed. Parents need education about the areas of stimulation that are withdrawn from their child during this time and instruction in ways to compensate for this deprivation. The fact that their child is born with a congenital anomaly may further impede the attachment process (Loeffel, 1985). The therapist assists the process by involving the parents in treatment as soon as possible and educating them about engaging and calming their child.

Toddlers who have cardiac surgery often recover very quickly and with few impairments. Anxiety over being left alone during the hospitalization may be the biggest problem interfering with function in this age group (Loeffel, 1985). The child may feel abandoned and react by becoming passive and apathetic or, conversely, by becoming aggressive. These behaviors are more commonly observed in the child who is in the hospital for the first time, such as the child with an atrial septal defect.

Toddlers tend to be limited more by their parents' restrictions than by their own physical limitations (Clare, 1985; Loeffel, 1985). Activity guidelines should be reviewed with parents on an ongoing basis; showing them by example may be even more helpful. Although it is beneficial to explain to the parents ahead of time what their child will experience, it may be helpful to wait to tell the toddler what is happening as it is happening.

Adolescents who have cardiac surgery may need to be encouraged to move and may need to be assisted to become active. The parents are often more reluctant than the child about early mobilization, including ambulation. They should be reassured that it is beneficial for their child to move as soon as possible. Adolescents may choose to assert their independence and try to do everything for themselves, or they may choose to become totally dependent on their parents and hospital staff. Whichever situation occurs, young persons benefit from early education about how to move and what they should be doing. This helps them realize what is expected of them. They should be informed of what they need to do and not given a choice when the task is not optional (van Breda, 1985).

CHRONIC DISABILITIES AND FUNCTIONAL LIMITATIONS

Various disabilities and functional limitations occur as a result of primary impairments incurred by children with congenital heart defects (see Table 28–1). The disabling process may start very early secondary to poor attachment between parent and infant (Goldberg et al., 1990b). Infants who had cardiac surgery showed less positive affect and engagement than normal babies, making it even more stressful for mothers who are already distressed (Gardner et al., 1996). Poor attachment can lead to poor social development. The overprotection and excessive activity restrictions imposed by some parents further compound this disability. Parents have stated that they were afraid to permit activity in their child with congenital heart disease (Gudermuth, 1975). If this attitude is allowed to persist, the child's developmental and functional level will surely suffer. It has also been observed that maternal perceptions of the child's disease severity were a stronger predictor of emotional adjustment than was disease severity (DeMaso et al., 1991). Emotional maladjustment may contribute to the poor self-esteem that is often noted in children with congenital heart defects. The limitations resulting from decreased activity, delayed development, poor self-esteem, overprotection by parents, and physical illness may all lead to poor peer interactions. This may further limit a child with congenital heart disease from interacting with society. These issues should be addressed with parents and the child as early as possible to try to limit the effect on developmental progression and functional capabilities. Subsequent sections elaborate on various aspects of the disabling process across childhood.

Infancy

In children with congenital heart disease, several contributing factors can lead to impairment and functional limitations in infancy. Common problems include poor feeding, poor growth, and developmental lag. Parents must constantly watch for signs and symptoms of congestive heart failure in their infant. These signs include the onset of rapid breathing, changes in behavior, edema, excessive sweating, fatigue, vomiting, and poor feeding (Clare, 1985; Zahr & Boisvert, 1990).

Parental frustration and stress can impair early attachment to the infant. It has been observed during the period of 1 year that securely attached infants showed greater improvements in health than did insecurely attached infants (Goldberg et al., 1991). Gardner and associates observed infants with cardiac defects to be consistently less engaging with their mothers when compared with infants without defects (Gardner et al., 1996). When compared with healthy infants and infants with cystic fibrosis, infants with congenital heart disease were the least attached to their mothers and their parents were the most stressed (Goldberg et al., 1990b). Normal attachment may be difficult, particularly with the very sick infant who is frequently hospitalized. The health care team should begin working with the parents as early as possible on how they can interact with their infant to facilitate attachment and avoid overstimulating their infant.

It is not uncommon for infants with congenital heart disease to be poor feeders, which further increases parental stress. An infant expends most of his or her energy during eating. In normal infants decreased ventilation is observed during feeding, creating a decrease in the partial pressure of oxygen and an increase in the partial pressure of carbon dioxide (Mathew, 1988; Mathew et al., 1985). This decrease in ventilation may seriously compromise the child with congenital heart disease compounded by the increase in metabolic rate observed. Not only does the child not eat well, but he or she also requires more calories to thrive (Gingell & Hornung, 1989).

Watching their child failing to thrive can be devastating to parents and can further increase their anxiety about feeding their child and trying to encourage adequate caloric intake (Gingell & Hornung, 1989). The prolonged feeding time can be frustrating to parents, as well as make them feel inadequate (Bruning & Schneiderman, 1983; Loeffel, 1985). If alternative feeding methods are used, such as nasogastric or gastrostomy tube feedings, parents should be educated not only in how to administer the feeding but also how to hold and nurture their child during the feeding (Loeffel, 1985). It may be helpful to tell parents that providing time for normal, nonstressful interaction may improve the parent-infant attachment and may ultimately improve the health of their infant.

It is also helpful to inform the parents that the overall time that supplemental feedings are necessary varies with each child. Some parents have stated that they were able to remove supplemental feedings within 1 week of leaving the hospital; others have stated that it took months for their child to take enough by mouth to be able to discontinue supplemental feedings. Many parents have stated to this author that their infant ate better at home, where it was possible to eat on demand and to have a more routine day.

Physical therapy assessment is sometimes needed to observe the infant feeding and parental interaction. There may be other problems unrelated to the poor endurance exhibited by the infant with congenital heart disease. If oral-motor dysfunction exists, it should be addressed with parents as soon as possible. Some parents need assistance in how best to handle and support their child during feeding. It can also be beneficial for the parents to observe that their child does not feed well for anyone.

Poor growth is closely associated with poor feeding. It has been observed that infants with cyanotic heart disease have poor growth in height and weight, whereas infants with acyanotic heart disease, specifically those with a large left-to-right shunt, are severely underweight secondary to the marked increase in metabolism (Gingell & Hornung, 1989). The child's growth improves after surgery but may not achieve normal parameters. This lack of catch-up growth is especially remarkable in children with cyanotic defects with a right-to-left shunt (Gingell & Hornung, 1989; Rosenthal, 1983).

Functional limitations, especially delayed achievement of basic motor skills, can be observed in the infant with cardiac disease. Decreased nutritional status and cardiac function may leave the infant too weak to expend the energy required for normal motor activity (Loeffel, 1985). Some cyanotic children preferentially scoot around on their buttocks and, even after extensive intervention at home, do not crawl. They often go on to walking without ever crawling (Johnson, 1991), probably because of the increased energy expenditure associated with use of both upper and lower extremities in crawling. Cyanotic children also tend to have an internal mechanism that permits them to do only what they are physically capable of doing, given their oxygen saturation (Clare, 1985). They often rest without cueing and can rarely be pushed beyond what they are willing to do. Intervention may or may not improve the child's functional abilities; however, it may do a great deal to relieve parental anxiety. Education should be focused on what the child is doing normally, such as using normal movement patterns, instead of on developmental lag based solely on age. Intervention should include parental education concerning areas the parent can work on with the child throughout the day, rather than in one focused block of time.

The presence of congestive heart failure is significantly associated with mental and motor developmental delay. Infants with congestive heart failure scored less well than expected on the Bayley Scales of Infant Development as early as at 2 months of age (Aisenberg et al., 1982). Haneda and associates (1996) observed a significant decrease in Gesell's developmental quotient score in infants and children who had circulatory arrest time greater than 50 minutes. This information is useful when working with parents to help them understand that their child is demonstrating typical developmental skills for a child with congenital heart disease. This does not mean that intervention does not improve the situation. Parents should be encouraged to work with their child on developmental tasks that are challenging. If functional limitations are minimized early, the effect of reparative surgery may be dramatic.

Neurologic impairment and functional limitations may also occur from external forces related to the surgical repair. Discrepancy exists among research study findings regarding the effect of deep hypothermia and circulatory arrest on the psychomotor and intellectual development of infants (Blackwood et al., 1986; duPlessis, 1997; Haka-Ikse et al., 1978; Messmer et al., 1976; Rossi et al., 1998; Settergren et al., 1982). Messmer and associates (1976) observed no delay in psychomotor and intellectual development in infants after deep hypothermia. In another study, the researchers did not observe neurologic impairment after surgery, but they did observe mild developmental delays, most profoundly in cyanotic infants (Haka-Ikse et al., 1978). Bellinger and associates (1997) observed that children who had total circulatory arrest during the arterial switch operation scored lower on the Bayley Scales of Infant Development at 1 year of age than the infants who had low-flow bypass. They were also observed to have expressive language difficulties at 2.5 years of age and exhibited more behavior problems (Bellinger et al., 1997). In light of this conflicting information, therapists should realize the potential for problems. Parents should be advised that their child might take longer than usual to accomplish developmental milestones.

Preschool Period

The preschool child with chronic disabilities caused by congenital heart disease has grown up in the medical environment. This may help alleviate some of the child's and the parents' anxieties. However, parental anxieties can be exacerbated during this period as they begin to realize the impact their child's cardiac disease has on growth and development. The child's symptoms could be worsening, and another surgery may soon be needed. The parents' response and interaction during this period are important; it should be recognized that parents already have the tendency to be overprotective of their child and that this may increase during the preschool period.

The emotional adjustment of the child has been observed to be affected by the mother's perception of the severity of the child's illness more than by its actual severity (DeMaso et al., 1991). If the mother perceives the child's disease to be more severe than it is and limits the child accordingly, the child's physical and social development may suffer. In acyanotic children, it has been observed that the intelligence quotient (IQ) was lower when associated with poorer adjustment, greater dependence, and greater maternal pampering and anxiety (Rasof et al., 1967). Functional limitations may be out of proportion compared with what the child is actually capable of doing. Intervention may need to be initiated to instruct parents on what activities the child is capable of performing, as well as how the child self-limits activity without parental intervention.

Children with congenital heart disease have been observed to have some developmental delay—especially those children with cyanotic disease (Bellinger et al., 1997; Feldt et al., 1969; Rasof et al., 1967). Cyanotic children scored significantly lower than acyanotic and normal children in all subscales of the Gesell Developmental Schedules (Haneda et al., 1996) and on Stanford-Binet and Cattell intelligence tests (Rasof et al., 1967). Cyanotic children were observed to sit and walk later than acyanotic and normal children and were slower in speaking phrases than were children without disabilities (Feldt et al., 1969; Rasof et al., 1967; Silbert et al., 1969). Curtailment of physical activity in the child with severe cardiac dysfunction interferes with the active manipulation of objects needed for the adequate development of early sensorimotor processes (Rasof et al., 1967; Silbert et al., 1969). This lack of opportunity may affect IQ scores and psychologic development. However, a study just completed by Caren Goldberg, MD, and colleagues at the University of Michigan Medical Center (not yet published) assessed neurodevelopmental outcome in 50 patients who had single ventricles and had undergone the Fontan operation and found them to be of normal intelligence and behavior.

Educating parents about what they should be allowing their child to do is as important as teaching them precautions pertaining to their child. Children were observed to have significant gross motor advances during the second year of life when parental warmth was combined with a decrease in parental restrictions. It was also observed that children with congenital heart disease performed better on IQ tests when their parents attempted to accelerate their child's development (Rasof et al., 1967). Parents should also be taught that children with cardiac disease, particularly cyanotic disease, limit their own activity and stop and rest when needed (Clare, 1985). Children with Down syndrome were also observed to score higher on developmental tests and achieve feeding milestones earlier if parents followed through appropriately with therapy instructions (Cullen et al., 1981).

School-Age Period

School adjustment and peer interaction have been observed to be altered in children with congenital heart disease. In a study by Youssef (1988), school absenteeism was high in these children and was proportional to the severity of their disease. It has been observed that a child's adjustment to school is affected more by the strain on the family than the child's physical limitations related to the congenital heart disease (Casey et al., 1996). Teachers have noted that children with congenital heart disease had more school problems, and more behavior problems were observed in boys. Children with more behavior problems had a lower self-esteem and more depression (Youssef, 1988). After surgical intervention, some of these problems may be alleviated; the child should miss less school and have an improved physical status and an increased activity level (Linde et al., 1970). Children may need rehabilitation after surgical repair, however, to teach them how much they are capable of doing and to help them deal with any functional limitations or inability to perform a task.

Surgical intervention that corrects a cyanotic defect plays an important role in the child's development. Improvement in IQ has been reported after surgery (Linde et al., 1970; O'Dougharty et al., 1985). The intellectual development was essentially normal in children after the Fontan operation (Uzark et al., 1998). Self-confidence, social confidence, and general adjustment have also improved after surgery (Linde et al., 1970). A significant improvement in self-perception was observed in children after they had their heart defect repaired (Wray & Sensky, 1998). If decreased experiences are a factor in developmental performance, a child who is no longer limited by disease should develop more normally.

Parental overprotectiveness can continue to prove more limiting to a child's development than the defect itself. Parents were found to underestimate their child's exercise tolerance in 80% of the cases studied by Casey and associates (1994). Parental restriction generally begins with the advice of the physician and proceeds from there (Clare, 1985; Kong et al., 1986). Social and emotional maladjustment in children with cardiac disease can be due to maternal maladjustment and guilt (Kong et al., 1986). Psychosocial or therapy intervention by professionals could be beneficial to preserving a more normal parent-child interaction. Some improvement in maternal interaction and attitude has been noted after surgical correction of the child's cardiac defect (O'Dougharty et al., 1985). In contrast to these reports is a recent study by Laane and associates (1997), which found that children with congenital heart defects reported a higher quality of life than healthy children.

Adolescence

Adolescents who have congenital heart disease and physical limitations show increased feelings of anxiety and impulsiveness (Kramer et al., 1989). Early professional intervention to assist the parents and child to cope best with the child's physical limitations may be helpful.

A delay in the onset of puberty in adolescents with congenital heart disease may further complicate their social development. The body structure of the adolescent with congenital heart disease was found to be noticeably different from that of normal adolescents. The weight and height were significantly less with the presence of cardiac disease. Adolescents with heart disease had head, neck, and shoulder measurements similar to those of healthy adolescents, but the thorax, trunk, pelvis, and lower extremities were significantly smaller. The anterior-posterior diameter of the pelvis was so reduced that it appeared almost flat (Angelov et al., 1980). Physical differences of this magnitude can only make adolescents with heart disease feel even more different and intensify their low self-esteem.

Intervention that encourages the adolescent to participate in physical activities, including guidelines on how to participate, may improve peer interaction and ultimately self-esteem. Children who participated in an exercise program were observed to have improvement in their self-esteem, as well as in their strength. Parents were found to be less restrictive and had less anxiety about their child after a formal exercise program (Donovan et al., 1983).

Physical activity is important for all children, including children with congenital heart disease. The defect and surgical intervention, as well as possible alterations in response to exercise, must be understood before prescribing an exercise program for a child with congenital heart disease. The American Heart Association has published an extensive review of exercise testing in the pediatric age group, including recommendations for those with various congenital heart defects (James et al., 1982).

Cardiac rehabilitation programs for children with cardiac disease have shown significant and beneficial changes in hemodynamics and improvement in exercise endurance and tolerance (Balfour et al., 1991; Bar-Or, 1985; Goldberg et al., 1981; Koch et al., 1988;

Mathews et al., 1983; Perrault & Drblik, 1989; Ruttenberg et al., 1983). Improvement from physical training allowed adolescents to function at nearly normal activity levels (Goldberg et al., 1981). The psychologic improvements were as noticeable and important as the physical improvements (Donovan et al., 1983; Koch et al., 1988; Mathews et al., 1983).

Adolescents who have undergone heart transplantation are able to achieve an increase in cardiac output in response to exercise; however, they do not achieve the same peak workloads or maximal oxygen consumption as do normal adolescents (Christos et al., 1992). During the early phase of rehabilitation, many children with transplanted hearts, lungs, or heart-lungs are so debilitated that they are unable to perform at an intensity that would raise their heart rate. The dyspnea index used as part of the Stanford heart transplant protocol is helpful in monitoring the child's physical tolerance during activity (Sadowsky et al., 1986). The child counts out loud to 15. The goal initially is to attempt to do this on one breath. At first, it may take three breaths to count to 15 while at rest. Exercise should increase the number of breaths to reach the count of 15 by only one or two breaths and should not be resumed until return to resting baseline. Most children progress quickly, usually reaching 15 on one breath within 1 week of beginning exercise. The dyspnea index is an easily used measure for self-monitoring of exercise tolerance at home (Johnson, 1991).

The patient who has had a heart-lung transplant also has an increased ventilatory response to exercise (Banner et al., 1988, 1989; Sciurba et al., 1988). The dyspnea index is again useful with these patients.

Heart, heart-lung, and lung transplant recipients have experienced marked rehabilitation after transplantation (Bolman, 1991). The author has found it highly beneficial for adolescents to be enrolled in a formal rehabilitation program after transplant to change their lifestyle, as well as condition them. The quality of life improves, with most children functioning at an age-appropriate level without developmental delays (Dunn et al., 1987; Lawrence & Fricker, 1987; Niset et al., 1988).

SUMMARY

This review of congenital heart defects, surgical and therapeutic intervention, and developmental consequences provides therapists with a foundation for treating this patient population. As surgical intervention occurs earlier and corrective techniques are performed sooner, it will be increasingly important to evaluate and monitor developmental progression. Children with congenital heart defects cannot be made to perform a developmental task that they do not have the energy to perform. The physical therapist plays an integral role in the habilitation and rehabilitation of children with congenital heart disease. A major part of this role involves parent education concerning typical developmental sequences in children with cardiac conditions and appropriate parent-child interaction.

Recommended Resources

Clough, P. The denervated heart. Clinical Management, 10:14–17, 1990.

Congenital Heart Anomalies—Support, Education, and Resources, Inc. (CHASER News)
2112 North Wilkins Rd.
Swanton, OH 43558
(419-825-5575)
Web site: http://www.csun.edu/~hfmth006/chaser/.

duPlessis, AJ. Neurologic complications of cardiac disease in the newborn. Clinics in Perinatology, 24:807–825, 1997.

Gardner, FV, Freeman, NH, Black, AM, & Angelini, GD. Disturbed mother-infant interaction in association with congenital heart disease. Heart, 76:56–59, 1996.

Leroy, S, Callow, L, & George, K. Hypoplastic left heart syndrome (HLHS): A guide for parents. Progress in Pediatric Cardiology, 5:65–69, 1996.

References

Aisenberg, RB, Rosenthal, A, Nadas, AS, & Wolff, PH. Developmental delay in infants with congenital heart disease. Pediatric Cardiology, 3:133–137, 1982.

Ali, J, Weisel, RD, Layug, AB, Kripke, BJ, & Hechtman, HB. Consequences of postoperative alterations in respiratory mechanics. American Journal of Surgery, 128:376–382, 1974.

Amitia, Y, Blieden, L, Shemtove, A, & Neufeld, H. Cerebrovascular accidents in infants and children with congenital cyanotic heart disease. Israel Journal of Medical Sciences, 20:1143–1145, 1984.

Angelov, G, Tomova, S, & Ninova, P. Physical development and body structure of children with congenital heart disease. Human Biology, 52:413–421, 1980.

Arciniegas, E. Ventricular septal defect. In Baue, AE, Geha, AS, Hammond, GL, Laks, H, & Naunheim, KS (Eds.), Glenn's Thoracic and Cardiovascular Surgery, 5th ed. Norwalk, CT: Appleton & Lange, 1991, pp. 1007–1016.

Asantila, R, Rosenburg, PH, & Scheinin, B. Comparison of different methods of postoperative analgesia after thoracotomy. Acta Anaesthesiologica Scandinavica, 30:421–425, 1986.

Austin, EH, III, Edmonds, HL, Jr, Auden, SM, Seremet, V, Niznik, G, Sehic, A, Sowell, MK, Cheppo, CD, & Corlett, KM. Benefit of neurophysiologic monitoring for pediatric cardiac surgery. Journal of Thoracic and Cardiovascular Surgery, 114(5):707–717, 1997.

Aziz, S, & Jamieson, S. Combined heart and lung transplantation. In Baue, AE, Geha, AS, Hammond, GL, Laks, H, & Naunheim, KS (Eds.), Glenn's Thoracic and Cardiovascular Surgery, 5th ed. Norwalk, CT: Appleton & Lange, 1991, pp. 1623–1638.

Bailey, LL, Assaad, AN, Trimm, RF, Nehlsen-Cannarella, SL, Kanakriyeh, MS, Haas, GS, & Jacobson, JG. Orthotopic transplantation during early infancy as therapy for incurable congenital heart disease. Annals of Surgery, 203:279–285, 1988.

Bailey, LL, & Gundry, SR. Hypoplastic left heart syndrome. In Gillette, PC (Ed.), The Pediatric Clinics of North America. Philadelphia: WB Saunders, 1990, pp. 137–150.

Balfour, IC, Drimmer, AM, Nouri, S, Pennington, DG, Hemkins, CL, & Harvey, LL. Pediatric cardiac rehabilitation. American Journal of Diseases of Children, 145:627–630, 1991.

Banasik, JL, Bruya, MA, Steadman, RE, & Demand, JK. Effect of position on arterial oxygenation in postoperative coronary revascularization patients. Heart and Lung, 16:652–657, 1987.

Banner, N, Guz, A, Heaton, R, Innes, JA, Murphy, K, & Yacoub, M. Ventilatory and circulatory responses at the onset of exercise in man following heart or heart-lung transplantation. Journal of Physiology, 399:437–449, 1988.

Banner, NR, Lloyd, MH, Hamilton, RD, Innes, JA, Guz, A, & Yacoub, MH. Cardiopulmonary response to dynamic exercise after heart and combined heart-lung transplantation. British Heart Journal, 61:215–223, 1989.

Bar-Or, O. Physical conditioning in children with cardiorespiratory disease. In Terjung, RL (Ed.), Exercise and Sport Science Review. New York: Macmillan, 1985, pp. 305–334.

Bartlett, RH. Pulmonary pathophysiology in surgical patients. Surgical Clinics of North America, 60:1323–1338, 1980.

Bartlett, RH. Respiratory therapy to prevent pulmonary complications of surgery. Respiratory Care, 29:667–677, 1984.

Bartlett, RH, Brennan, ML, Gazzaniga, AB, & Hanson, EL. Studies on the pathogenesis and prevention of postoperative pulmonary complications. Surgery, Gynecology and Obstetrics, 137:925–933, 1973a.

Bartlett, RH, Gazzaniga, AB, & Geraghty, TR. Respiratory maneuvers to prevent postoperative pulmonary complications. Journal of the American Medical Association, 224:1017–1021, 1973b.

Bauer, J, Dapper, F, Kroll, J, Hagel, KJ, Thul, J, & Zickmann, B. Heart transplantation in infants—experience at the children's heart center in Giessen. Zeitschrift fur Kardiologie, 87:209–217, 1998.

Bellinger, DC, Rappaport, LA, Wypij, D, Wernovsky, G, & Newburger, JW. Patterns of developmental dysfunction after surgery during infancy to correct transposition of the great arteries. Journal of Developmental and Behavioral Pediatrics, 18:75–83, 1997.

Blackwood, MJ, Haka-Ikse, K, & Steward, DJ. Developmental outcome in children undergoing surgery with profound hypothermia. Anesthesiology, 65:437–440, 1986.

Bolman, RM, Shumway, SS, Estrin, JA, & Hertz, MI. Lung and heart-lung transplantation. Annals of Surgery, 214:456–470, 1991.

Bonser, RS, & Jamieson, SW. Heart-lung transplantation. Clinics in Chest Medicine, 11:235–246, 1990.

Bott, J, Keilty, SE, Brown, A, & Ward, EM. Nasal intermittent positive pressure ventilation. Physiotherapy, 78:93–96, 1992.

Boutros, AR. Arterial blood oxygenation during and after endotracheal suctioning in the apneic patient. Anesthesiology, 32:114–118, 1970.

Brunberg, JA, Reilly, EL, & Doty, DB. Central nervous system consequences in infants of cardiac surgery using deep hypothermia and circulatory arrest. Circulation, 50(suppl II):60–67, 1973.

Bruning, MD, & Schneiderman, JU. Heart failure in infants and children. In Michaelson, CR (Ed.), Congestive Heart Failure. St. Louis: Mosby, 1983, pp. 467–484.

Byrum, CJ, Dick, M, Behrendt, DM, & Rosenthal, A. Repair of total anomalous pulmonary venous connection in patients younger than 6 months old. Circulation, 66(suppl I):208–214, 1982.

Callow, LB. A new beginning: Nursing care of the infant undergoing the arterial switch operation for transposition of the great arteries. Heart and Lung, 18:248–257, 1989.

Casey, FA, Craig, BG, & Mulholland, HC. Quality of life in surgically palliated complex congenital heart disease. Archives of Disease in Childhood, 70:382–386, 1994.

Casey, FA, Sykes, DH, Craig, BG, Power, R, & Mulholland, HC. Behavioral adjustment of children with surgically palliated complex congenital heart disease. Journal of Pediatric Psychology, 21:335–352,1996.

Castaneda, A, & Mayer, JE. Arterial switch operation for transposition of the great arteries. In Baue, AE, Geha, AS, Hammond, GL, Laks, H, & Naunheim, KS (Eds.), Glenn's Thoracic and Cardiovascular Surgery, 5th ed. Norwalk, CT: Appleton & Lange, 1991, pp. 1227–1235.

Christos, SC, Katch, V, Crowley, DC, Eakin, BL, Lindauer, AL, & Beekman, RH. Hemodynamic responses to upright exercise of adolescent cardiac transplant patients. Journal of Pediatrics, 121:312–316, 1992.

Chulay, M, Brown, J, & Summer, W. Effect of postoperative immobilization after coronary artery bypass surgery. Critical Care Medicine, 10:176–179, 1982.

Clare, MD. Home care of infants and children with cardiac disease. Heart and Lung, 14:218–222, 1985.

Clarke, CF, Beall, MH, & Perloff, JK. Genetics, epidemiology, counseling, and prevention. In Perloff, JK, & Child, JS (Eds.), Congenital Heart Disease in Adults. Philadelphia: WB Saunders, 1991, pp. 141–165.

Clough, P. The denervated heart. Clinical Management, 10:14–17, 1990.

Crane, LD. The neonate and child. In Frownfelter, DL (Ed.), Chest Physical Therapy and Pulmonary Rehabilitation. Chicago: Year Book, 1987, pp. 666–697.

Cullen, SM, Cronk, CE, Pueschel, SM, Schnell, RR, & Reed, RB. Social development and feeding milestones of young Down syndrome children. American Journal of Mental Deficiency, 85:410–415, 1981.

Davies, H, Kitchman, R, Gordon, I, & Helms, P. Regional ventilation in infancy. New England Journal of Medicine, 313:1626–1628, 1985.

Dean, E. Effect of body position on pulmonary function. Physical Therapy, 65:613–618, 1985.

de Leval, MR. Senning operation. In Baue, AE, Geha, AS, Hammond, GL, Laks, H, & Naunheim, KS (Eds.), Glenn's Thoracic and Cardiovascular Surgery, 5th ed. Norwalk, CT: Appleton & Lange, 1991, pp. 1211–1216.

DeMaso, DR, Campis, LK, Wypij, D, Bertram, S, Lipshitz, M, & Freed, M. The impact of maternal perceptions and medical severity on the adjustment of children with congenital heart disease. Journal of Pediatric Psychology, 16:137–149, 1991.

Donovan, EF, Mathews, RA, Nixon, PA, Stephenson, RJ, Robertson, RJ, Dean, F, Fricker, FJ, Beerman, LB, & Fischer, DR. An exercise program for pediatric patients with congenital heart disease: Psychological aspects. Journal of Cardiac Rehabilitation, 3:476–480, 1983.

Dull, JL, & Dull, WL. Are maximal inspiratory breathing exercises or incentive spirometry better than early mobilization after cardiopulmonary bypass? Physical Therapy, 63:655–659, 1983.

Dunn, JM, Cavarocchi, NC, Balsara RK, Kolff, J, McClurken, J, Badellino, MM, Vieweg, C, & Donner, RM. Pediatric heart transplantation, at St. Christopher's Hospital for Children. Journal of Heart Transplantation, 6:334–342, 1987.

duPlessis, AJ. Neurologic complications of cardiac disease in the newborn. Clinics in Perinatology, 24:807–825, 1997.

duPlessis, AJ, Chang, AC, Wessel, DL, Lock, JE, Wernovsky, G, Newburger, JW, & Mayer, JE, Jr. Cerebrovascular accidents following the Fontan operation. Pediatric Neurology, 12:230–236, 1995.

Egbert, LD, & Bendixon, HH. Effect of morphine on breathing pattern. Journal of the American Medical Association, 188:485–488, 1964.

Feldt, RH, Ewert, JC, Stickler, GB, & Weidman, WH. Children with congenital heart disease. American Journal of Diseases of Children, 117:281–287, 1969.

Ferry, PC. Neurologic sequelae of open-heart surgery in children. American Journal of Diseases of Children, 144:369–373, 1990.

Fox, MD, & Molesky, MG. The effects of prone and supine positioning on arterial oxygen pressure. Neonatal Network, 8:25–29, 1990.

Fox, WW, Schwartz, JG, & Shaffer, TH. Pulmonary physiotherapy in neonates: Physiologic changes and respiratory management. Journal of Pediatrics, 92:977–981, 1978.

Fricker, FJ, Trento, A, & Griffith, BP. Pediatric cardiac transplantation. In Brest, AN (Ed.), Cardiovascular Clinics. Philadelphia: FA Davis, 1990, pp. 223–235.

Gamsu, G, Singer, MM, Vincent, HH, Berry, S, & Nadel, JA. Postoperative impairment of mucous transport in the lung. American Review of Respiratory Disease, 114:673–679, 1976.

Gardner, FV, Freeman, NH, Black, AM, & Angelini, GD. Disturbed mother-infant interaction in association with congenital heart disease. Heart, 76:56–59, 1996.

Garson, A, Gillette, PC, Gutgesell, HP, & McNamara, DG. Stress-induced ventricular arrhythmia after repair of tetralogy of Fallot. American Journal of Cardiology, 46:1006–1012, 1980.

Giboney, GS. Ventricular septal defect. Heart and Lung, 12:292–299, 1983.

Gingell, RL, & Hornung, MG. Growth problems associated with congenital heart disease in infancy. In Lebenthal, E (Ed.), Textbook of Gastroenterology and Nutrition in Infancy, 2nd ed. New York: Raven Press, 1989, pp. 639–649.

Girlando, RM, Belew, B, & Klara, F. Coarctation of the aorta. Critical Care Nurse, 8:38–50, 1988.

Glanville, AR, Baldwin, JC, Hunt, SA, & Theodore, J. Long-term cardiopulmonary function after human heart-lung transplantation. Australian and New Zealand Journal of Medicine, 20:208–214, 1990.

Glanville, AR, Gabb, GM, Theodore, J, & Robin, ED. Bronchial responsiveness to exercise after human cardiopulmonary transplantation. Chest, 96:281–286, 1989.

Goldberg, B, Fripp, RR, Lister, G, Loke, J, Nicholas, JA, & Talner, NS. Effect of physical training on exercise performance of children following surgical repair of congenital heart disease. Pediatrics, 68:691–699, 1981.

Goldberg, S, Simmons, RJ, Newman J, Campbell, K, & Fowler, RS. Congenital heart disease, parental stress, and infant-mother relationships. Journal of Pediatrics, 119:661–666, 1991.

Goldberg, S, Washington, J, Morris, P, Fischer-Fay, A, & Simmons, RJ. Early diagnosed chronic illness and mother-child relationships in the first two years. Canadian Journal of Psychiatry, 55:726–733, 1990b.

Graham, TP, Bender, HW, & Spach, MS. Ventricular septal defect. In Adams, FH, Emmanouilides, GC, & Riemen Schneider, TA (Eds.), Moss's Heart Disease in Infants, Children, and Adolescents. Baltimore: Williams & Wilkins, 1989, pp. 189–208.

Griffith, BP, Hardesy, RL, Trento, A, Paradis, IL, Duquesnoy, RJ, Zeevi, A, Dauber, JH, Dummer, JS, Thompson, ME, Gryzan, S, & Bahnson, HT. Heart-lung transplantation: Lessons learned and future hopes. Annals of Thoracic Surgery, 43:6–16, 1987.

Gudermuth, S. Mothers' reports of early experiences of infants with congenital heart disease. Maternal-Child Nursing Journal, 4:155–164, 1975.

Haas, GS, Bailey, L, & Pennington, DG. Pediatric cardiac transplantation. In Baue, AE, Geha, AS, Hammond, GL, Laks, H, & Naunheim, KS (Eds.), Glenn's Thoracic and Cardiovascular Surgery, 5th ed. Norwalk, CT: Appleton & Lange, 1991, pp. 1297–1317.

Haka-Ikse, K, Blackwood, MA, & Steward, DJ. Psychomotor development of infants and children after profound hypothermia during surgery for congenital heart disease. Developmental Medicine and Child Neurology, 20:62–70, 1978.

Hammon, JW, & Bender, HW. Anomalous venous connection: Pulmonary and systemic. In Baue, AE, Geha, AS, Hammond, GL, Laks, H, & Naunheim, KS (Eds.), Glenn's Thoracic and Cardiovascular Surgery, 5th ed. Norwalk, CT: Appleton & Lange, 1991, pp. 971–993.

Haneda, K, Itoh, T, Togo, T, Ohmi, M, & Mohri, H. Effects of cardiac surgery on intellectual function in infants and children. Cardiovascular Surgery, 4(3):303–307, 1996.

Holden, KR, Sessions, JC, Cure, J, Whitcom, DS, & Sade, RM. Neurologic outcomes in children with post-pump choreoathetosis. Journal of Pediatrics, 132:162–164, 1998.

Huckabay, L, & Daderian, AD. Effect of choices on breathing exercises post-open heart surgery. Dimensions in Critical Care Nursing, 9:190–201, 1990.

Hussey, J. Effects of chest physiotherapy for children in intensive care after surgery. Physiotherapy, 78:109–113, 1992.

Hutter, JA, Despins, P, Higenbottam, T, Stewart, S, & Wallwork, J. Heart-lung transplantation: Better use of resources. American Journal of Medicine, 85:4–11, 1988.

Imle, PC. Percussion and vibration. In MacKenzie, CF, Ciesla, N, Imle, PC, & Klemic, N (Eds.), Chest Physiotherapy in the Intensive Care Unit. Baltimore: Williams & Wilkins, 1981, pp. 81–91.

James, FW, Blomqvist, CG, Freed, MD, Miller, WW, Moller, JH, Nugent, EW, Riopel, DA, Strong, WB, & Wessel, HU. Standards for exercise testing in the pediatric age group. Circulation, 66:1377A–1397A, 1982.

Jamieson, SW, Stinson, EB, Oyer, PE, Reitz, BA, Baldwin, J, Modry, D, Dawkins, K, Theodore, J, Hunt, S, & Shumway, NE. Heart-lung transplantation for irreversible pulmonary hypertension. Annals of Thoracic Surgery, 38:554–562, 1984.

Jarmakani, JM, & Canent, RV. Preoperative and postoperative right ventricular function in children with transposition of the great vessels. Circulation, 50(suppl II):39–45, 1974.

Johnson, AB, & Davis, JS. Treatment options for the neonate with hypoplastic left heart syndrome. Journal of Perinatal and Neonatal Nursing, 5:84–92, 1991.

Johnson, BA. Postoperative physical therapy in the pediatric cardiac surgery patient. Pediatric Physical Therapy, 2(1):14–22, 1991.

Kent, KM, & Cooper, T. The denervated heart: A model for studying autonomic control of the heart. New England Journal of Medicine, 291:1017–1021, 1974.

Koch, BM, Galioto, FM, Vaccaro, P, Vaccaro, J, & Buckenmeyer, PJ. Flexibility and strength measures in children participating in a cardiac rehabilitation exercise program. Physician and Sports Medicine, 116:139–147, 1988.

Kong, SG, Tay, JS, Yip, WC, & Chay, SO. Emotional and social effects of congenital heart disease in Singapore. Australian Paediatric Journal, 22:101–106, 1986.

Kopf, GS, Laks, H. Atrial septal defects and cor triatriatum. In Baue, AE, Geha, AS, Hammond, GL, Laks, H, & Naunheim, KS (Eds.), Glenn's Thoracic and Cardiovascular Surgery, 5th ed. Norwalk, CT: Appleton & Lange, 1991, pp. 995–1005.

Kramer, HH, Aswiszus, D, Sterzel, U, van Halteren, A, & Clafen, R. Development of personality and intelligence in children with congenital heart disease. Journal of Child Psychiatry, 30:299–308, 1989.

Krastins, IR, Corey, ML, McLeod, A, Edmonds, J, Levison, H, & Moles, F. An evaluation of incentive spirometry in the management of pulmonary complications after cardiac surgery in a pediatric population. Critical Care Medicine, 10:525–528, 1982.

Kriett, JM, & Kaye, MP. The registry of the International Society for Heart and Lung Transplantation: Eighth official report, 1991. Journal of Heart and Lung Transplantation, 10:491–498, 1991.

Laane, KM, Meberg, A, Otterstad, JE, Froland, G, & Sorland, S. Quality of life in children with congenital heart defects. Acta Paediatrica, 86:975–980, 1997.

Laks, H, & Breda, MA. Tetralogy of Fallot. In Baue, AE, Geha, AS, Hammond, GL, Laks, H, & Naunheim, KS (Eds.), Glenn's Thoracic and Cardiovascular Surgery, 5th ed. Norwalk, CT: Appleton & Lange, 1991a, pp. 1179–1201.

Laks, H, & Breda, MA. Tricuspid atresia. In Baue, AE, Geha, AS, Hammond, GL, Laks, H, & Naunheim, KS (Eds.), Glenn's Thoracic and Cardiovascular Surgery, 5th ed. Norwalk, CT: Appleton & Lange, 1991b, pp. 1259–1272.

Lawrence, KS, & Fricker, FJ. Pediatric heart transplantation: Quality of life. Journal of Heart Transplantation, 6:329–333, 1987.

Levitsky, S, & del Nido, P. Patent ductus arteriosus and aortopulmonary septal defects. In Baue, AE, Geha, AS, Hammond, GL, Laks, H, & Naunheim, KS (Eds.), Glenn's Thoracic and Cardiovascular Surgery, 5th ed. Norwalk, CT: Appleton & Lange, 1991, pp. 1017–1025.

Linde, LM, Rasof, B, & Dunn, OJ. Longitudinal studies of intellectual and behavioral development in children with congenital heart disease. Acta Paediatrica, 59:169–176, 1970.

Lloyd, TR. Prognosis of the hypoplastic left heart syndrome. Progress in Pediatric Cardiology, 5:57–64, 1996.

Locke, TJ, Griffiths, TC, Mould, H, & Gibson, GJ. Rib cage mechanics after median sternotomy. Thorax, 45:465–468, 1990.

Loeffel, M. Developmental considerations of infants and children with congenital heart disease. Heart and Lung, 14:214–217, 1985.

Markland, ON, Moorthy, SS, Mahomed, Y, King, RD, & Brown, JW. Postoperative phrenic nerve palsy in patients with open-heart surgery. Annals of Thoracic Surgery, 39:68–73, 1985.

Massery, M. Respiratory rehabilitation secondary to neurological deficits: Treatment techniques. In Frownfelter, DL (Ed.), Chest Physical Therapy and Pulmonary Rehabilitation. Chicago: Year Book, 1987, pp. 538–544.

Mathew, OP. Respiratory control during nipple feeding in pre-term infants. Pediatric Pulmonology, 5:220–224, 1988.

Mathew, OP, Clark, ML, Pronske, ML, Luna-Solarzano, HG, & Peterson, MD. Breathing pattern and ventilation during oral feeding in term newborn infants. Journal of Pediatrics, 106:810–813, 1985.

Mathews, RA, Nixon, PA, Stephenson, RJ, Robertson, RJ, Donovan, EF, Dean, F, Fricker, FJ, Beerman, LB, & Fischer, DR. An exercise program for pediatric patients with congenital heart disease: Organizational and physiologic aspects. Journal of Cardiac Rehabilitation, 3:467–475, 1983.

McWilliams, BC. Mechanical ventilation in pediatric patients. Clinics in Chest Medicine, 8:597–607, 1987.

Mee, RB. Current status of cardiac surgery in childhood. Progress in Pediatric Surgery, 27:148–169, 1991.

Messmer, BJ, Schallberger, Y, Gattiker, R, & Senning, A. Psychomotor and intellectual development after deep hypothermia and circulatory arrest in early infancy. Journal of Thoracic and Cardiovascular Surgery, 72:495–501, 1976.

Milgalter, E, & Laks, H. Truncus arteriosus. In Baue, AE, Geha, AS, Hammond, GL, Laks, H, & Naunheim, KS (Eds.), Glenn's Thoracic and Cardiovascular Surgery, 5th ed. Norwalk, CT: Appleton & Lange, 1991, pp. 1079–1987.

Morriss, JH, & McNamara, DG. Residua, sequelae and complications of surgery for congenital heart disease. Progress in Cardiovascular Diseases, 18:1–25, 1975.

Moulton, AL, & Malm, JR. Pulmonary stenosis, pulmonary atresia, single pulmonary artery and aneurysm of the pulmonary artery. In Baue, AE, Geha, AS, Hammond, GL, Laks, H, & Naunheim, KS (Eds.), Glenn's Thoracic and Cardiovascular Surgery, 5th ed. Norwalk, CT: Appleton & Lange, 1991, pp. 1131–1163.

Nakazawa, M, Okuda, H, Imai, Y, Takanashi, Y, & Takao, A. Right and left ventricular volume characteristics after external conduit repair (Rastelli procedure) for cyanotic congenital heart disease. Heart and Vessels, 2:106–110, 1986.

Niset, G, Coustry-Degre, C, & Degre, S. Psychosocial and physical rehabilitation after heart transplantation: 1-year follow-up. Cardiology, 75:311–317, 1988.

Noonan, JA. Syndromes associated with cardiac defects. In Engle, MA (Ed.), Pediatric Cardiovascular Disease. Philadelphia: FA Davis, 1981, pp. 97–115.

Norwood, SH, & Civette, JM. Ventilatory assistance and support. In Baue, AE, Geha, AS, Hammond, GL, Laks, H, & Naunheim, KS (Eds.), Glenn's Thoracic and Cardiovascular Surgery, 5th ed. Norwalk, CT: Appleton & Lange, 1991, pp. 45–66.

Norwood, WI. Hypoplastic left heart syndrome. Annals of Thoracic Surgery, 52:688–695, 1991a.

Norwood, WI. Hypoplastic left heart syndrome. In Baue, AE, Geha, AS, Hammond, GL, Laks, H, & Naunheim, KS (Eds.), Glenn's Thoracic and Cardiovascular Surgery, 5th ed. Norwalk, CT: Appleton & Lange, 1991b, pp. 1123–1130.

O'Dougharty, M, Wright, FS, Loewenson, RB, & Torres, F. Cerebral dysfunction after chronic hypoxia in children. Neurology, 35:42–46, 1985.

Page, GG. Tetralogy of Fallot. Heart and Lung, 15:390–400, 1986.

Pairolero, PC, & Payne, WS. Postoperative care and complications in the thoracic surgery patient. In Baue, AE, Geha, AS, Hammond, GL, Laks, H, & Naunheim, KS (Eds.), Glenn's Thoracic and Cardiovascular Surgery, 5th ed. Norwalk, CT: Appleton & Lange, 1991, pp. 31–43.

Peetz, DJ, Spicer, RL, Crowley, DC, Sloan, H, & Behrendt, DM. Correction of truncus arteriosus in the neonate using a nonvalved conduit. Journal of Thoracic and Cardiovascular Surgery, 83:743–746, 1982.

Pennington, DG, Noedel, N, McBride, LR, Naunheim, KS, & Ring, WS. Heart transplantation in children: An international survey. Annals of Thoracic Surgery, 52:710–715, 1991.

Perrault, H, & Drblik, SP. Exercise after surgical repair of congenital cardiac lesions. Sports Medicine, 7:18–31, 1989.

Peters, RM. Pulmonary physiologic studies of the perioperative period. Chest, 76:576–585, 1979.

Prakanrattana, U, Valairucha, S, Sriyoschati, S, Pornvilawan, S, & Phanchaipetch, T. Early extubation following open heart surgery in pediatric patients with congenital heart diseases. Journal of the Medical Association of Thailand, 80:87–95, 1997.

Puga, FJ. Surgical treatment of pulmonary atresia with ventricular septal defect. In Baue, AE, Geha, AS, Hammond, GL, Laks, H, & Naunheim, KS (Eds.), Glenn's Thoracic and Cardiovascular Surgery, 5th ed. Norwalk, CT: Appleton & Lange, 1991, pp. 1165–1177.

Rasof, B, Linde, LM, & Dunn, OJ. Intellectual development in children with congenital heart disease. Child Development, 38:1043–1053, 1967.

Razzouk, AJ, Chinnock, RE, Gundry, SR, & Bailey, LL. Cardiac transplantation for infants with hypoplastic left heart syndrome. Progress in Pediatric Cardiology, 5:37–47, 1996.

Risser, NL: Preoperative and postoperative care to prevent pulmonary complications. Heart and Lung, 9:57–67, 1980.

Rockwell, GM, & Campbell, SK. Physical therapy program for the pediatric cardiac surgical patient. Physical Therapy, 56:670–675, 1976.

Rosen, M, & Hillard, EK. The effects of negative pressure during tracheal suction. Anesthesia and Analgesia, 41:50–57, 1962.

Rosenthal, A. Care of the postoperative child and adolescent with congenital heart disease. In Barness, LA (Ed.), Advances in Pediatrics. Chicago: Year Book, 1983, pp. 131–167.

Rossi, AF, Seiden, HS, Sadeghi, AM, Nguyen, KH, Quintana, CS, Gross, RP, & Griepp, RB. The outcome of cardiac operations in infants weighing two kilograms or less. Journal of Thoracic and Cardiovascular Surgery, 116:28–35, 1998.

Rubin, M. The physiology of bedrest. American Journal of Nursing, 88:50–56, 1988.

Russell, IA, Zwass, MS, Fineman, JR, Balea, M, Rouine-Rapp, K, Brook, M, Hanley, FL, Silverman, NH, & Cahalan, MK. The effects of inhaled nitric oxide on postoperative pulmonary hypertension in infants and children undergoing surgical repair of congenital heart disease. Anesthesia and Analgesia, 87:46–51, 1998.

Ruttenberg, HD, Adams, TD, Orsmond, GS, Conlee, RK, & Fisher, AG. Effects of exercise training on aerobic fitness in children after open heart surgery. Pediatric Cardiology, 4:19–24, 1983.

Sadowsky, HS, Rohrkemper, KF, & Quon, SYM. Rehabilitation of Cardiac and Cardiopulmonary Recipients. An Introduction for Physical and Occupational Therapists. Stanford, CA: Stanford University Hospital, 1986.

Scheidegger, D, Bentz, L, Piolino, G, Pusterla, C, & Gigon, JP. Influence of early mobilisation on pulmonary function in surgical patients. European Journal of Intensive Care Medicine, 2:35–40, 1976.

Sciurba, FC, Owens, GR, Sanders, MH, Bartley, BP, Hardesty, RL, Paradis, IL, & Costantino, JP. Evidence of an altered pattern of breathing during exercise in recipients of heart-lung transplants. New England Journal of Medicine, 319:1186–1192, 1988.

Settergren, G, Ohqvist, G, Lundberg, S, Henze, A, Bjork, VO, & Persson, B. Cerebral blood flow and cerebral metabolism in children following cardiac surgery with deep hypothermia and circulatory arrest. Clinical course and follow-up of psychomotor development. Scandinavian Journal of Thoracic Cardiovascular Surgery, 16:209–215, 1982.

Silbert, A, Wolff, PH, Mayer, B, Rosenthal, A, & Nadas, AS. Cyanotic heart disease and psychological development. Pediatrics, 43:192–200, 1969.

Starnes, VA, Marshall, SE, Lewiston, NJ, Theodore, J, Stinson, EB, & Shumway, NE. Heart-lung transplantation in infants, children, and adolescents. Journal of Pediatric Surgery, 26:434–438, 1991.

Starnes, VA, Oyer, PE, Bernstein, D, Baum, D, Gamberg, P, Miller, J, & Shumway, NE. Heart, heart-lung, and lung transplantation in the first year of life. Annals of Thoracic Surgery, 53:306–310, 1992.

Stretton, CD, Mak, JCW, Belvisi, MG, Yacoub, MH, & Barnes, PJ. Cholinergic control of human airways in vitro following extrinsic denervation of the human respiratory tract by heart-lung transplantation. American Review of Respiratory Disease, 142:1030–1033, 1990.

Suoninen, P. Physical growth of children with congenital heart disease. Acta Paediatrica Supplement, 225:7–50, 1971.

Thoren, L. Post-operative pulmonary complications. Acta Chirurgica Scandinavica, 107:193–205, 1954.

Todd, TR. Early postoperative management following lung transplantation. Clinics in Chest Medicine, 11:259–267, 1990.

Trusler, GA. The Mustard procedure. In Baue, AE, Geha, AS, Hammond, GL, Laks, H, & Naunheim, KS (Eds.), Glenn's Thoracic and Cardiovascular Surgery, 5th ed. Norwalk, CT: Appleton & Lange, 1991, pp. 1203–1209.

Uretsky, BF. Physiology of the transplanted heart. In Brest, AN (Ed.), Cardiovascular Clinics. Philadelphia: FA Davis, 1990, pp. 23–55.

Uzark, L, Lincoln, A, Lamberti, JJ, Mainwaring, RD, Spicer, RL, & Moore, JW. Neurodevelopmental outcomes in children with Fontan repair of functional single ventricle. Pediatrics, 101:630–633, 1998.

van Breda, A. Postoperative care of infants and children who require cardiac surgery. Heart and Lung, 14:205–207, 1985.

Van De Water, JM, Watring, WG, Linton, LA, Murphy, M, & Byron, RL. Prevention of postoperative pulmonary complications. Surgery, Gynecology and Obstetrics, 135:229–233, 1972.

Vraciu, JK, & Vraciu, RA. Effectiveness of breathing exercises in preventing pulmonary complications following open heart surgery. Physical Therapy, 57:1367–1371, 1977.

Waldhausen, JA, Myers, JL, & Campbell, DB. Coarctation of the aorta and interrupted aortic arch. In Baue, AE, Geha, AS, Hammond, GL, Laks, H, & Naunheim, KS (Eds.), Glenn's Thoracic and Cardiovascular Surgery, 5th ed. Norwalk, CT: Appleton & Lange, 1991, pp. 1107–1122.

Ward, RJ, Danziger, F, Bonica, JJ, Allen, GD, & Bowes, J. An evaluation of postoperative maneuvers. Surgical Gynecology and Obstetrics, 66:51–54, 1966.

Warner, JO. Heart-lung transplantation: All the facts. Archives of Disease in Childhood, 66:1013–1017, 1991.

Webber, BA. Evaluation and inflation in respiratory care. Physiotherapy, 77:801–804, 1991.

Weinhaus, L, Canter, C, Noetzel, M, McAlister, W, & Spray, TL. Extracorporeal membrane oxygenation for circulatory support after repair of congenital heart defects. Annals of Thoracic Surgery, 48:206–212, 1989.

Weldon, CS, Behrendt, DM, & Haas, GS. Congenital malformations of the aortic valve and left ventricular outflow tract. In Baue, AE, Geha, AS, Hammond, GL, Laks, H, & Naunheim, KS (Eds.), Glenn's Thoracic and Cardiovascular Surgery, 5th ed. Norwalk, CT: Appleton & Lange, 1991, pp. 1089–1106.

Wells, FC, Coghill, S, Caplan, HL, & Lincoln, C. Duration of circulatory arrest does influence the psychological development of children after cardiac operation in early life. Journal of Thoracic and Cardiovascular Surgery, 86:823–831, 1983.

Whitehead, B, James, I, Helms, P, Scott, JP, Smyth, R, Higenbottam, TW, McGoldrick, J, English, TAH, Wallwork, J, Elliott, M, & de Leval, M. Intensive care management of children following heart and heart-lung transplantation. Intensive Care Medicine, 16:426–430, 1990.

Wilkinson, JL. Heart and heart/lung transplantation in children. Australian Paediatric Journal, 25:111–118, 1989.

Williams, WH. Rastelli's operation for "anatomic" repair of transposition of the great arteries with ventricular septal defect and left ventricular outflow tract obstruction. In Baue, AE, Geha, AS, Hammond, GL, Laks, H, & Naunheim, KS (Eds.), Glenn's Thoracic and Cardiovascular Surgery, 5th ed. Norwalk, CT: Appleton & Lange, 1991, pp. 1217–1226.

Wilson, RS. Anesthesia for thoracic surgery. In Baue, AE, Geha, AS, Hammond, GL, Laks, H, & Naunheim, KS (Eds.), Glenn's Thoracic and Cardiovascular Surgery, 5th ed. Norwalk, CT: Appleton & Lange, 1991, pp. 19–29.

Wray, J, & Sensky, T. How does the intervention of cardiac surgery affect the self-perception of children with congenital heart disease? Child: Care, Health and Development, 24:57–72, 1998.

Youssef, NM. School adjustment of children with congenital heart disease. Maternal-Child Nursing Journal, 17:217–302, 1988.

Zahr, LK, & Boisvert, J. Hypoplastic left heart syndrome repair. Dimensions in Critical Care Nursing, 9:88–96, 1990.

Zimmerman, AA, Burrows, FA, Jonas, RA, & Hickey, PR. The limits of detectable cerebral perfusion by transcranial Doppler sonography in neonates undergoing deep hypothermic low-flow cardiopulmonary bypass. Journal of Thoracic and Cardiovascular Surgery, 114:594–600, 1997.

SPECIAL SETTINGS AND SPECIAL CONSIDERATIONS

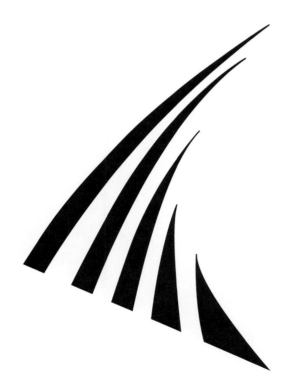

ROBERT J. PALISANO, PT, ScD

Section Editor

C H A P T E R
29

The Burn Unit

MERILYN L. MOORE, PT

Burn-related injuries are the leading cause of accidental death in children younger than age 2 years and the second leading cause of accidental death in children younger than age 14 years (Warden et al., 1988). Data accumulated by the National Burn Information Exchange, a voluntary registry established in 1964 (Feller, 1982), show that a disproportionately high number of burn accidents occur during the first 4 years of life and that boys are affected more often than girls. This age group alone incurs 52% of all pediatric burns. It is well recognized that child abuse is a common mechanism of injury in this age group. A recent study cites findings that, during a 24-month period, one third of 321 consecutive pediatric admissions, ages 3 years and under, were reported for abuse or neglect (Bennett & Gamelli, 1998).

During the first 2 years of life, 95% of the burn injuries occur indoors and the etiologic agent is a hot liquid in 80% of the patients (Feller, 1980). As the child gets older, the proportion of indoor injuries progressively declines and scalds become less frequent. During adolescence, 60% of the injuries occur outdoors and only 20% occur as a result of scalding (Green, 1984). The depth and extent of the burn also increase as the child gets older.

Great strides have been made in the management of thermal injuries, resulting in improvement in the survival rate of pediatric patients. In 1949, Bull and Squire reported a 50% mortality rate in children younger than 14 years of age with burns over 51% of the total body surface area. Forty-three years later Herndon and Rutan (1992a) reported a 50% mortality rate in children younger than 15 years of age with burns of greater than 95% of the total body surface area. Infants (younger than 12 months) with large (more than 30%) burns are reported to have poorer chances for survival than older children with similar injuries. However, recent experience with such infants has been positive (Sheridan et al., 1998).

Treatment of children with burns is concerned not only with skin coverage and prevention of infection but also with psychologic and social outcomes. Pediatric survivors often must live with permanent disfigurement and physical disabilities. A study by Doctor and co-workers (1997) suggests that people who survive a severe burn experience a stable and relatively good health status after their injury. Their health status, however, remains worse than that of the general population over time. Furthermore, people who survive a major burn indicate that vocation and psychosocial function are often troublesome. With decreased mortality rates and a marked reduction in length of hospitalization (Feller & Jones, 1984), the roles and responsibilities of various members of the burn team take on added importance. The purpose of this chapter is to describe the pathophysiology and medical management of burns, identify impairments and potential functional limitations of the child with a burn, and discuss physical therapy interventions and resources associated with quality care in the burn unit.

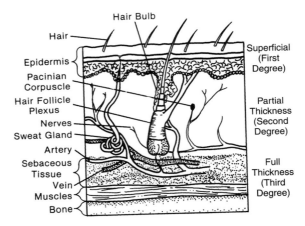

FIGURE 29–1. Depth of burn.

CLASSIFICATION AND PATHOPHYSIOLOGY OF BURNS

Burn injuries occur when energy is transferred from a heat source to the body. If heat absorption exceeds heat dissipation, cellular temperature rises above the point at which cell survival is possible. Tissue damage begins at temperatures of 40°C and increases logarithmically as the temperature rises. At 45°C, denaturation of tissue proteins ensues and leads to cellular necrosis (Carvajal, 1990). The extent of injury is related to (1) heat intensity, (2) duration of the exposure, and (3) tissue conductance (Achauer & Martinez, 1985).

Burns may be categorized into four types, according to the primary mechanism of injury: thermal, radiation, electrical, or chemical (Bayley, 1990). Thermal injuries include burns caused by contact with hot liquids (spills or immersion scalds), hot solid objects, or flames and make up approximately 95% of all burns treated (Solem, 1984). Chemical and electrical injuries make up about 5% of burns admitted to a regional burn center. Radiation injuries are extremely rare.

Burn injuries are classified as superficial, partial thickness, or full thickness according to the depth of tissue damage. Burn classification characteristics are depicted in Figure 29–1 and listed in Table 29–1. Deeper burns may at times extend into fascia, muscle, or bone. Burns involving tendon, muscle, or bone are most common on digits, hands, feet, and over bony prominences such as the iliac crest, patella, anterior tibia, and cranium, because these areas have only a thin covering of subcutaneous tissue (Solem, 1984).

Because skin varies in thickness in different parts of the body, application of the same intensity of heat for given periods of time results in different burn depth. Thus, in the young child in whom dermal

papillae and appendages have yet to develop fully, deeper burns result from heat of the same intensity that produces a moderate partial-thickness burn in the adult. The skin is thickest on the back and on the palm of the hands and is thinnest on the inner arm. Burned parts involving the thickest areas of skin regenerate faster.

Certain burn patterns are indicative of possible abuse, for example, burns of the buttocks, feet, and perineum when the backs of knees and anterior hip areas are not burned (Doane, 1989). This typically occurs when a child is placed in a tub of hot water. The child flexes into a protective position by curling up the knees and hips.

The extent of burn injury can be estimated in several ways. One approach is referred to as the "rule of nines" (Mikhail, 1988), which divides the body surface into areas, each representing 9% or a multiple of 9% of body surface area. This method is particularly unreliable in children younger than 15 years of age because it underestimates burned areas of the head and neck and overestimates burned areas of the legs (Solem, 1984). Another method, the Berkow chart (Feller & Jones, 1974), is modeled after Lund and Browder's work (1944), which recognizes that the proportion of body surface covering specific body parts changes with age. For example, the head and neck of an infant constitute 20% of the body surface compared with 9% in the adult.

Thermal destruction of the skin initiates a chain of physiologic changes in the local wound, as well as severe multiple systemic responses in almost all organ systems. The total amount of cell death and extracellular destruction is dependent on local chemical responses to the initial insult and on the systemic response to burn injury (Dimick, 1984). Important clinically apparent local responses in-

TABLE 29–1. **Classification of Burns**

	Superficial (First Degree)	Partial Thickness (Second Degree)		Full Thickness (Third Degree)
		Superficial	Deep	
Depth	Superficial epidermis	Epidermis and a small part of the dermis	Epidermis and a deeper portion of the dermis	Total destruction of the epidermis and dermis; may involve deeper tissue, muscle, or subcutaneous fat
Sensation	Painful	Increased sensitivity to pain and temperature	Increased sensitivity to pain and temperature	No pain or temperature sensation
Color	Bright red	Red	Marbled-white edematous appearance	White, brown-black charred appearance
Texture Blisters	Edematous Some, blanches with pressure	Normal or firm Large, thick walled, will usually increase in size	Firm Large, thick walled, will usually increase in size	Firm or leathery None, or if present will not increase in size

clude loss of the ability to regulate evaporative water loss, impairment of the body's first line of defense against infection, and the loss of massive amounts of body fluids through open wounds. The systemic effects of the burn injury on other organs are well described in the literature (Achauer & Martinez, 1985). The physiologic changes occurring in the skin and subadjacent tissues are addressed in the section on primary physical impairment later in this chapter.

THE BURN UNIT AND TEAM APPROACH TO CARE

Appropriate treatment decisions can be made after calculation of the severity of the burn by following the American Burn Association treatment guidelines. Patients with minor burns may be treated as outpatients. Moderately severe uncomplicated burns may be treated in a community hospital by an experienced surgeon or physician. Burns that should be referred to a burn unit include larger second-degree burns (greater than 25% in adults or 20% in children); all third-degree burns greater than 10%; burns of difficult areas such as the hands, face, eyes, ears, feet, and perineum; and burns with associated injuries, including inhalation or electrical injuries, fractures, or other trauma.

The burn unit is much like other intensive care units, but it also has unique characteristics. As in other units, it is a place characterized by high technology, specially trained staff, a team approach, and isolation, which may lead to a dehumanizing situation in which the patient is viewed in a fragmented and anatomic manner. The need for compassion, empathy, guidance, interest, and support is para-

mount. On the other hand, significant differences exist between the burn unit and other acute care units. The sights and smells characteristic of burn injury make for an obvious difference from other emergency care settings. Isolation of both staff and patient from the outside world is often more pronounced in the burn unit, primarily because of fear of infection. There is also the constant issue of pain management. Patients in burn centers stay longer than in other intensive care units, or indeed, any other hospital units. This results in a much more intense and prolonged patient-staff interaction.

A multidisciplinary team approach to burn care was developed in specialized burn treatment facilities established over the past 25 years. Presently burn teams usually consist of physicians and nursing personnel, physical therapists and occupational therapists, clinical nutritionists, social workers, psychiatrists or psychologists, child life specialists or recreational therapists, school teachers, and, when available, orthotists, prosthetists, and medical sculptors. With an integrated team approach, all team members work together and each plays a key role. The team members—rather than the patient—absorb the stress. This approach offers the patient an active role as the treatment is performed and includes the patient in the decision-making process. The integrated team approach has been shown to decrease predicted mortality and morbidity rates (Biggs et al., 1998). Successful outcomes of a sound interdisciplinary approach also include (1) the elimination of the duplication of services, (2) a decrease in the length of the patient's stay, (3) improved functional and cosmetic results, and (4) a decrease in the patient's temporary and permanent disability.

The team approach to burn management is based on a mutual respect and appreciation of each member's contribution to the overall care of the patient and a decision-making process that relies on the input of the child, family (on wound rounds and individually with staff), and all professional team members. Discussions at burn team conferences not only lead to improved patient care but also provide an opportunity for members to gain insights from the experiences of other team members who are caring for the same patient. Daily pressures the team must face include viewing mutilations and disfigurement, inflicting pain, dealing with emergency situations, and confronting death.

Medical Management of Burns

When a child is admitted to the appropriate facility, an estimate of the depth and surface area of the burn and the child's overall condition is first made. These decisions determine the need for immediate lifesaving measures, such as endotracheal intubation, ventilatory support, and intravenous fluid therapy (Hartford, 1984).

Shock is usual in children with burns affecting more than 12% of the surface area but can occur when the surface area is smaller if the burn is full thickness and when the child is younger than 1 year of age (Solomon, 1985). An intravenous line and a urinary catheter are placed and fluid delivery is begun. Until the capillary leak stops, intravenous fluid therapy is necessary to maintain the circulation and perfusion of tissues. After fluid resuscitation has been started and a detailed history and physical examination completed, attention is directed to care of the burn.

Escharotomy, incision through the burn, may be necessary to relieve the pressure caused by progressive edema in the extremities with circumferential deep burns. It is usually done when the tissue pressure exceeds 40 mm Hg. The incisions are made along the medial and lateral aspects of the limb. As the tissues are released, the subcutaneous fat bulges through the incision, tissue tension is relieved, and effective circulation is restored. Among patients with deep burns or high-voltage electrical injury involving muscle, fasciotomy may be necessary to relieve elevated pressure in fascial compartments unrelieved by simple escharotomy.

As soon as the patient's condition is stabilized, the wounds are assessed for the purpose of developing a plan for wound closure. Evaluation of the burn wound depth in pediatric patients is often difficult. A laser Doppler flowmeter with a temperature-controlled multichannel probe has been a useful tool for burn wound assessment in pediatric patients (Atiles et al., 1995). Necrotic tissue produced by the burn must be removed, either by daily mechanical debridement during wound care or, in deeper burns, by surgical excision either directly to fascia or tangentially (i.e., shaving sequential levels until viable tissue is exposed), and closure must be accomplished with autogenous split-thickness skin grafts.

Aggressive and thorough wound care is important to help delineate wounds before early surgical intervention, to protect and promote good granulation tissue until grafting, or to promote rapid healing in wounds that are healing without surgical intervention. There are three types of cleansing techniques: (1) local care of a particular wound or area (using a sterile container of water and cleansing agents at bedside or any convenient area); (2) spray hydrotherapy or nonsubmersion (using a shower head to allow the water to run intermittently over the burn wounds with the patient on a stretcher suspended over a tank or tub); and (3) submersion, which may or may not include agitation of the water (submerging the patient or burned extremity in a tub, tank, or whirlpool of water for up to 20 minutes). The choice depends on the depth of injury, extent and location of the wound, and medical condition of the patient (Head, 1984).

Most burn wound protocols call for daily or twice-daily dressing changes (Bayley, 1990). Various topical burn creams and solutions are available. No single topical agent has been demonstrated to be universally effective for burn care. Each has advantages and disadvantages, and the effectiveness of even a single agent may decrease after time. Different agents may be used on the same patient either concurrently, on different burned areas, or sequentially as the wound and its bacterial flora change. Each topical agent is applied with gauze dressings (type used is need specific). Gauze should be wrapped distally to proximally on burned extremities, and no two burn surfaces should be allowed to touch (e.g., fingers and toes should be wrapped separately, and burned ears should not touch the burned head). Such attention to detail helps prevent webbing caused by raw surfaces growing together. Wrapping digits individually also facilitates active and functional movements.

Excision may be initiated a few days after the burn or as soon as the patient is hemodynamically stable and edema has decreased (Heimbach, 1987). An autograft is immediately placed, or a temporary biologic or synthetic dressing is used until autografting can be done in a subsequent operation. Surgical excision is advantageous in contributing to decreased complications from invasive burn wound sepsis and a shorter time period from injury to wound closure and hospital discharge.

Full-thickness wounds require skin grafts unless they are small in size. Wounds of partial-thickness depth that do not heal spontaneously may be closed with a skin graft, if donor skin is available. Split-thickness skin grafts are used almost exclusively. This implies that the grafts are cut through a partial-thickness of depth of skin, leaving epidermal regenerative cells that cause reepithelialization of the donor site. Full-thickness skin grafts and flaps are occasionally used in primary repair of specific burn wounds (e.g., very deep electrical burns) but are primarily used later in some reconstructive procedures.

Skin grafts may be cut from virtually any area of the body except the face and hands. The foot as a skin donor source is generally impractical. The scalp is a superior donor site. It has excellent blood supply with deep, closely placed hair follicles that are able to effect reepithelialization in 4 or 5 days. Regrowth of scalp hair hides the donor site. Donor sites of the torso and extremities heal more slowly.

In the majority of instances, wounds of the hands, face, and neck take precedence for skin grafts. However, when there is limited donor skin, consideration must be given to covering larger areas to try to reduce the size of the wound to first preserve the patient's life. The next priority for skin grafts after the hands, face, and neck is the skin over joints.

Skin grafts must be undisturbed in order to take. Fibrin causes initial adherence. The cells of the graft are nourished by tissue fluid until inosculation (anastomosis) of blood vessels between the wound and the graft establishes a nutritive blood flow in the graft. Inosculation occurs in about 2 days. Joints must be held immobile until the take of the skin graft is ensured. Immobilization is usually accomplished by a splint or in some cases by skeletal traction.

In most cases there is enough tensile strength between the graft and the wound to permit active range of motion (ROM) on the fourth and certainly by the sixth day after skin grafting. Gentle passive ROM can be added on the sixth or seventh day.

Early massive excision of the burn wound has increased the median lethal dose to 98% of total body surface area burn but represents the problem of wound closure (Herndon & Rutan, 1992b). Autograft substitutes must be used for a large burn. Alternative methods of wound closure that are currently used include biologic dressings, biosynthetic dressings, artificial skin, and cultured skin. Alternative wound closure options are summarized in Table 29–2.

Biologic dressings consist of viable or once-viable tissues used to temporarily cover wounds in place

TABLE 29–2. Alternative Wound Closure Options

Type	Description	Advantages/Indications
Biologic	Viable or once-viable tissue	Short-term, several-day wound closure.
Allograft	Skin from living or recently deceased human	Tests bed for autograft preparedness.
Xenograft	Pig skin	Covers, protects, facilitates healing of interstices in widely meshed autografts.
Amnion	Human placenta	Pigskin left intact on partial-thickness scalds eliminates pain without impeding epithelialization.
Biosynthetic	Synthetic structure with biologic tissue added	Sterile, indefinite shelf life. Cheaper than biologic products. Offers pediatric patient immediate comfort and protection. Used to temporarily close excised full-thickness burns. Protective dressing over meshed autograft and donor sites.
Biobrane	Knitted elastic flexible nylon fabric bonded to a thin Silastic membrane coated with products of dermal collagen	
Dermagraft	Polyglycolic acid mesh impregnated with viable human neonatal fibroblasts	Fibroblasts secrete human collagen, growth factors, and other matrix proteins to form living dermal tissue.
Artificial skin	Bilayered membrane system	Provides matrix for development of neodermis.
Integra	Bovine tendon collagen matrix attached to Silastic outer layer	Provides wounds coverage after excision of large burns. Needs only very thin (0.005 inch) skin graft for final autograft coverage. Minimal hypertrophic scarring or contracture.
Cultured skin	Sheets of skin cultures from patient's cells	Requires only biopsy-size piece of unburned skin.
CEA	Cultured keratinocytes	Eliminates need for autografting.
CCA	Cultured keratinocytes attached to a dermal matrix	

of conventional dressings or leaving the wound exposed. Commonly used materials are partial-thickness grafts from living or recently deceased humans (hemografts or allografts), partial-thickness skin grafts from pigs (heterografts or xenografts), or amnion from the human placenta. All biologic dressings, viable and nonviable, can be used for short-term, several-day wound coverage. In a large burn, biologic dressings can be lifesaving by providing temporary wound closure until completion of autografting. Biologic dressings may also be effectively employed to protect wounds that have been covered by widely meshed graft. Used in this way, the wounds between the autografts are closed as well.

Problems with availability, sterility, and cost have led to the search for synthetic skin substitutes, which may eventually replace biologic dressings as temporary wound coverings (Bayley, 1990). One of these is Biobrane, a knitted elastic flexible nylon fabric that is bonded to a thin Silastic semipermeable membrane coated with products of dermal collagen. Sterile and semitransparent, Biobrane has an indefinite shelf life, allows the passage of some topical agents, and is cheaper than homograft or pig skin. Biobrane has been used to cover clean partial-thickness burns, temporarily to close excised full-thickness burns, and to dress meshed autograft and donor sites. Biobrane offers a number of advantages as a wound dressing for children. It does not require the use of surgical instruments, noisy distractions, painful manipulation of the wound, or regimented daily dressing changes. Biobrane offers the pediatric patient with burns immediate comfort and protection and enhances patient compliance and parental satisfaction (Bishop, 1995).

Dermagraft is a newly developed dermal substitute in early stages of clinical trials (Economou et al., 1993). It consists of polyglycolic acid mesh impregnated with viable human neonatal fibroblasts. Fibroblasts secrete native human collagen, growth factors, and other matrix proteins, forming a living, three-dimensional dermal tissue. It may be potentially useful as a synthetic dermal graft in large-area, full-thickness burns. There have been more advances in the availability of other dermal products. Integra artificial skin to provide a matrix for the development of a neodermis and other dermal replacement materials offer hope for more rapid wound healing and better functional and cosmetic outcomes (Clayton & Bishop, 1998; Helvig, 1997).

Recently, confluent sheets of epidermal cells (cultured epidermal autograft) have been grown successfully from a biopsy of the patient's own unburned skin (Clugston et al., 1991; Desai et al., 1991; Herndon & Rutan, 1992b). Cultured keratinocyte sheets lack a dermal component, however, and this is a potentially serious deficiency for achieving a successful replacement for full-thickness skin losses. Investigations are aimed at improving the engraftment and ultimate survival of cultured epidermal autograft.

Advances in technology continue to improve the potential for children to recover from severe burns. Two examples of treatments that have contributed to improved recovery are the clinical use of propranolol and growth hormone. Baron and Herndon (1993) reported safe administration of propranolol to 43 children with massive burns (mean percentage of total body surface area burn = $60 \pm 18\%$). Cardiac work was reduced by more than 70 beats per minute, and patient anxiety decreased. Herndon and colleagues (1990) and Gilpin and associates (1994) demonstrated a significant decrease in length of hospital stay as a result of increased healing rates of donor sites when recombinant human growth hormone was administered.

PRIMARY PHYSICAL IMPAIRMENT

Burn Scar

Regeneration of epithelial elements in partial-thickness injury comes from the epithelial cells lining every hair follicle and sweat gland. Healing of partial-thickness burns usually takes 14 days, but if the burn is sufficiently deep these burns may take 21 days for complete healing. As the epithelium grows, the normal pigmentation gradually and progressively returns. As the regenerated epithelium differentiates and forms the keratin layer, the function of the skin in maintaining and conserving core body temperature is restored.

Loss of capillary integrity is a pathophysiology of burn injury that leads to edema formation. This results in the outpouring of protein-rich intravascular fluid into the interstitium. This process occurs at all areas of partial-thickness burns and at areas adjacent to full-thickness burns. As the patient voluntarily limits movement at the injured part because of pain, and as a result of direct damage to the lymphatic systems, this edema fluid accumulates and persists in tissue spaces around tendons, joints, and ligaments. New collagen fibers form in this protein-rich edema fluid and eventually organize into unyielding adhesions and thickened support structures whose normal elasticity is lost.

Healing of deep dermal wounds also results in the replacement of normal integument with a mass of metabolically highly active tissues lacking the normal architecture of the skin (Parks et al., 1977). Several different processes appear to be at work in the healing wound. These processes include the following: mass production of large amounts of fused, highly disorganized collagen; replacement of the normal dermal elastic ground substance with inelastic chondroitin sulfate A; involuntary contraction of myofibroblasts; and inflammatory response with increased vascularity and localized lymphedema.

The bonds between the twisted collagen and firm inelastic ground substance, coupled with the simultaneous contraction of the myofibroblasts, contribute to the "heaped up" appearance of the hypertrophic scar. In addition, underlying voluntary skeletal muscle contraction reinforces the compaction of the collagen. The intensity and duration of the vascular response provides a visible clue to the likelihood of hypertrophic scarring and contracture formation (Larson et al., 1979). The hyperemia of the scar tissue signifies ongoing change within the closed wound. As long as this clinical characteristic persists, scar maturation has not been completed and hypertrophy is a possibility. The darker a patient's skin, the more predisposed that patient is toward hypertrophic scarring. Also, children are more susceptible to the development of hypertrophic scarring than adults (Deitch et al., 1983; Sullivan, 1990).

The active phase of scarring gradually subsides and will usually be completed in 1.5 to 2 years after the burn (Bayley, 1990; Dimick, 1984). In this regard, clinical reports indicate more rapid maturity for sheet graft compared with that reported for meshed grafts (Schwanholt et al., 1993). If appropriate measures are instituted during this active period, the scar tissue loses its redness and softens. Linares and coworkers (1973) have shown that "pressure induces loosening of collagen bundles and encourages parallel orientation of the collagen bundles to the skin surface with the disappearance of the dermal nodules." With the application of pressure there is a coincident restructuring of the collagen mass and a decrease in vascularity and cellularity. Larson and colleagues (1974) reported that at least 25 mm Hg pressure must be achieved to provide histologically and clinically significant pressure.

The position of comfort for most patients is that of flexion of the joints, which can lead to contracture. Maintenance of a flexed posture permits new collagen fibers in the wound to fuse together, resulting in contracture formation. Eventually the scar will mature, becoming a solid mass of fused collagen. The resulting mass of collagen will have a Swiss-cheese appearance as a result of continuing reabsorption of the collagen. The contracture, however, will remain because of fusion of some of the collagen fibers into the shortened position. Other impairments occur as a result of skin grafting required for full-thickness burns. When the skin is transplanted to the area of full-thickness burn, no hair follicles or sweat glands are included. Therefore, these grafted areas do not have the specialized skin appendages. Without these, the grafted area has none of the normal body oils, resulting in excessively dry skin. Another problem for patients with extensive skin grafting is created by the absence of sweat glands in grafted skin. The grafted areas are unable to dissipate the core body temperature if it is too high. Patients are cautioned about this problem and warned to avoid environments with high heat and humidity because they may have trouble dissipating excessive core body temperature.

Patients frequently report having other abnormal or odd sensations in their burn wounds, which are probably a result of regeneration of nerve endings into the burned areas. As the nerve endings grow through the areas of burned tissue, they frequently meet an obstruction that may cause an area of hypersensitivity, characterized by unusual or odd sensations. Small neuromas may occur in scattered areas throughout the burned area, causing hypersensitivity.

Scar formation is a natural sequela in the healing process of burned skin. It cannot be prevented, although current research suggests the potential for therapeutic use of interferons to down-regulate collagen production and inhibit wound contraction (Ghahary et al., 1993; Nedelec et al., 1995). The subjective assessment of scar appearance is a widely used method in the evaluation of burn outcomes and the effectiveness of treatment. A numeric scar-rating scale has been developed and has proved to be a useful tool for the evaluation of scar surface, thickness, border height, and color differences between a scar and the adjacent normal skin (Yeong et al., 1997).

Musculoskeletal Complications

In addition to burn scarring, many musculoskeletal complications are associated with immobility and inactivity during the acute phase of rehabilitation, including peripheral nerve involvement, exposed tendons and joints, heterotopic bone formation, and amputation. Peripheral nerve damage occurs in 15 to 29% of patients resulting from (1) electrical injury by passage of current through the nerve, (2) edema with elevated tissue pressure, (3) metabolic abnormalities and nutritional deficiencies, and (4) localized nerve compression or stretch injury from improper dressings or positioning.

Heterotopic bone formation around joints may cause a disabling complication in 2 to 3% of patients with burns who are hospitalized. The most common site of heterotopic calcification following burn injury is the elbow. The calcification is usually located posteriorly and medially with a bony bridge between the olecranon of the ulna and the medial epicondyle and intercondylar portion and posterior shaft of the humerus. Heterotopic bone formation is rare in children but may be evident in the adolescent population. Treatment consists of continuing physical therapy efforts at remobilization of the joint. Heterotopic bone disappears spontaneously in about one half of the cases. If excision is indicated, heterotopic ossification usually does not re-form after removal, and functional and often normal ROM is restored.

The patient with associated limb amputation presents a number of unique problems (Ward et al., 1990a), including intolerance of the stump to pressure or manipulation because of remaining open wounds, fragility of newly healed skin grafts, and wounds on other body surface areas. There is also an increased risk of developing joint contractures because of hypertrophic scarring and the inevitable loss of muscle strength from bed rest after surgery. Nevertheless, despite these problems, it appears that most patients with burns who require limb amputation can achieve successful prosthetic use (Ward et al., 1990b).

The impairments experienced by patients with severe burns who were grafted with cultured epithelial autografts have been outlined by Egan (1992). Cultured cells grow into very fragile skin that is highly susceptible to cuts and bruises and lacks tensile strength. These problems have persisted in patients grafted with cultured skin for as long as 2 years after initial treatment. Cultured skin also lacks any pigmentation and so is "blotchy white" and very susceptible to sunburn. Scarring occurs less often with cultured skin, but its fragility and lack of pigmentation present functional and cosmetic challenges, particularly to patients with black skin.

PHYSICAL THERAPY GOALS AND PROCEDURES

Examination, Evaluation, and Plan of Care

The purposes of the therapist's initial examination and evaluation are to determine the child's status, identify the rehabilitation needs, and anticipate the patient's potential problems. The first task is to ascertain the immediate postinjury status of the patient. The information necessary to make this determination includes an assessment of the circumstances of the injury; the duration, type, and extent of the burn; preexisting medical and rehabilitation problems; concurrent injuries; and ROM estimates. The developmental status of young children before the burn injury must be ascertained. The level of achievement of school-age children, both physically

and scholastically, should also be established to set realistic functional outcomes.

Identifying the rehabilitation needs of the child requires thorough evaluation of examination findings, as well as an understanding of the implications of different types of burns and their locations. For example, anticipated goals and outcomes will be achieved before the child's discharge home for burns that are likely to heal in 21 days. For deeper burns, whether or not the area is skin grafted, the child is likely to require outpatient physical therapy to ensure skin healing with minimal scarring and deformity with periodic team follow-up at the burn center. The expected clinical course and approximate length of stay of the patient should be estimated initially to anticipate potential emotional, physiologic, and rehabilitation problems.

Physical therapy examination in the postacute stage should consist of the following: burn scar assessment (scar mobility, turgor, and texture), ROM of joints adjacent to burned areas, pain, gait, and functional ability. Goals of the therapy program at this stage are based on the child's status, the effectiveness of the treatment procedures performed during the acute care period or after previous reconstructive operations, and the compliance of patient and family. Goals must be discussed with the child who is old enough to understand and in every case with the family.

The advent of managed health care has contributed to changes in the role of the physical therapist. In recent years, the role of the physical therapist has expanded from examination and intervention to reduce impairments such as edema, scarring, joint contracture, and muscle weakness and restore function to include prevention of disability in home, school, and work settings; establishment of a time frame for attainment of goals and outcomes; documentation of goals and outcomes; education of managed care personnel, families, employers, case managers, and the medical team; and coordination of care.

The emphasis of physical therapy is on functional outcomes that prevent or reduce disability (Fletchall & Hickerson, 1997). Outcomes, therefore, should be client focused and important for function. Client-focused outcomes to prevent or reduce disability for children include ability to perform self-care and mobility and engage in age-appropriate roles within the family and during play, school, and work. Establishment of functional outcomes for children who have difficulty communicating their needs and concerns can be challenging and is best performed within the context of family-centered care. Interviewing and clinical reasoning skills and the experience of the therapist are vital in evaluating the needs of a child and family and in determining outcomes that have a high probability of being achieved within a specific time frame.

The American Burn Association (1996) has published patient outcomes for the different phases of recovery (Staley & Richard, 1996). As part of this document, clinical indicators were established to assist service providers in evaluating patient progress in meeting desired outcomes. Having identified outcomes for burn care, the next step is the development of critical pathways that reflect best practice. Critical pathways can assist in identifying and quantifying differences between expected and actual outcomes. The functional-based outcomes that are the end points of a critical pathway are the focus of the rehabilitation program, including the following: examination, direct intervention, patient/client-related instruction and education, patient satisfaction, and cost containment. Program evaluation and clinical research are the means to evaluate the effectiveness of a critical pathway and make modifications when necessary.

The elements of patient/client management in the *Guide to Physical Therapist Practice* (American Physical Therapy Association 1997) describes a process for making clinical decisions for optimal intervention outcomes. Through the examination (history, systems review, and administration of tests and measures), the physical therapist identifies impairments, functional limitations, disabilities, or changes in physical function and health status to establish the prognosis (determination of the optimal level of improvement that might be attained and the amount of time required to reach that level) and to develop the plan of care (which specifies anticipated goals and desired outcomes, specific direct interventions, the frequency of visits, and criteria for discharge). The child, family, and caregivers participate by reporting activity performance and functional ability. The selection of examination procedures and the depth of the examination vary based on patient age; severity of the problem; stage of recovery; phase of rehabilitation; home, community, or work (job/school/play) situation; and other relevant factors. Examination procedures specific to a child with a burn include the following: assessment of the burn, including bleeding, signs of infection, and exposed anatomic structures; assessment of wound tissue, including epithelium, granulation, mobility, necrosis, slough, texture, and turgor; assessment of activities and postures that aggravate the wound or scar; and assessment of scar tissue, including banding, pliability, sensation, texture, and pigmentation. Integumentary preferred practice patterns C, D, and E describe the elements of patient/client management for burns (American Physical Therapy Association, 1997).

Once the examination and evaluation are completed, an individualized plan of care is established in collaboration with the child, family, and other members of the burn care team. The plan of care includes the goals and outcomes and direct interventions. The plan is developed with the primary focus on prevention of deformities, and interventions vary with the stages of wound recovery. Throughout implementation, the plan of care is coordinated closely with interventions provided by other team members, because outcomes are multidisciplinary. Success depends not on an individual discipline but rather on the cooperation and knowledge of each team member. Many patients hospitalized for care of burn injuries show transient psychologic distress independent of such factors as burn size and premorbid function. Patients with severe burns, resulting in extended hospitalization, are particularly vulnerable to development of psychologic distress. The repeated, intrusive, and aggressive nature of burn care, although necessary for survival, may contribute to feelings of loss of control. The symptoms seen in children include regression, anxiety, decreased physical activity, withdrawal, behavior problems, decreased social interaction and play, and other depressive symptoms. The quota system (Ehde et al., 1998) has been shown to be an effective new approach to helplessness behaviors and depressive symptoms that develop in some patients with burn injuries.

The deforming effects of burn scar contractures can be decreased by use of the following direct interventions: proper patient positioning and use of splints, ROM and graded resistive exercises, early ambulation, scar management techniques, and patient and family education regarding skin care and the rehabilitation program. Other modalities such as continuous passive motion, fluidotherapy, and paraffin all aid in increasing skin pliability and desensitizing the healed burn area. The plan of care should also include play activities and training in functional activities to facilitate the development of coping behavior. The child should be allowed as much self-care as is possible, depending on the stage of recovery. Participation in dressing changes, decision making when confronted with equal alternatives, and personal hygiene must be encouraged to give the child a sense of control. An overview of treatment options by body part burned is presented in Table 29-3.

Positioning and Splints

Positioning must be individualized to the child's need. A series of positions should be designed for each involved joint, whereby the child alternates positions every 2 to 4 hours, because static positioning is not well tolerated. When skin grafts or biologic

TABLE 29-3. **Treatment Options by Body Part**

Involved Area	Exercise	Positioning	Splinting	Pressure
Face, head	Massage Facial exercises, eye blinking Mouth opening, chewing Therabite	No pillow Elevate head of bed	Microstomia prevention Appliance Tongue blades Nasal splints	Custom elastomer mask Custom fabric hood Chin strap Clear mask with silicone
Neck	Neck ROM Wedge	No pillow Split mattress	Neck conformer Soft collar	Neck conformer Elastomer insert Silicone wrap
Axilla	Abduction/flexion exercises Overhead pulleys Finger ladder, wand exercises Wall weights Shoulder continuous passive motion (CPM)	Arm trough Papoose Sheepskin slings Bedside table	Axillary conformer	Padded figure-of-eight wrap Clavicle strap Custom vest Inserts
Elbow	Wall weights Barbells Pronation exerciser	Extension Supination	Anterior conformer Cast	Tubigrip Custom sleeve Silicone sleeve
Wrist, hand	Hand exercises Gripping devices Hand CPM	Elevation above heart Flexion wrap	Wrist cock-up splint Burn hand splint Pan extension splint	Coban Isotoner gloves Custom gloves Web spacers Silicone inserts
Trunk, buttock, hip	Ambulation Trunk stretches	Proning No pillow under knees Special beds	T-shirt splint Hip spica splint Bivalved cast	Custom pantyhose Bicycle shorts Breast plate Silicone patches
Knee	Ambulation Exercise bike Knee CPM Stairs	No pillow under knees Prevent frog lying	Knee conformer Knee immobilizer	Tubigrip Custom stockings
Ankle, foot	Ambulation Ankle circles Toe stretches Stairs	Foam heel protectors	Posterior foot splint Derotational splint Unna boot Toe flexion splint Burn shoe	Tubigrip Custom socks Toe web spacers Dorsal silicone inserts

dressings are required, accurate positioning contributes to good wound coverage. One of the many benefits of an early positioning program is reduction of edema in the extremities, allowing return of functional movement. Elevating the extremities allows reduction of edema, utilizing the pull of gravity. Proper positioning can help maintain ROM and counteract contracture by maintaining proper flexibility of connective tissue and skin. Methods of positioning are illustrated in Figure 29-2.

Children usually have difficulty understanding the long-range benefits of positioning procedures. Often, a splint is the most appropriate and effective method for proper positioning, especially during unsupervised periods and during sleep, when posi-

tions that contribute to deformity are often assumed. When the child is able to be active during the day, a night splint may be indicated to maintain ROM gained during the day. When voluntary movement is impaired, as in the presence of peripheral neuropathies, a splint must be worn continuously to avoid joint contracture. Wearing a splint 24 hours a day is also indicated to maintain slack on exposed tendons until wound closure occurs. Examples of splints used for children with burns are illustrated in Figure 29-3.

Clarke and colleagues (1990) noted that in children burns to the hand typically result from a different pattern of injury and respond differently to therapeutic intervention when compared with the adult

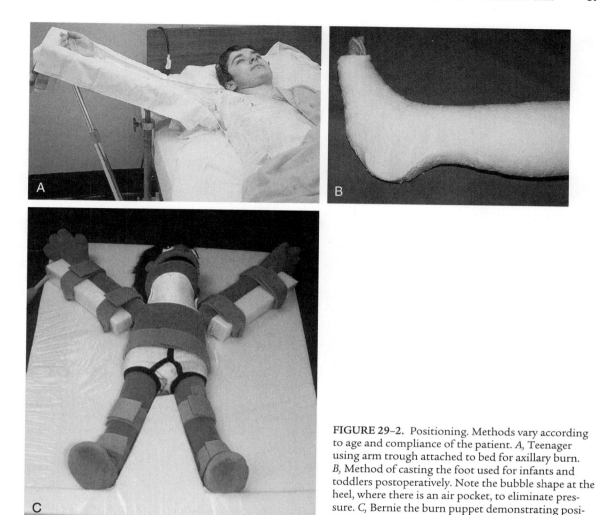

FIGURE 29–2. Positioning. Methods vary according to age and compliance of the patient. *A,* Teenager using arm trough attached to bed for axillary burn. *B,* Method of casting the foot used for infants and toddlers postoperatively. Note the bubble shape at the heel, where there is an air pocket, to eliminate pressure. *C,* Bernie the burn puppet demonstrating positioning in a foam papoose.

hand. Scald burns are most common in children. Children develop less stiffness in response to immobilization but tend to form more scar tissue compared with adults. Hand function therefore can be achieved in the majority of cases. However, deep flame injuries to the hand present a specific challenge to the rehabilitation team. The small size of the hands of young children and the lack of muscle strength to oppose the force of the contracting burn pose a challenge to splint fabrication.

These potential problems can be managed with the full participation of the burn team, the child, and the family. Warden and associates (1993) demonstrated that individuals with severe hand burns necessitating partial joint amputation or individuals with exposed joints and tendons can achieve functional outcomes during the initial acute hospitaliza-

tion when care is provided in a coordinated and efficient manner.

Factors to consider in a splint include construction, correct fit, application, and adjustment. A pliable, lightweight, low-heat thermoplastic material is desirable. Bulky dressings should be minimized because they interfere with the fit of the splint and compromise alignment. Splints must be checked at least once daily and necessary adjustments made. Pain, numbness, tingling, inflammation, or maceration of tissue indicates a poor-fitting or improperly applied splint, which can cause pressure necrosis of burned and unburned areas. Immediate adjustment is mandatory to prevent further damage.

Splints are also used to reduce contracture and thereby preclude or minimize the need for extensive reconstructive surgery. Children who are developing

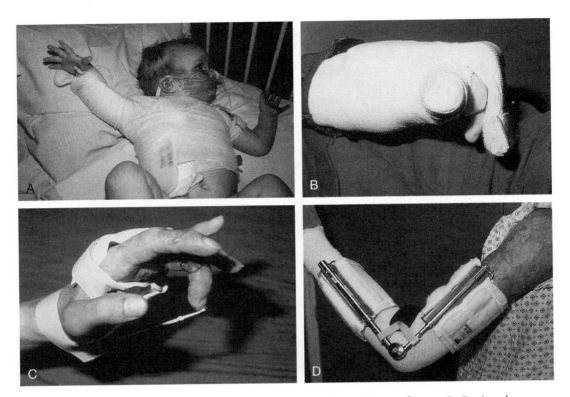

FIGURE 29–3. Splints used for children with burns. *A,* Custom-molded axillary conformer. *B,* Casting the metacarpopha-langeal joints into flexion. Note that this cast controls positioning of the first web space and allows for interphalangeal flexion of the fingers. *C,* Simple rubberband traction to provide gentle dynamic stretch to middle finger. *D,* Progressive stretch applied by dialing tension in this three-point elbow flexion dynasplint.

contractures or scar bands over the volar aspect of the hand, wrist, elbow, posterior knee, or dorsum of the ankle and foot are fitted with conforming splints to oppose contracture formation by producing a softening and flattening effect on the scar band, which then allows increased skin excursion. Frequently, these splints are worn at night only, and the child is encouraged to move actively during the day. As range of motion increases, the splint is remolded progressively until proper alignment of the part is achieved. The anterior surface of the neck is one area where a conforming splint worn at all times except for bath, meals, and exercise can be effective in maintaining ROM and skin contour.

Types of splints for different joints are described by Willis (1970), Pullium (1984), and Richard and Staley (1993). More recent studies describe innovative splint designs. The "T-shirt" splint, named for its appearance, is one method for prevention or reduction of postural deviations and ROM resulting from deep burns of the neck, chest, and axillae (Gilliam et al., 1993). An ankle-foot orthosis consisting of a footplate and two supports, one on the

medial and one on the lateral aspect of the leg, is described by Bennett and co-workers (1993). Using this design allows the calcaneal region to be free of pressure, decreasing the risk of skin breakdown.

Dynamic splints are the most effective method of reducing contractures involving the extensor surfaces of the wrist, hand, and posterior elbow. The proximity of the extensor tendons to the burned surface may result in scar adhesions forming around or attaching to the tendon. Dynamic splints that apply elastic tension in opposition to the contracture but allow controlled resisted motion force excursion of the tendon through the scar formation. Application of constant tension is necessary to elongate tissue. A dynamic elbow extension splint was reported as superior to a static splint when used to correct progressive loss of elbow range of motion (Richard et al., 1995). Dynamic orthoses, such as Dynasplint and Ultraflex Systems, have been reported as effective in patients with burns (Richard, 1986; Richard et al., 1988). These orthoses apply three-point pressure, are spring-loaded, and are designed to deliver a low-load, prolonged stretch to healing connective tissue. Pediatric sizes are available.

Serial casting may be a successful alternative when low-force dynamic splints cannot be sized small enough for a child or when patient compliance is unreliable. The goal in serial casting is gradual realignment of the collagen in a parallel and lengthened state by constant circumferential pressure from the cast, which cannot be removed by the patient. When casts are applied well and padded appropriately, there is little risk of pressure areas, because the casts are conforming and do not slip distally. Following serial casting for 7 days, the more traditional methods of treatment (paraffin, massage, ROM exercise, and splints) are continued to preserve the increased movement. Casts also delay or eliminate the need for surgical correction (Bennett et al., 1989). Serial casting has been shown to be highly effective in increasing ROM of the burned foot (Ridgway et al., 1991; Johnson & Silverberg, 1995) and the burned hand (Harris et al., 1993). The fabrication and use of removable digit casts to improve ROM at the proximal interphalangeal joint have also been described (Torres-Gray et al., 1993).

Severe fixed ankle and foot deformities may occur when optimal positioning is not possible, such as when air-fluidized beds are used. The typical deformities include ankle plantar flexion and varus (equinovarus) and forefoot adduction and supination. External fixators have been introduced in burn management. A clinical report by Metzger and coworkers (1993) describes the use of Brooker and Hoffman fixators, which can be used to arrest further deformity but do not allow for correction, and Ilizarov fixators, which allow a multidimensional application of force to achieve anatomically correct positioning. The use of fixators, and the Ilizarov fixator in particular, is superior to splinting because of the propensity for formation of decubiti when rigid splints are used.

Exercise and Activities

The child who has been burned tends to avoid movement, or, at best, moves rigidly and slowly. Structured exercise programs, therefore, are needed to prevent undesirable burn wound healing sequelae. Although physical therapists have primary responsibility for implementation of these programs, optimal physical restoration will largely depend on the combined and concentrated efforts of all team members, the child, and the family.

Many factors influence the therapist's ability to provide adequate exercise for children with burn injuries. Pain, surgical procedures, wound complications, and the child's and the family's adjustment to the injury affect therapy. The therapist's skill in determining when to initiate exercise, choosing the type of exercise, and transferring of care to the child and family are important determinants of function outcomes and the duration of the rehabilitation program.

Although children recovering from burns share common problems, the exercise program must be customized to each child's unique needs. Exercises for specific problems encountered by burn patients have been published (Nothdurft et al., 1984; Richard & Staley, 1993). Therapists often need to be creative with exercises. Written instructions are needed for parents to supervise young children and for older children to assume responsibility for their exercise program. Hayes-Lundy and associates (1993) performed a pilot study to test the usefulness of a computer-generated exercise program to create customized exercise programs for patients. Patients given computer-generated programs performed their exercises with an 88% success rate, compared with a 54% success rate for patients given handwritten programs. Several exercise software packages are available commercially.

Goals and the type of exercise needed for each stage of recovery are outlined in Table 29-4, and examples of exercises and activities are illustrated in Figure 29-4. The type and intensity of exercise are progressed according to the child's recovery status. During the emergent or resuscitative period, emphasis of treatment is placed on positioning and splinting. However, if the child is alert, he or she may be able to engage in some movement activities such as bed mobility and positioning of extremities for dressing applications. Exercise is initiated for most patients as soon as adequate signs of burn shock resuscitation have been observed, generally within the first 24 to 72 hours after injury. Escharotomies do not preclude exercise. Exercises that would compromise or dislodge lines and airways are withheld, and emphasis is placed on positioning.

As the child makes the transition from the emergent phase to the acute phase of burn rehabilitation, the physical treatment program must also change to meet the patient's needs. The acute phase generally refers to the time period after emergent care through wound coverage, when the foundations of scarring are just beginning to form. Joint contracture is a major threat during this period.

Exercises are performed with each joint separately, then with all joints combined in a gentle sustained stretch that elongates the burned area. This is especially important when the burn crosses more than one joint. Richard and colleagues (1994, 1999) reported that a measurable amount of forearm skin movement occurs to permit wrist extension. In

TABLE 29–4. **Exercise Goals for Each Stage of Recovery**

Stage	Exercise Goals	Methods
Emergent	1. Edema resolution 2. Maintenance of joint mobility 3. Prevention of respiratory complications	Slow, gentle active or active-assistive ROM 2–4 times/day
Acute	1. Stretch healing skin 2. Maintain full joint ROM 3. Preserve coordination of multiple joint movements 4. Promote functional independence 5. Minimize muscular atrophy	ROM exercises Functional activities Ambulation
Postacute/Rehabilitation	1. Increase joint ROM 2. Prevent/correct contracture 3. Strengthen and recondition 4. Maximize functional abilities	ROM/ADL/ambulation programs, incorporating stretching, coordination, strengthening, endurance, and conditioning

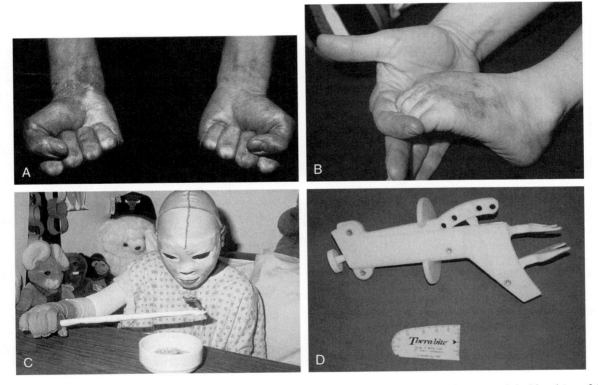

FIGURE 29–4. Exercise and activity. *A,* Full active ROM of hands. Note that fingernails cannot be seen and the blanching of the skin over the proximal interphalangeal joints. *B,* Full passive flexion of the toes, in combination with ankle plantar flexion, indicating full extensibility of the healing skin. *C,* Everyday activities maintain mobility achieved by ROM exercises. This child has been given an extended-length spoon handle to accommodate the flexion deficit from heterotopic bone at the elbow. *D,* The Therabite jaw exerciser has proved to be effective in maintaining a stretch of the oral commissures in all directions. It can be patient controlled or fixed and (shortened) used as a static splint. The unit allows normal motion of the temporomandibular joint.

addition, the position of the elbow influences the amount of elongation of skin tissue necessary for wrist extension. Multiple vigorous repetitions of movement should be avoided. Active and active-assistive ROM with terminal stretch aids in maintaining joint mobility and tissue pliability, as well as minimizing loss of strength. Many patients will lose ROM if left to do exercises on their own, despite verbal encouragement. This is particularly true with children. Burns around the mouth frequently result in contractures or microstomia. Over the years different orthoses have been used to stretch the mouth. In the past, the only true stretch achieved was horizontal. A device has been introduced that comfortably provides vertical and horizontal passive range of motion and can be adapted and used by children who demonstrate fair to good compliance (Ridgway & Warden, 1995).

Compared with adults, children exhibit increased pain reactions during exercise, often owing to fear and apprehension. Coordinating administration of pain medications with the nursing staff before exercise sessions greatly enhances the quality of exercise and amount of cooperation offered by the patient. It is also helpful for patient relaxation to initiate the exercise treatment with nonpainful or less painful exercises and gradually progress to the more painful exercises. Field (1995) reported that massage results in lower anxiety and stress hormones and improved clinical course. Patients with burns who received massage before debridement demonstrated specific immediate and longer-term effects (Field et al., 1998). The positive effects may be attributable to reduction in pain, anger, and depression.

Other specific management techniques used for pain control include anesthesia, hypnosis, and behavioral modification. The reinforcement given by way of reward for lack of negative response to pain has proved to be a successful management technique (Varni et al., 1980). Behavioral techniques such as desensitization, modeling, operant conditioning, and environmental manipulation have also been used successfully. Recent studies also discuss important developmental considerations regarding the adequate assessment of pain and distress (Foertsch et al., 1998). The importance of pain management cannot be overemphasized. Any safe and effective method should be used.

Play and group activities are fun and allow children increased control. Play is perhaps the best method to elicit desired active movement in young children. A report by Mahaney (1990) describes the loss of a severely burned child's ability to play and outlines the critical importance of play in the development of cognition, affectivity, and social learning (areas related to coping behavior). In addition,

implementing music therapy techniques during exercise sessions may provide an organizing structure within which rehabilitative and developmental gains can occur. Use of empathy, empowerment of caregivers, modeling, and coaching techniques encourages a positive working alliance with caregivers and allows for successful transfer of the intervention to the family (Badger et al., 1993).

If pain control, relaxation, and exercise techniques have failed to maintain joint range, ROM exercise performed while the patient is under anesthesia is sometimes recommended to determine the extent of joint restriction and as an adjunct to routine exercise sessions (Nicosia et al., 1979). This is a particularly beneficial procedure when assessing whether the child's fear, apprehension, or manipulative behavior is interfering with achieving the goals of exercise sessions.

After grafting, exercise to the grafted area is discontinued for approximately 5 days to encourage incorporation of the graft into the wound bed. Proper patient positioning is stressed at this time. Exercise is also withheld to joints proximal and distal to the grafted area, which, if exercised, might influence graft stability. Active and active-assistive ROM exercises to all other nongrafted areas are continued. On removal of staples or sutures, if the graft appears stable, exercise to the grafted area can be resumed with approval from the attending physician. It is wise for the therapist to observe dressing changes to identify areas of graft slough and possible tendon exposure.

It is typical that ROM decreases during the immobilization period after grafting. A general theory is that approximately 25% of the motion is lost during the postgraft stage (Artz et al., 1979). However, the patient who maintains essentially normal ROM during the pregrafting phase has a good prognosis to regain ROM. With most patients, full joint motion is expected 7 to 10 days after grafting.

As healing progresses, either spontaneously or after grafting, functional strengthening is introduced into the exercise program. Even if the child has open wounds and bandages, minimal manual resistance by the therapist is begun for initial strengthening. Resistance to isotonic contraction can be applied gently, or the child is asked to maintain a position and then resistance is applied.

The postacute rehabilitative phase begins when the catabolic state reverses and there are few unhealed burn areas. This is the difficult and lengthy phase of wound contracture and hypertrophic scarring in which physical function and appearance can be altered significantly. A child who heals initially with full ROM has the potential to develop severe deformities during the postacute period as the healed skin matures and hypertrophic scarring develops. Sustained stretching is one of the most effective exercise techniques for lengthening bands of scar tissue and increasing ROM. Active-assistive ROM with the therapist applying mild manual stretching at the extremes of motion is well tolerated. Skin should be stretched to the point of blanching. Holding the stretch for counts of 10 or 15 is recommended at the terminal point of stretch as tolerated. Whenever possible, overall patterns of motion are emphasized because scar tissue may cause profound limitations of motion when multiple joints are involved.

Coordinated movement is generally diminished after burn injury. It is essential that substitution patterns be recognized and altered before they become deeply ingrained as conditioned responses. Coordination exercises are extremely beneficial in eliminating the mechanical robot-like postures and movements frequently characteristic of patients with burns. In children, the application of neurodevelopmental treatment techniques provides a holistic means to address the goal of increased ROM by enhancing postural stability, mobility, and achievement of age-appropriate developmental milestones. By using this approach, Burne and colleagues (1993) have shown that therapeutic technique can be more easily incorporated into the child's home life through parent teaching, focusing on everyday activities, and consideration of the family's lifestyle.

Careful integration of physical conditioning with all other postacute rehabilitation exercise programs enhances the patient's restoration to a normal lifestyle. When possible, conditioning exercise incorporates activities enjoyable to the child, such as bicycling, dancing, or swimming, and provides the child not only with a sense of physical well-being but also with an opportunity for social interaction.

Ambulation

The ability to move about has a significant impact on the restoration of independence. Children begin to ambulate as soon as their physical condition warrants, usually by 48 to 72 hours after injury, when vital signs are stable and fluid resuscitation is complete. With proper precautions and necessary staff participation, children in the burn unit are assisted in ambulation to the limits of their physical endurance. Technical maneuvers and precautions have been developed by Hollowed and associates (1993) that ensure safety during ambulation of patients who are intubated. Beginning ambulation while the patient is still intubated was effective in reducing pulmonary complications and has increased the survival rate in patients with acute burns from 88 to 95%. The more involved case may require greater

planning. Transferring a child to a tilt table sometimes is the only way to progress the patient to weight bearing.

For nongrafted lower extremity burns, ambulation is initiated once the child is medically stable unless tendons or joint capsules are exposed, severe swelling or cellulitis is present, or the soles of the feet are severely burned. Mild to moderate burns of the feet do not preclude early ambulation. Dressings with extra padding and foam-soled slippers will protect the wounds and aid in reducing the discomfort of bearing weight. To avoid venous stasis in lower extremities and discomfort associated with upright positions, elastic bandages are applied from toe to groin before standing, and full weight bearing is encouraged. A figure-of-eight wrap is used, because this provides an even distribution of pressure and better support for the extremity than do circular wraps.

Assistive devices such as walkers, crutches, and canes are not encouraged, and use of a normal gait pattern is emphasized. However, young children often show regression in walking, particularly if they had been ambulating only a few weeks before the burn injury. Knowing what the child wants to play with or walk to may be the key to initiating ambulation (Johnson, 1984a). Toys such as Hot Wheels or tricycles can be great incentives. For the younger or smaller child, a circular walker allows the child to move around independently, but close supervision is needed for safe activity.

When to initiate ambulation after grafting is controversial. A prospective study by Schmitt and associates (1991) indicated a significant reduction (mean of 4.1 days) in length of hospital stay when patients who ambulated on postoperative day 7 were compared with patients who ambulated on postoperative day 11. Results of a study by Kowalske and colleagues (1993) found no difference in graft take or time to complete wound closure following lower extremity skin grafting between early (postoperative day 3 or 4) and late (postoperative day 7, 8, or 9) ambulators. Increased skin graft loss was, however, seen in patients whose physical conditions prohibited ambulation on the randomly assigned day.

The child with a less complicated burn can master the progression of walking with few problems. Dr. Paul Unna's "boot," a zinc oxide–calamine–gelatin bandage, has been marketed under various names such as Medicopaste (Graham-Field, Inc., Hauppage, NY 11788) and Primer (Glenwood, Inc., Tenafly, NJ 07670). It has been used with small wounds to allow patients to ambulate within 48 hours after grafting (Harnar et al., 1982). Wells and co-workers (1995) demonstrated a mean reduction in hospital stay from 12.9 days to 1.4 days, for a group of patients with uncomplicated noncircumferential lower extremity burns who were treated with split-thickness skin grafting and Unna paste. The Unna dressing has also proved to be effective in the outpatient management of skin grafts to the hands (Sanford & Gore, 1996).

Pressure Garments and Inserts

Hypertrophic scarring remains a major problem for the recovering patient. The mainstay of treatment is controlled pressure to the involved areas with Coban or Ace bandages and presized or custom-fit elastic garments. Inserts of rubber, foam, or gel materials have been used to improve the response to pressure. In the early 1970s, the use of pressure for the treatment of hypertrophic scars or keloids and severe contractures became a standard treatment in every burn facility. Historically, the use of controlled pressure originated and was promoted by the clinical and basic sciences approach developed by the wound healing team of the Shriners Burns Institute at Galveston, Texas (Linares et al., 1993). Although the exact mechanism of action is unknown, pressure appears clinically to enhance the scar maturation process (Staley & Richard, 1997).

The following guidelines on the characteristics of burn treatment can help the therapist select methods of pressure: (1) healing time of the burn, (2) size of the unhealed areas, (3) fragility or condition of the healed skin, (4) location of the burn, and (5) treatment cost (Johnson, 1984b). Briefly, all patients whose burns require 14 to 21 days to heal and who

have areas grafted with split-thickness grafts should have prophylactic pressure therapy. Lower extremity burns may require pressure not only to minimize scarring but also to minimize persistent edema and discoloration. Pressure should be applied as early as possible. The type of pressure, however, will depend on the fragility of the newly healed skin and remaining open areas.

Signs that the pressure program has been successful can be seen as early as 24 to 48 hours after the initial application. Immediately after the removal of the garment, evidence of clinically significant pressure includes blanching of scar tissue, flattening of the scar, increased softness, decreased edema, minimal blistering, and no tingling or numbness. If any of these effects are not observed, the therapist should consider the following reasons: (1) fit of garment— if the patient has gained or lost more than 10 pounds, this may be enough to decrease the pressure garment's effectiveness; and (2) condition of a garment—the wear life of pressure garments for the average patient is 3 months. If the garment loses its stretch and does not cause blanching of the scar, it has lost its effectiveness and new garments must be made. Studies indicate that the amount of pressure being provided by the garment can be measured easily and accurately (Mann et al., 1997). The I-Scan system, shown in Figure 29–5, simplifies the accurate measurement of garment-scar interface. Trouble spots receiving too much or too little pressure can be identified and altered.

When isolated areas of hypertrophy remain, sufficient pressure has not been applied. Areas where this

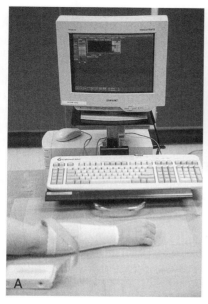
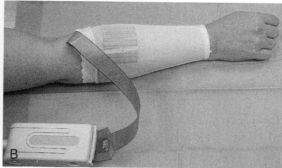

FIGURE 29–5. Measuring pressure. *A,* The I-Scan system has been developed to accurately record the amount of pressure provided by garments and other pressure devices. *B,* The I-Scan sensor shown in place under a custom forearm sleeve.

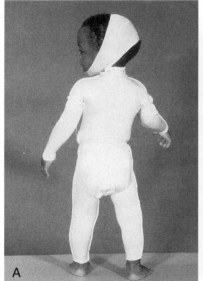
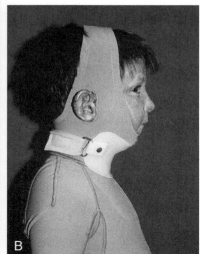

FIGURE 29–6. Pressure garments. A, Interim pressure can be provided by soft fabric standard-sized garments. B, Custom-fit garments. Extra pressure is often needed to further enhance effectiveness of the garments, as illustrated by the silicone pad under the elastic vest and application of the conforming neck splint.

commonly occurs include the sternum, face, volar aspect of the hand, angle of the mandible, web spaces, and across the flexor surfaces of the joint. Pressure garments frequently need to be supplemented by inserts in these areas to exert the needed pressure (Fig. 29–7). Characteristics to be considered in choosing the composition of the insert include its texture, flexibility, compressibility, and ability to conform. For effectiveness, an insert must be worn for the same amount of time as the pressure garment (23 hours per day). A multidisciplinary team representing physical therapy, computer-aided design and computer-aided manufacturing (CAD/CAM), biomedical engineering, and prosthetics has advanced the method of developing total-contact burn masks by use of human body electronic imaging, computer graphics, and numerically controlled milling processes. High-resolution surface scanning and CAD/CAM have been used successfully to accurately fabricate masks (Whitestone et al., 1995).

A thorough knowledge of properties of all available inserts is required to provide an effective pressure program. No single material suffices for all the situations in which an insert is indicated. Information regarding the qualities of various materials for pressure inserts is described by Alston and associates (1981), Perkins and colleagues (1987), and Ainsworth and co-workers (1993). Many patients and therapists report difficulties when using silicone or other types of inserts under garments. The most common problems include irritation of skin from the pad, limited joint motion, sweating, annoying

odor, and movement of the insert. One resourceful method used to apply a silicone elastomer pad beneath a pressure garment was described by Van den Kerckhove and colleagues (1991). Elastomer is molded on the patient between layers of Tubi-Grip. Another system for making a custom pocket has been described by Taylor (1993). Extra material in the form of a pocket can be stitched into the external vascular support to keep an insert from shifting its position and provide a soft, breathable, contact layer to the skin.

There appears to be consensus in the literature that silicone pads are especially effective in diminishing the thickness of the scar. Some authors suggest that this happens only in the body areas where high pressure was maintained (Van den Kerckhove et al., 1991). Others have reported that silicone products induce a positive effect on burn scars without pressure (Davey, 1997). Good results can be obtained even with old scars (Quin, 1987; Van den Kerckhove et al., 1991).

The face is particularly difficult to fit accurately, and face masks such as those shown in Figure 29–7 require frequent monitoring and modification. Caution and close monitoring of pressure garments is essential, particularly when face masks are used in the young growing child. Two studies suggest serious complications in children with head and neck burns. Fricke and colleagues (1999) demonstrated changes in growth direction of the mandible and maxilla after consistent application of the total face mask. In addition, Chester and associates (1993)

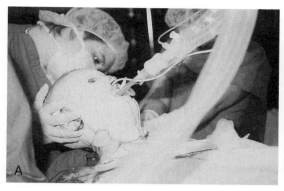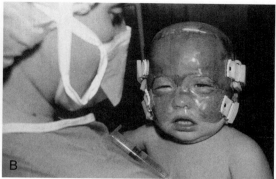

FIGURE 29-7. Face mask. Because of the many concavities on the face, custom-molded face masks are needed to provide pressure to the entire surface. *A,* Custom-molded silicone elastomer face mask being applied in the operating room, immediately following skin grafting. It is held in place with a modified featureless fabric hood. *B,* For long-term pressure, hard, clear, molded face masks can be used if the patient is able to keep frequent appointments for adjustments and modifications.

claim that the most common cause of obstructive sleep apnea is excessive pressure on the mandible by compression garments, particularly chin straps.

Compliance with wearing correctly applied pressure garments for effective scar control is crucial for burn survivors. External pressure support is prescribed to be worn 23 hours a day until the remodeling phase of healing is complete. Spurr and Shakespeare (1990) list the difficulties that arise with a pressure garment program. Pressure garment therapy is long lasting, inconvenient for patients, and relatively expensive. There is no guarantee that the child and parents will comply with the advice given to wear the garments. One study of adult patient compliance with pressure therapy determined that total compliance was less than 50% (Greenspan et al., 1993). Factors affecting compliance included patient's reported perception of the burn and garment, understanding of the pressure program and its effect, psychosocial influences, garment-specific factors, and the level of functional independence related to the burn and garment use. The identification of factors that affect garment use is therefore critical in formulating strategies to improve adherence.

A modification in garment design was introduced for patients who had cultured epithelial autograft (CEA) for the treatment of burn wounds (Wood et al., 1996). The garment design was changed to pay particular attention to reduction of shearing forces and dissipation of pressure. Hydrophobic fabric as a lining garment was introduced and is beneficial in reducing surface maceration and shearing injury.

An example of garment design modification to enhance compliance for children who wear diapers has been reported (Schwartz et al., 1993). Pediatric patients in diapers are difficult to fit with external vascular support garments. Soft diapers under a leotard decrease the amount of compression applied to buttock scars. Although the healing wound, donor site, or graft remains active, the scar tissue remains painful or pruritic whenever the garment is removed. If the infant excoriates the scars when the garment is off, the scars become thicker and more painful. The discomfort of frequent diaper changes stresses parents, contributing to poor compliance with garment application. A three-piece leotard was designed with detachable legs and an open crotch. The "brief" portion of the garment can be replaced without removing the stocking portions, and the open crotch allows ready diaper change without removing any portion of the garment. Repetitive shearing over fragile epithelium is minimized, and caregiver participation is enhanced, with subsequent optimal cosmetic and functional outcomes for the toddler. The introduction of colored pressure garments may increase social acceptance and contribute to better compliance (Thompson et al., 1992).

As scar tissue approaches maturity, the hyperemia fades and the scar flattens and becomes more pliable and soft. When these qualities persist for several weeks after removal of the pressure garments, the scar tissue is mature, and the garments and inserts may then be discontinued.

Other Modalities

Numerous modalities, each having a specific physiologic effect, are available in rehabilitation. Only the more commonly accepted modalities for the management of impairments of patients with burns will be addressed. These are paraffin, ultrasound, continuous passive motion, and fluidotherapy.

The combination of paraffin and sustained stretch usually is introduced late in the acute phase of rehabilitation after major healing has occurred, and it is generally continued throughout the patient's rehabilitation. The use of paraffin is particularly indicated when a painful and contracting scar limits joint ROM. The superficial heat and lubrication reduce scar pain and improve scar extensibility (Head & Helm, 1977; Nothdurft et al., 1984). The paraffin mixture is used when it reaches a temperature of 46° to 48°C or when a light skim covers the top of the mixture. Caution is suggested for newly healed scar tissue, which will blister easily if the standard paraffin bath temperature is used. Pouring or patting of the paraffin is done after the patient is positioned with the affected part in a sustained maximum stretch. The treatment time is 20 to 30 minutes. Patients report decreased joint pain, and objective measurements show a 5 to 10° increase in ROM after paraffin treatment. Claims that the results last up to 4 hours have been reported (Head & Helm, 1977).

Application of topical ultrasound directly to burn scars produces a rise in deep tissue temperature that is reported to increase extensibility of collagen and decrease pain associated with stretching (Belenger et al., 1969; Rozanova, 1979; Wright & Haase, 1971). However, a randomized blinded study by Ward and associates (1994) compared results of patients who received standard burn physical therapy and topical ultrasound with patients who received standard care alone. Statistical analysis revealed no differences in ROM or perceived pain between the two groups. Furthermore, there was no discernible trend toward subjective or objective improvements with ultrasound treatment.

Continuous passive motion has been shown to be beneficial in the rehabilitation of thermal injuries (Covey, 1988). This modality is limited to older children and adolescents, because infant- and pediatric-sized units have not been developed. In addition to the general effects of continuous passive motion (including delivery of a specific arc of motion at a specific speed and constant control of rate and degree of motion, which fosters patient relaxation and increased ROM), the autorange or continuous passive motion unit can be adjusted to maintain the extremity at the end of its available range for a regulated amount of time. Continuous passive motion should be used as an adjunct, and not as a replacement, for the traditional manual therapy techniques.

The fluidotherapy unit can be considered when seeking a thermotherapeutic agent to decrease pain or increase ROM in a body part, particularly a foot or a hand (Nothdurft et al., 1984). This high-intensity superficial heat modality consists of a dry whirlpool of finely divided solid particles suspended in a heated airstream. The use of fluidotherapy with burns is not well documented. The patient's skin durability and sensation must be evaluated before submersion in the unit. Periodic monitoring of the patient's skin responses while undergoing each treatment is imperative. The combination of the dry heat with the massaging solid particles, the allowance for active exercise while undergoing each treatment, and the fact that this unit can be used in the presence of open wounds (with protection of thin plastic or rubber gloves) are advantages of fluid therapy for the management of distal extremity problems in the older child or adolescent patient.

Family Education

It is crucial that the child's family understand the daily care that will be required at home. There may be extensive technical and medical information for parents to absorb, and it is best if the family begins early in the child's hospitalization to be instructed in all aspects of care and to ask questions, discuss treatments, and watch demonstrations. Some centers have found it helpful to create manuals to be reviewed with family members before discharge (Bochke, 1993; Reed & Heinle, 1993). In this way parents have a chance to absorb written material and to practice the child's care under supervision of the health care providers before discharge. Thus, when they arrive home with the child, they will feel more confident about their ability to carry out the required therapy. Special patient and family problems such as illiteracy, low learning levels, foreign languages, and deafness have also been addressed with customized guides, including pictorial guides, laminated flip charts, card file systems, audiotapes, videotapes, and photographic guides (Walling et al., 1993).

Indirect Services

Indirect services such as management, supervision, quality assurance, consultation, and research are also important components of the physical therapist's role in burn care (as have been described for occupational therapists by Kohlman-McGourty et al., 1985). Management is concerned with the delivery of effective care in a cost-efficient manner. Managed health care systems have affected burn care. Clients with managed health care insurance have experienced a lack of reimbursement for rehabilitation when functional outcomes are not achieved (Fletchall & Hickerson, 1997). Therapists must develop the ability to communicate and present data illustrating how therapy relates to costs, goals, outcomes, and time frames. Anticipating and developing rationales for burn rehabilitation can facilitate reimbursement, minimize delay between inpatient and outpatient therapy programs, and ensure optimal outcomes.

The quality and appropriateness of physical therapy services are monitored through the use of quality assurance programs, including participation in accreditation procedures. Technologic advances in the treatment of burn injuries offer ongoing opportunities for collaborative research to improve the quality of care of the child with burn injuries.

Outpatient Therapy and Follow-up

Perhaps the most difficult problem that a therapist faces during home care is the tendency for the child to manipulate his or her parents and thereby fail to carry out the prescribed home programs. This is particularly true if the parents feel guilty about the burn accident. Some children take advantage of feelings of guilt or sympathy and will resist therapy at home, even if they were cooperative while in the hospital. In conjunction with this, some parents also perceive their child to have more problems than the child or his or her teacher reports. Results of a study by Meyer and associates (1994) suggest that troubled parents may overestimate the difficulties of their child. Shelby and associates (1993) have identified additional family factors. Parents of children who sustained burns reported more depression and anxiety than spouses of adults who were burned. Higher somatic symptom reporting was associated with fewer social resources, higher anxiety, and depression. Lower somatic symptoms were seen in parents reporting high hardiness, esteem, and perceived family social support.

Most children continue to require daily therapy from a professional when they make the transition into postacute rehabilitation, although therapy services should serve a secondary role. Housinger and co-workers (1992) demonstrated that the success of pediatric outpatient rehabilitation is dependent on the dedicated effort of parents. Duration of sessions varies according to involvement and the child's tolerance. Moderate to major burns require anywhere from 1 to 5 hours of treatment per day, including rest periods. As the child demonstrates increased independence and goals are achieved, sessions are reduced to two to three times per week and eventually to weekly rechecks. Although therapy is demanding and crucial during this time, children should also be allowed time for other activities to make the transition to a normal lifestyle. Reybons (1992) stresses that leisure and recreation activities provide an opportunity for burn survivors to reestablish control over leisure time.

After discharge from the burn unit, settings for postacute rehabilitation are highly variable. In acute hospitals, the patient may continue to be seen in outpatient therapy settings. Burn centers sometimes transfer daily therapy care of children who travel from great distances to a community hospital and then follow the patient periodically in an outpatient burn clinic. Some burn centers have rehabilitation beds or step-down units that continue medical care until the patient is better able to handle the home situation. Other centers have transitional units, in which children and their families assume responsibility for care in a protective environment (Daugherty et al., 1993). Children with complicated injuries, amputations, large body surface area burns, or neurologic involvement may need several months in a designated rehabilitation center.

In most cases it is desirable for the child to return to the burn facility for follow-up outpatient clinic visits. Frequent checkups will allow the burn team to monitor the child's progress, see if the program is being followed, and alter the treatments when necessary. The checkups also enable the staff to detect any problems that may develop and to change the therapy program as necessary. As healing occurs, many questions regarding skin care will arise during therapy sessions and at outpatient clinic follow-up visits.

Common problems addressed in follow-up clinics include skin breakdown, maceration, dryness, itch, sun intolerance, and impaired thermoregulation. Other issues that may be addressed include physical activity level, continued use and fit of pressure garments and splints, maturation of scars, implementation of cosmetics use, and plan for further surgical procedures. If the family does not live near the primary care facility, local follow-up care can be arranged. In all cases, however, family members should be encouraged to contact the hospital when they have concerns or questions. With open communication, the development of secondary complications is minimized.

CHRONIC FUNCTIONAL LIMITATIONS

Typical Disabilities Identified

Persistent cutaneous inflexibility may result in tightening of underlying muscles, tendons, ligaments, joint capsules, fascia, and bone. Chronic limitation of motion, therefore, may continue to affect the physical ability of a child and become more noticeable with growth. Reconstructive procedures are often required after growth spurts and until bony growth is complete (Dado & Angelats, 1990). Aesthetically pleasing and good functional results may therefore be more difficult to achieve in children compared with adults. The child will require further intervention by the physical therapist after each reconstructive procedure for management of the new grafts.

In an article by Kramer and colleagues (1988), the incidence of surgical release of contractures was 4 times higher in children than in adults, even though burn wound size was similar in both populations. Areas associated with the highest incidence of contracture formation were the hand and the central body regions (head, neck, and axilla). Central body region contractures, plus contractures at sites that had been previously fascially excised, had the poorest outcome after surgical reconstruction. The review also concluded that reconstructive surgery should be delayed, when possible, until the burn scars have matured (consistent with findings by Alexander et al., 1981; Huang et al., 1978; and Parks et al., 1978). However, the study by Kramer and colleagues (1988) also suggests that early contracture release can be successfully performed in patients with severe contractures that significantly limit function.

Potential impairments for each body area are listed in Table 29–5. Surgical and rehabilitative goals for correction of chronic impairments vary according to the age and stated needs of each child. Consideration of length, sensibility, mobility, stability, strength, and, to a lesser extent, appearance dictate the reconstructive needs (Kurtzman & Stern, 1990). The emphasis on function versus appearance is different for children of each age group.

One of the more challenging areas requiring reconstruction after burn injury is the neck. High rates of contracture recurrence have also been documented. A study of pediatric burn patients by Waymack (1986) revealed recurrence rates of 81% after Z-plasty releases and 62% with split-thickness skin grafts. However, the use of a neck hyperextension splint for more than 1 year after skin grafting decreased the recurrence rate to 17%. Perineal contractures are also a frequent problem in the pediatric population. Pisarski and co-workers (1994) list several procedures for correction but report a high recurrence rate (46%), even with postoperative pressure garments, splints, and exercise.

In one study, the health care worker's perception of burn scars was compared with that of the patient (Prothman et al., 1993). Of scar variables, including color, texture, dryness, lack of hair, lack of stretch,

TABLE 29–5. Potential Impairments

Body Area	Impairment
Face	Facial disfigurement (contractures of eyelids, nose, mouth, ears, and adjacent facial skin)
	Inability to close eyes
	Loss of facial expression
	Teeth malalignment
	Drooling and inability to close lips
	Lower lip eversion
Neck	Loss of normal cervical spine ROM
	Limited visual fields
	Difficulties in anesthesia
Trunk	Protraction of shoulders
	Kyphosis
	Functional scoliosis
	Decreased respiratory function
	Breast entrapment
	Peroneal banding
Axilla	Type 1: either anterior or posterior contracture
	Type 2: anterior and posterior contracture with sparing of dome
	Type 3: anterior and posterior contracture and axillary dome
Hands	Metacarpophalangeal extension deformities
	Wrist extension deformities
	Proximal interphalangeal flexion deformities
	Interdigital web contractures
	Clawing of fourth and fifth digits
	Thumb contractures (adduction, opposition, flexion, and extension)
Arms and legs	Antecubital banding and flexion
	Posterior popliteal banding and flexion
	Anterior hip banding and flexion
	Medial and lateral malleolar scarring
Foot and ankle	Hyperextension of metatarsophalangeal joints
	Equinovarus
	Cavus foot
	Rocker-bottom deformity

wrinkles, height, and mesh appearance, only interrater scores for vascularity correlated positively with patient scores for scar appearance. Patients most often stated that nothing bothered them about the scar. However, when problems were reported, the scar variables that were most unattractive to the patient were often different from those that bothered the staff. This must be considered when planning reconstructive surgery.

Older children appear to have a much more difficult time accepting the residual scar. When faced with the burden of coping with disfigurement resulting from a burn injury, the adolescent's sense of self-esteem may be diminished. Providing adolescents the opportunity to learn makeup techniques that lessen the impact of their scars is an effective intervention for enhancing self-perception and their perception of how others view them. This was demonstrated in a study of 115 patients attending reconstructive makeup clinics (Beattie et al., 1993).

Assessment of Performance in Life Roles

Several factors are to be considered in the child's return to school and potential for future employment. These include preinjury status, changes in physical ability resulting from the burn injury, disfigurement, and the need for long-term and periodic treatment. Physical therapists, as part of the burn team, are often involved in the return-to-school process, both in assessment of the child's abilities (including treatment suggestions for school therapists or physical education specialists) and in preparing the teachers and students for the child's new abilities and needs (by means of individualized videotapes and, when necessary, on-site school visits). School reintegration programs have been developed to enhance a positive sense of self-worth in a child who has been burned.The premise of these programs is that cognitive and affective education about children with burns will diminish the anxiety of the child with a burn, the child's family, faculty and staff of the school, and the students. Five principles guide school reentry programs: (1) preparation begins as soon as possible, (2) planning includes the patient and family, (3) each program is individualized, (4) each patient is encouraged to return to school quickly after hospital discharge, and (5) burn team professionals remain available for consultation to the school (Blakeney, 1995). The student who has sustained a burn injury, the school's personnel, and the student's peer groups benefit from a school reentry program. Concrete, factual information about the burn injury helps open lines of communication between the returning student and peers. The concerns and expectations of school personnel are addressed (Bishop & Gilinsky, 1995).

Reybons (1992) has summarized the problems a person with a burn may experience in community reintegration as follows:

- Architectural barriers: stairs, ramps, escalators, doors
- Physical barriers: decreased ROM, contractures, decreased fine motor skills, decreased endurance, loss of hands
- Social barriers: facial disfigurement, feelings of "invasion of privacy," decreased initiation of contact with strangers

Over the long term, most patients do well and report a minimal impact of the burn injury in their lives and a satisfactory quality of life (Tarnowski et al., 1989). A 5-year study of physical and psychologic outcome after burns (Sheffield et al., 1988) resulted in the following significant findings:

- From 10 to 15% of patients have postburn courses complicated by psychiatric problems, noncompliance, and limited ROM.
- Patients who are more physically or psychologically impaired, or both, require longer follow-up treatment.
- Patients who do not adhere to intervention believe that the impact of the event on their lives is greater than others and report diminished quality of life.

A study reported by Blakeney and associates (1993) examined the psychologic adjustment of a group of children who survived the most severe burn injuries and the impact of such injury on the families. The conclusions were that children with burns affecting more than 80% of total body surface area develop positive feelings about themselves and appear no more troubled than a comparable group of children without burns. The impact on the families is significant, however, and must be considered of consequence in the rehabilitation of the child. In a follow-up study of the children who survived their burns and their parents, long-term psychosocial adaptation was within normal limits (Blakeney et al., 1998).

SUMMARY

Physical therapy for children with burns should begin at the time of injury and may extend for several years beyond the initial hospitalization. There is no single best physical therapy intervention for children with burns. Each child has unique problems, and specific procedures and techniques are incorporated into an individualized rehabilitation program developed by the team, the child, and the family. The recovery process is long and often complicated, but successful rehabilitation, based on a comprehensive psychologic, social, and physical view of the child, is extremely gratifying.

Recommended Resources

American Burn Association
Web Site: http://www.ameriburn.org.
Latarjet, J. A simple guide to burn treatment. International Society for Burn Injuries in collaboration with the World Health Organization. Burns, 21(3):221–225, 1995.
Linares, HA. From wound to scar. Burns, 22(5):339–352, 1996.
McLoughlin, E. A simple guide to burn epidemiology. International Society for Burn Injuries in collaboration with the World Health Organization. Burns, 21(3):217–220, 1995.

McLoughlin, E. A simple guide to burn prevention. International Society for Burn Injuries in collaboration with the World Health Organization. Burns, 21(3):226–229, 1995.

Pruitt, BA, Jr. The evolutionary development of biological dressings and skin substitutes. Journal of Burn Care and Rehabilitation, 18(1):S2–S5, 1997.

Saffle, JR, & Davis, BL. A simple guide to the burn registry. International Society for Burn Injuries in collaboration with the World Health Organization. Burns, 21(3):230–236, 1995.

Staley, M, & Richard, R. Critical pathways to enhance the rehabilitation of patients with burns. Journal of Burn Care and Rehabilitation, 17(6):S12–S14, 1996.

Staley, M, Richard, R, Warden, GD, Miller, SF, & Shuster, DB. Functional outcomes for the patient with burn injuries. Journal of Burn Care and Rehabilitation, 17(4):362–368, 1996.

Staley, M, & Serghiou, M. Casting guidelines, tips, and techniques: Proceedings from the 1997 American Burn Association PT/OT Casting Workshop. Journal of Burn Care and Rehabilitation, 19(3):254–260, 1998.

Ward, RS, & Saffle, JR. Topical agents in burn and wound care. Physical Therapy, 75(6):526–538, 1995.

References

Achauer, BM, & Martinez, SE. Burn wound pathophysiology and care. Critical Care Clinics, 1(1):47–58, 1985.

Ainsworth, P, Blache, C, Dyess, DL, & Luteman, A. Silipos gel, a new and improved gel insert for treatment of hypertrophic marring. Paper presented at the meeting of the American Burn Association, Cincinnati, March 1993.

Alexander, JW, MacMillan, BG, & Martel, L. Surgical correction of postburn flexion contractures of the fingers in children. Plastic and Reconstructive Surgery, 68:218–224, 1981.

Alston, DW, Kozerefski, P, Quan, PE, & Luterman, A. Materials for pressure inserts in the control of hypertrophic scar tissue. Journal of Burn Care and Rehabilitation, 1:40–43, 1981.

American Burn Association, Committee on the Organization and Delivery of Burn Care. Burn care outcomes and clinical indicators. Journal of Burn Care and Rehabilitation, 17(2):17A–39A, 1996.

American Physical Therapy Association. Guide to Physical Therapy Practice. Physical Therapy, 77(11):1557–1619, 1997.

Artz, CP, Moncrief, J, & Pruitt, B (Eds.). Burns: A Team Approach. Philadelphia: WB Saunders, 1979.

Atiles, L, Mileski, W, Spann, K, Purdue, G, Hunt, J, & Baxter, C. Early assessment of pediatric burn wounds by laser Doppler flowmetry. Journal of Burn Care and Rehabilitation, 16(6):596–601, 1995.

Badger, K, Gaboury, T, & Warden, GD. A collaborative effort: Music therapy and occupational/physical therapy in pediatric burn rehabilitation. Poster presented at the meeting of the American Burn Association, Cincinnati, March 1993.

Baron, P, & Herndon, DN. Chronic propranolol administration safely decreases cardiac work and anxiety in massively burned pediatric patients. Paper presented at the meeting of the American Burn Association, Cincinnati, March 1993.

Bayley, EW. Wound healing in the patient with burns. Nursing Clinics of North America, 25(1):205–222, 1990.

Beattie, DM, Chedekel, DS, & Krawczyk, T. Utilization of a reconstructive makeup clinic for self-image enhancement in burned adolescents. Paper presented at the meeting of the American Burn Association, Cincinnati, March 1993.

Belenger, M, Vanderelst, E, & Toussaint, JP. New contributions to treatment of localized burns of the hand. Annales de Chirurgie Plastique, 9:199, 1969.

Bennett, B, & Gamelli, R. Profile of an abused burned child. Journal of Burn Care and Rehabilitation, 19(1):88–94, 1998.

Bennett, GB, Helm, P, Purdue, GF, & Hunt, JL. Serial casting: A method for treating burn contractures. Journal of Burn Care and Rehabilitation, 10:543–545, 1989.

Bennett, MB, Epp, J, Boaz, M, Mani, M, & Varghese, G. An alternate to traditional ankle foot orthoses. Poster presented at the meeting of the American Burn Association, Cincinnati, March 1993.

Biggs, KS, de Linde, L, Banaszewski, M, & Heinrich, JJ. Determining the current roles of physical and occupational therapists in burn care. Journal of Burn Care and Rehabilitation, 19(5):442–449, 1998.

Bishop, B, & Gilinsky, V. School reentry for the patient with burn injuries: Video and/or on-site intervention. Journal of Burn Care and Rehabilitation, 16(4):455–457, 1995.

Bishop, JF. Pediatric considerations in the use of Biobrane in burn wound management. Journal of Burn Care and Rehabilitation, 16(3):331–333, 1995.

Blakeney, P. School reintegration. Journal of Burn Care and Rehabilitation, 16(2):180–187, 1995.

Blakeney, P, Meyer, W, Moore, P, Murphy, L, Robson, M, & Herndon, D. Psychosocial sequelae of pediatric burns involving 80% or greater total body surface area. Journal of Burn Care and Rehabilitation, 14(6):684–689, 1993.

Blakeney, P, Meyer, W, Robert, R, Desai, M, Wolf, S, & Herndon, D. Long-term psychosocial adaptation of children who survive burns involving 80% or greater total body surface area. Journal of Trauma, 44(4):625–632, 1998.

Bochke, I, Frauenfeld, A, Hartlieb, D, Zwicker, M, & Inkson, T. Patient and family education in burn care: Development of a series of teaching books by a multidisciplinary team. Poster presented at the meeting of the American Burn Association, Cincinnati, March 1993.

Bull, JP, & Squire, JR. A study of mortality in a burn unit: Standards for the evaluation of alternative methods of treatment. Annals of Surgery, 130(2):160, 1949.

Burne, BA, Hackencamp, TB, Pfabe-Wiggans, S, & Sprecht, D. The application of neurodevelopmental treatment in pediatric burns. Poster presented at the meeting of the American Burn Association, Cincinnati, March 1993.

Carvajal, HF. Burns in children and adolescents: Initial management as the first step in successful rehabilitation. Pediatrician, 17:237–243, 1990.

Chester, CH, Candlish, S, & Zuker, RM. Prevention of obstructive sleep apnea in children with burns of the head and neck. Paper presented at the meeting of the American Burn Association, Cincinnati, March 1993.

Clarke, HM, Wittpenn, GP, McLeod, AME, Candlish, SE, Guernsey, C J, Weleff, DK, & Zuker, RM. Acute management of pediatric hand burns. Hand Clinics, 6:221–232, 1990.

Clayton, MC, & Bishop, JF. Perioperative and postoperative dressing techniques for Integra artificial skin: views from two medical centers. Journal of Burn Care and Rehabilitation, 19(4):358–363, 1998.

Clugston, PA, Snelling, CFT, Macdonald, IB, Maledy, HL, Boyle, JC, Germann, E, Courtemanche, AD, Wirtz, P, Fitzpatrick, DJ, Kester, DA, Foley, B, Warren, RJ, & Cart, NJ. Cultured epithelial autografts: Three years of clinical experience with eighteen patients. Journal of Burn Care and Rehabilitation, 12:533–539, 1991.

Covey, M. Application of CPM devices with burn patients. Journal of Burn Care and Rehabilitation, 9:496–497, 1988.

Dado, DV, & Angelats, J. Management of burns of the hands in children. Hand Clinics, 6:711–721, 1990.

Daugherty, MB, DeSerna, C, Barthel, P, & Warden, GD. Moving patients and families toward independence: Establishing a transitional unit. Poster presented at the meeting of the American Burn Association, Cincinnati, March 1993.

Davey, RB. The use of contact media for burn scar hypertrophy. Journal of Wound Care, 6(2):80–82, 1997.

Deitch, EA, Wheelaham, TM, Rose, MP, Clotier, J, & Coltes, J. Hypertrophic burn scars: Analysis of variables. Journal of Trauma, 23:895–898, 1983.

Desai, MH, Mlakar, JM, McCauley, RL, Abdullah, KM, Rutan, R, Hall-Waymack, J, Robson, M, & Horndon, D. Lack of long-term durability of cultured keratinocyte burn-wound coverage: A case report. Journal of Burn Care and Rehabilitation, 12:540–545, 1991.

Dimick, AR. Pathophysiology. In Fisher, SV, & Helm, PA (Eds.), Comprehensive Rehabilitation of Burns. Baltimore: Williams & Wilkins, 1984, pp. 16–27.

Doane, CB. Children with severe burns. In Pratt, PN, & Allen, AS (Eds.), Occupational Therapy for Children. St. Louis: Mosby, 1989, pp. 524–534.

Doctor, JN, Patterson, DR, & Mann, R. Health outcome for burn survivors. Journal of Burn Care and Rehabilitation, 18(6):490–495, 1997.

Economou, TP, Kealey, GP, Lewis, RW, III, & Rosenquist, MD. An experimental study to determine the effects of Dermagraft on skin graft viability in the presence of bacterial wound contamination. Paper presented at the meeting of the American Burn Association, Cincinnati, March 1993.

Egan, M. Cultured skin grafts: Preserving lives, challenging therapists. OT Week, July 23, 1992, pp. 12–15.

Ehde, DM, Patterson, DR, & Fordyce, WE. The quota system in burn rehabilitation. Journal of Burn Care and Rehabilitation, 19(5):436–440, 1998.

Feller, I. Prevention of burns in 1 and 2 year olds. NBIE Newsletter, 1(2), 1980.

Feller, I. Burn epidemiology: Focus on youngsters and the aged. Journal of Burn Care and Rehabilitation, 3:285, 1982.

Feller, I, & Jones, CA. Nursing the Burned Patient. Ann Arbor, MI: Institute for Burn Medicine, 1974, p. 5.

Feller, I, & Jones, CA. Introduction: Statement of the problem. In Fisher, SV, & Helm, PA (Eds.), Comprehensive Rehabilitation of Burns. Baltimore: Williams & Wilkins, 1984, pp. 1–8.

Field, T. Massage therapy for infants and children. Journal of Developmental and Behavioral Pediatrics, 16(2):105–111, 1995.

Field, T, Peck, M, Krugman, S, Tuchel, T, Schanberg, S, Kuhn, C, & Burman, T. Burn injuries benefit from massage therapy. Journal of Burn Care and Rehabilitation, 19(3):241–244, 1998.

Fletchall, S, & Hickerson, WL. Managed health care: Therapist responsibilities. Journal of Burn Care and Rehabilitation, 18(1):61–63, 1997.

Foertsch, CE, O'Hara, MW, Stoddard, FJ, & Kealey, GP. Treatment-resistant pain and distress during pediatric burn-dressing changes. Journal of Burn Care and Rehabilitation, 19(3):219–224, 1998.

Fricke, NB, Omnell, ML, Dutcher, KA, Hollender, LG, & Engrav, LH. Skeletal and dental disturbances in children after facial burns and pressure garment use: A 4-year follow-up. Journal of Burn Care and Rehabilitation, 20(3):239–249, 1999.

Ghahary, A, Shen, YJ, Scott, PG, Gong, Y, & Tredget, EE. Enhanced expression of mRNA for transforming growth factor-beta, type I and type III procollagen in human post-burn hypertrophic scar tissues. Journal of Laboratory Clinical Medicine, 122(4):465–473, 1993.

Gilliam, KS, Hatler, B, Adams, S, & Helm, P. T-shirt splint for prevention of burn scar contracture of the neck, chest, and axillas. Poster presented at the meeting of the American Burn Association, Cincinnati, March 1993.

Gilpin, DA, Barrow, RE, Rutan, RL, Broemeling, L, & Herndon, DN. Recombinant human growth hormone accelerates wound healing in children with large cutaneous burns. Annals of Surgery, 220(1): 19–24, 1994.

Green, A. Epidemiology of burns in childhood. Burns, 10:368–371, 1984.

Greenspan, B, Johnson, J, Gorga, D, Goodwin, CW, & Naglet, W. Compliance with pressure garment use in burn survivors. Paper presented at the meeting of the American Burn Association, Cincinnati, March 1993.

Harnar, T, Engrav, L, Marvin J, Heimbach, D, Cain, V, & Johnson, C. Dr. Paul Unna's boot and early ambulation after skin grafting the leg. Journal of Plastic and Reconstructive Surgery, 69:359–360, 1982.

Harris, LD, Hatler, B, Adams, S, Gilliam, KS, & Helm, P. Serial casting and its efficacy in the treatment of the burned hand. Paper presented at the meeting of the American Burn Association, Cincinnati, March 1993.

Hartford, CE. Surgical management. In Fisher, SV, & Helm, PA (Eds.), Comprehensive Rehabilitation of Burns. Baltimore: Williams & Wilkins, 1994, pp. 28–63.

Hayes-Lundy, C, Ward, S, Mills, P, & Same, J. Use of computer-generated exercise programs to augment therapy programs. Poster presented at the meeting of the American Burn Association, Cincinnati, March 1993.

Head, MD. Wound and skin care. In Fisher, SV, & Helm, PA (Eds.), Comprehensive Rehabilitation of Burns. Baltimore: Williams & Wilkins, 1984, pp. 148–176.

Head, MD, & Helm, PA. Paraffin and sustained stretching in the treatment of burn contracture. Burns, 4:136–139, 1977.

Heimhach, DM. Early burn excision and grafting. Surgical Clinics of North America, 67:93, 1987.

Helvig, EI. Dermal replacement: An update. Seminars in Perioperative Nursing, 6(4):233–235, 1997.

Herndon, DN, Barrow, RE, Kunkel, KR, Brocmeling, L, & Rutan, RL. Effects of recombinant human growth hormone on donor-site healing in severely burned children. Annals of Surgery, 212:424–429, 1990.

Herndon, DN, & Rutan, RL. Have we improved burn care? In Carlson, RW, & Reines, HD (Eds.), Critical Care State of the Art, Vol. 13. Anaheim, CA: Society of Critical Care Medicine, 1992a, pp. 389–406.

Herndon, DN, & Rutan, RL. Use of dermal templates and cultured cells for permanent skin replacement. Wounds, 4(2):50–53, 1992b.

Hollowed, KA, Gunde, MA, Lewis, MS, & Jordon, MH. Ambulation of intubated burn patients. Poster presented at the meeting of the American Burn Association, Cincinnati, March 1993.

Housinger, T, Mortess, C, Dinkler, T, & Warden, GD. Outpatient therapy: Its efficacy in pediatric burns. Paper presented at the meeting of the American Burn Association, Salt Lake City, April 1992.

Huang, TT, Blackwell, SJ, & Lewis, SR. Ten years' experience in managing patients with burn contractures of axilla, elbow, wrist, and knee joints. Plastic and Reconstructive Surgery, 61:70–76, 1978.

Johnson, CL. Ambulating patients after lower extremity grafting. Journal of Burn Care and Rehabilitation, 5:114–115, 1984a.

Johnson, CL. Physical therapists as scar modifiers. Physical Therapy, 64(9):1381–1387, 1984b.

Johnson, J, & Silverberg, R. Serial casting of the lower extremity to correct contractures during the acute phase of burn care. Physical Therapy, 75(8):767–768, 1995.

Kohlman-McGourty, L, Givens, A, & Buddingh-Fader, P. Roles and functions of occupational therapy in burn care delivery. American Journal of Occupational Therapy, 39:791–794, 1985.

Kowalske, K, Purdue, G, Hunt, J, & Helm, P. Early ambulation following skin grafting of lower extremity burns: A randomized controlled trial. Paper presented at the meeting of the American Burn Association, Cincinnati, March 1993.

Kramer, MD, Jones, T, & Deitch, EA. Burn contractures: Incidence, predisposing factors, and results of surgical therapy. Journal of Burn Care and Rehabilitation, 9:261–265, 1988.

Kurtzman, LC, & Stem, PJ. Upper extremity burn contractures. Hand Clinics, 6:261–279, 1990.

Larson, DL, Abston, S, Willis, B, Linares, HA, Dobrkovsky, M, Evans, EB, & Lewis, SR. Contracture and scar formation in the burn patient. Clinics in Plastic Surgery, 1:653, 1974.

Larson, DL, Huang, T, Dobrkovsky, M, Bauer, PS, & Parks, DH. Prevention and treatment of scar contracture. In Artz, CP, Moncrief, JA, & Pruitt, B (Eds.), Burns: A Team Approach. Philadelphia: WB Saunders, 1979, pp. 466–491.

Linares, HA, Kischer, CW, Dobrkovsky, M, & Larson, DL. On the origin of the hypertrophic scar. Journal of Trauma, 13:70–75, 1973.

Linares, HA, Larson, DL, & Willis-Galstaum, BA. Historical notes on the use of pressure in the treatment of hypertrophic scars or keloids. Burns, 19:17-21, 1993.

Lund, CC, & Browder, NC. The estimation of areas of burns. Surgery, Gynecology and Obstetrics, 79:352, 1944.

Mahaney, NB. Restoration of play in a severely burned three-year-old child. Journal of Burn Care and Rehabilitation, 11:57-63, 1990.

Mann, R, Yeong, EK, Moore, ML, & Engrav, LH. A new tool to measure pressure under burn garments. Journal of Burn Care and Rehabilitation, 18(2):160-163, 1997.

Metzger, DJ, Cioffi, WG, Martin, S, McManus, WF, & Pruitt, BA. Ilizarov technique in the management of joint deformity in thermally injured patients. Paper presented at the meeting of the American Burn Association, Cincinnati, March 1993.

Meyer, W, Blakeney, P, Moore, P, Murphy, L, Robson, M, & Herndon, D. Parental well-being and behavioral adjustment of pediatric survivors of burns. Journal of Burn Care and Rehabilitation, 15(1):62-68, 1994.

Mikhail, NJ. Acute burn care: An update. Journal of Emergency Nursing, 14:1, 1988.

Nedelec, B, Shen, YJ, Ghahary, A, Scott, PG, & Tredget, EE. The effect of interferon alpha 2b on the expression of cytoskeletal proteins in an in vitro model of wound contraction. Journal of Laboratory Clinical Medicine, 126(5):474-484, 1995.

Nicosia, J, Stein, E, & Stein, J. The advantages of physiotherapy for burn patients under anaesthesia. Burns, 6:202-204, 1979.

Nothdurft, D, Smith, PS, & LeMaster, JE. Exercise and treatment modalities. In Fisher, SV, & Helm, PA (Eds.), Comprehensive Rehabilitation of Burns. Baltimore: Williams & Wilkins, 1984, pp. 96-147.

Parks, DH, Bauer, PS, & Larson, DL. Late problems in burns. Clinics in Plastic Surgery, 4:547, 1977.

Parks, DH, Evans, EB, & Larson, DL. Prevention and correction of deformity after severe burns. Surgical Clinics of North America, 58:1279-1289, 1978.

Perkins, K, Davey, RB, & Wallis, K. Current materials and techniques used in a burn scar management program. Burns, 13:406-410, 1987.

Pisarski, GP, Greenhalgh, DG, & Warden, GD. The management of perineal contractures in children with burns. Journal of Burn Care and Rehabilitation, 15(3):256-259, 1994.

Prothman, J, Engrav, L, & Cain, V. Evaluating appearance of burn scars: Patient vs. health care worker perceptions. Paper presented at the meeting of the American Burn Association, Cincinnati, March 1993.

Pullium, GF. Splinting and positioning. In Fisher, SV, & Helm, PA (Eds.), Comprehensive Rehabilitation of Burns. Baltimore: Williams & Wilkins, 1984, pp. 64-95.

Quin, KJ. Silicone gel in scar treatment. Burns, 13:133-140, 1987.

Reed, L, & Heinle, J. Meeting the challenge of education in a diversified patient population in a burn treatment center: Design of 2 patient handbooks. Poster presented at the meeting of the American Burn Association, Cincinnati, March 1993.

Reybons, MD. Community re-entry and leisure: Reuniting a lifestyle with a burn survivor. Progress Report, 4(3):20-22, 1992.

Richard, R, DerSarkisian, D, Miller, SF, Johnson, RM, & Staley, M. Directional variance in skin movement. Journal of Burn Care and Rehabilitation, 20(3):259-264, 1999.

Richard, R, Ford, J, Miller, SF, & Staley, M. Photographic measurement of volar forearm skin movement with wrist extension: The influence of elbow position. Journal of Burn Care and Rehabilitation, 15(1):58-61, 1994.

Richard, R, Shanesy, CP, III, & Miller, SF. Dynamic versus static splints: A prospective case for sustained stress. Journal of Burn Care and Rehabilitation, 16(3):284-287, 1995.

Richard, RL. Use of the Dynasplint to correct elbow flexion burn contracture: A case report. Journal of Burn Care and Rehabilitation, 7:151-152, 1986.

Richard, RL, Jones, LM, Miller, SF, & Finlay, RK, Jr. Treatment of exposed bilateral Achilles tendons with use of the Dynasplint. Physical Therapy, 68:989-991, 1988.

Richard, RL, & Staley, M. Burn Care and Rehabilitation Principles and Practice. Philadelphia: FA Davis, 1993.

Richard, RL, Staley, MF, Miller, SF, Warden, GD, & Finley, RK, Jr. Biomechanical basis for physical management of burn patients. Poster presented at the meeting of the American Burn Association, Cincinnati, March 1993.

Ridgway, CL, Daugherty, MB, & Warden, GD. Serial casting as a technique to correct burn scar contractures. Journal of Burn Care and Rehabilitation, 12:67-72, 1991.

Ridgway, CL, & Warden, GD. Evaluation of a vertical mouth stretching orthosis: Two case reports. Journal of Burn Care and Rehabilitation, 16(1):74-78, 1995.

Rozanova, EP. The use of ultrasonics for the prevention of contractures after burns. Orthopedia Traumatologia, 34:13, 1979.

Sanford, S, & Gore, D. Unna's boot dressings facilitate outpatient skin grafting of hands. Journal of Burn Care and Rehabilitation, 17(4): 323-326, 1996.

Schmitt, MA, French, L, & Kalil, ET. How soon is safe? Ambulation of the patient with burns after lower-extremity skin grafting. Journal of Burn Care and Rehabilitation, 12:33-37, 1991.

Schwanholt, C, Ridgway, C, Greenhalgh, D, Staley, M, Gaboury, T, Morress, C, Walling, S, & Warden, G. A prospective study of burn scar maturation in pediatrics: Does age matter? Paper presented at the meeting of the American Burn Association, Cincinnati, March 1993.

Schwartz, K, Rivers, E, Timming, R, Solem, L, & Ahrenholz, D. Improved outcomes for pediatric patients through the use of specialty three piece external vascular support leotards. Poster presented at the meeting of the American Burn Association, Cincinnati, March 1993.

Sheffield, CG, III, Irons, GB, Mucha, P, Malec, JF, Ilstrup, DM, & Stonnington, HH. Physical and psychological outcome after burns. Journal of Burn Care and Rehabilitation, 9:172-177, 1988.

Shelby, J, Groussman, M, Addison, C, Burgess, Y, Sullivan, J, & Saffie, J. Stress resiliency in close relatives of thermally injured patients. Paper presented at the meeting of the American Burn Association, Cincinnati, March 1993.

Sheridan, R, Remensnyder, J, Prelack, K, Petras, L, & Lyndon, M. Treatment of the seriously burned infant. Journal of Burn Care and Rehabilitation, 19(2):115-118, 1998.

Solem, LD. Classification. In Fisher, SV, & Helm, PA (Eds.), Comprehensive Rehabilitation of Burns. Baltimore: Williams & Wilkins, 1984, pp. 9-15.

Solomon, JR. Pediatric burns. Critical Care Clinics, 1(1):159-173, 1985.

Spurr, ED, & Shakespeare, PG. Incidence of hypertrophic scarring in burn-injured children. Burns, 16:179-181, 1990.

Staley, M, & Richard, R. Critical pathways to enhance the rehabilitation of patients with burns. Journal of Burn Care and Rehabilitation, 17(6):S12-S14, 1996.

Staley, MJ, & Richard, RL. Use of pressure to treat hypertrophic burn scars. Advances in Wound Care, 10(3):44-46, 1997.

Sullivan, T. Rating the burn scar. Journal of Burn Care and Rehabilitation, 11:256-260, 1990.

Tarnowski, KJ, Rasnake, LK, Linscheid, TR, & Mulick, JA. Behavioral adjustment of pediatric burn victims. Journal of Pediatric Psychology, 14:607-615, 1989.

Taylor, A. Pockets stitched into external vascular supports improve management of hypertrophic scars. Poster presented at the meeting of the American Burn Association, Cincinnati, March 1993.

Thompson, R, Summers, S, Dobbs, R, & Wheeler, T. Color-pressure garments: Perceptions from the public. Paper presented at the meeting of the American Burn Association, Salt Lake City, April 1992.

Torres-Gray, D, Johnson, J, Greenspan, B, Goodwin, CW, & Naglet, W. The fabrication and use of removable digit casts to improve range of motion at the proximal interphalangeal joint. Poster presented at the meeting of the American Burn Association, Cincinnati, March 1993.

Van den Kerckhove, E, Boeckx, W, & Kochuyt, A. Silicone patches as a supplement for pressure therapy to control hypertrophic scarring. Journal of Burn Care and Rehabilitation, *12*:361–369, 1991.

Varni, JW, Bessman, CA, Russo, DC, & Cataldo, MF. Behavioral management of chronic pain in children: A case study. Archives of Physical Medicine and Rehabilitation, *61*:375–379, 1980.

Walling, S, Walling, R, & Warden, GD. The development of home program instructional guides to accommodate the special needs of patients and families. Poster presented at the meeting of the American Burn Association, Cincinnati, March 1993.

Ward, RS, Hayes-Lundy, C, Reddy, R, Brockway, C, Mills, P, & Saffie, J. Evaluation of topical therapeutic ultrasound to improve response to physical therapy and lessen scar contracture after burn injury. Journal of Burn Care and Rehabilitation, *15*(1):74–79, 1994.

Ward, RS, Hayes-Lundy, C, Schnebly, WA, Reddy, R, & Saffle, JR. Rehabilitation of burn patients with concomitant limb amputation: Case reports. Burns, *16*(5):390–392, 1990a.

Ward, RS, Hayes-Lundy, C, Schnebly, WA, & Saffle, JR. Prosthetic use in patients with burns and associated limb amputations. Journal of Burn Care and Rehabilitation, *11*:361–364, 1990b.

Warden, GD, Brinkerhoff, C, Castellani, D, & Rieg, LS. Multidisciplinary team approach to the pediatric burn patient. Quality Review Bulletin, *14*:219–226, 1988.

Warden, GD, Lang, D, & Housinger, TA. Management of pediatric hand burns with tendon, joint and bone injury. Paper presented at the meeting of the American Burn Association, Cincinnati, March 1993.

Waymack, JP. Release of burn scar contractures of the neck in paediatric patients. Burns, *12*:422–426, 1986.

Wells, NJ, Boyle, JC, Snelling, CF, & Carr, NJ. Lower extremity burns and Unna paste: Can we decrease health care costs without compromising patient care? Canadian Journal of Surgery, *38*(6):533–536, 1995.

Whitestone, JJ, Richard, RL, Slemker, TC, Ause-Ellias, KL, & Miller, SF. Fabrication of total-contact burn masks by use of human body topography and computer-aided design and manufacturing. Journal of Burn Care and Rehabilitation, *16*(5):543–547, 1995.

Willis, B. The use of orthoplast splints in the treatment of the acutely burned child. American Journal of Occupational Therapy, *24*:187–191, 1970.

Wood, F, Liddiard, K, Skinner, A, & Ballentyne, J. Scar management of cultured epithelial autograft. Burns, *22*(6):451–454, 1996.

Wright, ET, & Haase, KH. Keloids and ultrasound. Archives of Physical Medicine and Rehabilitation, *52*:280, 1971.

Yeong, EK, Mann, R, Engrav, LH, Goldberg, M, Cain, V, Costa, B, Moore, M, Nakamura, D, & Lee, J. Improved burn scar assessment with use of a new scar-rating scale. Journal of Burn Care and Rehabilitation, *18*(4):353–355, 1997.

CHAPTER
30

The Special Care Nursery

LINDA KAHN-D'ANGELO, PT, ScD
RACHEL A. UNANUE, MSPT, PCS

This chapter describes the history and organization of the special care nursery and discusses which neonates and infants are at risk for central nervous system (CNS) dysfunction or developmental delay. Both a theoretic basis for and a discussion of physical therapy examination, evaluation, prognosis, and interventions for infants in the special care nursery are presented. The gestational and pathophysiologic conditions considered in this chapter are prematurity, hypoxic-ischemic encephalopathy, fetal alcohol syndrome, fetal abstinence syndrome, exposure to human immunodeficiency virus (HIV) infection, neonatal seizures, birth injuries related to the CNS, and spina bifida. The follow-up of infants after discharge from the special care nursery is addressed, and two case histories illustrate and integrate the material presented in this chapter.

HISTORY OF THE SPECIAL CARE NURSERY

Modern neonatal care was born with the development of the first incubator by Couveuse in France in 1880 (Hodgman, 1985). The first text on the premature infant, *The Nursling,* authored by Budin, a student of Couveuse, was published in 1900. Dr. Martin Couney, who was one of Budin's students, used these principles of treatment for the premature infant, and in a bizarre entrepreneurial twist, exhibited them to the public for a fee (Silverman, 1979). The main principles of neonatal care were support of body temperature, control of nosocomial infection, minimal handling, and provision of special nursing care. Interestingly, nurseries were quiet, and lights were dimmed at night. This exhibition was seen in Chicago by Dr. Julius Hess, who applied these principles in the late 1940s and achieved a neonatal mortality rate for preterm infants of 20%, which was respectable for the time. In response to the increased survival of premature infants reported by Hess, use of these principles of care spread across the United States.

During the 1950s, a number of cities developed centers for the care of premature infants and a number of states developed maternal mortality committees that gathered data to be used as a basis for planning activities directed at preventing maternal mortality. During the 1960s, Arizona, Massachusetts, and Wisconsin promulgated standards for maternity units and developed regional perinatal care centers. Reports from several professional organizations, including the American Medical Association, the American College of Obstetricians and Gynecologists, the American Academy of Pediatrics, and the Academy of Family Physicians, along with reports on data collected in the three states mentioned earlier, stimulated the development of the regional organization of perinatal services (Fanaroff & Graven, 1992).

By the late 1960s, ill full-term infants with health complications were also being treated in the neonatal nursery. Advances in microlaboratory techniques for biochemical determinations from minute quantities of blood and the development of miniaturized monitoring equipment, ventilatory support systems, and means to conserve body heat improved the care of the neonate with serious illness (Fanaroff & Graven, 1992). Expansion of neonatal pharmacology, widespread use of phototherapy for management of hyperbilirubinemia, and methods of delivery of high-caloric solutions parenterally when oral feeding was not possible also improved the chances for survival of the very sick neonate. In 1975, the emergence of the new subspecialties of neonatology and perinatology provided specialists in the field of caring for infants in the high-technology nursery.

During the past two decades there has been considerable progress in the treatment of neonates and children with critical illnesses. For example, there has been an increase in the survival rate of infants born at 23 to 25 weeks of gestational age from 1984–1989 to 1990–1995 of 27 to 42%, with most of the increase in disability being mild (Emsley et al., 1998). The improvement in survival and quality of life for these patients resulted from nationwide development of regional intensive care units in which an organized, highly specialized, multidisciplinary approach became the standard of care. The number of neonates needing close supervision and expert cardiorespiratory and metabolic support is large enough to make such units an essential component of a perinatal health care delivery system (Sarnaik & Preston, 1985). Currently, there are 700 neonatal intensive care units (NICUs) in the United States, which is a thirtyfold to fortyfold increase since the 1960s. It is well recognized that the increase in the number of NICUs is matched by a significant drop in neonatal and perinatal mortality rates of low birth weight (LBW) infants (Lubchenco et al., 1974; McDonald, 1981; Teberg et al., 1977). Long-term outcome of the very low birth weight (VLBW) infant, however, came under scrutiny with the suspicion that the typical nursery stay of several weeks may have a significantly detrimental effect on later behavioral performance (Hodgman, 1985).

Organization of Perinatal Services

Special care units are designed to meet a wide range of special needs, from the monitoring of apparently well infants at risk of serious illness to the intensive treatment of infants with acute illness. This range of services requires that the special care nursery be arranged for graduated care to meet the diverse and changing needs of infants (Whaley & Wong, 1991).

Because it is not economically feasible for every hospital to have the personnel and technology to care for neonates with complex needs, these services are organized on a regional basis.

The changing health care environment has led to a deterioration of perinatal regionalization in many areas, competition rather than cooperation among hospitals, and blurring of differences in levels of care so that levels of care are now as described in Box 30–1 (Kenner, 1998).

A broad-based Committee on Perinatal Health reconvened to analyze and redefine the future of perinatal care in the 1990s and beyond. The focus of perinatal care has shifted from hospital-based care to overall health awareness with emphasis on preventive health care, education, and counseling (Bagwell & Armstrong, 1998).

The Neonatal Intensive Care Unit Environment

The NICU is a busy, often crowded place, where the atmosphere is frequently high pressure (Pelletier & Palmeri, 1985). The amount and complexity of the equipment can be overwhelming to a newcomer. Each tiny patient lies in an incubator, an open warmer, or a crib, surrounded by and connected to ventilators and monitors, including heart, apnea, and oxygen monitors and infusion pumps (Fig. 30–1). Phototherapy lights; diagnostic transilluminators; and portable radiographic, electroencephalographic, and ultrasonographic units are also present in an NICU.

NICUs were designed to decrease neonatal morbidity and mortality rates. In an attempt to meet this goal, the NICU provides the neonate with a habitat for growth starkly different from the intrauterine environment. The intrauterine environment is replaced by bright lights, high noise levels, and the intrusive medical procedures characteristic

---

BOX 30–1. **In-Hospital Perinatal Services**

Basic Care: Surveillance and care of all patients admitted to obstetric service with triage to identify high-risk patients.

Specialty Care: Care of high-risk mothers and fetuses stabilization of ill newborns prior to transfer. Care of preterm infants with birth weight of 1500 g or more.

Subspecialty Care: Provision of comprehensive perinatal services for mothers and neonates of all risk categories. Research and educational support. Analysis and evaluation of regional data. Initial evaluation of new high-risk technologies.

Adapted from American Academy of Pediatrics, American College of Obstetricians and Gynecologists. Guidelines for Perinatal Care. 4th ed. Elk Grove Village, IL, Washington, DC: American Academy of Pediatrics, American College of Obstetricians and Gynecologists; 1997.

---

of high-technology treatment (Campbell, 1986; Gottfried, 1985).

Lighting

Typically, the ambient illumination within the NICU consists of daylight and artificial fluorescent lighting (Moseley et al., 1988). The American Academy of Pediatrics recommends a minimum light intensity of 100 foot-candles at the infant's level for adequate visualization by staff (Weibley, 1989). This same level of illumination may contribute to retinopathy of prematurity (ROP) (Glass et al., 1985; Kretzer & Hittner, 1986). No diurnal rhythmicity of light exists in the NICU, which some investigators believe may interfere with the infant's development of normal biologic rhythms. Glass and colleagues (1985) studied the effects of draping sunglass-filtering material over the incubators. They found that there was a significant increase in ROP in the infants in incubators without the filtering material, especially in the infants who weighed less than 1000 g. As a result of this study, an editorial in the journal that published the study recommended immediate diurnal cycling and dimming of lights (Weibley, 1989).

Sound

In the intrauterine environment, auditory stimuli include sound levels at about 85 dB consisting of rhythmic swooshing and bubbling sounds punctuated by the steady pulse of the maternal heartbeat (Gottfried, 1985; Gottfried & Hodgman, 1984). In the NICU the infant is surrounded by noise on a level comparable with that of auto traffic and, at times, heavy machinery. Highly exaggerated noise levels are present from trash receptacles, addressograph machines, centrifuges, telephones, and monitor alarms (Hilton, 1987). These harsh sounds can cause some infants to become hypoxic as part of a startle response (Thomas, 1989). Sound levels within the incubator are identical to those of the unit. The environment inside the incubator is characterized by continuous white noise and non-speech sounds. Harsh mechanical noises penetrate clearly, but speech sounds are indistinct and deflected (Newman, 1981). This lack of distinctness and the deflection of speech sounds may have negative effects on later interactive behavior if the infant learns to look away from the speaker to locate him or her. Drugs commonly used in the nursery are known from animal studies to potentiate noise-induced hearing loss (American Academy of Pediatrics, 1997; Perlstein, 1992). The American Academy of Pediatrics has recommended that noise levels be reduced to less than 70 dB, that manufacturers of incubators reduce the noise levels of motors below 58 dB, and that physicians limit the use of ototoxic drugs in neonates (Peabody & Lewis, 1985; Perlstein, 1992). Auditory evoked potential tests are typically done in every nursery before a neonate is discharged to establish risk for hearing loss. The American Academy of Pediatrics Committee on Environmental Health has issued recommendations for noise in the environment and its effects on the fetus and newborn, including the infant in the special care nursery.

Medical Procedures

In the NICU, the infant is placed on a flat mattress and is exposed to a dry, cool, air-filled environment. In the uterine environment the 28- to 32-week fetus sleeps 80% of the time. In contrast, premature infants were found to be disturbed an average of 132 times per day (Korones, 1976). The mean duration of undisturbed rest was 4 to 10 minutes.

Tactile input often heralds medical or technical events and causes sustained arousal, which exacts a physiologic toll on the infant. Unable to make sense of life-sustaining efforts, the infant begins to respond negatively to touch (Gottfried & Hodgman, 1984).

DEVELOPMENTAL CARE AND THE SPECIAL CARE NURSERY

In view of the research cited in the preceding sections about the iatrogenic effects of neonatal intensive care, and the shifting of emphasis from survival to the prevention and amelioration of the complications of prematurity, Als and co-workers (1986) have developed the concept of individualized, comprehensive, family-focused, developmentally supportive care for infants in the special care nursery. A growing body of literature supports this type of care (Als, 1986; Als et al., 1986, 1994; Buehler et al., 1995; Fleisher et al., 1995; Mouradian & Als, 1994; Parker et al., 1992). Whether or not this specific approach is used, more special care nursery staff members are incorporating a developmentally supportive environment and interventions such as diurnal light cycles; clustering care; specific rest time; interventions, including sponge baths, as needed rather than on a schedule; skin-to-skin contact, including "kangaroo" care; presentation of organizing environmental input such as music; the scent of the mother on clothing; and co-bedding of multiple-birth neonates

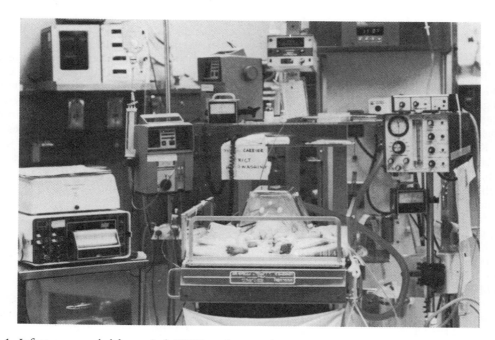

FIGURE 30–1. Infant surrounded by typical NICU equipment. (From Crane, L. Physical therapy for the neonate with respiratory disease. In Irwin, S, & Tecklin, JS [Eds.], Cardiopulmonary Physical Therapy, 2nd ed. St. Louis: Mosby, 1990, p. 400.)

(Bosque et al., 1995; delEstard, 1995; Standley & Moore, 1995; Tessier et al., 1998). Research on these methods has shown improvement in such dependent variables as weight gain, days on ventilator, oxygen saturation, days in hospital, infant state, and neuromotor behavior (delEstard, 1995; Mouradian & Als, 1994; Mueller, 1996).

WHO IS THE AT-RISK NEONATE/INFANT?

The meaning of the designation "high-risk infant" differs according to the area of expertise of the professional using the term. The neonatologist defines *risk* as related to morbidity or mortality, whereas psychologists, physical therapists, occupational therapists, and speech therapists may define the *at-risk infant* as one who has a high probability of manifesting developmental delay as a result of exposure to any one of a number of medical factors (Rossetti, 1986; Wilhelm, 1997). High-risk infants are classified according to birth weight, gestational age, and pathophysiologic problems (Whaley & Wong, 1991). Problems related to physiologic status are closely associated with the maturity of the infant and hypoxic episodes during the perinatal period, as well as with fetal exposure to alcohol and drugs and with HIV infection.

PREMATURITY AND LOW BIRTH WEIGHT

Infants born prematurely or who are small for gestational age (SGA) are divided into three major categories: LBW, from 1501 to 2500 g; VLBW, below 1501 g; and extremely low birth weight (ELBW), below 1000 g. Preterm delivery occurs in 8 to 10% of all live births in the United States in spite of current therapies to halt and prevent such deliveries (Harmon & Kenner, 1998). Approximately 75 to 80% of all neonatal morbidity and mortality is due to premature birth. More than 40,000 VLBW infants are born each year, and half of neonatal deaths occur in VLBW infants (Semmler, 1989). These high-risk infants are a heterogeneous group, including infants born preterm (less than 37 weeks of gestation) and those born at term but of reduced weight (Kleigman, 1992).

Black mothers are twice as likely as white mothers to deliver VLBW infants (Semmler, 1989). VLBW infants have an increased incidence of neurologic sequelae, delayed development, and lower intellectual and language abilities (Teberg, 1977; Volpe, 1995).

There have been several optimistic reports of prematurity prevention programs that include assessment of prenatal risk, weekly educational interventions, enhanced nutritional support, referral to a perinatologist when necessary, and pH self-measurements. These programs have shown a reduction in NICU admissions and preterm deliveries (Fangman et al., 1994; Joffe et al., 1995; Novy et al., 1995; Saling, 1997).

SGA infants are those whose birth weights are below the 10th percentile of published norms or whose ponderal index (ratio of birth weight to the cube root of the infant's length at birth) is low (Als et al., 1976). Term SGA infants demonstrate developmental problems such as behavioral and learning disorders, and preterm SGA infants may have an even greater prevalence of abnormal developmental problems than term SGA neonates (Kahn-D'Angelo, 1987).

The Clinical Assessment of Gestational Age in the Newborn Infant, developed by Dubowitz and colleagues (1970), is the test most often used to assess gestational age. The determination of gestational age is crucial for infants in the special care nursery to interpret neurologic and behavioral findings relative to the correct gestational age. This test includes 10 neurologic and reflex items and 11 external or superficial criteria that are scored on a four-point scale, and it is commonly administered by physicians or nurses in the newborn unit. The accuracy of gestational age is determined within 2 weeks on each assessment with a 95% confidence level. This test was standardized on 167 infants whose mothers were sure of the date of their last menstrual period. It has been used in the assessment of growth in early infancy and, in conjunction with the neurologic examination, to assess differences in development between twins, preterm infants with intraventricular hemorrhage (IVH), and the effects of eclampsia, placental abruption, and intrauterine growth retardation (Francis et al., 1987). Although gestational age is usually determined by physicians or nurses in the NICU, the physical therapist should be familiar with the Clinical Assessment of Gestational Age in the Newborn Infant and how gestational age is determined.

MEDICAL COMPLICATIONS AND TREATMENT IN PREMATURITY

Respiratory Distress Syndrome

Respiratory distress syndrome (RDS), or hyaline membrane disease, is the most common single cause of respiratory distress in neonates. The principal factors in the pathophysiology of RDS are pulmonary immaturity and deficiency of surfactant. Prematurity, low birth weight, low Apgar score at 1 and 5 minutes, maternal age over 34 years, and neonatal transport have been reported as risk factors for RDS (Rubaltelli et al., 1998; Shlossman et al., 1997). Low surfactant production results in increased surface tension, alveolar collapse, diffuse atelectasis, and decreased lung compliance. These factors cause an increase in pulmonary artery pressure that leads to extrapulmonary right-to-left shunting of blood and ventilation-perfusion mismatching (Carlo & Chatburn, 1988; Sweeney & Swanson, 1990; Walsh et al., 1988). Infants with RDS also demonstrate higher heart rates and reduced heart rate variability compared with full-term neonates, indicating that premature birth has an influence on cardiac function for up to 6 months after birth (Henslee et al., 1997).

Intervention for infants with RDS depends on the severity of the disorder and includes oxygen supplementation, assisted ventilation, surfactant administration, and extracorporeal membrane oxygenation (ECMO). Prophylactic surfactant administration of intubated infants less than 30 weeks of gestational age has been shown to be correlated with an initial improvement in respiratory status and a decrease in the incidence of RDS, pneumothorax, bronchopulmonary dysplasia (BPD), and mortality (Soll, 1998). Administration of multiple doses of natural surfactant extract results in improved clinical outcome and appears to be the most effective method of administration. Continuous distending-pressure ventilators, either positive or negative pressure, are used in the management of RDS. The positive-pressure ventilator is used more often; the negative-pressure ventilator assists ventilation by creating a negative pressure around the thorax and abdomen. Nasal and nasopharyngeal prongs are used for these ventilators (Carlo et al., 1992; Crane, 1990). (See Chapter 25 for a more detailed description of ventilators.) Partial liquid ventilation or perfluorocarbon-associated gas exchange has been used experimentally in conjunction with surfactant administration and has resulted in improved clinical course in a small sample of infants with severe respiratory distress syndrome (Leach et al., 1995). It has been suggested that this technology will provide a strong addition to available treatments for preterm infants and that there will be a resultant decrease in barotrauma and in BPD (Donovan et al., 1998).

The prognosis of infants with RDS varies with the severity of the original disease (Carlo & Chatburn, 1988). The mortality rate is about 10%, and RDS is the leading cause of neonatal mortality and morbidity. Infants who do not require assisted ventilation recover without sequelae, but the clinical course of the very immature infant may be complicated by air leaks in the lungs and BPD. Infants who survive severe RDS often require frequent hospitalization for upper respiratory tract infections and have an increased incidence of neurodevelopmental sequelae.

ECMO is a technique of cardiopulmonary bypass modified from techniques developed for open-heart surgery that are used to support heart and lung function (for review of ECMO and implications for pediatric physical therapy see Caron & Berlandi, 1997, and Pax Lowes & Palisano, 1995). In newborns with respiratory failure, the immature lungs are allowed to rest and recover to avoid the damaging effects of artificial ventilation. Because of the need for systemic heparinization and the resultant risk of systemic and intracranial hemorrhage, ECMO is reserved for use with infants who are at least 34 weeks of gestational age, weigh more than 2000 g, have no evidence of intracranial bleeding, required less than 10 days of assisted ventilation, and have reversible lung disease (Stork, 1992). ECMO is now used with considerable frequency in support of neonates with severe but reversible respiratory failure, including complicating meconium aspiration, congenital diaphragmatic hernia, sepsis, persistent fetal circulation, and RDS (Martin & Fanaroff, 1992). High-frequency oscillatory ventilation has been used as a bridge to conventional ventilation from ECMO in cases where conventional ventilation was not successful at first (Schexnayder et al., 1995).

Bronchopulmonary Dysplasia

Infants with BPD or chronic lung disease include those who, after requiring mechanical ventilation during the first week of life, remain dependent on oxygen for more than 28 days and have persistent areas of increased densities on chest radiographs (Abman & Groothius, 1994; Carlo & Chatburn, 1988). The overall incidence varies from 13 to 69% of infants weighing less than 1500 g and requiring ventilation, depending on diagnostic criteria and the neonatal population being studied (Mitchell, 1996).

Pathophysiologic features of BPD include interstitial fibrosis resulting from absorption of intraalveolar exudate by the alveolar wall during the resolution of RDS. Alveolar collapse may cause parts of the lung to become airless and solid. These nonaerated regions form scars of condensed lung tissue and become fibrotic. Mucosa of the bronchioles becomes dysplastic and inflamed, and there is hypertrophy of the smooth muscle of bronchioles and arterioles. Pulmonary function testing reveals severe maldistribution of ventilation in these infants. They have increased airway resistance, decreased dynamic compliance, and a large increase in the work of breathing.

Prematurity, barotrauma from high pressures used in assisted ventilation, and pulmonary oxygen toxicity are accepted as key causal components of BPD (Bancalari, 1992). Also, the endotracheal tube itself hinders drainage of tracheal secretions and increases both dead space and resistance to airflow. Other factors that may contribute to the pathogenesis of BPD are infection, pulmonary edema resulting from a patent ductus arteriosus or excessive fluid administration, and increased airway resistance. Immaturity of the pulmonary antioxidant systems and neutrophil-generated toxic oxygen radicals have also been implicated as part of the multifactorial etiology of BPD (Mitchell, 1996).

Treatment strategies for BPD are aimed at preventing or inhibiting the events that trigger the cascade of pathogenic mechanisms (Goetzman, 1986). Other medical treatments include respiratory support, fluid and nutrition management, infection control, bronchodilator, and steroid therapy (Kenner, 1998). Respiratory support includes use of mechanical ventilation only when needed and the use of the lowest peak airway pressure necessary to maintain adequate ventilation. Duration of mechanical ventilation should be limited (Bancalari, 1992). Intermittent mandatory ventilation, which allows the infant to breathe spontaneously between a set number of mechanical breaths per minute, may also be used (Carlo & Chatburn, 1988; Platzker, 1988).

Because infants with BPD are prone to developing cor pulmonale, congestive heart failure, and pulmonary edema, chronic diuretic therapy is instituted. The infant or child with BPD must also be closely monitored for infections, especially those caused by bacteria and fungi. Steroids are used to decrease inflammatory responses and improve lung functions through reduction in pulmonary edema, bronchial edema, and bronchospasm (Kenner, 1998). Other treatments for bronchospasm include inhaled bronchodilator and theophylline therapy (Bancalari, 1992; Davis et al., 1990). Stimulus reduction is also recommended in the nursing care of the infant with BPD (Kenner, 1998).

Chest physical therapy is a component of the care of an infant with BPD for airway clearance problems caused by submucosal and peribronchial smooth muscle hyperplasia, oxygen therapy, and the presence of frequent lower respiratory tract infections (Crane, 1987; Dean, 1987; Hazinski & Pacetti, 1988).

The incidence of developmental disability, such as mental retardation and cerebral palsy, in infants and children with BPD has been reported to be 29 to 34% (Robertson et al., 1991; Vidyasagar, 1985; Vohr et al., 1991). The important predictors for these disabilities are intracranial hemorrhage and periven-tricular echodensity, rather than severity of the BPD (Luchi et al., 1991). Transient neuromotor delays have been documented for infants with BPD because of prolonged periods of increased work of breathing, frequent infections, and recurrent hospitalizations (Mitchell, 1996).

Periventricular Leukomalacia

Periventricular leukomalacia is the principal ischemic lesion of the premature infant (Volpe, 1998). The lesion is caused by a reduction in cerebral blood flow in the highly vulnerable periventricular region of the brain where the arterial "end zones" of the middle, posterior, and anterior cerebral arteries meet. Systemic hypotension with resuscitative difficulties after birth may be a major causal factor. Patent ductus arteriosus and severe apneic spells are other contributing factors, particularly after the first week of life (McMenamin et al., 1984; Sweeney & Swanson, 1990).

Serial ultrasonography, computed tomography, magnetic resonance imaging, and positron emission tomography are useful diagnostic tools for periventricular leukomalacia (Sinha et al., 1990). With the increased availability of high-resolution cranial ultrasonography, ultrasonographic white matter echodensities and echolucencies (both abnormal findings) in LBW infants suggest later disabilities, especially cerebral palsy, more accurately than any other antecedent (Leviton & Paneth, 1990; Miller & Murray, 1992). Serial ultrasonographic studies are important because the evolution of periventricular echodensity is related to prognosis. Early periventricular echodensity that resolves during the first weeks of life is not correlated with later major disabilities; development of cysts as a result of dissolution of brain tissue secondary to infarction, however, is correlated with later cerebral palsy and cognitive deficits (Mantovani & Powers, 1991). Cerebral palsy occurs in infants who develop bilateral cysts larger than 3 mm in diameter in the parietal or occipital areas in more than 90% of the cases.

Medical management includes maintenance of adequate ventilation. The area affected includes the white matter through which long descending motor tracts travel to the spinal cord from the motor cortex. Because the motor tracts involved in the control of leg movements are closest to the ventricles, and therefore more likely to be damaged, spastic diplegia is the most common clinical sequela (Fig. 30–2). If the lesion extends laterally, the arms may be involved, with resulting spastic quadriplegia. Visual deficits may also result from damage to the optic radiations (Catto-Smith et al., 1985; Papile, 1997).

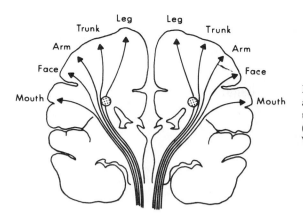

FIGURE 30–2. Diagram of corticospinal tracts. Dotted circular areas indicate periventricular leukomalacia that would be expected to affect descending fibers for control of the lower extremity. (From Volpe, JJ. Neurology of the Newborn, 2nd ed. Philadelphia: WB Saunders, 1987, p. 314.)

Germinal Matrix–Intraventricular Hemorrhage and Periventricular Hemorrhage

Germinal matrix–intraventricular hemorrhage (GM-IVH) is the most common type of neonatal intracranial hemorrhage and is characteristic of the premature infant of less than 32 weeks of gestational age and weighing less than 1500 g. An inverse relationship exists between gestational age and incidence of GM-IVH. The average incidence has been reported at 18% in preterm infants who are in the aforementioned categories for gestational age and weight (Volpe, 1995). Most hemorrhages occur within the first 2 postnatal days, and virtually all occur within 1 week of birth (Papile, 1997). This lesion involves bleeding into the subependymal germinal matrix, which is a gelatinous area that contains a rich vascular network supplied mainly by Heubner's artery, a branch of the anterior cerebral artery. This matrix is prominent from 26 to 34 weeks of gestation and is usually gone by term. The vessels that traverse the matrix are primitive in appearance, with a single layer of endothelium without smooth muscle, elastin, or collagen, and the area is devoid of supportive stroma. The site of origin of hemorrhage is from these primitive capillaries. In a small number of preterm infants, hemorrhage may occur from the choroid plexus or roof of the fourth ventricle (Fig. 30–3). GM-IVH pathogenesis includes fluctuating cerebral blood flow, a decrease or an increase in cerebral blood flow, an increase in cerebral venous pressure, and platelet and coagulation disturbance (Volpe, 1995).

Neuropathologic complications of IVH are hydrocephalus, germinal matrix destruction, cyst formation, and accompanying hypoxic-ischemic lesions. A four-level grading scale based on ultrasound scan has been developed by Papile to classify hemorrhages (Papile et al., 1983). Grade I is an isolated germinal matrix hemorrhage. Grade II is an IVH with normal-sized ventricles that occurs when hemorrhage in the subependymal germinal matrix ruptures through the ependyma into the lateral ventricles. Grade III includes an IVH with acute ventricular dilation, and grade IV involves a hemorrhage into the periventricular white matter. It has recently been shown that the cause of periventricular hemorrhage is not a simple extension of blood into the cerebral white matter from the germinal matrix, but that the lesion is a hemorrhagic venous infarction with the major cause being obstruction of blood flow in the terminal vein caused by GM-IVH (Volpe, 1998). Periventricular hemorrhagic infarction is nearly invariably unilateral or markedly asymmetric, and grossly hemorrhagic.

Ultrasound scan is the procedure of choice in the diagnosis, identification, grading, and timing of GM-IVH because of high-resolution imaging, portable instrumentation, lack of ionizing radiation, and relative affordability (Papile, 1997; Volpe, 1995). Computed tomography scanning is useful for identification of complicating lesions such as posterior fossa lesions.

Treatment includes support of cerebral perfusion by maintaining arterial blood pressure and avoidance of cerebral hemodynamic disturbances caused by rapid volume expansion, pneumothorax, increased arterial blood pressure, and hypoxemia. Serial ultrasound scans to monitor ventricular size and ventriculostomy or shunting for hydrocephalus are also important treatment components (Volpe, 1995). Prophylactic measures include transport of the infant in utero to a level III nursery, limiting noxious handling, optimal management of labor and delivery, and medications such as phenobarbital, indomethacin, and pancuronium (a neuromuscular blocking agent). Ethamsylate (to reduce capillary

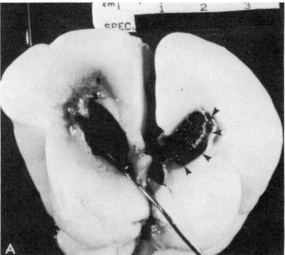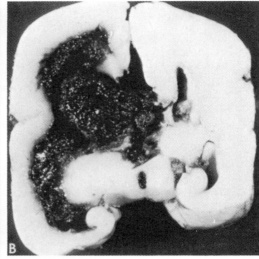

FIGURE 30–3. Coronal section of the cerebrum showing intraventricular hemorrhage. (From Volpe, JJ. Neurology of the Newborn, 2nd ed. Philadelphia: WB Saunders, 1987, p. 314.)

bleeding) and vitamins E and K are currently under investigation. When hemorrhage has occurred, medical management includes maintenance of cerebral perfusion through control of blood pressure and decrease in intracranial pressure through lumbar puncture and ventricular drainage.

The outcome of the infant with GM-IVH depends largely on the degree of associated parenchymal injury rather than the quantity of intraventricular blood. Volpe (1995) reported that for neonates with parenchymal injury greater than 1 cm, the mortality rate was 59% and the rate of major neurologic sequelae such as spastic hemiparesis or asymmetric spastic quadriplegia was 87%. In addition, 73% of the survivors had cognitive impairments. The risk of major neurologic disability in LBW preterm infants increases with each higher grade of IVH (McMenamin et al., 1984). The incidences of neurologic sequelae for grades I, II, and III are 15, 30, and 40%, respectively (Volpe, 1995). Dubowitz and Dubowitz (1981a, 1981b) have noted that a tight popliteal angle (130° or less in infants up to 31 weeks of gestation and 110° or less at 32 to 35 weeks of gestation) is a sign of IVH.

HYPOXIC-ISCHEMIC ENCEPHALOPATHY

Hypoxic-ischemic encephalopathy (HIE) is the major perinatal cause of neurologic morbidity in both the premature and full-term infant (Vannucci, 1997). Perinatal asphyxia results in hypoxemia (reduced amount of oxygen in the blood) and ischemia,

with ischemia being the most important form of oxygen deprivation. The period of reperfusion is when many of the complications that affect the metabolism, function, and structure of the brain occur. The relative importance of antepartum, intrapartum, and postnatal hypoxic-ischemic insults is difficult to determine. Major signs of HIE include seizures and abnormalities in state of consciousness, tone, posture, reflexes (especially disturbed suck, swallow, gag, and tongue movements), respiratory pattern, and autonomic function. Conditions associated with increased risk for fetal asphyxia are altered placental exchange, reduced maternal blood flow to the placenta, and decreased maternal oxygen saturation. Altered placental exchange may result from abruption, placenta previa, postmaturity, prolapsed umbilical cord, umbilical cord around the neck, and placental insufficiency. Maternal hypotension may reduce the blood flow to the placenta, and maternal hypoventilation, hypoxia, or cardiopulmonary disease may decrease maternal oxygenation. Intrapartum insults include those related to traumatic delivery, prolonged labor, and acute placental or cord problems. Prolonged partial asphyxia from any cause sets into motion a spiral of cytotoxic edema, with impaired cerebral blood flow, which leads to cerebral necrosis or ulegyria (Fig. 30–4). Infants with HIE commonly have disturbances of pulmonary, cardiovascular, hepatic, and renal functions.

Therapeutic care of an infant at risk for development of HIE includes careful monitoring by serial neurologic assessments, detection of reduced cerebral perfusion pressure, and assessment of the struc-

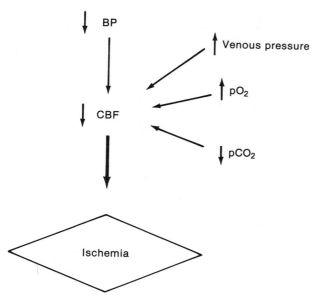

FIGURE 30–4. Model for production of cerebral edema. Decreased blood pressure (BP) leads to decreased cerebral blood flow (CBF) and ischemia. (From Campbell, SK: Clinical decision making: Management of the neonate with movement dysfunction. In Wolf, SL [Ed.], Clinical Decision Making in Physical Therapy. Philadelphia: FA Davis, 1985, p. 299.)

tural status of brain with computed tomography, ultrasound, magnetic resonance imaging, magnetic resonance spectroscopy, technetium scan, and electroencephalography or evoked potential tests (Brann & Schwartz, 1992a; Volpe, 1997, 1998). Treatment principles include prevention of intrauterine asphyxia; maintenance of adequate ventilation, perfusion, and blood glucose levels; and control of seizures and brain swelling.

Preventive measures for intrauterine asphyxia include antepartum assessment and identification of the high-risk pregnancy, electronic fetal monitoring, fetal blood sampling, and cesarean section when necessary. Maintenance of adequate oxygenation is essential to prevent additional injury. Volume expansion with the use of pressor agents to increase blood pressure is used to maintain cerebral blood flow. Partial exchange transfusion may be done if the infant's hematocrit is low to decrease hyperviscosity and enhance tissue oxygenation. Sodium bicarbonate and glucose are administered to treat severe, persistent metabolic acidosis and hypoglycemia, respectively. The use of barbiturates is being studied because they reduce the energy requirements of the brain and have been shown to decrease intracranial pressure in adults. Phenobarbital is the drug of choice for seizure control, with lorazepam as adjunctive therapy.

Sarnat and Sarnat (1976) identified three stages of encephalopathy after asphyxia. Stage 1 lasts less than 24 hours and is characterized by hyperalertness, low-threshold Moro and stretch reflexes, and normal muscle tone and electroencephalogram. The dura-

tion for stage 2 is approximately 5 days; clinical signs include lethargy, mild hypotonia, hyperactive stretch reflexes, strong distal flexion, hyperactive stretch reflexes, weak suck and Moro reflexes, strong tonic neck reflex, and multifocal seizures. Stage 3 is stupor, which lasts from a few hours to 4 weeks, with flaccidity alternating with decerebrate posturing, absent reflexes, response only to strong noxious stimuli, occasional seizures, and an isopotential electroencephalogram.

When the infant with hypoxic-ischemic insult has a normal neurologic examination by 1 week of age, sequelae are minimal. Those who continue to have an abnormal neurologic examination by 3 weeks of age, however, are at risk of developing major neurologic sequelae (Harper & Yoon, 1987). The neurologic sequelae of HIE include motor deficits with or without mental retardation, seizures, or both. Neuropathologic classifications of HIE include selective neuronal necrosis, status marmoratus, parasagittal cerebral injury, and focal ischemic brain necrosis (Volpe, 1995).

Selective Neuronal Necrosis

Selective neuronal necrosis, the most common type of HIE, is the death of neurons in a widespread but characteristic pattern and commonly accompanies the other manifestations of HIE. The major sites of neuronal necrosis include the hippocampus of the cerebral cortex and parts of the diencephalon, basal ganglia, pons, medulla, cerebellum, and spinal cord (Box 30–2, Table 30–1, and Fig. 30–5) (Cabanas et al., 1991). The pathogenesis of selective neuronal

BOX 30–2. Selective Neuronal Necrosis in Neonatal Hypoxic-Ischemic Encephalopathy—Major Sites

Cerebral cortex—hippocampus, supralimbic cortex
Diencephalon—thalamus, hypothalamus, and lateral geniculate body
Basal ganglia—caudate, putamen, and globus pallidus
Midbrain—inferior colliculus, oculomotor and trochlear nuclei, red nucleus, substantia nigra, and reticular formation
Pons—motor nuclei of trigeminal and facial nerves; dorsal, ventral cochlear nuclei; reticular formation; and pontine nuclei
Medulla—dorsal motor nucleus of vagus nerve, nucleus ambiguus, inferior olivary nuclei, cuneate and gracilis nuclei
Cerebellum—Purkinje cells, dentate, and other roof nuclei

From Volpe, JJ. Neurology of the Newborn, 2nd ed. Philadelphia: WB Saunders, 1987, p. 213.

TABLE 30–1. Sites of Particular Predilection for Apparent Hypoxic-Ischemic Selective Neuronal Injury in Premature and Term Newborns*

Brain Region	Premature	Term
Cerebral neocortex		+†
Hippocampus		
Sommer's sector		+
Subiculum	+	
Basal ganglia/thalamus	=†	=
Brainstem		
Cranial nerve nuclei	=	=
Pons (ventral)	+	
Inferior olivary nuclei	+	
Cerebellum		
Purkinje cells		+
Internal granule cells	+	
Spinal cord		
Anterior horn cells (alone)		+
Infarction (including anterior horn cells)	+	

*See text for references.
†+, Relatively more common in term versus premature newborn (or vice versa); =, equally common in term and premature newborns.

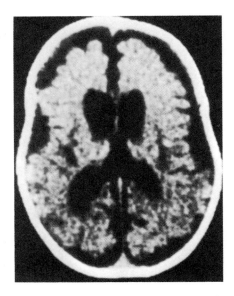

FIGURE 30–5. Computed tomography scan of selective cortical neuronal necrosis of a 4-week-old infant who experienced severe perinatal asphyxia. Note cortical atrophy and white matter injury. (From Volpe, JJ. Neurology of the Newborn, 2nd ed. Philadelphia: WB Saunders, 1987, p. 245.)

necrosis includes regional vascular factors because neuronal injury is more marked in vascular border zones, regional metabolic factors, and the regional distribution of glutamate receptors (Volpe, 1995, 1997, 1998). Clinical findings include stupor, coma, seizures, hypotonus, and problems in oculomotor, sucking, and tongue movement. Long-term sequelae include mental retardation, spastic quadriparesis, seizure disorder, ataxia, bulbar and pseudobulbar palsy, hyperactivity, impaired attention, and atonic quadriparesis.

Status Marmoratus

Status marmoratus is neuronal loss, gliosis, and hypermyelinization of the basal ganglia and thalamus. Impairments are not fully manifested until the latter part of the first year of life, although injury occurs in the perinatal period (Volpe, 1987). The pathogenesis of this lesion is related primarily to glutamate-induced neuronal death, as well as regional circulatory and metabolic factors (Volpe, 1995, 1998). Neonatal findings are unknown at this time, but long-term clinical sequelae include choreoathetosis, mental retardation, and spastic quadriplegia.

Parasagittal Cerebral Injury

Parasagittal cerebral injury results in a lesion of the cerebral cortex and subcortical white matter. This injury is usually bilateral and symmetric, with the parietal-occipital regions most affected (Volpe, 1995). The areas of necrosis are the border zones between the end fields of the major cerebral arteries. Clinical signs in the neonatal period include proximal limb weakness, especially in the upper extremities. Long-term sequelae include spastic quadriparesis and specific intellectual deficits such as delay in development of language, visuospatial abilities, or both.

Focal Ischemic Brain Necrosis and Cavitation

The category of focal ischemic brain necrosis includes large, localized areas of neuronal death in the distribution of single or multiple major blood vessels in the cerebral cortex and subcortical white matter. Most of these lesions are unilateral and involve the middle cerebral artery. The focal ischemic brain necrosis occurs perinatally as the result of cerebrovascular insufficiency secondary to malformation of vessels, arterial obstruction due to thrombi or emboli, or systemic circulatory insufficiency near the end of the second trimester. Resolution of neuronal necrosis results in the formation of cavities. Neurologic features during the neonatal period include hemiparesis, quadriparesis, and stereotyped and nonhabituating reflex responses. This lesion results in spastic hemiparesis in the case of a limited focal lesion, mental retardation, and seizure disorder (Volpe, 1995).

Necrotizing Enterocolitis

Necrotizing enterocolitis (NEC) is an acute inflammatory disease of the bowel that occurs most frequently during the first 6 weeks of life in premature infants weighing less than 2000 g (Whaley & Wong, 1991). Although the precise cause of the disease is not known, several factors appear to play a role in the pathogenesis of NEC. These factors include intestinal ischemia, infectious agents and toxins, and enteral alimentation. Diagnosis is made by physical examination, laboratory studies, and radiography. Vomiting, abdominal distention, bloody stools, lethargy, and alterations in respiratory status are signs of this condition (Dolgin et al., 1998). Medical care of infants with NEC includes parenteral alimentation, gastric suction, and administration of broad-spectrum antibiotics (Cressinger et al., 1992). Laboratory findings include anemia, leukopenia, and electrolyte imbalance. Breath hydrogen measurements have been found to be 99% effective in detecting absence of the disease and are suggested as an aid to diagnosis of NEC (Cheu et al., 1989). Abdominal radiographs are performed every 6 to 8 hours to detect progressive intestinal obstruction or possible perforation. Surgical intervention is indicated when there is radiographic evidence of fixed, dilated intestinal loops accompanied by intestinal distention (Cressinger et al., 1992). Surgical procedures include intestinal decompression by nasogastric tube placement or gastrostomy, resection of necrotic bowel, and diversion of the proximal fecal stream by ileostomy, jejunostomy, or colostomy. Although enterostomy is a lifesaving procedure, it has been reported to be a major cause of morbidity (O'Connor & Swain, 1998).

NEC is the most common cause of death in neonates undergoing surgery. The average mortality rate after surgery is 30 to 40%. Stricture formation, which is abnormal narrowing of the intestines, occurs in 25 to 35% of the survivors of medical or surgical treatment and causes failure to thrive, feeding abnormalities, diarrhea, or bowel obstruction (Cressinger et al., 1992).

Retinopathy of Prematurity

Retinopathy of prematurity (ROP) is a developmental vascular retinopathy that occurs in the incompletely vascularized retina of premature infants (Phelps, 1992). It is characterized by severe vascular constriction and followed by hypoxia of the immature vasculature of the retina. Subsequently, there is vascular proliferation of retinal capillaries into the hypoxic area. New vessels proliferate toward the lens, and the aqueous humor and then the vitreous humor become turbid. The retina becomes edematous, and hemorrhages separate the retina from its attachment. The outcome of the disease ranges from normal vision to total loss of vision if there is advanced scarring from the retina to the lens resulting in retinal detachment (Whaley & Wong, 1991). ROP was called retrolental fibroplasia in the early 1940s and was virtually eliminated with the severe restriction of oxygen use between 1950 and 1970. The condition has recurred as one of the major causes of disability in preterm infants as a result of the increased survival of VLBW infants. The incidence of ROP increases with lower gestational age, lower birth weight, and BPD (Holmstrom et al., 1998). Hyperoxia, shock, asphyxia, hypothermia, vitamin E deficiency, and light exposure have been implicated as possible pathogenic factors (Kretzer & Hittner, 1986). Antenatal dexamethasone administration appears to be associated with a decreased incidence of development of ROP of stage 2 or higher (Higgins et al., 1998). Light reduction was not shown to be effective in altering the incidence of ROP (Reynolds et al., 1998).

Prevention and treatment include oxygen administration at Pao_2 between 50 and 70 mm Hg, administration of vitamin E (which is still under investigation), and surgery, such as laser photocoagulation, cryotherapy, vitrectomy, and scleral buckling (Kretzer & Hittner, 1986). Supplemental oxygen with target oxygen saturation of 99% with Po_2 of no higher than 100 mm Hg was associated with regression of prethreshold ROP, without appearing to arrest retinal vascular maturation (Gaynon, 1997). Outcome of surgery ranges from complete recovery or mild myopia to blindness, depending on the extent of the disease, which is rated in stages 1 through 4 based on funduscopic examination: 1—demarcation line separating the posterior vascularized retina from the anterior nonvascularized retina; 2—intraretinal ridge formation; 3—intraretinal ridge plus fibrovascular proliferation; and 4—retinal detachment (Kingham, 1986). Whether there is "plus" disease for each of these stages (e.g., 3+) is also determined. Plus disease occurs when the retinal arteries and veins become tortuous and dilated as a result of shunting from arterioles to veins in the peripheral retina with active ROP (White et al., 1991). Screening for ROP has been recommended for infants less than 35 weeks of gestation or less than 1500 g (Wright, 1998).

Hyperbilirubinemia

Hyperbilirubinemia, or physiologic jaundice, is the accumulation of excessive amounts of bilirubin in the blood. Bilirubin is one of the breakdown products of hemoglobin from red blood cells. This condition is seen commonly in premature infants who have immature hepatic functions, an increased hemolysis of red blood cells as a result of high concentrations of circulating red blood cells, a shorter life span of red blood cells, and possible polycythemia from birth injuries (Whaley & Wong, 1991). The primary goal in treatment of hyperbilirubinemia is the prevention of kernicterus, which is the deposition of unconjugated bilirubin in the brain, especially in the basal ganglia and hippocampus. LBW infants of less than 2000 g receive phototherapy at 24 hours of life for 96 hours, regardless of bilirubin concentration. Phototherapy is administered by banks of 8 to 10 fluorescent lamps placed 12 to 16 inches above the unclothed infant in an open radiant warmer or incubator (Gartner & Lee, 1992). The infant's eyes are shielded by patches to avoid retinal damage. Studies show that on/off cycles of more than 1 hour are as effective as continuous treatment. A technique of fiberoptic phototherapy uses light from a halogen lamp transmitted through a fiberoptic bundle to a blanket that is wrapped around the infant (Biliblanket) (Gartner & Lee, 1992).

If phototherapy is not effective in reducing the total serum bilirubin concentrations to acceptable levels, or if there is a rapidly rising bilirubin level, exchange transfusion is done (Shaw, 1998). In this technique, approximately 85% of the infant's red blood cells are replaced. Initial human trials have shown beneficial effects of tin mesoporphyrin and tin protoporphyrin used as prophylaxis and treatment to reduce hyperbilirubinemia. These are inhibitors of heme oxygenase, which is an enzyme in the synthesis of bilirubin that limits the rate of degradation of heme to bile (Gartner & Lee, 1992; Kenner, 1998).

NEONATAL SEIZURES

Neonatal seizures are the most frequent and distinct neurologic signs that occur in the neonatal period (Brann & Wiznitzer, 1992). Seizures are the most frequent overt sign of neurologic disorders (Volpe, 1995). Most occur between the second and fifth days of life, and 85% occur in the first 15 days of life. A seizure during the neonatal period is a medical emergency, because it may indicate a life-threatening disease or disorder that can produce immediate and irreversible brain damage. Neonatal seizures may also result in decreased DNA content and brain cell number.

The causes of neonatal seizures include hypoxic-ischemic encephalopathy secondary to perinatal asphyxia. Seizures are also caused by intracranial hemorrhage, hypoglycemia, hypocalcemia, intracranial infection, developmental defects, and drug withdrawal (Volpe, 1995). Clinical manifestations of seizures in neonates differ greatly from those in older infants and children because of the immaturity of the brain. Clinical signs in the neonate include facial, oral, lingual, and ocular movements and autonomic manifestations such as apnea and changes in blood pressure, heart rate, and pupil size (Box 30-3). Abnormal movements and alteration of tone in the trunk and extremities, including rowing and bicycling movements, are also clinical signs of neonatal seizure (Mizrahi & Kellaway, 1987). Treatment includes administration of anticonvulsants such as

---

BOX 30-3. Characteristics of Subtle Seizures in Premature and Full-Term Infants

Ocular-tonic horizontal deviation of eyes (jerking) and sustained eye opening with ocular fixation
Eyelid blinking or fluttering
Sucking, smacking, drooling, and other oral-buccal-lingual movements
"Swimming," "rowing," and "pedaling" movements
Apneic spell

From Volpe, JJ. Neurology of the Newborn, 2nd ed. Philadelphia: WB Saunders, 1987, p. 134.

phenobarbital, phenytoin, and diazepam to control seizures and intravenous glucose for hypoglycemia.

Approximately 15 to 20% of all infants with neonatal seizures later exhibit mental retardation, motor impairment, or both. Seizures that occur in conjunction with perinatal asphyxia, severe IVH, intracranial infection, and prematurity with prolonged hypoglycemia have poor prognoses, with possible permanent neurologic sequelae such as cerebral palsy or mental retardation. Seizures that occur with subarachnoid hemorrhage without asphyxia or as a result of metabolic disorders have good prognoses if treatment begins early (Volpe, 1995).

FETAL ALCOHOL SYNDROME

Chronic alcohol exposure in utero may result in a multitude of symptoms at birth, including withdrawal symptoms of irritability, tremors, apnea, and seizures (Volpe, 1995; West et al., 1998). When severe, phenobarbital or paregoric (morphine) may be used to control withdrawal symptoms (Harper & Yoon, 1987). Alcohol rapidly crosses the placenta and the blood-brain barrier of the fetus, and there is a dose-dependent relationship between maternal alcohol intake in the first weeks of pregnancy and the occurrence of features of the fetal alcohol syndrome (FAS).

The full manifestation of FAS, one of the most common causes of mental retardation in the world, is characterized by a triad of symptoms composed of growth deficiency; cardiac defects; and CNS disturbance, such as microcephaly, mental retardation, and dysmorphology (including facial, genital, and joint abnormalities) (Barbour, 1990; Volpe, 1995).

In utero alcohol exposure is related to a wide continuum of effects ranging from full FAS to partial FAS, also referred to as fetal alcohol effects, to more subtle effects, such as neurologic disorders without dysmorphology (Scott et al., 1991). These subtle neurologic effects include hyperactivity, delayed language development, fine and gross motor problems, slowed reaction time, and problems with judgment and comprehension (Autti-Ramo & Granström, 1991; Scott et al., 1991). Long-term effects of prenatal alcohol exposure include deficits in several areas of intellectual functioning, including information processing, short-term memory, encoding, and preacademic skills (Coles et al., 1991; Little et al., 1989). Streissguth (1986) reported that 24% of children born to binge drinkers and 15% born to nonbinge drinkers were receiving special education services at 7.5 years of age. In addition to cognitive deficits, behavioral and communication problems lead to maladaptive social functioning, including impulsive behavior, anxiety, and dysphoria (Volpe, 1995).

FETAL ABSTINENCE SYNDROME

Maternal use of narcotics during pregnancy leads to the development of dependency on that drug by the fetus. The most commonly used drugs are heroin, methadone, and cocaine, and there is often maternal use of several drugs during pregnancy (Finnegan, 1988). The fetus experiences withdrawal when the mother is withdrawn from her drug or drugs or when the fetus is delivered. Symptoms of withdrawal are similar to those of withdrawal from alcohol and include irritability, tremors, seizures, apnea, increased muscle tone, inability to sleep, hyperactive deep tendon reflexes, incoordination, hyperactive sucking soon after birth and then ineffective sucking and swallowing, and shrill crying (Dixon, 1989; Hayford et al., 1988; Volpe, 1995). Premature delivery, meconium aspiration, low birth weight, small for gestational age, decreased head circumference, and abruptio placentae are common complications of labor and delivery (Chasnoff, 1988; Handler et al., 1991). Microcephaly is the most common brain abnormality in infants born to cocaine-using mothers. Disturbances in the behavioral organization and interactive abilities of these neonates make early bonding and attachment difficult (Hume et al., 1989). Follow-up studies indicate growth retardation, long-term intellectual impairment, and learning difficulties in children exposed to drugs in utero (Bauman & Levine, 1986; Davis & Templer, 1988; Free et al., 1990; Hume et al., 1989; Lewis et al., 1989).

EXPOSURE TO HUMAN IMMUNODEFICIENCY VIRUS

The risk of infants born to women with a positive HIV titer developing HIV infection is estimated to be 10 to 40% (Volpe, 1995). Infants are usually asymptomatic at birth, and the infection may not become evident until the child is 12 to 18 months old, with the median age at onset of symptoms being 9 months (Pizzi & Harris-Hinds, 1990). Infection early in fetal development may lead to microcephaly, cerebral atrophy, basal ganglia and white matter calcification, calcific vasculopathy of the CNS, spinal cord myelin loss, and facial anomalies (Volpe, 1995). Infants exposed to HIV should be monitored for signs of infection, such as failure to thrive, weight loss, temperature instability, and diarrhea, and assessed for opportunistic infections, such as herpes simplex virus infection, cytomegalovirus infection, lymphoid interstitial pneumonia, and viral, fungal, or protozoal infections. Because neonates with HIV infection are usually asymptomatic, they are not admitted to the NICU unless there are problems unrelated to HIV. It should be noted, however, that infants who were seropositive exhibited significantly lower scores on the Bayley Scales of Infant Development than seronegative infants (Aylward et al., 1992).

BIRTH INJURIES RELATED TO THE NERVOUS SYSTEM

Birth injuries are those sustained during labor and delivery and represent an important cause of neonatal morbidity (Mangurten, 1992). The most common traumatic lesions related to the nervous system include caput succedaneum, linear skull fracture, and brachial plexus palsy.

Caput Succedaneum

Caput succedaneum is hemorrhagic edema caused by compression of a portion of the scalp from the pressure of the uterus or vaginal wall during a vertex delivery. The clinical manifestation is a soft swelling usually a few millimeters thick. The edema is external to the periosteum and crosses suture lines. The lesion steadily resolves over the first days of life, and no intervention is necessary.

Linear Skull Fracture

Linear skull fractures are relatively common in newborns and are caused by direct compression of the head during a prolonged labor and delivery and use of forceps during delivery. Uncomplicated linear skull fractures are diagnosed by radiographs and require no treatment.

Brachial Plexus Palsy

Brachial plexus palsy is a paralysis or weakness involving the muscles of the upper extremity after mechanical trauma to the spinal roots of the fifth cervical (C5) through the first thoracic (T1) nerves during birth. Brachial plexus palsies are classified into three types: Erb's, or upper arm, paralysis (involving C5 and C6); Klumpke's, or lower arm, paralysis (involving C8 and T1); and Erb-Klumpke, or whole arm, paralysis. Approximately 90% of brachial plexus palsies involve the upper arm corresponding to Erb's palsy (Volpe, 1995). Most cases of brachial plexus palsy follow a prolonged and difficult labor. The infant is often of high birth weight, sedated, and hypotonic, rendering the arm vulnerable to separation of bony segments, overstretching, and soft tissue injury (Mangurten, 1992; Scoles, 1992; Shepherd, 1991). Traction on the shoulder during delivery of the head in a breech presentation, and lateral traction of the head and neck while delivering the shoulders in a vertex presentation, can injure the C5 and C6 roots. More forceful traction may result in paralysis of the whole arm. Forceful elevation and abduction of the arm, stretching the lower plexus under and against the coracoid process of the scapula, may be the cause of the less common lower palsy. The birth trauma that injures the brachial plexus may also be associated with other lesions. Associated lesions may include injury to the facial nerve, fractures of the clavicle or humerus, subluxation of the shoulder, torticollis, or a hemiparalysis of the diaphragm by injuring the phrenic nerve at C4.

In most infants with brachial plexus injury, the nerve sheath is torn and the nerve fibers are compressed by hemorrhage and edema. Clinical manifestations include a characteristic arm position of adduction, internal rotation with extension of the elbow, pronation of the forearm, and flexion of the wrist (Fig. 30-6). Passive abduction of the extremity results in it falling limply. The Moro, biceps, and radial reflexes are absent; grasp is intact.

Treatment of brachial plexus injury includes rest for 7 to 10 days after injury to allow hemorrhage and edema to decrease. During this time, partial immobilization is accomplished by positioning the limb gently across the upper abdomen (Volpe, 1995). Physical therapy begins after the initial period of immobilization. The goals of treatment are to maintain range of motion (ROM) by gentle passive exercising, to stimulate muscle function as neural regeneration occurs, and to encourage active movement (Fig. 30-7) (see Shepherd, 1991, for a comprehensive physical therapy assessment and treatment plan). Splinting is controversial, and continuous splinting in the "Statue of Liberty" splint is no longer recommended because it results in formation of abduction contractures and subsequent hypermobility of the shoulder. Intermittent splinting of the wrist and stabilization of the fingers are recommended by some health care professionals for lower arm palsy (Mangurten, 1992; Volpe, 1995).

SPINA BIFIDA

Spina bifida includes a continuum of congenital anomalies of the spine that range from failure of fusion of the posterior vertebral arch or arches to open spinal defects such as myelomeningocele (Edwards & Derechin, 1988) (see Chapter 23 for a full discussion of myelodysplasia). Approximately 80% of all lesions in infants with myelomeningocele occur in the lumbar area, which may reflect the fact

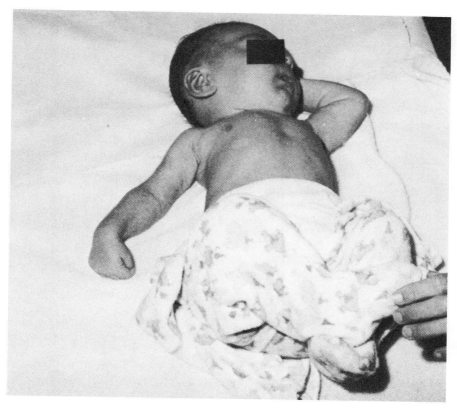

FIGURE 30–6. Four-week-old infant with partial paralysis of right arm as a result of brachial plexus injury. (From Shepherd, RB. Brachial plexus injury. In Campbell, SK [Ed.], Pediatric Neurologic Physical Therapy. New York: Churchill Livingstone, 1991, p. 107.)

that this is the last region of the neural tube to close (Noetzel, 1989; Volpe, 1995). When an open defect is present, early closure of the back lesion is performed during the first 24 to 48 hours after birth to prevent infections such as meningitis or ventriculitis and to prevent trauma to the exposed tissue and stretching of the other nerve roots, which can lead to a loss of motor function. There are proponents, however, for the delay of sac closure to allow for further assessment of neurologic function, intellectual potential, and extent of complications. These proponents also believe that delaying closure results in improved tolerance of the procedure, allows for better epithelialization of the sac, and permits easier mobilization of skin for closure (Charney et al., 1985). If prophylactic antibiotics are administered from 24 hours of life until surgery, infection rates are low. The most prudent course seems to be prompt closure after rational decision making by the parents and physicians (Volpe, 1995). The objective of sac closure is to replace the neural tissue into the vertebral canal, cover the spinal defect, and achieve a flat and watertight closure of the sac (Huttenlocher, 1987).

Hydrocephalus is a common complication of myelodysplasia. The incidence of hydrocephalus varies according to the site of the lesion (Noetzel, 1989; Volpe, 1995). With lesions involving the thoracolumbar, lumbar, or lumbosacral areas, the incidence of hydrocephalus is approximately 90%. With occipital, cervical, thoracic, or sacral lesions, the incidence of hydrocephalus is 60%. Ventriculoperitoneal shunting is performed when there are clinical or diagnostic signs of hydrocephalus. Clinical signs include full anterior fontanelle and split cranial sutures. Hydrocephalus is most commonly associated with overt clinical signs 2 to 3 weeks after birth. Serial computed tomography and ultrasonography are tools used to diagnose hydrocephalus.

Physical Therapy Examination and Intervention

Physical therapy examination of the neonate with myelodysplasia in the special care nursery may be done before or after closure of the back, or both before and after. This assessment is important to

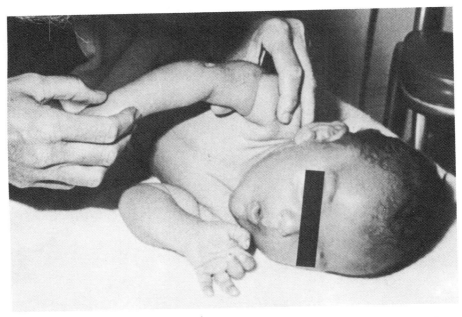

FIGURE 30–7. Therapist attempting to elicit activity in the deltoid muscle by encouraging hand-to-face movement. (From Shepherd, RB. Brachial plexus injury. In Campbell, SK [Ed.], Pediatric Neurologic Physical Therapy. New York: Churchill Livingstone, 1991, p. 112.)

evaluate skeletal alignment, ROM, the level of motor and sensory functioning, reflex development, and behavioral organization. The neonate with myelomeningocele may have joint deformities as the result of imbalance of muscle action and positioning in utero. Intermittent taping, positioning, ROM exercising, and splinting are techniques used by the physical therapist to treat joint deformities. Intermittent taping is more adaptable to the nursery setting and is reported to be more effective than ROM exercises to improve mobility (Sweeney & Swanson, 1995). A thorough knowledge of arthrokinematic principles and techniques is necessary to position the joint in a corrected position before taping. An external skin protection solution is applied under the tape, and an adhesive removal solution is used when the tape is removed. The therapist who performs taping must carefully observe skin condition and vascular tolerance when developing a taping schedule. Taping schedules begin with 1 hour and increase by 1 hour as tolerated. Positioning may also help improve or maintain skeletal alignment, such as prone positioning to maintain hip joint ROM and encourage development of the extensor muscles. Side lying can be used to encourage a symmetric posture. The supine position should be avoided because of the effects of gravity. Splinting or serial casting may also be used to improve skeletal alignment (Schneider, Krosschell, & Gabriel, 1995).

Range of Motion

ROM testing of the newborn with spina bifida is indicated to identify impairments and, if necessary, to take advantage of the neonatal period of hyperplasticity of ligaments, resulting from transplacental transfer of relaxin and estrogen from the mother (Hensinger, 1977; Sweeney & Swanson, 1995). The therapist must be aware of normal neonatal physiologic flexion of the hips and knees and the possibility of hip dislocation. Because of the latter, it is recommended that hip adduction be tested only to the neutral position. Limitations in ROM are not an indication for aggressive stretching. ROM exercises should be performed slowly and gently to avoid fractures of paralyzed lower extremities. Common limitations in muscle extensibility for neonates with spina bifida include tightness of hip flexors, hip adductors, and dorsiflexors or evertors of the ankle (Mazur & Menelaus, 1991; Tappit-Emas, 1999). ROM exercises should be done with hands placed close to the joint being moved with a brief hold at the end of the range preventing unnecessary stress to soft tissue and joint structures (Tappit-Emas, 1999).

Manual Muscle Testing

Muscle testing is performed by the physical therapist to determine the level of muscle innervation. Obviously, conventional methods of muscle testing are not appropriate for the neonate. Schneider, Krosschell, and Gabriel (1995) offer some strategies for eliciting muscle contraction that include carefully considering the state of the infant, tickling, holding the extremities in positions such as hip and knee flexion, and holding a limb in an antigravity position to stimulate the infant to move or hold a limb. Movements of the extremities may be observed, and contractions may be palpated. Gentle resistance may be given to elicit a stronger response (Tappit-Emas, 1999). Muscle strength may be graded as present, absent, or trace. Repeated assessment is recommended to obtain as accurate a picture as possible of muscle function.

Sensory Testing

Sensory testing should be performed when the neonate is in a quiet, awake state in order to determine the level of sensation. The skin is stroked with a pin or other sharp object to determine the neonate's reaction to pain, such as facial grimacing. The therapist begins at the anal area, the lowest sacral innervation level, and strokes across the buttocks, down the posterior thigh and leg, up the anterior surface of the leg and thigh, and across the abdominal musculature to determine reaction to pain (Schneider, Krosschell, & Gabriel, 1995). The neonate's response should be recorded for each dermatome.

Reflex and Behavioral Assessment

The physical therapist may also include reflex and behavioral testing such as the Brazelton Neonatal Behavioral Assessment Scale in the evaluation of the neonate with spina bifida (Brazelton, 1984). The purpose of this part of the assessment is to evaluate reflex activity such as sucking and swallowing and to determine the current status of the infant's organization of physiologic response to stress, state control, motor control, and social interaction (Schneider, Krosschell, & Gabriel, 1995). The physical therapist notes the neonate's strengths, as well as the problems the neonate is having. Repeated behavioral testing may help monitor progress in organization and reflect recovery. When performing a reflex or behavioral assessment, it is important to ascertain that the neonate's performance is not affected by CNS-depressant drugs.

PAIN

The neonate's ability to perceive pain has become a focus of clinical and research attention (Pigeon et al., 1989). Previously, it was assumed that the neonate's nervous system functioned at a decorticate level, with insufficient myelinization of pain tracts and centers to perceive, feel, or remember pain (Franck, 1987; Shiao et al., 1987; Whaley & Wong, 1997). Increased knowledge of the capabilities of the newborn brain and advances in neonatal pharmacology have fostered a concern for the importance of protecting the neonatal CNS from stresses in the NICU environment. Evidence exists that pain pathways, cortical and subcortical centers of pain perception, and neurochemical systems associated with pain transmission and modulation are intact and functional in the neonate (Anand, 1998; Franck, 1992). Slow conduction speed is the result of less myelinization, but it is balanced by shorter interneuronal distances traveled by painful nerve impulses and the fact that most nociceptive impulses are transmitted by nonmyelinated C fibers (Anand & Hickey, 1987). However, the endorphin system, which mediates analgesia, may not be completely functional, leaving the preterm infant more sensitive to pain than term or older infants (Stevens & Franck, 1995).

Although it is difficult to assess pain in the neonate, the physical therapist working with neonates and infants in the special care nursery should be aware of the methods used to assess pain and be able to perform the nonpharmacologic procedures to alleviate pain. Both physiologic and behavioral responses of the neonate to nociceptive or painful stimuli have been identified. Physiologic manifestations of pain include increased heart rate, blood pressure, and respirations, with evidence of decreased oxygenation. Skin color and character when pain is present include pallor or flushing, diaphoresis, and palmar sweating. Other indicators of pain are increased muscle tone, dilated pupils, and laboratory evidence of metabolic or endocrine changes (Whaley & Wong, 1991). Neonatal behavioral responses to nociceptive input include sustained and intense crying; facial expression of grimaces, furrowed brow, quivering chin, or eyes tightly closed; motor behavior such as limb withdrawal, thrashing, rigidity, flaccidity, and fist clenching; and changes in state (Pigeon et al., 1989). An infant may, however, be experiencing pain when lying quietly with closed eyes (Shapiro, 1989).

Several neonatal pain measurement instruments have been developed, including the Neonatal Facial Coding System (Gruneau & Craig, 1987; Gruneau et al., 1990); the Neonatal Infant Pain Scale (Barrier et al., 1989); the Modified Behavioral Pain Scale (Taddio et al., 1995); and the Premature Infant Pain Profile (Stevens et al., 1995).

Nonpharmacologic methods to alleviate pain include decreasing stimulation, swaddling, nonnutritive sucking, tactile comfort measures, rocking, containment, and music (Abad et al., 1996; Burke et al., 1995; Franck, 1987; Whaley & Wong, 1997).

Preterm neonates showed a significantly lower mean heart rate, shorter crying time, and shorter mean sleep disruption after heel stick with facilitated tucking (containing the infant with hands softly holding the infant's extremities in soft flexion) than without (Corff et al., 1995). Morphine, fentanyl, and topical mixture of a local anesthetic cream (EMLA) are the most commonly used analgesics in the NICU (Stevens & Franck, 1995).

FAMILY RESPONSE TO PREMATURE BIRTH

Although medical interventions are critical to the survival of the premature infant, there is an increased awareness of the importance of recognizing the needs of parents and providing supports. Taking on the parenting role is a major life task that is greatly complicated by the crisis of a critically ill newborn. Families react to this crisis in different and individual ways. Common emotions include anxiety, guilt, fear, resentment, feelings of inadequacy, and anger (Berns & Brown, 1998). Als and colleagues (1992) propose that the normal emotional preparation for parenting is interrupted by preterm birth. The desynchronization of emotional unpreparedness compounded by fear for the life of the infant often leads parents to experience feelings of helplessness, anger, grief, and sometimes prolonged depression. These experiences pose significant barriers to regaining confidence in oneself and daring to become invested in and committed to the infant. The costs to the other family members also must be considered. Als and colleagues (1992) suggest that goals for developmental care in the special care nursery include the following: (1) supporting parents as active partners; (2) helping parents learn how to observe their infant's stress and comfort signs; (3) assisting parents to develop competence in helping their infant to self-comfort, regulate, and organize behavior; and (4) reinforcing parents' feelings of their importance and effectiveness in caring for their infant.

Parents should progress in the care of their infant at their own pace. Parents should be supported by staff, counseling, and parent group meetings. Coordination of care and parent education and support are essential at transfer and discharge time. Several studies report benefits of both hospital and home-based family-centered intervention after discharge (Cusson & Lee, 1993).

THEORETIC FRAMEWORK FOR NEONATAL PHYSICAL THERAPY

The theoretic basis for neonatal physical therapy may be conceptualized from general and specific frameworks. The model of the disablement process developed by the National Center for Medical Rehabilitation Research (National Advisory Board on Medical Rehabilitation Research, 1993) describes pathophysiologic condition, impairment, functional limitation, disability, and societal limitation as being the dimensions of a disability. The infant in the special care nursery is at risk for disability that includes the interaction of all of these dimensions. High-risk neonates frequently demonstrate impairments in muscle tone, ROM, elicited reflexes, and automatic postural reactions. Functional limitations may include problems in feeding, visual and auditory responsiveness, and motor abilities, such as head control and movement of hands to mouth. Neonates may also demonstrate functional limitations in breathing and feeding. For some infants, the combination of pathologic conditions such as IVH and seizures and impairments creates an increased risk of long-term functional limitation or disability.

The purpose of the physical therapy examination and evaluation is to identify the presence of and risk for impairment, functional limitation, and disability. A focus of intervention is to prevent or minimize impairment and functional limitations and thereby decrease the risk of long-term disability. Outcomes are assessed by documenting the infant's attainment of physical therapy goals and objectives and through scientific methods such as single-subject designs (Campbell, 1985; Heriza & Sweeney, 1990a, 1990b) (see Chapter 7).

Sweeney and Swanson (1990) have described a theoretic framework specific to neonatal physical therapy that incorporates concepts of pathokinesiology, neonatal behavioral organization, and crisis intervention. Neonatal behavioral organization concepts of this model are those proposed in the synactive model of behavioral organization (Als, 1986). This model describes how newborn infants interact with the environment through five behavioral systems: autonomic, motor, state, attentional, and self-regulatory. The five systems are in continuous interaction with one another (synactive). The synactive model is useful when trying to determine the risk-benefit ratio for intervention, including the tolerance of a neonate to developmental examination and direct intervention procedures. For example, a neonate who reacts to examination procedures with autonomic and visceral stress signals such as gagging, tremors, or irregular respirations is demonstrating physiologic instability resulting from a negative interaction of subsystems. These reactions indicate a higher risk than benefit from this developmental assessment. The neonate who reacts to the same assessment with smooth respirations, pink color, well-regulated tone, and smooth movements is tolerating the procedure with a beneficial interaction of subsystems. Determination of the risk-benefit ratio and tolerance of the neonate to developmental assessment and intervention is an important part of the theoretic framework proposed by Sweeney and Swanson (1990).

Physical therapists who work in special care nurseries should base their intervention strategies on current knowledge of neonatal development and intervention (Fetters, 1986). Models that address characteristics of the infant and the environment, such as the two presented, provide a theoretic framework for the development of guidelines for intervention in the NICU. These models also allow for generation of hypotheses that may be examined through clinical research.

The physical therapist who has expertise in neonatal care has much to offer as a member of a developmental team in the prevention and treatment of impairments in ROM, posture, respiration, and state organization that occur in high-risk neonates. It has been recommended that physical therapists working in the NICU complete continuing education in neonatal medicine, fetal development, assessment and development in early infancy, parental education, early intervention, and interdisciplinary interaction in the specialized setting of the special care nursery (Campbell, 1985; Sweeney & Swanson, 1990). Knowledge of current theories of motor control and early motor learning is also beneficial. Other recommendations include a supervised preceptorship in an NICU, which may include training in the use of neonatal assessments such as the Neonatal Individualized Developmental Care and Assessment Program (NIDCAP) (Als, 1984) and the Neonatal Behavioral Assessment Scale (NBAS) (Brazelton, 1984). These assessments are discussed in the section on developmental physical therapy examination. For additional information on preparation for providing service in the NICU, the reader is referred to the American Physical Therapy Association, Section on Pediatrics, policy statement on competencies for the physical therapist in the NICU (Scull & Dietz, 1989). Currently, the competencies for the physical therapist in the NICU are in the process of being revised and updated.

PULMONARY FUNCTION

Examination of pulmonary function in the special care infant includes observation, inspection, and auscultation (Crane, 1995; Parker, 1985). Percussion is generally not appropriate for small infants (Crane, 1995). Observation and inspection include assessing signs of respiratory distress, chest configuration, skin color, breathing patterns, coughing, and sneezing. Signs of respiratory distress include retractions, nasal flaring, expiratory grunting, inspiratory stridor, use of accessory respiratory muscles (manifested by head bobbing), and bulging of intercostal muscles during expiration (Fig. 30–8) (Crane, 1995). Abnormal chest configurations include barrel-shaped chest and pectus excavatum. Cyanosis around the lips and mouth is a significant sign of hypoxemia (Crane, 1995).

Irregularity of respiration is normal in a neonate, and respiratory rates should be counted over a period of 60 seconds to account for this (Crane, 1995). The auscultation of an infant is an inexact procedure because of the thin chest wall, proximity of structures, and easy transmission of sounds (Fig. 30–9). This is also confounded by mechanical ventilation. During auscultation, the therapist is listening for normal, abnormal, and adventitious breath sounds. In infants, the specific location of the sound does not always correlate with the underlying lung segment. For this reason, auscultatory findings must be correlated with radiologic evidence. Palpation of the mediastinum and the trachea in the suprasternal notch is performed to ascertain if there is subcutaneous emphysema, edema, or rib fracture (Crane, 1986, 1987, 1995).

Chest Physical Therapy

The primary goal of chest physical therapy in the special care nursery is to improve airway clearance, thereby improving ventilation and decreasing the work of breathing. Chest physical therapy is indicated for RDS, meconium aspiration syndrome, neonatal pneumonia, and BPD (Crane, 1995; Hough, 1991). All these conditions involve problems with airway clearance of secretions (Crane, 1995; Hough, 1991). Many precautions and contraindications for chest physical therapy exist. Caution should be taken in performing chest physical therapy on vulnerable extremely preterm infants because of possible neurologic complications such as cerebral lesions resembling hemorrhagic infarcts (Harding et al., 1998). Because ill neonates respond to many procedures with hypoxemia and increased oxygen consumption (Long et al., 1980; Yeh et al., 1984), chest physical therapy procedures should be performed only when clearly indicated for a specific problem or to prevent a potential problem (Crane, 1995) such as increased secretions, changes on x-ray, and anticipated extubation (Harding et al., 1998). The most appropriate and safest combination of chest physical therapy procedures should be individually chosen for each infant in the NICU (Crane, 1995). The therapist must be constantly aware of the effects of chest physical therapy on heart rate, oxygenation, blood pressure, and state control. The chest physical therapy procedures appropriate for infants include positioning, chest percussion, vibration, and airway suctioning (Crane, 1995).

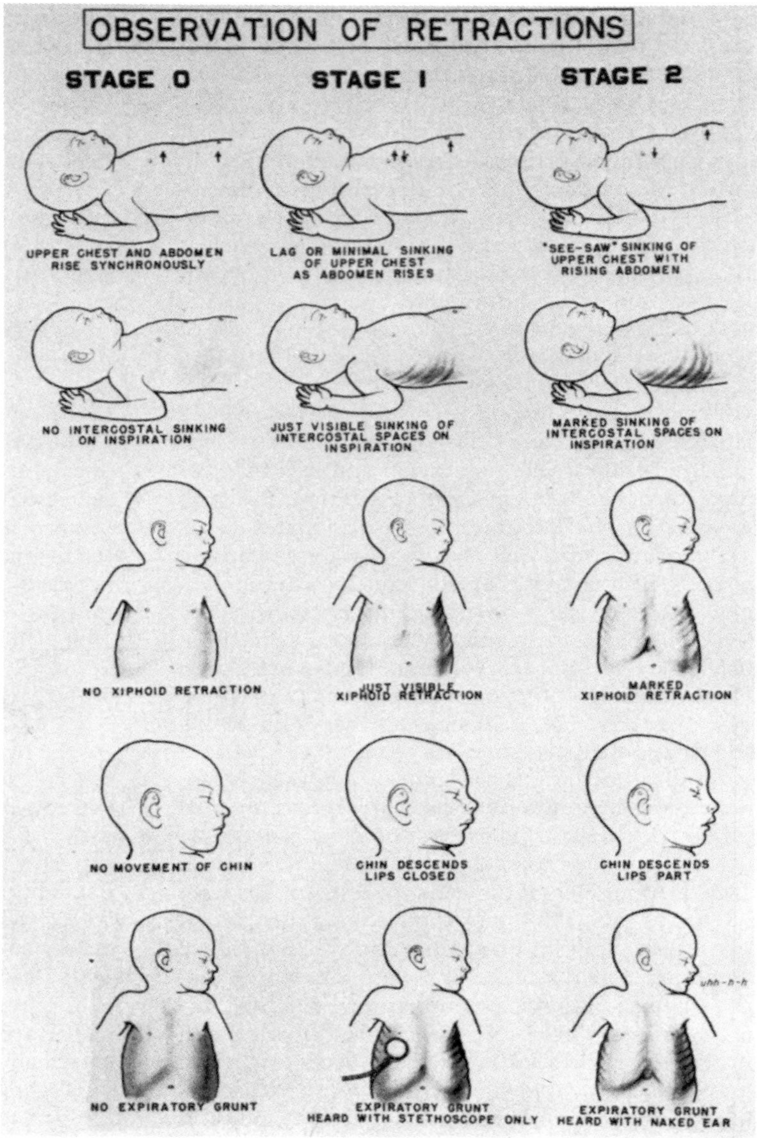

FIGURE 30-8. Observation and scoring of respiratory retractions. (Reproduced with permission from Silverman, WA, & Andersen, DH. Controlled clinical trial of water mist on obstructive respiratory signs: Death rate among premature infants. Pediatrics, *17*:1–10, 1956. Copyright 1956.)

Positioning

Positioning is indicated to enhance ventilation-perfusion ratios and to drain bronchopulmonary segments. Advantages of the prone position include improving oxygenation, lung compliance, state of alertness, and vital signs, whereas the primary advantage of the semierect position is to improve oxygenation (Crane, 1995; Martin et al., 1979; Wagoman et al., 1979). Positioning for postural drainage may need to be modified because of precautions and contraindications to certain positions in the neonate (Table 30–2). For example, the prone position is contraindicated by an untreated tension pneumothorax, and the head-down Trendelenburg position is contraindicated when there is an IVH of grades III and IV, acute congestive heart failure, or cor pulmonale (Crane, 1995).

Percussion and Vibration

Chest percussion and vibration are used with postural drainage to facilitate the loosening and movement of secretions and mucous plugs in the conducting airway. Percussion and vibration may be used separately or together, as indicated by the condition and tolerance of the infant. In neonates with

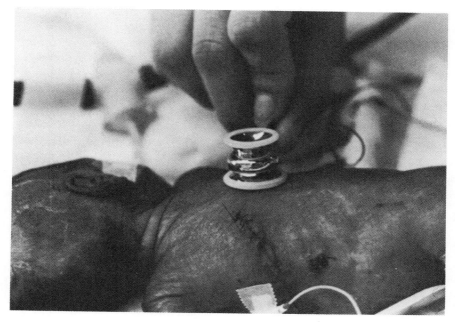

FIGURE 30–9. Auscultation of infant's lungs with neonatal stethoscope. (From Crane, L. Physical therapy for the neonate with respiratory disease. In Irwin, S, & Tecklin, JS [Eds.], Cardiopulmonary Physical Therapy, 2nd ed. St. Louis: Mosby, 1990, p. 402.)

TABLE 30–2. **Precautions and Contraindications for Postural Drainage in a Neonate**

Position	Precaution	Contraindication
Prone	Umbilical arterial catheter Continuous positive airway pressure in nose Excessive abdominal distention Abdominal incision Anterior chest tube	Untreated tension pneumothorax
Trendelenburg position (head down)	Distended abdomen SEH/IVH* (grades I and II) Chronic congestive heart failure or cor pulmonale Persistent fetal circulation Cardiac dysrhythmias Apnea and bradycardia Infant exhibiting signs of acute respiratory distress Hydrocephalus Less than 28 weeks of gestational age	Untreated tension pneumothorax Recent tracheoesophageal fistula repair Recent eye or intracranial surgery Intraventricular hemorrhage (grades III and IV) Acute congestive heart failure or cor pulmonale

From Crane, L. Physical therapy for the neonate with respiratory disease. In Irwin, S, & Tecklin, JS (Eds.), Cardiopulmonary Physical Therapy, 2nd ed. St. Louis: Mosby, 1990, p. 406.
*Subependymal hemorrhage/intraventricular hemorrhage.

pulmonary disease, percussion and vibration have been shown to improve oxygenation, decrease the incidence of postextubation atelectasis, and increase the volume of removed secretions (Crane, 1995). Once again, there are precautions and contraindications for these techniques (Boxes 30–4 and 30–5).

Several hand positions and a variety of devices can be used for percussion. All hand positions use a cupping gesture and include the full hand, three or four fingers, or the thenar and hypothenar eminences (Figs. 30–10 through 30–12). The therapist must avoid percussing over the liver, spleen, and

BOX 30-4. Precautions and Contraindications for Chest Percussion of a Neonate

Precautions	Contraindications
Poor condition of skin	Intolerance to treatment
Coagulopathy	as indicated by low
Presence of a chest tube	TcPo$_2$ values
Healing thoracic incision	Rib fracture
Osteoporosis and rickets	Hemoptysis
Persistent fetal circulation	
Cardiac dysrhythmias	
Apnea and bradycardia	
Signs of acute respiratory	
distress	
Increased irritability during	
treatment	
Subcutaneous emphysema	
Bronchospasm, wheezing,	
rhonchi	
Subependymal hemor-	
rhage/intraventricular	
hemorrhage	
Prematurity (less	
than 28 weeks of	
gestational age)	

From Crane, L. Physical therapy for the neonate with respiratory disease. In Irwin, S, & Tecklin, JS (Eds.), Cardiopulmonary Physical Therapy, 2nd ed. St. Louis: Mosby, 1990, p. 408.

BOX 30-5. Precautions and Contraindications for Vibration of a Neonate

Precautions	Contraindications
Increased irritability/crying	Untreated tension
during treatment	pneumothorax
Persistent fetal circulation	Intolerance to treatment
	as indicated by low
	TcPo$_2$ values
Apnea and bradycardia	Hemoptysis

From Crane, L. Physical therapy for the neonate with respiratory disease. In Irwin, S, & Tecklin, JS (Eds.), Cardiopulmonary Physical Therapy, 2nd ed. St. Louis: Mosby, 1990, p. 408.

kidneys and limit the areas percussed to within the borders of the lungs (Crane, 1995). Devices used for percussion include baby bottle nipples and small anesthesia masks. Vibration may be administered by manual vibratory motion transmitted through the therapist's fingers to the infant's chest wall or by mechanical vibrators such as an electric toothbrush with padded bristles (see Box 30–5). No conclusive evidence supports the use of the mechanical vibrator over manual techniques.

The time necessary for effective drainage of a lung area is a minimum of 3 to 5 minutes when using postural drainage, percussion, and vibration. If only postural drainage is used, drainage time in each position must be at least 20 to 30 minutes. All positions should not be used during a treatment session if time in each position will be significantly reduced. Areas of greatest involvement should be treated first. Less involved areas should be treated with short, frequent treatments in order to adequately treat all areas of the lung requiring drainage (Crane, 1995).

Suctioning

Airway suctioning is usually needed to help the infant clear the secretions loosened by bronchial drainage (Crane, 1987, 1995). Therapists working with infants with pulmonary dysfunction should know how to suction or how to assist (Crane, 1995). Deep tracheal suctioning is most effective and safe when performed through an artificial airway such as a nasotracheal or tracheostomy tube (Crane, 1995; Hubbell & Webster, 1986). A recommended procedure for suctioning includes first hyperventilating the infant with a self-inflating bag and then increasing the oxygen concentration by 10 to 20%. The catheter is then wet in sterile saline, inserted with no suction into the airway until resistance is met, and then retracted slightly; the catheter is then slowly turned while being withdrawn, and intermittent suction is applied for 10 seconds. Suctioning can be potentially harmful to the infant. These risks can be reduced when proper procedures are used and precautions are taken (Crane, 1995).

DEVELOPMENTAL EXAMINATION AND EVALUATION

The purposes of the developmental physical therapy examination and evaluation are to identify the following: (1) neuromuscular, neuromotor, and feeding impairments that require intervention; (2) methods of positioning and handling; and (3) how to adapt the environment to optimize development. Based on examination findings, the physical therapist also evaluates the risk for functional limitations in development and parent-infant attachment. During examination procedures, the therapist must be aware of signs that the infant is undergoing stress, such as hypoxemia, excessive increase in heart rate, gagging, choking, and gasping. The therapist may need several brief sessions to fully assess the infant who is medically fragile (Sweeney, 1986). If the infant is too fragile for physical handling, observation of postures and spontaneous motor behavior may be useful.

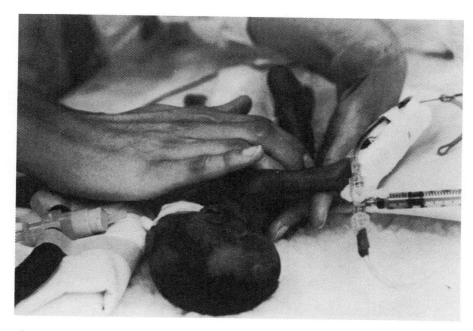

FIGURE 30–10. Chest percussion using three fingers with middle finger tented. (From Crane, L. Physical therapy for the neonate with respiratory disease. In Irwin, S, & Tecklin, JS [Eds.], Cardiopulmonary Physical Therapy, 2nd ed. St. Louis: Mosby, 1990, p. 411.)

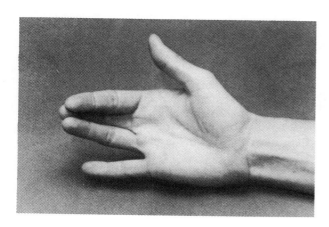

FIGURE 30–11. Palmar view of three fingers cupped for percussion with middle finger tented. (From Crane, L. Physical therapy for the neonate with respiratory disease. In Irwin, S, & Tecklin, JS [Eds.], Cardiopulmonary Physical Therapy, 2nd ed. St. Louis: Mosby, 1990, p. 409.)

Tests and measures appropriate for the premature infant include the Neurologic Assessment of the Preterm and Full-Term Newborn Infant (Dubowitz & Dubowitz, 1981a, 1981b), the NIDCAP (Als, 1984), the Neurobehavioral Assessment for Preterm Infants (NAPI) (Korner et al., 1991), and the Test of Infant Motor Performance (TIMP) (Campbell et al., 1993; Kolobe et al., 1992).

Tests and measures designed for at-risk full-term infants include the Neonatal Behavioral Assessment Scale (Brazelton, 1984) and the Morgan Neonatal Neurobehavioral Examination (Morgan et al., 1988).

These measures may be used with preterm infants once they reach 38 weeks of conceptional age, but criteria for scoring are based on the development of full-term infants.

Observation of movement is an important component of the physical therapist's examination and is included in many of the standardized assessments. Ferrari and colleagues (1990) have developed a method of systematic analysis of qualitative characteristics of general spontaneous movements from sequential videotape recordings. These authors used videotape recordings to document the early

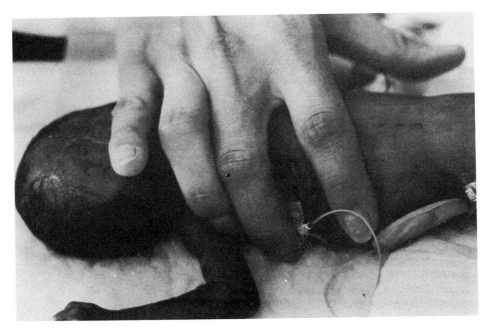

FIGURE 30–12. Manual chest vibration. (From Crane, L. Physical therapy for the neonate with respiratory disease. In Irwin, S, & Tecklin, JS [Eds.], Cardiopulmonary Physical Therapy, 2nd ed. St. Louis: Mosby, 1990, p. 412.)

evolution of different types of cerebral palsy in infants with brain lesions. Characteristics of general movements such as amplitude, speed, character (cramped or floppy), sequencing, fluency, and subtle distal movements are used to arrive at a global evaluation. Cramped synchronized movement and lack of fluency and complexity are indicative of the development of infants with cerebral palsy. Conversely, the development of infants who do not have CNS insults is characterized by rotational movements in combination with extension and flexion of the limbs (Ferrarri et al., 1990). Kakebeeke and colleagues (1997) developed a 10-point scale to rate the fluency and spatiotemporal variability of arm and leg movements and sequencing of general movement patterns. Significant differences were found for these three movement quality parameters among term, low-risk preterm, and high-risk preterm infants.

Neurologic Assessment of the Preterm and Full-Term Newborn Infant

The Neurologic Assessment of the Preterm and Full-Term Newborn Infant is a systematic, quickly administered, neurologic and neurobehavioral assessment developed by Dubowitz and Dubowitz (1981a, 1981b; Dubowitz, 1988). The test was developed to document changes in neonatal behavior in the preterm infant after birth, to compare preterm neonates with full-term neonates, to detect devia-

tions in neurologic signs, and to document patterns of resolution in neurologic deficits (Sweeney, 1986). The test includes multiple neurobehavioral items of the Brazelton NBAS (Brazelton, 1984) using the six behavioral states. The neurobehavioral items include habituation to light and sound while sleeping, auditory and visual orientation responses, quality and duration of alertness, defensive reaction to cloth over face, peak of excitement, irritability, and consolability. The 15 neurologic items were taken from the Clinical Assessment of Gestational Age by Dubowitz and colleagues (1970), the Neurologic Examination of the Newborn (Prechtl & Beintema, 1964), and the neurologic examination of the full-term infant and the abnormal inventory protocol by Saint-Anne Dargassies (1977). The Neurologic Assessment of the Preterm and Full-Term Newborn Infant was tested on more than 500 infants during a 2-year period. The test takes 15 minutes or less to administer. Scoring is done by looking at patterns of response rather than by determining a summary or total score.

In a prospective study of the predictive validity of the Neurologic Assessment of the Preterm and Full-Term Newborn Infant, Dubowitz and colleagues (1984) found that 91% of premature infants who were classified as normal at 40 weeks of gestation were normal according to detailed neurologic assessment and the Griffiths Mental Development Scale at 1 year. Sixty-five percent of infants classified as abnormal at 40 weeks of gestation, including those with cerebral palsy, dystonia, global delays, clumsiness, and hearing or visual deficit, were considered abnormal at 1 year.

Although reliability has not been determined, this examination has great potential for physical therapists who work in the NICU because of its brief administration time and systematic method of recording. Caution must be used when administering this assessment because it has been documented that medically stable preterm infants demonstrated an increase in heart rate during and after this examination (Sweeney, 1986).

Neonatal Individualized Developmental Care and Assessment Program

The NIDCAP was developed to provide developmental observation and assessment training for neonatal health care professionals and includes Naturalistic Observation of Newborn Activity (Als, 1984). This involves systematic observation—without the observer manipulating or interacting—of the preterm or full-term infant in the nursery or at home during caregiving and handling. A behavior observation checklist based on the concepts of the Assessment of Preterm Infant Behavior (APIB) (Als et al., 1982) includes environmental characteristics such as light, sound, and positioning apparatus. The self-regulatory ability of the infant is recorded, with some of the signs of stress being irregular respirations, color other than pink, tremors, startles and twitches, and visceral signs, including spitting up, gagging, hiccoughing, grunting, and gasping. Other signs of stress that can be recorded include flaccidity, frequent extensor movements of extremities, arching, tongue thrusts, finger splaying and fisting, fussing, yawning, and eye averting. Physiologic signs include heart rate below 120 or above 160 beats per minute, respiratory rate below 40 or above 60, and transcutaneous Po_2 below 55 or above 80 mm Hg. Suggestions for caregiving modifications that may reduce stress for the infant are developed from the summary. These suggestions may pertain to lighting, noise level, activity level, bedding, aids to self-regulation, interaction, timing of manipulations, and facilitation of transitions from one activity to another. A list of training centers may be obtained from the National NIDCAP Training Center, 320 Longwood Ave., Boston, MA 02115.

The Neurobehavioral Assessment for Preterm Infants

The NAPI was developed by Korner and colleagues (1991) to assess longitudinally the neurobehavioral development of preterm infants. The NAPI is designed for use with infants from 32 weeks of conceptional age to term and is used primarily to measure the relative maturity and function of preterm infants at different ages. Specific purposes for administration include the following: (1) to monitor the neurobehavioral development of preterm infants, (2) to document developmental progress over repeated examinations, and (3) to evaluate the effects of intervention and changes in infant care. The NAPI may also be used as an outcome measure for clinical research or to collect normative data on the neurobehavioral development of preterm infants (Korner et al., 1991).

Most test items overlap with those used in other neurobehavioral examinations with the difference existing in the theoretic and developmental rationale underlying the choice of items, scoring, and data analysis. An invariant sequence of item presentation is used that incorporates a sequence of rousing, soothing, and alerting. This maximizes the ability to test various functions in appropriate behavioral states. Test items are clustered together based on conceptual cohesion and face validity. The NAPI assesses seven neurobehavioral dimensions: (1) motor development and vigor, (2) alertness and orientation, (3) scarf sign, (4) popliteal angle, (5) irritability, (6) percent of asleep ratings, and (7) vigor of crying. Test-retest reliability coefficients for these dimensions range from .60 to .85, except asleep ratings, which have a test-retest reliability of .43. The mean interrater reliability is .85 with a range of .64 to .98.

Test of Infant Motor Performance

The TIMP is the first test designed specifically for use by physical and occupational therapists (see Chapter 1) to test infants from 32 weeks of postconceptional age to 4 months postterm (Campbell et al., 1993; Kolobe et al., 1992). The construct of the TIMP is postural alignment and selective control necessary for functional movements in early infancy. The TIMP requires approximately 36 minutes to administer and score (Campbell et al., 1995). Spontaneous and elicited movements are assessed with separate subscales. The Observed Scale consists of 28 dichotomously scored behaviors (Murney & Campbell, 1998). The observed behaviors reflect the infant's spontaneous attempts to change positions or to orient the body, to selectively move individual body segments, and to perform qualitative movements such as ballistic or oscillating movements. Examples of observed behaviors include bringing hands together in midline, lifting the head while prone, and aligning the head in midline while supine. The Elicited Scale includes 25 items scored on a four-, five-, or six-point hierarchic scale (Murney & Campbell, 1998). Elicited behaviors reflect the infant's response to positioning and handling in a variety of spatial orientations and to visual and auditory stimuli. Examples include rolling prone with head righting when the leg is rotated across the body and turning the head to follow a visual stimulus or to search for a sound in prone, supine, and supported sitting positions.

Construct validity of the TIMP has been established, specifically the ability of the TIMP to discriminate on the basis of both medical complications and maturation (Campbell et al., 1995). Scores on the TIMP increase with increasing postconceptional age. Infants with a greater number of medical complications do less well than infants of the same age (Campbell et al., 1995). A study has also been performed that looks at the relationship between environmental demands placed on infants during caregiving activities, including play, and the demands placed on the infant during the administration of the Elicited Scale items of the TIMP (Murney & Campbell, 1998). During caregiving activities, approximately 50% of the demands placed on the infants corresponded to items on the TIMP. In addition, 98% of the TIMP Elicited Scale items corresponded to observed environmental demands (Murney & Campbell, 1998). These findings suggest that the demands placed on infants when administering the TIMP are representative of typical environmental demands.

The Neurologic Examination of the Full-Term Newborn Infant

The Neurologic Examination of the Full-Term Newborn Infant was developed by Prechtl and Beintema to identify abnormal neurologic signs in the newborn period (Prechtl, 1977; Prechtl & Beintema, 1964). This examination was standardized on 1500 neonates who were born between 38 and 42 weeks of gestational age. Prechtl reported interrater reliability coefficients to be in the range of .80 to .96. The test includes an observation period and a screening examination to determine if the full 30-minute assessment of posture, tone, reflexes, and spontaneous movement is required. Prechtl's examination includes observation of behavioral state changes, threshold of reactions to stimuli, and intensity of responses. Different patterns of findings led Prechtl to identify four clinical syndromes. The comatose syndrome includes absent or minimal arousal to pain or other stimuli and abnormal respiratory patterns. The apathetic syndrome consists of a very high stimulatory threshold for response and frequently occurs before manifestation of the hemisyndrome,

which includes three asymmetric findings. The hyperexcitable syndrome includes instability of behavioral states, prolonged crying, tremor, hypertonus, increased deep tendon reflexes, and hyperkinesis.

Bierman–van Eedenburg and co-workers (1981) and Njiokiktjien and Kurver (1980) have attempted to analyze the predictive ability of this examination. In the first study a high rate of false-positive findings was reported. In the latter report, the suboptimal group differed significantly on a few of the behavioral and neurologic items when infants were evaluated at 21 to 23 months of age, suggesting that subtle neurologic differences were maintained across time. Harris and Brady (1986) pointed out that these investigators did not examine predictive validity in the true statistical sense.

Neonatal Behavioral Assessment Scale

Brazelton (1984) developed the NBAS to document individual differences in the behavior of full-term infants and to score the infant's available responses to and effect on his or her environment (Als et al., 1977). The NBAS assesses interactive ability, motor behavior, behavioral state organization, and physiologic organization. Interactive ability items include response to auditory and visual animate and inanimate stimuli, consolability, and alertness. Motor items include observation of hand-to-mouth activity, head control during pull-to-sit, response to cloth over face, and reflex items taken from Neurologic Examination of the Full-Term Newborn Infant (Prechtl, 1977). Behavioral state items include the infant's ability to transition through the various states and to habituate to auditory, visual, and tactile stimuli during sleep states. Clusters of behavior indicative of problems with interactive, motor, and organizational behavior have been described (Brazelton et al., 1987). This assessment tool has also been used as a parent teaching intervention and, when used as such, may lead to positive effects in the infant-parent interaction and later cognitive and fine motor development (Francis et al., 1987).

The NBAS has not been formally standardized. Interrater reliability has been reported to be .85 to 1.00 (Francis et al., 1987). Recommended training includes viewing a training film that describes the scale, observation of a demonstration examination performed by a certified examiner, practice training in examining at least 20 infants, and then determining reliability with a certified examiner to a set criterion for certification (Brazelton et al., 1987). Certification for use of the Brazelton NBAS in research is offered in many university health science centers and university-affiliated child development centers, including the Children's Hospital in Boston, Massachusetts.

Morgan Neonatal Neurobehavioral Examination

The Morgan Neonatal Neurobehavioral Examination (NNE) was designed to quantify the neurobehavioral abilities of infants between 37 and 40 weeks of conceptional age (Morgan et al., 1988). The authors stated that a quantitative rather than a qualitative assessment would be valuable in identification of infants at risk for developmental disabilities and would also provide a research tool for evaluating early intervention protocols. The test was constructed from items taken from the work of Brazelton (1984) and Dubowitz and Dubowitz (1981a). The 27 assessment items are organized into sections on tone and motor patterns, primitive reflexes, and behavioral responses. Interestingly, the response decrement items of the Brazelton scale were not included because the authors believed that high-risk infants must habituate themselves to noxious sounds and lights because they are continuously exposed to them in an NICU. A three-point scoring system is used for each item, with the highest total score being 81 and the lowest possible score being 27.

The NNE was standardized on 54 healthy full-term infants at 2 days of age and on 298 high-risk infants at 37 to 40 weeks of conceptional age (gestational age at birth plus chronologic age) or at discharge, whichever came first. Scores fell into three clusters for the high-risk infants, which correlated with conceptional age and not with severity of illness or gestational age at birth. These clusters represented performance at greater than 36 weeks, 32 to 36 weeks, and less than 32 weeks of gestational age. This suggests that the NNE reflects gestational maturation and quantitatively represents neurobehavioral status. Intertester reliability is reported as 88% agreement by item and 95% agreement by total score (Morgan et al., 1988). Validity studies are in progress. Lee and colleagues (1989) reported that the NNE can be used to predict motor outcome for high-risk infants born at or below 1500 g or between 37 and 42 weeks of gestation.

Oral-Motor Examination

Oral-motor examination is another competency of the neonatal therapist. Two useful measures are the Neonatal Oral-Motor Assessment Scale (NOMAS) (Braun & Palmer, 1985/1986), which has been updated (Gaebler & Hanzlik, 1996), and the Nursing Child Assessment Feeding Scale (NCAFS) (Barnard & Eyres, 1979). The NOMAS measures components of nutritive and nonnutritive sucking. Variables assessed during sucking include rate, rhythmicity, jaw excursion, tongue configuration, and tongue movement. A pilot study determined cutoff scores for oral-motor disorganization and dysfunction. The NCAFS assesses parent-infant feeding interaction and evaluates responsiveness of parents to their infant's cues, signs of distress, and social interaction during feeding.

There are also instruments to study the pressure generated by each suck and the length of sucking bursts such as the Kron Nutritive Sucking Apparatus (Medoff-Cooper & Gennaro, 1996) and the Actifier (Finan & Barlow, 1996), which can also be used as a method for stimulation of intraoral tissue in neonates.

High-Risk Profiles

Examination and evaluation may lead to identification of the infant as having one of three basic high-risk profiles described by Sweeney and Swanson (1990). Although not all neonates fit the behaviors described in the high-risk profiles, the profiles address the need for individualized levels of stimulation and approaches to the management of infants with abnormal tone and movement (Sweeney & Swanson, 1990). The profiles represent the extremes in sensorimotor and interactional behavior. The profiles identify abnormalities in muscle tone, behavioral characteristics, and interactional styles associated with motor status and therefore have implications for the development of individualized goals, outcomes, and intervention strategies.

The infant who is irritable and hypertonic is often in a state of overstimulation, with poor self-quieting abilities. Extensor patterns of posture and movement predominate, with little antigravity flexion available. Movement is disorganized and tremulous, with poor midline orientation. Feeding is difficult as a result of increased tone in the oral musculature. Visual tracking is also difficult.

The infant who is hypotonic is lethargic even at feeding time. Crying is weak and of short duration. Hypotonicity is noted in the trunk, intercostal, and neck accessory musculature, with decreased respiratory capacity. An infant who fits this profile demonstrates paucity of movement, weak and uncoordinated sucking, and poor interactive capability.

The infant who is disorganized demonstrates fluctuating tone and movement and is easily overstimulated. An infant who fits this profile remains passive when left alone but responds well to swaddling. When calm, the infant interacts and feeds well; but when distracted and overstimulated, the infant becomes hypertonic and irritable.

DEVELOPMENTAL INTERVENTIONS

Neonatal physical therapy is a subspecialty of pediatric physical therapy that emerged in the mid-1970s (Sweeney & Chandler, 1990). As specialists in the NICU, it is important to know the evidence guiding and supporting our practice. Several studies have shown support for developmental intervention in the NICU. Scarr-Salapatek and Williams (1973) reported greater developmental progress at 4 weeks and 12 months in infants who received developmental intervention that included visual, tactile, and kinesthetic stimulation in the nursery. Leib, Benfield, and Guidubaldi (1980) reported that an intervention program consisting of visual, tactile, kinesthetic, and auditory stimulation enhanced the quality of development for high-risk preterm infants. In addition, Field and co-workers (1986) demonstrated that preterm infants benefited from a program of tactile and kinesthetic stimulation in the NICU. Parker and colleagues (1992) reported the positive benefits of a developmental intervention program in the NICU for infants of mothers of low socioeconomic status. Als and co-workers (1994) have also demonstrated the positive effects of individualized developmentally supportive care. Although physical therapists were not involved in these studies, the interventions are those typically performed during physical therapy intervention in the NICU.

Although there is evidence to support developmental interventions for preterm infants in the NICU, stimulation in the form of tactile, kinesthetic, visual, and auditory stimulation has the potential to be harmful. Physical therapists, therefore, must carefully monitor infants during intervention. Monitoring includes oxygen saturation, heart rate, respiratory rate, and identification of behavioral signs indicating stress. Careful monitoring of infants during intervention is essential to avoid potentially adverse physiologic effects.

The goals of physical therapy for neonates may include reduction or prevention of impairments in muscle tone, ROM, postural adaptation, and control of extremity movements. Outcomes include improved regulation and organization of motor behavior, interactions with caregivers and the environment, and family attachment (Campbell, 1985; Sweeney & Swanson, 1990). Parents, primary nurses, and other caregivers should be involved in the development of goals and outcomes and coordination of the care plan. Specific intervention strategies, whether direct or by consultation, include modification of the environment, positioning, promotion of efficient movement, and modulation of sensory input (e.g., oral-motor stimulation, hydrotherapy, and the use of water mattresses). Parent education and support regarding the development and input appropriate for neonates is an important aspect of intervention (Gottwald & Thurman, 1990).

The design for a care plan should be individualized based on infant and caregiver needs. Factors to consider include the infant's postconceptional age, physiologic abilities, and behavioral abilities. These individualized care plans should include the provision of social interaction stimuli during alert periods, avoidance of handling during quiet sleep periods, and immediate termination or alteration of stimulation producing avoidance responses (Campbell, 1985). Avoidance responses include vomiting, sneezing, coughing, hiccoughing, gagging, sighing, respiratory changes, and changes in tone (Als, 1986). While the neonate is in the NICU, the environment should be modified to avoid overstimulation by excessive light, noise, or physical handling (Avery & Glass, 1989; Field, 1990). Caregivers should provide tactile and kinesthetic stimuli that are contingent on the neonate's responses to alleviate stress, if possible, or to help the infant prepare for, or adapt to, stress-producing stimuli.

Positioning

Positioning has already been mentioned in relation to improving oxygenation. Positioning is also important to promote state organization, stimulate the flexed midline positions typical of the full-term infant, and maintain ROM (Sweeney & Swanson, 1990). The premature infant does not have the opportunity to develop physiologic flexion and may demonstrate hypotonia (Fig. 30–13). The preterm infant must also contend with ventilatory and infusion equipment, which often exaggerates extension of the neck, trunk, and extremities. Hypotonic extended limbs may also be fixed to padded boards to protect intravenous lines (Fetters, 1986). Prolonged hyperextension may lead to neck extensor muscle contracture (Sweeney & Swanson, 1990) (Fig. 30–14).

The prone position, with the head in midline and elevation of the head at 30°, has the beneficial effects of decreasing intracranial pressure, gastroesophageal reflux, and aspiration and increasing stomach emptying (Semmler, 1989; Wolfson et al., 1992). Many different methods are used for placing the infant in prone and side-lying positions, including blanket or diaper rolls, sandbags, customized foam inserts, buntings, and nests (Creger & Browne, 1995; Semmler, 1989; Sweeney & Swanson, 1990) (Figs. 30–15 through 30–17). The desired posture includes neck flexion or chin tucking, trunk flexion, shoulder protraction, posterior pelvic tilt, and symmetric flexion of legs. When supine positioning is used, the head is positioned in midline and blanket rolls may

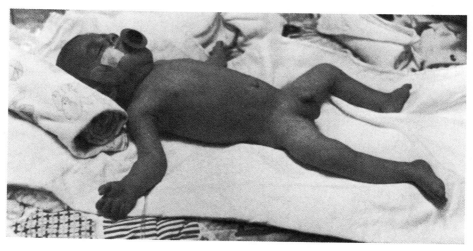

FIGURE 30–13. Characteristic hypotonic posture with minimal movement against gravity in a premature infant at 4 months of age. (From Sweeney, JK, & Swanson, MW. At-risk neonates and infants: NICU management and follow-ups. In Umphred, DA [Ed.], Neurological Rehabilitation, 2nd ed. St. Louis: Mosby, 1990, p. 218.)

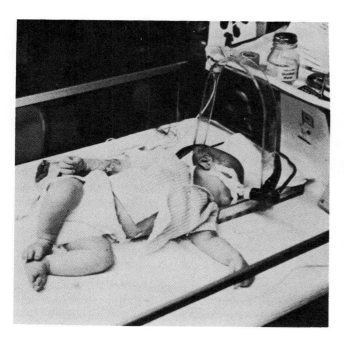

FIGURE 30–14. Neck hyperextension posture exaggerated by position of the endotracheal tube. (From Sweeney, JK, & Swanson, MW. At-risk neonates and infants: NICU management and follow-ups. In Umphred, DA [Ed.], Neurological Rehabilitation, 2nd ed. St. Louis: Mosby, 1990, p. 201.)

be placed along the infant's sides and under the shoulder girdle for support, as well as under the knees. Supported semierect positions while the infant is swaddled may also be beneficial to elicit the alert state, head righting, and visual and auditory tracking.

Hammocks and water mattresses are also used in conjunction with positioning. Water mattresses are soft, and the surface intermittently oscillates, providing gentle vestibular and proprioceptive stimulation. Water mattresses have proved effective in decreasing apnea, reducing position-induced head flattening, and improving skin conditions (Deiriggi, 1990; Piecuch, 1988; Sweeney & Swanson, 1990; Taylor & Dalbec, 1989). Positions should be changed throughout the day, especially for infants with respiratory problems involving increased secretions (Crane, 1987).

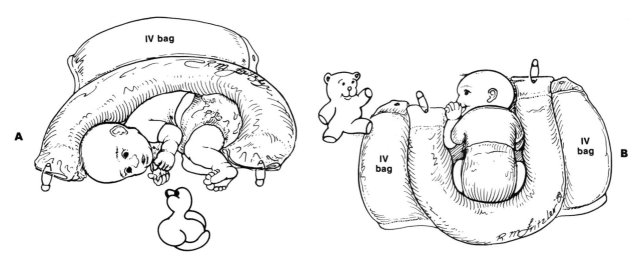

FIGURE 30–15. Positioning in flexion using a long blanket roll reinforced by a sand or intravenous bag. (From Sweeney, JK, & Swanson, MW. At-risk neonates and infants: NICU management and follow-ups. In Umphred, DA [Ed.], Neurological Rehabilitation, 2nd ed. St. Louis: Mosby, 1990, p. 201.)

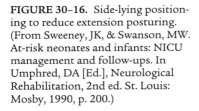

FIGURE 30–16. Side-lying positioning to reduce extension posturing. (From Sweeney, JK, & Swanson, MW. At-risk neonates and infants: NICU management and follow-ups. In Umphred, DA [Ed.], Neurological Rehabilitation, 2nd ed. St. Louis: Mosby, 1990, p. 200.)

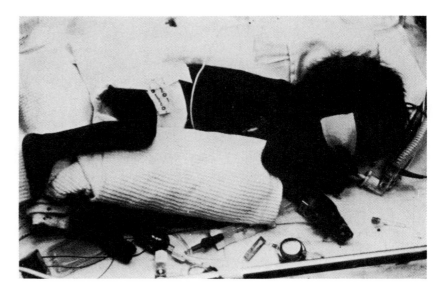

Sensorimotor Stimulation

Physical therapy intervention includes appropriate interaction with the neonate, which involves sensory input. Psychologists and nurses have studied the effect of supplemental stimulation on weight gain, visual responsiveness, growth, development, and sensorimotor functions (Fetters, 1986; Field, 1980; Heriza, 1989; Mueller, 1996). Most of these studies have involved the relatively healthy premature infant weighing more than 1000 g at birth. Little research has been published on the effects of supplemental stimulation of the sicker, VLBW, or asphyxiated newborn (Campbell, 1985). The majority of supplemental stimulation studies used predetermined, packaged, nonindividualized treatments (Harris et al., 1988). In a few studies, sensory stimulation interventions have been individualized and based on behavioral cues from the infant (Als, 1986; Berns, 1993; Fetters, 1986; Heriza, 1989). Mueller (1996) has published an integrated review of research on multimodal stimulation of premature infants. Interestingly, she included developmental care as

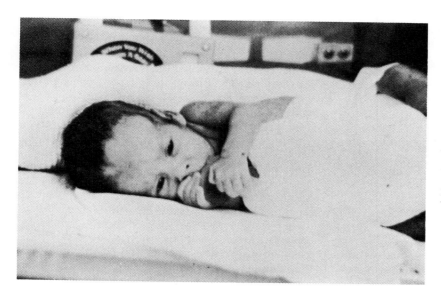

FIGURE 30–17. Use of anterior roll and pacifier promotes flexed position. (From Sweeney, JK, & Swanson, MW. At-risk neonates and infants: NICU management and follow-ups. In Umphred, DA [Ed.], Neurological Rehabilitation, 2nd ed. St. Louis: Mosby, 1990, p. 200.)

one type of multimodal stimulation. In this context, sensorimotor stimulation would include any sensory input, such as the visual input of the therapist's face, tactile input, physical handling, positioning, offering visual or auditory stimuli, and social interaction.

The purposes of providing contingent sensorimotor stimulation to infants in the NICU include improving behavioral organization, promoting integration of the sensory systems, enhancing development of motor and interactive abilities, and supporting parent-infant attachment. Sensory input must be provided in a graded manner that is contingent on the infant's behavioral cues. Gradual introduction of unimodal sensory stimulation may be necessary at first to allow the infant to maintain physiologic and state control. Once the infant is able to maintain state control, multimodal stimuli may be used.

Techniques to aid the infant's state organization, self-consolation, and orienting include encasement (gentle tactile contact with infant's head or soles of feet in a gently flexed position), swaddling, and firm tactile input to the soles of the feet. Constant vigilance must be practiced to weigh the costs and benefits of any intervention. The therapist must be constantly aware of changes in heart rate, blood pressure, and oxygen levels, as well as state control or organization changes during and after intervention.

Using the high-risk infant assessment profiles of Sweeney and Swanson (1990) as a point of reference, it is obvious that strategies of intervention should be individualized. The infant who is lethargic and hypotonic needs stimulation to reach the alert state and facilitation of proximal neck and trunk musculature, whereas the infant who is irritable and hypertonic needs calming to the alert state and inhibition of increased tone.

Als (1986) found that infants who were dependent on a respirator and at high risk for BPD improved self-regulation capabilities after a series of procedures were implemented. These procedures included inhibition through firm tactile input to the soles of the feet, encasement of the infant's trunk and back of the head in the caregiver's hand, the tactile input of a finger to squeeze or suck, and nonnutritive sucking of a finger or a "suckel" (something for the infant to suck on). By contrast, sensory inputs such as rocking, stroking, and talking were not well tolerated by infants.

Methods of calming an infant who is irritable and hypertonic include swaddling, that is, wrapping the infant in a blanket or using a bunting. If swaddling is done with flexed, midline extremity positioning, there may be facilitation of flexor tone, increased hand-to-mouth awareness, and decreased jittery and disorganized movements. Vestibular stimulation in a horizontal position with the infant swaddled has a calming effect.

Procedures used to promote an alert state include positioning in supported sitting, swaddling, and using a bunting or tactile containment. In the infant who is more robust, carefully graded, arrhythmic vestibular input, such as quick rocking in the upright position, and light touch may be used for state arousal. Once the alert state is reached and maintained, sensory input such as visual or auditory stimuli may be added one at a time and modified as indicated by the infant's response. Visual stimuli include the therapist's face, a black-and-white bull's-eye target, and a red ball. Auditory stimuli include classical instrumental music, calling the infant's name, and a soft rattle (Brazelton et al., 1987; Burke, 1995; Collins & Kuck, 1991). Once the infant can maintain an alert state and can fixate on an object, visual tracking may be attempted.

Early movement experiences such as hand-to-mouth contact, shoulder protraction and retraction, pelvic tilt, movement of extremities against gravity, and holding of the head in midline may also be facilitated (Campbell, 1985). Hand-to-hand, hand-to-knee, and hand-to-foot activity are encouraged to provide tactile stimulation and flexion input.

Oral-Motor Therapy

The infant in the special care nursery often exhibits feeding difficulties related to neurologic immaturity, abnormal muscle tone, depressed oral reflexes, or prolonged use of endotracheal tubes for mechanical ventilation (Sweeney & Swanson, 1990). Decreased tongue mobility, tongue thrusting, poor seal on nipple due to weak lip closure, weak sucking, or hypersensitivity of the oral area may also have a negative impact on feeding (Semmler, 1989).

Nonnutritive sucking should be encouraged early with the immediate aim of self-consolation and the long-term goal of normal oral-motor development (Gaebler & Hanzlik, 1996; Pickler et al., 1996). Achieving a quiet alert state and positioning the infant in supported sitting with semiflexion of the neck may also enhance feeding behavior. Methods of tactile stimulation of facial muscles and intraoral structure and external support to the infants' cheeks have been described and have resulted in weight gain and decreased hospital stay for infants in level II special care (Anderson, 1986; Gaebler & Hanzlik, 1996; Harris, 1986; Sweeney & Swanson, 1990). Waber and colleagues (1998) reported that once infants were able to breast or bottle feed, they fed on demand rather than on a schedule, showed more feeding cues, and had a shorter hospital stay.

DEVELOPMENTAL FOLLOW-UP AFTER DISCHARGE FROM THE SPECIAL CARE NURSERY

Developmental follow-up of infants after discharge from the special care nursery varies from state to state and with the particular problems or risk factors of each infant. Primary care is usually provided by a pediatrician in private practice, through a hospital, or through a community-based clinic. An interdisciplinary program such as an early intervention program also provides assessment, monitoring, and direct intervention, as well as a support group for parents (Hack, 1992; Leonard, 1988). Because many early intervention programs have waiting lists for physical therapy and occupational therapy, services initially may be provided by the community visiting nurse association or other home care agencies.

Level III nurseries typically have a developmental follow-up clinic for high-risk infants. Clinics vary in staffing and their criteria for follow-up care. Factors such as birth weight, gestational age, Apgar scores, time on a ventilator, IVH, seizures, and environmental factors such as maternal drug or alcohol use are useful criteria. Results of developmental assessments administered at the follow-up clinic are useful in determining whether specialized therapy services are necessary beyond the provision of general recommendations for development and parent education. Specialized referral for nutrition, audiology, and ophthalmology also is made when necessary.

The physical therapist has a role in the follow-up care of infants as a member of an early intervention program, a visiting nurse association, or a follow-up clinic. As a team member, the therapist plays an important role in the examination and monitoring of sensorimotor development and pulmonary function in order to prevent or decrease the risk of impairment or functional limitation and provide parent education and anticipatory guidance (Platzker et al., 1988; Resnick et al., 1987; Rothberg, 1991; Thom, 1988). Interventions such as positioning, sensory stimulation, and facilitation of movement are also provided when necessary. The physical therapist also assists families in coordination of care and initiates referrals to other professionals and community agencies when appropriate.

CASE HISTORY

The following two hypothetical case histories serve as examples of the neonates seen in the special care nursery and illustrate the physical therapy examination, evaluation, and intervention. Several other excellent case histories have been published (Campbell, 1985; Fiterman, 1987; Heriza, 1989).

Case History: Thomas

Thomas was born at 28 weeks of gestation with a birth weight of 1260 g (2 lb 12.5 oz). Maternal complications included severe preeclampsia and excessive weight gain during the last month of pregnancy. Thomas had Apgar scores of 2 at 1 minute and 5 at 5 minutes, and he was blue and limp at birth. He did not respond to bag mask ventilation and was treated with mechanical ventilation for 2 weeks after birth. Perinatal medical problems included asphyxia, RDS, hyperbilirubinemia, and a grade II IVH.

Thomas was referred to physical therapy at 3 weeks of chronologic age because of irritability and hypertonicity. The physical therapist performed a chart review and spoke with the primary nurse before observing Thomas during routine nursing care using the Naturalistic Observation of Newborn Activity (Als, 1984). He demonstrated a low tolerance to handling and was frequently in a state of overstimulation with signs of stress such as irregular respiration, startling, and grunting. The therapist also noted that Thomas' parents visited him daily.

As part of the examination process, the physical therapist administered the Neurologic Assessment of the Preterm and Full-Term Newborn Infant (Dubowitz & Dubowitz, 1981b). This measure was selected because of its ease of administration and scoring and its inclusion of behavioral, movement, muscle tone, and reflex sections. Findings included poor habituation to light and rattle stimuli and postures and movements that were predominantly in extension, tremulous, and disorganized. The therapist also noted that Thomas showed poor midline orientation and limited antigravity movement into flexion. Visual tracking was impaired, and frequent consoling by the examiner was needed. The therapist also spoke with both parents and found that they were anxious and apprehensive of interacting with their son but were highly invested in him and willing to learn how to respond appropriately to him.

The therapist developed a care plan that included swaddling, positioning, and sensory input in response to Thomas' cues. Direct intervention was implemented three times a week for the duration of Thomas' hospital stay. Goals for Thomas included the following: (1) maintenance of an alert state during treatment; (2) visual fixing and tracking left and right; (3) auditory tracking; (4) increasing antigravity movements into flexion; (5) ability to self-calm; and (6) parents' independence in reading Thomas' behavioral cues. Swaddling, or using a bunting with the infant in a flexed, midline extremity position, provided neutral warmth and an organizing effect on state and movement. Positioning Thomas prone with his head elevated 30° promoted the development of flexor posture and decreased intracranial pressure. When he was placed supine, a roll inserted under his knees promoted flexion. Use of a hammock facilitated a flexed position, and a water mattress helped reduce irritability.

Appropriate sensory inputs included the use of an appropriately sized pacifier along with swaddling, bunting, or hand containment techniques. Stimulation to maintain an alert state included swaddling and gentle vestibular rocking in a horizontal position. Once Thomas was able to maintain an alert state, the therapist began using unimodal stimuli such as the visual stimulus of her face or voice only to engage visual and auditory tracking. She also used a black, white, and red picture to facilitate visual tracking.

The therapist taught many of these techniques to the parents, who became more and more comfortable in interacting with Thomas once they learned how to read his cues (Harrison, 1989). The therapist also recommended several books for the parents to read, including those by Harrison and Kositsky (1983) and Manginello and DiGeronimo (1991).

The therapist constantly monitored Thomas' physiologic and state responses to her interaction with him. She also communicated daily with the primary nurse and several times a week with the parents. The therapist continued to treat Thomas when he was transferred to the step-down facility, and she assisted in his discharge planning, which included referrals to a local visiting nurse association and early intervention program, as well as the hospital's premature infant follow-up clinic.

At discharge, Thomas had achieved many of his goals. He was visually tracking left and right approximately 30°. He would turn his head right and left in response to auditory stimuli. Thomas moved his extremities in small ranges against gravity. His movements continued to be jerky. Thomas was able to bring his hands to midline and to mouth. He was easily consoled with rocking, hands to mouth, and sucking on a pacifier. Thomas was able to consistently clear his face in prone and was beginning to make attempts at head control while in supported sitting. Thomas' parents were able to read his behavioral signs and respond appropriately to them. They felt comfortable taking him home.

Case History: Susan

Susan is a former 3300 g (7.26 lb) full-term infant born to a 32-year-old mother whose pregnancy was uncomplicated. Susan was born with the cord wrapped around her neck and was blue and limp. Her Apgar scores were 2 at 1 minute and 6 at 5 minutes. She received bag mask ventilation, but did not require intubation in the delivery room. Shortly after her transfer to the NICU, Susan began having seizures with associated decreases in respiratory rate requiring bagging. The neurologic examination noted that Susan had absent suck and gag reflexes and was slow to respond to stimuli.

Susan was referred for a physical therapy examination on day 2 of life. The physical therapist used practice pattern 5A: Impaired Motor Function and Sensory Integrity Associated with Congenital or Acquired Disorders of the Central Nervous System in

Infancy, Childhood, and Adolescence (American Physical Therapy Association, 1997) to guide her examination, evaluation, and intervention. The physical therapist reviewed Susan's medical history during the chart review and spoke to nursing about any concerns noted during routine caregiving activities. The physical therapist observed Susan before, during, and after a routine nursing activity using the Neonatal Individualized Developmental Care and Assessment Program (NIDCAP) (Als, 1984). Susan demonstrated poor handling tolerance with an increase in stress signs. Stress signs included a decrease in respiratory rate, startles, arching, and cry. Susan also demonstrated an inability to maintain an awake state and poor state transitions. She quickly transitioned from being lethargic to a hyper-alert state to cry without any intervening quiet alert states. In addition, Susan was not able to calm herself by using self-regulatory behaviors such as hand to mouth, hands to midline, and sucking.

A family-focused approach to physical therapy was used in the NICU. This approach incorporates the family's goals and needs into the care plan. As part of this, the physical therapist spoke with Susan's parents, explaining the role of the physical therapist in Susan's care. Both parents appeared very interested in Susan, although they did voice concerns about her poor handling tolerance and sudden changes from being asleep to crying. Both parents were interested in activities they could do with Susan and appropriate methods to calm her down.

As part of the examination process, the physical therapist performed the Morgan Neonatal Neurobehavioral Examination (NNE) (Morgan et al., 1988). The NNE was chosen because (1) it has been standardized on full-term and high-risk infants; (2) it is quick and easy to administer; and (3) the items include muscle tone and motor patterns, reflexes, and behavioral responses. Susan demonstrated low tone, poor head and trunk control, weak suck, and delayed or absent reflexes. Susan received a total score of 60 on the test. This indicates that she was performing below that of typical full-term infants.

In addition to administering the NNE, the therapist observed Susan's postures, movements, state control, and interactive behaviors. Susan's strengths included brief response to voice and calming with tight swaddling and rocking. Susan did not have any limitations in ROM in her arms or legs. When Susan did move her arms and legs, she was able to move them in very global patterns through her available range. When supine, Susan postured with her lower extremities in a frog-leg position and her upper extremities abducted and externally rotated. Susan was either lethargic with eyes closed or crying during the examination and was very difficult to console. The therapist also noted that Susan was unable to bring her hands to midline or to mouth. She displayed minimal movements of the arms and legs. Movements were jerky and into extension. Susan did not focus on or track objects left or right.

The physical therapist developed a care plan for Susan that included positioning, handling tolerance, and sensory stimulation. Physical therapy was provided three to five times a week to Susan's tolerance or up to 30 minutes. This episode of care was for the duration of Susan's stay in the hospital. As part of the care plan, positioning was done to encourage midline and symmetry, to bring her shoulders forward (prevent abduction and external rotation), and to promote hip flexion with neutral rotation. Pictures of side-lying, supine, and prone positions were posted at bedside for both nursing and the family.

Handling tolerance was increased using swaddling with gentle sensory stimulation such as rocking. As handling tolerance increased, Susan transitioned to a cry state less often. With this decrease in crying, the therapist worked on state transitions to an awake alert state. Along with the development of handling tolerance, the therapist worked on self-calming behaviors such as hands to midline and hands to mouth. Slowly, visual stimulation was brought into the plan to work on fixing and following.

The physical therapist wrote specific outcomes to guide her physical therapy intervention with Susan. These goals focused on the limitations that were noted during Susan's evaluation. The goals included the following: (1) transitions to a quiet alert state and maintenance of this state for increasing periods of time; (2) ability to briefly self-calm using hands to mouth, holding onto clothes, or sucking on hand or pacifier; (3) visual fixing on an object for a brief time with increasing duration over time; (4) developmental activities such as lifting head to clear face in prone or briefly (1 to 2 seconds) holding head vertical in midline in supported sitting; and (5) parents independent in caring for her physical needs at home. Although the therapist wrote five outcomes for Susan, they were not all addressed within each session.

Weekly updates were posted at the bedside for both parents with activities to improve response to handling, improve self-calming, and encourage an alert state. Susan's mother visited daily. The physical therapist included Susan's mother in all treatment sessions in which she was present. This was at least once or twice per week. The physical therapist explained all activities during Susan's treatment session. In addition, the therapist actively involved Susan's mother in handling and self-calming activities. All activities discussed and demonstrated during a treatment session with Susan's mother were written down and pictures included for the mother's reference. The therapist also communicated with nursing daily. The physical therapist requested a referral for occupational therapy to work on oral motor skills. The therapist reexamined Susan weekly to update her care plan. The therapist was involved in her discharge planning, which included a referral to an early intervention program, as well as the hospital's NICU follow-up clinic.

After discharge from the NICU, Susan showed improvements, achieving several of her outcomes. Her parents were independent in her caregiving and felt very comfortable with the activities the therapist gave them. Susan was tolerating handling for longer periods of time, approximately 15 to 20 minutes. She was able to transition to a quiet alert state for a brief period of time, up to 5 minutes. She still was easily overstimulated, which caused her to transition to a cry state and decreased her handling tolerance. She began fixing on stationary objects, such as a black-and-white picture. She did not follow objects left or right. In addition, Susan inconsistently cleared her face while prone, continued to have a complete head lag with pull-to-sit, and did not make attempts to maintain her head vertically in midline while in supported sitting. Susan began receiving home physical therapy through a local early intervention program with frequent visits to the follow-up clinic for monitoring of her progress.

ACKNOWLEDGMENTS

Special thanks and acknowledgment are extended to Patricia Carvajal, PT, Rehabilitation Clinical Specialist at Brigham and Women's Hospital, Boston, Massachusetts, for her willingness to share her expertise.

References

Abad, F, Diaz, NM, Domenech, E, Robayna, M, & Rico, J. Oral sweet solution reduces pain-related behavior in preterm infants. Acta Paediatrica, 85:854–858, 1996.

Abman, S, & Groothius, J. Pathophysiology and treatment of bronchopulmonary dysplasia. Respiratory Medicine, 41:277–307, 1994.

Als, H. Neonatal Individualized Developmental Care and Assessment Program (NIDCAP). Boston: Children's Hospital, 1984.

Als, H. A synactive model of neonatal behavioral organization: Framework for the assessment of neurobehavioral development in the premature infant and for support of infants and parents in the neonatal intensive care environment. Physical and Occupational Therapy in Pediatrics, 6(3/4):3–54, 1986.

Als, H. Individualized, family-focused developmental care for the very low-birth weight preterm infant in the NICU. In Friedman, SL, & Sigman, MD (Eds.), The Psychological Development of Low Birthweight Children, Advances in Applied Developmental Psychology, vol 6. Norwood NJ: Ablex Publishing, 1992.

Als, H, Lawhon, G, Brown, E, Gives, R, Duffy, F, McAnulty, G, & Blickman, J. Individualized behavioral and environmental care for the very low birth weight preterm infant at high risk for bronchopulmonary dysplasia: Neonatal intensive care unit and developmental outcome. Pediatrics, 78:1123–1132, 1986.

Als, H, Lawhon, G, Duffy, H, McAnulty, G, Gibes-Grossman, R, & Blickman, G. Individualized developmental care for the very low-birth-weight preterm infant. Journal of the American Medical Association, 272:853–858, 1994.

Als, H, Lester, BM, Tronick, E, & Brazelton, TB. Towards a research instrument for the assessment of preterm infants' behavior (APIB). In Fitzgerald, HE, & Yosman, MW (Eds.), Theory and Research in Behavioral Pediatrics, Vol. 1. New York: Plenum Press, 1982, pp. 35–63.

Als, H, Tronick, E, Lester, B, & Brazelton, TB. The Brazelton Neonatal Behavioral Assessment Scale. Journal of Abnormal Psychology, 5:215–231, 1977.

Als, H, Tronick, E, Adamson, L, & Brazelton, TB. The behavior of the full-term yet underweight newborn infant. Developmental Medicine and Child Neurology, 18:590–602, 1976.

American Academy of Pediatrics. Noise: A hazard for the fetus and newborn. Pediatrics, 100:724–727, 1997.

American Academy of Pediatrics, American College of Obstetricians and Gynecologists. Guidelines for Perinatal Care, 4th ed. 1997, pp. 4–6.

American Physical Therapy Association. Guide to physical therapist practice. Physical Therapy, 77(11):1371–1382, 1997.

Anand, KJ. Clinical importance of pain and stress in preterm neonates. Biology of the Neonate, 73:1–9, 1998.

Anand, KJ, & Hickey, P. Pain and its effects in the human neonate and fetus. New England Journal of Medicine, 317:1321–1329, 1987.

Anderson, J. Sensory intervention with the preterm infant in the neonatal intensive care unit. American Journal of Occupational Therapy, 40(1):19–26, 1986.

Autti-Ramo, I, & Granström, ML. The effect of intrauterine alcohol exposition in various durations on early cognitive development. Neuropediatrics, 22:203–210, 1991.

Avery, GB, & Glass, P. The gentle nursery: Developmental intervention in the NICU. Journal of Perinatology, 9(2):204–206, 1989.

Aylward, EH, Butz, AM, Hutton, N, Joyner, ML, & Vogelhut, JW. Cognitive and motor development in infants at risk for human immunodeficiency virus. American Journal of Diseases of Children, 146:218–222, 1992.

Bada, HS, Korones, SB, Perry, EH, Arheart, KL, Ray, JD, Pourcyrous, M, Magill, HL, Runywan, W, III, Somes, GW, & Clark, FC. Mean arterial blood pressure changes in premature infants and those at risk for intraventricular hemorrhage. Journal of Pediatrics, 117(4):607–614, 1990.

Bagwell, G, & Armstrong, V. Regionalization of care. In Kenner, C, Lott, J, & Flandermeyer, A (Eds.). Comprehensive Neonatal Nursing: A Physiologic Perspective. Philadelphia: WB Saunders, 1998, pp. 144–151.

Bancalari, E. Neonatal chronic lung disease. In Fanaroff, AA, & Martin, RJ (Eds.), Neonatal-Perinatal Medicine: Diseases of the Fetus and Infant. St. Louis: Mosby, 1992, pp. 861–875.

Barbour, BG. Alcohol and pregnancy. Journal of Nurse-Midwifery, 35(2):78–85, 1990.

Barnard, KE, & Eyres, SJ. Feeding scale. In Child Health Assessment (DHEW Publication No. HRA 79-25). Hyattsville, MD: US Department of Health, Education, and Welfare, Health Resources Administration, Bureau of Health Manpower, Division of Nursing, 1979.

Barrier G, Attia, J, Mayer, Amiel-Tison, CL, & Shnider, SM. Measurement of postoperative pain and narcotic administration in infants using a new clinical scoring system. Intensive Care Medicine, 15:S37–S39, 1989.

Bauman, P, & Levine, S. The development of children of drug addicts. International Journal of Addiction, 21(8):849–863, 1986.

Berns, S, & Brown, L. The changing family. In Kenner, C, Lott, J, & Flandermeyer, A (Eds.). Comprehensive Neonatal Nursing: Physiologic Perspectives. Philadelphia: Saunders, 1998, pp. 61–68.

Bierman-van Eedenberg, M, Jurgens-van der Zee, AD, & Olinga, AA. Predictive value of neonatal neurological examination: A follow-up study at 18 months. Developmental Medicine and Child Neurology, 2:296–305, 1981.

Bosque, E, Brady, J, Affonso, D, & Wahlberg, V. Physiologic measures of kangaroo versus incubator care in a tertiary-level nursery. Journal of Obstetric, Gynecologic, and Neonatal Nursing, 24:219–226, 1995.

Brann, AW, Jr, & Schwartz, JF. Assessment of neonatal neurologic function. In Fanaroff, AA, & Martin, RJ (Eds.), Neonatal-Perinatal Medicine: Diseases of the Fetus and Infant. St. Louis: Mosby, 1992a, pp. 691–699.

Brann, AW, Jr, & Schwartz, JF. Developmental anomalies and neuromuscular disorders. In Fanaroff, AA, & Martin, RJ (Eds.), Neonatal-Perinatal Medicine: Diseases of the Fetus and Infant. St. Louis: Mosby, 1992c, pp. 734–752.

Brann, AW, Jr, & Wiznitzer, M. Seizures. In Fanaroff, AA, & Martin, RJ (Eds.), Neonatal-Perinatal Medicine: Diseases of the Fetus and Infant. St. Louis: Mosby, 1992, pp. 729–733.

Braun, MA, & Palmer, MM. A pilot study of oral-motor dysfunction in "at-risk" infants. Physical and Occupational Therapy in Pediatrics, 5(4):13–25, Winter 1985/1986.

Brazelton, TB. Neonatal Behavioral Assessment Scale, 2nd ed. Clinics in Developmental Medicine, No. 88. Philadelphia: JB Lippincott, 1984.

Brazelton, TB, Nugent, NK, & Lester, BM. Neonatal Behavioral Assessment Scale. In Osofsky, JD (Ed.), Handbook of Infant Development, 2nd ed. New York: Wiley, 1987, pp. 780–817.

Budin, P. Le Nourisson. Paris: Octave Doin, 1900. (English translation by Maloney, WJ. The Nursling. London: Caxton, 1907.)

Buehler, D, Als, H, Duffy, F, McAnulty, G, & Liederman, J. Effectiveness of individualized developmental care for low-risk preterm infants: Behavioral and electrophysiologic evidence. Pediatrics, 96: 923–932, 1995.

Burke, M, Walsh, J, Oehler, J, & Gingras, J. Music therapy following suctioning: Four case studies. Neonatal Network: Journal of Neonatal Nursing, 14:41–49, 1995.

Cabanas, F, Pellicer, A, Perez-Higueras, A, Garcia-Alix, A, Roche, C, & Quero, J. Ultrasonographic findings in thalamus and basal ganglia in term asphyxiated infants. Pediatric Neurology, 7:211–215, 1991.

Campbell, SK. Clinical decision making: Management of the neonate with movement dysfunction. In Wolf, SL (Ed.), Clinical Decision Making in Physical Therapy. Philadelphia: FA Davis, 1985, pp. 295–324.

Campbell, SK. Organizational and educational considerations in creating an environment to promote optimal development of high-risk neonates. Physical and Occupational Therapy in Pediatrics, 6(3/4):191–204, 1986.

Campbell, SK, Kolobe, THA, Osten, ET, Lenke, M, & Girolami, GL. Construct validity of the Test of Infant Motor Performance. Physical Therapy, 75:585–596, 1995.

Campbell, SK, Osten, E, Kolobe, THA, & Fisher, A. Development of the Test of Infant Motor Performance. Physical Medicine and Rehabilitation Clinics of North America, 4(3):541–550, 1993.

Carlo, WA, & Chatburn, RL. Assisted ventilation of the newborn. In Carlo, WA, & Chatburn, RL (Eds.), Neonatal Respiratory Care. Chicago: Year Book, 1988, pp. 320–346.

Carlo, WA, Martin, RJ, & Fanaroff, AA. Assisted ventilation and the complications of respiratory distress. In Fanaroff, AA, & Martin, RJ (Eds.), Neonatal-Perinatal Medicine: Diseases of the Fetus and Infant. St. Louis: Mosby, 1992, pp. 820–833.

Caron, E, & Berlandi, J. Extracorporeal membrane oxygenation. Advances and Emerging Topics in Perioperative Pediatric Nursing, 32:125–140, 1997.

Catto-Smith, AG, Yu, VYH, Bajuk, B, Orgill, AA, & Astbury, J. Effect of neonatal periventricular haemorrhage on neurodevelopmental outcome. Archives of Disease in Childhood, 60:8–11, 1985.

Charney, EB, Weller, SC, Sutton, LN, Bruce, DA, & Schut, LB. Management of the newborn with myelomeningocele: Time for a decision-making process. Pediatrics, 75:58–64, 1985.

Chasnoff, IJ. Drug use in pregnancy: Parameters of risk. Pediatric Clinics of North America, 35:1403–1412, 1988.

Cheu, HW, Brown, DR, & Rowe, M. Breath hydrogen excretion as a screening test for the early diagnosis of necrotizing enterocolitis. American Journal of Diseases of Children, 143:156–159, 1989.

Coles, CD, Brown, RT, Smith, IE, Platzman, KA, Erickson, S, & Falek, A. Effects of prenatal alcohol exposure at school age. Neurotoxicology and Teratology, 13:357–367, 1991.

Collins, SK, & Kuck, K. Music therapy in the neonatal intensive care unit. Neonatal Network, 9(6):23–26, 1991.

Corff, K, Seideman, R, Venkataraman, P, Lutes, L, & Yates, B. Facilitated tucking: A nonpharmacologic comfort measure for pain in preterm neonates. Journal of Gynecologic and Neonatal Nursing, 24:143–147, 1995.

Crane, LD. Cardiorespiratory management of the high-risk neonate: Implications for developmental therapists. Physical and Occupational Therapy in Pediatrics, 6(3/4):255–282, 1986.

Crane, LD. The neonate and child. In Frownfelter, DL (Ed.), Chest Physical Therapy and Pulmonary Rehabilitation, 2nd ed. Chicago: Year Book, 1987, pp. 666–698.

Crane, LD. Physical therapy for the neonate with respiratory disease. In Irwin, S, & Tecklin, JS (Eds.), Cardiopulmonary Physical Therapy, 2nd ed. St. Louis: Mosby, 1990, pp. 486–515.

Crane, LD. Physical therapy for the neonate with respiratory disease. In Irwin, S, & Tecklin, JS (Eds.), Cardiopulmonary Physical Therapy, 3rd ed. St. Louis: Mosby, 1995, pp. 486–515.

Creger, PJ, & Browne, JV. Developmental Interventions for Preterm and High-Risk Infants. Tucson, AZ: Therapy Skill Builders, 1995, pp. 97–144.

Cressinger, KD, Ryckman, FC, Flake, AW, & Balistreri, WF. Necrotizing enterocolitis. In Fanaroff, AA, & Martin, RJ (Eds.), Neonatal-Perinatal Medicine: Diseases of the Fetus and Infant. St. Louis: Mosby, 1992, pp. 1068–1074.

Cusson, R, & Lee, A. Parental interventions and the development of the preterm infant. Journal of Gynecologic and Neonatal Nursing, 23:60–68, 1993.

Davis, DD, & Templer, DI. Neurobehavioral functioning in children exposed to narcotics in utero. Addictive Behaviors, 13:275–283, 1988.

Davis, JM, Sinkin, RA, & Aranda, JV. Drug therapy for bronchopulmonary dysplasia. Pediatric Pulmonology, 8:117–125, 1990.

Dean, E. The intensive care unit: Principles and practice of physical therapy. In Frownfelter, DL (Ed.), Chest Physical Therapy and Pulmonary Rehabilitation. Chicago: Year Book, 1987, pp. 377–442.

Deiriggi, PM. Effects of waterbed flotation on indicators of energy expenditure in preterm infants. Nursing Research, 39:140–146, 1990.

delEstard, K, & Lennox K. Developmental care: Making your NICU a gentler place. Canadian Nurse, 2:23–26, 1995.

Dixon, SD. Effects of transplacental exposure to cocaine and methamphetamine on the neonate (specialty conference). Western Journal of Medicine, 150:436–442, 1989.

Dolgin, SE, Shlasko, E, Levitt, MA, Hong, AR, Brillhart, S, Rynkowski, M, & Holzman, I. Alterations in respiratory status: Early signs of necrotizing enterocolitis. Journal of Pediatric Surgery, 33:856–858, 1998.

Donovan, E, Schwartz, J, & Moles, L. New technologies applied to the management of respiratory dysfunction. In Kenner, C, Lott, J, & Flandermeyer, A (Eds.), Comprehensive Neonatal Nursing: Physiologic Perspectives, 1998, pp. 268–289.

Dubowitz, L. Neurologic assessment. In Ballard, RA (Ed.), Pediatric Care of the ICN Graduate. Philadelphia: WB Saunders, 1988, pp. 59–85.

Dubowitz, L, & Dubowitz, V. The Neurological Assessment of the Preterm and Full-Term Newborn Infant. London: Heinemann, 1981a.

Dubowitz, L, & Dubowitz, V. The Neurological Assessment of the Preterm and Full-Term Newborn Infant. Clinics in Developmental Medicine, No. 79. Philadelphia: JB Lippincott, 1981b.

Dubowitz, L, Dubowitz, V, & Goldberg, C. Clinical assessment of gestational age in the newborn infant. Journal of Pediatrics, 77: 1–10, 1970.

Dubowitz, L, Dubowitz, V, Palmer, PG, Miller, G, Fawer, CL, & Levene, MI. Correlation of neurologic assessment in the preterm newborn infant with outcome at 1 year. Journal of Pediatrics, 105:452–456, 1984.

Edwards, MSB, & Derechin, ME. Neurosurgical problems in the infant. In Ballard, RA (Ed.), Pediatric Care of the ICN Graduate. Philadelphia: WB Saunders, 1988, pp. 196–204.

Emsley, HC, Wardle, SP, Sims, DG, Chiswick, ML, & Souza, SW. Increased survival and deteriorating developmental outcome in 23 to 25 week old gestation infants, 1990–4 compared with 1984–9. Archives of Disease in Childhood, Fetal and Neonatal Edition, 78:99–104, 1998.

Fanaroff, AA, & Graven, SN. Perinatal services and resources. In Fanaroff, AA, & Martin, RJ (Eds.), Neonatal-Perinatal Medicine: Diseases of the Fetus and Infant. St. Louis: Mosby, 1992, pp. 12–21.

Fangman, JJ, Marj, PM, Pratt, L, & Conway, KK. Prematurity prevention programs: An analysis of successes and failures. American Journal of Obstetrics and Gynecology, 170:744–750, 1994.

Ferrari, F, Cioni, G, & Prechtl, HFR. Qualitative changes of general movements in preterm infants with brain lesions. Early Human Development, 23:193–231, 1990.

Fetters, L. Sensorimotor management of the high-risk neonate. Physical and Occupational Therapy in Pediatrics, 6(3/4): 217–230, 1986.

Field, T. Supplemental stimulation of preterm neonates. Early Human Development, 4:301–314, 1980.

Field, T. Alleviating stress in newborn infants in the intensive care unit. Clinics in Perinatology, 17(1):1–9, 1990.

Field, TM, Schanberg, SM, Scafidi, F, Bauer, CR, Vega-Lahr, N, Garcia, R, Nystrom, J, & Kuhn, CM. Tactile/kinesthetic stimulation effects on preterm neonates. Pediatrics, 77(5):654–658, 1986.

Finan, DS, & Barlow, S. The actifier: a device for neurophysiological studies of orofacial control in human infants. Journal of Speech and Hearing Research, 39:833–838, 1996.

Finnegan, L. Management of maternal and neonatal substance abuse problems. National Institute on Drug Abuse Research Monograph Series, 90:177–189, 1988.

Fiterman, C. Physical therapy in the NICU. In Connolly, BH, & Montgomery, PC (Eds.), Therapeutic Exercise in Developmental Disabilities. Chattanooga, TN: Chattanooga Corporation, 1987, pp. 29–41.

Fleisher, B, VandenBerg, K, Constantinou, J, Heller, C, Benitz, W, Johnson, A, Rosenthal, A, & Stevenson, D. Individualized developmental care for very-low-birth-weight premature infants. Clinical Pediatrics, 34:523–529, 1995.

Francis, PL, Self, PA, & Horowitz, FD. The behavioral assessment of the neonate: An overview. In Osofsky, JD (Ed.), Handbook of Infant Development, 2nd ed. New York: Wiley, 1987, pp. 723–779.

Franck, LS. A national survey of the assessment and treatment of pain and agitation in the neonatal intensive care unit. Journal of Gynecological and Neonatal Nursing, Nov/Dec 1987, pp. 387–393.

Franck, LS. The influence of sociopolitical, scientific, and technological forces on the study and treatment of neonatal pain. Advanced Nursing Science, 15:11–12, 1992.

Free, T, Russell, F, Mills, B, & Hathaway, D. A descriptive study of infants and toddlers exposed prenatally to substance abuse. Maternal Child Nursing, 15:245–249, 1990.

Gaebler, C, & Hanzlik, R. The effects of prefeeding stimulation program on preterm infants. American Journal of Occupational Therapy, 50:184–192, 1996.

Gartner, LM, & Lee, KS. Unconjugated hyperbilirubinemia. In Fanaroff, AA, & Martin, RJ (Eds.), Neonatal-Perinatal Medicine: Diseases of the Fetus and Infant. St. Louis: Mosby, 1992, pp. 1075–1103.

Gaynon, MW, Stevenson, DK, Sunshine P, Fleisher, BE, & Landers, MB. Supplemental oxygen may decrease progression of prethreshold disease to threshold retinopathy of prematurity. Journal of Perinatology, 17:434–438, 1997.

Glass, P, Avery, GB, Siva Subramanian, KN, Keys, MP, Sostek, AM, & Friendly, DS. Effect of bright light in the hospital nursery on the incidence of retinopathy of prematurity. New England Journal of Medicine, 313:401–404, 1985.

Goetzman, BW. Understanding bronchopulmonary dysplasia. American Journal of Diseases of Children, 140:332–334, 1986.

Gottfried, AW. Environment of newborn infants in special care units. In Gottfried, AW, & Gaiter, JL (Eds.), Infant Stress Under Intensive Care. Baltimore: University Park Press, 1985, pp. 23–54.

Gottfried, AW, & Hodgman, J. How intensive is newborn intensive care? An environmental analysis. Pediatrics, 74:292–294, 1984.

Gottwald, SR, & Thurman, SK. Parent-infant interaction in neonatal intensive care units: Implications for research and service delivery. Infants and Young Children, 2(3):1–9, 1990.

Gruneau, RVE, & Craig, KD. Pain expression in neonates: Facial action and cry. Pain, 28:395–410, 1987.

Gruneau, RVE, Johnston, CC, & Craig, KD. Neonatal facial and cry responses to invasive and non-invasive procedures. Pain, 42:295–305, 1990.

Hack, M. Follow-up for high-risk neonates. In Fanaroff, AA, & Martin, RJ (Eds.), Neonatal-Perinatal Medicine: Diseases of the Fetus and Infant. St. Louis: Mosby, 1992, pp. 753–758.

Handler, A, Kistin, N, & Davis, F. Cocaine use during pregnancy: Perinatal outcomes. American Journal of Epidemiology, 133:818–825, 1991.

Harding, JE, Miles, FKI, Becroft, DMO, Allen, BC, & Knight, DB. Chest physiotherapy may be associated with brain damage in extremely premature infants. Journal of Pediatrics, 132:440–444, 1998.

Harmon, J, & Kenner, C. High-risk pregnancy. In Kenner, C, Lott, J, & Flandermeyer, A (Eds), Comprehensive Neonatal Nursing: Physiologic Perspective. Philadelphia: WB Saunders, 1998, pp. 144–151.

Harper, RG, & Yoon, JJ. Handbook of Neonatalogy, 2nd ed. Chicago: Year Book, 1987.

Harris, MB. Oral-motor management of the high-risk neonate. Physical and Occupational Therapy in Pediatrics, 6(3/4): 231–254, 1986.

Harris, SR, Atwater, SW, & Crowe, TK. Accepted and controversial neuromotor therapies for infants at high risk for cerebral palsy. Journal of Perinatology, 8:3–12, 1988.

Harris, SR, & Brady, DK. Infant neuromotor assessment instruments: A review. Physical and Occupational Therapy in Pediatrics, 6(3/4): 121–154, 1986.

Harrison, H, & Kositsky, A. The Premature Baby Book: A Parent's Guide to Coping and Caring in the First Years. New York: St. Martin's Press, 1983.

Harrison, LL. Teaching stimulation strategies to parents of infants at high risk. Maternal Child Nursing, 14:125, 1989.

Hayford, SM, Epps, RP, & Dahl-Regis, M. Behavior and development patterns in children born to heroin-addicted and methadone-addicted mothers. Journal of the National Medical Association, 80:1197–1200, 1988.

Hazinski, MF, & Pacetti, AS. Nursing care of the infant with respiratory disease. In Carlo, WA, & Chatburn, RL (Eds.), Neonatal Respiratory Care. Chicago: Year Book, 1988, pp. 154–235.

Hensinger, RN. Orthopedic problems of the shoulder and neck. Pediatric Clinics of North America, 24:889, 1977.

Henslee, JA, Schechtman, VL, Lee, MY, & Harper, RM. Developmental patterns of heart rate and variability in prematurely-born infants with apnea of prematurity. Early Human Development, 47:35–50, 1997.

Heriza, CB. The neonate with cerebral palsy. In Scully, R, & Barnes, ML (Eds.), Physical Therapy. Philadelphia: JB Lippincott, 1989, pp. 1238–1257.

Heriza, CB, & Sweeney, JK. Effects of NICU intervention of preterm infants: I. Implications for neonatal practice. Infants and Young Children, 2(3):31–47, 1990a.

Heriza, CB, & Sweeney, JK. Effects of NICU intervention on preterm infants: II. Implications for movement research. Infants and Young Children, 2(4):29–41, 1990b.

Higgins, RD, Mendelsohn, AL, DeFeo, MJ, Ucsel, R, & Hendricks-Munoz, KD. Antenatal dexamethasone and decreased severity of retinopathy of prematurity. Archives of Ophthalmology, 116:601–605, 1998.

Hilton, A. The hospital racket: How noisy is your unit? American Journal of Nursing, January 1987, pp. 59–61.

Hodgman, JE. Introduction. In Gottfried, AW, & Gaiter, JL (Eds.), Infant Stress Under Intensive Care. Baltimore: University Park Press, 1985, pp. 1–6.

Holmstrom, G, Broberger, U, & Thomassen, P. Neonatal risk factors for retinopathy—A population-based study. Acta Ophthalmologica Scandinavica, 76:204–207, 1998.

Hough, A. Physiotherapy in Respiratory Care. San Diego: Singular Publishing, 1991, pp. 194–203.

Hubbell, KM, & Webster, HF. Respiratory management of the neonate. In Streeter, NS (Ed.), High-Risk Neonatal Care. Rockville, MD: Aspen, 1986, pp. 107–162.

Hume, RF, Jr, O'Donnell, KJ, Stanger, CL, Killam, AP, & Gingras, JL. In utero cocaine exposure. Observations of fetal behavioral state may predict neonatal outcome. American Journal of Obstetrics and Gynecology, 161:685–690, 1989.

Huttenlocher, PR. The nervous system. In Behrman RE, Vaughn, VC, & Nelson, WE (Eds.), Nelson Textbook of Pediatrics, 13th ed. Philadelphia: WB Saunders, 1987, pp. 1274–1330.

Joffe, GM, Symonds, R, Alverson, D, & Chilton, L. The effect of comprehensive prematurity prevention program on the number of admissions to the neonatal intensive care unit. Journal of Perinatology, 15:305–309, 1995.

Kahn-D'Angelo, L. Is the small for gestational age, term infant at risk for developmental delay? Physical and Occupational Therapy in Pediatrics, 7(3):69–73, 1987.

Kakebeeke, TH, Von Siebenthal, K, & Largo, LH. Differences in movement quality at term among preterm and term infants. Biology of the Neonate, 71(6):367–378, 1997.

Kennell, JH, & Klaus, MH. Care of the parents. In Carlo, WA, & Chatburn, RL (Eds.), Neonatal Respiratory Care. Chicago: Year Book, 1988, pp. 212–235.

Kenner, C. Complications of respiratory management. In Kenner, C, Lott, J, & Flandermeyer, A (Eds.), Comprehensive Neonatal Nursing: A Physiologic Perspective. Philadelphia: Saunders, 1998, pp. 290–305.

Kingham, JD. Classification of retinopathy of prematurity. In McPherson, AR, Hittner, HM, & Kretzer, FL (Eds.), Retinopathy and Prematurity. Toronto: BC Decker, 1986, pp. 17–26.

Kleigman, R. Bioethics of the mother, fetus and newborn. In Fanaroff, AA, & Martin, RJ (Eds.), Neonatal-Perinatal Medicine: Diseases of the Fetus and Infant. St. Louis: Mosby, 1992, pp. 22–35.

Kolobe, THA, Campbell, SK, Osten, ET, Girolami, GL, & Lenke, M. Development of the Test of Infant Motor Performance (Abstract). Pediatric Physical Therapy, 4:4, 1992.

Korner, AF, Constantinou, J, Dimiceli, S, Brown, BW, Jr, & Thom, VA. Establishing the reliability and developmental validity of a neurobehavioral assessment for preterm infants: A methodological process. Child Development, 62:1200–1208, 1991.

Korones, SB. Disturbance and infants' rest. In Moore, T (Ed.), Iatrogenic Problems in Neonatal Intensive Care, Report of the 69th Ross Conference on Pediatric Research. Columbus, OH: Ross Laboratories, 1976.

Kretzer, FL, & Hittner, HM. Human retinal development: Relationship to the pathogenesis of retinopathy of prematurity. In McPherson, AR, Hittner, HM, & Kretzer, FL (Eds.), Retinopathy and Prematurity. Toronto: BC Decker, 1986, pp. 27–52.

Leach, CL, Greenspan, JS, Rubenstein, SD, Shaffer, TH, Wolfson, MR, Jackson, JC, DeLemos, R, & Fuhrman, BP. Partial liquid ventilation with perflubron in premature infants with severe respiratory distress syndrome. The LiquiVent Study Group. New England Journal of Medicine, 335:761–767, 1996.

Lee, VL, Morgan, A, & Ling, W. Predictability for the Neonatal Neurobehavioral Examination at 6 and 18 months corrected age. Physical Therapy, 69:362, 1989.

Leib, SA, Benfield, G, & Guidubaldi, J. Effects of early intervention and stimulation on the preterm infant. Pediatrics, 66(1):83–90, 1980.

Leonard, CH. High-risk infant follow-up programs. In Ballard, RA (Ed.), Pediatric Care of the ICN Graduate. Philadelphia: WB Saunders, 1988, pp. 17–23.

Leviton, A, & Paneth, N. White matter damage in preterm newborns: An epidemiologic perspective. Early Human Development, 24:1–22, 1990.

Lewis, KD, Bennett, B, & Schmeder, NH. The care of infants menaced by cocaine abuse. Maternal Child Nursing, 14:324–329, 1989.

Little, RE, Anderson, KW, Ervin, CH, Worthington-Roberts, B, & Clarren, SK. Maternal alcohol use during breast-feeding and infant mental and motor development at one year. New England Journal of Medicine, 321:425–430, 1989.

Long, JG, Philip, AGS, & Lucey, JF. Excessive handling as a cause of hypoxemia. Pediatrics, 65:203–207, 1980.

Lubchenco, LO, Bard, H, Goldman, AL, Coyer, WE, McIntyre, C, & Smith, DM. Newborn intensive care and long-term prognosis. Developmental Medicine and Child Neurology, 16:421–431, 1974.

Luchi, JM, Bennett, FC, & Jackson, JC. Predictors of neurodevelopmental outcome following bronchopulmonary dysplasia. American Journal of Diseases of Children, 145:813–817, 1991.

Manginello, FP, & DiGeronimo, TH. Your Premature Baby. New York: Wiley, 1991.

Mangurten, HH. Birth injuries. In Fanaroff, AA, & Martin, RJ (Eds.), Neonatal-Perinatal Medicine: Diseases of the Fetus and Infant. St. Louis: Mosby, 1992, pp. 346–371.

Mantovani, JF, & Powers, J. Brain injury in premature infants: Patterns on cranial ultrasound, their relationship to outcome, and the role of developmental intervention in the NICU. Infants and Young Children, 4(2):20–32, 1991.

Martin, RJ, & Fanaroff, AA. The respiratory distress syndrome and its management. In Fanaroff, AA, & Martin, RJ (Eds.), Neonatal-Perinatal Medicine: Diseases of the Fetus and Infant. St. Louis: Mosby, 1992, pp. 810–819.

Martin, RJ, Herrell, N, Rubin, D, & Fanaroff, A. Effect of supine and prone positions on arterial oxygen tension in the preterm infant. Pediatrics, 63:528–531, 1979.

Mazur, JM, & Menelaus, MB. Neurologic status of spina bifida patients and the orthopedic surgeon. Clinical Orthopedics, 264:54–64, 1991.

McDonald, AD. Survival and handicap in infants of very low birthweight. Lancet, 2:194–198, 1981.

McMenamin, JB, Shackelford, GD, & Volpe, JJ. Outcome of neonatal intraventricular hemorrhage with periventricular echodense lesions. Annals of Neurology, 15:285–290, 1984.

Medoff-Cooper, B, & Gennaro, S. Prediction of developmental outcomes of infants of very low birth weight. Nursing Research, 45(5):291–296, 1996.

Medoff-Cooper, B, Weininger, S, & Zukowsky, K. Neonatal sucking as a clinical assessment tool: Preliminary findings. Nursing Research, 38:162–165, 1989.

Miller, MJ, & Murrary, GS. Noninvasive diagnostic techniques. In Fanaroff, AA, & Martin, RJ (Eds.), Neonatal-Perinatal Medicine: Diseases of the Fetus and Infant. St. Louis: Mosby, 1992, pp. 700–702.

Mitchell, S. Infants with bronchopulmonary dysplasia: A developmental perspective. Journal of Pediatric Nursing, 11:145–151, 1996.

Mizrahi, EM, & Kellaway, P. Characterization and classification of neonatal seizures. Neurology, 37:1837–1844, 1987.

Morgan, AM, Koch, U, Lee, V, & Aldag, J. Neonatal Neurobehavioral Examination. Physical Therapy, 68:1352–1358, 1988.

Moseley, MJ, Thompson, JR, Levene, MI, & Fielder, AR. Effects of nursery illumination on frequency of eyelid opening and state in preterm neonates. Early Human Development, 18:13–26, 1988.

Mouradian, L, & Als, H. The influence of neonatal intensive care unit caregiving practices on motor functioning of preterm infants. America Journal of Occupational Therapy, 48:527–533, 1994.

Mueller, C. Multidisciplinary research of multimodal stimulation of premature infants: An integrated review of the literature. Maternal-Child Nursing Journal, 24:18–31, 1996.

Murney, ME, & Campbell, S. The ecological relevance of the Test of Infant Motor Performance Elicited Scale items. Physical Therapy, 78:479–489, 1998.

National Advisory Board on Medical Rehabilitation Research. Research Plan for the National Center for Medical Rehabilitation Research (NIH Publication No. 93-3509). Rockville, MD: National Institutes of Health, 1993.

Newman, LF. Social and sensory environment of low birth weight infants in a special care nursery. Journal of Nervous and Mental Disease, 169:448–455, 1981.

Njiokiktjien, C, & Kurver, P. Predictive value of neonatal neurological examination for cerebral function in infancy. Developmental Medicine and Child Neurology, 22:736–747, 1980.

Noetzel, MJ. Myelomeningocele: Current concepts of management. Clinics in Perinatology, 16:311–329, 1989.

Northway, WH, Jr, Moss, RB, Carlisle, KB, Parker, BR, Popp, RL, Pitlick, PT, Eichler, I, Lamm, RL, & Brown, BW, Jr. Late pulmonary sequelae of bronchopulmonary dysplasia. New England Journal of Medicine, 323:1793–1799, 1990.

Novy, MJ, McGregor, J, & Iams, JD. New perspectives on the prevention of extreme prematurity. Clinical Obstetrics and Gynecology, 38:790–808, 1995.

O'Connor, A, & Sawin, RS. High morbidity of enterostomy and its closure in premature infants with necrotizing enterocolitis. Archives of Surgery, 133:875–880, 1998.

Papile, LA. Periventricular-intraventricular hemorrhage. In Fanaroff, AA, & Martin, RJ (Eds.), Neonatal-Perinatal Medicine: Diseases of the Fetus and Infant. St. Louis: Mosby, 1997, pp. 891–899.

Papile, L, Munsick-Bruno, G, & Schaefer, A. Relationship of cerebral intraventricular hemorrhage and early childhood neurological handicaps. Journal of Pediatrics, 193:273–277, 1983.

Parker, A. Chest physiotherapy in the neonatal intensive care unit. Physiotherapy, 71(2):63–65, 1985.

Parker, S, Zahr, L, Cole, J, & Brecht ML. Outcome after developmental intervention in the neonatal intensive care unit for mothers of preterm infants with low socioeconomic status. Journal of Pediatrics, 120:780–785, 1992.

Pax Lowes, L, & Palisano, RJ. Review of medical and developmental outcome of neonates who received extracorporeal membrane oxygenation. Pediatric Physical Therapy, 7:215–221, 1995.

Peabody, JL, & Lewis, K. Consequences of newborn intensive care. In Gottfried, AW, & Gaiter, JL (Eds.), Infant Stress Under Intensive Care. Baltimore: University Park Press, 1985, pp. 199–226.

Pelletier, JM, & Palmeri, A. High risk infants. In Clark, PN, & Allen, AS (Eds.), Occupational Therapy for Children. St. Louis: Mosby, 1985, pp. 292–311.

Perlstein, PH. Physical environment. In Fanaroff, AA, & Martin, RJ (Eds.), Neonatal-Perinatal Medicine: Diseases of the Fetus and Infant. St. Louis: Mosby, 1992, pp. 401–419.

Phelps, DL. Retinopathy of prematurity. In Fanaroff, AA, & Martin, RJ (Eds.), Neonatal-Perinatal Medicine: Diseases of the Fetus and Infant. St. Louis: Mosby, 1992, pp. 1391–1395.

Pickler, RH, Frankel, HB, Walsh, KM, & Thompson, NM. Effects on nonnutritive sucking on behavioral organization and feeding performance in preterm infants. Nursing Research, 45:132–135, 1996.

Piecuch, R. Cosmetics: Skin scars, and residual traces of the ICN. In Ballard, RA (Ed.), Pediatric Care of the ICN Graduate. Philadelphia: WB Saunders, 1988, pp. 50–56.

Pigeon, HM, McGrath, PJ, Lawrence, J, & MacMurray, SB. Nurses' perceptions of pain in the neonatal intensive care unit. Journal of Pain Symptom Management, 4:179–183, 1989.

Pizzi, M, & Hinds-Harris, M. Infants and children with HIV infection: Perspectives in occupational and physical therapy. Physical and Occupational Therapy in Pediatrics, 10(4):103–123, 1990.

Platzker, ACG. Chronic lung disease of infancy. In Ballard, RA (Ed.), Pediatric Care of the ICN Graduate. Philadelphia: WB Saunders, 1988, pp. 129–156.

Platzker, ACG, Lew, CD, Cohen, SR, Thompson, J, Ward, SLD, & Keens, TG. Home care of infants with chronic lung disease. In Ballard, RA (Ed.), Pediatric Care of the ICN Graduate. Philadelphia: WB Saunders, 1988, pp. 289–294.

Prechtl, H. The Neurological Examination of the Full-Term Newborn Infant, 2nd ed. Clinics in Developmental Medicine, No. 63. Philadelphia: JB Lippincott, 1977.

Prechtl, H, & Beintema, D. The Neurological Examination of the Newborn Infant. Clinics in Developmental Medicine, No. 12. London: Heinemann Educational Books, 1964.

Resnick, MB, Eyler, FD, Nelson, RM, Eitzman, DV, & Bucciarelli, RL. Developmental intervention for low birth weight infants: Improved early developmental outcome. Pediatrics, 80:68–74, 1987.

Reynolds, JD, Hardy, RJ, Spencer, R, van Heuven, WA, & Fiedler, AR. Lack of efficacy of light reduction in preventing retinopathy of prematurity. Light reduction in retinopathy of prematurity cooperative group. New England Journal of Medicine, 338:1572–1576, 1998.

Robertson, CM, Etches, PC, Goldson, E, & Kyle, JM. Eight-year school performance, neurodevelopmental, and growth outcome of neonates with bronchopulmonary dysplasia: A comparative study. Pediatrics, 89:365–372, 1991.

Rossetti, LM. High-Risk Infants: Identification, Assessment, and Intervention. Boston: Little, Brown, 1986.

Rothberg, AD, Goodman, M, Jacklin, LA, & Cooper, PA. Six-year follow-up of early physiotherapy intervention in very low birth weight infants. Pediatrics, 88:547–552, 1991.

Rubaltelli, F, Bonafe, L, Tangucci, M, Spagnolo, A, & Dani, C. Epidemiology of neonatal acute respiratory disorders. A multicenter study on incidence and fatality rates of neonatal acute respiratory disorders according to gestational age, maternal age, pregnancy complications and type of delivery. Italian Group of Neonatal Pneumology. Biology of the Neonate, 74:7–15, 1998.

Saint-Anne Dargassies, S. Neurological Development in the Full-Term and Premature Neonate. New York: Excerpta Medica, 1977.

Saling, E. Prevention of prematurity. A review of our activities during the last 25 years. Journal of Perinatal Medicine, 25:406–417, 1997.

Sarnaik, AP, & Preston, G. The organization of a pediatric critical care service. In Vidyasagar, D, & Sarnaik, AP (Eds.), Neonatal and Pediatric Intensive Care. Littleton, MA: PSG, 1985, pp. 339–344.

Sarnat, HB, & Sarnat, MS. Neonatal encephalopathy following fetal distress: A clinical and electroencephalographic study. Archives of Neurology, 33:696, 1976.

Scarr-Salapatek, S, & Williams, ML. The effects of early stimulation on low-birth-weight infants. Child Development, 44:94–101, 1973.

Schexnayder, SM, Torres, A, Binns M, Anders, M, & Heulitt, MJ. High frequency oscillatory ventilation as a bridge from extracorporeal membrane oxygenation in pediatric respiratory failure. Respiratory Care, 40:44–47, 1995.

Schneider, JW, Krosschell, K, & Gabriel, KL. Congenital spinal cord injury. In Umphred, DA (Ed.), Neurological Rehabilitation, 3rd ed. St. Louis: Mosby, 1995, pp. 454–483.

Scoles, PV. Neonatal musculoskeletal disorders. In Fanaroff, AA, & Martin, RJ (Eds.), Neonatal-Perinatal Medicine: Diseases of the Fetus and Infant. St. Louis: Mosby, 1992, pp. 1396–1403.

Scott, KG, Urbano, JC, & Boussy, CA. Long-term psychoeducational outcome of prenatal substance exposure. Seminars in Perinatology, 15:317–323, 1991.

Scull, S, & Dietz, J. Competencies for the physical therapist in the neonatal intensive care unit (NICU). Pediatric Physical Therapy, 1:11–14, 1989.

Semmler, CJ. A Guide to Care and Management of Very Low Birth Weight Infants: A Team Approach. Tucson, AZ: Therapy Skill Builders, 1989.

Shapiro, C. Pain in the neonate: Assessment and intervention. Neonatal Network, 8(1):7–21, 1989.

Shaw, N. Assessment and management of hematologic dysfunction. In Kenner, C, Lott, J, & Flandermeyer, A (Eds.), Comprehensive Neonatal Nursing: A Physiologic Perspective. Philadelphia: Saunders, 1998, pp. 520–563.

Shepherd, RB. Brachial plexus injury. In Campbell, SK (Ed.), Pediatric Neurologic Physical Therapy, 2nd ed. New York: Churchill Livingstone, 1991, pp. 101–130.

Shiao, SPK, Chang, Y, Lannon, H, & Yarandi, H. Meta-analysis of the effects on nonnutritive sucking on heart rate and peripheral oxygenation: Research from the past 30 years. Issues in Comprehensive Pediatric Nursing, 20:11–24, 1997.

Shlossman, PA, Manley, JS, Sciscione, AC, & Colmorgen, GH. An analysis of neonatal morbidity and mortality in maternal (in utero) and neonatal transports at 24–34 weeks gestation. American Journal of Perinatology, 14:449–456, 1997.

Silverman, WA. Incubator-baby side shows. Pediatrics, 64:127–141, 1979.

Sinha, SK, D'Souza, SW, Rivlin, E, & Chiswick, ML. Ischaemic brain lesions diagnosed at birth in preterm infants: Clinical events and developmental outcome. Archives of Disease in Childhood, 65:1017–1020, 1990.

Soll, RF. Prophylactic synthetic surfactant in preterm infants. The Cochrane Library (Oxford), 3(13p), 1998.

Standley, J, & Moore, R. Therapeutic effects of music and mother's voice on premature infants. Pediatric Nursing, 21:509–512, 1995.

Stevens, B, & Franck, L. Special needs of preterm infants in the management of pain and discomfort. Journal of Gynecologic and Neonatal Nursing, 24:856–861, 1995.

Stork, EK. Extracorporeal membrane oxygenation. In Fanaroff, AA, & Martin, RJ (Eds.), Neonatal-Perinatal Medicine: Diseases of the Fetus and Infant. St. Louis: Mosby, 1992, pp. 876–882.

Streissguth, AP. The behavioral teratology of alcohol: Performance, behavioral, and intellectual deficits in prenatally exposed children. In West, JR (Ed.), Alcohol and Brain Development. New York: Oxford University Press, 1986, pp. 3–44.

Sweeney, JK. Physiologic adaptation of neonates to neurological assessment. Physical and Occupational Therapy in Pediatrics, 6(3/4):155–170, 1986.

Sweeney, JK, & Chandler, LS. Neonatal physical therapy: Medical risks and professional education. Infants and Young Children, 2(3):59–68, 1990.

Sweeney, JK, & Swanson, MW. Neonatal care and follow-up for infants at neuromotor risk. In Umphred, DA (Ed.), Neurological Rehabilitation, 3rd ed. St. Louis: Mosby, 1995, pp. 203–262.

Taddio, A, Nulman, I, Koren, BS, Stevens, B, & Koren, G. A revised measure of acute pain in infants. Journal of Pain and Symptom Management, 6:456–463, 1995.

Tappit-Emas, E. Spina bifida. In Tecklin, JS (Ed.), Pediatric Physical Therapy, 3rd ed. Philadelphia: Lippincott/Williams & Wilkins, 1999, pp. 163–222.

Taylor, KJ, & Dalbec, S. Use of a pressure-reducing cushion in a neonatal setting. Journal of Enterostomal Therapy, 16:137–138, 1989.

Teberg, A, Hodgman, JE, Wu, PYK, & Spears, RL. Recent improvements in outcome for the small premature infant. Clinical Pediatrics, 16:307–313, 1977.

Tessier, R, Cristo, M, Velez, S, Giron, M, & De-Calume, ZF. Kangaroo mother care and the bonding hypothesis. Pediatrics, 102:e17, 1998.

Thom, VA. Physical therapy: Follow-up of the special-care infant. In Ballard, RA (Ed.), Pediatric Care of the ICN Graduate. Philadelphia: WB Saunders, 1988, pp. 86–93.

Thomas, KA. How the NICU environment sounds to a preterm infant. Maternal Child Nursing, 14:249–251, 1989.

Vannucci, R. Hypoxia-Ischemia: Clinical aspects. In Fanaroff, AA, & Martin, RJ (Eds.), Neonatal-Perinatal Medicine: Diseases of the Fetus and Infant. St. Louis: Mosby, 1997, pp. 856–876.

Vidyasagar, D. The organization of a neonatal intensive care unit. In Vidyasagar, D, & Sarnaik, AP (Eds.), Neonatal and Pediatric Intensive Care. Littleton, MA: Publishing Sciences Group, 1985, pp. 344–347.

Vohr, BR, Coll, CG, Lobato, D, Yunis, KA, O'Dea, C, & Oh, W. Neurodevelopmental and medical status of low-birthweight survivors of bronchopulmonary dysplasia at 10 to 12 years of age. Developmental Medicine and Child Neurology, 33:690–697, 1991.

Volpe, JJ. (Ed.) Neurology of the Newborn, 2nd ed. Philadelphia: WB Saunders, 1987.

Volpe, JJ. (Ed.). Neurology of the Newborn, 3rd ed. Philadelphia: WB Saunders, 1995.

Volpe, JJ. Brain injury in the premature infant: Neuropathology, clinical aspects, and pathogenesis. MRDD Research Review, 3:3–12, 1997.

Volpe, JJ. Neurologic outcome of prematurity. Archives of Neurology, 55:297–300, 1998.

Waber, B, Hubler, EG, & Padden, ML. Clinical observations. A comparison of outcomes in demand versus schedule formula-fed premature infants. Nutrition in Clinical Practice, 13:132–135, 1998.

Wagoman, MJ, Shutack, JG, & Moomjian, AS. Improved oxygenation and lung compliance with prone positioning of neonates. Journal of Pediatrics, 94:787–791, 1979.

Walsh, MC, Carlo, WA, & Miller, MJ. Respiratory diseases of the newborn. In Carlo, WA, & Chatburn, RL (Eds.), Neonatal Respiratory Care. Chicago: Year Book, 1988, pp. 260–288.

Weibley, TT. Inside the incubator. Maternal Child Nursing, 14:96–100, 1989.

West, JR, Perrotta, DM, & Erickson, CK. Fetal alcohol syndrome: A review for Texas physicians. Texas Medicine, 94:61–67, 1998.

Whaley, LF, & Wong, DL. Nursing Care of Infants and Children, 4th ed. St. Louis: Mosby, 1991.

White, GL, Jr, Trainor, SF, Kivlin, JD, & Wood, SD. Identification and treatment of retinopathy of prematurity: An update and review. Southern Medical Journal, 84:475–478, 1991.

Wilhelm, IJ. The neurologically suspect neonate. In Campbell, SK (Ed.), Pediatric Neurologic Physical Therapy, 2nd ed. New York: Churchill Livingstone, 1991, pp. 67–100.

Wolfson, MR, Greenspan, JS, Deoras, KS, Allen, JL, & Shaffer, TH. Effect of position on the mechanical interaction between the rib cage and abdomen in preterm infants. Journal of Applied Physiology, 72:1032–1038, 1992.

Wright, K, Anderson, ME, Walker, E, & Lorch, V. Should fewer premature infants be screened for retinopathy of prematurity in the managed care era? Pediatrics, 102:31–34, 1998.

Yeh, TF, Lilien, LD, Leu, ST, & Pildes, RS. Increased O_2 consumption and energy loss in premature infants following medical care procedures. Biology of the Neonate, 46:157–162, 1984.

C H A P T E R
31

Family-Centered Intervention

THUBI H.A. KOLOBE, PT, PhD
JOYCE SPARLING, PT/OT, PhD
LINDA EZELLE DANIELS, MS, PT

Childrearing is a family affair. Research and theory in child development have maintained that families have distinctive interactive patterns and styles that formulate children's development and behavior over time (Bricker & Squires, 1989; Bronfenbrenner, 1986; Gallagher, 1990; Parker et al., 1992; Sameroff, 1986). Because intervention directed at families has been linked to significant outcomes in child development and family functioning, programmatic initiatives and research focusing on families have increased considerably in the past 15 years. With the reauthorization of the Individuals with Disabilities Education Act of 1997 (IDEA '97) (PL 105-17 Parts B and C), the federal government has clarified the mandated recognition of the importance of families in the care of children in decision making at various levels of service provision (Individuals with Disabilities Act Amendments of 1997, *Federal Register,* April 1998). This gradual shift toward recognizing parents as being knowledgeable about their children and as being resourceful partners in the provision of services to children with special needs continues to redefine the role of therapists and other health care professionals. Not only do therapists require an understanding of the scientific basis of a child's disorder and financial aspects of the health care system, but they now need to comprehend the scientific and sociocultural context within which the child develops and performs.

To provide a perspective on the family involvement context and how it differs from other approaches, *family-centered intervention* must be defined

881

and explained. Several definitions of the concept of family-centered intervention have been presented (Dunst et al., 1991; Shelton et al., 1994). A common thread in the definitions is that family-centered care is a philosophical approach with many facets; it is a combination or constellation of beliefs, attitudes, and practices to care and is family driven. For the purposes of this chapter, the definition by Dunst and associates is adopted: "a combination of beliefs and practices that define particular ways of working with families that are consumer-driven and competency enhancing" (1990, p. 115). Perhaps the most important difference between family-centered and the "traditional" medical approach is that the professional's role is defined by each family's resources and priorities, as opposed to the child's biologic deficits. Initially, the less defined role may be unsettling to professionals, whose professional education and expertise is biased toward identification and treatment of impairments and functional limitations among children with special needs.

The National Center for Family-Centered Care (1990) has proposed key elements of family-centered care that should influence provision of services to families and children (Shelton et al., 1994). They include the following:

- Recognition of the family as the constant in a child's life
- Facilitation of family-to-family networking
- Promotion of parent-professional collaboration at all levels of health care
- Incorporating developmental needs of children into health care systems
- Implementation of programs and policies that provide emotional and financial support to meet the needs of the family
- Honoring diversity (racial, cultural, socioeconomic, ethnic)
- Designing health care services that are accessible, flexible, and responsive to families' needs

These elements and other aspects of the family-centered care approach appear to be common sense, and often conceal the complexity of the practical application of the approach. Within professions with a history of working with children with disability, service providers may be inclined to regard this as not being different from what they have always practiced. Implicit in the family-centered approach is that the role of the family extends beyond involvement in the care of the child, to being beneficiaries of interventions (Sparling, 1991a). The underlying tenet is that optimal family functioning promotes optimal child development and not necessarily the other way around. In this approach, the informational, educational, and health needs of the family are addressed in concert with those of the child even though the individual is the "ultimate target" of intervention (U.S. Department of Health and Human Services, 1990). To employ family-centered care, health care professionals are challenged to extend their knowledge base to include understanding of the multidimensional aspects of family functioning, the family's adaptations to internal and external influences such as limited resources, access to and utilization of support, perceptions about childrearing practices, and cultural factors, and to apply this new knowledge to intervention with families. Collaboration and partnership with families extends beyond teaching parents a home program, engaging in home-based therapy, obtaining the child's developmental history from parents, or obtaining parental consent for various interventions.

Systematic study of families and family functioning has not been commonly included in physical therapy educational curricula. According to one survey (Cochrane et al., 1990), physical therapists reported that they are not conversant with the scientific basis of practice related to the family. Representatives of 87% of responding entry-level and postprofessional programs believed that they needed further course instruction in family-centered intervention. This result is not unique to the profession of physical therapy; it is also characteristic of occupational therapy (Humphry & Link, 1990) and speech and language pathology (Crais & Leonard, 1990).

The purpose of this chapter is to describe the scientific and clinical rationale for therapists to focus on the childrearing context of child development and to suggest processes of care that can be used collaboratively with contemporary families for the benefit of the child. There are various ways to approach the subject of family-centered care. We have chosen to focus on the ecologic, family, and social systems perspectives of child development. In this chapter, we base our recommendations of processes of care for therapists on evidence from studies in the areas identified previously. The contemporary family unit is described in this chapter so that the contextual stressors that families and their children may experience and their coping strategies can be recognized. Transactional family functioning is briefly discussed to highlight broader contexts that regulate family behavior and create individuality. Contextual support in terms of the family, community, and society is presented to illuminate utilization patterns of available services, and the impact of culture on childrearing is presented to demonstrate the challenge involved in meeting the needs of families. An enumeration of physical therapy and caregiver competencies, necessary for formulation of collaborative partnerships, leads into a delineation of the intervention process with contemporary families. Although family-centered care tends to be used in the context of early intervention for children ages 0 to 3 years, the concepts described in this chapter encompass all pediatric populations.

THE CONTEMPORARY FAMILY AND CHANGE

The household structure and composition is a variable that has been observed to influences the type of care received by the child (Rohner, 1975). Families may either be mother-child or father-child households (single-parent families), nuclear families (mother, father, and children), extended households (grandparents and aunts and cousins), or foster families. The nuclear family is common in only a small proportion of all human societies (Whiting & Whiting, 1975). Given the changing demographics in the United States, definitions of what constitutes a family and family roles are changing, giving way to a more blended or contemporary family. The contemporary family consists of "those significant others who profoundly influence the personal life and health of the individual over an extended period of time" (Sparling, 1992a, p. 71) (Fig. 31–1). Because parents are interactive with their child in utero (Cranley, 1993), this definition applies to families of fetuses, as well as neonates, infants, and school-age children. Understanding the issues of contemporary family life, such as single parenting, dual ca-

reers, and cultural diversity within members of families, is central to effective interaction with families. For example, in extended households the infant may be indulged by a large number of adults. As a result, the demand on the infant to be independent in areas such as self-help may not be high. In other instances the other member of the family may influence the parents to place high expectations on the child.

Families with Single Parents

The statistics related to paternal- and maternal-headed families with a single parent describe these families as one of the most common family units with which therapists will interact (U.S. House of Representatives, 1989). The total number of single-parent–headed families in the United States increased from 9% in the 1960s to 24% in the 1980s (Burns, 1992). This trend exists in other industrialized societies and appears to be related to changes in divorce laws and marriage attitudes. Because of divorce, separation, or a parent having never been married, or being widowed, approximately 50% of children in the United States will at one time or another live in a single-parent family. At least 20% of these family units live in poverty, suggesting an at-risk status for future generations. To meet these challenges, policies to promote further educational opportunities for these parents have been created to alleviate their poverty and enhance their self-esteem.

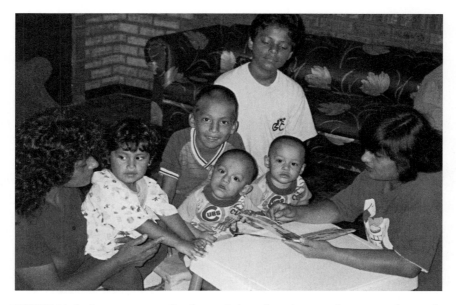

FIGURE 31–1. A contemporary family consisting of cousins, grandparents, and an uncle.

These programs have proved successful (Burns, 1992), but access to them requires availability of child care, which presents a barrier for single parents.

In a review of U.S. census data from 1969 to 1972, McHanahan (1983) noted that single mothers experience more chronic life strains, more major life events, and greater withdrawal of social and psychologic supports than their married male counterparts. This study did not report single-male–headed family data because, according to the author, there were so few single-father–headed households in the early 1970s. Recent statistics reveal that the number of single-father–headed households in the United States is markedly increasing. The U.S. House of Representatives Select Committee on Children, Youth, and Families (1989) estimates a 142% increase from 1970 to 1988 in children living with fathers only. This figure suggests that study and concern for male-headed families with a single parent should be supported and problems of single fathers identified (Sparling, 1992a). Hamner (1985) has described some of these problems as loss of self-esteem, loneliness, difficulty in creating meaningful social relationships, and extensive role responsibilities, including work and child care.

Other reviews (Sparling, 1991a) document these worrisome trends related to children and their families in the United States and suggest the need for "two-generational" intervention (Smith, 1991), in which the focus is on the caregiver as well as the child. This approach becomes particularly relevant in intervention with children with special needs (Gallagher, Beckman, & Cross, 1983), as well as with families with single parents. Sharing information and facilitating the education of single mothers and siblings may have an impact on the family with a child with a developmental disability, in addition to providing direct therapeutic services for the child (Fig. 31–2).

Families with Dual-Career Parents

Families with dual careers are also becoming more prevalent. Dual-career families are a modification of the nuclear family and are characterized by both parents pursuing a career and maintaining a family, often including children (Gilbert, 1985). These families may include part-time workers and full-time workers who share family responsibilities. Although having dual careers may enhance financial status and self-esteem, these families also may experience family and work role conflicts, energy depletion, time constraints on the pursuit of interaction and the maintenance of social support systems, and cultural discrepancies related to role responsibilities (Farber, 1988).

Although they may not perceive their work in terms of careers, families living at the poverty level may also have two working parents and experience many similar stressors. Breslau and associates (1982) conducted a study of the impact of child disability on the participation of women in the labor force. Based on information from 369 families with children with impairments such as cerebral palsy and

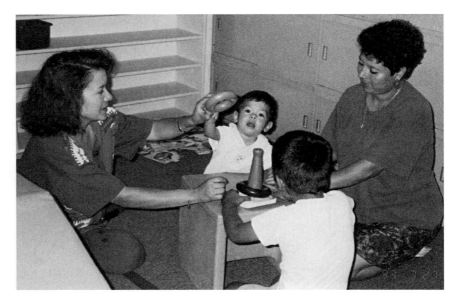

FIGURE 31–2. A sibling is participating in the intervention program.

myelodysplasia and a comparison group of 456 families with children without impairment, these investigators reported a differential effect of the child on labor-force participation according to race and income. Those mothers of two-parent working families with low incomes and who were black were affected the most. They either dropped out of the labor force because of the poor income it provided compared with the severity of their child's needs, or they had to work longer hours at a low-paying job to meet their basic survival requirements.

The impact of long work hours on families living in poverty is described by Farran and Ramey (1980) in reporting the results of a longitudinal study with mothers living in poverty and middle-class mothers. Between 6 and 20 months of age, children become more mobile and verbal, placing an added stress on their mothers. During this period, low-income mothers in this study tended to withdraw from interaction, whereas middle-class mothers engaged in more interaction. Results of developmental testing revealed a negative effect on developmental performance of children of low-income mothers. Whether withdrawal resulted from increased fatigue related to longer work hours, as suggested by Breslau and associates (1982), is unknown. It does appear that availability of the caregiver for interaction is a major factor in learning. Intervention studies suggest that low-income mothers could benefit from training in ways to access the health care system and develop communication skills (Cosper & Erickson, 1985).

Families Living in Poverty

One in every five children lives in poverty, a rate suggesting future economic problems for American families and their children (Eggebeen & Lichter, 1991). Curtailed adult educational and socioeconomic achievements are often concomitants of these high poverty rates. The combination of these factors leads to higher infant mortality rates (Tresserras et al., 1992) and potentially to lower health status of the children who do survive.

An interaction effect exists for families with single parents or two workers and families living in poverty. In 1990, nearly 14% of the total U.S. population was officially designated as poor, a dramatic increase over the previous 30 years. At present, approximately 40% of our nation's poor are children (Sidel, 1992). In 1959, 23% of those living in poverty were single mothers; in 1990, nearly 52% of those living in poverty in the United States were single-mother families. These conditions are worse for African-American and Latina women. Nearly 74% of poor African-American families are headed by a woman, and 47% of poor Latino families are headed by a woman with

no male present (Sidel, 1992). Follow-up data suggest that those children who are vulnerable at birth as a result of poverty and single-parent status are more likely than those not living in these conditions to require special education placement (Goldberg et al., 1990). When poverty and minority status coincide with motor involvement, structuring appropriate intervention becomes even more complex. Environmental risks to the family and child are manifested in various ways, such as material and social constraints; nonfinancial barriers to health care (Lewis-Epstein, 1991), such as psychologic factors that compromise parents' ability to meet the needs of the child (e.g., lack of social networks) (Musick & Stott, 1990); living in communities with poor transportation and safety concerns (Halfon et al., 1995); and limited parental understanding of child development and knowledge of resources, resulting in isolation (Breslau et al., 1982).

For contemporary families, providing for a child with special needs may be only one aspect of family life that demands the family's attention or competes for the family's resources at any given time. Evidence suggests that the way the family perceives a problem is as important as what it does about it (Vuchinich & De Baryshe, 1997). The challenge for professionals is in understanding the caregiving environment and the competing priorities and in providing the necessary support. Evening or weekend meetings and both written and verbal information may be necessary intervention accommodations for these families. The therapist may become involved in helping establish household schedules and task responsibilities to fit in needed health-related activities. The identification of support persons with similar interests, the provision of respite care, and the facilitation of role sharing are major mediating variables in the adaptation of these families.

FAMILY STRUCTURE AND FUNCTION

Family structure and function provide an important context for the child's developmental variations (Sameroff & Fiese, 1990; Seifer et al., 1995). Family units consist of subsystems that represent different levels of interactions (Dickstein et al., 1998). Levels may represent the characteristics of an individual member of the family or a parent-parent, a parent-child, and child-child dyads. A parent or a child in any given situation is but one subsystem of the family unit; therefore interventions directed at a child without regard to other subsystems may be limited. The interplay within each family's subsystems is also complex and requires careful consideration when gathering information from families.

Family functioning refers to the family's ability to conduct and accomplish everyday activities across various situations (Hayden et al., 1998). Efforts to categorize family behaviors and conditions have been depicted in models developed by psychologists and those in related fields. These models assist us in understanding more about family interaction, but most require specialized training for application to a specific family (Ackerman, 1984; Beavers et al., 1985; Morris, 1990; Olson, 1986; Reiss, 1981). Some categorize families according to interaction styles and attitudes that are based on a variety of assumptions related to demographic variables and stressor conditions. These models do not always address the continuum of family characteristics and interactions and the unique ways in which individual families interact with their children at different periods in their life. Because of the innumerable variables involved in family functioning, each family exhibits a different composite of concerns and needs.

To express this point more vividly, the initial physical therapy decision-making process will be described for two families who could be placed in a similar functional category according to Olson's Circumplex Model (Olson, 1986) but who in reality functioned very differently. The Olson model describes 16 types of family systems characterized on dimensions of adaptability and cohesion. Either low or high scores on these two dimensions describe families who function in the extreme. The two children for whom physical therapy was requested for developmental delay were 6 months of age, had no siblings, and lived in a single-parent family that included a maternal grandmother. One family lived in the rural south, and the other lived in the urban north. In both situations the mothers were in their late teens and had dropped out of school before the birth of their sons.

On initial assessment at 6 months of age, Charles was 2 months delayed in gross motor skills, did not explore his environment, and had a "flat" affect. During physical therapy sessions, the mother was quiet and hesitant to interact with the therapist. The grandmother assumed primary responsibility for decision making regarding Charles. Six weeks after the initiation of physical therapy, Charles' grandmother contacted the home health agency to report the disappearance of Charles and his mother. The grandmother contacted the police and stated that she intended to find her daughter and fight for the custody of her grandson. Approximately 2 weeks after this contact, Charles' mother called the agency and stated that she and her son were living with Charles' father, who was providing emotional and financial support. She requested that their whereabouts not be shared with the grandmother. In addition, the mother requested that home intervention be resumed. During these interventions, both parents were present and were attentive and interactive. After several visits, Charles' mother revealed that as a child she had not had a close relationship with her own mother and characterized her original family by behaviors that Olson might label as "low" in cohesion and "high" on the dimension of adaptability. Her present nuclear family appeared "connected" on cohesion and "structured" on adaptability, placing them in a "balanced" category. After the move, and with support of his father, Charles demonstrated steady progress in the development of gross motor skills, testing within a low normal range at 16 months of age when physical therapy was terminated. At this time, his social progress was dramatic, as evidenced by babbling, laughing, and age-appropriate toy play.

In contrast, Greg's family provided a different developmental context. Greg was referred to and assessed at an urban early intervention center at 6 months of age with a diagnosis of tetralogy of Fallot and developmental delays. Greg lived with his mother, Maria, his uncles, and his grandmother. Since birth, Greg's grandmother reportedly had made most of the decisions regarding his operations and other medical interventions and had accompanied Maria and Greg to the initial evaluation. At the individualized family service plan (IFSP) meeting, Greg's mother attended alone and explained to the team that her mother wanted her to establish relationships with the team and believed that this would not happen if she were present as she had been in the past. Although Maria expressed her developmental goals for Greg and identified some of the areas with which she needed help, she was often hesitant. After the team reassured her that the IFSP could be changed after she discussed the contents with Greg's grandmother, she became more relaxed. These behaviors suggest that the family was moving from an enmeshed family functioning at one extreme to a more balanced or "flexibly connected" family.

This greater balance was noted during the next 6 months as the grandmother drove Maria and Greg to the center, sometimes participating in the sessions and sometimes dropping them off at the center and running errands. During one of the meetings, Greg's grandmother expressed her desire to have her daughter return to school. To make this possible she offered to help look after Greg daily during school hours. The team in turn agreed to schedule one morning appointment every month to enable the grandmother to participate in Greg's therapy session. Maria showed more independence and began to participate in other center activities, such as attending parent groups once a month. In these activities she displayed confidence in managing Greg's needs, while Greg's grandmother and a friend continued to be available to her for support. Nine months later, Greg was enrolled in a child care center for children of teenage mothers who were returning to school and Maria had returned to school and continued to take turns with her mother in bringing Greg to the center.

These young children and their families initially appeared to be similar and could be described or labeled with similar categorical terms, yet they were very different. They varied in numerous characteristics, including reciprocity, degrees of dependence, and confidence in making choices. Attempts to categorize these families according to categorical variables, therefore, were thwarted just as are attempts to categorize children with special needs. As complex systems that change over time, families have different structures and developmental histories; as a result, families function differently depending on perceptions of their respective roles, internal and external factors, and desired outcomes (Vuchinich & De Baryshe, 1997). According to Brazelton (1982), the success of intervention with a family is directly related to the interventionist's perception of that family as a unique unit.

Extrinsic and Intrinsic Factors That Affect Family Functioning

Research and clinical observation suggest that a family's perception of stressor events and the social support that is available during periods of change interact with a family's typical pattern of response. These factors describe a complexity of behavior that obfuscates attempts to develop simple solutions to family dilemmas and intervention. The confluence of stressors and support in contemporary families defines the uniqueness of each family and demands

an individual approach to addressing a family's needs, concerns, and priorities. Bricker (1989) has outlined these factors in a global perspective appropriate for guiding intervention with contemporary families experiencing change themselves and change in relation to their children with special needs. This model (shown in Fig. 31–3) emphasizes the importance of stressors and social support in early intervention. These factors are central to contemporary intervention within an ecologic perspective.

All contemporary families experience unique stressors. Families react to these stressors according to the family's perception of them, the number of stressful events they are experiencing simultaneously, the family's resources for managing the stressors, and characteristics of the stressor events themselves (McCubbin & Patterson, 1982). Unlike McCubbin and Patterson (1982), who categorized responses to stress in terms of either good or bad adaptation, Boss (1985) has described outcomes more realistically in terms of a continuum. To study this continuum of adjustment, Petersen and Wikoff (1987) assessed 105 mothers of children with a disability on a combination of home environment and family adjustment variables. Using statistical analysis, the investigators determined that the mere presence of a child with a disability in the family was not sufficient to elicit maladaptation. The number of child-related stressors and the amount and quality of family resources, such as social support, were the most significant variables in the adjustment of the family. This study suggests that the interventionist must be aware of the real and perceived stressors and the unique resources or support available to each family unit, because these factors relate to adaptation and to the potential involvement of the family in the health care of the child. Adaptation appears to be a continuous variable depending on the unique combination of these stressors and resources.

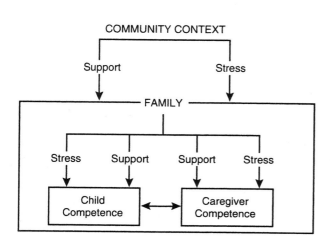

FIGURE 31–3. Transactional model in environmental context. (Redrawn from Bricker, DD. Early Intervention for At-Risk and Handicapped Infants, Toddlers, and Preschool Children, 2nd ed. Palo Alto, CA: VORT Corporation, 1989. Copyright © 1989 Diane D. Bricker by permission of VORT Corp.)

Many factors influence how the family responds to demands from within and without. In this section, only selected factors that may be unique to families with children with disabilities and that have been demonstrated to influence family functioning will be discussed (e.g., transitions, health care needs, support, and caregiver characteristics). For a broader discussion on these and other factors the reader is referred to other sources (e.g., Minuchin, 1985, 1988; Walsh, 1982).

Transitions

Children without developmental delays and their families experience life-cycle transitions that affect child development and family functioning. Children with disabilities and their families experience additional transition challenges. Supreme among these are transitions related to the receipt of services from various agencies in the United States, as described in the provisions of PL 102-119 (Parts H and B) (1991), (Rapport, 1996), or IDEA '97 (Parts B and C) (Individuals with Disabilities Act Amendments of 1997, *Federal Register,* April 1998). These agencies vary in philosophy, funding regulation, and staffing patterns, facts that may cause confusion and stress for the family (Dunn et al., 1989). Transitions and change related to them create uncertainties and stress and require the assumption of new roles (Turnbull & Turnbull, 1986). Concerns about the appropriateness of a setting, adaptation of the child to the setting, and the child's ability to cope with being separated from the family, making friends, being accepted, and receiving appropriate education and related services all contribute to stress during transitions. Families experiencing contemporary stressors of other types may be particularly vulnerable to changes in service delivery settings, a situation described in the case of Gertrude.

Gertrude is a 14-year-old girl with myelomeningocele and hydrocephalus. She lives with her parents, two older brothers (ages 17 and 15.5 years), and one younger sister (age 10 years). Gertrude's mother, Lisa, is a homemaker and the children's primary caregiver. Gertrude is in a special class studying at the ninth-grade level. Since 3 months of age, she has been receiving weekly physical therapy at school and weekly physical and occupational therapy in a children's rehabilitation center. Gertrude ambulates with crutches and bilateral ankle-foot orthoses. Her therapeutic program consists mainly of strengthening and endurance exercises. In addition, the condition of her feet is monitored and adaptive equipment is provided.

Until a year ago, Lisa had been a very capable mother, had a good relationship with Gertrude, was active in the parents' group, and sometimes volunteered at Gertrude's school. When Gertrude graduated from junior high school a year ago, her parents wanted her to be mainstreamed into a regular classroom near her home despite the fact that the school principal and teacher did not believe that Gertrude would benefit from being placed in a regular classroom. During that summer, Gertrude's attitude changed, her relationship with her mother deteriorated, and her interaction with her siblings was minimal. She often refused to come to therapy and walked less. At this time the mother reported behavior problems in Gertrude's younger sister and requested counseling for her. After several sessions, the psychotherapist on the team requested that all services be temporarily discontinued because the parents were experiencing marital discord, in addition to the crises with Gertrude's siblings. After several sessions with the family and with Gertrude, the psychotherapist reported that Gertrude expressed that she did not want to change schools and lose her friends. Her younger sister, although close to Gertrude, apparently did not want her to come to her school because she thought the other children would make fun of her. After the team agreed that Gertrude would stay at her old school for as long as she wanted, Gertrude's attitude became more positive, her interactions with therapists and her sister improved, and she resumed regular therapy.

Gertrude's situation demonstrates the need for an individualized transition plan for each child and family. Such a specific plan, including implementation steps, must be described in each child's IFSP. To meet this federal mandate, families need support in developing their own strategies for managing transitions (Turnbull & Turnbull, 1986). The family and child in collaboration with professionals should explore transitional options as early as possible in the process. Some anxiety can be alleviated by giving families appropriate information to come to an understanding about the transition, to allay their fears about making inappropriate decisions, and to assist them in becoming effective advocates for their children. For Gertrude, the professionals overlooked the importance of including siblings and children in decision making and involving the whole family in the transition process.

Another form of transition that disrupts continuity of services to families and is often overlooked occurs among service providers and between institutions. Parents have identified the practice of staff rotation between units of care, often implemented in hospitals, and lack of communication among staff when infants are discharged from neonatal care units, or when a staff member resigns, as stressful. To facilitate communication, discussions about transition should be initiated early and interim forms of support should be identified and implemented until the child is established in a new program or agency.

Health Care Financial System

The type of health care coverage the family has may influence the family's pattern of interaction with stressors or support services or the family's perceptions of needs. The potential effects of family resources on their ability to meet the needs of their children include access to health care as well. Health care coverage for children, particularly those with special needs, is unique. Many of these children tend to require specialized services at some stage during their development (Slilagyi, 1998), and depending on the family's health care plan, the family may encounter barriers such as out-of-pocket expenditure or a limited number of treatment sessions.

As part of their coordination and communication role, pediatric therapists should be aware of how managed care plans affect accessibility and quality of health services provided to the children with special health needs. Although managed care is supposed to improve access to care while containing costs, the results of the few studies that have focused on children are inconclusive (Hughes & Luft, 1998; Slilagyi, 1998). The availability of preventive care is an advantage; however, children from impoverished communities, who tend to receive care at the neighborhood health center, may find exclusion of these centers from the managed care plan a barrier. Also, some of the recipients of Medicaid are not given the option to enroll in plans other than managed care. A few studies on managed care associated with Medicaid coverage reveal restrictions in access to specialty services and the number of visits for children who are chronically ill (Fox et al., 1993; Reid et al., 1996). Children likely to require assistive devices and technology are particularly affected. The results of a recent study indicate that parents of children with special health needs in fee-for-service plans are significantly more satisfied than parents in managed care health plans, with coverage for specialty services, access to pediatric specialists, access to other health professionals, and the ability to obtain a second opinion (O'Neil et al., 1999). Although options for health care coverage are mostly employment based, therapists can educate families on the natural progression of the disabling condition a child may expect, if known, so that parents can make informed decisions whenever possible. In addition, therapists can assist families in advocating for their children by providing proper documentation of evaluation reports, functional goals, and timely progress notes.

Support

Support represents the relationship between the need perceived by an individual and the appropriateness of the response. Two forms of support have been described in the literature: social and professional, or informal and formal (Dunst & Trivette, 1990). The need for professional and social support has been well documented even before the birth of a child. Professional support offered through prenatal exercise classes has been shown to be related to the amount of medication requested during labor and the request by mothers for breast feeding (Bennett et al., 1985). In an earlier study (Sosa et al., 1980), mothers who had a support person with them during labor had significantly fewer perinatal problems and interacted more with their child after birth than mothers without support. An important source of professional support is information sharing. Positive child and family outcomes have been associated with interventions that focus on providing parents with information pertaining to child development, caregiving for a child with special needs or a chronic disease, and linking families to community resources (Moxley-Haegert & Serbin, 1983; Seitz & Provence, 1990). Therapists are an important source of information for parents in many areas of development, particularly on issues related to mobility and assistive devices.

Social support refers to mutually rewarding personal interactions from which an individual derives feelings of being valued and esteemed. Social support is a dynamic need of special children and their families that varies throughout the life course. Darling (1979) has described the shift in type of support as the child matures from professional support, to family support, to support from friends. Previous studies have suggested that the caregivers of younger children rely on spouse interaction (Flynt et al., 1992) and physician information for support, whereas caregivers of older children rely more on friends and community members (Darling, 1979). The impact of social support on parent, child, and family functioning has been studied extensively by Dunst and associates (Dunst & Trivette, 1990). Overall the findings reveal that adequacy of various forms of support enhances positive caregiver interaction styles, positive perception of the child, and family well-being. According to Dunst and Trivette (1990), "an indicated need for support is a necessary condition for support to have positive influences on family functioning" (p. 327), thus supporting the importance of identifying and understanding the family's needs. The authors also discuss various ways of assessing social support.

In addition to personal support in mediating stressors, support may be financial, intellectual, or religious (Heifitz, 1987). Not only is support offered in different ways and perceived to have different meanings by families, but the theoretic foundation of the concept of support is differentially construed by a variety of professionals. Stewart (1989) describes five social support theories that can be clinically applied and, therefore, are germane to our discussion. Attribution theory relates to motives for helping, the process of gaining or giving support, and the negative as well as positive aspects of support. Coping theory refers to the cognitive aspects of support and its costs to those involved. Equity theory describes the reciprocal nature of support, loneliness theory emphasizes the affective aspects of support, and social-comparison theory addresses the effects of peer support.

Combining these perspectives, Stewart (1989) proposes several major concepts to enhance intervention. Health care professionals and persons providing support must be in agreement about their intervention approach if the intervention is to be effective. Team members must understand that support can foster adaptation to stress and prevent health disorders and that therapists have a role in understanding the sources of, if not in providing, support. Therapists can ascertain whether their patients have a social network that mediates potential loneliness and ultimately helps in modifying their health problems. According to Stewart, recognition by a health care professional of the reciprocal role of social support may encourage the professional to share information and offer support to decrease the patient's sense of isolation.

The reciprocal nature of support is reminiscent of the transactional approach described in Bricker's model (see Fig. 31–3), in which stressors and the support needed to mediate them are major intervention determinants for the child, caregiver, family, and community. In this model, individual child and caregiver competencies are expressed through a decision-making process. The outcome of this process defines to a large degree the competency of the family as it meets its own and society's demands within a unique community context. To provide intervention without considering these factors diminishes the potential effectiveness of the intervention.

Childrearing Attitudes, Expectations, and Beliefs

Several parental psychologic and economic factors that influence childrearing attitudes have received tremendous attention from researchers over the past 20 years (Simmons et al., 1993). These factors include parental attitudes (Greenspan et al., 1987; Luster et al., 1989; Rauh et al., 1990), beliefs (Goodnow, 1988; Kochanska, 1990; Sigel, 1985), ma-

ternal expectations (Fox, 1995), maternal education level and socioeconomic status (Kelley et al., 1992), and maternal age (Ragozini et al., 1982; Whitman et al., 1987). Although these factors are related to child behavior, the nature of their interaction is not well understood. Investigations in this area continue to identify conditions under which interventions geared toward families are effective (Rauh et al., 1990). Some, but not all, research findings indicate that change in these intrinsic attributes is often related to change in the child's development or behavior (Kochanska et al., 1989; Parke, 1986). Earlier studies with families of children with multiple risk factors have focused on changing these factors through parent education and support programs. Overall the findings supported the effectiveness of family-focused intervention.

PARENTAL CHILDREARING ATTITUDES

The relationship between parental childrearing attitudes and childrearing practices has also been the topic of research for many years (Kochanska et al., 1997; Kolobe, 1983; Power & Chapieski, 1986; Shaefer & Bell, 1958). Findings suggest that positive childrearing attitudes are related to positive developmental outcomes in children, and negative outcomes are predictive of developmental delays or disorders.

Despite the value of literature on parental childrearing attitudes, lack of consensus on the definition of childrearing attitudes among researchers makes direct application of the findings to practice difficult. For example, some researchers do not make a distinction between parental attitudes and parental beliefs, expectations, and knowledge (Holden & Edwards, 1989). Assessment tools such as the Adult-Adolescent Parenting Inventory (AAPI) that include several constructs associated with attitude have been found to be more useful clinically (Bavolek, 1984). The scale is available in both English and Spanish and takes approximately 20 minutes to administer (see Appendix I). Therapists may find this scale helpful in situations where the parent's attitude toward the child's behavior is a concern. Results of longitudinal studies suggest that parental attitudes can change over time (Holden & Edwards, 1989; Milner & Crouch, 1997), making them amenable to interventions.

PARENTAL BELIEFS AND PERCEPTIONS

Childrearing attitudes alone may not accurately reflect parental behaviors a child is likely to experience. Therefore, it is important to understand parents' beliefs about their children. Few researchers have examined the relationships between parental childrearing beliefs and parental actions (Goodnow, 1988; Kochanska et al., 1989; Kochanska, 1990). Kochanska and associates (1989) found an association between a mother's self-reported childrearing beliefs and her socialization behaviors. Two types of parental beliefs were observed—those related to endorsed methods of childrearing, and those that expressed affective attitudes toward parenting and childrearing experience. The authors reported higher prediction of maternal behavior by the first type of belief compared with the second, and the second type of belief was associated with the degree of difficulty experienced by mothers in childrearing. Therapists may find scales such as the Perceptions of Parental Role Scales useful if concerned about this aspect of parent behavior. Caution should be taken in interpreting the results because this scale was developed on white middle-class working parents employed in a university setting. The questionnaire, however, assessed 13 parental areas in three domains of caregiving—teaching, providing for basic needs, and family as an interface with society—that have relevance to physical therapy.

The intrinsic factors may be easy to observe during interactions between parents and their child or children, but they may be difficult to quantify. Unlike the extrinsic factors, parents may not always be open to discuss or admit negative attitudes or difficulty with caregiving unless it is related to the child's biologic limitations. Standardized questionnaires with sound psychometric properties could be used to assess maternal childrearing beliefs, expectations, attitudes, and perceptions. Self-report measures, however, have problems associated with their use. First, the measures are subject to distortions (Milner & Crouch, 1997). Parents who engage in less than optimal interactions with their children may either exaggerate or minimize their responses. Therefore, in selecting the measures to be used in a given program, preference should be given to those with known psychometric properties: high internal consistency among scales, high reliability and construct validity, and those that have been used extensively in research (see Appendix I).

CULTURAL CONSIDERATIONS IN FAMILY-CENTERED CARE

Major contemporary stressors are often sociocultural and are related to the developmental transitions experienced by families. The family's cultural background has a strong influence on the family's perception of stressors and the family's ability to cope, adapt, or access resources. Cultures tend to preserve their value system, particularly through childrearing practices (Brown, 1981). From the first days of life, the parents' caretaking behaviors shape their children into the culture to which they belong (Lynch, 1992). Examples of childrearing practices

that are influenced by culture are use of visual and auditory stimuli, provision of stimulation to calm an infant, feeding schedules, use of praise and punishment, and expectations regarding self-help and achievement (Clark, 1981). For contemporary families, these childrearing practices may further be altered by factors such as poverty or role conflicts that are unique to these families.

Family-centered intervention is a cross-cultural encounter of the culture of the professional and that of the family (Hanson, 1992). This cross-cultural encounter is particularly crucial when one considers the demographics of families in the United States. It is estimated that by the year 2000, 38% of U.S. children younger than age 18 years will be nonwhite (Research and Policy Committee of the Committee for Economic Development, 1987). As cited in Hanson (1992), there will be 2.4 million more Latino children, 1.7 million more African-American children, 483,000 more children of other races, and 66,000 more white children than there were in 1985. Also according to Hanson (1992), as of July 1988, 18.5 million of the nearly 64 million children in the United States were younger than age 5 years. Using a conservative estimate of 3%, 555,000 of these 18.5 million children will have identified disabilities. This means that the number of children from nondominant cultures who require services will increase and the programs serving the children and their families will continue to be predominantly staffed by professionals from the dominant culture, resulting in cultural mismatch. According to Green, "it is when individuals confront others with different cultures that a sense of cultural distinctiveness becomes important" (Green, 1982, p. 12). For some contemporary families, intervention services and outcome proposed by professionals from the larger culture may be inconsistent with the family's expectations.

The concept of cultural identity must be considered when interacting with families. Families become more or less enculturated as situations demand, and cultural pluralism is a view that is gaining acceptance (Anderson, 1986; Chan, 1990; Green, 1982; Lynch, 1992; McGoldrick et al., 1982). Unlike the melting-pot view, cultural pluralism views children and their families as different but equal. Some families may practice both the dominant and nondominant cultures (bicultural or multicultural), choose to maintain their cultural roots, or assimilate values of the dominant culture (Green, 1982). These differences are supposed to contribute strength and not weakness to various communities (Green, 1982). The case of Ricky illustrates the complexity of planning appropriate interventions with culturally diverse parents and the importance of cultural competency.

The family of an 18-month-old child, Ricky, with congenital rubella syndrome was referred to a community-based early intervention center. Ricky's mother (Elsa) spoke Spanish only, and his father was bilingual. The child had been receiving intervention at an outpatient center of a large hospital since he was 3 months of age. He received weekly physical therapy and speech therapy, as well as other medical interventions. During the evaluation session at the center, Elsa reported that the child had not responded to these treatments and that she did not follow through with home programs because the child was very irritable and often threw up food. Asked if she had communicated her observations to the therapists and physicians, she said "No." Asked if she was going to continue with therapy there, she said "Yes," because her child needed more therapy. Ricky was very irritable during the arena assessment, even with Elsa handling the child under the directions of the team members. Following the session, the team met with Elsa to discuss the family's major concerns and priorities, to share their observations with Elsa, and to develop an interim IFSP. Because of his irritability and poor sleeping and eating behaviors, home-based intervention was agreed on, with monthly physical, occupational, and speech therapies, and weekly visits by a parent-infant educator. The educator was always accompanied by one of the professionals. At the 3-month review, the team determined that the child's progress was very slow and too much professional time was expended on the family (the family lived 45 to 60 minutes from the center). A physical therapy consultant working with the team on family-centered interventions advised the team to focus only on caretaking tasks, which had been listed by the family as "major concerns" in the child's IFSP. The therapist also recommended that the team select an older, more experienced Mexican-American educator to work with the family for 3 months. The temporary plan was discussed with the family, and they gladly embraced it. By the end of the second month, Ricky had made tremendous progress in all areas of development. His mother was in charge of the home program and chose to discontinue outpatient therapy at the hospital. She initiated introduction of semisolid and chunky foods and proudly related Ricky's improved sleeping and eating habits, social interactions, and motor abilities to the therapist consultant and the team. She highly praised the parent-infant educator.

What was different about this second situation? Many factors obviously contributed to the success of the intervention, among which may be the facts that (1) the parent-infant educator was from the same ethnic group and country of origin as the parents; (2) the parent-infant educator spoke the mother's language and shared some of the mother's cultural

values in childrearing practices; and (3) the intervention team *acknowledged* the limitations of its intervention strategies in this situation. The educator, although not a health care professional, helped the mother regain her pride as a mother, as opposed to teaching her activities that her son rejected and that created tension between them and feelings of inadequacy. These services were presented to the family in a way that was culturally acceptable to them. Each family's view about the cause of the disability will influence the choice of intervention. In some cases, professional help (e.g., early intervention) may be sought as a last resort. The family's definition of criteria for problem resolution also has to be taken into consideration when working with culturally diverse families. Resolution for some families may be when the intervention and the family's understanding of it match (Green, 1982; Mead, 1956; Taft, 1977).

Culturally sensitive interventions with contemporary families require an awareness of one's individual and professional culture (Lynch, 1992). According to the authors, "when we [professionals] are out of touch with our own culture and its influence on us, it is impossible to work effectively with people whose cultures differ from our own. Only when we examine the value, beliefs, and patterns of behavior that are a part of our own cultural identity can we distinguish truth from tradition" (Lynch, 1992, p. 21). Brownlee (1978) suggested that "outside health workers who have poor understanding of their own culture, that of the society where they are working and the differences between them, are likely to give assistance that may actually do more harm than good. When intervention fails, the tendency is to fault the professional's skills and knowledge; seldom is the appropriateness of the intervention for the intended families questioned" (p. v). Therapists should be aware of where the power is within each contemporary family; in many families, the father is the decision maker. When learning about cultures, it is better to seek knowledge from members of that culture because most of the cultural practices are passed on verbally, through modeling and social interactions. Therapists may also consult with professionals from other ethnic and cultural backgrounds who are able to articulate the diverse lifestyles of their communities (Green, 1982). Language can be a barrier to cross-cultural communication, but speaking the same language does not guarantee effective communication (Lynch, 1992). Intervention in a cross-cultural encounter is a reciprocal process between families and therapists, a process in which both parties teach and learn.

Caregiving by older siblings should not be overlooked (Zuniga, 1992; Whiting & Whiting, 1975). Structured and unstructured teaching through play is largely provided by older siblings in other cultures, even though the siblings may not be expected to take care of the infant's or toddler's other needs. Because infants and toddlers acquire a considerable amount of social and cognitive skills through play, the sibling-child interaction may be related to the child's development in these areas, depending on the degree of sibling involvement. Research findings indicate that children of immigrants appear to adapt more rapidly to the culture of the host family than their parents (Landau-Stanton, 1990). This increases the likelihood for cultural "clashes" and differences in expectations and interactional styles. Considering the cultural expectations of caregiving by parents, and contributions of siblings to childrearing in these families, the siblings' styles of interaction with the children receiving intervention should be examined. Intervention models for these families that incorporate sibling education may have a greater impact on the family as a whole than those that neglect siblings (see Fig. 31–2).

PHYSICAL THERAPY COMPETENCIES

Collaboration

Specific professional competencies are suggested for effective practice by pediatric physical therapists, and specific educational practices are mandated by federal law. According to the literature on professional competencies, physical therapists can and should provide family-centered care (Chiarello et al., 1992; Effgen et al., 1991; Harris, 1990; Kolobe, 1991, 1992; Phillips, 1990; Sparling, 1992b). Physical therapists should be able to interpret the results of assessments for parents, consider the family's needs and concerns in establishing short-term and long-term objectives for their child, and work collaboratively in implementing and evaluating these program objectives. Developing a partnership between professional and parent is a stated competency for pediatric physical therapists and is one that continues to be influential in the family's adaptation process (Featherstone, 1980). Recognition of family stressors and a commitment to facilitating the process of obtaining support to alleviate these stressors is a logical and necessary component of pediatric physical therapy practice. Fundamental to the enactment of these family competencies is an understanding of the laws supporting family-centered intervention as described in Chapters 32 and 34.

Interviewing and Observation Skills

Interviewing and observation skills are paramount when assessment is conducted in a family-centered context. Effective interaction with the family unit in a therapeutic context is characterized by the ability to observe in an unbiased manner, ask pertinent questions, and listen. Observation is a well-developed skill of therapists, a skill that should be extended to include the observation in the caregiving context and its effect on the developing child. The long-term benefits that accrue from the therapeutic understanding of the milieu of the child can be dramatic, albeit time consuming.

The interview process related to early intervention has been described by several authors (Patton, 1990; Sullivan, 1970; Winton & Bailey, 1988). Depending on the designation of the service coordinator, who may be the caregiver or even the therapist, the physical therapist may be in a position to conduct initial interviewing. This potential suggests that each therapist should gain an understanding of and experience in interviewing family members to develop skill in ascertaining their changing concerns and needs.

Specific behaviors essential to effective interviewing have been identified by Winton and Blow (1991). These include nonverbal behaviors such as the maintenance of eye contact, attempts to elicit and explore parental concerns and interests, questions and comments that are nonjudgmental and understandable, provision of relevant and well-timed information, and attention to parental solutions and strategies. The way in which questions are asked can determine the information obtained. Winton and Bailey (1988) have described three major types of questions, each of which can be used to obtain different kinds of information. One type is the linear question that is used to obtain specific information or a "yes" or "no" response. A second type is an open-ended question that is used to facilitate elaboration on an issue. A third type is circular, in which every response facilitates or dictates an additional response. At times the therapeutic use of silence is more helpful than questioning. Realini and associates (1992) have developed a scale to assess the use of silence in a medical interview. This tool is extremely helpful in recognizing the importance of silence and the ways in which silence can be used to enhance the therapeutic interview.

Observation of interactive skills and asking questions to learn of family concerns and needs are skills seldom taught in entry-level educational programs. Listening to the concerns of the caregiver and, when indicated, to other family members becomes a major role of the contemporary developmental therapist. Therapeutic agendas may be more readily accepted by the caregiver if the agendas are responsive to the unique concerns and characteristics of both the family as a whole and the child. The therapist is expected to comprehend the child's functioning within the various subsystems of human ecology (familial, community, and societal) that affect the child's developmental processes (Bronfenbrenner, 1986) and to develop competency in addressing the child's interactional skills across the various levels such as familial, community, or societal.

CAREGIVER COMPETENCIES

The family-centered approach elevates and expands the role of the family, particularly parents. On one hand parents are expected to use their existing parenting skills and resources to meet the needs of their family. On the other hand they must learn new skills that are related to taking care of a child with special needs, such as advocacy, negotiation, collaboration, and intervention strategies. Because of the fragmented child health system, parents also have to coordinate services not only within one component such as developmental services offered within communities or schools, but also primary health care centers and public health programs such as perinatal outreach programs. Each of these components is independently financed. Although most families may demonstrate the necessary skills and coping in accessing and utilizing the necessary services, some may need more support.

This level of involvement may not be appropriate for all parents or caregivers. Some parents will elect not to be involved at all. The appropriateness of variations in involvement for individual family members is in keeping with the intent of federal law and suggests a continuum rather than a hierarchy of involvement. Components of this continuum are depicted in Figure 31–4. Although this is only a skeletal description of caregiver involvement, use of this model rather than a hierarchic model (Simeonsson & Bailey, 1990) emphasizes that caregivers have a right to select the way in which they will be involved. The model also suggests a responsibility of the caregiver to define the level of his or her own involvement and in this way acts as a contract.

A major component of family-centered intervention is the sharing of information to enhance the decision-making process. Because the physical therapist no longer is the sole decision maker, he or she is now challenged to empower (Dunst et al., 1989) the parent or other caregivers to collaborate in and even direct the decision-making process.

Parents are change agents (Halpern, 1990). Empirical findings reveal long-term maintenance in optimal infant behavior with change in parenting (Hutcheson et al., 1997; Stein & Jessop, 1991). Family-centered intervention directed at parents, therefore, should be viewed as a form of an investment. To this end parents must be given tools that they can use and modify when situations demand. Parents and professionals may have to revisit some of the various approaches to adult learning, changing attitudes, and skill acquisition and explore ways in which they could be incorporated into family-centered intervention.

THE INTERVENTION PROCESS

Intervention with children who have special needs is determined by federal law and available resources. Within the law, the child with special needs is recognized as a system that is embedded within the larger family, sociocultural, and health care systems. All four systems are characterized by and respond to intrinsic and extrinsic stressors, many of which relate to available resources. The role of the pediatric physical therapist, therefore, is not a simple one and can no longer be a unilateral one with the therapist assessing child needs and providing child intervention. The multidimensionality of family functioning makes it difficult to isolate factors that would influence positive or desired outcome. Pediatric physical therapists are challenged to extend their expertise beyond the target child to include factors that we now know have an impact on child outcome. Besides environmental factors and state and federal laws, economic factors associated with managed care also mandate a different kind of intervention and an even greater professional responsibility than existed previously.

A growing body of literature describes processes of service provision, all of which attempt to address various elements of family-centered care (Caro & Derevensky, 1991; Durnst et al., 1988; Law et al., 1998; Shelton et al., 1994). Some intervention processes have focused on empowering families, some on providing support, others on providing parent education and comprehensive care through service coordination, and others on exploring a model of family-centered functional therapy. Because of the

FIGURE 31–4. Continuum of caregiver involvement.

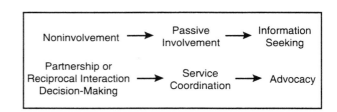

paucity of research and conceptual frameworks to guide practical application and program development, variations of family-centered intervention models will continue in many settings serving children and their families. More recently Rosenbaum and associates (1998) have described a framework that incorporates basic assumptions and principles underlying family-centered care and elements that "represent provider behaviors" (p. 5). All components on which the framework is based are described in the literature and have been discussed in this chapter.

In this chapter, processes of intervention are presented rather than intervention steps or models because physical therapy services to families are sometimes provided by independent practitioners (e.g., hospital outpatients), by therapists who provide team-based services from community-based centers, or by individual therapists who are members of multidisciplinary teams from one agency (e.g., home health or schools). Currently, no theoretic frameworks guide the application of family-centered intervention. It is hoped that therapists will use these processes in developing intervention programs or services. Although the major steps of this complex process can still be conceptualized in terms of the areas of assessment, program development, implementation, and evaluation, within the family-centered context they may never be enacted exactly as stated because those who are the focus of the intervention and those enacting the intervention are each different, develop differently, and perform differently. The processes, however, are biased toward information gathering because intervention is as good as the methods used to gather the information guiding it. The process of information gathering also provides a good opportunity for the therapist to educate himself or herself about the family.

Eight major steps of the early intervention process with families are described. These steps are guidelines to encourage continued dialogue about the intervention process and in doing so ultimately elevate the child with special needs to a higher level of function and to an equal status with other members of society. Activities within these steps are construed as essential to intervention and at times necessitate that the physical therapist will assume aspects of another discipline's role to provide appropriate and comprehensive intervention. This concept is antithetical to therapists' typical disciplinary training and to cultural emphasis on the rights of the individual. If the maternal and child health goals for the United States as expressed in *Healthy Children 2000* (U.S. Department of Health and Human Services, 1990) are to be met, however, and intervention is to be provided to children in the rural and urban areas, flexibility, adaptability, and accountability must be-

come professional characteristics. The process areas are outlined in Box 31-1.

These steps have the potential to help the therapist gain an insight into the child's and family's caregiving environment, the family's perspective, and the development of meaningful intervention strategies with the family. They may assist caregivers in extending their knowledge of their child's potential functional capabilities and in creating a responsive caregiving environment. Traditionally, physical therapists have competently fulfilled the demands of steps D and G, informally observed and questioned the family (C), and evaluated their intervention plans (H) (see Box 31-1). In response to the increase in empirical evidence supporting the ecologic and transactional frameworks of child and family functioning (Farran, 1990; Gallaher, 1990), the family-centered care approach (Rosenbaum et al., 1998), and the goals for children for the year 2005, the other steps are now suggested as essential intervention concerns that, if not addressed by another team member, must be addressed by the physical therapist.

The caregivers of a child are identified before any intervention, thereby emphasizing their importance in the intervention process. No preconceived ideas can be held about the caregiver role, because this role might be filled by foster parents, biologic parents, youthful or aging grandparents, or siblings. In the case of Charles and Greg, the grandparents were the major caregivers initially, and in the case of Lisa, the mother was.

Determination of Caregivers' Concerns, Priorities, and Resources

Determination of caregivers' concerns and resources is in many ways the first step toward the development of the individualized family service plan (IFSP) and formation of collaborative partnerships. On one end of the spectrum this step could be

---

BOX 31-1. Processes of Intervention

A. Determination of the caregivers' concerns, priorities, and resources
B. Assessment of the caregiving environment
C. Initial observation of interactions between the child and the caregivers
D. Examination of the child's competencies
E. Determination of caregiver involvement with the child
F. The IFSP process
G. Implementation of the intervention plan
H. Evaluation of the intervention plan and caregiving environment

accomplished relatively quickly by assigning the task to the receptionist who gathers the information using institutional questionnaires. On the other end a professional with expertise in interviewing skills who is comfortable working with diverse populations may be assigned to each family. The method used in gathering the information is as important as the type of data obtained, hence the importance of the therapist's skills in interviewing and culturally competent communication.

Determining the family's concerns and resources is not analogous to the medical step of history taking in which the family is questioned about the prenatal, perinatal, and postnatal history, medication, and so on. The process expands beyond the mother and child to gathering information on how concerns and stressors affect family functioning now and in the foreseeable future. In addition, this process allows families to articulate these and available resources in their own words.

Therapists have expressed frustration at the difficulty of getting some parents to articulate their family's concerns, the child's needs, and goals for intervention. This may be particularly true during IFSP or Individual Educational Plan (IEP) meetings where some parents have also reported feeling intimidated and "outnumbered" by professionals, who parents consider to be "experts with answers" (communication from a parent who served as faculty in an early intervention project at UIC, 1997). The consensus from these parents is that this information should be solicited during the initial stages of the intervention process to increase the likelihood of family concerns and goals driving evaluation and intervention aspects of the process. This step is particularly important for families with children who have chronic problems. Some parents may prefer interviews, some self-reported questionnaires, some both (Davis & Gettinger, 1995). Several tools that may be used to help gather this information are described in Appendix I.

Assessment of the Caregiving Environment

The capacity of children to influence and be influenced by their social environment necessitates looking beyond the individual to the environment. A child's environment has several components: the physical, interactive, and relational elements, all of which influence childrearing practices that sustain and enhance development (Minuchin, 1985; Sameroff & Fiese, 1990). The physical environment includes the actual space where the family and child spend most of their time, toys, accessibility, and safety (Bradley, 1993). The interactive environment pertains to amount and type of stimulation (social, cognitive, etc.) the child receives from members of the family (Barnard & Kelly, 1990). Relational pertains to roles of members within the family such as those that influence decision making, marital and child-parent relationships, and roles pertaining to caregiving (Hayden et al., 1998). Understanding the caregiving environment helps one to focus on the dynamics between the child and her or his environment and may help clarify why parents behave, perceive, structure, or make the choices they do, thus promoting one's competency in collaborating and designing interventions that are meaningful to each individual family. Although assessment of factors is not the focus of the physical therapist's education, these "avenues of influence" (Humphry, 1989) often have a direct impact on the motor performance of the child. Assessment of the caregiving environment is particularly useful when the process includes a home visit, in addition to any other methods therapists may choose to use.

The child's home also offers the therapist an opportunity to put interactions in context. For example, during a home interview with the parents of the 4-week-old infant with Down syndrome, the child's age-appropriate patterns of movement and posture were noted in her initial antigravity neck flexion, homolateral reaching and arm extension, initial attempts at moving from prone to side lying, and difficulty with tongue retraction. A reciprocal exchange of sounds with the father was so powerful that the sibling, mother, and therapist felt a momentary exclusion and at the same time a respect for the child's and father's interactive ability. Their enjoyment and skill in interaction suggested a technique to enhance intervention. Evaluation in the home may provide additional information for developing an intervention plan. Type of floor surface, limited space, and curbs and steps may need to be considered as barriers to the use of adaptive equipment and wheelchairs and should be addressed in the IFSP.

Identification of the contexts in which children live, such as those related to decreased nutrition, clothing, and shelter, can make an intervention program more realistic. When these basic needs are not addressed, exercise regimens appear to be superfluous and are seldom sustained, resulting in the professional's designation of parental noncompliance (Coy, 1989; Hunt et al., 1989). The home program model described by Rainforth and Salisbury (1988) emphasizes embedding program goals and regimens into existing family routines, thus decreasing the potential for noncompliance. Although details of these family conditions are within the practice domain of the social worker, physical therapists unconcerned about these basic needs cannot provide realistic intervention for such children.

There are well-known assessments to evaluate the contexts in which children live (Caldwell & Bradley, 1984; Harms & Clifford, 1980). The Home Observation for Measurement of the Environment (HOME) is particularly useful in gathering information about the caregiving environment. Numerous family-oriented assessments measure aspects of social support, such as the Inventory of Socially Supportive Behaviors (Berrera, 1981), the Family Needs Survey (Bailey & Simeonsson, 1988), and perceptions of family roles and responsibilities (the Family Routines Inventory) (Gallagher et al., 1983). Efforts have been made to make these assessments unbiased according to ethnicity and other social factors. The scales provide a method of collecting information in a systematic manner. See Appendix I for descriptions of some of the scales.

Initial Observation of the Interaction between the Child and Caregivers

The parable of three youths and their transition from scholarly to clinical wisdom, as paraphrased by Patton (1990), is particularly applicable to the belief in the expenditure of clinical time devoted to observation and interview. Three youths were sent into the world for 6 months to observe human interactions. Upon returning to their mentor after 6 months, the youths reported on their observations. The first youth stated that he learned that all people behave the same: they come to the market place, conduct business and pleasurable interactions, and leave. The second youth stated that he understood that life was simple in its organization: all people were in search of the basic necessities of life and their activities reflected this search. The third youth reported that he was uncertain in his knowledge: he kept wondering about the people he saw, where they came from, where they were going and why, and what they were trying to achieve. In reporting this information, he believed he had failed in his observation of the human condition. Instead, his mentor informed him that he had learned the most of the three youths. In observing and asking questions about his observations, he had learned the most about the meaning of another person's experience (Patton, 1990).

The approach used by the third youth is suggested as appropriate in the therapeutic intervention with families. By presenting themselves to families first as understanding listeners and keen observers of their child's functional activities, therapists communicate to the caregivers the fact that their concerns are central to intervention.

Substantial evidence from studies of infants and toddlers suggests that the quality of parent-child interaction, particularly mother-child interactions, is a crucial factor in determining the caregiving provided by the parent. In addition, parent-child interaction is an important predictor of the child's development (Barnard et al., 1988; Farel et al., 1991). The contributions of the parent and child competencies to parent-child interaction styles have been demonstrated (Gross et al., 1993; Kang et al., 1995; Ramey et al., 1992). Observations of parent-child relationships (interactions) are also widely used to demonstrate correspondence between parental reports of beliefs and attitudes with childrearing practices (Kochanska et al., 1989).

Assessment of parent-child interaction requires a framework that considers the adaptive capacities of the child over time because the infant's capacity to read and give cues is crucial to parental responses and adaptations (Barnard et al., 1988). The framework of infants' capacities described by Greenspan (1990) provides a useful context. It allows one to identify changes in interactional styles that may result from increasing demands children place on the caregiver as they grow. For example, at certain ages the child may be expected to show emerging interest in the environment through the use of sight, smell, taste, sound, and touch; at other ages, the child develops complex patterns of communication with the primary caregivers (Greenspan, 1990). Research findings from the few studies that have included observations of parent-child interactions over time suggest that interactions may be based on parents' beliefs about the *onset* of developmental milestones (Greenspan, 1987). For intervention purposes, therefore, categorizing the pattern of interaction as normal or abnormal may not be as useful as understanding the parent's perception. Although therapists have sometimes incorporated observations of parent-child interactions in their initial assessment procedures, this practice must be done consistently and in a systematic manner to permit comparisons across time. For a review of instruments that may be used to quantify patterns of parent-child interactions, therapists may find the chapter by Barnard and Kelly (1990) helpful. Chiarello and Palisano (1998) also describe a model of physical therapy intervention that promotes mother-child interaction through play.

Determination of some unique needs of members of the family can also be accomplished during the initial observation. At the end of the interaction, these concerns can be summarized and prioritized, but initially the concerns need expression without imposing an order on them. In the hour-long interview with the family of the child with Down syndrome, the need for the father to take a time-out from the interview and from the realities of his new responsibilities was clear and was afforded him by the changing of diapers. The need of the mother for specific information was identified by her questions about the process of motor development. Essential stressors and resources for managing them were observed by the therapist but not verbalized by the family.

Previous research has suggested the prenatal period as a time of adaptation with prenatal exercise classes (Cranley, 1993) or high-risk clinics (Sparling et al., 1988) offering initial support and an opportunity to develop rapport between therapist and parent before the needed attendance to the child's needs in the neonatal period. Postnatal interaction with a first-time parent must take into consideration that the parents' expectations of a normal child have not been met. Cowan and co-workers (1991) have identified five domains critical in facilitating the adaptation to parenthood: assessment of each individual in the family; parental relationships, especially related to communication and division of labor; caregiver relationship with the child; intergenerational relationships; and relationships with other family and community members. This perspective is consistent with the ecologic view that is fundamental to family-centered intervention.

Examination of the Child's Competencies

The child's initial assessment provides a window through which professionals gain an understanding of the child's developmental abilities and needs. In family-centered intervention, professionals and the family negotiate and agree on the type of assessment, the format of assessment, and the location and time of assessment (Leviton et al., 1992). In addition, most states require that at least one developmental test, which includes all areas of development, be used for every child during the initial assessment, to determine the child's functional levels. Therapists have to be competent, therefore, in the administration and scoring of tests required by the state in which they practice.

Assessment of the child's physical abilities must be expanded to include three levels of functioning. Level I describes the assessment of impairment that includes the child's motor control during movement, passive and active range of motion, amount of force created by specific muscles, sensory perception, and biomechanical alignment of the body during movement and static postures. Level II describes the assessment of function that may include attributes such as the child's ability to perform purposeful transitional movements and the child's endurance and speed and energy requirements in performing age-appropriate gross motor activities. Level III describes the assessment of the child's functional abili-

ties with the environment and may include factors related to the child's ability to use community resources that are available to children without disabilities. In family-centered assessment, the therapist extends the evaluation beyond level II to include the extent to which motor skills exhibited by the child foster or hinder caregiving or limit the child's ability to integrate into environments in which children without disabilities develop and function. In addition, assessment helps determine the activities the child enjoys, the way these activities fit into the family's interaction patterns and daily life, and potential benefits the child can gain from other community resources such as a swimming program or gymnastic program at the local YMCA. The therapist, therefore, must be knowledgeable about community resources available to children.

One type of assessment that is consistent with family-centered intervention is arena assessment. This approach permits professionals and caregivers to observe the spontaneous behavior of the child under different situations and is consistent with the transdisciplinary approach (Linder, 1990). In the arena assessment model, a facilitator may serve as a primary tester while other members of the team observe and score discipline-specific aspects of the assessment (Wolery & Dyk, 1984). The physical therapist is expected to assess sensorimotor areas and may serve as a facilitator of the assessment, depending on the child's primary area of need. Other members of the team may assist the facilitator during the assessment. Parents may also serve as facilitators, particularly if the child is hesitant to participate in the process. The play-based assessment fits very well into the arena model.

The arena model has been rated by parents as superior to assessment within the interdisciplinary model (Wolery & Dyk, 1984). In a study comparing these two approaches to assessment, the majority of the parents rated the arena model as more thorough and accurate in describing their child's abilities and as less time consuming than assessment within the interdisciplinary approach. Professionals rated the arena model as more effective, more conducive to team interaction, and more appropriate for small children and all children with severe disabilities than for older children with mild disabilities. Professionals rated both approaches as equal in efficiency.

Advantages of the arena model have been summarized by Wolery and Dyk (1984). They include reduction of the number of professionals handling the child, reduction of redundant testing and parent questioning, provision of a more holistic view of the child, increase in team interaction and learning, greater consensus on the outcome of the assessment than when each discipline tests the child independently, and decrease in child fatigue. The arena approach requires active observation by all team members, provides an opportunity for a team member to clarify test items or child responses for the family members, and permits the family to administer items to achieve the child's best response. More detailed qualitative assessment of the child's functional status or control of movement and posture can be obtained through additional observation or standardized assessment as described for infants in Chapters 1 and 2 of Wilhelm (1992) and in chapters on specific impairments in disabling conditions in this text.

In addition to observational and standardized assessment of sensorimotor development, the physical therapist may be responsible for noting other health care needs such as cardiorespiratory status, growth parameters, and state control. Consultation with other team members, such as the nurse, will be essential to a comprehensive assessment of the child.

Determination of Caregiver Involvement

Caregiver involvement has been a major concern since 1975 with the enactment in the United States of Public Law 94-142 and its mandated opportunity for caregiver involvement in intervention with his or her children. A continuum of involvement already has been described (see Fig. 31–4) to emphasize the various needs of caregivers. An understanding that all caregivers do not want to, or cannot, participate directly in the care of their child may not be forthcoming during initial stages of interactions with families when trust is being formulated. This may particularly be the case with families from impoverished backgrounds or underserved areas. However, this information can be determined through sensitive contextual observation or during informal and formal conversations with family members. As with all assessments, determination of the family's involvement must be undertaken only with the family's permission.

Professional involvement is another concern. To conduct a comprehensive assessment and develop an appropriate intervention plan for the child, best practice dictates a team approach. According to Dunn and colleagues (1989), a team can consist of only a therapist and a caregiver. Ideally, the makeup of a team should reflect the unique needs of each family. Further information on team models can be found in Chapters 19 and 32. Professional involvement may also be constrained by the logistics of providing services to family recipients of managed care. The IFSP meeting can be used to negotiate this issue with all concerned.

The IFSP Process

The culmination of all the information gathering (from the family, the environment, and about the child) is the development of the individualized family service plan. Although the IFSP for children between birth and 3 years of age is mandated by federal law, each family of a child with special needs requires a service plan specifically developed to address the child's needs. The principle underlying an IFSP is that families have diverse needs based on their individual structure, values, and coping styles. For intervention to be meaningful for the child, therefore, the individuality of their contemporary family must be established (Kjerland & Kovach, 1987). As stated previously, the IFSP process should begin during the initial stages of information gathering.

All the practical aspects of service provision to the family should be addressed during IFSP process. The IFSP process provides an opportunity for important negotiations and collaborations between the family and professionals about key issues that are likely to affect service provision. These include the determination of an appropriate setting and timing for intervention, prioritization of goals and professional support, interagency coordination (if needed), financial issues such as managed coverage, service coordination, communication, and transition. Issues related to assistive devices such as ankle-foot orthoses or wheelchairs are also best discussed at this time for two reasons: (1) the emotional turmoil that some families experience in making decisions around this issue and (2) the cost involved, particularly in light of financial constraints imposed by most managed care plans. Availability of personnel resources reflecting the current staffing patterns of the program or agency must also be discussed in a candid and open manner so that other options can be explored. The idea of focusing only on goals and activities identified by parents must be supported; however, problems may arise when parents identify goals that their children may not be ready for, or never attain, or where professional involvement is limited by the family's insurance coverage (American Academy of Pediatrics, 1998; Hughes & Luft, 1998). Further exploration of why specific goals are important to the family and detailed explanations and information about the child's disabling condition may be helpful in moving negotiations toward compromises. Periodic IFSP reviews allow for renegotiations, or revisions of the service plan, as well as monitoring of goal attainment.

For families to negotiate for the types of support they need, and to ensure equal partnership and ownership in this process, the family should be provided with information that will enable them to make informed decisions and choices *before* the IFSP meeting (or any meeting that culminates in a service plan). This information may be shared with the family during the information-gathering stages, in the form of a postevaluation interpretive conference, or in writing in the form of an evaluation report. When feasible, questions the family may have pertaining to the evaluation results should also be addressed before the IFSP meeting, so that questions related to the logistics of service provision can be fully discussed during the meeting. This will also help reduce the prolonged process that sometimes characterizes IFSP or IEP meetings.

Another benefit to sharing the information at least a few weeks before the IFSP meeting is that the family can decide on whom they want to invite to the meeting, something that families consider to be a valuable form of support during this stage. Therapists may find the information in the *Federal Register,* April 1998, on who should be at the IFSP or IEP meeting helpful. The suggested family-centered approach to service planning may represent a shift from therapists' traditional decision-making roles of determining the child's needs, appropriate services, and family responsibilities. Therapists may find the book by McGonigel and colleagues (1991) helpful in developing collaborative goals and in addressing some of the challenges of the practical aspects of the IFSP process.

Implementation of the Intervention Plan

The way in which information is shared with caregivers, whether written or verbal, and the way treatment goals are collaboratively established with caregivers (Bazyk, 1989) often determines the success of physical therapy. Similarly, the physical therapist's skill is a treatment factor, as are the models under which treatment is provided. Therefore, parent-professional collaboration with a skilled and knowledgeable therapist will have far-reaching intervention outcomes. A carefully planned physical therapy intervention plan has the potential to affect at least five major areas of influence on child development and behavior: (1) the parents' cultural beliefs about child development and attitudes about childrearing; (2) the quality of interaction between the parents and child, siblings and child, or other "secondary" caregivers within the family; (3) the child's current developmental status; (4) the quality of the child's home environment; and (5) formal and informal support networks and family resources.

Does family-centered treatment represent a departure from current practices employed by therapists? In our estimation, perhaps not completely. The actual treatment strategies therapists use to ad-

dress impairments underlying functional limitations, and activities used to promote functional mobility, may be the same. What are different, however, are adaptations that must be made to these activities right from the beginning, to accommodate the family's role and environmental resources. In some cases this may involve a compromise between "hands-on" activities and activities that, to the therapist, may appear to be "common sense." In other cases the use of certain equipment or toys may have to be curtailed in order to enhance the family's use of the child's own environment in promoting development and function. The difficulty of changing the environment, or using the child's environmental resources, is probably the most challenging aspect of treatment, particularly when working with families from impoverished backgrounds. The model proposed by Chiarello and Palisano (1998), which involves using the toys found in the home, is useful in this regard. Research findings suggest that this aspect of intervention does not "always manifest itself immediately or in direct proportion to the intensity of the intervention" (Bradley, 1993, p. 478).

One of the historical questions related to treatment is parent participation. An early paper by Farber and Lewis (1975) suggested that parents are requested to participate in the education of their child because school personnel have abrogated their responsibility in this area. This argument is not as tenable as it was in 1975 because of the passage of the federal laws mandating parental involvement. With the family-centered approach, however, similar questions arise about the extent of caregiver responsibility. The practical answer is not easy. On one hand parents are supposed to choose their level of involvement (Turnbull & Turnbull, 1986; Viscardis, 1998). On the other hand research on efficacy of parent teaching and theories of skill learning suggest that interventions are effective when there is a fairly high level of involvement by parents (Farran, 1990; Stein & Jessop, 1991).

The concept of compliance is a related issue. Caregivers can be under stress for a variety of reasons and often cannot maintain the regimens established by therapists. To intimate noncompliance in such cases suggests that therapists are performing as experts and parents are passive recipients of their authoritative instruction. These issues represent some of the many challenges that must be faced when providing family-centered intervention and building collaborative partnerships.

Providing family-centered treatment to culturally diverse families is another challenge. Most treatment adaptations and strategies that have been proposed in the literature were not put together in a conceptual framework and therefore have never been tested for their effectiveness. We propose that the unique-ness of a culturally sensitive family-centered inter-vention should be in the timing, structuring, and sequencing of interventions for each family, in addi-tion to the "usual" developmental program or activi-ties. Timing, sequencing, and structuring are partic-ularly important in working with families whose cultural values and beliefs are different from those of the mainstream population. For example, if a fami-ly's belief is that "children should be seen and not heard," the timing and sequencing of educating the parents on this issue will be different. In other words, instead of directly teaching a family to listen to a child, the topic would be introduced at a much ear-lier stage (before the child can talk), so as to allow the family to get used to the idea (timing). Structuring educational experiences plays a role in creating shared versus isolated educational experiences. For example, whether the topic should be addressed in a group versus individually would be an important consideration because parents who do not permit their child to talk or ask too many questions may be acting in conformity with cultural beliefs held by other members of the community. Thus a shared educational experience with other parents may allow them to make adaptations without a concern for being an seen as "exceptions," thus minimizing the "peculiarity" of their adaptations. The shared experi-ence could also be structured in such a way that it includes other members of the family, or both par-ents (Fig. 31–5). Finally, sequencing plays a role in when and where developmental and educational ex-periences take place.

Another issue that often comes up in discussions of family-centered treatment is that of the setting in which intervention is provided. A setting in which therapy takes place in and of itself is not a reflection of the family-centeredness of a program. In some cases, the most appropriate place to intervene with the child may be in the home, particularly with med-ically fragile infants; in others, center-based interven-tion may be appropriate. Children and families who receive home-based intervention often receive less frequent and less intensive intervention because of extensive travel times and lack of staff availability. Studies comparing clinic and home-based nursing management of children with failure to thrive report no differences in child outcomes at the end of the first year of intervention, but remarkable advantages, particularly in motor and cognitive skills, among children receiving home intervention (Black et al., 1995; Hutcheson et al., 1997). Because clinic visits for nursing checkups are not similar to center visits for therapy, studies comparing the effectiveness of center- versus home-based physical therapy are needed. Cost is usually a primary determinant where services are offered; however, the overall cost-effectiveness of any therapy services should also be considered in terms of the child and family out-comes (Lieu & Newman, 1998).

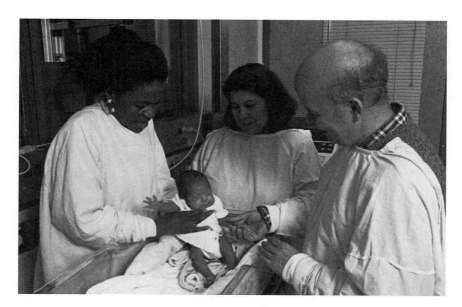

FIGURE 31–5. Therapist showing both parents various ways of handling their premature infant, a process aimed at shared experiences.

Evaluation of the Intervention Plan and the Caregiving Environment

The logical first step in evaluating the effectiveness of a family-centered intervention is to determine the extent to which goals stated in the IFSP or service plan are met (Individuals with Disabilities Act Amendments of 1997, *Federal Register,* April 1998). To be useful, however, the goals must be stated in observable and measurable format. Parents' input is particularly valuable in this regard because they know how the child performs during functional activities at home. Because parents are supposed to have a copy of their child's IFSP, they could be asked to rate progress made based on the IFSP before the IFSP review meeting. The meeting could, therefore, be used to cross-check and compare the ratings, to discuss barriers limiting progress, and to modify or change goals (Fig. 31–6).

The effects of family-centered intervention may not always be limited to the goals identified on the IFSP or the child's functional status. Other factors, such as ease of access to care, intrinsic parental factors (e.g., attitudes), and self-efficacy, may also be positively influenced (Lieu & Newman, 1998). Unfortunately, these factors are hard to measure, particularly if they were not the focus of intervention.

Patient satisfaction is increasingly being used to measure outcome of many health interventions, including family-centered care (Godley, Fiedler, & Funk, 1998; Lieu & Newman, 1998; Sitzia & Wood, 1997; Williams, 1994). It has been increasingly used by managed care organizations to represent the qual- ity of services, although the link between the two is weak (Williams, 1994). Measures of parent satisfaction have been used in early intervention programs to determine the extent to which families believe the programs meet their needs (Kjerland & Kovach, 1987). Although these measures offer important information for improvement of services and provider behaviors, the results do not provide information about the effectiveness of interventions. Another method of assessing the extent to which services to families are provided in a family-centered manner has been described by King and associates (1998). This method involves assessment of parents' and service providers' perceptions using the Measures of Processes of Care (MPOC) (see Appendix I). The resulting information is particularly useful in program evaluation and staff development, particularly if the two surveys are conducted during the same period.

Studies are needed to assess the effectiveness of family-centered physical therapy. Therapists may contribute to the establishment of large data sets needed to support improvement by developing systematic methods of data collection for all the children and families enrolled in their programs or on their caseloads.

CONCLUSION

A challenge to pediatric therapists is to determine strategies for providing the best practice given less than adequate health care and educational resources. This challenge is complicated by characteristics of

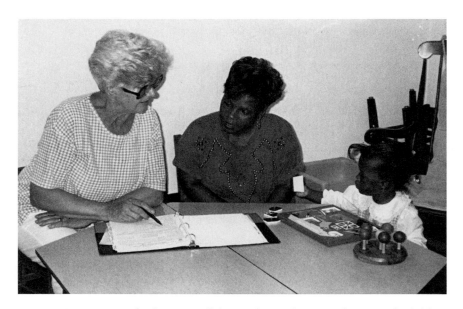

FIGURE 31–6. A parent and a therapist collaborate during the 6-month review of a child's IFSP.

contemporary family life that involve change. Understanding conditions necessitating change, however, can facilitate interaction and foster the development of decision-making and collaborative skills. In other words, the therapist can use the findings from ecologic and family systems frameworks to help develop effective negotiation skills and successful professional-parent partnerships, which are important long-term goals of family-centered intervention. In this approach, the therapist, together with the family, identifies the stressors; examines the ability of the caregiving environment to meet the needs of the child, including the support available to the family; and addresses the functional limitations of the child based on an understanding of the pathophysiology of the child's diagnosis. This marriage of pathophysiologic and sociocultural knowledge is critical for the physical therapist based on research related to motor development and functional independence (Campos et al., 1982; Cassidy, 1986; Cintas, 1992; Clydesdale et al., 1990) and education (Bricker, 1989). In keeping with this perspective, Haley and Baryza (1990) have challenged physical therapists to develop a hierarchy of psychosocial factors to accompany their motor outcome model that is initiated at the level of spontaneous movement and terminates in motor skills and adaptive motor function.

Recognizing the importance of the immediate family and larger sociocultural environments for the developing child supports effective intervention for children of all ages. Family and contextual variables that support child motor outcome goals vary over the course of development. One factor may take precedence over another at any one time, but at no time can child, family, or sociocultural variables be excluded from the therapist's considerations. Physical therapists who search for family-oriented outcomes related to the child's movement, and collaborate with families on the process of care, are engaging in best practice for children and their families.

ACKNOWLEDGMENTS

Dr. Kolobe wishes to thank Cathy Franks, Susan Klepper, and Bob Palisano for their suggestions, and Maggie O'Neil for her input on managed care.

References

Ackerman, NJ. A Theory of Family Systems. New York: Gardner Press, 1984.

American Academy of Pediatrics (Committee on Children with Disabilities). Managed care and children with special needs: A subject review. Pediatrics, *102*(3):657–660, 1998.

Anderson, L. Ethnicity and illness experience: Ideological structures and the health care delivery system. Social Sciences and Medicine, *22*:1277–1283, 1986.

Bailey, DB, & Simeonsson, RJ. Assessing needs of families with handicapped infants. Journal of Special Education, *22*(1):117–127, 1988.

Barnard, KE. Nursing Child Assessment Feeding Scale. Seattle: University of Washington, 1978a.

Barnard, KE. Nursing Child Assessment Teaching Scale. Seattle: University of Washington, 1978b.

Barnard, KE, Booth, CL, Mitchell, SK, & Telzrow, R. Newborn nursing models: A test of early intervention to high-risk infants and families. In Hibbs, E (Ed.), Children and Families: Studies in Prevention and Intervention. Madison, CT: International Universities Press, pp. 63–81, 1988.

Barnard, KE, Hammond, MA, Booth, CL, Mitchell, SK, & Spieker, SJ. Measurement and meaning of parent-child interaction. In Morrison, FJ, Lord, CE, & Keating, DP (Eds.), Applied Development Psychology, Vol. 3. New York: Academic Press, 1989.

Barnard, KE, & Kelly, JF. Assessment of parent-child interaction. In Meisels, SJ, & Shonkoff, JP (Eds.), Handbook of Early Childhood Intervention. New York: Cambridge University Press, pp. 278–302, 1990.

Bavolek, SJ. Handbook for the Adult-Adolescent Parenting Inventory (AAPI). Eau Claire, WI: Family-Development Resources, Inc., 1984.

Bazyk, S. Changes in attitudes and beliefs regarding parent participation and home programs: An update. American Journal of Occupational Therapy, *43*:723–728, 1989.

Beavers, R, Hampson, R, & Hulgus, Y. Commentary: The Beavers' system approach to family assessment. Family Process, *24*:398–405, 1985.

Bennett, A, Hewson, D, Booker, E, & Holliday, S. Antenatal preparation and labor support in relation to birth outcomes. Birth, *12*(1):9–16, 1985.

Berrera, M, Jr. Social support in the adjustment of pregnant adolescents. In Gottlieb, BH (Ed.), Social Networks and Social Support. Beverly Hills: Sage, 1981, pp. 69–96.

Black, MM, Dubowitz, H, Hutcheson, J, Berenson-Howard, J, & Starr, RH. A randomized clinical trial of home intervention for children with failure to thrive. Pediatrics, *95*(6):807–814, 1995.

Boss, P. Family stress: Perception and context. In Sussman, MB, & Stemmetz, S (Eds.), Handbook on Marriage and the Family. New York: Plenum Press, 1985, p. 704.

Bradley, RH. Children's home environments, health, behavior, and intervention efforts: A review using the HOME inventory as a marker measure. Genetic, Social, and General Psychology Monographs, *119*(4):439–490, 1993.

Brazelton, TB. Early intervention: What does it mean? In Fitzgerald, HE, Lester, BM, & Yogman, MW (Eds.), Theory and Research in Behavioral Pediatrics, Vol. 1. New York: Plenum Press, 1982, pp. 1–34.

Breslau, N, Salkever, D, & Staruch, KS. Women's labor force activity and responsibilities for disabled dependents: A study of families with disabled children. Journal of Health and Social Behavior, *23*:169–183, 1982.

Bricker, D. Early Intervention for At-risk and Handicapped Infants, Toddlers and Preschool Children, 2nd ed. Palo Alto, CA: VORT Corporation, 1989.

Bricker, D, & Squires, J. Low cost system using parents to monitor the development of at-risk infants. Journal of Early Intervention, *13*(1):50–60, 1989a.

Bricker, D, & Squires, J. The effectiveness of parental screening of at-risk infants: The infant monitoring questionnaires. Topics in Early Childhood Special Education, *9*(3):67–85, 1989b.

Bronffenbrenner, U. Ecology of the family as a context for human development research perspectives. Developmental Psychology, *22*:723–742, 1986.

Brown, MS. Culture and childrearing. In Clark, AL (Ed.), Culture and Childrearing. Philadelphia: FA Davis, 1981, pp. 3–35.

Brownlee, AJ. Community, Culture, and Care: A Cross-cultural Guide for Healthworkers. St. Louis: Mosby, 1978.

Burns, A. Mother-headed families: An international perspective and the case of Australia. Social Policy Report, *6*(1):1–23, 1992.

Caldwell, BM, & Bradley, RH. Manual for the Home Observation for Measurement of the Environment, Rev. ed. Little Rock: University of Arkansas, 1984.

Campos, J, Svejda, M, Campos, R, & Bertenthal, B. The emergence of self-produced locomotion: Its importance for psychological development. In Bricker, D (Ed.), Intervention with At-risk and Handicapped Infants. Baltimore: University Park Press, 1982, pp. 195–216.

Caro, P, & Derevensky, JL. Family-focused intervention model: Implementation and research findings. Topics in Early Childhood and Special Education, 11(3):66–80, 1991.

Cassidy, J. The ability to negotiate the environment: An aspect of infant competence as related to quality of attachment. Child Development, 57:331–337, 1986.

Chan, SQ. Early intervention with culturally diverse families of infants and toddlers with disabilities. Infants and Young Children, 3(2): 78–87, 1990.

Chiarello, L, Effgen, S, & Levinson, M. Parent-professional partnerships in evaluation and the development of individualized family service plans. Pediatric Physical Therapy, 4:64–69, 1992.

Chiarello, LA, & Palisano, RJ. Investigation of the effects of a model of physical therapy on mother-child interactions and the motor behaviors of children with motor delay. Physical Therapy, 78(2):180–194, 1998.

Cintas, HM. The relationship of motor skill level and risk-taking during exploration in toddlers. Pediatric Physical Therapy, 4:165–170, 1992.

Clark, AL. Childrearing in matrix America. In Clark, AL (Ed.), Culture and Childrearing. Philadelphia: FA Davis, 1981, pp. 37–54.

Clydesdale, TT, Fahs, IJ, Kilgore, KM, & Splaingard, ML. Social dimensions to functional gain in pediatric patients. Archives of Physical Medicine and Rehabilitation, 71:469–472, 1990.

Cochrane, CG, Farley, BG, & Wilhelm, IJ. Preparation of physical therapists who work with handicapped infants and their families: Current status and training needs. Physical Therapy, 70:372–380, 1990.

Cosper, M, & Erickson, M. The psychological, social and medical needs of lower socioeconomic status mothers of asthmatic children. Journal of Asthma, 22:145–148, 1985.

Cowan, CP, Cowan, PA, Heming, G, & Miller, NB. Becoming a family: Marriage, parenting, and child development. In Cowan, PA, & Hetherington, M (Eds.), Family Transitions. Hillsdale, NJ: Lawrence Erlbaum Associates, 1991, pp. 79–109.

Coy, JA. Autonomy-based informed consent: Ethical implications for patient noncompliance. Physical Therapy, 69:826–833, 1989.

Crais, ER, & Leonard, CR. PL 99-457: Are speech-language pathologists prepared for the challenge? Journal of the American Speech-Language and Hearing Association, 32:57–61, 1990.

Cranley, M. The origins of the mother-child relationship: A review. Physical and Occupational Therapy in Pediatrics, 12(2/3):39–51, 1993.

Darling, RB. Families Against Society: A Study of Reactions to Children with Birth Defects. Beverly Hills: Sage, 1979, p. 78.

Davis, SK, & Gettinger, M. Family-focused assessment for identifying family resources and concerns: Parent preferences, assessment information, and evaluation across three methods. Journal of School Psychology, 33:99–121, 1995.

Dickstein, S, Seifer, R, Hayden, LC, Schiller, M, Keitner, G, Miller, I, Matzko, M, Sameroff, AJ, Rasmussen, S, & Magee, KD. Levels of family assessment: II. Impact of maternal psychopathology on family functioning. Journal of Family Psychology, 12(1):23–40, 1998.

Dunn, W, Campbell, PH, Oetter, PL, Hall, S, Berger, E, & Strickland, LR. Guidelines for Occupational Therapy Services in Early Intervention and Preschool Services. Rockville, MD: American Occupational Therapy Association, 1989.

Dunst CJ, & Trivette, CM. Assessment of social support in early intervention programs. In Meisels, SJ, & Shonkoff, JP (Eds.), Handbook of Early Childhood Intervention. New York: Cambridge University Press, 1990, pp. 327–369.

Dunst, CJ, Trivette, CM, Gordon, NJ, & Pletcher, LL. Building and mobilizing informal family support networks. In Singer, GHS, & Irwin, LK (Eds.), Support for Caregiving Families: Enabling Positive Adaptation to Disability. Baltimore: Paul H Brookes, 1989, pp. 121–141.

Dunst, C, Johanson, C, Trivetter, C, & Hamby, D. Family oriented early intervention policies: Family centered or not? Exceptional Child, 21(11):115–118, 1991.

Effgen, SK, Bjornson, K, Chiarello, L, Sinzer, L, & Phillips, W. Competencies for physical therapists in early intervention. Pediatric Physical Therapy, 3:77–80, 1991.

Eggebeen, DJ, & Lichter, DT. Race, family structure, and changing poverty among American children. American Sociological Review, 56:801–817, 1991.

Epstein, NB, Baldwin, LM, & Bishop, DS. The Me Master Family Assessment Device. Journal of Marriage and Family Therapy, 9:171–177, 1983.

Farber, R. Integrated treatment of the dual-career couple. American Journal of Family Therapy, 16(1):46–57, 1988.

Farber, B, & Lewis, M. The symbolic use of parents: A sociological critique of educational practice. Journal of Research in Development and Education, 8(2):34–43, 1975.

Farel, AM, Freeman, VA, Keenan, NL, & Huber, CJ. Interaction between high-risk infants and their mothers: The NCAST as an assessment tool. Research in Nursing and Health, 14(2):109–118, 1991.

Farran, DC. Effect of intervention with disadvantaged and disabled children: A decade review. In Meisels, SJ, & Shonkoff, JP (Eds.), Handbook of Early Childhood Intervention. New York: Cambridge University Press, 1990, pp. 501–539.

Farran, DC, & Ramey, CT. Social class differences in dyadic involvement during infancy. Child Development, 51:254–257, 1980.

Featherstone, H. A Difference in the Family: Life with a Disabled Child. New York: Basic Books, 1980.

Flynt, SW, Wood, TA, & Scott, RL. Social support of mothers of children with mental retardation. Mental Retardation, 30:233–236, 1992.

Fox, HB, Wicks, LB, & Newacheck, PW. Health maintenance organizations and children with special needs. A suitable match? American Journal of Diseases of Children, 147:546–552, 1993.

Fox, RA. Parent Behavior Checklist. Brandon, VT: Clinical Psychology, 1994.

Fox, RA. Maternal factors related to parenting practices, developmental expectations, and perceptions of child behavior problems. Journal of Genetic Psychology, 156(4):431–441, 1995.

Gallagher, JJ. The family as a focus for intervention. In Meisels, SJ, & Shonkoff, JP (Eds.), Handbook of Early Childhood Intervention. New York: Cambridge University Press, 1990, pp. 540–559.

Gallagher, J, Beckman, P, & Cross, A. Families of handicapped children: Sources of stress and its amelioration. Exceptional Children, 50:10–19, 1983.

Gilbert, LA. Men in Dual Career Families: Current Realities and Future Prospects. Hillsdale, NJ: Lawrence Erlbaum Associates, 1985.

Godley, SH, Fiedler, EM, & Funk, RR. Consumer satisfaction of parents and their children with child/adolescent mental health services. Evaluation and Program Planning, 21:31–45, 1998.

Goldberg, S, Morris, P, Simmons, JM, & Levison, J. Chronic illness in infancy and parenting stress: A comparison of three groups of parents. Journal of Pediatric Psychology, 15:347–358, 1990.

Goodnow, JJ. Parents' ideas, actions, and feelings: Models and methods from developmental and social psychology. Child Development, 59:296–320, 1988.

Green, JW. Cultural Awareness in the Human Services: Ethnicity and Social Services. Englewood Cliffs, NJ: Prentice-Hall, 1982, pp. 3–27.

Greenspan, SI, Wieder, S, Lieberman, A, Nover, R, Lourie, R, & Robinson, M (Eds.). Clinical Infant Reports: No. 3. Infants in Multi-risk Families: Case Studies in Preventive Intervention. New York: International Universities Press, 1987.

Greenspan, S. Comprehensive clinical approaches to infants and their families: Psychodynamic and developmental perspectives. In Meisels, SJ, & Shonkoff, JP (Eds.), Handbook of Early Childhood Intervention. New York: Cambridge University Press, 1990.

Gross, D, Conrad, B, Fogg, L, Willis, L, & Garvey, C. What does the NCATS (Nursing Child Assessment Teaching Scale) measure? Nursing Research, 42(5):260–265, 1993.

Haley, SM, & Baryza, MJ. A hierarchy of motor outcome assessment: Self-initiated movements through adaptive motor function. Infants and Young Children, 3:1–14, 1990.

Halfon, N, Inkelas, M, & Wood, D. Nonfinancial barriers to care for children and youth. Annual Review of Public Health, 16:447–472, 1995.

Halpern, R. Community-based early intervention. In Meisels, SJ, & Shonkoff, JP (Eds.), Handbook of Early Childhood Intervention. New York: Cambridge University Press, 1990, pp. 469–498.

Hamner, TJ, & Turner, PH. Parenting in Contemporary Society. Englewood Cliffs, NJ: Prentice-Hall, 1985.

Hanson, MJ. Ethnic, cultural, and language diversity in intervention settings. In Lynch, EW, & Hanson, MJ (Eds.), Developing Cross-cultural Competence: A Guide for Working with Young Children and Their Families. Baltimore: Paul H Brookes, 1992, pp. 1–18.

Harms, T, & Clifford, RM. Early Childhood Environment Rating Scale. New York: Teachers College Press, 1980.

Harris, SR. Efficacy of physical therapy in promoting family functioning and functional independence for children with cerebral palsy. Pediatric Physical Therapy, 2:160–164, 1990.

Hayden, LC, Schiller, M, Dickstein, S, Seifer, R, Sameroff, AJ, Miller, I, Keitner, G, & Rasmussen, S. Levels of family assessment: I. Family, marital, and parent-child interaction. Journal of Family Psychology, 12(1):7–22, 1998.

Heifitz, LJ. Integrating religious and secular perspectives in the design of disability services. Mental Retardation, 25:127–131, 1987.

Holden, GW, & Edwards, LA. Parental attitudes toward child rearing: Instruments, issues, and implications. Psychological Bulletin, 106: 29–58, 1989.

Hughes, DC, & Luft, HS. Managed Care and Children: An Overview. The Future of Children, 8(2):25–38, 1998.

Humphry, R. Early intervention and the influence of the occupational therapist on the parent-child relationship. American Journal of Occupational Therapy, 43:738–742, 1989.

Humphry, R, & Link, S. Preparation of occupational therapists to work in early intervention programs. American Journal of Occupational Therapy, 44(9):828–833, 1990.

Hunt, LM, Jordan, B, Irwin, S, & Browner, CH. Compliance and the patient's perspective: Controlling symptoms in everyday life. Culture, Medicine and Psychiatry, 13:315–334, 1989.

Hutcheson, JJ, Black, MM, Talley, M, Dubowitz, H, Howard, JB, Starr, RH, & Thompson, BS. Risk status and home intervention among children with failure-to-thrive: Follow-up at age 4. Journal of Pediatric Psychology, 22(5):651–668, 1997.

Individuals with Disabilities Act Amendments of 1997. Federal Register, Final Rules, April 1998. 34 CFR Part 303.

Kang, R, Barnard, K, Hammond, M, Oshio, S, Spencer, C, Thibodeau, B, & Williams, J. Preterm infant follow-up project: A multi-site field experiment of hospital and home intervention programs for mothers and preterm infants. Public Health Nursing, 12(3):171–180, 1995.

Kelley, MA, Pauer, TG, & Wimbush, DD. Determinants of disciplinary practices in low income black mothers. Child Development, 63: 573–582, 1992.

King, G, Law, M, King, S, & Rosenbaum, P. Parents' and service providers' perceptions of the family-centredness of children's rehabilitation services. Physical and Occupational Therapy in Pediatrics, 18(1):21–40, 1998.

King, S, Rosenbaum, P, & King, G. The Measures of Processes of Care (MPOC): A Means to Assess Family-Centered Behaviors of Health Care Providers. Neurodevelopmental Clinical Research Unit, McMaster University, Hamilton, Ontario, Canada, 1995.

Kjerland, L, & Kovach, J. Structure for Program Responsiveness to Parents. Eagan, MN: Project Dakota, 1987.

Kochanska, G. Maternal beliefs as long-term predictors of mother-child interaction and report. Child Development, 61(6):1934–1943, 1990.

Kochaska, G, Clark, LA, & Goodman, MS. Implications of mothers' personality for their parenting and their young children's developmental outcomes. Journal of Personality, 65(2):387–420, 1997.

Kochanska, G, Kuczynski, L, & Radke-Yarrow, M. Correspondence between mothers' self-reported and observed child-rearing practices. Child Development, 60:56–63, 1989.

Kolobe, THA. The relationship between maternal characteristics and the ability to follow through with home-based intervention program for her handicapped infant. South African Society of Physiotherapy Journal, 39:59–65, 1983.

Kolobe, THA. Family-focused early intervention. In Campbell, SK (Ed.), Pediatric Neurologic Physical Therapy, 2nd ed. New York: Churchill Livingstone, 1991, pp. 397–432.

Kolobe, THA. Working with families of children with disabilities. Pediatric Physical Therapy, 4:57–63, 1992.

Kuhlthau, K, Walker, D, Perrin, JM, Bauman, L, Gortmaker, SL, Newachek, PW, & Stein, REK. Assessing managed care for children with chronic conditions. Health Affairs, 17(4):42–52, 1998.

Landau-Stanton, J. Issues and methods of treatment for families in cultural transition. In Marian, MP (Ed.), The Social and Political Contexts of Family Therapy. Boston: Allyn & Bacon, 1990, pp. 251–275.

Law, M, Darrah, J, Pollock, N, King, G, Rosenbaum, P, Russell, D, Palisano, R, Hams, S, Armstrong, R, & Walt J. Family-centred functional therapy for children with cerebral palsy: An emerging practice model. Physical and Occupational Therapy in Pediatrics, 18(1):83–102, 1998.

Leviton, A, Mueller, M, & Kauffman, C. The family-centered consultation model: Practical application for professionals. Infants and Young Children, 4(3):1–8, 1992.

Lewis-Epstein, N. Determinants of regular source of care in black, Mexican, Puerto Rican, and non-Hispanic white populations. Medical Care, 29:543–557, 1991.

Lieu, TA, & Newman, TB. Issues in studying the effectiveness of health services for children. Health Services Research, 33(4):1041–1058, 1998.

Linder, TW. Transdisciplinary Play-based Assessment: A Functional Approach to Working with Young Children. Baltimore: Paul H Brookes, 1990.

Luster, T, Rhoades, K, & Haas, B. The relation between parental values and parenting behavior: A test of the Kohn hypothesis. Journal of Marriage and the Family, 51:139–147, 1989.

Lynch, EW. Developing cross-cultural competence. In Lynch, EW, & Hanson, MJ (Eds.), Developing Cross-cultural Competence: A Guide for Working with Young Children and their Families. Baltimore: Paul H Brookes, 1992, pp. 35–64.

McCubbin, HI, & Patterson, JM. Systematic Assessment of Family Stress, Resources and Coping. St. Paul: University of Minnesota, 1982, pp. 7–15.

McGoldrick, M, Pearce, J, & Giordano, J. Ethnicity and Family Therapy. New York: Guilford Press, 1982, pp. 3–30.

McGonigel, MJ, Kaufmann, RK, & Johnson, BH (Eds.). Recommended Practices for the Individualized Family Service Plan. Bethesda, MD: Association for the Care of Children's Health, 1991.

McHanahan, SS. Family structure and stress: A longitudinal comparison of two-parent and female-headed families. Journal of Marriage and the Family, 65:345–357, 1983.

Mead, M. Understanding cultural patterns. Nursing Outlook, 4:260–262, 1956.

Milner JS, & Crouch JL. Impact and detection of response distortions on parenting measures used to assess risk for child physical abuse. Journal of Personality Assessment, 69(3):633–650, 1997.

Minuchin, P. Relationships within the family: A systems perspective on development. In Hinde, RA, & Stevenson-Hinde, J (Eds.), Relationships Within Families: Mutual Influences. New York: Oxford University Press, 1988.

Minuchin, P. Families and individual development: Provocations from the field of family therapy. Child Development, 56:289–302, 1985.

Morris, TM. Culturally sensitive family assessment: An evaluation of the Family Assessment Device used with Hawaiian-American and Japanese-American families. Family Process, 29:105–116, 1990.

Morriset, CE, Barnard, KE, Greenberg, MT, Booth, CL, & Spieker, SJ. Environmental influences on early language development: The context of social risk. Development and Psychopathology, 2:127–149, 1990.

Moxley-Haegert, L, & Serbin, LA. Developmental education for parents of delayed infants: Effects on parental motivation and children's development. Child Development, 54:1324–1331, 1983.

National Center for Family-Centered Care. What is family-centered care? Bethesda, MD: Association for the Care of Children's Health, 1990.

Olson, DH: Circumplex model VII: Validation studies and FACES III. Family Process, 25:337–351, 1986.

O'Neil, M, Farel, A, & Palisano, R. Parents' perspectives of managed care: Implications for pediatric physical therapy. Pediatric Physical Therapy, 11:24–32, 1999.

Parker, SJ, Zahr, LK, Cole, JG, & Brecht, ML. Outcomes after developmental interventions in the neonatal intensive care unit for mothers of preterm infants with low socioeconomic status. Journal of Pediatrics, 120:780–785, 1992.

Patton, MQ. Qualitative Evaluation and Research Methods, 2nd ed. Newbury Park, CA: Sage, 1990, pp. 277–368.

Petersen, P, & Wikoff, RL. Home environment and adjustment in families with handicapped children: A canonical correlation study. Occupational Therapy Journal of Research, 7:67–82, 1987.

Phillips, WE. Stress and coping in the family of the child with cerebral palsy: The role of the physical therapist. Pediatric Physical Therapy, 2:166–168, 1990.

Power, TG, & Chapieski, ML. Childrearing and impulse controls in toddlers: A naturalistic observation. Developmental Psychology, 22:271–27, 1986.

Public Law 94-142, Education for All Handicapped Children Act, 1975.

Public Law 102-119, Individuals with Disabilities Education Amendments of 1991.

Ragozini, AS, Basham, RB, Crnic, KA, Greenberg, MT, & Robinson, NM. Effects of maternal age on parenting role. Developmental Psychology, 18:627–634, 1982.

Rainforth, B, & Salisbury, CL. Functional home programs: A model for therapists. Topics in Early Childhood Special Education, 7(4):33–45, 1988.

Ramey, CT, Bryant, DM, Wasik, BH, Sparling, JJ, Fendt, KH, & LaVange, LM. Infant health and development program for low birth weight, premature infants: Program elements, family participation, and child intelligence. Pediatrics, 89(3):454–465, 1992.

Rapport, MJ. Laws that shape therapy in educational environments. Physical and Occupational Therapy in Pediatrics, 15(2):5–32, 1995.

Rauh, VA, Wasserman, GA, & Brunelli, SA. Determinants of maternal child-rearing attitudes. Journal of the American Academy of Child and Adolescent Psychiatry, 29(3):375–381, 1990.

Realini, A, Kalet, A, & Sparling, J. Silence in the medical interaction: II. A means of encouraging patient participation in the interaction. Paper presented at the American Academy of Family Physicians 44th Annual Scientific Assembly, San Diego, CA, October 15–18, 1992.

Reid, RJ, Hurtado, MP, & Starfield, B. Managed care, primary care, and quality for children. Current Opinion in Pediatrics, 8:164–170, 1996.

Reiss, D. The Family's Construction of Reality. Cambridge, MA: Harvard University Press, 1981.

Research and Policy Committee of the Committee for Economic Development. Children in Need: Investment Strategies for the Educationally Disadvantaged. New York: Committee for Economic Development, 1987.

Rohner, RP. They love me, they love me not: A world-wide study of the effect of parental acceptance and rejection. New Haven, CT: HRAF Press, 1975.

Rosenbaum, P, King, S, Law, M, & Evans, J. Family-centred service: A conceptual framework and research review. Physical and Occupational Therapy in Pediatrics, 18(1):1–20, 1998.

Sameroff, AJ. Environmental context of child development. Journal of Pediatrics, 109:192–200, 1986.

Sameroff, AJ, & Fiese, BH. Transactional regulation and early intervention. In Meisels, SJ, & Shonkoff, JP (Eds.), Handbook of Early Childhood Intervention. New York: Cambridge University Press, 1990, pp. 119–149.

Shaefer, ES, & Bell, RQ. Development of a parental attitude research instrument. Child Development, 29:339–361, 1958.

Seifer, R, Schiller, M, Sameroff, AJ, Resnick, S, & Riordan, K. Attachment, maternal sensitivity, and temperament during the first year of life. Developmental Psychology, 32:12–25, 1995.

Seitz, V, & Provence, S. Caregiver-focused models of early intervention. In Meisels, SJ, & Shonkoff, JP (Eds.), Handbook of Early Childhood Intervention. New York: Cambridge University Press, 1990, pp. 400–427.

Shelton, TL, & Stepanek, JS. Family-centered care for children needing specialized health and developmental services, 3rd ed. Bethesda, MD: Association for the Care of Children's Health, 1994.

Sidel, R. Women and children first: Towards a US family policy. American Journal of Public Health, 82:664–665, 1992.

Sigel, IE. A conceptual analysis of beliefs. In Sigel, IE (Ed.), Parental Belief Systems: The Psychological Consequences for Children. Hillsdale, NJ: Erlbaum, 1985, pp. 345–371.

Simeonsson, RJ, & Bailey, DB. Family dimensions in early intervention. In Meisels, SJ, & Shonkoff, JP (Eds.), Handbook of Early Childhood Intervention. New York: Cambridge University Press, 1990, p. 428.

Simmons, RL, Beaman, J, Conger, RD, & Chao, W. Childhood experience, conceptions of parenting, and attitudes of spouse as determinants of parental behavior. Journal of Marriage and Family, 55:91–106, 1993.

Sitzia, J, & Wood, N. Patient satisfaction: A review of issues and concepts. Social Science and Medicine, 45(12):1829–1843, 1997.

Smith, S. Two-generation program models: A new intervention strategy. Social Policy Report, 5(1):1–4, 1991.

Sosa, R, Kennell, J, Klaus, M, Robertson, S, & Urrutia, J. The effect of a supportive companion on perinatal problems, length of labor, and mother-infant interaction. New England Journal of Medicine, 303:597–600, 1980.

Sparling, JW. The cultural definition of the family. Physical and Occupational Therapy in Pediatrics, 11(4):17–29, 1991a.

Sparling, JW. Brief report: Infantile autism: A prospective report from pregnancy to four years. Journal of Autism and Developmental Disabilities, 21(2):229–236, 1991b.

Sparling, JW. Embedding Family Information into an Entry-level Physical Therapy Curriculum. Chapel Hill, NC: Frank Porter Graham Child Development Center, 1992a.

Sparling, JW. Assessment of family resources and needs. In Wilhelm, IJ, (Ed.), Physical Therapy Assessment in Early Infancy. New York: Churchill Livingstone, 1992b, pp. 71–104.

Sparling, JW, Berger, B, & Biller, M. Fathers: Myth, reality and PL 99-457. Infants and Young Children, 4(3):9–19, 1992a.

Sparling, JW, Seeds, JW, & Farran, DC. The relationship of obstetrical ultrasound to parent and infant behavior. Obstetrics and Gynecology, 72:902–907, 1988.

Sparling, JW, & Sekerak, DK. Embedding the family perspective in an entry level physical therapy curriculum. Pediatric Physical Therapy, 4:116–122, 1992.

Stein, REK, & Jessop KD. Long-term mental health effects of a pediatric home care program. Pediatrics, *88*:490–496, 1991.

Stewart, MJ. Social support: Diverse theoretical perspectives. Social Science and Medicine, *28*:1275–1282, 1989.

Sullivan, HS. The Psychiatric Interview. New York: WW Norton, 1970.

Szilagyi, PG. Managed care for children: Effect of access to care and utilization of health services. Future of the Children, *8*(2):39–59, 1998.

Taft, R. Coping with unfamiliar cultures. In Warren, N (Ed.), Studies in Cross Cultural Psychology. San Diego, CA: Academic Press, 1977, pp. 121–153.

Tresserras, R, Canela, J, Alvarez, J, Sentis, J, & Salleras, L. Infant mortality, per capita income, and adult illiteracy: An ecological approach. American Journal of Public Health, *82*:435–437, 1992.

Turnbull, A, & Turnbull, H. Families, Professionals, and Exceptionality: A Special Partnership. Columbus, OH: Merrill, 1986.

U.S. Department of Health and Human Services. Healthy Children 2000: National Health Promotion and Disease Prevention Objectives Related to Mothers, Infants, Children, Adolescents, and Youth. Washington, DC: Public Health Service, 1990.

U.S. House of Representatives Select Committee on Children, Youth, and Families. U.S. Children and Their Families: Current Conditions and Recent Trends, 3rd ed. Washington, DC: U.S. Government Printing Office, 1989.

Viscardis, L. The family-centred approach to providing services: A parental perspective. Physical and Occupational Therapy in Pediatrics, *18*(1):41–53, 1998.

Vuchinich, S, & De Baryshe, B. Factor structure and predictive validity of questionnaire reports on family problem solving. Journal of Marriage and the Family, *59*(11):915–927, 1997.

Walsh, F. Conceptualizations of normal family functioning. In Walsh, F (Ed.), Normal Family Processes. New York: Guilford Press, 1982.

Whiting, BB, & Whiting, JWM. Children of six cultures: A psychocultural analysis. Cambridge, MA: Harvard University Press, 1975.

Whitman, TL, Borkowski, JG, Schellenbach, CJ, & Nath, PS. Predicting and understanding developmental delay of children of adolescent mothers: A multidimensional approach. American Journal of Mental Deficiency, *92*:40–56, 1987.

Wilhelm, IJ (Ed.). Physical Therapy Assessment in Early Infancy. New York: Churchill Livingstone, 1992.

Williams, B. Patient satisfaction: A valid concept? Social Science and Medicine, *38*(4):509–516, 1994.

Winton, PJ, & Bailey, DB. The family-focused interview: A collaborative mechanism for family assessment and goal-setting. Journal of the Division of Early Childhood, *12*:195–207, 1988.

Winton, PJ, & Blow, C. Family Interview Performance Rating Scale. Chapel Hill, NC: Frank Porter Graham Child Development Center, 1991.

Wolery, M, & Dyk, L. Arena assessment: Description and preliminary social validity data. The Association for Persons with Severe Handicaps, *9*:231–235, 1984.

Zuniga, M. Families with Latino Roots. In Lynch, EW, & Hanson, MJ (Eds.), Developing Cross-Cultural Competence: A Guide for Working with Young Children and Their Families. Baltimore: Paul H Brookes, 1992, pp. 151–179.

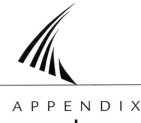

APPENDIX

I

Measures of Family Support and Caregiving

The *Inventory of Socially Supportive Behaviors* (ISSB) is a 40-item measure developed by Berrera (1981). Although this assessment was developed for use with pregnant adolescents, it is applicable to other populations. The assessment describes the supportive behavior, requests how often the behavior has been performed for the individual in the last week, and then asks who provided the support. By using this assessment, the extent of support for the individual or family can be readily determined.

The *Family Routines Inventory* (Gallagher et al., 1983) can be conducted as a family interview. Family members can score it separately, or it can be used as the focus of a family interview. Determining caregivers' perceptions of family roles and responsibilities relates directly to the balance of work assumed by family members and to the perceived dimensions of caregiving in the family.

The *Family Needs Survey* (Bailey & Simeonsson, 1988) includes eight items related to social support. In assessing 34 two-parent families receiving home-based intervention services with this survey, the authors found that 74% of the mothers and 50% of the fathers wanted information about other parents who had a child with a similar condition to their child. At times, a brief assessment such as this may help the therapist to clarify unique family needs or the readiness for interaction of individual family members.

The *Home Observation for Measurement of the Environment (HOME)* (Caldwell & Bradley, 1980) measures the quantity and quality of stimulation in the home environment. The 45 binary items on the HOME are organized into six subscales, which are scored using semistructured interviews and observa-

tions of mother-child interactions during a home visit. The HOME is widely used in research and interventions. It has sound psychometric properties.

The *Measures of Processes of Care (MPOC)* (King et al., 1995) is a 56-item self-report measure designed to examine the way care is delivered and the influence of service delivery to children with disabilities and their families. The MPOC consists of five subscales that assess the following areas: enabling and partnership, providing general information, providing specific information, coordinated and comprehensive care for the child and family, and respectful and supportive care. Extensive testing was done in the development of the measure.

MEASURES OF PARENTING AND CHILDREARING

The *Adult-Adolescent Parenting Inventory (AAPI)* developed by Bavolek (1984) is a 32-item questionnaire designed to assess high-risk parenting and childrearing attitudes among adults and adolescents. The AAPI consist of four subscales that assess constructs associated with maladaptive parenting: (1) inappropriate expectations, (2) lack of empathy, (3) belief in corporal punishment, and (4) reversing parent-child family roles. The inventory is a self-report and takes approximately 20 minutes to complete. A table of norms is available in the manual and may be used for scoring. The AAPI is available in both English and Spanish.

The *Perceptions of Parental Role Scales (PPRS)* is a 78-item questionnaire that is used to assess 13 parental areas in three domains of caregiving: teaching, providing for basic needs, and family as an interface with society. Subscales within the teaching domain are (1) cognitive development, (2) social skills, (3) handling of emotions, (4) physical health, (5) norms and social values, (6) personal hygiene, and (7) survival skills. In the basic needs domain, subscales are (1) health care, food, clothing, and shelter; (2) child's emotional needs; and (3) child care. The family as an interface with society domain consists of two subscales: (1) social institutions and (2) the family unit itself. The PPRS takes approximately 10 minutes to complete. A high score on each scale reflects greater levels of perceived responsibility. Although the PPRS was developed from responses of white middle-class working parents employed in a university setting and therefore is not representative of the perceptions of individuals from different social, ethnic, or cultural backgrounds, the subscales tap attributes that are associated with culture.

The *Parenting Behavior Checklist (PBC)* (Fox, 1994) is a 100-item Likert-type scale that assesses behaviors and developmental expectations of parents of young infants (ages 1 to 4 months). The PBC consists of three subscales, which measure parents' developmental expectations (expectation factor), parents' discipline strategies (discipline factor), and how parents promote their children's psychologic growth (the nurturing factor). Rating scales for each item are used with A = always/almost always, F = frequently, S = sometimes, and N = never/almost never. The PBC demonstrates sound psychometric properties. Another strength of the PBC is that items reflect descriptions of actual parenting behaviors as opposed to parenting attitudes.

The *Nursing Child Assessment Feeding Scale (NCAFS)* and *Nursing Child Assessment Teaching Scale (NCATS)* (Barnard, 1978a, 1978b) have been used widely in research to measure parent-child interactions (Barnard & Kelly, 1990; Morriset, 1990). The scales were developed based on a model of parent-child reciprocity and mutual adaptation (Barnard Child Health Assessment Interaction Model and Sameroff Transactional Child Development Model). The Barnard Child Health Assessment Interaction Model focuses on three factors: the caregiver, the child, and the environment. The model is based on the assumption that caregivers and infants have certain responsibilities to keep interaction going in a reciprocal manner, with patterns of mutual adaptations.

The NCATS is a binary scale consisting of 73 items designed to assess interactions between the caregiver and child. The parent subscales measure parent-child interaction in four conceptual domains: (1) sensitivity to a child's cues, (2) response to a child's distress, (3) socioemotional growth-fostering behavior, and (4) cognitive growth-fostering behavior. Two domains are also assessed in the child's subscales: the child's clarity of cues and responsiveness to the mother. The NCATS and NCAFS have sound psychometric properties and have been used extensively in research and practice. The scales also have demonstrated predictive validity for developmental outcomes in children through preschool age. An NCATS normative sample data bank of white, black, and Hispanic subjects is available for comparisons of optimal interaction scores. To use the scales for research purposes, certification by NCATS faculty at the University of Washington School of Nursing is required. Training before reliability certification is provided by an NCATS instructor or the NCATS faculty at the University of Washington.

CHAPTER 32

The Educational Environment

SUSAN K. EFFGEN, PT, PhD

Almost from the start of physical therapy in the United States, physical therapists have worked in educational environments. The Civil Rights Movement of the 1960s and federal legislation of the 1970s, however, marked the beginning of major changes in services for all children with special needs in educational environments. In this chapter the history of the delivery of physical therapy in educational environments is reviewed along with a discussion of federal legislation and significant court cases that have changed how children with special needs are educated and receive physical therapy. The focus is on key issues related to physical therapy in educational environments such as inclusive education, models of team interaction, service delivery models, the individualized educational plan (IEP), the individualized family service plan (IFSP), and intervention strategies. Management issues and critical issues facing school-based physical therapists are also discussed.

BACKGROUND

Although the history of physical therapy in the United States is traced to "reconstruction aides" serving the injured of World War I, it can also be traced to the service of "crippled children," especially those with poliomyelitis. These children were served in hospitals and special settings. Special schools and classes began to appear early in the twentieth century in major cities. The children had a variety of diagnoses, including poliomyelitis and spastic paralysis (Cable et al., 1938; Givins, 1938), cardiac disorders, "obstetrical arms," bone and joint tuberculosis, clubfeet, and osteomyelitis (Batten, 1933; Cable et al., 1938; Mulcahey, 1936). By the 1930s, numerous articles had been published describing the delivery of physical therapy in these special schools (Batten, 1933; Mulcahey, 1936; Sever, 1938; Vacha, 1933).

The role of physical therapy in schools has continued to expand throughout the century. Epidemics of poliomyelitis increased the need for special schools and physical therapists. After the vaccine for poliomyelitis was developed in the 1950s, the need for special schools was temporarily reduced, until public awareness increased regarding of the needs of other children with disabilities.

Most children in special schools had normal or near-normal intelligence. Many schools required children to be toilet trained, and some required children to walk independently. This trend to serve only those with physical disabilities and normal intelligence continued in many areas of the United States until schools were federally mandated in 1975 to serve all children with disabilities by the enactment of Public Law (PL) 94-142, the Education for All Handicapped Children Act.

FEDERAL LEGISLATION AND LITIGATION

A number of social and political events paved the way for the enactment of PL 94-142, the Education for All Handicapped Children Act. In 1954, the historic Supreme Court decision regarding segregated schools, *Brown v. Board of Education of Topeka,* was decided. Separate-but-equal schools were found inherently unequal. This Supreme Court decision was to end the segregated education of African-American children. The principles and grounds of this case could apply to segregated schools for those with disabilities. The call for social equality had begun and would eventually include those with disabilities. President Kennedy's personal experience helped lead him to establish a President's Panel on Mental Retardation in 1961. Television documentaries exposed institutions in New York, and Blatt and Kaplan's book, *Christmas in Purgatory: A Photographic Essay on Mental Retardation* (1966), raised national concern for the care and treatment of individuals with disabilities. Leaders such as Wolfensberger (1971) were influential proponents of deinstitutionalization and normalization. Cruickshank (1980, p. 65) noted that "as is usually the case with major changes in social policy, the normalization trend is not based on empirical data showing greater effectiveness or efficiency of the changes proposed by its advocates." The normalization trend was, rather, an emphasis on civil rights of individuals, a prevailing antiinstitutional attitude—especially governmental institutions—and a commitment "to the democratic, the individualistic, and the humanitarian" (Cruickshank, 1980, pp. 65–66). The federal Developmental Disabilities Assistance and Bill of Rights Act of 1975 (PL 94-103) included a provision that states had to develop and incorporate a "deinstitutionalization and institutional reform plan" (Braddock, 1987, p. 71). Advocacy groups had gained power, and they used the judicial system to win their rights.

The *Pennsylvania Association for Retarded Citizens (PARC) v. Commonwealth of Pennsylvania* (1971) was the historic, decisive court case establishing the uncompromising right to an education for all children with disabilities. This was a class-action suit filed on behalf of 14 specifically named children and all other children who were in a similar "class" to those with trainable mental retardation. In Pennsylvania, these children were excluded from public school if a psychologist or mental health professional certified that a child could no longer profit from attendance at school. The local school board could refuse to accept or retain a child who had not reached the mental age of 5 years. Children who were classified as trainable mentally retarded, therefore, were unable to get a public education in Pennsylvania. The court sided with the children.

In *PARC v. Commonwealth of Pennsylvania,* the court found that all children, between 6 and 21 years of age, regardless of degree of disability, were to be given a "free and appropriate public education (FAPE)." Children with disabilities were to be educated with children without disabilities in the least restrictive environment (LRE). The educational system was ordered to stop applying exclusionary laws; parents were to become involved in the child's program; and reevaluations were to be done. This landmark court case established many important principles that were later incorporated into the Education for All Handicapped Children Act.

Simultaneous with PARC case other important court cases were being decided. *Mills v. Board of Education of the District of Columbia* (1972) was filed on behalf of all children excluded by public schools for a disability of any kind, including behavioral problems. The major result of this case was that all children, no matter how severe their mental retardation, behavioral problem, or disability, were educable and must be provided for suitably by the public school system. Related services, including physical therapy, were to be part of their educational program.

In *Maryland Association for Retarded Citizens v. Maryland* (1972) it was ruled that children have the right to tuition subsidies, the right to transportation, and the right to be educated with children who are not disabled. These cases and others across the nation began to establish the right of all children to a "free and appropriate public education." It was in this climate that PL 94-142 was enacted.

PL 94-142: EDUCATION FOR ALL HANDICAPPED CHILDREN ACT

Provisions

On November 29, 1975, PL 94-142, the Education for All Handicapped Children Act, was passed by the U.S. Congress. The law included the elements won in individual court cases across the nation and provided for a "free and appropriate public education" for all children with disabilities from ages 6 to 21 years (age 5 years if this is the age at which a state begins to provide public education to children without disabilities). The major provisions of PL 94-142 concern the concepts of zero reject, education in the least restrictive environment, right to due process, nondiscriminatory evaluation, individualized educational plan, parent participation, and the right to related services, which include physical therapy.

Zero Reject

All children are to receive an education, including children with severe or profound disabilities. These children were initially to receive priority for service because they were probably not receiving appropriate service at that time.

Least Restrictive Environment

Public agencies are to ensure the following:

To the maximum extent appropriate, children with disabilities, including children in public or private institutions or other care facilities, are educated with children who are not disabled, and special classes, separate schooling, or other removal of children with disabilities from the regular educational environment occurs only when the nature or severity of the disability of a child is such that education in regular classes with the use of supplementary aids and services cannot be achieved satisfactorily.

PL 105-17, 111 Stat. 61, Part B, Sec. 612, (a) (5) (A)

Right to Due Process

The law provides parents with numerous rights. Parents have the right to an impartial hearing, the right to be represented by counsel, and the right to a verbatim transcript of a hearing and written findings. They can appeal and get an independent evaluation. Later, under PL 99-372, the Handicapped Children's Protection Act [1986, 20 USC 1415 (e) (4), (f)], parents would be able to get reimbursed for legal fees if they prevailed in a court case.

Nondiscriminatory Evaluation

Several court cases had noted the discriminatory nature of the testing and placement procedures used in many school systems. Nondiscriminatory tests were to be used, and no one test could be the sole criterion used for placement. Nondiscriminatory testing is critical in the cognitive and language domain; however, physical therapists should also be careful to determine that their tests are not biased. When possible, standardized tests that have norms for different racial and cultural groups should be used.

Individualized Educational Plan

Every child receiving special education must have an IEP. This is the comprehensive plan outlining the specific special educational and related services the child is to receive. It includes annual goals and objectives. The IEP is developed annually at an IEP meeting.

Parent Participation

Active participation of parents is encouraged under PL 94-142. Parents are the individuals responsible for the continuity of services for their child and should be the child's best advocates. Parents are major decision makers in the development of the IEP: they must give permission for an evaluation, they can restrict the release of information, they have access to their child's records, and they can request due process hearings.

Related Services

Related services, such as transportation, speech pathology, audiology, psychologic services, physical therapy, occupational therapy, recreation, and medical and counseling services, are to be provided "as may be required to assist a handicapped child to benefit from special education" (PL 99-142, 89 Stat. 775). This quotation from the law has been interpreted in many different ways. Physical therapy "to assist a handicapped child to benefit from special education" in some school systems is limited to only those activities that help the child write or sit properly in class. Other school systems more appropriately interpret the law to mean physical therapy that can help the child explore the environment, perform activities of daily living, improve function in school, prepare for vocational training, and improve physical fitness so as to be better prepared to learn and prepare for life after school.

PL 99-457: EDUCATION OF THE HANDICAPPED ACT AMENDMENTS OF 1986; PL 102-119: INDIVIDUALS WITH DISABILITIES EDUCATION ACT AMENDMENTS OF 1991; PL 105-17: INDIVIDUALS WITH DISABILITIES EDUCATION ACT AMENDMENTS OF 1997

PL 94-142 must be reauthorized by Congress at set intervals. PL 99-457, the Education of the Handicapped Act Amendments of 1986, is critical not only because of the reauthorization of PL 94-142, but because this act extended services to infants, toddlers, and preschoolers with disabilities and their families. On October 7, 1991, PL 94-142 and PL 99-457 were reauthorized and amended as PL 102-119, the Individuals with Disabilities Education Act Amendments of 1991, or IDEA. The most recent reauthorization, PL 105-17, was signed into law on June 4, 1997. The key elements of this reauthorization, really a refinement and reorganization of the previous amendments, consists of four parts.

Part A: General Provisions

Congress found that "disability is a natural part of the human experience and in no way diminishes the right of individuals to participate in or contribute to society. Improving educational results for children with disabilities is an essential element of our national policy of ensuring equality of opportunity, full participation, independent living, and economic self-sufficiency for individuals with disabilities" [PL 105-17, 111 Stat. 38, Part A, Sec. 601 (c)]. The recognition that education is not merely the three "R's," but that it is intended to prepare children for independent living and self-sufficiency, is critical for therapists. This expands what goals and objectives could be considered "educationally relevant."

Part B: Assistance for Education of All Children with Disabilities

Part B outlines the right to a free appropriate public education to all children ages 3 to 21 years. Children 3 to 5 and 18 to 21 years of age might not be served if inconsistent with state law. States are mandated to identify, locate, and evaluate all children with disabilities. Children eligible for special education and related services are those having one or more of the disabilities listed in Box 32-1.

Children 3 to 5 years of age are to have IEPs, as are school-age children; however, the 1991 reauthorization, PL 102-119, allowed states the option of using IFSPs for preschool-age children. The use of IFSPs is supported by the Council for Exceptional Children, Division of Early Childhood Education (1990), and the American Physical Therapy Association, Section on Pediatrics (1991). Many professionals believe the problems of preschoolers and their families are more similar to those of infants and toddlers than they are to those of school-age children.

Least Restrictive Environment

The education of children with disabilities in the LRE to the maximum extent appropriate continues to be an important element of IDEA. Funding mechanisms must support rather than hinder use of the LRE. Children are not merely to be "placed" in general education, but they are to fully participate and have goals related to their curricular and social advancement.

Transition

Because transition planning to the next highest level of services is often neglected, it has been more specifically addressed in PL 105-17. Transition plans must be included in the IFSP and IEP. Consideration must be given to transition from early intervention to preschool, from preschool to school, at critical points during school, and especially from age 14 years to exit from school. Physical therapists and other related service personnel are to be involved in the transition planning for postschool activities, as appropriate.

Assistive Technology

Assistive technology devices and assistive technology services allow the child to fully benefit from her or his educational environment.

An assistive technology device means any item, piece of equipment, or product system whether acquired commercially off the shelf, modified, or customized, that is used to increase, maintain, or improve the functional capabilities of a child with a disability...assistive technology service means any service that directly assists a child with a disability in the selection, acquisition, or use of an assistive technology device.

PL 105-17, 111 Stat. 42, Part A, Sec. 602

BOX 32-1. Federal Definitions of Children with Disabilities

Autism: A developmental disability significantly affecting verbal and nonverbal communication and social interaction, generally evident before age 3, that adversely affects a child's educational performance. Other characteristics often associated with autism are engagement in repetitive activities and stereotyped movements, resistance to environmental change, change in daily routines, and unusual responses to sensory experiences. The term does not apply if a child's educational performance is adversely affected primarily because the child has a serious emotional disturbance.

Deaf-blindness: Concomitant hearing and visual impairments, the combination of which causes such severe communication and other developmental and educational problems that they cannot be accommodated in special education programs solely for children with deafness or children with blindness.

Deafness: A hearing impairment that is so severe that the child is impaired in processing linguistic information through hearing, with or without amplification, that adversely affects a child's educational performance.

Developmental delay: "The term *child with a disability* for a child aged 3 through 9 may, at the discretion of the State and local educational agency, include a child . . . experiencing developmental delays, as defined by the State and as measured by appropriate diagnostic instruments and procedures, in one or more of the following areas: physical development, cognitive development, communication development, social or emotional development, or adaptive development, and who, for that reason, need special education and related services" [PL 105-17, 111 Stat. 43, Sec. 602 (3) (B)].

Hearing impairment: An impairment in hearing, whether permanent or fluctuating, that adversely affects a child's educational performance but that is not included under the definition of deafness.

Mental retardation: Significantly subaverage general intellectual functioning existing concurrently with deficits in adaptive behavior and manifested during the developmental period that adversely affects a child's educational performance.

Multiple disabilities: Concomitant impairments (e.g., mental retardation–blindness, mental retardation–orthopedic impairment) the combination of which causes such severe educational problems that they cannot be accommodated in special education programs solely for one of the impairments. The term does not include deaf-blindness.

Orthopedic impairment: A severe orthopedic impairment that adversely affects a child's educational performance. The term includes impairments caused by congenital anomaly (e.g., clubfoot, absence of some member), impairments caused by disease (e.g., poliomyelitis, bone tuberculosis), and impairments from other causes (e.g., cerebral palsy, amputations, and fractures or burns that cause contractures).

Other health impairment: Having limited strength, vitality, or alertness, because of chronic or acute health problems (e.g., heart condition, tuberculosis, rheumatic fever, nephritis, asthma, sickle cell anemia, hemophilia, epilepsy, lead poisoning, leukemia, diabetes), that adversely affects a child's educational performance.

Serious emotional disturbance: A condition exhibiting one or more of the following characteristics over a long period of time and to a marked degree that adversely affects a child's educational performance: (1) an inability to learn that cannot be explained by intellectual, sensory, or health factors; (2) an inability to build or maintain satisfactory interpersonal relationships with peers and teachers; (3) inappropriate types of behavior or feelings under normal circumstances; (4) a general pervasive mood of unhappiness or depression; or (5) a tendency to develop physical symptoms or fears associated with personal or school problems. The term includes schizophrenia. The term does not apply to children who are socially maladjusted, unless it is determined that they have a serious emotional disturbance.

Specific learning disability: A disorder in one or more of the basic psychologic processes involved in understanding or in using language, spoken or written, that may manifest as an imperfect ability to listen, think, speak, read, write, spell, or do mathematical calculations. The term includes such conditions as perceptual disabilities, brain injury, minimal brain dysfunction, dyslexia, and developmental aphasia. The term does not apply to children who have learning problems that are primarily the result of visual, hearing, or motor disabilities; of mental retardation; of emotional disturbance; or of environmental, cultural, or economic disadvantage.

Speech and language impairment: A communication disorder such as stuttering, impaired articulation, a language impairment, or a voice impairment that adversely affects a child's educational performance.

Traumatic brain injury: An acquired injury to the brain caused by an external physical force, resulting in total or partial functional disability or psychosocial impairment, or both, that adversely affects a child's educational performance. The term applies to open- or closed-head injuries resulting in impairments in one or more areas, such as cognition; language; memory; attention; reasoning; abstract thinking; judgment; problem solving; sensory, perceptual, and motor abilities; psychosocial behavior; physical functions; information processing; and speech. The term does not apply to brain injuries that are congenital or degenerative or brain injuries induced by birth trauma.

Visual impairment including blindness: An impairment in vision that, even with correction, adversely affects a child's educational performance. The term includes both partial sight and blindness. (From *Federal Register,* September 29, 1992, pp. 44801–44802.)

The assistive technology services include evaluation, selection, purchasing, and coordination with education and rehabilitation plans and programs. This is an important area for physical therapists, who frequently provide assistive devices to minimize disability and encourage function. Therapists adapt seating so children can function better and safely in the classroom. They assist other team members in devising the most functional communication systems along with providing access to switching devices and computers. Ambulation devices (e.g., walkers, crutches, and canes) are frequently necessary to allow the child to walk throughout the school. Power mobility devices allow the child with severe impairments and functional limitations to independently access the school building and grounds and thereby minimize disability. The extent of assistive technology services and the purchasing of devices vary among school systems. For additional information, see Chapter 24 on assistive technology.

Part C: Infants and Toddlers with Disabilities

Part C outlines the policy for assistance to states to

(1) develop and implement a statewide, comprehensive, coordinated, multidisciplinary, interagency system that provides early intervention services for infants and toddlers with disabilities and their families;
(2) facilitate the coordination of payment for early intervention services from federal, state, local, and private sources (including public and private insurance coverage);
(3) enhance their capacity to provide quality early intervention services and expand and improve existing early intervention services being provided to infants and toddlers with disabilities and their families; and
(4) encourage States to expand opportunities for children under 3 years of age who would be at risk of having substantial developmental delay if they did not receive early intervention services.

PL 105-17, 111 Stat. 135, Part C, Sec. 631

Infants and toddlers with disabilities are those under age 3 years or 36 months "who would be at risk of experiencing a substantial developmental delay if early intervention services were not provided" [PL 105-17, 111 Stat. 106, Part C, Sec. 632 (1)]. Early intervention services are developmental services provided under public supervision and "at no cost except where federal or state law provided for a system of payments" [PL 105-17, 111 Stat. 107, Part C, Sec. 632 (4) (B)]. Intervention is not, however, without limits, and the extent of services varies from state to state. Early intervention services and providers are listed in Box 32-2.

> **BOX 32–2. Early Intervention Services and Providers**
>
> Early Intervention Services:
>   (i)   family training, counseling, and home visits;
>   (ii) special instruction;
>   (iii) speech-language pathology and audiology services;
>   (iv) occupational therapy;
>   (v)   physical therapy;
>   (vi) psychologic services;
>   (vii) service coordination services;
>   (viii) medical services only for diagnostic or evaluation purposes;
>   (ix) early identification, screening, and assessment services;
>   (x)   health services necessary to enable the infant or toddler to benefit from the other early intervention services;
>   (xi) social work services;
>   (xii) vision services;
>   (xiii) assistive technology devices and assistive technology services; and
>   (xiv) transportation and related costs that are necessary to enable an infant or toddler and the infant's or toddler's family to receive another service.
>
> Qualified service providers include:
>   (i)   special educators;
>   (ii) speech-language pathologists and audiologists;
>   (iii) occupational therapists;
>   (iv) physical therapists;
>   (v)   psychologists;
>   (vi) social workers;
>   (vii) nurses;
>   (viii) nutritionists;
>   (ix) family therapists;
>   (x)   orientation and mobility specialists; and
>   (xi) pediatricians and other physicians.

From PL 105-17, 111 Stat. 107, Part C, Sec. 632 (4) (E) & (F).

Early intervention services "are designed to meet the developmental needs of the infant or toddler with a disability in any one or more of the following areas—...physical development...cognivitive development...communication development...social or emotional development; or...adaptive development" [PL 105-17, 111 Stat. 107, Part C, Sec. 632 (4) (C)]. The amount of developmental delay or impairment required to receive services is determined by each state.

The law describes the details of comprehensive early intervention services. Each child must have a timely, comprehensive, multidisciplinary evaluation of his or her functioning and a family-directed identification of the needs of each family to appropriately assist in the development of the infant or toddler. A written IFSP must be developed by the multidisciplinary team, including the parent or guardian. The specifics of the IFSP and other service delivery issues are discussed under Program Development later in this chapter.

Section 504 of the Rehabilitation Act

Section 504 of the Rehabilitation Act of 1973 (PL 93-112) is a broad antidiscrimination statute designed to ensure that federal funding recipients—including schools—treat people with disabilities the same as nondisabled people (Discipline Under Section 504, 1996). It has been used to broaden a student's eligibility for related services in school. Educational agencies that receive federal funds are not allowed to exclude qualified individuals with disabilities from participation in any program offered by the agency. The definition of "qualified handicapped person" under Section 504 is broader than it is in IDEA. Under Section 504,

"handicapped persons means any person who (i) has a physical or mental impairment which substantially limits one or more major life activities. ... Major life activities means functions such as caring for one's self, performing manual tasks, walking, seeing, hearing, speaking, breathing, learning, and working."

Federal Register, Sec. 1043 (j), 1988.

Thus it is possible that a child who does not require special education under the accepted definitions of disabilities, but who is a "qualified handicapped person," might be able to receive all the aid and services necessary to receive a free and appropriate public education (National Information Center for Children and Youth with Disabilities, 1991).

PL 101-336: AMERICANS WITH DISABILITIES ACT

The Americans with Disabilities Act (ADA) (PL 101-336) was signed into law on July 26, 1990. It "extends to individuals with disabilities comprehensive civil rights protection similar to those provided to persons on the basis of race, sex, national origin, and religion under the Civil Rights Act of 1964" (*Federal Register,* July 26, 1991, p. 3540). The regulations cover employment; public service, including public transportation, public accommodations, and telecommunications; and miscellaneous provisions. Although the law is not specific in reference to issues related to children in school, its provisions assist children with disabilities, especially those in day care centers and transition to employment (Pax Lowes & Effgen, 1996). Public buildings, including schools, must be accessible, and children should be able to use public transportation to get to school, work, and

social activities. Children with disabilities should expect to use the skills learned at school in an accessible workplace. The Americans with Disabilities Act is discussed in Chapter 34.

CASE LAW

A law as comprehensive and complex as IDEA was bound to lead to some controversy. All possible situations could not be anticipated, and some issues were expected to be resolved by the courts. As a result, a number of significant court cases have helped define the scope of the law.

Related Services

Tatro v. Texas (1980) was one of the early major cases involving PL 94-142. Amber Tatro had spina bifida and required clean intermittent catheterization several times during the school day. Amber's parents wanted assistance with catheterization at school. The school officials refused, saying catheterization was a medical procedure and Amber could not attend school unless her parents handled the procedure. The parents then initiated what turned out to be a 10-year legal battle. During the legal process, they were told that although catheterization was necessary to sustain Amber's life, it was not necessary to benefit from education; the school system, therefore, was not obligated to provide the service. After a complicated course though the court system, the case was heard by the U.S. Supreme Court. Amber attempted to attend the Supreme Court proceedings, only to discover that the Supreme Court was not readily accessible.

The Supreme Court ruled that clean intermittent catheterization was a related service that enabled the child to benefit from special education:

A service that enables a handicapped child to remain at school during the day is an important means of providing students with the meaningful access to education that Congress envisioned. The Act makes specific provision for services, like transportation, for example, that do no more than enable a child to be physically present in class.

Martin, 1991, p. 45; *Tatro v. Texas,* 1980, at 891.

This case led to the "bright-line" physician-nonphysician rule that the services of a physician (other than for diagnostic and evaluation purposes) need not be provided by the school system, but that services that can be given by a nurse or qualified layman must be provided by the school. This case is important to physical therapists because the realm of related services was expanded, as was the meaning of "required to benefit from special education."

More recent court cases regarding related services have involved children who are medically fragile and require extensive services of a nurse and others. Some states advocate the use of an extent/nature test. In the extent/nature test, decision making focuses on the individual case and considers the complexity and need for services. The decision of the U.S. Supreme Court in *Cedar Rapids Community School District v. Garret F.,* 25 IDELR 439, will provide major direction for the educational provision of related services to children with complex health care needs.

Best Possible Education

Rowley v. Board of Education of Hendrick Hudson Central School District (1982) involved Amy Rowley, who was deaf. She had a special tutor, her teachers were trained in basic sign language, and she was provided with a sound amplifier. After experimenting with an interpreter in general education class, the school system decided she did not need the service. Her parents believed she needed the interpreter and went through due process to continue the interpreter. A district court held that Amy was not receiving a free and appropriate public education because she did not have "an opportunity to achieve her full potential commensurate with the opportunity provided to other children." The school system appealed, and the case eventually went to the U.S. Supreme Court. The 1982 Supreme Court decision held that Congress did not intend to give children with disabilities a right to the best possible education (i.e., education that would "maximize their potential"); it rejected the standard used by the lower courts that children with disabilities are entitled to an educational opportunity "commensurate with the education available to nonhandicapped children" and set two standards, namely, that a state is required to provide meaningful access to an education for each child with a disability and that sufficient supportive and related services must be provided to permit the child to benefit educationally from special education instruction.

When the Supreme Court applied these standards in *Rowley* it found that Amy did not need interpreter services because she was making "exemplary progress in the regular education system" with the help of the extensive special services. The Supreme Court was careful to point out that merely passing from grade to grade does not mean a child's education is appropriate.

The *Rowley* decision has had a significant impact on the provision of related services, including physical therapy. Unfortunately, in some school systems the *Rowley* decision has been used to limit the amount of physical therapy provided on the premise that schools are not obligated to provide the "best services." What must be remembered is that Amy was receiving extensive services and was making "exemplary progress in the regular education system." Therapists must recognize that "exemplary progress" may be a reason to terminate physical therapy unless significant educational need for physical therapy can be substantiated.

Extended School Year

As children with special needs began to benefit from 9-month educational programs, some parents realized that their children's skills were regressing during the summer and that it took several months to regain those skills when the children returned to class in the fall. Because the U.S. Congress had realized that more than the traditional 12 years of schooling might be necessary for children with disabilities to reach their potential, perhaps it could be inferred that if a child regressed during the summer, extended school year services might be necessary (Martin, 1991).

Several court cases addressed this issue. In both *Battle v. Commonwealth of Pennsylvania* (1981) and *Georgia Association of Retarded Citizens v. McDaniel* (1981), parents sought to extend the school year. In Pennsylvania, it was found that the state's policy of defining a school year as 180 days could not be used to prevent the provision of an extended school year. In Georgia, the court ruled that an extended school year must be based on individual cases. The child must show significant regression, the extended year must be part of the IEP, and an extended year does not mean 5 days a week for 52 weeks but must be based on a program to attain goals.

Eligibility for extended school year services is now based on several criteria. These include "individual need, nature and severity of the disability, educational benefit, regression and recoupment, self-sufficiency and independence, and failing to meet short-term goals and objectives" (Rapport & Thomas, 1993, p. 16). The possibility of receiving services for the entire year has many implications for physical therapy. The children most likely to require extended school year services are usually those with the most serious disabilities, often requiring physical therapy. One criterion used to qualify for extended school year services is documentation of regression during vacation and the length of time it takes to recoup or relearn former skills. It is therefore vital for physical therapists to do an examination and evaluation before and after school breaks. Documentation of regression, especially during short breaks, might enable a child to receive physical therapy during the summer. Using the child's status at the end of the summer as the basis for extended school year physical therapy services might be confounded if parents obtain private physical therapy during the summer and regression is prevented.

An ethical dilemma can arise for some physical therapists over the extended school year issue. Some school therapists provide private physical therapy during the summer and might prefer that the school system not provide the service. Others might not want the obligation of having to provide services during the summer, either through the school or privately. Therapists must be careful to recognize this potential conflict of interest.

Least Restrictive Environment

Not only has the issue of LRE or inclusion generated much discussion, it has also generated many due process hearings and lawsuits. The outcomes have been mixed. During the early 1990s, the party seeking inclusion, usually the parent, prevailed in a series of court cases, the most noted being *Oberti* (3d Cir. 1993) and *Daniel R.R.* (5th Cir. 1989) (Zirkel, 1996). Later cases ruled against inclusive, general education placements as the LRE for students who were past elementary school age and had severe disabilities (Special Educator, 1996). A rational approach must prevail in issues regarding inclusion. There must be a continuum of locations and types of services available to the child that can and should change over time.

EDUCATIONAL MILIEU

Physical therapists are not new to special educational environments but have only recently begun serving children with disabilities in the general education setting. Educational administrators and teachers may not be familiar with the role of physical therapy, just as the physical therapist may not be familiar with the educational milieu. Hence, there is the need for open communication and collaboration. Physical therapists must take the time to develop relationships and to understand the written and unwritten rules of the educational environment to create an effective working environment.

Least Restrictive Environment

Education of all children in the LRE, no matter how severe their disability, is what the federal laws and "best practices" indicate we must strive to achieve (Meyer et al., 1991; PL 105-17; Rainforth & York-Barr, 1997; Taylor, 1988). The conceptual framework for education in the least restrictive environment started in the 1960s. Reynolds (1962) advocated a continuum of placement options from most restrictive to least restrictive. Deno (1970) termed this the *cascade* of educational placements. The cascade of environments, from most to least restrictive, includes the residential setting, homebound services, special schools, special classes in neighborhood schools, general classes with resource assistance in neighborhood schools, and general classes in the neighborhood school with children without assistance. Terminology used to describe LRE has evolved from *mainstreaming*, to *integrated*, to *inclusive;* the difference is more than merely a change in language.

Placement in the LRE is not necessarily as widely accepted as one might hope. General educators are often concerned about having children with special needs placed in their classrooms without appropriate support services. Administrators are often concerned about the cost to the educational system. Parents sometimes believe that segregated environments have better services for their children. Taylor (1988), an advocate for total integration of people with severe disabilities, proposes that the focus of service systems must change from the development of programs in which people must fit to the provision of services and supports necessary for full participation in community life.

These shifts in focus, which are occurring to varying degrees across the nation, present some challenges for physical therapists. Therapists must be prepared to work in all schools with professionals who may know little about children with disabilities. Therapists will miss contact with peers and professional discussions and peer review. They might also have far to travel to see a single child, and scheduling services and times to meet with teachers is difficult. Physical therapists and teachers must work together so that collaboration and effective service can be achieved in the general education environment. The reader is encouraged to read further for a more in-depth discussion of inclusion (Falvey et al., 1995; Peck, Odom, & Bricker, 1993; Rainforth & York-Barr,1997; Taylor, 1988).

Models of Team Interaction

There has been an evolution in team interaction during the past two decades. The hierarchy of team interaction is presented in Box 32-3. The unidisciplinary model is not a team model and should rarely, if ever, be used in school settings. The multidisciplinary model involves several professionals doing independent evaluations and then meeting to discuss their evaluations and determine goals, objectives, and a plan of action. The meaning of multidisciplin-

---

BOX 32-3. Models of Team Interaction

Unidisciplinary

Professional works independently of all others.

Intradisciplinary

Members of the same profession work together without significant communication with members of other professions.

Multidisciplinary

Professionals work independently but recognize and value the contributions of other disciplines. "Little or no interaction or ongoing communication occurs among professionals" (Thurman & Wilderstrom, 1990, p. 225). However, the Rules and Regulations (*Federal Register,* June 22, 1989, p. 26313) for PL 99-457 redefines multidisciplinary to mean "the involvement of two or more disciplines or professions in the provision of integrated and coordinated services, including evaluation and assessment."

Interdisciplinary

Individuals from different disciplines work together cooperatively to evaluate and develop programs. Emphasis is on teamwork. Role definitions are relaxed.

Transdisciplinary

Professionals are committed "to teaching, learning and working with others across traditional disciplinary boundaries" (Rainforth et al., 1992, p. 13). Role release occurs when a team member assumes the responsibilities of other disciplines for service delivery.

Collaborative

The team interaction of the transdisciplinary model is combined with the integrated service delivery model. Services are provided by professionals across disciplinary boundaries as part of the natural routine of the school and community.

BOX 32-4. Characteristics of Collaborative Teamwork

- Equal participation in the collaborative teamwork process by family members and service providers
- Consensus decision making in determining priorities for goals and objectives
- Consensus decision making about the type and amount of intervention
- All skills, including motor and communication skills, are embedded throughout the intervention program
- Infusion of knowledge and skills from different disciplines into the design and application of intervention
- Role release to enable team members to develop confidence and competence necessary to facilitate the child's learning

Adapted from Rainforth, B., & York-Barr, J. Collaborative Teams for Students with Severe Disabilities, 2nd ed. Baltimore: Paul H Brookes, 1997.

---

quency in meeting the child's needs. In a transdisciplinary model occasionally only one individual provides the intervention, thereby increasing consistency, decreasing handling of children by many individuals, and allowing rapport to be established with the child and family.

As the team process has developed, the use of the terms *collaboration* and *collaborative teams* has appeared. These are supportive terms and might incorporate a number of models of team interaction based on the needs of the team, child, and family. The defining characteristics of collaborative teamwork, as conceptualized by Rainforth and York-Barr (1997), are summarized in Box 32-4. They believe that significant benefits are gained because of the diverse perspectives, skills, and knowledge available from the individuals on the educational team. This combined talent is an enormous resource of problem solving and support. Collaborative teams are of vital importance when working with children having multiple disabilities or with those who are severely or profoundly disabled.

When joining a team, physical therapists should ask for a clarification and a definition of terms regarding models or expectations of team interaction. All individuals should have the same understanding to avoid miscommunication and conflict.

Models of Service Delivery

There is an array of models of physical therapy service delivery. Unfortunately, there is also an array of confusing, conflicting, and overlapping terms used to describe the various models. The models include direct, integrated, consultative, monitoring, and collaborative (Table 32-1).

ary has changed since 1986 because of its usage in PL 99-457. In the law, the term *multidisciplinary* is used to describe an interdisciplinary model, as noted in Box 32-3; therefore, there is frequently confusion when using this term.

The definition and application of the transdisciplinary model is also ambiguous. For some, the continuous sharing of information across disciplines is sufficient for a transdisciplinary model. For others, there must be complete role release. Role release involves not just the sharing of information but also the sharing of performance competencies. Team members teach each other specific interventions so that all can provide greater consistency and fre-

TABLE 32–1. Physical Therapy Service Delivery Models in Educational Settings

	Direct	Integrated	Consultative	Monitoring	Collaborative
Therapist's primary contact	Pupil	Pupil, teacher, parent, aide	Teacher, parent, aide, pupil	Pupil	Entire team, pupil
Environment for service delivery	Distraction-free environment (may need to be separate from learning environment) Specialized equipment needed	Learning environment and other natural settings Therapy area if necessary for a specific child	Learning environment and other natural settings	Learning environment Therapy area if necessary for a specific child	Learning environment and other natural settings
Methods of intervention	Educationally related functional activities Specific therapeutic techniques that cannot safely be delegated Emphasis on acquisition of new motor skills	Educationally related functional activities Positioning Emphasis on practice of newly acquired motor skills in the daily routine	Educationally related activities Positioning Adaptive materials Emphasis on adapting to learning environment and generalization of acquired skills	Emphasis on making certain child maintains status to benefit from special education	Educationally related activities
Amount of actual service time	Regularly scheduled sessions, generally at least weekly	Routinely scheduled Flexible amount of time depending on needs of staff or pupil	Intermittent or as needed, depending on needs of staff or pupil	Intermittent, depending on needs of pupil, may be as infrequent as once in 6 months	Ongoing intervention Discipline-referenced knowledge shared among team members so relevant activities occur throughout the day
Implementer of activities	PT, PTA	PT, PTA, teacher, parent, aide, OT, COTA	Teacher, parent, aide	PT	Team
Individualized education plan objectives	Specific to therapy programs as related to educational needs	Specific to educational program	Specific to educational program	Specific to being able to maintain educational program	Organized around life domains in an ecologic curriculum

Adapted from Iowa Guidelines for Educationally Related Physical Services. Des Moines, IA: Department of Education, 1996.
COTA, Certified occupational therapist assistant; OT, occupational therapist; PT, physical therapist; PTA, physical therapist assistant.

Direct Model

In the direct model, the therapist is the primary service provider to the child. This is the traditional model used to provide physical therapy. Direct intervention is given when there is emphasis on acquisition of new motor skills and when specific therapeutic techniques cannot be safely delegated. Rarely, if ever, should direct intervention be given without also instructing the child's teachers and parents. Hanft and Place (1996) note that even in a direct service "pullout" model where the child is removed from the natural environment, there should be ongoing consultation with teachers and other team members. It is not unusual for a child to receive direct intervention for a specific goal while other models of service delivery are used to achieve other goals. Rarely should only a direct service model be used. A combination of several models of service delivery is consistent with the integrated and collaborative service delivery models.

Integrated Model

The Iowa State Department of Education (1996) defines the *integrated model* as one in which the therapist's contact is not only the child but also the teacher, aide, and family; service delivery is in the learning environment; and many people are involved in implementation of the therapy program. This model may also include direct and consultative services and is the foundation for the collaborative model.

Dunn (1991) further classified the integrated model as consisting of peer integration, functional integration, practice integration, and comprehensive integration. Peer integration occurs when a child with a disability functions in a classroom or at a social event with children without disabilities. Functional integration occurs when a child can use a therapeutic strategy or newly acquired skill in the natural environment. Encouragement of functional integration is the rationale behind providing therapy in the natural environment, especially when the objectives involve fluency (refinement of skills) and generalization of the ability to perform the skills in multiple environments with different individuals and equipment. Practice integration involves the collaboration of professionals to meet a child's individual needs. Comprehensive integration combines all the areas of integration and is the level toward which we must strive.

The integrated model of service delivery can, and frequently does, include direct physical therapy. The therapist, however, must collaborate with all other key individuals serving the child. Goals and objectives should be jointly developed, and all individuals serving the child should be instructed in how to achieve these objectives within their capability. Direct services, if best for the child, are provided in the LRE. Only when it is in the best interests of the child should the intervention be in a restrictive environment, such as a special room, because generalization of skills learned in a treatment room do not necessarily generalize to other settings (Brown, Effgen, & Palisano, 1998). Common examples of when therapy might be acceptable in a more restrictive environment are when the child is taking mainly academic courses, when extensive equipment is required, when the child is highly distractable, or when it is necessary for the child's safety.

Consultative Model

In the consultative model, the therapist's contacts might be the entire educational team, including the parent and child. The service is provided in the learning environment, and activities are implemented by all personnel *except* the therapist. The therapist meets with, and demonstrates activities to, all appropriate staff. The responsibility for the outcome is with the consultee—the individuals, usually the teachers, receiving the consultation (Dunn, 1991).

Hanft and Place (1996) note that consultation in the school may be provided by a variety of service delivery models, such as integrated or monitoring, further blurring the lines between these models. Consultation may be child specific, as outlined in Table 32–1, but might also include programmatic consultation involving issues related to safety, transportation, architectural barriers, equipment, documentation, continuing education, and improvement of the program's quality (Lindsey et al., 1980). Programmatic consultation should be the major activity of a therapist at the beginning of each academic year. Issues related to safety, transportation, and positioning are frequently more important than child-specific goals and objectives. Once the environment is safe, the child is properly positioned throughout the day, and a safe means of mobility is determined, the specific intervention program can be initiated.

Monitoring Model

In the monitoring model of service delivery the team is instructed as appropriate, but the therapist, although not providing direct intervention, maintains regular contact with the child to check on status and remains responsible for the outcome of the intervention. Monitoring is important for follow-up of children who have impairments or functional limitations that might deteriorate over time. Monitoring allows the therapist to check on the need for modifications in adaptive equipment and assistive devices. Monitoring is also an important way to determine if a child is progressing as necessary for transition to the next level of educational or vocational services. Monitoring is useful for transition from direct or integrated services to no services. Monitoring gives the family, child, and therapist a sense of security that the child is being observed. Also, if the child should require physical therapy, it generally allows more rapid receipt of services because physical therapy is already listed on the IEP.

Collaborative Model

Not everyone would consider the collaborative model a model of service delivery; however, because it is defined as a combination of transdisciplinary team interaction and an integrated service delivery model, it is being discussed as part of service delivery (Rainforth & York-Barr, 1997). As noted in Box 32–4 and Table 32–1, services in a collaborative model are provided by all team members, as in an integrated model, but the degree of role release and crossing of disciplinary boundaries is greater. The team assumes responsibility for developing a consensus on the goals and objectives and the implementation of the program activities. The activities are educationally relevant and are implemented in the natural routine of the school and community. In the collaborative model, the amount of service delivery or practice of an activity should, theoretically, be greater than in other models because the entire team is carrying out the activities. In reality, this might not be the case because of the varied levels of skill of the implementors, insufficient "natural" opportunities to practice an activity, competition among activities, and the difficulty of some activities (Prieto, 1992; Soccio, 1991).

In the past, many believed that the state physical therapy practice acts prohibited school personnel from performing procedures used by physical therapists. This generally is not the case as long as the individual does not represent himself or herself as a physical therapist, does not bill for physical therapy, and does not perform a physical therapy evaluation (Rainforth, 1997). In fact, a study by Rainforth (1997) indicates few limitations on the delegation of procedures by others, especially of the nature likely to occur in an educational environment.

PROGRAM DEVELOPMENT

Examination and Evaluation

Throughout this text, language suggested by the *Guide to Physical Therapist Practice* (American Physical Therapy Association, 1997) has been used; however, federal education laws use slightly different terminology. Therefore, both sets of terms are used in this chapter as appropriate. Evaluations (examination and evaluation) are to be done "to determine whether a child is a child with a disability…and to determine the educational needs of such child…In conducting the evaluation, the local educational agency shall…use a variety of assessment tools and strategies to gather relevant functional and developmental information" [PL 105-17, 111 Stat. 81, Sec. 614, (a) (1) (B)]. The assessments are to be given by trained and knowledgeable personnel in accordance with instructions and in the child's native language without racial or cultural bias. Selection of standardized tests should be based on professional judgment and dictated by the characteristics of the individual child. Therapists should work with school personnel to identify appropriate tests and measures. The child's functional abilities should be assessed in the natural environment. This means that the therapist must see the child in the classroom, hallway, and other school settings. For infants, toddlers, and preschoolers, the therapist should visit the child at home, in the child care center, or in the preschool. If it is not feasible to assess the child in these natural environments, every attempt must be made to make the evaluation setting as close to the natural environment as possible. A test developed by Coster and co-workers (1998), the School Function Assessment, should be of great assistance in determining the functional skill level of children in school. Examination and evaluation should also include a full assessment of all body systems: musculoskeletal, neuromuscular, cardiopulmonary, and integumentary. Impairment of any of these systems can cause functional limitations. Reduction of impairment may be necessary before the child can improve in functional abilities. The IEP or IFSP includes the goals, objectives, or benchmarks related to attainment of functional abilities.

The examination and evaluation is critical in determining eligibility and the services needed and, later, in comparing the success of services and the need for extended school year programming. As noted, for school-age children, a motor delay or disability does not necessarily qualify a child for special education and related services. The children must first have an educational need for special education in one of the categories listed in Box 32–1. Once the child meets the criteria for special education in one of these categories, the related service needs are determined as "required to assist a child with a disability to benefit from special education." If a child is not eligible for special education, he or she may be eligible for related services under Section 504 of the Rehabilitation Act.

The need for related services must be based on the individual needs of the child, and there should be no set criteria to determine educational needs for physical therapy. Several school systems, however, have attempted to develop exclusionary criteria. One such criterion is the use of prerequisite skills that must be demonstrated before the child is considered likely to benefit from related services (Rainforth, 1991). This performance discrepancy criterion, also called cognitive referencing, has been attempted by some schools. In this system, the criteria do not allow for the treatment of children whose cognitive development is below their motor development (Carr, 1989, p. 506). This is based on a belief that there is a positive correlation between the development of cognition and motor skills. Under this interpretation, the child most appropriate for physical therapy has normal intellectual skills but delay in motor skills. Children whose cognitive and motor skills are similar would not be eligible for services. Aside from the major legal and ethical questions regarding cognitive referencing, research does not support this position (Baker, Cole, & Harris, 1998; Cole, Mills, & Harris, 1991).

For infants and toddlers, an established condition or a specific delay or impairment in physical or motor development qualifies them for early intervention services and, if appropriate, physical therapy. The amount of delay a child must display is determined by each individual state. Some states use solely test-based criteria and other states a combination of test-based and non–test-based criteria. Criteria for developmental delay include the following (Brown & Brown, 1993):

1. 15 to 50% delay in one or more developmental areas
2. 1.5 standard deviation below the mean in at least one area or 1 standard deviation below the mean in two areas
3. Moderate or severe sensory impairment
4. 1 year of age: minimum delay of 3 months
5. 1.5 years of age: minimum delay of 4 months
6. 2 years of age: minimum delay of 6 months
7. 2.5 years of age: minimum delay of 7 months

Infants might qualify for early intervention services in one state or community and not another. In addition, eligibility can be influenced by the tests used. The criteria on some tests are far more rigorous than on others, and a child is likely to score lower on a more rigorous test than on either a less rigorous test or one that allows scoring by parent report (Long, 1992).

In addition to the comprehensive assessment of the child, early intervention programs must conduct family assessments to determine the resources, priorities, and concerns of the family related to enhancing the development of their child. The physical therapist, due to the interrelationship of the child and family evaluation, might be required to participate in or perform a family assessment. The therapist should become knowledgeable in family assessment tools and seek appropriate training (Chiarello et al., 1992; Sparling, 1993).

Developing Goals and Objectives

To develop appropriate goals and objectives, desired outcomes must first be identified. Determining a desired outcome might be as simple as merely asking the child, or it might require several team meetings. Outcome statements do not need to be measurable, but they should be functional. Once the desired outcome is identified, the goals that are necessary to achieve the outcome must be expressed. Goals are written to be achieved in 1 year. McEwen and Shelden (1992) indicated that goals should be measurable, although others (Montgomery, 1987; Wilson, 1991) indicated that goals may be global statements that are not necessarily measurable. After the desired outcomes and goals are identified, the measurable objectives must be developed.

All objectives must contain a statement of the behavior to be achieved, under what conditions, and the criteria to be used (Effgen, 1991; Mager, 1962). These "objectives are developed based on a logical breakdown of the major components of the annual goals, and can serve as milestones for measuring progress towards meeting the goals" (*Federal Register,* September 29, 1992, p. 44838). Once a major objective is determined, it can be broken down into short-term objectives. Short-term objectives are based on a task analysis of the long-term objective or goal. When possible, each short-term objective should be functional and educationally relevant; however, there are situations when a short-term objective is reduction of an impairment that is limiting the child's achievement of the functional, long-term objective. The recognition and listing of such short-term objectives is important to document progress. Achievement of these objectives indicates progression toward the educationally relevant, functional objective. Teachers would agree that reading is a very important goal of education; however, few teachers would negate the importance of the child's first knowing the prerequisite alphabet. The situation is the same in physical therapy. Sitting is an important functional skill; however, without the prerequisite trunk muscle strength and hip range of motion, independent sitting is impossible.

An example of a desired outcome and the objectives involving independent stair climbing is given in Box 32–5. To climb stairs at school independently, a child should have 90° of knee flexion and good strength in the quadriceps muscles. The educationally relevant objectives go in the child's IEP, and the other short-term objectives, which may or may not be considered educationally relevant, would go in the therapist's plan. Documentation of achievement of each objective is important to report to the child and family. Attainment of short-term objectives should be recognized and rewarded in lieu of waiting for achievement of the long-term objective.

When doing a task analysis and developing the short-term objectives, several variables should be considered: (1) changes in the behavior itself, (2) changes in the conditions under which the behavior is performed, and (3) changes in the criteria expected for ultimate performance (Effgen, 1991). Changes in the behavior may reflect maturation of the behavior itself, progressing from basic skills to more complex skills, or increasing levels of functional activity. Changes in conditions may be from

---

BOX 32–5. Example of Desired Outcome and Objectives Involved in a Specific Task

Task

I want to be able to climb the steps to get into school.

Functional Long-Term Objective or Measurable Goal That Is Educationally Relevant

Jonathan will be able to walk up and down the school stairs independently without using the railing.

Functional Short-Term Objectives That Are Educationally Relevant

1. Jonathan will be able to climb up 8 stairs at school with minimal assistance using a railing.
2. Jonathan will be able to climb up 8 stairs at school with minimal assistance without using a railing.
3. Jonathan will be able to climb down 8 stairs at school with minimal assistance using a railing.
4. Jonathan will be able to climb down 8 stairs at school with minimal assistance without using a railing.
5. Jonathan will be able to climb up 8 stairs at school without assistance or a railing.
6. Jonathan will be able to climb down 8 stairs at school without assistance or a railing.

Short-Term Objectives That May or May Not Be Considered Educationally Relevant

These objectives are necessary to achieve the educationally relevant objectives and would be part of the therapist's intervention plan, not in the IEP.

1. Jonathan will progress from 30 to 50° of active right-knee flexion.
2. Jonathan will progress from a poor to a fair muscle-strength grade in his left quadriceps.
3. Jonathan will achieve 90° of active right-knee flexion.
4. Jonathan will achieve a good muscle-strength grade in his left quadriceps.

---

simple to complex, such as walking in an empty hallway to walking in a hallway filled with students. Progression of criteria may be qualitative or quantitative. The criterion might include the qualitative measure of hip extension during midstance, which helps make gait more efficient, or a more direct quantitative measure of the walking speed. Use of quantitative criteria, such as judgment by three of four trials or 80% of the time, should be considered carefully. Successfully crossing the street only 80% of the time can be fatal! Selection of the behavior, conditions, and criteria for judging attainment of each objective for each individual child must be based on sound professional judgment. Books, computer programs, or other materials that provide lists of potential objectives cannot replace professional judgment.

In addition to the task variables, consideration

should be given to the hierarchy of response competence (Alberto & Troutman, 1990). A behavior is first acquired; it is then refined as fluency or proficiency develops. The skill must then be maintained and finally generalized to multiple environments, individuals, and equipment. *Acquisition, fluency, maintenance,* and *generalization of behaviors* are the terms used by educators. Use of this terminology is important when there is a need to convey the rationale for providing services past the acquisition phase.

Therapists are also encouraged to consider using a prompting system as a strategy to achieve an objective and as a variable in writing the criteria for judging attainment of the objective. A systematic delivery of levels of prompting assistance may be implemented in two ways. One is the "system of maximum prompts," and the other is the "system of least prompts" (Alberto & Troutman, 1990; Effgen, 1991). The prompts are usually verbal or visual cues, demonstration or modeling, partial assistance or guiding, and maximum assistance. In the system of maximum prompts, the therapist first provides maximum assistance and then gradually, over successive sessions, reduces the amount of assistance as the child achieves more independence. This is a common technique used by therapists, and it allows for maximal success during learning. This system is best suited for acquisition, when it is important to avoid unsafe movement, and for a complex series of tasks such as some activities of daily living.

In the system of least prompts, the child is initially provided the least amount of assistance, usually a verbal or visual cue, and then progresses to model, guide, or maximal assistance as necessary. This approach allows the child to display his or her best effort before the therapist prematurely provides unnecessary assistance. The system of least prompts is best for tasks in which the child has some ability or is developing fluency or generalization to new settings, individuals, or equipment.

Individualized Educational Plan

The IEP is the document that guides the program of special education and related services for the school-age child, 5 to 21 years of age. It is also the document used in many states for the educational program of preschoolers ages 3 to 5 years. The IEP is developed at a meeting involving the child's parents; at least one regular educator (if the child is or will be participating in regular education); a representative of the local educational agency who is qualified to provide specially designed instruction and is knowledgeable about the curriculum and resources; an individual who can interpret the instructional implications of the evaluation; and "at the discretion of the parent or the agency, other individuals who have knowledge or special expertise regarding the child, including related services personnel as appropriate; and whenever appropriate, the child" [(PL 105-17, 111 Stat. 85, Sec. 614 (d) (1) (B) (vi) (vii)]. The physical therapist has a professional obligation to participate when decisions regarding physical therapy are being made. The physical therapy contribution to the IEP must relate to the educational needs of the child. Measurable annual goals, including benchmarks or short-term objectives, must be developed. Objectives should be functional, with implementation integrated in the child's overall program.

The IEP must include the following:

(i) *a statement of the child's present levels of educational performance, including—*
  (I) *how the child's disability affects the child's involvement and progress in the general curriculum; or*
  (II) *for preschool children, as appropriate, how the disability affects the child's participation in appropriate activities;*
(ii) *statement of measurable annual goals, including benchmarks or short-term objectives, related to—*
  (I) *meeting the child's needs that result from the child's disability to enable the child to be involved in and progress in the general curriculum; and*
  (II) *meeting each of the child's other educational needs that result from the child's disability;*
(iii) *a statement of the special education and related services and supplementary aids and services to be provided to the child, or behalf of the child and a statement of the program modifications or supports for school personnel that will be provided for the child—*
  (I) *to advance appropriately toward attaining the annual goals;*
  (II) *to be involved and progress in the general curriculum . . . and to participate in extracurricular and other nonacademic activities; and*
  (III) *to be educated and participate with other children with disabilities and nondisabled children;*
(iv) *an explanation of the extent, . . . if any, to which the child will not participate with non-disabled children in the regular class; . . .*
(v) (I) *a statement of any individual modifications in the administration of State or district wide assessments; . . .*
  (II) *if the IEP Team determines that the child will not participate . . . why that assessment is not appropriate . . . and how the child will be assessed;*
(vi) *the projected date for the beginning of services and modifications . . . and the anticipated frequency, location, and duration of those services and modifications.*

PL 105-17, 111 Stat. 83, 84, Sec. 614 (d) (1) (A)

In addition, beginning at age 14 years there must be a statement of the transition service needs of the child that focuses on the child's program of study. At age 16, there must be a statement of the transition services for the child that includes, as appropriate, the interagency needs and linkages. The IEP must also address behavior management for eligible children who exhibit behavior problems that interfere with their ability to learn or with the learning of others. This is a new requirement of IDEA. Discipline issues have been an area of serious discussion and concern in the reauthorization process and are an area still subject to federal changes. At present, if the child requires a behavioral management program, a functional behavioral assessment must be performed. Therapists should assist in the assessment and then the functional behavioral intervention plan as appropriate. Therapists should educate themselves in behavior management so that they do not hinder the management program and can appropriately collaborate with the team to facilitate acceptable behaviors in all settings.

The IEP is a written commitment by the educational agency of the resources necessary to enable a child with a disability to receive needed special education and related services. It is also a management tool and a compliance and monitoring document and serves as an evaluation tool in determining the child's progress toward meeting the projected outcomes. IDEA does not require that teachers or other school personnel be held accountable if a child with a disability does not achieve the goals and objectives set forth in the IEP.

The IEP goals, objectives, and stated frequency of services cannot be changed without initiating another IEP meeting. However, as long as there is no change in the overall amount of time, some adjustments in scheduling the services should be possible (based on the professional judgment of the service provider) without holding another IEP meeting (*Federal Register*, September 29, 1992, p. 44839). This clarification is helpful because it allows therapists to choose between blocked and distributed practice or group and individual sessions as long as the objectives and overall amount of time for service delivery for the individual child does not change.

Individualized Family Service Plan

The IFSP is developed for infants and toddlers and their families and, in some states, for preschool-age children and their families. The IFSP differs from the IEP in its conceptual framework. The family is central to the development of the young child and is therefore central to the IFSP. The philosophy of family-centered early intervention is consistent with current theories of infant development and family functioning.

The IFSP is developed by a multidisciplinary team, including the parent or guardian. Physical therapy is one of the primary early intervention services, and the need for physical therapy is based on the disability or delay in physical development. In early intervention, physical therapy is not a related service provided based only on the educational needs of the child.

The IFSP must be in writing and contain the following:

(1) *a statement of the infant's or toddler's present levels of physical development, cognitive development, communication development, social or emotional development, and adaptive development based on acceptable objective criteria;*

(2) *a statement of the family's resources, priorities, and concerns relating to enhancing the development of the family's infant or toddler with disability;*

(3) *a statement of the major outcomes expected to be achieved for the infant and toddler and the family, and the criteria, procedures, and timeliness used to determine the degree to which progress toward achieving the outcomes is being made and whether modifications or revisions of the outcomes or services are necessary;*

(4) *a statement of specific early intervention services necessary to meet the unique needs of the infant or toddler and the family, including the frequency, intensity, and the method of delivering services;*

(5) *a statement of the natural environments in which early intervention services shall appropriately be provided, including a justification of the extent, if any, to which the services will not be provided in a natural environment;*

(6) *the projected dates for initiation of services and the anticipated duration of the services;*

(7) *the identification of the service coordinator from the profession most immediately relevant to the infant's, toddler's, or family's needs (or who is otherwise qualified to carry out all applicable responsibilities under this part) who will be responsible for the implementation of the plan and coordination with other agencies and persons; and*

(8) *the steps to be taken to support the transition of the toddler with a disability to preschool or other appropriate services.''*

PL 105-17, 111 Stat. 111 & 112, Part C, Sec. 636 (d)

The IFSP is developed with the parents, and their informed written consent must be obtained before providing early intervention services. If the parents do not consent to some aspects of the services, the early intervention services to which there is consent are provided. The IFSP must be evaluated once a year and reviewed at 6-month intervals or more often, based on the needs of the child and family.

Intervention

Intervention must be based on the needs of the child, not the system or professionals. The content, objectives, frequency, location, and intensity of intervention services are decided at the IEP and IFSP meetings. The therapist, family, and entire team must decide on the most appropriate intervention strategies.

Best practice, research, and federal law indicate that most, if not all, intervention should occur in the natural environment (American Physical Therapy Association, Section on Pediatrics, 1987; Association for Those with Severe Handicaps, 1986; Effgen & Klepper, 1994; PL 105-17; Noonan & McCormick, 1993; Peck, Odom, & Bricker, 1993; Rainforth & York-Barr, 1997). Recent research continues to suggest that there is little generalization of gross motor skills learned in a physical therapy department to the more natural environments of the home or recreation room (Brown, Effgen, & Palisano, 1998).

In the school setting, the therapist should first ensure that the child is properly positioned on the bus and in the classrooms. The safety of the aisles for ambulation or wheelchair mobility should be assessed. Architectural barriers must be evaluated and appropriate actions taken to eliminate or lessen them. The teachers and family must be consulted regarding their concerns. They should be instructed in proper handling, positioning, and use of body mechanics.

Direct intervention, if indicated, should then start in the natural environment of the classroom or home. This is accomplished easily with preschoolers and those in special classes for children with severe or profound disabilities (Giangreco et al., 1989; Noonan & McCormick, 1993; Peck, Odom, & Bricker, 1993). It is more difficult for children whose educational programs consist primarily of academic subjects. Physical therapy in the algebra class or the reading room, after the initial consultation, is generally inappropriate. Common sense must prevail. Perhaps therapy can be given during gross motor time in a preschool or during physical education. This is not always appropriate, however, because this might be the only time the child has to engage in free play and physical activity with her or his peers. Taking this opportunity away from the child might affect motivation, cooperation, and the development of important social skills that occur during these activities.

Merely moving traditional intervention from a special room to a more natural environment is also not in the spirit of best practices. The therapist must adjust intervention to the unique opportunities afforded in the natural environment. Available furniture and household or classroom items should be used as opposed to bringing in special equipment. Use of these common objects increases the likelihood that the child might use them to practice and develop motor skills when the therapist is not present and allows the therapist to model their use for the parent or teacher.

In the integrated and collaborative service delivery models the teachers, staff, and parents are usually participants in the delivery of some aspects of the intervention. Their involvement may be as simple as using proper carrying techniques, or as complicated as facilitating the proper reciprocal creeping pattern. These individuals must first be instructed in proper positioning and use of adaptive equipment and then in how to encourage selected motor activities. It is probably best to have classroom staff encourage activities at the fluency or generalization stage of motor development. Frequently, motor activities at the initial acquisition stage are too difficult for untrained individuals or are unsafe without experienced guidance.

Selection of which activities to teach others is a professional decision that must be based on characteristics of the individual child, the specific activity, and the capabilities and interest of the other individuals. In a series of single-subject design studies, Prieto (1992) found that when teachers are properly instructed in gross motor activities the frequency with which they encourage children to perform those activities generally increases. Soccio (1991) performed a study to examine the frequency of opportunities to practice specific gross motor skills during physical therapy and group early intervention classes. There was no difference in the number of opportunities to practice head control when direct physical therapy was compared with integrated group sessions for a child with severe disabilities. However, two children with cerebral palsy had more opportunities to practice standing and ambulation activities during direct, individual physical therapy sessions than during integrated group sessions in the classroom. The results suggest that the opportunity to practice motor activities in the classroom varies based on the type of movement and the class routines. Therapists must carefully select those activities they expect others to assist with because active movement is more limited in classrooms than expected (Ott, 1995).

The specific type of treatment provided depends on the needs of the individual child and the education, training, and experience of the therapist. There is no one accepted intervention approach. Informa-

tion provided throughout this text should assist the therapist in providing state-of-the-art physical therapy. Physical therapy in an educational setting should be based on sound professional judgment and guided by the IEP. If the appropriate intervention cannot be provided for a school-age child because it is not educationally relevant and is not related to the objectives in the IEP, the therapist has a professional obligation to inform the parents. Once the parents are aware of the limitations of school-based physical therapy, they might obtain additional therapy elsewhere.

Physical therapists in educational settings need not write the daily notes required in other settings. In the United States, however, they must comply with their individual state practice acts. They must be careful to record objectively the child's status before and after short and long school breaks. This is important in determining the need for extended school year services. A simple but comprehensive system of data collection using self-graphing data collection sheets is recommended (Alberto & Troutman, 1990; Effgen, 1991). One example of recording prompting needed to achieve a motor skill is provided in Figure 32–1. The availability of laptop computers has also made data collection and its graphic presentation much easier for many therapists. Extensive documentation is also necessary to support the need to increase, decrease, or terminate intervention. Physical therapy is not a lifelong activity such as learning. Both therapists and parents must recognize that, after a period of no change in status, physical therapy should be terminated or the child placed on a monitoring service delivery system. A continued desire for ambulation or similar activity is not sufficient reason for continued therapy after due diligence in trying to achieve the objective.

MANAGEMENT OF PHYSICAL THERAPY SERVICES

An important factor in successful management and service delivery in an educational environment is recognition and understanding of the significance of the team process. The physical therapist is part of the educational or early intervention team. Physical therapists must focus on collaboration with members of all other disciplines and recognize their importance in the total well-being of the child. They cannot work in isolation if they expect maximal effectiveness. The team, including the child and family, must decide on the most appropriate services at each phase in the child's life.

Just as team leaders or case managers are needed in intervention teams, so too a manager or director of physical therapy is needed in school settings. The

Trials

Verbal Cue	1 2 3 4 5 6	1 2 3 4 5 6	1 2 3 4 5 6	1 2 3 4 5 ⑥	1 ②③④⑤⑥
Gesture	1 2 3 4 5 6	1 2 3 4 5 6	1 2 3 4 5 6	1 2 ③④ ⑤ 6	1 ② 3 4 5 6
Model	1 2 3 4 5 6	1 2 3 4 5 6	1 2 3 4 5 6	1 2/3 4/5 6	1/2 3 4 5 6
Prompt	1 2 3 4 5 6	1 2 3 ④⑤⑥	①②③④⑤⑥	①② 3 ④ 5 6	① 2 3 4 5 6
Guide	①②③④⑤⑥	①②③ 4 5 6	1 2 3 4 5 6	1 2 3 4 5 6	1 2 3 4 5 6
Incorrect	1 2 3 4 5 6	1 2 3 4 5 6	1 2 3 4 5 6	1 2 3 4 5 6	1 2 3 4 5 6
Date	7/24	7/25	7/26	7/27	7/28
Objective/task	Creep to swing	Creep to swing	Creep to swing	Creep to swing	Creep to swing
Cue(s)	Verbal cue: "Creep to the swing." Gesture—wave forward Model—therapist creeps Prompt—tap abdominal muscles Guide—support at abdomen and assist with arm and leg movement Use "least to maximum" prompting system.	Same as 7/24	Same as 7/24, except prompt was a quick tap to the abdominal muscles and triceps	Same as 7/26	Same as 7/26
Criterion and Conditions	Independently creep to swing, 12 feet away, with abdomen off the floor and elbows straight, 3 times	Same as 7/24	Same as 7/24	Same as 7/24	Same as 7/24
Comments	Required much assistance, did not appear interested in task.	Placed toy in swing, which appeared to stimulate interest; had difficulty with elbow extension.	Continues to have difficulty with elbow extension, especially on right.	Elbow extension improved bilaterally.	Ready to creep further distances; still concerned about ability to maintain elbow extension.

FIGURE 32–1. *Self-graphing data collection sheet.* (Adapted from Alberto, PA, & Schofield, P. Instructional interaction pattern for the severely handicapped. Teaching Exceptional Children, *12*:16–19, 1979. Copyright © 1979 by The Council for Exceptional Children. Reprinted with permission. From Effgen, SK. Systematic delivery and recording of intervention assistance. Pediatric Physical Therapy, *3*:63–68, 1991.)

majority of directors of physical therapy in school systems across the nation are not physical therapists or, indeed, any type of related service personnel (Effgen & Klepper, 1994). This has serious implications. To understand professional roles and responsibilities and how to nurture a professional, one must understand the profession. Many of the problems encountered in school systems could probably be prevented if supervision was provided by an experienced therapist. Therapist managers understand the profession and are able to professionally and appropriately address management issues.

Therapists, unlike teachers, are trained to work in a wide variety of settings and therefore have little, if any, opportunity to learn about educational settings. Therapists new to a school system must receive orientation, mentoring, and in-service education. The roles and responsibilities of the therapist and all support staff should be defined clearly in a detailed job description that complies with federal and state laws. Therapists should be introduced to the entire team of professionals with whom they will be working at all sites. They need to know whom to ask for equipment, space, and other items necessary for successful intervention. These introductions should be part of a planned orientation program. Therapists need to know how referrals are received and handled, how caseloads are determined, how team meetings are planned and when they are scheduled, written policies and procedures, how peer review or quality improvement is done, emergency procedures, and policy for continuing education, to name but a few issues. None of these are unusual requests; they can easily and cost-effectively be addressed in any system.

After the therapist is properly introduced and oriented to the system, administrators and therapists must continue to talk before problems arise. Frequent areas of discontent are the lack of continuing education opportunities, insufficient peer contact, lack of an identified place to work, lack of time allotted for administrative tasks and meetings, and too much travel (Effgen & Klepper, 1994). More time and effort should be spent in retention of physical therapists so that there is not a need for continuous recruitment.

A system for obtaining referrals from physicians, if dictated by state law, must be developed. The referral allows the therapist to examine and evaluate, and then determine and provide appropriate intervention for, the child. Most physical therapy state practice acts in the United States allow a therapist to examine and evaluate without a referral, and 32 states (American Physical Therapy Association, 1998) allow therapists to examine and evaluate and provide intervention without a referral. Depending on the complexity of the child's medical problems and the need for pertinent information, a therapist might still want a referral no matter what the state law. Collaboration with physicians and all members of the child's medical and educational team encourages optimal service delivery.

A method must be developed for determination of therapy caseloads, and a rational system must be created for determining who should receive intervention and how much intervention should be given. This can be a difficult task. The Florida Department of Exceptional Student Education (1987) developed a matrix that combines clinical judgment factors and a therapy profile to determine the amount of therapy a child should receive. The Iowa Guidelines for Educationally Related Physical Therapy Services (1996) relates the potential to benefit from intervention with factors such as critical periods for skill acquisition, the amount of the program that can be performed by others, and the extent that motor problems interfere with the educational program to determine the amount of physical therapy. Children with critical needs for therapy require more intense intervention than do those with lesser needs. A therapist whose caseload includes only children having

extensive needs for therapy is able to serve fewer children than a therapist whose caseload includes all children having minimal needs. Having a clear system to determine eligibility for services, amount of services, and termination of services provides needed documentation to support the complex, sensitive decisions regarding allocating services.

CRITICAL ISSUES

Shortage of Pediatric Physical Therapists

The shortage of qualified pediatric physical therapists has been an ongoing issue facing school-based physical therapy. The reasons for the shortage are numerous and include the low pay in schools, professional isolation, challenge of other areas of practice, and difficulty in working with children. Solutions are numerous and sometimes complex, but one of the easiest is often neglected. The best way to train and then recruit new physical therapists is to have them on clinical affiliations in an educational setting while they are students.

Therapists, especially new graduates and those new to pediatrics, should strive to achieve the competencies for physical therapists in early intervention (Effgen et al., 1991) or school-based physical therapy (American Physical Therapy Association, 1990) that have been developed and endorsed by the Section on Pediatrics of the American Physical Therapy Association. These competencies are being updated and are an excellent resource for therapists to identify minimal standards for practice, as well as for encouraging professional growth. The competencies may also be shared with administrators to help define the role of physical therapy and identify the resources necessary for effective service delivery. Therapists should continually read, participate in continuing education, take graduate courses, and engage in dialogue with colleagues. Therapists working in school systems and early intervention settings must be aware of the potential for professional isolation and seek opportunities for developing improved competence. Employers must support therapists' efforts at maintaining their professional skills (Effgen, 1988).

Service Delivery System

The shortage of therapists has also affected the type of service delivery system used and the roles assumed by personnel. The literature supports integrated or collaborative service delivery models (Dunn, 1991; Rainforth et al., 1992; Rainforth & York-Barr, 1997). The advantages of more frequent practice in the natural setting with the support of all personnel is obvious. An appropriately administrated therapy program in the natural environment might require more and certainly not less personnel. Training all personnel in a truly integrated or collaborative model requires a great deal of time for training and meetings (Giangreco et al., 1989; Rainforth et al., 1992; York et al., 1990). There are those, however, who incorrectly think these models can be used to decrease the time required for physical therapy. Instead of having a therapist provide the required intervention, unqualified staff might provide activities without adequate supervised instruction, or a teacher might be forced to provide an intervention for which he or she is not properly trained. Instead of providing the intervention in a room with necessary equipment, a classroom or hallway is used in the name of natural environment. Rarely are there sufficient empirical data to support any service delivery system. Educators and therapists alike must step back and ask if they are truly meeting the needs of each individual child.

Professional Roles

In systems in which there is full staffing, professionals can collaborate to decide on the specific roles of each team member. Overlap of professional roles is acknowledged, and divisions of responsibility are made that are best suited to the needs of the child, system, and professional staff (Fairfax, 1992). In general, the overlap in physical therapy, occupational therapy, and education is greatest when professionals from these disciplines are serving young children. For older children there is less overlap in professional roles. Areas of frequent overlap between occupational therapy and physical therapy include programs for strength and endurance, body awareness, classroom positioning and adaptations, and enhancement of motor experience (Fairfax, 1992). Areas of overlap between physical therapists and educators might include advanced gross motor skills, endurance training, and writing. In systems in which there is a critical shortage of physical therapists, the breadth of roles assumed by other staff members increases based on need and not necessarily on professional skill.

Educationally Relevant Physical Therapy

Educationally relevant versus non–educationally relevant physical therapy is a frequent topic of debate. In school systems committed to the comprehensive provision of services to children with disabilities and with adequate therapy staffing, the definition of *educationally relevant physical therapy* is frequently broad based and depends on the individual needs of the child addressed at the IEP meeting. The new IDEA clearly indicates that education is to prepare students for independent living and economic self-sufficiency.

Having goals and objectives that are mutually agreed on by the entire educational team helps make physical therapy more educationally relevant. The educational system was never meant to provide for all the child's therapy needs. Physical therapy can be provided out of the educational system as appropriate, and all therapists serving the child should collaborate and coordinate services. Therapists and parents must remember that therapy takes time away from other educational and social opportunities that are vital to the total well-being of the child.

Least Restrictive Environment

As more children are educated in the least restrictive environment, therapists must be willing to travel to meet the needs of those students. Unfortunately, travel to many schools is not the most time- and cost-effective method of service delivery. Therapists and administrators must be creative in their approach to serving children in their local schools. Materials such as *Choosing Options and Accommodations for Children: A Guide to Planning Inclusive Education* have been used successfully to encourage inclusive education (Giangreco et al., 1993b).

Reimbursement for Services

The cost of providing related services in educational environments and physical therapy in early intervention settings is a serious concern of program administrators. IDEA provides some federal funding, but it has never been sufficient to cover the full spectrum of services needed by children in special education and early intervention. To cover the costs of physical therapy, some school systems are charging third-party payers. This is a serious concern because of the lifetime cap on many insurance policies, limited therapy coverage, and the possibility of losing insurance if bills are too high. Parents are not required to have their insurance company pay for these services, and they should not be intimidated into thinking their child will not receive services without insurance payment. Medicaid has approved procedures allowing school systems to bill Medicaid directly for physical therapy.

SUMMARY

In the United States, physical therapy is mandated as part of federally sponsored programs to serve infants, toddlers, children, and youth with disabilities. For school-age children, physical therapy is a related service of the educational program for those children who require special education. Physical therapy is part of the early intervention services provided to infants who have disabilities or delay in physical development.

The provision of physical therapy in an educational environment is challenging for physical therapists. It is not the high-tech, health-focused environment of the modern hospital setting or the therapy-focused environment of the rehabilitation setting. In the educational environment, the therapist is a member of a team of professionals for whom therapy may or may not carry a high priority in the overall goals and objectives for an individual child. The educational needs of the child have the highest priority.

The therapist must learn to understand the educational milieu to provide the best possible services and be satisfied in the work environment. The federal, state, and local laws and rules and regulations that govern services in the educational environment must be understood and respected. Rules and regulations are meant to help serve the child and family, not hinder service provision.

Therapists who work in the educational environment have a true picture of the everyday lives of the children they serve. They see first hand the struggles children with special needs face and are asked daily to solve complex problems to make life better for these children and their families. The education setting is a rewarding and wonderful environment in which to work for those who are willing and able to adjust to its unique demands.

References

Alberto, PA, & Schofield, P. Instructional interaction pattern for the severely handicapped. Teaching Exceptional Children, 12:16–19, 1979.

Alberto, PA, & Troutman, AC. Applied Behavior Analysis for Teachers, 3rd ed. Columbus, OH: Merrill, 1990.

American Physical Therapy Association. Physical Therapy Practice in Educational Environments. Alexandria, VA: American Physical Therapy Association, 1990.

American Physical Therapy Association. Guide to physical therapist practice. Physical Therapy, 77:1163–1650, 1997.

American Physical Therapy Association. Practice Department Report. Alexandria, VA: American Physical Therapy Association, 1998.

American Physical Therapy Association, Section on Pediatrics. TASH Position Statement: On the Provision of Related Services to Persons with Severe Handicaps. Alexandria, VA: American Physical Therapy Association, 1987.

American Physical Therapy Association, Section on Pediatrics. Report of the Section on Pediatrics of the American Physical Therapy Association to the Senate Committee on Labor and Human Resources and the House of Representatives Committee on Education and Labor on Reauthorization of Part H of the Education of the Handicapped Act. Alexandria, VA: American Physical Therapy Association, 1991.

Association for Those with Severe Handicaps. Position Statement of the Related Services Subcommittee of the TASH Critical Issues Committee. Seattle, WA: Association for Those with Severe Handicaps, 1986.

Baker, BJ, Cole, KN, & Harris, S. Cognitive referencing as a method of OT/PT triage for young children. Pediatric Physical Therapy, 10: 2–6, 1998.

Batten, HE. The industrial school for crippled and deformed children. Physical Therapy Review, 13:112–113, 1933.

Battle v Commonwealth of Pennsylvania, 629 F2d 280 (3rd Cir 1981).

Blatt, B, & Kaplan, F. Christmas in Purgatory: A Photographic Essay on Mental Retardation. Boston: Allyn & Bacon, 1966.

Braddock, D. Federal Policy Toward Mental Retardation and Developmental Disabilities. Baltimore: Paul H Brookes, 1987, p. 71.

Brown v Board of Education of Topeka, 347 US 483 (1954).

Brown, DA, Effgen, SK, & Palisano, RJ. Performance following ability-focused physical therapy intervention in individuals with severely limited physical and cognitive abilities. Physical Therapy, 78:934–949, 1998.

Brown, W, & Brown, C. Defining eligibility for early intervention. In Brown, W, Thurman, SK, & Pearl, LF (Eds.), Family-centered Early Intervention with Infants and Toddlers. Baltimore: Paul H Brookes, 1993.

Cable, OE, Fowler, AF, & Foss, HS. The crippled children's guide of Buffalo, New York. Physical Therapy Review, 16:85–88, 1938.

Carr, SH. Louisiana's criteria of eligibility for occupational therapy services in the public school system. American Journal of Occupational Therapy, 43:503–506, 1989.

Chiarello, L, Effgen, SK, & Levinson, M. Parent professional partnership in evaluation and development of individualized family service plans. Pediatric Physical Therapy, 4:64–69, 1992.

Cole, KN, Mills, PE, & Harris, SR. Retrospective analysis of physical and occupational therapy progress in young children: An examination of cognitive referencing. Pediatric Physical Therapy, 3:185–189, 1991.

Coster, W, Deeney, T, Haltiwanger, J, & Haley, H. School function assessment. San Antonio: The Psychological Corporation, 1998.

Council for Exceptional Children, Division of Early Childhood Education. Statement of the International Division for Early Childhood of the Council for Exceptional Children to the Congress of the United States with Respect to Reauthorization of Part H and Amendments to Part B of the Education of the Handicapped Act Regarding Services to Children from Birth to Age Six Years. Reston, VA: Council for Exceptional Children, 1990.

Cruickshank, WM. Psychology of Exceptional Children and Youth, 4th ed. Englewood Cliffs, NJ: Prentice-Hall, 1980, pp. 65–66.

Deno, E. Special education as developmental capital. Exceptional Children, 37:229–237, 1970.

Discipline Under Section 504. Special Educator, November 22, 1996, p. 7.

Dunn, W. Integrated related services. In Meyer, LH, Peck, CA, & Brown, L (Eds.), Critical Issues in the Lives of People with Severe Disabilities. Baltimore: Paul H Brookes, 1991, pp. 353–378.

Effgen, SK. Preparation of physical therapists and occupational therapists to work in early childhood special education settings. Topics in Early Childhood Special Education, 7(4):10–19, 1988.

Effgen, SK. Systematic delivery and recording of intervention assistance. Pediatric Physical Therapy, 3:63–68, 1991.

Effgen, SK, Bjornson, K, Chiarello, L, Sinzer, L, & Phillips, W. Competencies for physical therapists in early intervention. Pediatric Physical Therapy, 3:77–80, 1991.

Effgen, SK, & Klepper, S. Survey of physical therapy practice in educational settings. Pediatric Physical Therapy, 6:15–21, 1994.

Fairfax County Public Schools. PT/OT, Education's Helping Hands. Fairfax, VA: Fairfax County Public Schools, 1992.

Federal Register, Part II, Department of Education, 34 CRF Parts 300 and 301, Assistance to States for the Education of Children with Disabilities Program and Preschool Grants for Children with Disabilities, Final Rule, Vol. 57, No. 189, September 29, 1992.

Federal Regulations, Section 104, 3(j), 1988.

Falvey, MA, Grenot-Scheyer, M, Coots, JJ, & Bishop, KD. Services for students with disabilities: Past and present. In Falvey, MA (Ed.), Inclusive and Heterogeneous Schooling: Assessment, Curriculum, and Instruction. Baltimore: Paul H Brookes, 1995, pp. 23–40.

Florida Department of Exceptional Student Education. OT/PT Reporting System. Evaluation Protocols for Occupational and Physical Therapists in Public School. Tallahassee, FL: Department of Exceptional Student Education, 1987.

Georgia Association of Retarded Citizens v McDaniel, 511 F Supp 1263 (Northern District of Georgia, 1981).

Giangreco, MF, Cloninger, CJ, Dennis, RE, & Edelman, SW. National expert validation of COACH: Congruence with exemplary practice and suggestions for improvement. Journal of the Association for Persons with Severe Handicaps, 18:109–120, 1993a.

Giangreco, MF, Cloninger, CJ, & Iverson, V. Choosing Options and Accommodations for Children: A Guide to Planning Inclusive Education. Baltimore: Paul H Brookes, 1993b.

Giangreco, MF, York, J, & Rainforth, B. Providing related services to learners with severe handicaps in educational settings: Pursuing the least restrictive option. Pediatric Physical Therapy, 1:55–63, 1989.

Givins, EV. The spastic child in the classroom. Physical Therapy Review, 18:136–137, 1938.

Hanft, BE, & Place, PA. The consulting therapist: A guide for OTs and PTs in schools. San Antonio, TX: Therapy Skill Builders, 1996.

Iowa Guidelines for Educationally Related Physical Services. Des Moines, IA: Department of Education, 1996.

Lindsey, D, O'Neal, J, Haas, K, & Tewey, SM. Physical therapy services in North Carolina's schools. Clinical Management in Physical Therapy, 4:40–43, 1980.

Long, TM. The use of parent report measures to assess infant development. Pediatric Physical Therapy, 4:74–77, 1992.

Mager, RF. Preparing Instructional Objectives. Belmont, CA: Fearon, 1962.

Martin, EW. Lessons from implementing PL 94-142. In Gallagher, JJ, Trohanis, PL, & Clifford, RM (Eds.), Policy Implementation and PL 99-457: Planning for Young Children with Special Needs. Baltimore: Paul H Brookes, 1989, pp. 19–32.

Martin, R. Extraordinary Children, Ordinary Lives: Stories Behind Special Education Case Law. Champaign, IL: Research Press, 1991, pp. 45–63.

Maryland Association for Retarded Citizens v Maryland, Equite No. 100/182/77676 (Cir Ct Baltimore County, 1972).

McEwen, I, & Shelden, M. Writing functional goals: A means to integrate related services in special education. Paper presented at conference of The Association for Persons with Severe Handicaps Annual Convention, San Francisco, November 1992.

McEwen, IR, & Shelden, ML. Pediatric therapy in the 1990s: The demise of the educational versus medical dichotomy. Occupational and Physical Therapy in Pediatrics, 15:33–45, 1995.

Meyer, LH, Peck, CA, & Brown, L (Eds.). Critical Issues in the Lives of People with Severe Disabilities. Baltimore: Paul H Brookes, 1991.

Mills v Board of Education of the District of Columbia, 348 F Supp 866 (DDC 1972).

Montgomery, PC. Treatment planning: Establishing behavioral objectives. In Connolly, BH, & Montgomery, PC (Eds.), Therapeutic Exercise in Developmental Disabilities. Chattanooga, TN: Chattanooga Corporation, 1987, pp. 21–26.

Mulcahey, AL. Detroit schools for crippled children. Physical Therapy Review, 16:63–64, 1936.

National Information Center for Children and Youth with Disabilities. Related services for school-aged children with disabilities. News Digest, National Information Center for Children and Youth with Disabilities, 1(2):8, 1991.

Noonan, MJ, & McCormick, L. Early intervention in natural environments. Pacific Grove, CA: Brooks/Cole, 1993.

Ott, DAD. Occurrence of gross motor activities in integrated and segregated preschool settings. Unpublished master's thesis, Medical College of Pennsylvania and Hahnemann University, Philadelphia, 1995.

Pax Lowes, L, & Effgen, SK. The Americans with Disabilities Act of 1990: Implications for pediatric physical therapist. Pediatric Physical Therapy, 8:111–116, 1996.

Peck, CA, Odom, SL, & Bricker, DD. Integrating young children with disabilities into community programs. Baltimore: Paul H Brookes, 1993.

Pennsylvania Association for Retarded Citizens v Commonwealth of Pennsylvania, Civil Action No. 71-42, 334 F Supp 1257 (ED Pa 1971), 343 F Supp 279 (ED Pa 1972).

Prieto, GM. Effects of Physical Therapist Instruction on the Frequency and Performance of Teacher Assisted Gross Motor Activities for Students with Motor Disabilities. Unpublished master's thesis, Hahnemann University, Philadelphia, 1992.

Public Law 93-112, Rehabilitation Act (1973), 29 USC Sec. 794.

Public Law 94-103, Developmental Disabilities Assistance and Bill of Rights Act (1975). US Statutes at Large 89, pp. 486–507.

Public Law 94-142, Education of All Handicapped Children Act (1975), 89 Stat. 773-796.

Public Law 99-372, Handicapped Children's Protection Act (1986), 20 USC 1415(e) (4) (f).

Public Law 99-457, Education of the Handicapped Act Amendments of 1986, 100 Stat. 1145-1177.

Public Law 101-336, Americans with Disabilities Act (1990), 42 USC Sec. 12101.

Public Law 102-119, Individuals with Disabilities Education Act Amendments of 1991, 105 Stat. 587-608.

Public Law 105-17, Individuals with Disabilities Education Act Amendments of 1997, 111 Stat. 37-157.

Rainforth, B. OSERS clarifies legality of related services eligibility criteria. TASH Newsletter, 17:8, 1991.

Rainforth, B. Analysis of Physical Therapy Practice Acts: Implications for role release in educational environments. Pediatric Physical Therapy, 9:54–61, 1997.

Rainforth, B, York, J, & MacDonald, C. Collaborative Teams for Students with Severe Disabilities. Baltimore: Paul H. Brooks, 1992.

Rainforth, B, & York-Barr, J. Collaborative Teams for Students with Severe Disabilities, 2nd ed. Baltimore: Paul H Brookes, 1997.

Rapport, MJ, & Thomas, SB. Extended school year: Legal issues and implications. Journal of the Association for Persons with Severe Handicaps, 18(1):16–27, 1993.

Reynolds, M. A framework for considering some issues in special education. Exceptional Children, 28:367–370, 1962.

Rowley v Board of Education of Hendrick Hudson Central School District, 458 US 176 (1982).

Sever, JW. Physical therapy in schools for crippled children. Physical Therapy Review, 18:298–303, 1938.

Soccio, CA. Direct-individual versus integrated-group models of physical therapy service delivery. Unpublished master's thesis, Hahnemann University, Philadelphia, 1991.

Sparling, JW. Assessment of family resources and needs. In Wilhelm, IJ (Ed.), Physical Therapy Assessment in Early Infancy. New York: Churchill Livingstone, 1993, pp. 71–104.

Special Educator. Court: Regular class not always LRE, 11(21):8, 1996.

State of Iowa. Iowa Guidelines for Educationally Related Physical Therapy Services. Des Moines, IA: State of Iowa, 1996.

Tatro v Texas, 625 F2d 557 (1980); on rem'd 516 F Supp. 968 (1981); aff'd 703 F 2d 823 (1983); S Ct. No. 83-558 (aff'd July 5, 1984).

Taylor, SJ. Caught in the continuum: A critical analysis of the least restrictive environment. Journal of the Association for Persons with Severe Handicaps, *13*(1):41–53, 1988.

Thurman, SK, & Widerstrom, AH. Infants and Young Children with Special Needs, 2nd ed. Baltimore: Paul H Brookes, 1990.

Vacha, VB. History of the development of special schools and classes for crippled children in Chicago. Physical Therapy Review, *13*:21–26, 1933.

Wilson, JM. Cerebral Palsy. In Campbell, SK (Ed.), Clinics in Physical Therapy: Pediatric Neurologic Physical Therapy, 2nd ed. New York: Churchill Livingstone, 1991, pp. 301–360.

Wolfensberger, W. Will there always be an institution? The impact of new service models. Mental Retardation, *9*:31–38, 1971.

York, J, Rainforth, B, & Giangreco, MF. Transdisciplinary teamwork and integrated therapy: Clarifying the misconceptions. Pediatric Physical Therapy, *2*:73–79, 1990.

Zirkel, P. Inclusion: Return of the pendulum? Special Educator, *12*(9):5, 9, 1996.

CHAPTER
33

Private Practice Pediatric Physical Therapy: A Quest for Independence and Success

VENITA S. LOVELACE-CHANDLER, PT, PCS, PhD
BENJAMIN R. LOVELACE-CHANDLER, PT, PCS, PhD

In the first edition of this text (Campbell, 1994), we described the health care climate of the 1960s and 1970s, when many physical therapists were opposed to the private enterprise arena and when private practice therapists were described in unprofessional terms (Guglielmo, 1988). We also described the changes of the 1980s and early 1990s, in which a strong, independent private sector had been accepted as an ideal rather than an abomination in physical therapy (Carlson, 1987). At that time, a profession was defined by autonomy, public image, and income more than specialty or discipline (Wood, 1986), and society's value of a professional service was judged by the extent of private practice (Cooper, 1982). The climate of the 1980s and early 1990s reflected the perception that the growth of practice had been slow and may have hindered the development of professionalism within physical therapy. We suggested that this issue is of particular concern to pediatric services because the number of physical therapists limiting their private practices to pediatrics, although unknown, was perceived to have been extremely small.

Of 1609 respondents to a 1992 survey on private practice (Private Practice Section, 1992), only 26.6% indicated that pediatric services were among the services offered by their practices. Furthermore, 10 of 13 clinical service areas were predicted to expand in the private practice to a greater extent than pediatric services, with only cardiopulmonary and mental health services predicted to have less growth. The 1996 survey on private practice (Private Practice Section, 1996) did not seek information relative to type of service. Membership in the Private Practice Section (PPS) of the American Physical Therapy Association (APTA) at that time was approximately 3600, having decreased from approximately 4300 in 1992. In December 1998, PPS membership was below 3000. The consistent decrease in membership may indicate a decrease in private practitioners, including pediatric private practitioners.

The motivators for establishing a private practice include greater patient contact, larger income, independence, fulfilling community or client needs, and prestige (Cole, 1986; Smoyak, 1986; Wood, 1986). Pediatric physical therapists should be interested in pursuing these goals. Our experience in pediatric private practice was initiated with motivations for independence in decision making and the desire to reduce the length of the chain of command. Each of us had held more than one employed physical therapy administrative position, yet neither of us had been satisfied with the control that existed at that level of authority. In every instance, a higher administrator determined staffing patterns, equipment purchases, funding for continuing education, and often the types and amount of physical therapy services to be offered. Frequently, services were selected for productivity rather than to address the best interests of clients or families, and rates were established to recover costs elsewhere in the institution rather than to reflect the costs of providing physical therapy. Often, we were thwarted in efforts to design services that were based on our philosophy of best practice.

In 1982, one of us was in an employed administrative position experiencing these negative factors when the decision was made to begin a private practice. The practice was established as a sole proprietorship with the therapist/owner who provided treatment and a spouse/therapist who volunteered as business manager, bookkeeper, and billing specialist. We selected a sole proprietorship, the legal title for a business with one owner (Wood, 1986), because the organizational structure is simple, the paperwork is minimal, and governmental restrictions are few. For example, our practice was opened by merely ordering business cards.

In our case, the spouse was satisfied in an employed position and provided financial security during the first 2 years of the practice, including health, dental, and life insurance. The spouse had 2 years of experience as an insurance filing clerk and the willingness to work part time for the practice. With sufficient resources and the desire to be independent in professional practice, the business was established and has flourished. Even during difficult periods, the owner experienced enormous control, independence, and job satisfaction, and both of us were delighted with the financial gain, which exceeded expectations.

More physical therapists must seek the private practice setting if increased recognition as a profession is to be achieved, and pediatric physical therapists must be among those practitioners who accept the risks and rewards that accompany private practice. A paucity of material related to pediatric private practice is available and may help to explain the small number of pediatric private practitioners. This chapter is written for the physical therapist who may be considering developing a pediatric private practice or for the student who may wish to learn about a possible work setting, that of the full-time independent pediatric practitioner. The purposes of this chapter are to (1) define the private practitioner, including characteristics and responsibilities; (2) provide information on risk management concepts for establishing and maintaining a private practice; (3) present current trends in private practice; and (4) provide insight into the uniqueness of a pediatric private practice through a description of one experience.

Most published research and information on topics related to private practice are specific to adults. In this chapter, information from other professions and adult services has been extrapolated for application to pediatric physical therapy, and no evidence can be offered for the appropriateness of this extrapolation. We hope that the chapter will provide informative reading and direction for the pediatric physical therapist beginning a private practice and will allow the reader to avoid many of the mistakes and problems of our early years. A revelation to us in preparing this chapter was the quantity of information available to the therapist interested in private practice relative to how little we knew as beginners. Our intent is for the entrepreneurial pediatric therapist or student to be encouraged and to use the information of this chapter in a quest for the independence and success available in private practice.

THE PRIVATE PRACTITIONER

History and Definition

Although the origin of physical therapy private practice is difficult to ascertain, evidence exists that a few therapists were engaged in such practices in the 1950s and that these therapists exchanged information regarding the private practice setting during a meeting at the 1954 Annual Conference of the APTA (Dicus, 1991). In 1955, the APTA responded to a request from private practice therapists by establishing a steering committee to make recommendations on the advisability of creating a Self-Employed

Section. The committee members perceived defining who constituted a self-employed therapist as one of the most difficult problems in the development of the section. Dicus (1991) noted that this difficulty in clearly delineating the private practitioner resulted in such problems as uncertainty regarding the philosophy of the section, a lack of common ground among members, diversity in educational needs, and misunderstanding of governmental regulations. The problems persisted during the section's formative years and during the evolution into the current PPS (renamed in 1975) (Reuss, 1991). In 1996, the section's board recommended a name change to the Section on Business Practice (PPS Impact, 1997). At the PPS General Business Meeting, members voted to retain the existing name. The 1996 survey (Private Practice Section, 1996) indicated a discrepancy regarding future focus of the PPS. Several members wanted to welcome corporation members, but the greatest majority were very independent and looked to the section to protect the interests of PT-owned independent practices (Valente, 1996).

Frazian (1985) notes that the definition of private practice is still disputed. Between the staff therapist, employed by an institution, and the independent therapist, owner of a practice or corporation, are innumerable therapists who are establishing lifestyles and professional private practices to meet the needs of society and themselves. Examples of the variety of private practices include performing a few hours of home health care services in addition to a full-time employed position, working part time in an employed position and part time as owner of a practice, and providing numerous hours through several contractual arrangements. Contracting denotes assuming responsibility for providing clinical services in a particular setting for a fixed payment (Bernstein, 1986). Contractors are self-employed and have differing financial processes in regard to income tax, Social Security tax, and retirement funds, but little difference may be noted in the actual provision of clinical services by employees or contractors.

Although Brown (1992) questions the use of the term *private practice* and alludes to every physical therapist as an independent practitioner with a high level of decision-making ability and professionalism, the guidelines in this chapter are directed to a very specific practitioner whom we have defined as follows: *The private practice physical therapist has autonomy, uses minimal bureaucracy, practices according to professional values, and takes risks to achieve financial and professional independence and success.*

Autonomy

A frequent misconception is that any therapist contracting for services is a private practitioner (Faust & Meaker, 1991). Private practice is more than having a contract with an agency or a facility. The first requirement of self-employment is the ability to function in an autonomous manner as a businessperson. When one giant corporation enters into a business relationship with another corporation, autonomous practice is absent, and this arrangement is no more a private practice than the per diem therapist who engages in a contractual relationship with a large health care institution. Selker (1995) cautions that the managed care system has the goal of health care increasingly ruled by managerial issues rather than the issues of professional autonomy. He asks whether autonomy needs to be shared. Pediatric physical therapists must be willing to assume autonomy in managing the practice, designing and offering services, implementing marketing strategies, billing for services, establishing relationships with children and families, and consulting with other professionals and agencies, but these practitioners may need to be flexible in sharing autonomy in order to maintain business success.

Minimal Bureaucracy

Private practice is characterized by low levels of internal bureaucracy as opposed to the management style of a typical corporation (Faust & Meaker, 1991). Private practitioners are free to choose a streamlined bookkeeping system and may have less paperwork than that required by agencies. Within the boundaries established by licensure laws, the rules and standards for continuing education, promotion, supervision and delegation, and collegial consultation can be established without approval from other administrative bodies. Decisions regarding equipment purchases, budgeting, and secretarial support are made by the owner, often the sole practitioner, but may in larger practices include input from other appropriate employees. Pediatric therapists must be willing to exercise independent decision making and must understand that supervisors, department directors, and administrators are usually not available to assist (or resist) the private practitioner's decisions.

Professional Practice

Professional values and norms direct the behavior of the private practice organization. Corporations, including health agencies, often use marketing forces and business perspectives to determine organizational structure and behavior. Although knowledge and use of business principles are essential to survival in private practice, the services must be offered in a manner in which professional standards are paramount and supersede financial considerations. Wood (1986) suggests that private practice is more a philosophy than a work setting and that professional success can be achieved without financial success, but we believe that financial success in private practice cannot be achieved without quality services. The pediatric physical therapist in private practice will find that the business will be successful only when professionalism and quality coexist with financial concerns to offer the consumer a service worth purchasing. The *Guide to Physical Therapist Practice* (APTA, 1997b) is essential for the pediatric therapist. The *Guide* describes the elements of accepted practice, standardizes practice terminology, and provides preferred practice patterns. The practice patterns are based on expert opinion and describe acceptable intervention strategies and procedures (Hack, 1998).

Risk Taking

The great risks involved in initiating a private practice, including costs and the potential for mistakes, have been cited by several authors (Cole, 1986; Flower, 1986; Kooper & Sullivan, 1986; McClain et al., 1992; Parish, 1986; Walker, 1977; Wood, 1986; Woody, 1986). Many practicing therapists are not interested in management and avoid the business responsibilities and attention to detail required in private practice (Deaton, 1992b; Walker, 1977). Many small businesses with marketable services or products fail because the initial financial resources are exhausted before income can be produced (Walker, 1977) or because business responsibilities have been mismanaged.

One characteristic of private practice is the personal assumption of risk and the realization that service delivery within private enterprise carries the opportunity to fail (Wood, 1986). Areas of potential risk include financial, professional, personal relationships, and legal aspects. Pediatric private practitioners must have sufficient general knowledge of business management to understand basic principles and to seek qualified counsel when needed. Although many risks will be present at the onset of the practice, additional risks are associated with expansion of an established practice, whether the expansion involves purchasing equipment, hiring additional personnel, or changing office space (Cole, 1986). Three important considerations before starting a private practice are that (1) risk taking involves the possibility of either negative or positive outcome; (2) risk management fosters positive outcome and allows entering risky situations with hope as opposed to avoiding risky situations for fear of negative results; and (3) methods for minimizing risks have been identified and are available for use by new private practitioners (McFadden & Hanschu, 1985).

Baskin (1997) describes starting a practice in 1992 when many private practitioners were joining corporations or closing practices. He indicates 4 years later that private practice gives the therapist the highest level of accountability and that the greatest risks result in the largest rewards. Pediatric physical therapists still have options for initiating private practices, but consideration of risk factors must be paramount.

Personal and Professional Characteristics

Although Walker (1977) advocates that only experienced physical therapists should consider entering private practice, a setting he considers unsuited for the novice, physical therapy will not achieve increased recognition as a profession until more practitioners seek the private practice setting. New graduates and other therapists may enter this arena if personal characteristics and professional skills are compatible with private practice. The person drawn to private practice is attracted primarily by the opportunity to be self-governed and by the desire to be one's own boss (Cole, 1986). The private practitioner is focused on self-control, independence, self-governance, and diversity of tasks. Expertise or specialization is necessary to the success of a practice. Wood (1986) offers the following two very direct statements that should be carefully considered by the therapist interested in private practice: "If you don't have anything to market, stay out of the marketplace" (p. 6), and "It is impossible to be too blunt with yourself when assessing your skills and expertise" (p. 7).

Walker (1977) suggests that the physical therapist in private practice must possess the following seven traits:

1. The therapist needs good physical and mental health to sustain the long hours, work stress, coping mechanisms, and interference with routine often associated with a new private practice.

2. The ability to develop strong relationships with clients, physicians, and other health care personnel is essential to the business aspects of the practice, and the ability to maintain a supportive relationship with family and friends is essential to personal well-being.

3. Self-discipline, including adherence to a self-imposed schedule, timely devotion to business details, and self-initiation skills, is crucial to the private practitioner. The therapist who functions best when responsible for someone else's schedule and goals should remain in an employed position.

4. An interest in business management and such subjects as accounting, bookkeeping, and economics is necessary for financial success. The ability to han-

dle personal finances and to promptly manage personal bank accounts, tax files, real estate issues, insurance coverage and claims, and savings accounts might provide insight into the probability of successful business management.

5. Good oral and written communication skills are important to successful interaction with clients, physicians, third-party payers, and other health care personnel. Private practitioners must be comfortable with face-to-face professional contacts with the intent of securing referrals, with technical report writing to enhance reimbursement, and with difficult situations such as collecting payment from clients.

6. Professional training and experience must be adequate for the services to be marketed. Self-advancement and self-directed learning are essential to building a successful private practice.

7. Dedication and determination to address the problems as well as the promises of a private practice are necessary for successful risk management.

The Committee on Private Practice of the American Speech-Language-Hearing Association (ASHA) (1991) provides 13 personal characteristics that should be considered when initiating a private practice: necessary experience, an established reputation, good clinical skills, an affinity for the work, willingness and ability to work long hours for a few years, handling a challenge, learning what is not known, acceptance of no or low income for a period of time, desire for a private practice, family support, stress management, strong self-image, and a network or support system. Physical therapy private practitioners also will find these characteristics to be essential.

Cole (1986), writing about speech-language pathology and audiology but offering advice applicable to any private practitioner, cautions that individuals should examine their professional practice attitudes and personal characteristics in relation to the roles that must be assumed as business owner, manager, and clinician. The business aspects of owning and managing a private practice are often shocking to therapists who consider their work as a service to be given to clients. Therapists must be willing to regard services as a product to be sold for a profit but realize that most of the time and energy for the first year or more will be devoted to building the practice without experiencing any profit.

All health care professionals who engage in private practice probably do so for similar professional reasons. Smoyak (1986) noted that private practice offers psychiatric nurses the advantages of maximal autonomy for patients and professionals with little bureaucratic red tape and interference with profes-

sional judgment. The author offers the following comment:

> Patients, if they can afford it, or have insurance that will allow it, can freely select the practitioner of their choice, using such criteria as age, sex, race, credentials, style, location, availability, cost, educational background, and recommendation of others. Theoretically, this freedom to select the therapist may increase the probability that the treatment will be helpful. Similarly, the therapist's freedom to concentrate on specific treatments and kinds of patients should enhance their clinical skills. A fee-for-service system, with practitioners earning income by hours spent in treating patients, tends to maximize productivity and minimize time spent on paperwork, meetings, and other non–revenue producing functions (Smoyak, 1986, p. 22).

Parsons (1986) refers to private practitioners as "heroes" and "politicians" who develop expertise through specialization and let others know about their expertise through marketing. The individual practitioner is able to use specialization for visibility and clarity about capabilities and limitations. For example, the practice may be limited to a specific age range, such as infants and toddlers, preschoolers, or adolescents, or to a diagnostic category, such as developmental disabilities or orthopedics. The therapist should learn how services are perceived by different segments of the community where the practice will be established and market services that address consumer needs. The ability to develop referral sources depends on others' perceptions of the therapist's competence, which is influenced by professional visibility and charisma. Building a caseload requires offering unique services, accepting third-party payment, providing flexible scheduling, meeting with physicians and other health care professionals, being competent, giving speeches, meeting local health needs, cultivating personal referral sources, and achieving professional visibility. Speaking to community groups, giving workshops, publishing, and participating in professional activities increase visibility. In our practice, free services were provided to clients who had no funding in order to establish relationships with physicians who were sending referrals to pediatric centers that required reimbursement. Calling the physicians regarding client issues, writing thorough reports, and providing follow-up letters to referral sources were practices that contributed to the rapid expansion of our referral base. After only 1 month, client referrals were sufficient to meet operating costs of the practice and to provide a very minimal salary.

The Small Business Administration (SBA) is a federal funding entity that provides support to owners of small businesses. The SBA provides a list of basic survival skills needed to run a business (Roussel & Epplin, 1987). These skills include a working knowledge of basic record keeping; financial management; personnel management; market analysis; breakeven analysis; product or service knowledge; federal, state, and local taxes; legal structure; and communication skills. Of these basic skills, the typical therapist will possess service knowledge and communication skills.

Deaton (1992a), a frequent speaker at the annual meetings of the PPS, has complimented physical therapists in private practice. He indicated the respect he had for the education and body of knowledge of physical therapy. As new graduates, therapists enter a complex health care system with a maze of administrative, reimbursement, social, and clinical issues. Therapists survive the maze, providing quality services to clients with a wide range of impairments and functional limitations. As if this feat were not enough, an increasing number of therapists decide to enter the private enterprise arena. The skills required to be a successful business owner are not possessed (or even known).

Deaton's description certainly fit our business adventure. The owner and spouse possessed several but not all of the professional characteristics recommended as essential. Clinical skills in the area of pediatrics were varied and advanced. We both had 11 years of pediatric experience, master's degrees that included coursework in pediatric physical therapy, doctoral degrees in health education, and certification in specific clinical techniques such as neurodevelopmental treatment. The owner had administrative experience from serving as a physical therapy department director in an outpatient pediatric physical therapy center, as director of physical therapy at a residential facility for 1200 clients with developmental disabilities, and as the director of rehabilitation at an urban children's medical center. An interest in business management, accounting, bookkeeping, and economics was absolutely lacking, and the business aspects of owning and managing the practice were shocking to us. We were anxious to implement our philosophy of care and anticipated the outstanding services that we would offer children and families, but we never considered cash flow problems, third-party payers who provided reimbursement but only after months of delay, families who received payment from third-party payers and spent the funds on personal expenditures, parents who were offended when asked for payment, and funding agencies who refused to reimburse for outpatient services provided by a private practitioner in an office or home when identical outpatient services were reimbursable if provided in a hospital or center by the same practitioner.

The spouse had 2 years of experience in insurance processing, and all billing was done in evening hours. For the first 12 years, only one client who was expected to pay failed to do so. Our collection rate was incredible, but the toll on personal lives, marriage, and children cannot be overestimated. If we had been aware of the business aspects of private practice and our obvious deficiencies in management, the practice would still have been initiated, but we would have sought assistance from others earlier and would not have considered ourselves as failures because of the reimbursement, tax, accounting, and record-keeping problems. Physical therapists who desire to enter private practice in pediatrics must develop business skills or purchase business services from others if professional and personal satisfaction is to be optimal. Prior authorization in order to receive reimbursement for services has become a factor during the last several years of our practice. Now, for us, most reimbursement issues are between our corporation and third-party payers. Families are rarely involved in the reimbursement process except occasionally to advocate with their reimbursement entity if payment for services is being denied.

Jayaratne and colleagues (1991) found that although the need for a continuous supply of clients and concerns over the business aspects of a private practice may produce stress in social workers, the private practice setting created less strain than agency settings. Social workers in private practice reported fewer psychologic and health strains, higher levels of performance, and better feelings about their life circumstances. These authors suggested that individuals who seek private practice may differ from employed individuals by being healthier from the beginning, having characteristics that foster health, serving kinds of clients that produce less stress in the practitioner, or experiencing different psychosocial aspects of business in the private practice arena. We believe that the private practice environment has afforded more happiness and better mental health for the owner than any previous employed position. The spouse has been able to experience many of the rewards of the practice through a sense of accomplishment, less marital stress, and greater financial gains.

Personal and Professional Responsibilities

Standards of practice, preferred practice patterns, and statements of ethical principles and conduct have been developed by the APTA (1991a, 1991b, 1996, 1997a, 1997b, 1997c). Although these standards and statements apply universally to members of that association and may be adopted by non-member physical therapists and physical therapist assistants, ethical behavior is situational, and specific circumstances may determine the manner in which the ethical principles are applied. We have perceived that employed therapists have greater ethical expectations of private practitioners than of themselves or other employed therapists. Flower (1986) determined that speech-language pathologists and audiologists perceive private practice as entailing unique ethical considerations and responsibilities that are more challenging than the ethical concerns of employed therapists, suggesting that increased expectations for private practitioners are not unique to the profession of physical therapy. He suggests that although private practitioners may engage in unethical practices such as treating clients with dubious prognoses, maintaining clients endlessly in treatment programs, making recommendations without regard for economic impact, and failing to obtain informed consent, employed therapists commit the same unprofessional behaviors. Ethical considerations remain similar regardless of the delivery system, and personal and professional responsibilities for quality services at reasonable cost are not limited to the private practice environment.

Wood (1986) notes that certain aspects of professional morality underlie the spirit of ethical principles and that these aspects include responsibility, integrity, and competence. Institutions frequently provide administrative leadership that reduces individual professional responsibility, or at least perceived responsibility, and institutions are able to compensate for limited professional competence in one practitioner through supervision by or use of other practitioners. In institutions, several therapists may collaborate on difficult ethical decisions and produce a superior decision, but poor ethical decisions by one therapist may also be concealed and the therapist protected by other staff members. Concerns regarding ethical practice should be heeded by physical therapists because sheltering and protection are not usually available to private practitioners in any profession.

Flower (1986) suggests six areas of frequent ethical dilemmas for private practitioners that, if monitored appropriately, produce ethical practices: professional competence (practitioner and employees), confidentiality and informed consent, fees and financial activities, marketing and advertisement, relationships, and product recommendation and dispensing. The reader is referred to Flower's work for a comprehensive discussion of each area.

We suggest that the pediatric physical therapist in private practice may ethically provide services to any patient unless a misfit exists between the patient's needs and the therapist's skills. A sole practitioner may be more limited in treatment strategies than therapists in a hospital or group practice. A practitioner should seek advice or make referral to another therapist if other strategies are warranted. Private practitioners are cautioned that pride, an unwillingness to limit a practice, and fear of economic loss may prevent admission of shortcomings.

The Code of Ethics of the APTA (1991a) and the guides for conduct (APTA, 1991b, 1996, 1997a) are valuable resources for all private practitioners. Additionally, the Section on Pediatrics of the APTA offers documents to assist pediatric practitioners in offering ethical and appropriate services (Scull & Deitz, 1989; Task Force on Early Intervention, 1991). Both the Section on Pediatrics and PPS provide sources for articles, commentaries, and other information of value to private practitioners through such publications as *Pediatric Physical Therapy*, *PPS Impact*, and *Advance for Directors in Rehabilitation*. Adhering to the regulations regarding state licensure and pursuing development through continuing education will assist in maintaining ethical and competent practice.

RISK MANAGEMENT IN ESTABLISHING A PRIVATE PRACTICE

Starting a Practice

Walker (1977) notes that no clear-cut "how to" methods exist for establishing a professional office, but several considerations and procedures are recommended. Knowledge of the process might lessen the mistakes, risks, and costs, thereby increasing the rewards for the pediatric therapist beginning a private practice. Sims (1992) suggests identifying and building the practice desired by the individual therapist, not the practice everyone else thinks should be built. Pediatric private practitioners must determine the ages and types of disabilities of children for whom services will be provided. A subspecialty practice within the broader pediatric specialty may be appropriate. Niche practices are increasingly prevalent and have been suggested as a method for maintaining a private practice as managed care reimbursement policies affect fiscal security (Huelskamp, 1997). A niche market may be a narrowly focused effort, a place or use that is unique, or a small area of specialization. Remember that the practitioner must possess the skills and expertise for the planned practice and that a niche in the marketplace must exist if success is to be obtained.

Our practice was envisioned as an office-based practice that would provide services for young children with developmental disabilities, probably from birth to 12 years of age. The office practice never flourished as well as desired, and in the early years, few infants and toddlers were referred. A niche in the marketplace did not exist for office services for young children because most families could obtain this type of physical therapy service from a variety of outpatient treatment centers that also provided social services, educational classes for preschoolers, and other therapies. Our business became particularly successful because services were provided at schools, child care centers, or client homes as was necessary to provide ecologically based services to children. Our niche in the marketplace developed by addressing special situations such as contracting with school districts to relieve the shortage of school-based therapists, serving the children of working parents in the everyday environment of the child, providing treatment to clients receiving educational services at home, and traveling to the homes of families without transportation or to small, nearby towns where several families resided but where no services were available. Contracts with school districts sustained the practice at first, but because the school districts wanted employees rather than autonomous practitioners, the contracts were discontinued as the practice grew with individual clients.

During the first 2 years, our practice was not the business we had envisioned, but autonomy, low bureaucracy, and our philosophy of care were present. Within a few years, the practice was shaped into the desired business, but even during the early years, the practice was limited to clients younger than 21 years of age. The owner declined adult clients, even though numerous referrals were received for adults with neurologic involvement. Continued success has been the result of blending the wishes of the owner with the needs in the marketplace.

Selecting a Legal Structure

Every business organization must have a legal structure (Hampton, 1986). Numerous potential legal structures exist and should be considered by the therapist initiating a private practice. The tax obligations, financial advantages, applicable laws and liabilities, and employer and employee benefits for each legal entity are determined by federal and state regulations. An attorney and an accountant, both with expertise in small businesses, should be consulted to determine the legal form most appropriate for the planned practice. The county clerk and the state licensing board can provide information about the legal forms available in a specific geographic location (ASHA, 1991). Generally, an individual practice consists of a single therapist providing services for a fee through a small business, an associate private practice consists of professional and technical staff members employed and directed by one therapist, and a

partnership has two or more co-owners (McClain et al., 1992). The specific legal form for each of these organizational patterns may vary. For example, a single practitioner may be a sole proprietor or the owner of a corporation.

The three common and most appropriate legal structures for a professional practice are sole proprietorship, partnership, and corporation (Hampton, 1986; Parish, 1986; Wood, 1986). As indicated previously, the sole proprietorship is the simplest form of legal structure. Additionally, this form is used by more than half of all business organizations, and almost half of all sole proprietorships are service organizations (Hampton, 1986).

Partnerships have two or more owners who enter into business together (Hampton, 1986). Parish (1986) notes that a partnership is similar to a marriage and that this form of legal structure requires partners who are personally compatible and possess complementary abilities. One partner must have controlling interest in the business, or final decisions may be difficult to achieve. If the partnership is split equally among partners, disputes are resolved only by compromise or defeat. When disputes cannot be resolved, dissolution of the partnership may be required and also may be similar to a marriage that ends in divorce. A buy-sell agreement established at the initiation of the partnership indicates the mechanism for dissolving the partnership by allowing one partner to buy the percentage of the business held by other partners or to sell the partner's percentage to other partners or someone else. Partnerships are the least common legal structure for businesses, making up less than 10% of all organizations (Hampton, 1986).

Corporations form the most complex type of legal structure, and an attorney will be needed to prepare the articles of incorporation (Parish, 1986). The corporation is a legal entity, and the owner who incorporates a company becomes an employee of the corporation. Income tax is paid on the profits of the corporation separately from the individual taxes paid by the owner and employees. Income levels that exceed $50,000 may indicate the need for a corporate structure to maximize tax benefits (Sullivan, 1986). Several types of corporations exist (Hampton, 1986), and an attorney or accountant can assist in determining the correct type for the planned business. Costs of incorporating a business range from $500 to $1500, according to the geographic location and the type of corporate structure (Sullivan, 1986). About 20% of all businesses are corporations, but the vast majority of business income is generated by this type of legal structure (Hampton, 1986).

For 6 years, our business was operated as a sole proprietorship, but we incorporated the practice during the seventh year. A lawyer advised that incorporation would assist in several of the tax complications relating to contracting with other therapists and would provide better liability protection for the owner. In a sole proprietorship, our home and cars could be taken to settle a business debt in the event of litigation, and we believed that our personal assets had to be safe from the liabilities of the business. The private practice pediatric therapist should seek advice from a lawyer, a tax consultant, and a financial advisor to determine the most suitable organizational structure for the proposed practice.

Hampton (1986) suggests that the private practitioner will have the final decision regarding the legal structure of the business and that the decision will be based on personal or professional needs. In our experience, we did not have the expertise to determine the best legal structure and were forced to rely on an accountant we trusted. Our accountant has changed the type of corporation once since we incorporated to better reflect the financial status of our business. Parish (1986) warns that the complexity of the tax structure for corporations requires that accountants and attorneys will be needed for the foreseeable future. We are unable to intelligently read our incorporation documents or our corporate tax forms even though the spouse had tax preparation experience and filed all tax documents for the sole proprietorship without assistance from an accountant. We accept the premise that changes in the practice in subsequent years and changes in tax law may require adjustment in the legal structure of the business. Periodic review of the status of any pediatric private practice is recommended. Table 33–1 provides the features of each of the three common organizational structures (Hampton, 1986; Parish, 1986; Sullivan, 1986; Wood, 1986).

Developing a Business Plan

A business plan is the key to obtaining financing and to business success and should be developed as soon as the type of practice has been determined (Sims, 1992). A fundamental task in business planning is to set goals and objectives for development of the practice. Formulating strategies and establishing alternative courses of action to achieve the goals must be accomplished and must include the financial, physical, and human resources necessary for goal attainment (Dillon & Duke, 1991).

PLANNING FOR FINANCIAL RESOURCES

The financial aspects of the business plan include the initial or start-up costs for the entire practice (Sims, 1992). All expected expenses should be arranged within a monthly, quarterly, and yearly spending budget. Projected revenues for the practice should be compiled using the same time periods. Reviewing the finances and writing a short narrative on how the pediatric practice fits into the physical therapy market in the projected area will prepare the therapist to discuss the plan with other persons. Bankers, accountants, and businesspersons are able to review the feasibility of the plan. Two forms of the financial plan might be designed (Driskell, 1988). The short form should be designed to provide the lender an overview of the business. The long form complements the short form by providing detailed information to allow the practitioner to answer all questions. The two forms have the same format, but more detail is included in the longer form. The lender will need information on physical therapy in general, licensure and legal considerations, and the growth of physical therapy services. Include the types of services you will offer, referral sources, the available market, and information on your education and work experience. Provide the same information for other staff you intend to use. Explain how the loan will be used and the proposed method of repayment.

Professional assistance is recommended when designing the financial plan. Aydelotte and associates (1988) inferred that nurse entrepreneurs in private practice who sought assistance from sources other than nurses made higher incomes than nurses who sought assistance from other nurses when initially establishing a practice. These authors suggested that further research is needed to determine if assistance from sources other than nurses leads to higher income levels for private practice nurses. However, the inference is sufficient to suggest that expertise in business is critical to accurate development of a financially sound business plan and that physical therapists may not possess the knowledge necessary for financial planning for a pediatric private practice. We suggest that new practitioners seek sufficient advice to minimize financial risks.

Therapists with a written plan and an understanding of the financial risk should apply for the needed capital from a bank. Aydelotte and associates (1988) found that nurses who used sources of venture capital other than personal savings received higher gross income than nurses who used individual savings. No explanation was offered by the authors, but the possibility exists that true entrepreneurial ventures and subsequent income might be restricted if only existing savings are considered in planning. However, the loan application for a novice businessperson may be denied by the bank, and the plan and presentation may need to be adjusted before proceeding to the next bank (Sims, 1992). The banker may want a financial projection for 1 to 5

TABLE 33–1. Characteristics of the Three Major Legal Structures of a Business

Sole Proprietorship	Partnership	Corporation
Easiest to initiate, sell, or dissolve; taxed on business profits that are considered personal income; owner personally liable for the debts; owner's personal assets at risk if sued (Parish, 1986)	Two or more people share costs and profits; each partner is liable; each partner is taxed personally; should involve written agreement that describes control of business, insurance, time, functions and duties of each partner, division of profits and loss; buy-sell agreement needed; all partners liable for the actions of each other (Parish, 1986)	Identity separate from the owner; owner may be an employee; business is taxed separately from the owner as an employee (Parish, 1986)
Simplest, most common form of legal structure; more than 70% of all business organizations are sole proprietorships, but only 8% of total gross income of businesses is from sole proprietorship (Hampton, 1986)	May restrict liability by being a limited partner if one partner has unlimited liability; written agreement not required but recommended (Hampton, 1986)	Variations in type of corporation (Hampton, 1986)
Owner has full responsibility for conducting business; owner reaps the profits; can minimize liability risks through careful financial management (Sullivan, 1986)	Each partner carries risk of personal property; allows for maximizing assets to start the business; capital costs may be divided among partners; the impact of debt, illness, or lack of ability in a particular aspect of the business is reduced (Sullivan, 1986)	Personal assets are protected unless personal negligence of the officers; owners personally guarantee loans for the corporation; state laws for corporation may differ from federal tax law (Sullivan, 1986)
Subject to the fewest governmental restrictions; provides the greatest autonomy; owner pays self-employment tax; usually uses Social Security number as business taxpayer identification number; must pay quarterly tax estimates; fringe benefits are not always deductible; employees may be hired or contracts with other practitioners may be developed on an as-needed basis (Wood, 1986)	Partners share control and authority; one partner's reputation extends to other partners; partners must compromise; philosophies of all partners must agree for successful partnership; any number of persons can form a partnership; the overhead costs for several or all partners may be less than for each practitioner separately; individual goals may change, leading to partner incompatibility; several types of partnerships (Wood, 1986)	Close governmental regulations; expensive to form because of legal and filing fees; adaptable to both small and large practices; deductible fringe benefits may be available to corporate employees; may enhance image of the business; the act of incorporating helps produce guidelines for dealing with problems (Wood, 1986)

years, which is a difficult task for many new private practitioners. Nevertheless, adequately capitalizing for the needs of the practice at the beginning and adhering to a budget will minimize financial pressures (Walker, 1977).

Money must flow into the practice if the business is to continue. The business plan should include obtaining enough income to cover salaries for 4 to 6 months. The bank will assist in establishing a line of credit so that only the amount of money needed for expenses will be borrowed. The base of referrals is the financial foundation to a practice, and time will be required to establish a referral base in a community. Be innovative in marketing the services of the practice, and do not rely on referrals from one or two sources to maintain the practice. A maximum of 5% of referrals from any one source will avoid financial pressures should the source terminate referrals. Initially, the private practitioner may need to accept referrals from any source, but the goal of diversity among referral sources should be sought as the practice develops (Sims, 1992).

While speaking to a group of students regarding private practice, Finch (1982) remarked that if he terminated his practice of approximately 15 years, he could still receive an income for 2 to 3 years from his outstanding accounts. Cash flow may be very slow in the initial stages of a practice, and numerous accounts will require several months or more for collection. We experienced very minimal cash flow for the first 2 years of the practice, and accounts receivable mounted. We now average $125,000 to

$150,000 in accounts receivable at any given time. A major third-party payer once delayed payment of a large account for 3 years. We have found that many insurance companies will require numerous requests before payment is sent. Learn how to bill and collect for your services by recognizing what different insurance companies require for claim submission, as well as what each will pay when billed. A universal billing form (Form HCFA-1500) is acceptable to many insurance companies and is available for purchase. (Refer to Appendix I for the address for ordering the universal billing form.) The Health Care Financing Administration in cooperation with the American Medical Association periodically reviews and modifies the form, and the practitioner should be aware of the need to obtain the most recently approved form.

Medicaid is a federally funded program administered by a state agency to provide reimbursement for medical services for low-income clients and includes physical therapy services. Many pediatric clients will have Medicaid funding, and billing for these clients can be accomplished through electronic billing on a computer. The state provides the necessary software and in-service training on electronic billing, and this method is superior in processing and collection. Presently, insurance companies accept electronic billing but also seek copies of all intervention documentation. We do not find the electronic billing process helpful with most private insurance companies.

Our practice was opened with no established referral base. Miraculously, four clients were referred after contact with pediatricians and orthopedic surgeons and formed the income source for the first few weeks. The owner moonlighted on weekends at a general hospital to pay the costs of the business for the first 4 months. Contracts with school districts and other agencies were negotiated, and additional clients were referred to the office. Several contracts with state-supported centers for children with developmental disabilities have been available at various times. These centers desire their own employees but contract with the practice when necessary. Most of our client base for several years has been for individual care.

The determination of fees to be charged for services may be simple or complex. The fee schedule may be based on the general fee structure of other service providers in the geographic area, but if the private practitioner has lower overhead costs than agencies or other providers, the fees may be appropriately lower. Major insurance companies will have established "usual and customary" rates, and payment for pediatric physical therapy services will be based on those rates regardless of the established fees

of the practice. Practitioners should charge only for services rendered, should establish fees commensurate with the costs of providing the services, should disclose the schedul of fees, and should learn to discuss fees with potential clients or their caretakers (Bernstein, 1986).

PLANNING FOR PHYSICAL RESOURCES

Office space is an important consideration when preparing the business plan. The space should meet the needs of both clients and staff and provide for the placement of needed equipment so that an efficient flow can occur (Sims, 1992). Walker (1977) suggests listing space and utility requirements and drawing a tentative floor plan before shopping for office space. He notes that the needs of the practice will change and growth should be anticipated. An office might be considered a luxury at first but will become a necessity as the practice grows. A waiting area is nonproductive space but will be necessary to meet the needs of clients and families. Restrooms also are a necessity, and local and state codes may determine whether employees and clients may use the same restroom facilities and whether the space may be used by both genders. Remember to note parking and accessibility needs when planning or selecting space. Water supply, storage closets and cabinets, cleaning and maintenance, utility costs, convenience for the targeted market, and the option to extend the lease are other important considerations in acquiring space.

We chose to rent a two-room office with a 3-year lease. The rent was satisfactory and the location was one of convenience to the owner's home, but no market survey or other consideration was given to the location as a marketing tool to acquire clients. No lawyer reviewed the lease, and although the specifics of the lease were adequate, the time frame proved too long for our needs. We were unaware of the advice to allow for growth, and we desired larger space before the lease expired. Luckily, the company that held the lease was able to offer us an office with more space at a nearby location. Because the move was profitable for the company, we were allowed to terminate the first lease with no penalty.

For the initial office, a handmade divider separated the waiting area from the "office" in one room, and the second room was used for treatment. We shared restroom space with another office. This arrangement was never satisfactory because of the need to modify the restroom for pediatric clients. Private practices for adult clients may have individual treatment rooms, partitioned areas within a larger treatment area, or a large gym area with no cubicles. In a pediatric office, the treatment area for infants and toddlers might be separate from treatment areas for older children, but our experience has not indicated the need for numerous treatment rooms or cubicles. We eventually needed a room for a billing office, a room for staff desks, and a room for casting. The space we selected at that time also had three additional rooms that were used for treatment, but one large space would have been adequate. Although individual treatment areas provide privacy for clients and diversity of design to meet specific client needs, the requirements for additional electrical wiring, ventilation, lighting, decorating, and equipment increase costs. If the tentative floor plan is drawn to scale and incorporates the planned use of the space for ambulation, exercise, play, or other activities, the practitioner should be able to identify space requirements. A realtor will be helpful in locating suitable space, in negotiating the price, and in arranging for structural changes in the space if warranted for the practice, and a lawyer should review the lease.

Some practitioners interested in private practice will find themselves in an employed position with a contract that prohibits competing with the employer in a certain geographic area or for a specific period of time following employment. This restriction may limit the choice of locations. Burch and Iglarsh (1988) suggest that at least 5 miles and probably 7.5 to 10 miles should exist between the practice location and other competitors and that this distance usually satisfies legal issues regarding competition clauses. Pediatric therapists with no legal encumbrances to geographic location will want to consider the distance between the private practice and other pediatric service providers. Pediatric therapists, however, may have a smaller percentage of a market area as potential clients than other specialists and may need to draw from a larger geographic base. The uniqueness of the private practice environment may allow competition with other pediatric service providers.

Our practice was initiated in a city with a population of approximately 200,000 persons and with two established pediatric outpatient agencies and a children's hospital that provided outpatient services. At the time we established the service, no other pediatric private practices existed, but we were not certain that a city of that size could support a practice limited to pediatrics. As indicated previously, we had to revise our practice goals to accommodate the marketplace, but the practice was very successful. Over the next several years, numerous physical therapists engaged in pediatric private practice and occupational therapists also established practices limited to pediatrics. Although we have changed locations several times since the practice began, the market for

our practice continues to be the entire city (which now has a population of approximately 250,000 persons), surrounding smaller towns, and a few sites in other areas of the state. The current office is located in close proximity to several pediatric physician offices, but these offices do not form a strong referral base for the practice. Proximity to other providers and to a physician referral base are suggestions for the locations of adult practices in larger cities or states, but we are unable to determine if these suggestions apply to pediatric practices.

Equipment needs include both office equipment and physical therapy equipment. Office equipment may cost up to $10,000 (Sims, 1992), and estimates for physical therapy equipment offered to us by private practitioners engaged in orthopedic practice varied from $100,000 to $300,000. Pediatric private practitioners are able to initiate a practice with much less funding. The specific disabilities of the clients who will be served will influence the selection of physical therapy equipment, but an office that provides play-based therapy for clients who are developmentally challenged might require only mats, therapeutic balls, bolsters, mirrors, toys, and a standing/ambulation area. Bernstein (1986) notes that crayons, dolls, blocks, and brand-name toys may serve the needs of younger children, but games and more sophisticated entertainment are required for older children.

An office practice providing services to pediatric clients with orthopedic or other disabilities would have specific equipment needs, and equipment requirements are mandated by at least one major funding source for pediatric clients. If the practice provides services for clients funded by Medicaid, you will need to be Medicare certified, which is interpreted to mean that all physical therapy treatments could be provided by the practice. Each state has enormous latitude in deciding how the regulations will be interpreted and which services will be reimbursable. Heat, cold, electrotherapy, and other physical agents may be required by the specific official who inspects the office for compliance with Medicare requirements. The state agency should be contacted to obtain a list of the requirements for certification before final equipment costs are determined. Even if you do not see clients with diagnoses that would require physical agents, you must be able to provide those services if you are seeking Medicaid reimbursement for any clients.

Our initial office was very modest with minimal furniture and office equipment. The treatment room consisted of a mat placed on the floor, a large wall mirror, and numerous toys. Although the initial cost for these items was only several hundred dollars, the office was not certified for Medicaid clients at that time. The current office contains a large, carpeted treatment room with floor mat, therapeutic balls, bolsters, shelves, and toys. One small treatment room contains a floor mat, a large mirror, shelves, and toys, and the other small treatment room contains a platform mat and large mirror. The hall and large treatment room provide space for walking, as does the outdoor sidewalk and lawn areas in good weather. The waiting room is very small. The casting room contains a sink and cabinets; the billing office has a desk, desk chair, side chair, telephone, and computer; and the staff office contains several desk areas, a reception area with a window opening into the waiting room, telephone, lamp, computer, typewriter, copier, and other office equipment. Although the equipment assets of the practice now total several thousand dollars, these assets were obtained over several years. The typical pediatric physical therapy practice will never experience equipment costs in the hundred thousand dollar range. We chose to add audiology to our practice, and the audiology booth was in excess of $60,000.

PLANNING FOR HUMAN RESOURCES

A practitioner may employ other therapists and staff or contract for other services if needed. The solo practitioner will have difficulty attending continuing education programs, taking vacation time, or using sick leave unless help is available. Burch and Iglarsh (1988) recommend finding a therapist who can be trusted with the practice to offer relief to the solo practitioner. Employing or contracting with other therapists and support staff requires an understanding of laws and regulations for personnel. The services of the lawyer and tax consultant for the practice can be used to determine the best plan for obtaining the services of other persons.

Planning for needed support staff must be as deliberate as planning for other aspects of the business (Sims, 1992). Office staff must have the equipment necessary to accomplish the required tasks, must be clearly informed of the job responsibilities, and must be given time to learn the equipment and the management systems for the practice. Some practices use a medical billing and collecting firm to manage accounts receivable if the staff does not have expertise in billing.

An administrative assistant may provide the expertise in business management not typically possessed by the physical therapist owner. Private practices have differing needs, and the administrative assistant may be an on-the-job trained office manager or a certified public accountant and financial planner (Wilson, 1992). The owner must determine the needs of the practice, seek an administrative assistant with the skills necessary to meet needs, and

relinquish the responsibilities and tasks to the administrative assistant. The administrative assistant may have responsibility for any task that is not directly treatment related, but all administrative assistants should have experience with preparation and collection of accounts receivable. Lynch (1992) suggests that the administrative assistant should mirror the practitioner/owner in personality, image, competence, and commitment. The PPS has supported the development of the Private Practice Physical Therapy Administrative Assistants group, which has bylaws and publishes a newsletter. This group meets at annual meetings of the PPS and provides excellent information and support for administrative assistants and private practitioners.

Salaries for yourself and other staff, if employed, are the major expense of a service business. A friend with a long-standing adult orthopedic private practice suggested establishing a 3-year goal for the owner to reach the salary that was abandoned to start the practice. The first-year salary for the owner for our practice was set at $15,000, the amount necessary to supplement the spouse's salary for our personal expenses. As previously noted, the spouse provided billing services and no other staff were employed. The telephone answering machine served as receptionist when a client was being treated. All bills and the salary as established were paid, and the net loss for the first year was $97.00. During the second year, an additional therapist was hired as an independent contractor, and the salary available to the owner exceeded the salary originally determined to be the 3-year goal. The salary level for the owner grew at a rapid rate, and competitive salaries were soon offered to therapists employed by the practice.

As a practice grows, a decision will have to be made on whether to keep the practice small or to allow growth and to offer exclusively physical therapy services or to expand into other services. During the first 10-year period, our practice expanded to include 14 physical therapists, 1 full-time and 1 part-time secretary, and 1 administrative assistant. In retrospect, the administrative assistant should have been employed earlier and responsibilities for billing should have been delegated from the beginning. Several sources offer suggestions for recruiting and retaining quality staff in a physical therapy private practice (Deaton & Gutterud, 1992; McNeil, 1990, 1991).

RISK MANAGEMENT IN MAINTAINING A PRIVATE PRACTICE

Resource development and availability are importance aspects of the business plan. As the practice matures, the practitioner will need to continually assess the strengths and weaknesses of the practice, take advantage of change, and exhibit management control (Dillon & Duke, 1991). Management control involves using resources in an effective manner to accomplish the goals and objectives of the practice. Dillon and Duke (1991) suggest the use of critical success factors, the crucial components of a business, to achieve success. The owner should identify the specific key components and measure performance by focusing on these components through information gathering and reporting. Deaton (1992a) noted that therapists in private practice often use computer programs to collect and produce lengthy reports that do not highlight the crucial components of the business. For example, information on the number of units of service for each referring physician would not be useful in a practice in which the therapists determine the frequency and type of treatment procedures to be provided. Information on the number of units of service generated each month would be useful in determining peak service months and in planning for vacations and staffing.

Dillon and Duke (1991) provide several questions that may assist the owner in identifying the critical success factors for the practice. Measurable indicators for each critical success factor must be determined and used for management control. Indicators should allow comparison to a desired level of performance, use staff input to enhance compliance and cooperation, be reliable, provide timely information, and allow for simple identification of problem areas.

We did not employ risk management concepts using critical success factors or any other type of control processes when the business was initiated, nor for the first several years. Experience in accounts receivable collection enhanced success, but luck was a primary factor in maintaining the practice. Eventually, we realized the need to gather information on the number of patients treated in each facility and at the office; the collection rate for different insurance companies; the cost of each employee, including vacation time, sick time, and continuing education time and expenses; the revenue generated by each employee; and the cost of supplies and casting materials. We perceived this information as comprising the critical success factors for our business, and as control over these crucial components was established and maintained, the profit for the practice increased significantly. As when planning a practice, the financial, physical, and human resources should be considered in maintaining a successful practice.

Maintaining Financial Resources

Efficient collection of outstanding accounts and determination of when to refer an account to an attorney or a collection agency for assistance in bringing the account current are important but difficult tasks. As previously mentioned, many accounts will be outstanding for lengthy periods of time. Prompt and consistent billing of new charges and reminders of outstanding charges will allow for continual collections after the first year or so of practice. The owner must establish standards by which credit is extended to clients and by which sufficient information is obtained to enable collection of an account should delinquency occur. In addition to the demographic information obtained from clients at the initiation of treatment, the owner or staff member responsible for billing should find out where the individual responsible for payment of the charges is employed and where banking is done. If possible, a copy of the bank account number should be obtained by copying one of the checks (Merry, 1992), and the insurance or Medicaid card should be copied. Figure 33-1 provides an example of the form we used to gather client information. Merry (1992) provides suggestions on contracts with clients, collecting debt, terminating services for clients with delinquent accounts, and using an attorney to collect accounts. He notes that failure to implement and follow collection practices will be costly to a private practice. Newell (1988) provides samples of a payment policy statement, a reminder letter, and a final notice letter, as well as suggestions for collecting accounts by telephone.

We require the party responsible for payment to authorize payment of benefits to the practice (see Fig. 33-1). This necessitates that all billing be done by the practice rather than having clients submit claim forms, but we are comfortable with the collection rate obtained through the use of assignment of benefits to the practice. Occasionally, an insurance company will reimburse the client for services. If an authorization for payment to the practice is on file, however, the insurance company will pay the practice and assume responsibility for recovery of the payment from the client.

Financial resources may be compromised by unethical staff. Deaton (1992a) asked a large audience of private practice physical therapists to indicate the incidence of stealing by staff. Over 50% of the practitioners indicated that staff had taken funds from the practice. In our practice, we believe that billing specialists managed to divert several thousand dollars into personal accounts on two separate occasions. Staff members are able to bill for relatives who never received services and for fictitious clients using a false address. A second bank account may be established for deposits. The owner may never know that the false billing has occurred. An accountant will be able to assist in planning to prevent stealing and in designing safeguards for the owner who is not competent in the business aspects of the practice.

CLIENT:	ADDRESS:	PHONE #:	SS #:	DATE OF BIRTH:	SEX: Male ——— Female ———	DIAGNOSIS:		
PHYSICIAN:	PHYSICIAN'S ADDRESS:	PHYSICIAN'S PHONE #:	PARENT'S NAMES and SS #: Father: SS#: Mother: SS #:	PARENT'S ADDRESS:	PARENT'S PHONE #: Home: Work:			
INSURANCE INFO: Primary Insurance Company:	Employer:	Employee:	ID #:	Group #:	OTHER INSURANCE: Secondary Insurance Company:	Employer:	Employee:	ID #:

ASSIGNMENT OF BENEFITS

I authorize payment of medical benefits be paid directly for services rendered.

_____
Signature

AUTHORIZATION FOR TREATMENT

I authorize treatment be given as ordered by my physician.

_____
Signature

AUTHORIZATION TO RELEASE MEDICAL INFORMATION

I authorize release of any medical information to another physician or insurance company to assist in treatment or claim processing.

_____
Signature

FIGURE 33–1. Example of a client information sheet and assignment form for a private practice.

Ball and Lindquist (1998) report that government and law enforcement agencies are intensely scrutinizing health care practices. They suggest developing and implementing a compliance program with internal policies consistent with the business and with the law. The compliance program will allow identification of potentially volatile situations and avoid activities that could expose you to charges of fraud.

Our practice referral base is largely through the state system of case management coordinators, and well over 50% of our clients have Medicaid funding. Despite awareness of the recommendation that no more than 5% of referrals should occur from one referral source, we are unable to alter our referral base. Many pediatric therapists will find that current laws and regulations ensure services to infants and toddlers through mechanisms funded by the state, and that referral source will form a substantial portion of the revenue for a practice. We experienced a severe cash flow problem in the tenth year of business when the state funding for Medicaid was jeopardized by low state revenues. Very quickly, the state owed more than $100,000, and the business experienced the only true threat to continuation. The funds were eventually paid in full, but we learned that a successful business could be at risk if a major funding source was eliminated.

Likewise, if the business continues to grow, cash flow problems will recur. Employees will often be paid several months before the funds generated by the employees are received. Each owner will have to determine the desire for growth and the tolerance for cash flow difficulties. An established practice will be able to maintain an ongoing line of credit with the bank and to pay bills and employees while experiencing growth. Dobrin (1991) cautions that loans for growth may be difficult to obtain unless an existing base of clients is evident.

Fonte (1998) and Cohen (1998) have suggested strategies to avoid the influence of managed care on financial resources. Many adult practices are becoming cash-only practices or are only accepting clients with private-pay insurers. Pediatric therapists will need to monitor the environment to determine if these strategies can be successful for pediatric clients.

Maintaining Physical Resources

Although physical resources, particularly office space and location, may change with growth of the practice, few pediatric therapists will have yearly purchases of expensive equipment as is the case for therapists engaged in practice areas using ever-advancing, high-technology equipment. In our practice, the purchase of tests and measures, electrotherapy equipment, casting supplies, and equipment for ambulation have resulted in expenditures in the area of physical resources. Mats, therapeutic balls and bolsters, and equipment for therapists who provide services outside the office have been purchased. Much of the initial equipment is still in use after 16 years of practice, and few major equipment expenses have occurred with the exception of the expansion of our practice into audiology services. Toys and expendable play supplies represent the largest portion of expenses for the practice beyond salaries, health insurance, mileage reimbursement, and continuing education.

Maintaining Human Resources

A challenge for private practitioners is attracting and retaining qualified physical therapists (Deaton & Gutterud, 1992). In 1990, McNeil suggested that the gap between supply and demand was still increasing at an intimidating rate and that private practices experience employee turnover of up to 40% annually. New and experienced therapists and assistants are seeking the best employment offer, and owners must offer a salary and benefit package that is competitive (Deaton & Gutterud, 1992). An increase in the number of schools, the number of graduates, and the number of graduates interested in pediatrics has occurred in the last several years, and we find filling positions much easier. McNeil (1990) notes that role modeling, having a defined philosophy of management, gaining credibility with employees, and offering opportunities for growth and development are some key points in reducing turnover in physical therapy private practices. In order to retain the best possible employees, we believe that we must adhere to good management practices regardless of the availability of practitioners.

Most of the therapists and physical therapist assistants in our practice work in relative isolation, meeting only weekly for a staff conference or for supervisory sessions between therapists and assistants. This isolation is common in private practice but presents a particular challenge for pediatric therapists who are accustomed to center-based practices. New graduates in our practice have had fewer adjustment difficulties than experienced therapists, and this phenomenon was a surprise to the owner, who was hesitant to employ new graduates in a private practice with so many isolated activities. One explanation for the success with new graduates may be that educational programs are preparing graduates for diverse practice environments. All of the new graduates employed in recent years have held the entry-level master of science degree. New graduates receive orientation and mentoring on a planned basis, and all therapists and assistants have access to their co-workers by telephone. Social activities are included in the weekly staff meetings to promote a sense of belonging and collegiality.

Student affiliation agreements are maintained with one physical therapist assistant and four physical therapist educational programs. Students participate in all aspects of the practice and serve as a source for recruitment, as well as motivators for the staff. Students often provide in-service presentations and perform unique projects that stimulate therapists, assistants, and clients.

Continued education and opportunities for growth are of primary importance in our practice. Information regarding specialized skills, such as inhibitive casting or family-guided services, are shared freely among practitioners either through consultation or in-service education. The practice supports graduate or other formal education experiences. Tuition reimbursement is available to therapists and physical therapist assistants who seek further academic education. Achievement of specialization is fostered, and therapists in addition to the owner and co-therapist have become certified pediatric specialists.

Attracting therapists who would travel to multiple locations, including some potentially unsafe home environments, was also a challenge for our practice. We have attempted to balance this challenge with the practical benefit of reimbursing mileage costs and with philosophic advantages. Each therapist is offered the opportunity to provide services within a philosophy of private practice including maximal autonomy, self-governance, reduced bureaucracy, and independence in exercising professional judgment. Each assistant is afforded similar opportunity within the constraints of supervision and delegation. The result has been a good retention rate.

Between 1982 and 1998, our practice grew to more than 40 employees, including occupational therapists, speech-language pathologists, audiologists, a nurse, and four separate offices. The state Medicaid funding changes of 1998 and managed care payers forced the need to downsize the practice and salaries (which were highly competitive) or increase the productivity of each employee. Several therapists matured into practitioners who were willing to take risks in their own private practices rather than take potential decreases in salary, and left the practice. Our success in getting these practitioners to adopt the philosophy of private practice resulted in an eventual loss to the practice and increased competition as new practices developed. A common discussion at meetings of the PPS is that good employees must be made partners or they will eventually become competitors. We have chosen to remain as owners without partners and accept the risks that are inevitable with that decision. We expect the practice to remain smaller at least until the full impact of managed care allows for more accurate forecasting of financial risks.

TRENDS IN PRIVATE PRACTICE

Issues identified by the Private Practice Section of the APTA as potentially harmful to private practitioners include the rapid growth of non–physical therapist corporate-owned practices and cost-containment measures that provide inequitable constraints on physical therapists. The Private Practice Section has acknowledged that physical therapists need to take a proactive stance in addressing these issues. Pediatric physical therapy is not exempt from these concerns, and many pediatric therapists are not reimbursed for services or are reimbursed at a lower rate if services are provided in a private practice setting rather than in a hospital or rehabilitation center.

Most therapists, including those in private practice, do not have a business background, and the Private Practice Section participates in a monthly publication, *Advance for Directors in Rehabilitation*, to provide information on business as well as clinical issues. The annual meeting of the Private Practice Section is designed to provide additional educational opportunities for private practitioners, and regional meetings are held each year.

The Section on Pediatrics of the APTA has recognized some movement toward private practice among section members. The movement appears to be primarily for increased autonomy and because of disenchantment with practice settings in which pediatric therapists perceive themselves as "revenue generators" for a facility rather than as caregivers for clients (Dasch & Finney, 1991).

Current trends indicate the need for physical therapists to move into environments such as health maintenance organizations, preferred provider arrangements, and point-of-service plans and less often into individual practice settings. One projection is that physical therapist–owned practices using a group mode will be more common as the base for practice than the solo mode (Moffat, 1991). Faust and Meaker (1991) suggest that a group private practice can have the three key elements: (1) high autonomy, (2) strong professional identity, and (3) low bureaucracy. These authors note that therapists tend to distance themselves from the important topics of reimbursement, business, and administration. Group practice might allow several therapists to combine resources to address these business needs and to meet the essential practice roles of clinical services, management, administration, and professional activities.

Moffat (1991) also recommends using the skills of the physical therapist assistant to complement practice and to free therapists to maximize their own skills. Assistants have traditionally been encouraged to seek general hospital experiences (Infante et al., 1976; Larson & Davis, 1975; Physical Therapy Assistant Program, 1975). Settings providing specialized health care have been suggested as appropriate for employment of the assistant (Lovelace-Chandler & Lovelace-Chandler, 1979).

The private practice arena offers numerous opportunities for appropriate use of physical therapist assistants. Understanding the academic preparation of the assistant and adhering to the ethical guidelines of the APTA (1991b, 1996) and the legal restrictions of the state are important prerequisites to determining the appropriate roles of assistants in any practice arena. Our philosophy includes the belief that no treatment techniques performed in the duties of the practice are inconsistent with the qualifications of the assistant. Tasks related to treatment are delegated only after a therapist performs the initial examination and establishes a care plan. We have identified factors, including individual patients' differences, unique circumstances, individual assistants' competencies, and acute or severe problems, that might restrict the delegation of tasks (Lovelace-Chandler & Lovelace-Chandler, 1979). We also have suggested how to develop a job description for the physical therapist assistant, determine the skills of an assistant, and provide education or remediation if skills are lacking. We have experienced a general reluctance on the part of pediatric physical therapists to use the skills of the physical therapist assistant. The pediatric therapist in private practice must recognize that effective use of assistants is essential to providing high-quality services at the lowest cost.

Health care reforms will require more emphasis on prevention and on health restoration (Moffat, 1991). The low level of bureaucracy of private practice provides the unique opportunity to quickly respond to shifts in public policy and to play a major role in prevention. Pediatric therapists must assume responsibility for accident prevention among clients and families. Education on safety should be provided to families and caregivers for all of the child's environments and to older children who can assume responsibility for accident prevention. For example, children who use a wheelchair must learn independent mobility without compromising the safety of themselves or those around them. Education on safety should also include parents, siblings, teachers, and classmates. Physical therapists in private practice might contract with the state child care licensing agency or the state insurance carrier to provide instruction to personnel in state-supported child care centers in appropriate lifting and handling techniques for children with disabilities.

The promotion of patient and family education is important in all aspects of therapy (Moffat, 1991), but pediatric therapists must be particularly responsive to the legislative mandates for family-guided care. Private practitioners must seek methods that allow reimbursement for educational activities with clients. Group practices might include health educators, case managers, or other persons with expertise in client and family education.

Economic trends of the next millenium may hinder growth for private practitioners. Dobrin (1991) suggests that physical therapists may counteract this trend by marketing in a concerted manner to promote the practice. Brown and Morley (1986) suggest that four factors are essential to developing a marketing plan:

1. Determine the needs and wants of your clients (in the case of pediatric physical therapy, the needs and wants of the families) and examine your practice from the viewpoint of the client. A consumer survey may be effective in determining the perspectives of families and of older clients served by your practice.

2. The marketing philosophy and methods of marketing should be shared with and accepted by all staff.

3. Ethical methods of marketing are a necessity. The responsibilities and ethics of the professional transcend the quest for economic survival. A good marketing plan will reinforce and enhance the socially responsible principle of providing high-quality, cost-effective care that is in the best interest of the client and family.

4. The marketing plan must be executed in a cost-effective manner. The public will not begrudge efforts to increase profit through marketing if the profits are viewed as reasonable and the service meets health care needs. Momberg (1988) recommends that physical therapists spend 5% to 10% of any anticipated increased profits on advertising. The higher percentage is expended during the initial aspects of establishing the business or in marketing a new service, and the lower percentage is recommended for ongoing advertising.

Trzecki (1988) recommends the VIP method of visibility, image, and promotion for marketing physical therapy services. When conducted correctly, promotion highlights visibility and enhances image. Money directed to marketing is directed away from client services (Barone, 1988), and only the amount needed to market the practice in a dignified and professional manner should be expended. The ethics of marketing is unquestioned if the practitioner believes that the practice offers the highest quality of services and that these services are equal to or exceed the quality of services provided by competitors (Brown & Morley, 1986). Failure to market the services would deprive potential clients of access to quality care. Ensuring dignity and responsibility for marketing and advertisement rests with the individual practitioner. "Communicate your passion, caring and expertise and your market will break down your doors" (Barone, 1988, p. 47). Numerous resources exist to assist the pediatric private practitioner in planning marketing strategies (Abeln, 1993; Adams, 1993; Baum, 1992; Davidson, 1987; Dohallow, 1993; Klehfoth, 1993; Nosse & Friberg, 1992; Patin & Adams, 1991; Schunk, 1989; Schunk & Jaffe, 1993).

THE UNIQUE PHILOSOPHY OF PEDIATRIC PHYSICAL THERAPY

Any practitioner considering a private practice limited to pediatric physical therapy must be cognizant of the uniqueness of pediatrics as a specialty. Cherry (1991) has summarized the philosophy, the scientific components, and the quantitative and qualitative differences that must be considered in selecting treatment techniques that meet the needs of children. Albeit evolved from the philosophy and techniques of the wider field of physical therapy, pediatric physical therapy is distinguished by a distinct philosophy. Inherent in this philosophy are the beliefs that a child is viewed as a whole person existing in the context of the family and with natural ecologic settings, that the developmental characteristics of children require unique knowledge of existing and future development, and that children require advocacy.

The natural ecologic settings for children are the home and school (Cherry, 1991). Other common settings include child care centers, churches or other religious environments, and settings where leisure activities are enjoyed. Therapists in private practice must be willing to provide services within natural settings, using the natural activities of the settings as the intervention strategies. Private practitioners must accept family members, in addition to the child, as clients with wishes and needs, and be responsive to those wishes and needs. Otherwise services will be sought from facilities or practitioners who identify and implement family goals. Family-focused therapy became prominent in the United States after the passage of PL 99-457, and the private practitioner has numerous resources available to assist in service design using family theory (see Chapter 31).

Developmental science, pediatric medical pathology, examination, and management of children with developmental disabilities form the scientific bases of pediatric physical therapy. Intervention strategies and procedures for children may be adapted from adult treatment or may be specific to the young client (Cherry, 1991). Private practitioners wishing to offer services to children must possess the unique knowledge and skills necessary for the practice of pediatrics.

RECOMMENDATIONS FOR BEST PRACTICE

The following recommendations summarize our beliefs regarding best practice in private practice physical therapy. We have not always followed these recommendations, but the business would probably have been more successful if we had done so. You will be able to determine which recommendations meet your philosophy of care and your needs regarding the financial, physical, and human resources of the practice.

1. Possess advanced skill in the specialty area of pediatrics. Although recognized specialization such as that awarded by the American Board of Physical Therapy Specialists (ABPTS) should not be a requirement for initiating a pediatric practice, any clinician who is not acquiring the skills essential to that credential should not be in pediatric private practice.

2. Gain knowledge of all appropriate laws, regulations, policies, and position statements that affect pediatric physical therapy. Federal laws have greatly influenced the practice of pediatric physical therapy in recent years, and state laws and regulations determine which pediatric therapy services are allowable and will be reimbursed. State and city laws and regulations affect the operation of the business.

3. Have persons with business skills available to the practice. The owner/therapist does not need to have knowledge of accounting, taxes, bookkeeping, and management, but this knowledge must be accessible to the business through the use of lawyers, accountants, bankers, and billing specialists. Business sense is required to achieve business cents (translate dollars).

4. Provide services that are needed in the marketplace. The trends in health care cost containment and private practice service provision will increase competition among health care providers. Pediatric therapists must be responsive to the needs and wants of clients and families.

5. Identify the quantity of services you can provide. Do not exceed that quantity, or quality will suffer.

6. Design the appropriate practice setting. If an office practice is used, the space and decor should reflect the clients you serve. Employ staff who support your philosophy and image.

7. Purchase the proper supplies. Experienced pediatric therapists will know that diapers, tissues, crayons, toys, games, holiday decorations, and stickers are more important purchases than massage lotion. Vendors who serve practices for adults may not be able to recommend the correct supplies for new pediatric practitioners.

8. Know how to interact and play with the clients you serve. New graduates may not have knowledge of play activities commensurate with their knowledge of therapeutic techniques. Seek continuing education or consultation for areas of service provision in which you are lacking.

9. Understand the natural environments for children. The work of children is their play, and children function within the context of family life, preschool, or school. Design the practice to fit into the lives of children and families.

10. Offer family-guided physical therapy in the private enterprise arena. Understand the context of the family and the advocacy role of the family. Develop cultural competence for the families you serve. Learn about the language, food, holiday, religious, childrearing, and discipline preferences of your clients. Accept the closeness you will develop with families and children. In private practice, professional distance is reduced. Demonstrate affection or even love for your clients. Aloofness and professional demeanor are inconsistent with the intimacy found in most private practices.

SUMMARY

The pediatric physical therapist in private practice has autonomy, uses professional values, and takes risks with a minimum of bureaucracy to achieve independence and success. The roles of owner, business manager, and clinician must coexist, and the private practitioner must seek services from such resources as accountants, bankers, lawyers, realtors, and other therapists to augment the knowledge and skills required for private practice. Personal and professional characteristics and responsibilities have been suggested by numerous authors, and possession or development of these attributes will diminish risk and liability. A private practice is established and maintained through selection of an appropriate legal structure and consideration of the necessary financial, physical, and human resources. Societal trends offer private practitioners the opportunity for creative business activities when services are envisioned

through the unique philosophy of pediatric physical therapy and with regard for best practices. Professionalism in pediatric physical therapy will be enhanced as an increased number of therapists enter the private practice arena.

References

Abeln, SH. A payer-based marketing approach. Physical Therapy Today, 16(1):25-29, 1993.

Adams, C. Preproduced marketing tools. Physical Therapy Today, 16(1):42-44, 1993.

American Physical Therapy Association. Code of Ethics. Alexandria, VA: APTA, 1991a.

American Physical Therapy Association. Standards of Ethical Conduct for the Physical Therapist Assistant. Alexandria, VA: APTA, 1991b.

American Physical Therapy Association. Guide for Conduct of the Affiliate Member. Alexandria, VA: APTA, 1996.

American Physical Therapy Association. Guide for Professional Conduct. Alexandria, VA: APTA, 1997a.

American Physical Therapy Association. Guide to physical therapist practice. Physical Therapy, 77:1163-1650, 1997b.

American Physical Therapy Association. Standards of Practice for Physical Therapy and the Criteria. Alexandria, VA: APTA, 1997c.

American Speech-Language-Hearing Association. Considerations for establishing a private practice in audiology and/or speech-language pathology. ASHA, 33(suppl 3):10-21, 1991.

Aydelotte, MK, Hardy, MA, & Hope, KL. Nurses in Private Practice: Characteristics, Organizational Arrangements, and Reimbursement Policy. Kansas City, MO: American Nurses' Foundation, 1988.

Ball, JA, & Lindquist, SC. Searching for fraud: Will your practice be the next target? Advance for Directors in Rehabilitation, 7(8):43-44, 1998.

Barone, DL. Being market-wise. Physical Therapy Today, 11(3):46-47, 1988.

Baskin, W. Making a move. Advance for Directors in Rehabilitation, 6(8):37, 39, 1997.

Baum, N. Marketing Your Clinical Practice Ethically, Effectively, Economically. Gaithersburg, MD: Aspen, 1992.

Bernstein, DK. Part-time private practice in speech-language pathology and audiology. In Butler, KG (Ed.), Prospering in Private Practice: A Handbook for Speech-Language Pathology and Audiology. Gaithersburg, MD: Aspen, 1986, pp. 13-46.

Brown, S. Sorry—I'm not in private practice. Clinical Management, 12(1):14-15, 1992.

Brown, SW, & Morley, AP. Marketing Strategies for Physicians: A Guide to Practice Growth. Oradell, NJ: Medical Economics Books, 1986.

Burch, EA, & Iglarsh, A. A conversation about starting a private practice. Physical Therapy Today, 11(4):37-42, 1988.

Campbell, SK. Physical Therapy for Children, 1st ed. Philadelphia: WB Saunders, 1994.

Carlson, T. Tom Carlson, 1987 Robert G. Dicus award winner. Whirlpool, 10:35-37, 1987.

Cherry, DB. Pediatric physical therapy: Philosophy, science, and techniques. Pediatric Physical Therapy, 3(2):70-75, 1991.

Cohen, RS. Running a cash-only practice: Tips to keep the minnows swimming upstream. Advance for Directors in Rehabilitation, 7(5):57-58, 63, 1998.

Cole, PR. Private practice: Personal prerequisites and potential. In Butler, KG (Ed.), Prospering in Private Practice: A Handbook for Speech-Language Pathology and Audiology. Gaithersburg, MD: Aspen, 1986, pp. 3-11.

Cooper, E. The state of the profession and what to do about it. ASHA, 24:931-936, 1982.

Dasch, D, & Finney, M. The future and specialty practice. Clinical Management, 11(6):26–33, 1991.

Davidson, JP. Advanced marketing techniques: Becoming your own press agent. Whirlpool, 10(1):38–42, 1987.

Deaton, WC. Do you know where your practice is tonight? Paper presented at the 1992 Private Practice Section Annual Conference and Exposition, Dallas, TX, November 11–15, 1992a.

Deaton, WC. Running your practice by the numbers. Physical Therapy Today, 15(2):31–35, 1992b.

Deaton, WC, & Gutterud, SR. Attracting and retaining quality staff: Using fringe benefits and incentive compensation. Physical Therapy Today, 15(3):44–47, 1992.

Dicus, RG. Origins of the self-employed section. Physical Therapy Today, 14(4):19–20, 22, 1991.

Dillon, RD, & Duke, PJ. Planning for success. Clinical Management, 11(5):28–32, 1991.

Dobrin, J. Private practice: Big, small, or not at all. Physical Therapy Today, 14(3):52, 54, 56, 1991.

Dohallow, J. A physical therapist's guide to marketing a private practice. Physical Therapy Today, 16(1):46–48, 1993.

Driskell, C. Planning for success: Developing a business plan to secure financing. Physical Therapy Today, 11(1):40–41, 1988.

Faust, L, & Meaker, MK. Private practice occupational therapy in the skilled nursing facility: Creative alliance or mutual exploitation? American Journal of Occupational Therapy, 45:621–627, 1991.

Finch, J. Private Practice Physical Therapy: Presentation for Physical Therapy Students. Conway, AR, 1982.

Flower, RM. Ethical concerns in private practice. In Butler, KG (Ed.), Prospering in Private Practice: A Handbook for Speech-Language Pathology and Audiology. Gaithersburg, MD: Aspen, 1986, pp. 101–123.

Fonte, AM. Boutique PT: How to succeed without managed care. Advance for Directors in Rehabilitation, 7(11):51–52, 1998.

Frazian, BW. Tidal surge and private practice: The historic eighties. In Cromwell, FS (Ed.), Private Practice in Occupational Therapy. New York: Haworth Press, 1985, pp. 7–13.

Guglielmo, FX. The 1988 Robert G. Dicus award recipient. Physical Therapy Today, 11(4):18–24, 1988.

Hack, LM. History, purpose, and structure of part two: Preferred practice patterns. PT Magazine, 6(6):72–79, 1998.

Hampton, D. Establishing and equipping an audiology private practice. In Butler, KG (Ed.), Prospering in Private Practice: A Handbook for Speech-Language Pathology and Audiology. Gaithersburg, MD: Aspen, 1986, pp. 135–148.

Huelskamp, S. Finding your niche: Niche marketing—an answer to staying competitive. Advance for Directors in Rehabilitation, 6(3):37, 39, 1997.

Infante, MS, Speranza, KA, & Gillespie, PW. An interdisciplinary approach to the education of health professional students. Journal of Allied Health, 5(4):13–22, 1976.

Jayaratne, S, Davis-Sacks, ML, & Chess, WA. Private practice may be good for your health and well-being. Social Work, 36(3):224–229, 1991.

Klehfoth, K. Public relations: The key to a profitable small practice. Physical Therapy Today, 16(2):34, 36, 1993.

Kooper, JD, & Sullivan, CA. Professional liability: Management and prevention. In Butler, KG (Ed.), Prospering in Private Practice: A Handbook for Speech-Language Pathology and Audiology. Gaithersburg, MD: Aspen, 1986, pp. 59–79.

Larson, CW, & Davis, ER. Following up the physical therapist assistant graduate: A curriculum evaluation process. Physical Therapy, 55:601–606, 1975.

Lovelace-Chandler, V, & Lovelace-Chandler, B. Employment of physical therapist assistants in a residential state school. Physical Therapy, 59(10):1243–1246, 1979.

Lynch, R. Selection of an administrative assistant. Physical Therapy Today, 15(2):50–51, 1992.

McClain, L, McKinney, J, & Ralston, J. Occupational therapists in private practice. American Journal of Occupational Therapy, 46:613–618, 1992.

McFadden, SM, & Hanschu, B. Risk taking in occupational therapy. In Cromwell, FS (Ed.), Private Practice in Occupational Therapy. New York: Haworth Press, 1985, pp. 3–6.

McNeil, LL. The people part of practice management. Physical Therapy Today, 13(1):34–35, 37–38, 40, 1990.

McNeil, LL. Employee turnover: Do we have a problem? Physical Therapy Today, 14(3):57–60, 1991.

Merry, TR. Ten commonly asked questions in dealing with accounts receivable: What every private practice owner would like to ignore but can't. Physical Therapy Today, 15(1): 59–62, 64–65, 1992.

Moffat, M. Beyond 2000: Who will you be? Clinical Management, 11(6):8–9, 1991.

Momberg, WA. Budgeting your advertising dollars. Physical Therapy Today, 11(3):48, 1988.

Newell, D. Collecting accounts receivable by telephone. Physical Therapy Today, 11(2):28–31, 1988.

Nosse, LJ, & Friberg, DG. Management Principles for Physical Therapists. Baltimore: Williams & Wilkins, 1992, pp. 177–191.

Parish, R. Constraints and commitments: An introduction to the financial aspects of private practice. In Butler, KG (Ed.), Prospering in Private Practice: A Handbook for Speech Language Pathology and Audiology. Gaithersburg, MD: Aspen, 1986, pp. 81–99.

Parsons, L. Planning and initiating a private practice in nursing psychotherapy. In Durham, JD, & Hardin, SB (Eds.), The Nurse Psychotherapist in Private Practice. New York: Springer, 1986, pp. 75–86.

Patin, S, & Adams, C. The marketing plan: An integrative tool for the future. Physical Therapy Today, 14(3):68, 70, 72, 1991.

Physical Therapy Assistant Program. Physical therapy assistant program evaluation. Charlotte, NC: Central Piedmont Community College, 1975.

Private Practice Section. 1992 profile of a private practice physical therapist. Physical Therapy Today, 15(3):60–69, 1992.

Private Practice Section. 1996 Member Needs and Assessment Survey. Washington, DC: PPS, APTA, 1996.

Private Practice Section. PPS Membership Votes to Retain Section Name and Mission Statement. PPS Impact, February 1997.

Reuss, R. The maturation of the private practice section. Physical Therapy Today, 14(4):24–26, 28–32, 34–36, 38–48, 1991.

Roussel, FJ, & Epplin, R. Thinking About Going into Business? Management Aid Number 2.025. Fort Worth, TX: U.S. Small Business Administration, 1987.

Schunk, C. The referral within: Marketing to your peers. Physical Therapy Today, 12(4):52–53, 1989.

Schunk, C, & Jaffe, RL. Teamwork: The marketing management tool. Physical Therapy Today, 16(1):31–32, 34, 37, 40, 1993.

Scull, S, & Deitz, J. Competencies for the physical therapist in the neonatal intensive care unit (NICU). Pediatric Physical Therapy, 1(1):11–14, 1989.

Selker, LG. Human resources in physical therapy: Opportunities for service in a rapidly changing health system. Physical Therapy, 75(1):31–37, 1995.

Sims, D. Wishing you continued success. Physical Therapy Today, 15(1):7–11, 1992.

Smoyak, SA. The nurse psychotherapist as unique practitioner. In Durham, JD, & Hardin, SB (Eds.), The Nurse Psychotherapist in Private Practice. New York: Springer, 1986, pp. 21–23.

Sullivan, CA. Business and management aspects of private practice in speech-language pathology and audiology. In Butler, KG (Ed.), Prospering in Private Practice: A Handbook for Speech-Language Pathology and Audiology. Gaithersburg, MD: Aspen, 1986, pp. 149–165.

Task Force on Early Intervention, Section on Pediatrics, APTA. Competencies for physical therapists in early intervention. Pediatric Physical Therapy, 3(2):77–80, 1991.

Trzecki, KJ. Considering marketing? Be a VIP. Physical Therapy Today, *11*(3):42–45, 1988.

Valente, CM. Member needs and assessment survey results. PPS Impact, June, 1996.

Walker, RC. Over My Shoulder: Reflections on Beginning a Private Practice in Physical Therapy. Cedar Rapids, IA: RC Walker, 1977.

Wilson, FD. Administrative assistants: What role should they play? Physical Therapy Today, *15*(2):47–49, 1992.

Wood, ML. Private Practice in Communication Disorders. Boston: College-Hill, 1986.

Woody, RH. Legal issues for private practitioners in speech language pathology and audiology. In Butler, KG (Ed.), Prospering in Private Practice: A Handbook for Speech-Language Pathology and Audiology. Gaithersburg, MD: Aspen 1986, pp. 47–57.

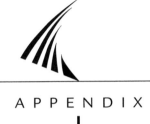

Resources for Information for the Pediatric Private Practitioner

American Physical Therapy Association
1111 N. Fairfax Street
Alexandria, VA 22314
1-800-999-APTA

Private Practice Section, APTA
1101 17th Street, NW, Suite 1000
Washington, DC 20036
202-457-1115

Pediatric Section, APTA
1111 N. Fairfax Street
Alexandria, VA 22314
1-800-999-APTA

Consult the U.S. Government section in the telephone directory for the Small Business Administration (SBA) office nearest you, or call 1-800-U ASK SBA.

A free SBA list of publications and videotapes may be obtained from

Small Business Directory
P.O. Box 1000
Ft. Worth, TX 76119

The Universal Billing Form (HCFA-1500) may be purchased at the following address:

American Medical Association
c/o The Order Department
P.O. Box 2964
Milwaukee, WI 53201

CHAPTER
34

Medicolegal Issues
in the United States

WENDY E. PHILLIPS, PT, PCS, MA, MS
MICHAEL L. SPOTTS, JD

OVERVIEW

The implementation of federal legislation along with increased litigation related to patient care and outcome in a rapidly evolving medical system increases the likelihood of an interaction between pediatric physical therapists and the legal system. A conceptual understanding of public laws, such as the Individuals with Disabilities Education Act (IDEA) (PL 105-17) and the Americans with Disabilities Act (ADA) (PL 101-336), is required of the practicing clinician or student who will be working with children and adolescents with disabilities and their families. Similarly, a familiarity with the litigation process as it is relevant to issues,

such as medical malpractice and petitions for the determination of appropriate medical treatment, is useful.

The purpose of this chapter is to provide an overview of IDEA and ADA. Also provided is an overview of the process of litigation as it is relevant to pediatric patients, using case histories as examples. The physical therapist's responsibility in reporting cases of child abuse and neglect is also included along with related ethical issues. The clinical implications of the federal legislation discussed are presented in several chapters of this book, particularly Chapter 32 on the educational environment and Chapter 31 on family-centered intervention.

Individuals with Disabilities Education Act

The Individuals with Disabilities Education Act is a federal law passed in 1975 (PL 94-142), reauthorized in 1990 (PL 101-476) and amended in 1997 (PL 105-17). It mandates that all children receive a free, appropriate public education regardless of the level or severity of their disability. It provides funds to assist states in the education of students with disabilities and requires that states ensure that such students receive an individualized education program. The student's individualized education program is to be based on the student's unique needs and is to be provided in the least restrictive environment possible. IDEA provides guidelines for determining what related services are necessary. This chapter reviews those sections of the law that are particularly relevant to the practice of physical therapy.

Americans with Disabilities Act

In an attempt to rectify past discrimination against individuals with physical and mental disabilities related to housing, employment, and other areas, the ADA (PL 101-336) was enacted. Although the ADA may appear to be related to the adult population of persons with disabilities, various provisions are directly or indirectly applicable to families who have children with disabilities. Aspects of the law that are particularly relevant to children and families will be discussed in this chapter.

For example, parents are protected from discrimination with respect to employment hiring practices based on their status as parents of a child with a disability. The act ensures that a parent cannot be denied health insurance for the family because of the child's condition. These and other provisions of the act that may affect children and families served by the pediatric physical therapist are discussed.

Child Abuse and Neglect

Although laws with respect to child abuse and neglect vary in the United States from state to state, their purpose is consistent: to protect children whose health and welfare are adversely affected and further threatened by the conduct of those responsible for their care and protection. The law dictates that certain persons, including hospital or medical personnel, report all suspected cases of abuse and neglect to the appropriate state agency. Failure to report a suspected case of abuse or neglect results in a misdemeanor charge.

Physical abuse, sexual abuse, and neglect are all conditions that by law must be reported. Child and adult behaviors associated with physical and sexual abuse may not be easily identified by the physical therapist. For example, the behaviors associated with child sexual abuse, including enuresis, nightmares, a decline in academic performance, secretiveness, and helpless behavior, may not routinely be identified as possibly related to suspected child sexual abuse. This section includes a description of child and adult behavior that may be associated with abuse, as well as a general protocol for the documentation and reporting of suspected abuse. Appropriate referrals to other professionals in situations of suspected abuse are also considered.

Litigation

Although litigation is an unsavory topic to many pediatric physical therapists, it has become common in the U.S. health care system. As the number of lawsuits increases, so does the probability that the pediatric physical therapist's examination and intervention documentation may be subpoenaed for use in court.

There are various reasons for an emphasis on objective and comprehensive documentation, including determination of progress and change and the evaluation of the effectiveness of intervention. When records may be reviewed or interpreted by persons who do not share the physical therapist's vocabulary and who are not familiar with specific treatment techniques, use of objective data and valid tests and measures is essential. With the use of a case history format, this chapter considers the usefulness and relevance of various types of documentation and includes a situation where the physical therapist's documentation was important in determining the outcome of the case.

Medical Technology

Technologic advances in medical treatment have increased the rate of survival of infants and children who are medically fragile. Increasingly, differences of opinion among medical professionals or between parents and medical professionals regarding the choice of treatment and the continuation or deceleration of medical support have been decided in the courts. An estimate of a child's present functional status or future outcome may be a consideration in the determination of a plan of appropriate medical care. Estimated functional outcome may be determined by the clinical opinion of the physician, psychologist, or physical therapist.

Formulation of an opinion or a functional prognosis for a child with a central nervous system deficit or congenital anomaly may not be a familiar task for the pediatric physical therapist. Should an opinion be requested, the pediatric physical therapist will require skills, including the ability to draw from past experience with similar cases and from the results of outcome-focused research studies, and in the presentation of the results of the assessment, which may include the use of standardized measures. A case history is presented in this chapter as an illustration.

A related issue involves the pediatric physical therapist's ability to identify any personal values and beliefs that may affect objectivity in the formulation of an opinion regarding a child's functional abilities and outcome. Consideration of the relationship between belief systems and decision making, as well as the influence of the therapist's ethical standards, is included in this chapter.

INDIVIDUALS WITH DISABILITIES ACT

Background and Purpose

The purpose of the Individuals with Disabilities Education Act is to ensure that all children with disabilities have access to free and appropriate educational services. This includes special educational services and related services that meet each child's unique needs. Physical therapy is considered one such related service. The act seeks to protect the rights of children and their parents while assisting states and localities in providing education for all children with disabilities. IDEA attempts to ensure the effectiveness of efforts to educate children with disabilities. The focus of this section of the chapter is to summarize the Individuals with Disabilities Act Amendments of 1997 (PL 105-17) that are particularly relevant to pediatric physical therapy.

The purposes for the 1997 amendments are as follows [20 USCS 14319 (b)]:

1. Develop and implement a statewide comprehensive, coordinated multidisciplinary interagency system that provides early intervention services for infants and toddlers with disabilities and their families

2. Facilitate the coordination of payments for early intervention services from federal, state and local and private sources (including public and private insurance coverage)

3. Enhance the capacity to provide quality early intervention services and expand and improve existing early intervention services being provided to infants and toddlers with disabilities and their families

4. Encourage states to expand opportunities for children under 3 years of age who would be at risk for having substantial developmental delay if they did not receive early intervention services

The background section of the amendments, based on a review of research, lists ways that programs providing special education services for children may be further strengthened and improved. Those suggestions include supporting the role of parents and ensuring that families have the opportunity to participate in their children's education, providing special education and related services in the regular classroom, and supporting high-quality professional development for all personnel.

Additionally, the issue of the effect of the changing cultural demographics on the educational environment of children with disabilities is raised. The rate of population increase for groups of people who are considered "minorities" in the United States is greater than that for white Americans. For example, between 1980 and 1990, the rate of increase in the population for white Americans was 6%, while the rate of increase for racial and ethnic minorities was much higher: 53% for Hispanics, 13.2% for African-Americans, and 107.8% for Asians. By the year 2000, the United States will have 275,000,000 people, nearly one of every three of whom will be African-American, Hispanic, Asian-American, or American Indian.

The effect of these population changes on public school systems is noted. Children from cultural groups that are considered minorities in the United States make up the majority of students in urban school systems. For example, in 1993 percentages of children from minority groups in public schools were 84% in Miami, 89% in Chicago, 78% in Philadelphia, 84% in Baltimore, 88% in Houston, and 88% in Los Angeles.

Many of these children have limited proficiency for communication in English, are more likely to be referred to special education services, and are more likely to drop out of school than white students. The number of teachers from "minority" cultural groups is also disproportionately low. Possible interventions to consider evolving student needs are addressed among funding priorities and a protocol for nondiscriminatory procedures to be used in testing and evaluation.

Services for Infants and Toddlers

Title I of IDEA relates to delivery of early intervention services, including physical therapy, to children younger than 3 years of age. Important definitions include the following:

1. At risk infant or toddler:
   The term "at risk infant or toddler" means an individual under 3 years of age who would be at risk of experiencing a substantial developmental

delay if early intervention services were not provided to the individual.

2. Council:

    The term "council" means a state interagency coordinating council established under section 1441 of this title.

3. Developmental delay:

    The term "developmental delay" when used with respect to an individual residing in a State, has the meaning given such term by the State under section 1435 (a) (1) of this title.

4. Early intervention services:

    The term "early intervention services" means developmental services that:

    A. are provided under public supervision;

    B. are provided at no cost except where Federal or State law provides for a system of payments by families, including a schedule of sliding fees;

    C. are designed to meet the developmental needs of an infant or toddler with a disability in any one or more of the following areas:
        i. physical development
        ii. cognitive development
        iii. communication development
        iv. social or emotional development
        v. adaptive development

    D. meet the standards of the State in which they are provided, including the requirements of this subchapter;

    E. include:
        i. family training, counseling, and home visits;
        ii. special instruction;
        iii. speech-language pathology and audiology services;
        iv. occupational therapy;
        v. physical therapy;
        vi. psychological services;
        vii. service coordination services;
        viii. vision services;
        ix. assistive technology devices and assistive technology;
        x. transportation and related costs that are necessary to enable an infant or toddler and the infant's or toddler's family to receive another service described in this paragraph;

    F. are provided by qualified personnel, including:
        i. special educators
        ii. speech-language pathologists and audiologists
        iii. occupational therapists
        iv. physical therapists
        v. psychologists
        vi. social workers
        vii. nurses
        viii. nutritionists
        ix. family therapists
        x. orientation and mobility specialists
        xi. pediatricians and other physicians

    G. to the maximum extent appropriate, are provided in natural environments, including the home, and community settings in which children without disabilities participate; and

    H. are provided in conformity with an individualized family service plan adopted in accordance with section 1436 of this title.

5. Infant or toddler with a disability:

    The term "infant or toddler with a disability":

    A. means an individual under 3 years of age who needs early intervention services because the individual:
        i. is experiencing developmental delays, as measured by appropriate diagnostic instruments and procedures in one or more of the areas including cognitive development, physical development, communication development, social or emotional development, and adaptive development; or
        ii. has a diagnosed physical or mental condition which has a high probability of resulting in developmental delay; and

    B. may also include at a state's discretion, at risk infants and toddlers. (20 USC 1432 et al.)

The inclusion of pediatric physical therapy as an early intervention service is related to the identification of physical development, including gross motor skill development, as one of the areas in which an infant with disabilities may receive intervention. Physical therapists are the professionals who are best qualified to examine and provide services to children with disabilities affecting motor development and their families.

The revision identifies a wide range of professionals who will also provide coordinated services in partnership with an infant or toddler and her or his family. The pediatric physical therapist who works in early intervention will need to develop a style of interaction and communication that allows him or her to work with those professionals on the multidisciplinary team who best address the infant or toddler and family's needs. In early childhood, areas of development are interrelated, and children may not require direct services from all members of the team. Pediatric physical therapists, therefore, may need to broaden their skills in order to provide support in areas of development not ordinarily considered their area of expertise (see Chapter 31).

The fact that the revision allows individual states

to determine the magnitude of delay that will allow an infant or toddler to qualify to receive early intervention services will influence the pediatric physical therapist's plans for examination. Pediatric physical therapists should be sure the tests and measures they use are easily interpreted in light of the state's definition of developmental delay. For example, if delay is defined by the state in terms of standard deviations below the mean for age, the pediatric physical therapist will need to use an instrument on which performance scores may be presented as standard deviations varying around the mean score for the child's age.

Amendments Related to the Individual Educational Plan

The revision guarantees a free, appropriate public education to children ages 3 to 21 with disabilities, including children who have previously been suspended from school. A system for locating children with disabilities who live in the state and offering such students special education services is outlined in the revision. The requirement for an Individual Educational Plan (IEP) as the document that guides the child's participation in special education programs is stated.

Parents, regular and special education teachers, and, when appropriate, the child with a disability are identified as members of the IEP team. Although the physical therapist is not required to attend the IEP meeting, participation is encouraged when physical therapy will be included in the IEP or when there are issues regarding the need for physical therapy. The physical therapist may also be included on the IEP team at the request of a parent or other members of the team because of his or her knowledge or special expertise regarding the student.

Children with disabilities are to receive their education in the same environment as children who are not disabled to the maximum extent that is appropriate. A child should be removed from the regular education environment only when the nature or severity of a child's disability does not allow participation in regular classes, even if supplementary aids and special education services are offered.

The IDEA revision gives states the authority to refer children with disabilities to a private school or facility if a free, appropriate public education is not otherwise available. This referral must be in conformance with the IEP, and the private school or facility must provide special education services. The child will attend the private school or facility at no cost to the parents. The school or facility must meet the state educational agency and the local educational agency's standards and requirements. The child in

this facility has all of the rights of a child with a disability who is served by a public agency.

If a child with a disability is placed in a private school or facility by the parents, the public agency is not required to pay for the child's education at the private school or facility. The public agency, however, must make services available to the child. Children with disabilities who attend private schools are to receive special education and related services in accordance with an IEP. Services may be provided on the premises of private and parochial schools.

An emphasis of the IDEA amendments on providing the opportunity for children with disabilities to receive their education in regular education settings will influence the contexts in which pediatric physical therapists practice. In the past, pediatric physical therapists working in school systems have practiced in schools where the majority of students had disabilities. As the revisions to the IDEA are implemented, pediatric physical therapists will work primarily in settings that are inclusive of all students. Children with disabilities are likely to receive services in private, parochial, and public school settings (see Chapter 32).

The emphasis on including children with disabilities in the general education curriculum in their neighborhood school has direct implications for the provision of physical therapy services. A therapist's caseload may involve students from several schools, necessitating time for travel between schools. Therapy goals focus not only on a child's ability to function independently within the physical structure of the school, but also on learning motor skills necessary to participate in activities that are part of the general education curriculum. Therapists will plan therapeutic activities using materials that are readily available in schools or easily transported to a student's school. Coordination, communication, instruction, and consultation with teachers and other school personnel are important roles of the physical therapist who provides services to students in educational settings.

Evaluation

The 1997 amendments include guidelines for evaluation to be used by all personnel involved in the evaluation of children with disabilities. The term *evaluation* as used in federal laws is similar to *examination* as defined in the *Guide to Physical Therapist Practice* (American Physical Therapy Association, 1997). Following the guidelines established by the IDEA ensures that the physical therapist will fairly and thoroughly evaluate an infant, toddler, or student and will ensure that the therapist adheres to best practice standards.

The IDEA amendment requires the following:

1. The person performing an evaluation will use a variety of tests and measures to gather information relevant to a child's function and development, including information provided by the parent, that may assist in determining whether the child qualifies for services, and the child's IEP, including information related to a child's ability to participate in the general curriculum or, for preschool children, to participate in appropriate activities.

2. The person performing an evaluation will not use the results of any single test or measure as the sole criterion for determining whether a child qualifies for services or for determining an appropriate educational program for the child.

3. The person performing an evaluation will use technically sound instruments that may assess the relative contribution of cognitive and behavioral factors, in addition to physical or developmental factors.

Additionally, there are requirements to help prevent discrimination against children from varied cultural backgrounds during the evaluation process. Specifically, the amendment requires that

A. tests and other materials used to evaluate a child are:
   i. selected and administered so as not to be discriminatory on a racial or cultural basis; and
   ii. provided and administered in the child's native language or other mode of communication, unless it is clearly not feasible to do so; and
B. standardized tests that are given to the child:
   i. have been validated for the specific purpose for which they are used;
   ii. are administered by trained and knowledgeable personnel; and
   iii. are administered in accordance with any instructions provided by the authors of the tests;
C. the child is assessed in all areas of suspected disability; and
D. the tests and measures used provide relevant information that assists persons in determining the educational needs of the child. (Title 20, Sec. 1414 b)

Eligibility determination is to be made by a team of qualified professionals, which may include the pediatric physical therapists and also includes the parents of the child. The team must be sure that a child is not determined to have a disability solely because of a lack of proper educational instruction or because of limited English proficiency. Eligibility determination must take into consideration existing evaluation data, classroom-based observations, teacher and related service provider observations, and input from the child's parents.

Nondiscriminatory Procedures

In addition to federal requirements, each state must include procedural safeguards to ensure that testing and evaluation materials and procedures are not racially or culturally discriminatory. The parent must be fully informed of all information relevant to the evaluation in his or her native language. The evaluation materials of procedures shall be provided and administered in the child's native language or mode of communication, unless it is clearly not feasible. No single procedure should be the sole criterion for determination of an appropriate educational program for a child.

In accordance with the guidelines for evaluation outlined in the revision, physical therapists must carefully consider selection of tests and evaluation procedures. Instruments used for evaluation must have been standardized on children who are similar to the child being evaluated. In order for findings to be valid, a child must be evaluated using tests or measures that have been standardized or normed on children of the same cultural group and economic level.

Consideration of the child's developmental experiences and culture is essential when deciding on the appropriate tests given the diverse cultural backgrounds of today's student population. The physical therapist must be sure that assumptions about the developmental experiences of the child being evaluated are accurate. For example, authors of a test may assume that preschool-age children have had experiences on riding toys and that riding a tricycle will be a familiar experience for a 3-year-old child. The performance of a child who has recently immigrated to the United States from a Southeast Asian refugee camp and has never ridden on a tricycle cannot be considered a valid indicator of gross motor and coordination skills. Similarly, if a test item is based on the assumption that preschool-age children have experience eating with a spoon, administration of the item to a child from a family that uses bread held in the fingers to scoop and eat food may not be valid.

The IDEA amendments require that no one instrument or score be used alone to determine eligibility and that observation of the child's functioning in the school environment be included as part of the evaluation. The use of information and data from multiple sources (child, teacher, parent, direct observation) will help the physical therapist consider various aspects of the child's functional abilities in the evaluation process and will decrease the possibility that the therapist will make erroneous conclusions concerning the child's true abilities.

State Advisory Panel

Each state shall establish a state advisory panel on the education of children with disabilities. The advisory panel must be appointed by the governor or any other state official authorized under state law to make those appointments. The advisory panel must be composed of persons involved in or concerned with the education of children with disabilities. The membership must include at least one person representative of each of the following groups:

Individuals with disabilities
Teachers of children with disabilities
Parents of children with disabilities
State and local education officials
Special education program administrators

The majority of the advisory panel should be individuals with disabilities or parents of children with disabilities. The function of the advisory panel is to advise the state educational agency of needs within the state in education of children with disabilities. The advisory panel is to comment on promulgated rules and policies with regard to children with disabilities and assist the state in developing and reporting information to the federal government.

Personnel Standards

The state must establish standards to ensure that personnel necessary to serve children with disabilities are appropriately and adequately prepared. The standards are based on the highest requirements in the state applicable to the profession or discipline in which a person is providing special education or related services. The state must have policies and procedures relating to the establishment and maintenance of standards to ensure that personnel are appropriately and adequately prepared and trained.

The formulation of the state advisory panel and the development of personnel standards are intended to ensure that professionals are adequately trained and possess the skills required to meet the educational needs of children with disabilities and their families. Physical therapists are identified in the IDEA as professionals who are appropriate to work with infants, toddlers, and children with disabilities. Along with the requirement that professionals intervening with this population are trained at the highest level required by the state, this ensures that physical therapy services are provided by or under the direction of licensed physical therapists. The formulation of the state advisory panel further ensures that problems with the provision of educational services to this population are identified and corrected.

CASE HISTORY
HECTOR

Sara, a physical therapist who works in the school system, is preparing to evaluate a 6-year-old boy to help determine his eligibility for special education and related services. The child, Hector, comes from a family in which only Spanish is spoken. Hector's family comes from a small village in Guatemala. In Hector's village, there are few schools, recreational materials, or play materials.

Sara decides to use a standardized test that includes instructions, toys, and play materials common to children in the United States. While administering the test, Sara notices that Hector does not seem to understand the directions she gives him. Using gestures, Sara is able to communicate her requests for Hector to perform various skills and activities.

After administering the test, Sara estimates Hector's performance on the items he seemed confused about. Sara scores the test and finds Hector's performance to be nearly age appropriate. Sara concludes that Hector does not have a delay in motor development, and she does not recommend physical therapy as part of his individual educational plan.

Response

Sara's evaluation of Hector does not comply with the evaluation procedures set out in the statute. In conducting the evaluation, Sara should never use a single procedure as a sole criterion for determining whether or not a child has a disability, nor should it determine an appropriate educational program for Hector. This one test did not allow her to develop strategies necessary to gather relevant functional and developmental information. She failed to gather information from Hector's family concerning his life before his arrival in the United States. She also failed to gather any information that may have assisted her in determining whether Hector has a disability.

The test and other evaluation materials used to assess Hector should be selected and administered so as not to be discriminatory on a racial or cultural basis. Because Hector is from Guatemala, there should be a consideration of language barriers. Instructions should have been given in Spanish or another (indigenous) language if necessary.

AMERICANS WITH DISABILITIES ACT

Although the Americans with Disabilities Act is frequently considered to be most closely related to employment and public access for individuals with disabilities, sections of the law are particularly relevant to families of children with disabilities. The purpose of this section is to summarize portions of this law that are useful to physical therapists in their role as advocates for families of children with disabilities. Illustrative case examples are included.

Employment

The Americans with Disabilities Act prevents an employer from denying an employment opportunity or benefit because of an individual's association with a person who has a disability. The law protects a parent from being denied a job because she or he has a child with a disability. An employer cannot assume that because an employee is the parent of a child with a disability, the employee may be unavailable or unreliable with respect to job requirements.

The law also prohibits discrimination related to health insurance benefits that are offered as a fringe benefit of employment. An employer cannot deny an applicant a job or refuse to hire a parent of a child with a disability because the employer anticipates an increase in insurance costs, nor can an employer subject an employee who has a child with a disability to different terms or conditions of insurance. Although the parent of a child with a disability is protected from discrimination in the areas of hiring and insurance, the employer is not obligated to modify work schedules to facilitate child care.

The Americans with Disabilities Act also protects parents from discrimination related to association with other individuals with disabilities or to working with organizations associated with persons with disabilities. For example, a parent who does volunteer work for a service organization for acquired immunodeficiency syndrome cannot be discriminated against in employment opportunities or in benefits of employment such as health insurance.

Enforcement Provisions

Parents who believe that they have been discriminated against related to hiring or insurance can file a charge with the Department of Justice. Parents may also file a charge if they believe that retaliation has occurred as a result of filing a charge or opposing a discriminatory practice.

The Department of Justice investigates charges of discrimination. If the Department of Justice believes that discrimination has occurred, an attempt at resolution will be made. If conciliation fails, the Department of Justice will file suit or issue a "right to sue" letter to the person who filed the charge. Remedies for violations of the Americans with Disabilities Act related to employment include hiring, reinstatement, promotion, the payment of back pay and front pay, and restoration of benefits, including health insurance.

The Americans with Disabilities Act covers all activities of state and local governments regardless of the government entity's size or receipt of federal funding. The act requires that state and local governments give people with disabilities an equal opportunity to benefit from all of their programs, services, courts, and activities (e.g., public education, employment, transportation, recreation, health care, social services, courts, voting, and town meetings).

Complaints of Americans with Disabilities Act violations may be filed with the Department of Justice within 180 days of the date of discrimination. In certain situations, cases may be referred to a mediation program sponsored by the Department of Justice. The Department of Justice may bring a lawsuit when it has investigated a matter and has been unable to resolve violations.

Transportation

The Americans with Disabilities Act protects individuals with disabilities from discrimination with respect to participation in any public services, programs, or activities. Public transportation, including buses and rapid rail systems, is included under the rubric of "public services." According to the law, new buses and rail cars purchased after July 26, 1990, as well as stations constructed after this date, must be accessible to individuals with disabilities who may require wheelchairs or other assistive devices for mobility or who may have a visual impairment.

Public transportation services for individuals with disabilities must be available on a schedule that is comparable to that provided for persons without a disability. Available transportation may include transportation that is accessible to a person who does or does not require a wheelchair lift for transportation. The law provides for assistance with transportation to regular public transportation stops for those who are unable to reach these stops without assistance. The law also provides for transportation of an accompanying assistant for the individual with a disability as long as the assistant's seat is not needed for another person with a disability.

Parents of children with disabilities who live in areas served by public transportation should expect increased availability of accessible transportation services. Bus service, for example, should be available on the same schedule as service for persons without a disability. Public transportation service may also become available at a family's residence, should a child be unable to get to a regular transportation stop independently. On intercity and commuter rail systems, at least one rail car per train must be accessible to individuals with disabilities.

Physical Structures

The Americans with Disabilities Act also protects individuals with disabilities from discrimination related to limited access to public accommodations. Public accommodations may include hotels, restaurants, food and retail stores, and shopping malls. Recreational facilities, such as amusement parks, zoos, and museums, are also included. Educational facilities, such as nurseries, elementary or secondary schools, and public and private undergraduate and graduate colleges and universities, must also be accessible.

State and local governments are required to follow specific architectural standards in the new construction and alteration of their buildings. They also must relocate programs or otherwise provide access in inaccessible older buildings and communicate effectively with people who have hearing, vision, or speech disabilities. Public entities are not required to make modifications that would involve undue financial and administrative burdens. They are required to make reasonable modifications to policies, practices, and procedures where necessary to avoid discrimination, unless they can demonstrate that doing so would fundamentally alter the nature of the service, program, or activity being provided.

Families of children with disabilities may expect greater access to structures in their communities related to education, shopping, and recreation. Greater access for persons who require assistance or devices for mobility should facilitate the integration of these individuals into all areas of the community.

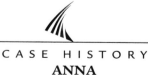

CASE HISTORY
ANNA

Ms. Jones is the single parent of a child, Anna, who has Down syndrome. Ms. Jones is a licensed ultrasound technologist and worked until the birth of her daughter. She planned to return to work 3 months after her daughter's birth; however, because of the medical complications Anna experienced, Ms. Jones decided to remain at home, forfeiting her past position. By the time Anna was 8 months old, she was doing well medically, and Ms. Jones applied for a job with a small, private company that contracted out ultrasonography services to local hospitals and physicians' offices.

During the employment interview, the personnel director commented favorably on Ms. Jones' excellent work record and references from her past employer. He inquired regarding the reason that Ms. Jones decided not to return to her old position. When Ms. Jones related the circumstances of her daughter's birth and disability, the tone of the interview changed. The personnel director questioned Ms. Jones regarding her ability to meet her daughter's medical needs and the demands of a full-time job and interjected his personal experience with a family in his neighborhood who had a child with a disability. In that family, the mother's decision to remain at home was considered a necessity.

Ms. Jones believed when she left the interview that she would probably not be offered the job. Her suspicion was confirmed when she received a letter stating that the job was offered to another qualified applicant. Ms. Jones was puzzled when the company continued to advertise the position. She contacted the personnel director again and was able to convince him of her ability to handle both the job and the care of her daughter. After considerable negotiation, she was offered the position under the stipulation that she accept a lower amount of health insurance coverage than the company's other employees and pay a slightly higher rate. Ms. Jones questioned the personnel manager's right to make such an offer and wondered if she should seek the opinion of an employment rights specialist.

Response

Ms. Jones should seek the opinion of an employment rights specialist. Under the employment component of the Americans with Disabilities Act, the actions of this employer are illegal. In a hiring situation, it is illegal even to consider a dependent who has a disability. This act attempts to level the playing field for parents of children with disabilities. Questions as to the health of dependent children are not related to the job and, therefore, are prohibited under ADA.

Second, Ms. Jones is entitled to the same benefits as the company's other employees. It is illegal under ADA to require Ms. Jones to contribute more for health insurance or to provide her with less coverage. The employer cannot pass the extra cost of the insurance on to the parent.

CHILD ABUSE AND NEGLECT

The subject of child abuse and neglect is discussed more openly and freely at the present time than in the past. A possibly related phenomenon is the increase in the number of reported cases of child abuse

(De Jong et al., 1983; Hampton & Newberger, 1985). Because physical therapists may provide services to children who are at risk for or have experienced abuse or neglect, a review of the signs of abuse and the physical therapist's responsibility with respect to reporting suspected abuse is provided in this section.

Neglect

Child abuse and neglect are defined by the Child Abuse Prevention and Treatment Act of 1974 as "the physical or mental injury, sexual abuse, negligent treatment or maltreatment of a child under the age of eighteen by a person who is responsible for the child's welfare under circumstances which indicate that the child's health and welfare are harmed or threatened hereby" (PL 93-247, p. 247). Child abuse and neglect may occur in various forms, including, but not limited to, severe physical injury that may be fatal or life threatening.

Neglect occurs when a child's basic needs are not being met by an adult who is responsible for the child's care. Neglectful situations may involve inadequate or unstable shelter or inadequate or inappropriate nutrition. Neglect may also occur related to lack of needed medical or dental care. Concerning medical neglect, the pediatric physical therapist may be the member of the health care team who observes and documents a pattern of missed appointments or noncompliance with instructions that results in a deterioration in the child's status. In such a situation, the physical therapist is responsible for reporting the suspected neglect to the proper authorities.

A difficulty in the determination of neglect is related to willfulness. Neglect need not be a willful act on the part of the adult responsible (Newberger et al., 1987). Neglect may be related to a parent's inability to meet a child's needs because of extreme environmental stresses or may be related to a parent's limited knowledge base concerning appropriate stimulation and behavior management for children.

Neglect that is not willful may be distressing to report from the physical therapist's perspective. Filing a report may be associated with blaming the parents for the child's situation. An important consideration in a case of nonwillful neglect is the ultimate effect on the child: If the child is not thriving because nutritional, medical, or other physical or emotional needs are not being met, intervention is needed. Examples of situations in which neglect may be present are listed in Box 34-1.

Physical Abuse

The symptoms associated with physical abuse have been collectively termed the *battered child syndrome* (Kempe et al., 1962). Associated physical inju-

---

BOX 34-1. Signs and Situations Associated with Child Neglect

Evidence of poor nutrition
Reports of hunger
Nutritionally inadequate diet
Evidence of poor hygiene
Soiled clothing
Soiled skin, body odors
Skin breakdown in diaper area
Dental caries
Lack of compliance with medical or therapy appointments
Excessive cancellations
Frequent "no shows"
Lack of follow-through with home program instructions, resulting in a decline in the child's status

---

ries may be detected by a child's pediatrician, an emergency department physician, or a school nurse. The physical manifestations include injury to bone and soft tissue, as well as affective changes. Signs and symptoms associated with the battered child syndrome are listed in Box 34-2.

Because a child's clothing is routinely removed during physical therapy sessions, signs of physical abuse may be more readily and naturally observed during treatment than in other settings, such as the school classroom. When symptoms are observed, the suspected abuse must be reported to the proper authorities. The fact that symptoms commonly associated with abuse may also be related to other medical conditions or common childhood accidents deserves careful consideration. A differential diagnosis can be made only by a physician. Questionable symptoms require further investigation by a physician.

Sexual Abuse

The signs of sexual abuse that may be observed by the pediatric physical therapist are likely to be manifested behaviorally. Psychosomatic or behavioral illnesses, behavioral alterations, and acting-out behaviors may accompany sexual child abuse (Gommes-Schwartz et al., 1985). Somatization, or the expression of emotional conflicts as symptoms of physical illness, frequently occurs in association with sexual child abuse (Rosenfeld, 1982; Rosenfeld & Sarles, 1986). The occurrence of behavioral disorders such as anorexia nervosa or bulimia and enuresis or encopresis may signal sexual abuse. Abdominal pain without an organic cause is an example of a psychosomatic problem that may be associated with sexual abuse. Behavioral changes such as an alteration in school performance, atypical shyness, and extroverted or hostile behavior may be associated

---

BOX 34–2. Signs and Symptoms of Physical Abuse: Battered Child Syndrome

Bony fractures
Soft tissue injuries
Burns
Hematomas
Welts
Internal injuries
Contusions

---

with sexual abuse (Rosenfeld, 1982; Rosenfeld & Sarles, 1987).

Psychosomatic and behavioral problems, however, may be associated with problems other than sexual abuse, and such symptoms and signs require further evaluation by a professional such as a medical social worker, psychologist, or physician. Sexual acting-out behavior, sexual aggression toward other children, or an overly sophisticated knowledge of sexual activities and practice are salient signs of sexual abuse.

Child sexual abuse accommodation syndrome (Summitt, 1982) describes the behaviors associated with a child's attempt to adapt to sexual abuse that occur over time. As a young child attempts to cope with feelings of disbelief, rejection, helplessness, and self-blame associated with victimization by sexual abuse, long-lasting behavioral changes may be noted. Secrecy; helplessness; entrapment and accommodation; delayed, conflicted, and unconvincing disclosure of incidents; and retraction of reported abuse are all behaviors associated with child sexual abuse accommodation syndrome.

A physical therapist who observes a child behaving in a manner that may be associated with ongoing sexual abuse should give such behavior careful consideration. Secrecy regarding relationships with certain adults or conflicting reports about incidents that are suspicious may be indicators of a child's victimization by sexual abuse. A physical therapist who suspects sexual abuse may work together with a social worker, psychologist, or physician to further evaluate the child's situation and make necessary reports to the appropriate authorities.

Legal Obligation to Report

A review of state laws in various geographic regions of the United States reveals that health care professionals, including physical therapists, are unequivocally required to immediately report suspected child abuse to the proper agency (III Illinois Annotated Statutes; Official Code of Georgia, Annotated). Each state or county has an established proto-

col for the reporting of suspected abuse. Protocols describe the routing of reports of abuse, the consideration of factors in the determination of the child's risk status, and a plan for removal from the home, if necessary (California Penal Code). Protocols are available for examination through county departments of family and children's services and agencies such as state councils on child abuse.

Failure to report suspected child abuse is a misdemeanor in most states. Associated penalties include monetary fines, imprisonment, or both. Failure to report suspected abuse may also result in the revocation or suspension of a professional license or the denial of licensure renewal.

Many state statutes protect an individual who reports suspected abuse from civil action related to a lack of substantiation of the report (Official Code of Georgia, Annotated). Such a statute frees the individual making the report from undue concern over retaliation on the part of the accused party should the report be unconfirmed. State statutes also address the situation in which individuals knowingly make false reports of abuse (23 Illinois Annotated Statutes). A consideration of the repercussions for failure to report suspected abuse reflects the seriousness of this crime and its effect on children.

If abuse is suspected, the physical therapist should call the proper authorities immediately. Delaying a call could place a child at further risk. The physical therapist need not know for certain that abuse or neglect has occurred to make a report. The therapist need only suspect that there is a risk that abuse or neglect may occur to make a report.

The physical therapist should not investigate the circumstances for child abuse. The responsibility for investigation rests with the proper authorities. Any investigation by persons other than a child protection worker or a police officer may prejudice efforts to protect the child.

The following case history taken from the experience of one of the authors is presented as an illustration of issues related to the reporting of suspected child abuse by health care professionals in general and by pediatric physical therapists specifically.

CASE HISTORY
JERRY

Amy, a pediatric physical therapist working in an early intervention program, makes routine home visits to infants and their families. A considerable proportion of Amy's caseload is with families who are indigent. One of Amy's patients is Jerry, an 18-month-old infant with spina bifida. Jerry's defect is at the upper thoracic level of his spine. Jerry demonstrates some functional use of his upper extremities but no volitional movement in his lower extremities.

Jerry lives with his parents, Mr. and Mrs. Smith, and two older siblings. Mrs. Smith was in junior high school when her eldest child was born. She is now 18 years old. Mrs. Smith has attempted to complete her high school education, but her course work has been interrupted by Jerry's frequent hospitalizations. In a conversation with Amy, Mrs. Smith related that she does not receive much support from Mr. Smith, who believes that Jerry will somehow eventually recover from his disability. She also told Amy about Mr. Smith's history of substance abuse and her own history of having been abused during her childhood. At the present time, Mrs. Smith appears listless, and Amy believes that Mrs. Smith is depressed.

On her visits to Jerry's house, Amy has been concerned about Jerry's care. He is not usually bathed and dressed by the time she visits at 1 o'clock in the afternoon. His diaper is usually wet, and his pajamas smell of urine. He often acts hungry and weak. Mrs. Smith frequently reports that she has fed Jerry "a few bites from her own plate," but not a full meal of his own.

One occasion when Amy worked with Jerry in his own bedroom, she noticed that one of the railings of his crib was missing, leaving an open space. Amy was also concerned because on one of her visit days, she had met Mrs. Smith walking home from the store and Mrs. Smith reported that Jerry was not at home and said that Amy should not come in. Amy believed that she had heard Jerry's voice inside the home.

During Amy's most recent visit to Jerry's home, she discovered a small decubitus ulcer forming in the sacral region of Jerry's spine. Amy was concerned about Jerry's health and safety but at the same time did not want to blame Mrs. Smith. Amy believed that Mrs. Smith was probably doing the best she could, considering her depression, her lack of resources, and lack of support from Jerry's father. Amy decided that she needed to try to determine her responsibility in informing an outside agency about her concerns for Jerry's welfare.

Response

The state laws usually require that all cases of suspected abuse and neglect be reported immediately to the proper authorities. The key word here is "suspected" abuse and neglect. The law does not require a case of neglect to be proven before being reported. It requires that any information that would tend to indicate that a child is abused or neglected be reported.

It is important that the physical therapist document specific findings and report a case to the authorities. Many states make failure to report a case of suspected abuse or neglect a misdemeanor punishable by up to 12 months in jail.

LITIGATION

Although litigation is an area in which pediatric physical therapists may not wish to be involved, issues related to medical malpractice are permeating all areas of the health care system. Medically related lawsuits are increasing rapidly in our society. Pediatric physical therapists must be aware of the process of litigation and of how they may willingly or unwillingly be involved. In this section, issues relevant to litigation are presented from an attorney's perspective to make the pediatric physical therapist aware of how components of practice, such as medical documentation, fit in the scheme of medically related litigation.

O'Sullivan (1975) has outlined the process for review of the medical record in preparation for the presentation of a medical malpractice case in court. Consistency in chart records is considered to be a primary point of evaluation of a medical record. A medical record should, according to O'Sullivan, be straightforward and flow smoothly from beginning to end. Chart records should be consistent, and inconsistencies in charting are "red flags" for further scrutiny by the attorney involved. Among noted inconsistencies are discrepancy between diagnoses and selected therapy or intervention and chronologic inconsistencies between objective findings and corresponding changes in intervention. Improper use of forms and improper reporting of information or incidents to authorities are also examples of inconsistencies. Even the smallest of inconsistencies is considered relevant, particularly to the attorney whose client alleges hospital liability or negligence on the part of the health care provider.

Progress notes should include documentation of changes in patient status. Notes are expected to include changes in symptoms, complaints, objective signs, and the results of tests that contribute to the understanding of the diagnosed condition. When progress notes are complete, "there is no reason to evaluate other records" (O'Sullivan, 1975, p. 125).

Documentation serves as the interface between the physical therapist and the attorney in legal cases. Clear, objective, and accurate documentation is an essential component of quality treatment, regardless of whether it is ever evaluated by an attorney or outside party. However, in the event that records are subpoenaed, organized, clear, and objective records will serve both to protect the pediatric physical therapist from liability and to provide an accurate account of the status and progress of the patient.

When a medical record may be evaluated by

an outside party who is not an expert in the characteristics and usual physical therapy treatment of a child with a specific developmental disability, documentation such as progress notes or evaluations should be written in terms that are understandable and meaningful, even for individuals who are not physical therapists or who have not received training in a particular treatment approach or theoretic orientation.

Documentation of progress by a method that is meaningful to outsiders also poses a challenge for pediatric physical therapists. The use of norm-referenced, standardized measures may provide data concerning a child's motor performance in comparison with peers that is easily understood by others. The description of a child's motor performance on a standard measure may be useful for purposes of assessment, as well as for documentation of change.

MEDICAL TECHNOLOGY

Another potential interface between pediatric physical therapists and the legal system involves children who are dependent on medical technology for survival. As medical technology has become more sophisticated, the ability to support children whose illnesses or injuries would, in other times, have been fatal has increased (see Chapter 25).

The point at which the continuation of technologic life support compromises the quality of a child's life is not easily determined. Because individual physicians, health care professionals, and families differ in their beliefs about issues related to quality of life and preservation of life, differences of opinion regarding the extent to which technologic life-support measures should be employed have occurred. At times, disagreements between parents and physicians and other members of the health care team, such as nurses and social workers, have been so extreme that decisions regarding the appropriateness of medical interventions have been made by the court system (National Center for State Courts, 1991).

One of the considerations in the determination of whether technologic life support should continue for a particular child may be the child's prognosis with respect to the expected future level of functioning. Although physicians have formulated prognoses for children in court cases in the past, it is not unlikely that the pediatric physical therapist may be asked to contribute a clinical opinion regarding a child's developmental outcome. The following case provides an example of a physical therapist's involvement in a health care team decision regarding the continuation of technologic life support for an in-

fant. Although this particular case was not decided in court, it is representative of the type of situation in which pediatric physical therapists may increasingly be involved.

CASE HISTORY
KENNY

Kenny is an infant delivered at 23 to 24 weeks of gestational age at a birth weight of 770 g. Kenny's mother is a single parent who received no prenatal care. His father was involved in an emotional relationship with his mother; however, their relationship was physically abusive. One child previously was removed from the home by the Department of Family and Children's Services.

Kenny experienced multiple neonatal complications, including necrotizing enterocolitis, severe bronchopulmonary dysplasia, and several unsuccessful attempts to permanently wean him from ventilator support. Kenny's other medical complications include metabolic bone disease, intrahepatic cholestasis, and multiple bouts of sepsis. He also experienced a grade III intraventricular hemorrhage. His head circumference is significantly less than would be expected for his age and other anthropometric measurements, probably as a result of cerebral atrophy.

At 10 months chronologic age, Kenny's physical therapist, Sharon, estimated Kenny's level of motor functioning to be at 1 month. At this time, he began to experience a slow deterioration of his cardiopulmonary system, including congestive heart failure. Related to the deterioration of his health status, Sharon reported that it was difficult to follow through with the physical therapy intervention plan because the infant was frequently too ill to tolerate treatment. He was infrequently alert and did not demonstrate visual observation of faces or other interactive behavior. Active movements were athetoid in quality. Just before a significant decline in his status, including congestive heart failure, Kenny experienced a few days in which he was able to tolerate handling and treatment out of his crib on a mat.

Subsequently, Kenny experienced a decline in his status and was reintubated and ventilated. Kenny's primary physician, a pediatric intensive care specialist, and other members of Kenny's health care team began to consider the appropriateness of the repeated intubation and ventilation and other technologic support measures. Kenny's mother frequently inquired about his prognosis and level of functioning and was willing to consider a deceleration in his care. Kenny's father, however, was not in agreement with such a plan.

Kenny's doctor approached Sharon with questions about Kenny's current level of motor functioning and his expected outcome in future years should the infant's medical condition become more stable. In light of this request, the therapist had to determine a strategy for the development of a clinical opinion regarding Kenny's present status and future level of functioning.

Response

In a situation such as Kenny's, the physical therapist, Sharon, could integrate information from a variety of sources in the formulation of her opinion. She could use her own clinical judgment, based on experience with other infants who had similar characteristic motor patterns and shared a similar medical history. Fortunately, Sharon had several years of pediatric experience with toddlers and older children in addition to her work in a neonatal intensive care unit. In this case, Kenny's lack of behavioral interaction, severely delayed motor skills, and athetoid movements were considered in the formulation of Sharon's opinion.

Sharon also considered the results of outcome research studies on infants who experienced some of the same neonatal complications that Kenny experienced. In her review of outcome studies, Sharon found that grade III intracranial hemorrhage and cerebral atrophy were associated with poor neurodevelopmental outcomes. Based on assessment and observations, past experience with infants with motor performance similar to Kenny's, and a review of the literature concerning neurodevelopmental outcome, Sharon was able to formulate an opinion regarding Kenny's developmental prognosis. Sharon expected that Kenny would have significant motor impairment.

Because Kenny died before the issues related to technologic support were resolved, this case did not reach the court system. Nevertheless, Sharon's strategy for the formulation of an opinion could have been used in a legal case. Sharon's use of her past experience together with a review of the outcome literature helped her to formulate an opinion. Although not used in this instance, results of a norm-referenced standardized measure of motor development would also have been helpful.

Ethical Concerns

Although not a consideration in this case, the formulation of an opinion about Kenny might have presented an ethical dilemma for Sharon. For example, if Sharon's personal beliefs regarding the continuation or removal of technologic support for critically ill patients had not been congruent with that of the family and other members of the health care team, the formulation of an opinion might have been difficult. Health care professionals' personal beliefs regarding the sources of health improvement in their patients are as likely to contribute to the formulation of their clinical decisions as is past experience or a review of the literature.

In the development of their measurement tool, the Child Health Improvement Locus of Control scales, DeVellis and colleagues (1985) considered the relation between parental beliefs and behavior associated with their child's illness. The Child Health Improvement Locus of Control scales assess parental beliefs related to the source of control over a child's recovery and outcome. DeVellis and colleagues (1985) found that factors related to the child, parents, and professionals; to chance; and to divine influence are also related to parents' beliefs regarding locus of control for health improvement in their children.

Research using the Child Health Improvement Locus of Control scales demonstrated that parents may ascribe different amounts of responsibility for child health improvement to factors such as the child himself or herself, health care professionals, parents, chance, or divine influence as determinants of their child's recovery. For example, whereas one parent may believe that professionals are primarily responsible for their child's recovery, another may attribute recovery to divine intervention or to chance.

Health care professionals, like parents, may attribute health improvement in infants and children to various factors. Health care professionals' locus of control with respect to health improvement in children may influence their decision making in cases such as the one previously described. For example, had Sharon attributed an improvement in Kenny's health to divine influence and had another member of the team attributed Kenny's improvement to intervention by professionals, Sharon's clinical opinion would have been influenced by factors related to her own belief system that were different from those of her colleague.

CONCLUSION

Although not often acknowledged, a pediatric physical therapist's belief system may influence decision making or may be a source of personal stress when it is not congruent with that of other members of the health care team. Identification of the therapist's own beliefs with respect to locus of control for health improvement in children and identification of how beliefs may influence decision making increase the objectivity of clinical decision making and the formation of opinions related to expected outcomes for children.

References

American Physical Therapy Association. Guide to physical therapist practice. Physical Therapy, *77*:1163–1650, 1997.
California Penal Code, Section 11166 (G).

De Jong, AR, Hervada, AR, & Emmett, GA. Epidemiological variations in childhood sexual abuse. Child Abuse and Neglect, 7:155-162, 1983.

DeVellis, SR, DeVellis, SBM, Revcki, DA, Lurie, SJ, Runyan, DIC, & Bristol, M. Development and validation of the Child Health Improvement Locus of Control (CHILC) scales. Journal of Social and Clinical Psychology, 3:307-324, 1985.

Gommes-Schwartz, B, Horowitz, JM, & Sauzier, M. Severity of emotional distress among sexually abused preschool, school aged and adolescent children. Hospital Community Psychiatry, 11:503-508, 1985.

Hampton, RH, & Newberger, EH. Child abuse incidence and reporting by hospitals: Significance of severity, class and race. American Journal of Public Health, 75:56-64, 1985.

23 Illinois Annotated Statutes. 2053, Sec. 4.

III Illinois Annotated Statutes. 4267-0.

Kempe, CH, Silverman, FW, Steele, BF, Droegemueller, W, & Silver, HK. The battered child syndrome. Journal of the American Medical Association, 181:17-24, 1962.

National Center for State Courts. Guidelines for state court decision making in authorizing or withholding life-sustaining medical treatment, Vol. 18, No. 10. Williamsburg, VA: National Center for State Courts, 1991, pp. 253-275.

Newberger, EH, Hyde, JN, Jr, Holter, JC, & Rosenfeld, A. Child abuse and neglect. In Hoekelman, RA, Blatman, S, Friedman, SB, Nelson, NM, & Seidel, HM (Eds.). Primary Pediatric Care. St. Louis: Mosby, 1987, pp. 629-638.

Official Code of Georgia, Annotated. Title 19, Chapter 7. 5(2)F.

O'Sullivan, DD. Evaluation of the medical record. Medicine Trial Technique Quarterly. Chicago: Callaghan, 1975.

Public Law 93-247, Child Abuse Prevention and Treatment Act of 1974, 42 USCS 5101-5106.

Public Law 94-142, Education of All Handicapped Children Act (1975), 20 USCS 1400.

Public Law 99-457, Education of the Handicapped Act Amendments of 1986, 20 USCS 1400.

Public Law 101-336, Americans with Disabilities Act (1990), 42 USCS 12102.

Public Law 101-476, Individuals with Disabilities Education Amendments of 1990. 20 USCS 1400.

Public Law 102-119, Individuals with Disabilities Education Act Amendments of 1991, 105 Stat. 587-608.

Public Law 105-17, Individuals with Disabilities Education Act Amendments of 1997, 111 Stat. 37-157.

Rosenfeld, A. Sexual abuse of children: Personal and professional responses. In Newberger, E (Ed.), Child Abuse. Boston: Little, Brown, 1982, pp. 57-74.

Rosenfeld, A, & Sarles, RM. Sexual misuse of children. In Hoekelman, RA, Blatman, S, Friedman, SB, Nelson, NM, & Seidel, HM (Eds.). Primary Pediatric Care. St. Louis: Mosby, 1986, pp. 642-651.

Summit, RC. The child sexual abuse accommodation syndrome. Child Abuse and Neglect, 7:177-193, 1982.

INDEX

Page numbers in italics indicate illustrations; page numbers followed by *t* indicate tables.